FISIOLOGIA DO ESPORTE E TRATAMENTO DE LESÕES
UMA ABORDAGEM INTERDISCIPLINAR

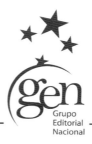

O GEN | Grupo Editorial Nacional – maior plataforma editorial brasileira no segmento científico, técnico e profissional – publica conteúdos nas áreas de ciências da saúde, exatas, humanas, jurídicas e sociais aplicadas, além de prover serviços direcionados à educação continuada e à preparação para concursos.

As editoras que integram o GEN, das mais respeitadas no mercado editorial, construíram catálogos inigualáveis, com obras decisivas para a formação acadêmica e o aperfeiçoamento de várias gerações de profissionais e estudantes, tendo se tornado sinônimo de qualidade e seriedade.

A missão do GEN e dos núcleos de conteúdo que o compõem é prover a melhor informação científica e distribuí-la de maneira flexível e conveniente, a preços justos, gerando benefícios e servindo a autores, docentes, livreiros, funcionários, colaboradores e acionistas.

Nosso comportamento ético incondicional e nossa responsabilidade social e ambiental são reforçados pela natureza educacional de nossa atividade e dão sustentabilidade ao crescimento contínuo e à rentabilidade do grupo.

FISIOLOGIA DO ESPORTE E TRATAMENTO DE LESÕES
UMA ABORDAGEM INTERDISCIPLINAR

Dr. Stuart Porter
PhD, BSc(Hons), SFHEA, PGCAP, GradDipPhys, MCSP, SRP, CertMHS, MLACP
Lecturer in Physiotherapy, University of Salford, Manchester, UK.
Visiting Lecturer, Corpus Christi College, Cambridge, UK.
Senior Fellow of the Higher Education Academy.
Visiting Lecturer, Universidade Paulista, Sao Paulo, Brazil.

Johnny Wilson
MSc, PGCE, BSc(Hons)
Clinical Director, 108 Harley Street.
Managing Director, Nottingham Physio.
MSC Sport & Exercise Medicine.
MACP Advanced Manual Therapy Practitioner.

Revisão Técnica
Ricardo Ambrosio
Mestre no Programa de Pesquisa em Cirurgia pela Faculdade de Ciências Médicas da Santa Casa de São Paulo (FCMSCSP).

Tradução
Dilza Campos

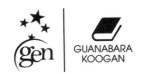

- Os autores deste livro e a editora empenharam seus melhores esforços para assegurar que as informações e os procedimentos apresentados no texto estejam em acordo com os padrões aceitos à época da publicação. Entretanto, tendo em conta a evolução das ciências, as atualizações legislativas, as mudanças regulamentares governamentais e o constante fluxo de novas informações sobre os temas que constam do livro, recomendamos enfaticamente que os leitores consultem sempre outras fontes fidedignas, de modo a se certificarem de que as informações contidas no texto estão corretas e de que não houve alterações nas recomendações ou na legislação regulamentadora.

- Data do fechamento do livro: 29/09/2022

- Os autores e a editora se empenharam para citar adequadamente e dar o devido crédito a todos os detentores de direitos autorais de qualquer material utilizado neste livro, dispondo-se a possíveis acertos posteriores caso, inadvertida e involuntariamente, a identificação de algum deles tenha sido omitida.

- **Atendimento ao cliente:** (11) 5080-0751 | faleconosco@grupogen.com.br

- Traduzido de:
  A COMPREHENSIVE GUIDE TO SPORTS PHYSIOLOGY AND INJURY MANAGEMENT: AN INTERDISCIPLINARY APPROACH, FIRST EDITION.
  Copyright © 2021, Elsevier Limited. All rights reserved.
  This edition of *A Comprehensive Guide to Sports Physiology and Injury Management: An Interdisciplinary Approach, 1st edition*, by Stuart Porter and Johnny Wilson, is published by arrangement with Elsevier Inc.
  ISBN: 978-0-7020-7489-9
  Esta edição de *A Comprehensive Guide to Sports Physiology and Injury Management: An Interdisciplinary Approach*, 1ª edição, de Stuart Porter e Johnny Wilson, é publicada por acordo com a Elsevier Inc.

- Direitos exclusivos para a língua portuguesa
  Copyright © 2023 by
  GEN | GRUPO EDITORIAL NACIONAL S.A.
  Publicado pelo selo Editora Guanabara Koogan Ltda.
  Travessa do Ouvidor, 11
  Rio de Janeiro – RJ – CEP 20040-040
  www.grupogen.com.br

- Reservados todos os direitos. É proibida a duplicação ou reprodução deste volume, no todo ou em parte, em quaisquer formas ou por quaisquer meios (eletrônico, mecânico, gravação, fotocópia, distribuição pela Internet ou outros), sem permissão, por escrito, do GEN | Grupo Editorial Nacional Participações S/A.

- Capa: Bruno Gomes

- Imagem da capa: © master1305 (iStock)

- Editoração eletrônica: Viviane Nepomuceno

Nota

Este livro foi produzido pelo GEN | Grupo Editorial Nacional, sob sua exclusiva responsabilidade. Profissionais da área da Saúde devem fundamentar-se em sua própria experiência e em seu conhecimento para avaliar quaisquer informações, métodos, substâncias ou experimentos descritos nesta publicação antes de empregá-los. O rápido avanço nas Ciências da Saúde requer que diagnósticos e posologias de fármacos, em especial, sejam confirmados em outras fontes confiáveis. Para todos os efeitos legais, a Elsevier, os autores, os editores ou colaboradores relacionados a esta obra não podem ser responsabilizados por qualquer dano ou prejuízo causado a pessoas físicas ou jurídicas em decorrência de produtos, recomendações, instruções ou aplicações de métodos, procedimentos ou ideias contidos neste livro.

- Ficha catalográfica

CIP-BRASIL. Catalogação na Publicação
Sindicato Nacional dos Editores de Livros, RJ

P878f

Porter, Stuart
  Fisiologia do esporte e tratamento de lesões : uma abordagem interdisciplinar / Stuart Porter, Johnny Wilson ; tradução Dilza Campos ; revisão técnica Ricardo Ambrosio. - 1. ed. - Rio de Janeiro : GEN | Grupo Editorial Nacional S.A. Publicado pelo selo Editora Guanabara Koogan Ltda., 2023.
  488 p. : il. ; 28 cm.

  Tradução de: A comprehensive guide to sports physiology and injury management : an interdisciplinary approach
  Inclui bibliografia e índice
  ISBN 978-85-9515-939-6

  1. Exercícios físicos - Aspectos fisiológicos. 2. Esportes - Aspectos fisiológicos. 3. Lesões esportivas. I. Wilson, Johnny. II. Campos, Dilza. III. Ambrosio, Ricardo. IV. Título.

22-78742
CDD: 617.1027
CDU: 612.766.1:616-001

Meri Gleice Rodrigues de Souza - Bibliotecária - CRB-7/6439

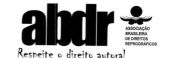

Odiei cada minuto de treinamento, mas disse: "Não desista. Sofra agora e viva o resto de sua vida como um campeão."

Muhammad Ali, 1942-2016
Campeão mundial dos pesos-pesados

Dedicamos este livro a esportistas de todas as idades, habilidades e orientações que se esforçam para se destacar e merecem o melhor apoio possível de nós, profissionais médicos, para alcançar seus objetivos.

Colaboradores

Ademola Adejuwon
Consultant Sports and Exercise Medicine, Institute of Sports, Exercise and Health, London (ISEH). Honorary Consultant University College London Hospitals NHS Foundation Trust. 10 years lead club doctor for English Premiership Rugby Club. Founding member of the multi-disciplinary Complex Concussion Clinic at the Institute of Sports Exercise Health, London.

Nikhil Ahluwalia, MBBS, BSc (Hons), MSc in Sports Cardiology
Cardiology Specialty Registrar at St Bartholomew's Hospital, London, UK. Nikhil's clinical subspecialty interests are in arrhythmias and devices. He has an active research interest in atrial fibrillation and early electrophysiological manifestations associated with exercise in amateur athletes.

Jill Alexander, MSc, BSc (Hons), MSST, MSMA, RFU, FHEA
Senior Lecturer and Course Lead for the BSc Sports Therapy programme and module leads on the MSc Football Science and Rehabilitation course at the University of Central Lancashire. Jill is working towards completing her PhD investigating mechanisms of cryotherapy in elite sport. Jill has worked in semi and professional rugby for several years at national and county level and most recently with the France national team at the U20's World Cup. Jill has publications in the area of cryotherapy and her research focuses around the effects of cryotherapy and whole-body cryotherapy in sport through several performance parameters including biomechanical, physiological, psychological markers. Jill currently supervises postgraduate research students across several scopes of elite sport performance, injury, rehabilitation and decision making. Although not limited to this area she has publications in elite performance and injury recovery; and her research interests include current projects in the remit of elite equine and rider performance through kinematic analysis.

Nick Allen, PhD, MSc (Sports Med), BSc (Hons)
Clinical Director, Birmingham Royal Ballet, Honorary Lecturer for Queen Mary's University London. Nick has over 20 years' experience in elite sports and performance. Alongside his work at the ballet he has worked as an external consultant to various professional and Olympic organizations. Prior to joining Birmingham Royal Ballet he was Head of Medical Services for a premiership rugby club. He lectures on the MSc in Sports Medicine at QMUL and Nottingham University. He is on the Sports Advisory Group for the Centre for Sport, Exercise and Osteoarthritis Research Versus Arthritis.

Brent Arnold, PhD, ATC, FNATA
Professor and Chair, Department of Health Sciences, School of Health and Human Sciences, Indiana University (IUPUI). Prior to Indiana University, Dr. Arnold was the Director of the Sports Medicine Research Laboratory and of Graduate studies in the Department of Kinesiology at Virginia Commonwealth University. He was also on the Kinesiology faculty at the University of Virginia and was a practicing athletic trainer at Princeton University. His research has focused on balance and proprioceptive deficits in individuals with chronic ankle instability.

Marcus Bateman, MSc (Physiotherapy),
BSc (Hons) (Physiotherapy)
Consultant physiotherapist at Derby Shoulder Unit, University Hospitals of Derby & Burton NHS Foundation Trust, Derby, UK. Marcus is a Copeland Fellow of the British Elbow and Shoulder Society. He has a special interest in atraumatic shoulder instability and designed the Derby Shoulder Instability Rehabilitation Programme which is now used worldwide. Marcus is involved with numerous clinical research trials and lectures internationally on the subject of the assessment and management of shoulder disorders.

Mike Beere, MSc, BSc, ASCC (Accredited Strength and Conditioning Coach with UKSCA)
Senior Strength and Conditioning Coach at Cardiff City Football Club. Mike is focused on the performance enhancement and preparation of football players, and on the role of strength and conditioning practices in rehabilitation, with a key area of interest in hamstring (posterior chain) and calf performance. Mike is currently working for a PhD on strength and conditioning practices in elite football, and how practices can be incorporated into periods of fixture congestion to help maintain and improve performance; and on the use of isometric force testing as a key monitoring and predictive tool for lower limb performance.

Marc Beggs, MSc (Sports and Exercise Medicine),
BSc (Hons) Physiotherapy
First Team Physiotherapist, Munster Rugby. Marc has been involved in professional rugby in a range of different roles, including Ulster Rugby, Welsh Rugby and Irish Rugby. Marc's work focuses on the long-term rehabilitation of players as well as the monitoring of previously injured players following their return to play. He has a particular interest in the rehabilitation of upper limb injuries in rugby.

Paco Biosca
Specialist in Orthopaedic Surgery; former President of both the European Federation of Orthopaedic and Sports Trauma and the Spanish Society of Sports Trauma; Professor Titular Anatomia at University of Lleida (INEF-C); Head of Chelsea FC Medical Department.

Lyndsey M. Cannon, BSc, GSR, FAFS
Lecturer in Sport Rehabilitation, School of Sport, Health & Applied Sciences at St Mary's University, Twickenham, London, UK. Lyndsey studied sport rehabilitation at St Mary's, after which she worked in private practice, within professional national sport and taught at St Mary's as a visiting lecturer. Lyndsey has recently become a Fellow of Applied Functional Science after completing her studies with the American functional movement specialists, Gray Institute.

Dean Chatterjee, MBBS, PgDip Clin Ed
Club doctor for Nottingham Rugby and team doctor for the England U18s men's football team. Dean is also an event doctor for England athletics and British gymnastics. He has a keen interest in pitch-side emergency care, sports cardiology and concussion.

David M. Clancy, MSc (Sports Medicine),
BSc (Physiotherapy), MISCP
Founder and strategic director of Hauora Ltd., a whole-person wellbeing and healthcare company, based in Dublin, Ireland; Consultant for medical and performance services for the European players of the Brooklyn Nets and the San Antonio Spurs of the NBA. David is the founder and host of the podcast Sleep Eat Perform Repeat, which focuses on what makes high-performing individuals succeed in sport and business. He was involved in research in the Royal College of Surgeons (Dublin, Ireland) as part of a research group investigating injury surveillance and

load management in schoolboys rugby in Dublin. He is a guest lecturer at Florida International University. David's work focuses on injury prevention strategies, movement analysis, load management of tendons and the rehabilitation of injuries such as ACL, shoulder instability and hamstring strains. He has written articles in The Times (UK) as a sports medicine opinion expert.

Nicholas Clark, PhD, MSc, MCSP, MMACP, CSCS
Physiotherapy Lecturer and Researcher in the School of Sport, Rehabilitation and Exercise Sciences, University of Essex, UK, External Examiner for masters and doctoral degree programmes in the United Kingdom, Knee Consultant Physiotherapist. As a chartered physiotherapist with more than 21 years of clinical experience, Nick has practiced in London NHS teaching hospitals, at Saracens Rugby Union Football Club, with the British Army Infantry and Parachute Regiments, and in private practice. Nick's teaching roles have included Visiting Lecturer and External Examiner to the MSc Manual Therapy and MSc Sports Physiotherapy degrees at University College London, Clinical Tutor and Examiner for the Musculoskeletal Association of Chartered Physiotherapists (MACP), teaching exercise rehabilitation instructors and physiotherapists for the Ministry of Defence, and teaching on sports medicine masters and doctoral degrees in the United States. Nick also serves as a manuscript reviewer for scientific and clinical journals.

Paul Comfort, BSc (Hons) Sports Science, MSc Exercise and Nutrition Science, PhD in Sports Biomechanics and Strength and Conditioning, PGCAP
Reader in Strength and Conditioning and programme leader for the MSc Strength and Conditioning, University of Salford, UK. Professional Member British Association of Sport and Exercise Sciences (BASES) Certified Strength and Conditioning Coach, recertified with Distinction (CSCS*D) with the National Strength and Conditioning Association (NSCA); Accredited Strength and Conditioning Coach (ASCC) with the United Kingdom Strength and Conditioning Association (UKSCA), Founder Member of the UKSCA. During his time at the University of Salford, Paul has consulted with numerous professional rugby league, rugby union and football teams, in addition to coordinating the sports science support and strength and conditioning for England Men's Lacrosse (2008–2012). He has co-authored >150 peer reviewed journal articles and is on the editorial boards for the Journal of Strength and Conditioning Research, Sports Biomechanics and the European Journal of Sport Science.

Paulina Czubacka, BSc Sport Rehabilitation and Exercise Science, BASRaT-reg
Paulina graduated from the University of Nottingham in 2017 and following her elective placement at the club, she joined Notts County FC as a First Team Sport Rehabilitator. Currently Paulina works at Nottingham Trent University as a lead therapist for Women's and Men's Football Programme, Men's Basketball Programme, as well as Nottingham Forest Women's Football Club. She is also working in the private sector at a Physiotherapy & Sport Rehabilitation Clinic – Nottingham Physio. Paulina's work is primarily focused around lower limb rehabilitation. She is passionate about end stage and return to play rehab.

Eamonn Delahunt, PhD, BSc, MISCP
Professor, University College Dublin, Dublin, Ireland. Eamonn is recognized nationally and internationally as a leading academic sports physiotherapist. He has published >120 peer-reviewed articles.

Carrie Docherty, PhD, LAT, ATC
Dr. Docherty is the Executive Associate Dean in the School of Public Health – Bloomington at Indiana University. She is also a Professor in the Department of Kinesiology and the Program Director of the Graduate Athletic Training Program. Her research focuses on rehabilitation sciences, specifically how chronic ankle instability affects the ability to participate in physical activity and health related quality of life. She is an internationally recognized scholar and educator in athletic training.

Jon Fearn, MSc, MACP, MCSP
First Team Physiotherapist, Chelsea Football Club. Jon's career in professional football spans over 20 years, with the past 10 years at Chelsea FC. Jon's work is primarily involved in managing the rehabilitation of first team players after injury and overseeing the Medical Department in the Academy. He also speaks on a number of postgraduate MSc courses and occasionally represents the Chelsea medical team at international conferences.

Ian Gatt, MSc, OMT, MAACP, MCSP, SRP, BSc (Hons)
Head of Performance Services and Lead Physiotherapist for GB Boxing. Ian has been a sport physiotherapist for over 20 years, working predominately in Olympic and Professional boxing. He is an Upper Limb Injury specialist with the prestigious English Institute of Sport (EIS), providing an advisory role particularly on Hand-Wrist injuries. Ian has lectured on Sporting Upper Limb biomechanics and injuries through various platforms, as well as collaborating on several publications. He is currently a PhD candidate with Sheffield Hallam University on wrist kinematics in boxing.

Michael Giakoumis, MSc (Exercise Science S&C), MSc (Sports Physiotherapy), BSc (Physiotherapy)
Sports Physiotherapist and Medical Research and Innovation Lead at British Athletics, the Centre for Health and Human Performance (CHHP), and Total Performance UK. Michael's career has involved working across Australian rules and European football, the NBA, and international athletics. His work focuses on the diagnosis, management and rehabilitation of lower limb injuries, with a particular interest in the hip and groin, and lower limb tendon and muscle injuries.

Mark Glaister, BSc, PhD, FACSM
Reader in Exercise Physiology, HEA Senior Fellow, Faculty of Sport, Health and Applied Sciences, St Mary's University, Twickenham, UK. Mark gained his doctorate from the University of Edinburgh and is currently working and researching at St Mary's University, Twickenham. His research interests are in physiological responses to multiple sprint work as well as the effects of various ergogenic aids, particularly caffeine.

Paul Godfrey, MSc, PGDMT(Aus), Grad Dip Phys, MACP, AACP, ACPSEM(Gold), HCPC
Head of Medical & Performance Services at Coventry City FC. Paul is a Chartered Manipulative Physiotherapist and Physiologist with extensive clinical experience of working with individuals and teams across a number of sporting codes and performance genres at national and international levels in the UK and abroad. He has worked with elite athletes in a variety sports for the English Institute for Sport (EIS), UK Athletics (UKA) and a number of professional football teams across all four divisions. Paul has also worked with artistic athletes from Cirque du Soleil and West End productions. Currently, his role involves the management and co-ordination of all the medical, rehabilitation and performance requirements of the club's first team & U23 players.

Neil Greig, PGDip (SEM), BSc (Hons) (Sports Therapy)
Head of the Medical Department, Brentford Football Club. Neil's career within professional sport has spanned 15 years, predominantly within elite football. His work focuses mainly on the rehabilitation of lower limb sports injury, with particular interests in knee pathologies and criteria-guided return to sport.

Tom Hallas, BSc
Tom currently works at Nottingham Forest academy as performance and rehabilitation therapist. In his role Tom liaises with the entire sports science and medicine team to deliver the rehabilitation programmes for injured U16-U23 players. Previously, Tom held the role of first team

sports therapist at Notts County FC for five years. Tom has a keen interest in the area of rehabilitation of lower limb sporting injuries and is also a member of BASRAT.

Charlotte Häger, PhD (Neurophysiology), BSc (Physiotherapy)

Professor at the Department of Community Medicine and Rehabilitation, Physiotherapy, Umeå University, Sweden. Charlotte's research spans the study of basic movement functions in health and in pathological conditions to intervention studies and research on how to study and assess human movements reliably. She is head of the U-motion analysis laboratory and has a clinical affiliation to the Orthopaedic Clinic of Umeå University Hospital. Charlotte and her research group have published extensively on ACL injuries, particularly in relation to consequences of injury on movement patterns and strategies.

Kim Hébert-Losier, PhD, BSc (Physiotherapy)

Senior Lecturer for *Te Huataki Waiora* School of Health, Division of Health, Engineering, Computing and Science, University of Waikato, New Zealand. She is the lead biomechanics researcher at the University of Waikato Adams Centre for High Performance. Dr Hébert-Losier's work focuses on the objective quantification of human movement in health and sport, with a particular emphasis on the prevention of musculoskeletal injuries of the lower limb, sports performance, and clinical assessment methods.

Jackie Hindle, MSc, MMACP, MCSP

Senior Lecturer at Manchester Metropolitan University, Manchester, UK. Jackie is also a private practitioner. Jackie has been a member of the Musculoskeletal Association of Chartered Physiotherapists since 2002.

Jonathan Hobbs, BSc (physiotherapy), MSc (acupuncture), MCSP, FHEA

A physiotherapist with over 20 years clinical experience practising acupuncture and dry needling within the NHS, private sector and professional sport. He is a Fellow of the Higher Education Academy and Chairman of the Acupuncture Association of Chartered Physiotherapists. A previous school principal of physiotherapy he currently lectures internationally and consults for physiotherapists from the English Institute of Sport, Sport Wales, Premiership and Championship football clubs as well as the Ministry of Defence and the NHS.

Shivan Jassim, MBBS, BSc (Hons), MRCS, MSc (Sports & Exercise Medicine), FRCS (Tr & Orth)

Senior Orthopaedic Fellow in Melbourne, Australia. Shivan completed his specialist training on the Stanmore Rotation in London. He has worked as a pitch side Rugby Union doctor at International Level in the Men's and Women's games. He has a specialist interest in shoulder and elbow surgery and has just completed the Melbourne Orthopaedic Group Upper Limb Fellowship, which involved the treatment of several elite athletes in Australian Rules Football and Rugby League.

Lester Jones, BSc, MScMed, PGCE

Inaugural Chair of National Pain Group, Australian Physiotherapy Association. Lester is a pain physiotherapist with a wealth of experience spanning 25 years in education and clinical practice. He has worked in a range of clinical settings, including interdisciplinary clinics, with an emphasis on psychologically-informed assessment and treatment of pain. He is coauthor of the Pain and Movement Reasoning Model, a clincial reasoning tool that has been adapted and adopted to assist health practitioners assess pain in a range of settings, including pain associated with the musculoskeletal system, the pelvic region, with breastfeeding and in people who have survived torture or other traumatic experiences.

Paul A. Jones, PhD, MSc, BSc (Hons), CSCS*D, CSci, BASES Accredited

Lecturer in Sports Biomechanics/Strength and Conditioning at the University of Salford, UK. Paul earned a BSc (Hons) and MSc in Sports Science both from Liverpool John Moores University and a PhD in Sports Biomechanics at the University of Salford. He is a Certified Strength and Conditioning Specialist recertified with distinction (CSCS*D) with the National Strength and Conditioning Association (NSCA), an Accredited Sports and Exercise Scientist with the British Association of Sports and Exercise Sciences (BASES) and a Chartered Scientist (CSci) with The Science Council. Paul has over 18 years' experience in Biomechanics and Strength and Conditioning support to athletes and teams, working in sports such as athletics, football and rugby and was a former sports science support co-ordinator for UK disability athletics (2002–2006). Paul has authored/co-authored over 80 peer reviewed journal articles and is a member of the BASES Accreditation committee.

Dimitrios Kalogiannidis, MBBS, FRCEM, MsC SEM

First Team Club Doctor Chelsea Football Club, Emergency Medicine consultant and sport medicine doctor. Has been working at Chelsea FC for the past 6 years and has been involved with Chelsea Women's team, the Academy and Men's First Team. Dimitris's work is primarily now with managing day to day injuries and illnesses of athletes and preparation of Emergency Action plan. He is also currently covering medical care on all home and away games.

Simon Kemp

Associate Professor Simon Kemp is a Specialist Sports Medicine Doctor and the Medical Services Director for the Rugby Football Union, the National Governing Body for the game in England. He worked as a team physician in Rugby, Soccer (Fulham Football Club) and Basketball (English Basketball Team) from 1995 to 2013 and was the England team doctor for the Rugby World Cup campaigns in 2003 and 2007. He was the Tournament Medical Director for the 2015 Rugby World Cup. He has over 20 years of experience from clinical, research and policy perspectives in head injury management. He is a member of World Rugby's Medicine, Science and Research and Concussion working groups and the Football Association Independent Head Injury and Concussion Expert Panel.

Roger Kerry, PhD, MSc, BSc (Hons) Physiotherapy

Associate Professor, Faculty of Medicine and Health Sciences at the University of Nottingham, UK. Roger is a qualified chartered physiotherapist, and an Honorary Fellow of the UK's Musculoskeletal Association of Chartered Physiotherapists. His interests are in adverse events and physiotherapy interventions of the head and neck, particularly on the causal nature of interventions.

Jason Laird, PG Dip (Advanced Musculoskeletal Physiotherapy), MSc (Physiotherapy), BSc (Sport Rehabilitation)

Lead Physiotherapist, British Gymnastics and English Institute of Sport, Lillieshall National Sports Centre, Shropshire, UK. Jason is an experienced sports physiotherapist currently working for the English Institute of Sport as the Lead Physiotherapist for British Gymnastics. Prior to his work in Gymnastics, he worked for British Judo as the Lead Physiotherapist during the Rio 2016 cycle. Jason has extensive experience of elite performance environments having previously worked at the Chelsea FC Academy and the Royal Ballet Company.

Etienne Laverse, MBBS, BSc (Hons), MRCP (UK) (Neurology)

Research Fellow in Traumatic Brain Injury at UCL Institute of Neurology, Queen Square, UK and a Consultant Neurologist in the NHS.

Elaine Lonnemann, PT, DPT, OCS, MTC, FAAOMPT Adv MSC PT

Doctor of Physical Therapy, BS in Physical Therapy; Program Director for the Transitional Doctor of Physical Therapy program, University of Louisville University of St Augustine for Health Sciences; Associate Professor at Bellarmine University in Louisville, Kentucky. Elaine has been involved in teaching in the distance education programme with the University of St Augustine since 1998. She has worked as a physical therapist at Northside Hospital and Sullivan Center in East Tennessee, Flagler Hospital, University of Louisville Hospital, and Roane Physical Therapy in Rockwood, Tennessee. She is a member and a fellow of AAOMPT, and a member of the American Physical Therapy Association (APTA), chair of the AAOMPT's international monitoring and educational standards committee and a member of the board of directors of Physiopedia. She was the 2017 recipient of the John McMillan Mennell Service of AAOMPT.

Tommy Lundberg, PhD Sports Science
Lecturer and researcher at the Division of Clinical Physiology, Karolinska Institutet, Stockholm, Sweden. Tommy's ongoing research project relates to nonsteroidal antiinflammatory drugs and muscle adaptations to exercise regimes. Given the need for effective countermeasures to combat muscle atrophy within the clinical setting (sarcopenia, various muscle disorders, etc.) these studies could have a significant impact on exercise and/or medical prescriptions for maintaining muscle health.

Marc-André Maillet, MSc (Coaching Education & Sports Pedagogy)
Founder and Chief Education Officer at Beyond Pulse in Portland, Oregon USA. Former Ohio University lecturer. Marc-André is dedicated to help improve coaching behavior in youth sports.

Aneil Malhotra, MB BChir, MA, MRCP(UK), MSc, PhD, FESC
Aneil is a Presidential Senior Lecturer, University of Manchester, and Consultant Cardiologist, Wythenshawe Hospital and Manchester Royal Infirmary and Manchester Institute of Heath and Performance.

Simon Marsh, BA, MB BChir, MA, MD, FRCSEng, FRCSGen Surg
Consultant Surgeon and Surgical Director of the Gilmore Groin and Hernia Clinic, London, UK. Simon trained at Trinity College Cambridge and the Clinical School, Addenbrooke's Hospital, and was one of the few students to be awarded the William Harvey Studentship in consecutive years. He qualified in 1987, receiving the London FRCS in 1992. In 1996 he was awarded an MD by the University of Cambridge and received the Intercollegiate Fellowship in General Surgery. In 1999, he joined the Gilmore Groin and Hernia Clinic and has been Surgical Director since 2010. Working with Jerry Gilmore, he has modified, and improved, the original Gilmore's groin repair technique into what is now known as a groin reconstruction (the Marsh modification of the Gilmore technique).

Karen May, MSc Sports Med, PGCE LTHE, FHEA, MCSP, HCPC
Principle Lecturer and Academic Lead for Performance Medicine, the School of Medicine, University of Central Lancashire, UK. Prior to joining the University of Central Lancashire, Karen worked as a lead physiotherapist for both professional and semiprofessional sports covering rugby league Super League in England and Australia, rugby union, club, county and international U21 and England junior women's basketball and UK Athletics multi-events team. She continues to work with Olympic skiers, GB mountain & fell runners, and ultra distance runners. Karen has 25 years of experience of working with musculoskeletal and sports injuries and has focused her clinical research with published papers on whole-body cryotherapy and the effects of localized cryotherapy on joint position sense.

Bruno Mazuquin, PhD, MSc, BSc (Physiotherapy)
Research Fellow in Physiotherapy, Clinical Trials Unit, University of Warwick and Department of Health Professions, Manchester Metropolitan University, UK. Bruno's work is focused on the rehabilitation of musculoskeletal disorders, especially on shoulders. His work also involves the clinical application of biomechanics, evidence-based practice development and epidemiology.

Steve McCaig, BSc Physiotherapy (Hons), MSc Manipulative Therapy
Athlete Health Consultant, English Institute of Sport, Loughborough, UK. Steve has worked as a physiotherapist in elite sport for over 14 years. Previously he was a senior physiotherapist at the England and Wales Cricket Board. He has been involved in research in a number of areas including injury surveillance, workload, bowling biomechanics and low back pain in cricketers. He is currently completing a PhD in throwing arm pain in cricketers.

Christopher J. McCarthy, PhD, PGDs Biomechanics, Man. Therapy, Physiotherapy, FCSP, FMACP
Consultant Physiotherapist and Spinal Fellow, Department of Health Professions, Manchester Metropolitan University, Manchester, UK. After qualifying as a physiotherapist in 1989 Chris undertook postgraduate training in biomechanics and manipulative therapy before undertaking a PhD in rehabilitation within the Faculty of Medicine at Manchester University. Following postdoctoral studies investigating the subclassification of nonspecific low back pain, he joined Imperial College Healthcare. He now teaches and runs the clinical facility of Manchester School of Physiotherapy and teaches internationally on manual therapy, specifically on combined movement theory. He regularly reviews and publishes papers in the academic field of manual therapy. He was awarded a Fellowship of the MACP for advances in manual therapy in 2010 and a Fellowship of the Chartered Society of Physiotherapy in 2011.

Ruth MacDonald
Senior lecturer in physiotherapy at Manchester Metropolitan University, UK. Ruth completed her MSc in Manual Therapy in 2007 and became a member of the MACP in 2004. She continues to work in private practice.

David McKay, B.S. Sports Medicine and Exercise Science, CSCS, USSF A license, UEFA B license
First team assistant coach/performance coach for the Philadelphia Union. He previously served as the director of fitness for Orlando City Soccer Club and assistant fitness coach for Sporting Kansas City.

Jamie McPhee, PGCAP, FHEA, PhD Skeletal Muscle and Exercise Physiology, BSc, Sport and Exercise Science
Deputy Director of University Alliance Doctoral Training Alliance in Applied Biosciences for Health, member of the Management Board at Manchester Interdisciplinary Centre for Research into Ageing (MICRA), Manchester, UK. Jamie is also an expert advisor to several public health groups on falls prevention, Physical Deputy Director of Musculoskeletal Sciences Research, Lead of the Neuromuscular and Skeletal Ageing Research Group, Lead BSc Applied and Environmental Physiology.

Akbar de Medici, MBBS, BSc (Hons), PhD MRCS
Dr de Medici is an Honorary Associate Professor at UCL/UCLH and supported the creation of the Institute of Sport Exercise and Health (ISEH), a major legacy of the 2012 Olympic Games. Akbar has worked closely with the CMO of the NFL, supporting medical provisions for the London games since 2015. He also is the founding partner of Cavendish Health - a leading international health management company.

Said Mekary, PhD in Exercise Physiology
Dr Said Mekary is the Director of the Acadia Active Aging program, an associate professor and exercise physiologist in the School of Kinesiology at Acadia University. He is an emerging scholar with a broad background in the biological and cardiovascular health sciences who has established himself as an up-and-coming leader in the field of exercise physiology, cardiovascular aging and cognition studies in Canada. Dr Mekary was recently awarded the Acadia University Faculty of Professional Studies Outstanding Research Project Award for his work on the role of pulmonary physiology and exercise. Dr Mekary also continues to have applied research interests in the outcomes of exercise interventions in athletes, aging populations, and those with chronic disease and disability.

Claire Minshull, PhD, BSc, PGCHE
Claire is Principal Researcher at the RJAH Orthopaedic Hospital, UK and Director and founder of Get Back To Sport, an education and training company for healthcare professionals. Claire completed her PhD

in neuromuscular physiology and exercise science at the University of Wales, Bangor in 2004. She has worked for over 20 years years in academia, research and in practice, including as Senior Lecturer at Nottingham Trent University; collaboration lead between between Universities in Edinburgh and the Royal Infirmary of Edinburgh on physiotherapy-focused clinical trials and, in a rehabilitation role with individual patients and athletes. Claire's research and teaching interests include the influences of exercise and conditioning on rehabilitation endeavours and in the management of osteoarthritis.

James Moore, MPhtySt (Manips), MSc App Biomechanics, BSc (Hons), CSCS

Founder and Director of Sports and Exercise Medicine for the Centre for Health and Human Performance (CHHP), London, UK. James has had an expansive career in sport both as a clinician and a leader. He has worked in cricket for 5 years, with England Rugby Elite Performance Squad in the preparation for the Rugby World Cup 2011, and with Saracens RFC as Head of Medical Services. He has also been involved in four Olympic cycles, culminating in being Deputy Chef De Mission for Performance Services for Team GB at the Olympic Games Rio 2016, the most successful games to date for the British Olympic Association. James has lectured on hip and groin and hamstring injuries, as well as lower limb biomechanics for over 15 years, and is currently a PhD candidate with University College London for modelling the hip.

Puneet Monga, MBBS, MS (Orth.), DNB, MRCS, Dip Sports Med (GB&I), MSc, FRCS (Tr & Orth.), MD

Consultant Orthopaedic Surgeon at Wrightington Hospital, Wigan, UK. Puneet has a specialist clinical practice focusing on shoulder problems. His surgical practice focuses on arthroscopic shoulder surgery, sports injuries and shoulder replacement surgery. His research interests include biomechanics of the shoulder, assessment of surgical outcomes and the application of modern technology, including the use of 3D printing to improve surgical treatment.

Jim Moxon, MB ChB, MRCGP, MSc (MSK ultrasound), MFSEM

Head of Football Medicine and Fitness, Liverpool FC Academy, Liverpool, UK. Jim's research work is focused on the application of shear-wave elastography to muscles and tendons.

Ali Noorani, MBBS, BSc (Hons), MRCS, FRCS (Trauma & Orth)

Consultant Trauma & Orthopaedic Surgeon in shoulder, elbow and upper limb surgery at St Bartholomew's and the Royal London Hospital, Barts Health NHS Trust, London, UK. Ali is also the Medical Director of an elite group of surgeons called Orthopaedic Specialists and also the Medical Director of Harley Street Specialist Hospital. He has specialist interests in sports injuries and joint preservation of the shoulder and elbow.

Aidan O'Connell

High Performance Manager with Cork GAA. Formerly Strength and Conditioning Coach with Munster Rugby and the IRFU from 2001–2019. Aidan graduated with a Sport Science Degree from the University of Limerick in 1997 and received his Masters in Coaching Studies from the University of Edinburgh in 2001.

Des O'Shaughnessy

Bachelor of Applied Science (Physiotherapy), Masters of Science Module, ESP for the Allied Health Professional, Masters of Public Health Module. Des works in the Alice Springs Pain Clinic and in private practice, Connections Physical Therapy. Des graduated over 20 years ago from the University of Sydney, and worked in Sydney and Alice Springs. Over half of his clinical experience has been in the UK including as the Clinical Specialist Lead for the Islington Primary Care Trust Musculoskeletal Outpatients Service. He has also worked in the community development field working with indigenous communities of Central Australia addressing their levels of disadvantage.

Jason Palmer, B.H.M.S.(Ed.) Hons., B.Phty.

Jason is an Australian born and trained physiotherapist with more than 25 years' experience working in professional sport. Jason moved to the UK in 2001 to join Fulham Football Club's Medical staff as they entered the English Premiership, before moving to Chelsea Football Club in 2008 where he remains a consultant physiotherapist.

Ioannis Paneris

Ioannis qualified as a physiotherapist in 2006 and completed his MSc in manual therapy in 2013. He has more than 20 years of clinical experience as a physiotherapist in the NHS with the last 19 years in neuro-musculoskeletal care. Since 2008 he has worked as an Advanced Practitioner in central Manchester. He has lectured in manual and neuro-musculoskeletal postgraduate courses for a number of UK universities and he has made chapter contributions in a number of neuro-musculoskeletal physiotherapy and rehabilitation publications. He is an associate lecturer at Manchester Metropolitan University.

Amanda Parry, BSc (Hons) Radiography, PGDip Medical Ultrasound (Aust), PGCert MSK Ultrasound

Amanda is currently studying for MSc in Ultrasound. Amanda is a sonographer with a special interest in musculoskeletal ultrasound; she has been practising for 20 years both in the UK and Australia, in the public and private sector. She currently works within the NHS, alongside sports physicians, orthopaedic surgeons, radiologists and other allied health practitioners.

Nic Perrem, BSc, MSc (Sports Injury Management), BSc (Hons) (Sports Therapy), MSST (Member of the Society of Sports Therapists)

Lecturer in Sport Rehabilitation, St Mary's University, London, UK. Nic is a graduate sports therapist who holds full membership of the Society of Sports Therapists alongside associate membership of the British Association of Sport and Exercise Medicine (BASeM) and professional membership of the British Association of Sport and Exercise Sciences (BASES). Nic holds professional qualifications in manual and manipulative therapy, acupuncture and dry needling, kinesiology taping (RockDoc certified), pitch-side emergency trauma, nutrition and personal training. He has also worked in private practice with varied patient case load. At St Mary's Nic teaches at both undergraduate and postgraduate levels. He is currently engaged in a number of research projects examining factors related to lower limb injury and motor control and is an active member of the Knee Injury Control and Clinical Advancement (KICCA) research group.

Jim Richards, PhD, MSc, BEng

Professor of Biomechanics and Research Lead, Allied Health Research Unit, University of Central Lancashire, UK. Jim's work includes the clinical application of biomechanics, the development of new assessment tools for chronic disease, conservative and surgical management of orthopaedic and neurological conditions and development of evidence-based approaches for improving clinical management and rehabilitation.

James Rowland, PGDip (Sports Physiotherapy), BSc (Hons) Physiotherapy

Senior 1st Team Physiotherapist, Cardiff City Football Club. James has worked in professional football for 10 years, operating from the Premier League to League Two. He has particular interest in the delivery and design of return-to-play protocols, with research interests in isometric posterior chain strength and fatigue-profiling during fixture congested schedules.

Diane Ryding, MSc, BSc (Hons) (Physiotherapy)

Head Physiotherapist for the Foundation and Youth Development Phases at Manchester United FC. Diane has been involved in academy football since 2004. Her role is to ensure that paediatric injuries are managed appropriately whilst considering growth and maturation and ensuring that the long-term athletic development of the player takes precedent over short-term gains. She also teaches on sports trauma management courses.

James Selfe, DSc, PhD, MA, GradDipPhys, FCSP
Professor of Physiotherapy, Manchester Metropolitan University, Manchester, UK. James led the first group to develop an anatomically based method to define a region of interest for thermal imaging analyses. He and his team have used this method to investigate skin temperature response to a variety of low-cost localized cryotherapy interventions which patients and healthcare professionals can apply in domestic environments. They have also used this method to investigate optimum treatment time dosage in whole-body cryotherapy.

Rohi Shah, BMBS, BMedSci, MRCS, MSc SEM
Trauma and Orthopaedic Specialty Registrar at the East Midlands South Deanery. Rohi has been the Club Doctor for Notts County Football Club for 6 years. He has a keen interest in pitch-side emergency care and has been at the forefront of developing and refining the Emergency Action Protocol. His surgical subspecialty interests include soft-tissue reconstruction and trauma surgery.

Adam Sheehan, MSc (Strength & Conditioning) BBUS
Head of Conditioning and Sport Science at Munster Rugby, Munster, Eire. Adam's work is focused on repeated high-intensity efforts in rugby union, specifically at peak game demands and effect on passage duration with respect to repeated high-intensity efforts. His work also involves athletic development and sport science integration.

Natalie Shur, MBChB, BMedSci (Hons), MRes, MRCP(UK)
Sport and Exercise Medicine Registrar and Clinical Research Fellow, University of Nottingham, UK. Dr Shur is currently undertaking a PhD at the University of Nottingham investigating the maintenance of muscle metabolic health in relation to immobilization and injury, before completing her specialty training in sport and exercise medicine.

Graham Smith, GradDipPhys, FCSP, DipTP, CertED
Rehabilitation and Sports Injury Consultant, Fellow of the Chartered Society of Physiotherapy and Chairman of the Society of Sports Therapists (UK). Graham is responsible for setting up and running the Football Association National Rehabilitation Centre at Lilleshall and has worked with British Olympic and representative teams, as well as in professional football. He now runs a clinic and consultancy in Glasgow, and lectures nationally and internationally on the treatment and rehabilitation of musculoskeletal injuries and sports injury management.

Paul Sindall, BSc, MSc, PhD, FHEA
Senior Lecturer at the University of Salford, UK. Paul is a member of the Peter Harrison Centre for Disability Sport and a member of the European Research Group in Disability Sport (ERGiDs). His PhD and masters studies were in exercise physiology, working in the field of disability sports testing and training. Paul has extensive practice-based and managerial experience in the health and fitness industry, and in the provision of sports science support services to athletes in a range of disability and able-bodied sports. He is interested in the role of exercise and physical activity in the prevention and treatment of disease.

Neil Sullivan, MSc, BSc (Hons), chartered physiotherapist, MCSP, MSST
Neil has over 16 years of experience in professional football, leading medical departments at Derby County, Oxford United and Peterborough FC. More recently Neil has focused on private practice and consultancy roles in Elite sports. He has a special interest in pelvic dysfunction and its implications to pain and performance.

Michael Sup, PhD
Michael is a Co-Founder of Beyond Pulse serving as the VP of Sports Education and Research. Michael has a coaching background and has served as an Academy Coach at Luton Town FC as well as a host of different coaching positions in the USA. Michael's research interests involve developing best practices in youth sports development and coaching education.

Richard Sylvester, MB BCh, PhD, FRCP
Consultant Neurologist at the National Hospital of Neurology and Honorary Lecturer at University College London specializing in the management of brain injury and cognitive disorders. Lead of the complex concussion clinic at the Institute of Sport Exercise and Health, UCL. Member of the traumatic brain injury advisory expert group of the Association of British Neurologists and English Football Association's Concussion Expert panel.

Alan J. Taylor, MSc, MCSP, HCPC
Physiotherapy Assistant Professor, Faculty of Medicine and Health Sciences at the University of Nottingham, UK. Alan is a qualified chartered physiotherapist, and a former professional cyclist. He also works as a medico-legal expert witness. His interests are in sports medicine, rehabilitation and haemodynamics. He has written widely on the topic of adverse events linked to physiotherapy interventions of the head and neck.

Mick Thacker, PhD, MSc, GradDipPhys, GradDipMan NMSD, FCSP
Associate Professor, Department of Allied Health Sciences Centre of Human & Aerospace Physiological Sciences, South Bank University, London, UK. Mick is also the director of the Pain: Science and Society MSc course at King's College London.

Keith Thornhill, MSc Exercise Science, BSc (Hons) Physiotherapy
Senior First Team Physiotherapist, Munster Rugby. Since graduating in 2007, Keith has worked in a variety of sporting environments, including Leeds Rhinos and currently Munster Rugby. Keith's current role focuses on the management of acute, short-term and ongoing injuries occurring within the squad. Keith has a particular interest in the promotion of injury reduction strategies and building robustness in a team environment.

Cari Thorpe, BSc, PGcert, MCSP, HCPC
Senior Lecturer in Physiotherapy, Manchester Metropolitan University, UK. Cari has a postgraduate certificate in advanced physiotherapy and is currently working towards her PhD, the focus of which is injury prevention in touch (rugby). This involves reviewing recovery strategies and the use of cryotherapy in the reduction of symptoms and enhancement of performance of elite touch players within a tournament situation. Cari has been the Head of Medical Services of England Touch (Rugby) for the past 5 years. This includes the management of a multidisciplinary team of sport science and physiotherapy staff, updating protocols for preseason screening, injury management and recovery to prevent and minimize the effect of injury.

Tony Tompos, PgDip (Physiotherapy), BSc Hons (Sports Rehabilitation)
Sports Physiotherapist. Tony has worked in professional football for more than 7 years, both in the English Football League and the Scottish Premiership. In 2017 Tony was awarded the Scottish League Award at the Football Medical Association annual awards ceremony for his role in improving the management of concussion protocols during football league matches. Tony has a keen interest in the rehabilitation of hamstring and ACL injuries.

Anna Waters, CPsychol AFBPsS, PhD, MSc, BSc
Director at Chimp Management Ltd., Anna has over 15 years' experience of working within professional and Olympic sports, as well as with performers in the arts, including ballet dancers, actors, singers and classical musicians. Anna's research has focused on understanding the role of psychology in athletic injury and developing psychological interventions to facilitate return to sport.

Tim Watson, PhD, BSc(Hons), FCSP
Professor of Physiotherapy, University of Hertfordshire, Hatfield, UK. Tim trained as a physiotherapist before moving into academic work. He taught at Brunel University before taking up his current post. He is also a freelance consultant and provider of postgraduate education programmes, author and researcher. Tim was honoured with a Fellowship of the Chartered Society of Physiotherapy in 2013. His primary research interests are linked to Tissue Repair and Electrophysical modalities.

Daniel Williams, MBChB BSc (Hons), FRCS (Trauma and Ortho)
Research Fellow, Brisbane Hand and Upper Research Institute, Australia. Daniel completed his specialist training on the Percival Pott Rotation in London. He has a specialist interest in upper limb surgery and is currently undertaking a fellowship with the Brisbane Hand and Upper Research Institute, Australia.

Mark Wilson
UEFA A Licensed Coach, NSCAA DOC Diploma, Co-Founder of Beyond Pulse. Mark is a former professional football player who had a 16 year career. Mark played for Manchester United, Middlesborough, FC Dallas and represented England at U16–U21 levels. Post playing Mark was a Director of coaching for a multi-franchise USA youth soccer club overseeing 500 players and 65 staff. More recently Mark co-founded the Beyond Pulse EDTech platform and product in 2017 which now hosts 7500 players and hundreds of coaches across the USA and Canada. As a keynote speaker and TV football pundit, Mark enjoys sharing his thoughts and perceptions in the public domain.

Prefácio

Este livro didático poderá ser usado repetidamente como obra de referência e como auxílio à educação, sem perder seu impacto e sua relevância. Nesta primeira edição, *Fisiologia do Esporte e Tratamento de Lesões: Uma Abordagem Interdisciplinar* conta com 43 capítulos escritos por renomados autores de todo o mundo, cada um com sua expertise em seu campo de atuação.

Dividimos o livro em duas partes: a primeira aborda os principais conceitos básicos do esporte e do desempenho do corpo humano; e a segunda concentra-se em aplicações clínicas, adotando uma abordagem regional e, às vezes, patológica. O livro contém ainda ilustrações totalmente atuais e gráficos de última geração, além do conteúdo baseado em evidências.

Reconhecemos que todos precisam de uma plataforma sólida a partir da qual possam desenvolver novas habilidades, e o material apresentado nesta obra possibilita isso. No entanto, também desafiamos o leitor a tirar as próprias conclusões, por meio de suas habilidades de raciocínio clínico. O objetivo é atrair alunos de graduação e pós-graduação, esperando conquistar também um público internacional, sobretudo nos países onde o esporte tem sido adotado de modo mais holístico.

Embarcar neste projeto foi emocionante e assustador na mesma medida. Gostaríamos de agradecer à Elsevier por nos confiar essa grande responsabilidade; esperamos ter produzido algo de valor. Agradecemos também aos colaboradores, que sempre responderam às nossas educadas insistências com dignidade e profissionalismo quando o tempo de publicação estava próximo. Nossos agradecimentos ainda a Helen Leng, Poppy Garraway e Gill Cloke, da Elsevier, por seu apoio durante o processo editorial.

Mudança é o resultado final de todo verdadeiro aprendizado.
Leo Buscaglia

Stuart Porter
Johnny Wilson

Sumário

Parte 1 Conceitos Básicos Importantes em Esportes, 1

1 Forma e Função do Músculo... 1
Jamie McPhee e Tommy Lundberg

2 Adaptações Musculares e Fadiga.................................. 7
Tommy Lundberg e Jamie McPhee

3 Fisiologia do Desuso, da Imobilização
e de Ambientes de Baixa Carga.......................... 13
*Nicholas C. Clark, Mark Glaister, Lyndsey M. Cannon
e Nic Perrem*

4 Força e Condicionamento: Aspectos Científicos,
Incluindo Princípios de Reabilitação........................ 21
Paul Jones e Paul Comfort

5 Biomecânica das Lesões Esportivas, Manejo
e Considerações Clínicas...................................... 41
*Jim Richards, Carrie Docherty, Brent Arnold, Kim Hébert-Losier,
Charlotte Häger, Bruno Mazuquin e Puneet Monga*

6 Agentes Eletrofísicos: Fisiologia e Evidências........... 53
Tim Watson

7 Crioterapia: Fisiologia e Novas Abordagens............. 65
James Selfe, Cari Thorpe, Karen May e Jill Alexander

8 Fisiologia da Recuperação Esportiva e Atlética........ 79
Tony Tompos

9 Como Entender a Dor na Fisioterapia Esportiva:
Aplicação do Modelo de Raciocínio para a Dor
e o Movimento.. 87
Des O'Shaughnessy e Lester E. Jones

10 Fisiologia da Terapia Manual...................................... 99
*Christopher J. McCarthy, Elaine Lonnemann, Jackie Hindle,
Ruth MacDonald e Ioannis Paneris*

11 Fisiologia da Analgesia por Acupuntura.................. 105
Jonathan Hobbs

12 Determinantes Fisiológicos para o Desempenho
de Resistência: Consumo Máximo de Oxigênio –
Teste, Treinamento e Aplicação Prática................... 111
Paul Sindall

13 Imagem de Ultrassonografia em Lesões na Virilha....131
Amanda Parry

Parte 2 Aplicação Clínica, 139

Seção 1 Problemas Regionais

14 Manejo Conservador de Lesões Agudas
e Crônicas na Virilha.. 139
James Moore e Michael Giakoumis

15 Tratamento Cirúrgico de Lesões
Esportivas na Virilha.. 151
Simon Marsh

16 Quadril Esportivo.. 159
James Moore

17 Disfunção Lombopélvica na População Esportiva:
o "o Que", o "Porquê" e o "Como"........................ 169
Neil Sullivan

18 Reabilitação do Desempenho para Lesões dos
Isquiotibiais – Abordagem de
Sistemas Multimodais.. 177
Johnny Wilson, Paulina Czubacka e Neil Greig

19 Manejo de Ruptura dos Músculos Gastrocnêmico
e Sóleo em Jogadores de Futebol Profissional........ 193
Paul Godfrey, Mike Beere e James Rowland

20 Lesões no Joelho no Futebol Profissional............... 207
Jon Fearn, Paco Biosca, Dimitris Kalogiannidis e Jason Palmer

21 Tornozelo Esportivo: Entorse Lateral do
Tornozelo – a Lesão Musculoesquelética
de Membro Inferior mais Comum.......................... 215
Eamonn Delahunt

22 Reabilitação do Ombro no Rúgbi: Proposta
de Abordagem para o Manejo................................ 223
Keith Thornhill e Marc Beggs

23 Avaliação do Ombro Esportivo............................... 243
Marcus Bateman

24 Cotovelo Esportivo... 251
Daniel Williams, Shivan Jassim e Ali Noorani

25 Lesões nas Mãos e nos Punhos: Boxe em Foco...... 261
Ian Gatt

26 Coluna Cervical: Avaliação de Risco e Reabilitação.. 277
Alan J. Taylor e Roger Kerry

27 Manejo de Lesões na Cabeça.................................. 291
*Etienne Laverse, Akbar de Medici, Richard Sylvester,
Simon Kemp e Ademola Adejuwon*

28 Abordagem de Alto Desempenho para Otimizar
uma Pré-Temporada da Liga Principal de Futebol... 299
David McKay

29 Introdução ao Trabalho em uma Academia de
Futebol de Elite... 307
Diane Ryding

30 Ossos em Crescimento: Anatomia e Fraturas......... 315
Diane Ryding

31 Ossos em Crescimento: Osteocondroses
e Condições Pediátricas Graves............................. 323
Diane Ryding

32 Evento Cardíaco no Atleta Jovem........................... 335
Dean Chatterjee, Nikhil Ahluwalia e Aneil Malhotra

33 Como Desenvolver Qualidades de Velocidade
em Atletas Jovens.. 341
*Johnny Wilson, Michael Sup, Mark Wilson, Marc-André Maillet
e Said Mekary*

Fisiologia do Esporte e Tratamento de Lesões: Uma Abordagem Interdisciplinar

34 Condicionamento para a Batalha do Momentum: Uso Prático da Tecnologia GPS para Estratégias de Condicionamento....................................349
Adam Sheehan

35 Gerenciamento do Atleta *Overhead*.........................357
Steve McCaig

36 Tratamento e Manejo de Lesões em Tecidos Moles... 369
Graham Smith

37 Programa de Força Durante a Temporada: Uma Perspectiva Profissional do Rúgbi – Programação ao Longo da Temporada....................375
Aidan O'Connell

38 Análise de Movimento: a Ciência Encontra a Prática.......................................385
David M. Clancy

39 Eficácia do Condicionamento: Roteiro para Otimizar os Resultados na Reabilitação com Base no Desempenho 399
Claire Minshull

40 Atleta "Versátil": Principais Considerações de Desempenho para o Manejo de Lesões Relacionadas com Tornozelo, Tronco e Tendão em Ginastas do Sexo Feminino.......................................409
Jason Laird

41 Introdução à Medicina da Dança............................419
Nick Allen

Seção 2 Considerações Práticas

42 Preparação para Responder a uma Emergência......429
Natalie Shur, Paulina Czubacka, Jim Moxon, Rohi Shah, Tom Hallas e Johnny Wilson

43 O Que é Reabilitação sem Aceitação do Paciente? Importância da Psicologia na Reabilitação de Lesões Esportivas..439
Anna Waters

Índice Alfabético...**449**

xvi

Encarte

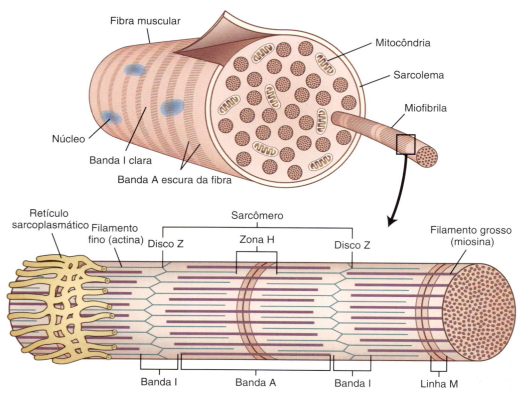

Figura 1.1 Microestrutura do músculo esquelético humano.

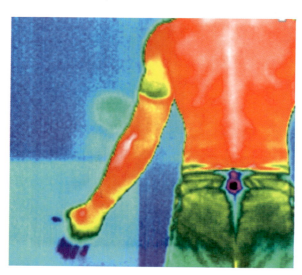

Figura 7.1 Imagem térmica infravermelha mostrando o gradiente de temperatura da pele do membro superior (*vermelho* mais quente do que *azul*) em sujeito adulto saudável do sexo masculino.

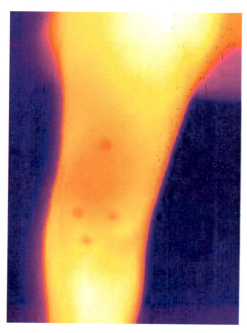

Figura 7.2 Imagem térmica infravermelha com quatro marcadores anatômicos termicamente inertes no local, mostrando uma temperatura da pele mais fria (*laranja*) sobre um joelho saudável.

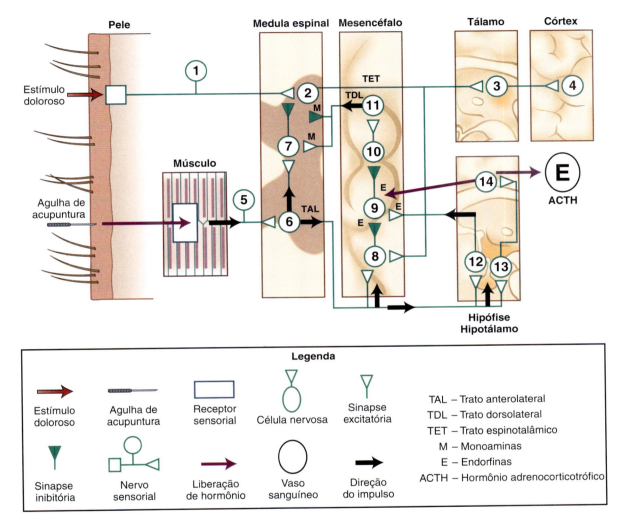

Figura 11.1 Mecanismo de analgesia por acupuntura. Dor: estímulo doloroso de pequenas fibras nervosas aferentes Aδ e C (*1*) fazem sinapse no corno dorsal da medula espinal (*2*) antes de subir do trato espinotalâmico (*TET*) para o tálamo (*3*) e terminar no córtex (*4*) onde a dor pode ser percebida em um nível consciente. Agulhamento: agulhamento do músculo estimula as fibras Aδ (*5*) que fazem sinapse na medula espinal (*6*) e estimulam a célula (*7*) onde a encefalina é liberada causando inibição pré-sináptica da célula (*1*). A célula (*6*) também faz sinapses com o trato anterolateral (*TAL*) para o mesencéfalo, estimulando células (*8*) e (*9*) na substância cinza periaquaductal (CPA) que liberam β-endorfina para excitar a célula (*10*) do núcleo da rafe e a célula (*11*), desencadeando impulsos ao longo do trato dorsolateral (*TDL*) para liberar monoaminas (*M*) nas células (*2*) e (*7*) da medula espinal. A célula (*1*) é inibida pré-sinapticamente por M (serotonina) por intermédio da célula (*7*), enquanto a célula (*2*) é inibida pós-sinapticamente por M (norepinefrina). O estímulo de TAL nas células (*12*) e (*13*) dentro do complexo hipotalâmico hipofisário libera hormônio adrenocorticotrófico (*ACTH*) e β-endorfina na circulação em medidas iguais. O ACTH modula a resposta anti-inflamatória. A estimulação da célula (*8*) pela célula (*2*) via TET também causa analgesia pelo mecanismo de controle inibitório nocivo difuso (CIND), onde um estímulo nocivo pode inibir outro.

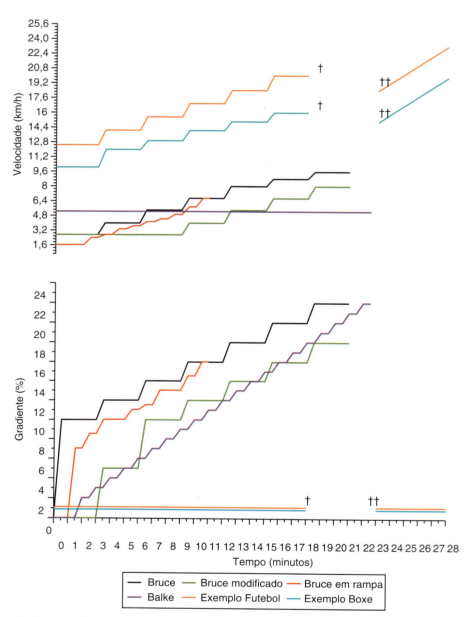

Figura 12.2 Comparação de protocolos incrementais de esteira motorizada (velocidade e gradiente) para avaliação do consumo de oxigênio durante o exercício. Protocolos comuns (Bruce, Bruce modificado, Bruce em rampa e Balke) são apresentados contra dois exemplos de protocolos usados com jogadores de futebol profissional e boxeadores. †, fim do teste graduado submáximo seguido por um período de recuperação de 5 minutos antes de ††, início do teste de pico até a exaustão.

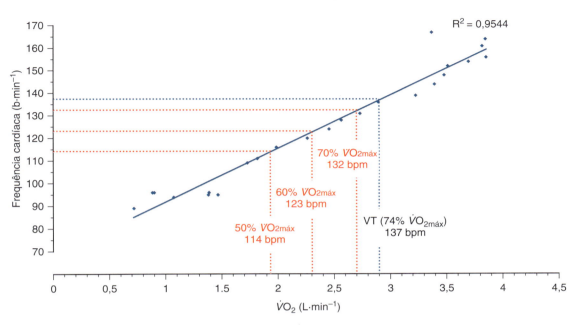

Figura 12.3 Regressão linear simples da frequência cardíaca (FC) e $\dot{V}O_{2máx}$ **durante o teste de exercício graduado em laboratório.** A *linha pontilhada vermelha* indica o processo de extrapolação da FC (y) a partir do $\dot{V}O_{2máx}$ (x) usando porcentagens fixas. A *linha pontilhada azul* indica o limiar ventilatório (LV), conforme definido pela análise separada das respostas respiratórias ao trabalho incremental até a exaustão. *bpm*, batimentos por minuto.

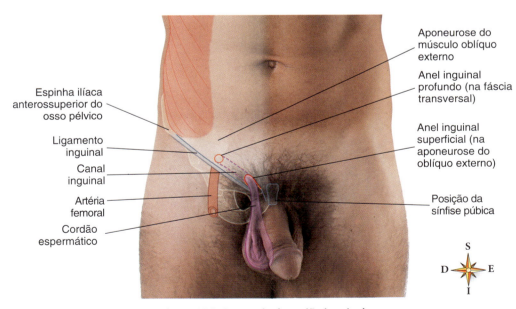

Figura 13.2 Anatomia da região inguinal.

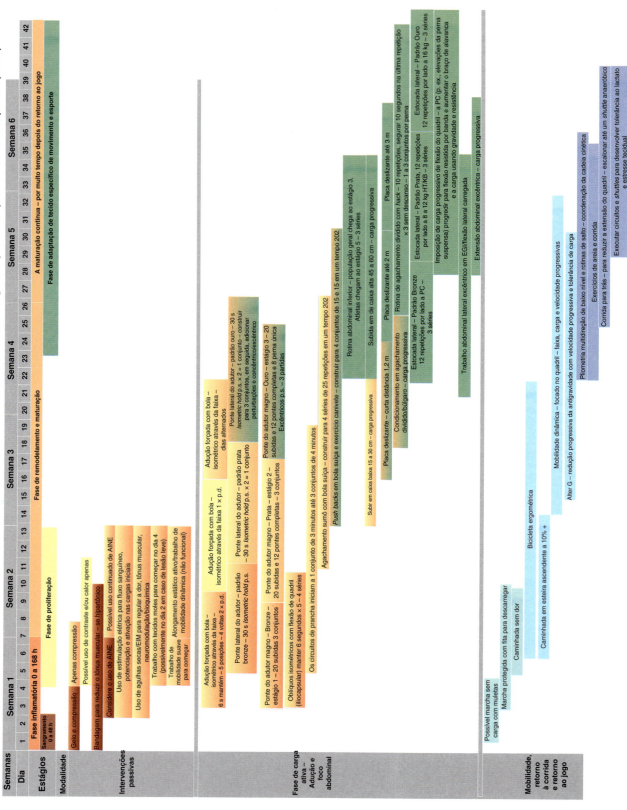

Figura 14.1 Protocolo de lesão do músculo adutor. *AINE*, anti-inflamatórios não esteroidais; *EGI*, elevação do glúteo-isquiotibiais; *EIM*, estimulação intramuscular; *HT*, halteres; *KB*, kettlebell; *PC*, peso corporal; *p.d.*, por dia; *p.s.*, por série.

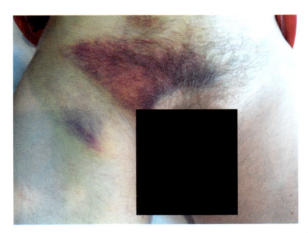

Figura 15.1 Padrão de hematoma que ocorre em uma lesão grave na virilha. Nesse paciente, jogador de futebol profissional, o hematoma delineia os limites anatômicos da região inguinal, acima da do sulco inguinal, além de demonstrar ruptura adutora concomitante com hematoma na parte superior da coxa. Em casos como este, não é apropriado operar na presença de hematomas significativos, pois os planos do tecido terão sido obliterados. Na verdade, esse paciente se recuperou completamente em um período de 8 semanas e não precisou de cirurgia.

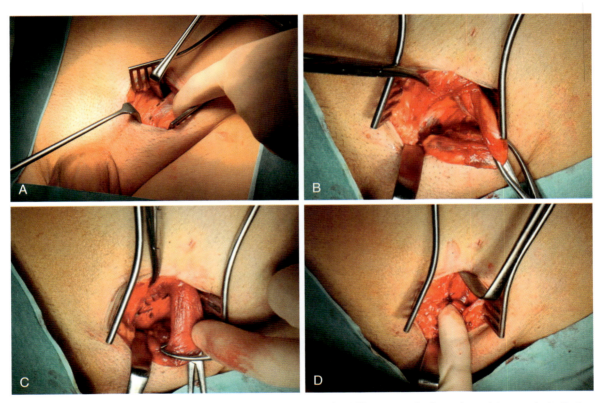

Figura 15.2 Fotografias operatórias durante a cirurgia de reconstrução da virilha esquerda. Em todas as fotos, a orientação é a mesma: a cabeça está voltada para o topo da foto com a perna esquerda voltada para o canto inferior direito. **A.** Aponeurose externa atenuada. **B.** Cordão espermático sendo retraído lateral e inferiormente, mostrando a ruptura muscular da parede posterior, visto como a área branca à esquerda do cordão. **C.** A mesma área após a parede posterior ter sido reparada – o músculo oblíquo interno foi recolocado no ligamento inguinal para que o defeito fosse fechado. **D.** Reparo completo com o anel inguinal superficial reconstituído.

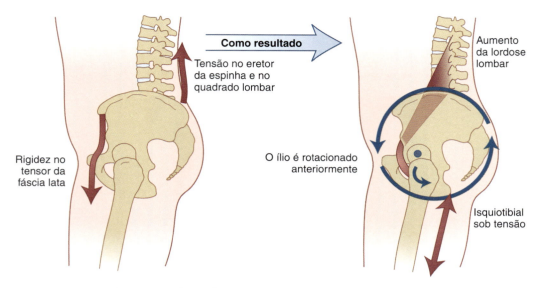

Figura 17.3 Efeitos da musculatura tensa no alinhamento da pelve.

Exercício funcional linear
Exercício funcional linear simples

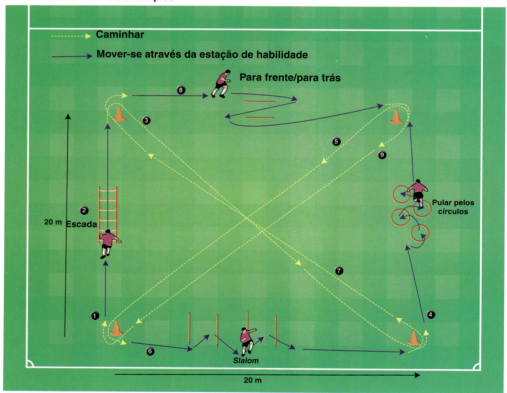

Exercício de movimento funcional linear (sem bola):

- O jogador começa em um cone *(1)* e então se move através da primeira estação de exercício *(2)*
- Uma vez que o jogador chega ao cone na outra extremidade, desacelera o giro ao redor dele, caminhando pela grade até o próximo *(3)*
- No próximo cone o jogador vira e se move pela próxima estação de exercício *(4)*, repetindo o ciclo de giro e andando pela grade *(5)* para recuperação
- O ciclo continua até que as quatro 4 estações de exercício tenham sido executadas. Esse exercício pode ser realizado em intensidades variadas durante a fase de trabalho e pode ser repetido 2 a 3 vezes como um único ciclo de quatro estações com 60 a 90 segundos de descanso entre cada ciclo, ou o jogador pode realizar o circuito 2 a 3 vezes seguidas conforme seu progresso de função e reabilitação.

Figura 20.3 Diagrama de um exercício linear inicial.

Exercício complexo de ataque   **Exercício de ataque**

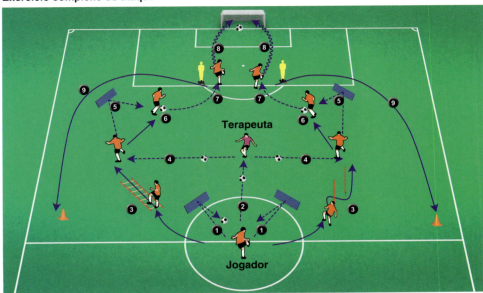

Exercício de ataque: O jogador fica no círculo central e passa alternadamente pelas duas placas de rebatidas próximas a ele *(1)*. Após 5 a 8 segundos, o terapeuta fala "esquerda" ou "direita", e o jogador reage passando a bola para o terapeuta *(2)* e se move na direção indicada pela estação de habilidade sem a bola *(3)*. Conforme o jogador sai da estação de habilidade, o terapeuta passa a bola para o jogador *(4)*. O jogador controla a bola e passa a bola para fora do segundo quadro *(5)*, controla a bola que rebate (6) e ataca o manequim mais próximo *(7)*, chutando ao passar *(8)*. Então, imediatamente após o chute, o jogador corre em velocidade de volta para o cone próximo à linha do meio *(9)*.

Esse exercício pode ser executado de 4 a 6 vezes em direções variadas, com um bom período de recuperação (60 a 90 segundos) entre cada execução para que a qualidade e a intensidade da execução sejam otimizadas.

Figura 20.4 Diagrama de um exercício de campo controlado mais avançado para um jogador de futebol de ataque.

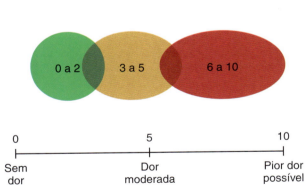

Figura 21.1 Escala numérica de classificação de dor "semáforo". *Verde*, provavelmente seguro para continuar o exercício; *laranja*, é necessário cuidado, pois o exercício pode exceder a tolerância dos tecidos carregados; *vermelho*, provavelmente inseguro para continuar o exercício, pois a tolerância dos tecidos carregados provavelmente foi excedida.

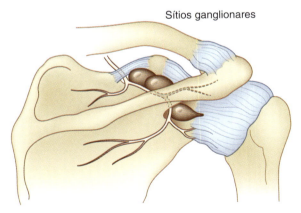

Figura 23.4 Diagrama mostrando como um gânglio pode comprimir o nervo supraescapular em diferentes locais ao longo de seu curso. (Adaptada de Moore T. P., Hunter R. E., 1996. Suprascapular nerve entrapment. Operative Techniques in Sports Medicine 4 [1], 8-14.)

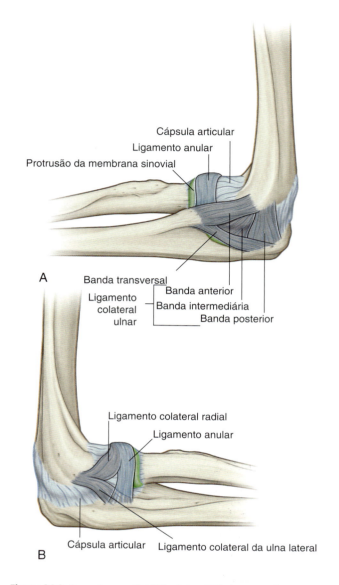

Figura 24.2 Aspectos medial (A) e lateral (B) do cotovelo esquerdo mostrando a cápsula articular e os ligamentos colaterais radial e ulnar.

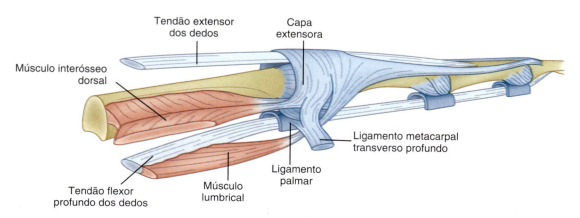

Figura 25.2 Anatomia do dedo com capa extensora (bandas sagitais) da articulação.

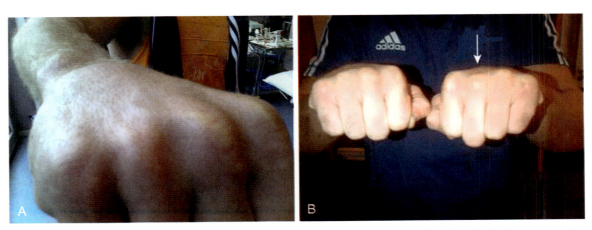

Figura 25.6 Apresentação da lesão carpometacarpal (CMC). **A.** Edema nas costas da mão. **B.** Efeito de tecla de piano ocorrendo no terceiro dedo ou CMC do dedo médio na mão esquerda (nó do dedo médio visto caindo com relação aos outros nós da mão).

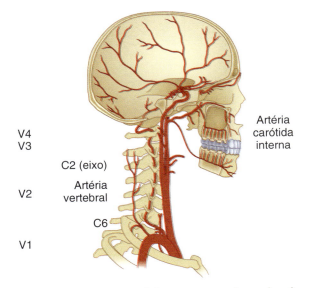

Figura 26.1 Anatomia normal dos vasos sanguíneos da cabeça e do pescoço. (Reproduzia com autorização de McCarthy, C. 2010. Combined Movement Theory. Churchill Livingstone, Edinburgh.)

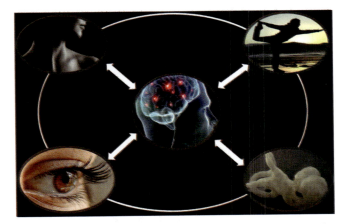

Figura 26.5 Entradas e saídas dos sistemas de propriocepção, visual, vestibular e de equilíbrio do pescoço que estão envolvidos na disfunção sensorimotora.

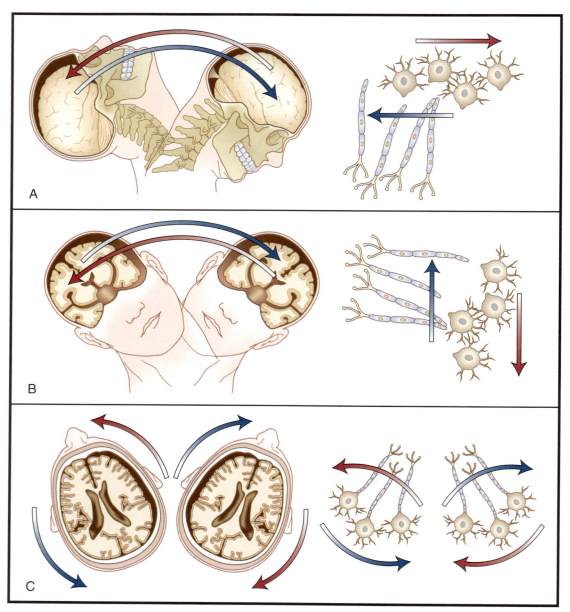

Figura 27.2 Lesão cerebral traumática: axonal e de cisalhamento. A aceleração angular ou linear do cérebro pode resultar em cisalhamento e disfunção neuronal.

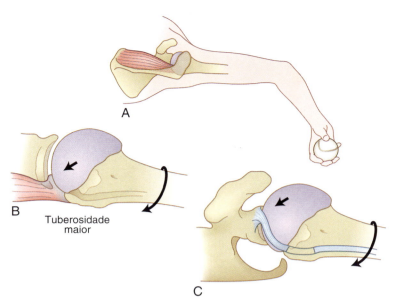

Figura 35.1 Impacto interno e o fenômeno de "descascar". **A.** Ombro em rotação externa máxima durante a fase de elevação **B.** Choque interno. **C.** Fenômeno de "descascar". (Adaptada de Chang, I.Y., Polster, J.M., 2016. Pathomechanics and magnetic resonance imaging of the thrower's shoulder. Radiologic Clinics of North America 54 [5], 801-815.)

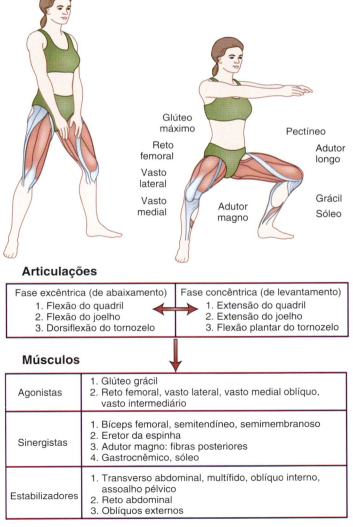

Figura 38.1 Ações articulares e musculares que ocorrem durante o agachamento.

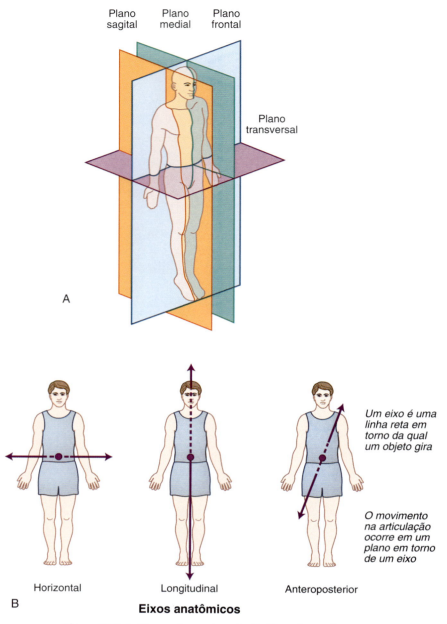

Figura 38.2 A. Planos do movimento. B. Eixos do movimento.

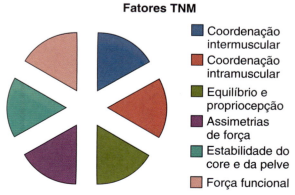

Figura 38.13 Fatores de padrão de movimento que podem contribuir para um padrão motor incorreto. Deve-se desenvolver um programa amplamente individualizado que aborde todos ou alguns desses aspectos. Um foco na taxa de desenvolvimento de força (a rapidez com que a força pode ser produzida), rápida ativação neural e coordenação muscular geral são imperativos.

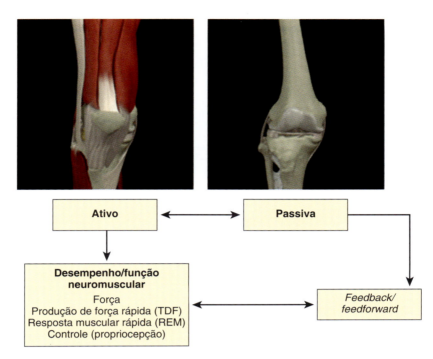

Figura 39.1 Modelo conceitual para estabilidade da articulação do joelho. *REM*, retardo eletromecânico; *TDF*, taxa de desenvolvimento de força.

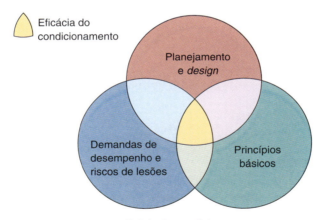

Figura 39.3 Eficácia do condicionamento.

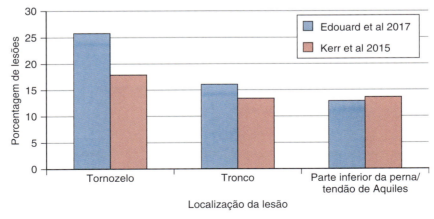

Figura 40.2 Localizações das lesões em estudos de epidemiologia da ginástica artística feminina. Fonte: (From Edouard, P., Steffen, K., Junge, A., Leglise, M., Soligard, T., Engebretsen, L., 2017. Gymnastics injury incidence during the 2008, 2012 and 2016 Olympic Games: analysis of prospectively collected surveillance data from 963 registered gymnasts during Olympic Games. British Journal of Sports Medicine 52 (7), 475-481; Kerr, Z.Y., Hayden, R., Barr, M., Klossner, D.A., Dompier, T.P., 2015. Epidemiology of National Collegiate Athletic Association women's gymnastics injuries, 2009–2010 through 2013–2014. Journal of Athletic Training 50 (08), 870-878.)

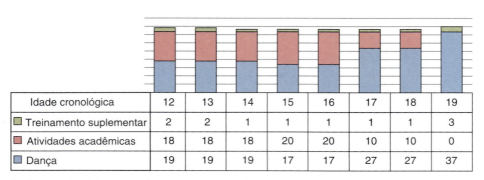

Figura 41.2 Exemplo de carga horária semanal em uma escola profissionalizante de dança. (Adaptada de Injuries and adolescent ballet dancers: Current evidence, epidemiology, and intervention, PhD Thesis, Nico Kolokythas, 2019.)

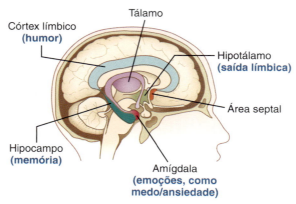

Figura 43.2 Sistema límbico.

Parte | 1 | Conceitos Básicos Importantes em Esportes

Capítulo | 1 |

Forma e Função do Músculo

Jamie McPhee e Tommy Lundberg

Controle neuromuscular do movimento

A incrível variedade de movimentos voluntários que os humanos podem realizar é possibilitada por interações neuromusculares eficazes. O controle dos movimentos é complexo e requer a cooperação do sistema nervoso central (SNC) e do sistema nervoso periférico (SNP). O SNC inclui o cérebro e a medula espinal, enquanto o SNP inclui todas as células nervosas fora do SNC e é subdividido em porções sensoriais e motoras.

O início do movimento voluntário começa com a criação de um esboço do movimento planejado nas áreas motivacionais do cérebro. O plano de movimento é enviado ao cerebelo e aos núcleos da base para conversão do escoamento em ordens de excitação mais precisas. Esses programas motores são enviados para o córtex motor, depois para os neurônios espinais e, por fim, transmitidos do SNC para os neurônios alfamotores do SNP. Algumas modificações ainda são possíveis ao longo desta cadeia de comando em resposta às entradas dos centros subcortical e espinal. Por exemplo, uma sequência de movimento planejada pode ser ajustada com base no *feedback* sensorial aferente de fusos musculares, órgãos tendinosos de Golgi e terminações nervosas livres, conhecidas como proprioceptores, que detectam sensação de dor e alongamento muscular, tensão e metabólitos.

Nós controlamos os movimentos aumentando a quantidade de unidades motoras recrutadas ou suas taxas de disparo individuais. Uma unidade motora consiste em um único neurônio alfamotor e todas as fibras musculares que ele inerva. Normalmente, os músculos dos membros possuem centenas ou milhares de unidades motoras que variam em tamanho, com algumas pequenas e outras muito grandes no mesmo músculo (Buchthal et al., 1959). Em músculos menores ou onde o controle motor fino é necessário, a quantidade de fibras por unidade motora (taxa de inervação) é pequena, enquanto em músculos grandes e poderosos a taxa de inervação pode chegar a 2 mil fibras para cada neurônio motor (Buchthal et al., 1959). O "princípio do tamanho" descreve um recrutamento altamente organizado de unidades motoras de acordo com seu tamanho, desde a menor progressivamente até a maior, de modo que as forças produzidas correspondam adequadamente às demandas da tarefa (Henneman et al., 1965).

Estrutura do músculo esquelético

Músculos inteiros

Existem mais de 600 músculos estriados esqueléticos no corpo humano, e suas massas combinadas são responsáveis por 40 a 50% do peso corporal total em adultos saudáveis (Al-Gindan et al., 2014) e por mais de 60% em muitos atletas. Os músculos esqueléticos geram as forças necessárias para os movimentos voluntários e o controle postural, contribuem para a termorregulação secundária ao gerar calor a partir das contrações, desempenham um papel fundamental no metabolismo de todo o corpo e servem às funções endócrinas e parácrinas, liberando hormônios de crescimento e outros fatores que regulam a função de outros órgãos do corpo.

Músculos inteiros são compostos de muitas células musculares individuais, conhecidas como *fibras musculares*. Eles são caracteristicamente longos, geralmente cilíndricos e envolvidos por uma camada de tecido conjuntivo conhecida como *endomísio*. Uma camada de tecido conjuntivo chamada de *perimísio* envolve grupos de fibras organizando-os em *fascículos*. Ao redor de todo o músculo está a camada mais externa de tecido conjuntivo, chamada de *epimísio*, e uma *fáscia* de tecido conjuntivo separa os músculos uns dos outros. Vários outros tipos de células e tecidos também são encontrados dentro dos músculos inteiros, incluindo (mas não se limitando a) vasos sanguíneos, capilares, células do sistema imunológico e outros componentes do sangue, bem como nervos sensoriais e motores.

As fibras musculares individuais e o tecido conjuntivo associado se conectam aos tendões em ambas as extremidades. O tendão proximal é conhecido como *origem*, e o distal, como *inserção*, ou, respectivamente, *origem proximal* e *origem distal*. Um princípio básico é que, quando ativados, os músculos esqueléticos encurtam para produzir força (observe que os músculos também podem se alongar sob tensão, controlando o processo de "des-recrutamento" das fibras musculares). Como todo o músculo encurta durante a contração, a origem permanece relativamente fixa na posição ancorada a um osso, enquanto a inserção é conectada a uma região proximal de um osso posicionado distalmente à articulação em rotação e é puxada pelo tendão para causar movimento.

Arranjos musculares

Os músculos são organizados em grupos de músculos opostos: aqueles que reduzem um ângulo articular são conhecidos como *flexores* e aqueles que estendem um ângulo articular são *extensores*. Por exemplo, durante a extensão do joelho, o grupo de músculos quadríceps aumenta o ângulo da articulação do joelho, enquanto os isquiotibiais se alongam passivamente para permitir que a extensão do joelho ocorra. O grupo de músculos ativos é conhecido como *agonista* (quadríceps), enquanto o grupo inativo é o *antagonista* (isquiotibiais). Outros músculos podem ajudar a estabilizar as articulações durante os movimentos, os quais são chamados de *sinergistas*.

O arranjo do fascículo varia de músculo para músculo. Alguns músculos têm um arranjo *fusiforme* em que as fibras musculares individuais são quase paralelas e estão diretamente em série com os tendões de origem e inserção, como o bíceps braquial. Muitos dos músculos grandes dos membros têm arranjo de fascículos *penados*, nos quais os fascículos são oblíquos ao tendão. Por exemplo, os músculos vastos do quadríceps têm fascículos penados que se interceptam com a camada profunda de tecido conjuntivo do músculo em ângulos de cerca de 10 a 20°. Os músculos *bipenados*, como o reto femoral do quadríceps, têm um filamento central de tecido conjuntivo espesso que atravessa a barriga do músculo e os fascículos se estendem obliquamente para fora (um pouco como as farpas da pena de um pássaro se estendendo da pena). Outros arranjos de fascículos mais complexos também estão presentes, incluindo o *triangular* (como o peitoral) e o *circumpenado* ou cilíndrico (tibial anterior), e alguns músculos *multipenados* aparecem compartimentados, com diferentes arranjos de penação dependendo da região observada, como o deltoide. A orientação fascicular pode influenciar na intensidade da força e na taxa de contrações (Narici et al., 2016).

Microestrutura e proteínas contráteis

Independentemente dos arranjos fasciculares, todas as fibras musculares esqueléticas compartilham a mesma microestrutura (Figura 1.1). Geralmente, elas são cilíndricas, finas, alongadas e podem abranger o comprimento de todo o músculo ou podem começar ou terminar dentro do fascículo. A membrana da célula fibrosa é chamada de *sarcolema* e o interior da célula é o *sarcoplasma*, onde todas as proteínas contráteis e organelas estão localizadas. As fibras têm muitos núcleos que contêm todo o conjunto de genes e expressam os genes necessários para manter a estrutura e função da fibra muscular. Tipos especializados de células-tronco chamadas de *células-satélite* contribuem para o crescimento, desenvolvimento e reparo das fibras musculares (Pallafacchina et al., 2013).

As proteínas que regulam a contração muscular são as proteínas mais abundantes e respondem por cerca de 85% do volume da fibra. Outras proteínas sarcoplasmáticas e proteínas mitocondriais respondem por cerca de 10 e 5% do volume da fibra, respectivamente (Lüthi et al., 1986). As proteínas contráteis são organizadas ao longo das *miofibrilas*, que aparecem como filamentos longos e repetitivos de unidades funcionais menores em série e em paralelo, conhecidas como *sarcômeros*. Os sarcômeros são as menores unidades contráteis e são compostos principalmente pelas proteínas contráteis *actina* e *miosina*, organizadas ao longo de *filamentos finos* e *grossos*, respectivamente, e têm uma aparência estriada. O filamento fino também inclui tropomiosina e troponina. Uma extremidade de cada filamento fino é ancorada a um disco Z, o qual une sarcômeros sucessivos em série.

Contração muscular e energia para o movimento

Teoria do filamento deslizante para a contração muscular

Teoria do filamento deslizante descreve nosso entendimento geral de como ocorre a contração muscular. Quando uma fibra muscular é ativada pelo sistema nervoso, os íons de cálcio são liberados no sarcoplasma e a miosina, no filamento grosso, pode formar uma *ponte cruzada* com a actina no filamento fino. A cabeça da miosina "gira" para produzir o *golpe de força*, fazendo com que filamentos finos "deslizem" através dos filamentos grossos em direção ao centro do sarcômero. Esse processo usa a energia liberada pelas ligações de alta energia do trifosfato de adenosina (ATP), deixando como resíduos um fosfato inorgânico (Pi) e um difosfato de adenosina (ADP).

Energia para o movimento

O ATP é sintetizado a partir da energia química na forma de gorduras, carboidratos e proteínas que são consumidos como parte da dieta, e os músculos transformam essa energia química em energia mecânica durante as contrações. A gordura é o estoque de energia mais abundante, e 1 g contém aproximadamente 9 kcal de energia; em comparação, os carboidratos e as proteínas contêm cerca de 4 kcal de energia por grama. Os carboidratos são armazenados como cadeias de glicose, chamadas de *glicogênio*, no fígado e em outras células, com os maiores estoques nos músculos esqueléticos. As reservas de glicogênio do fígado são usadas para repor os níveis de glicose no sangue quando estão baixos, e o glicogênio muscular fornece grandes reservas locais de glicose imediatamente disponíveis para alimentar as contrações. A proteína tem uma contribuição direta menor para o estoque geral de energia, mas os aminoácidos constituintes são intermediários metabólicos importantes durante o metabolismo energético e, em momentos de necessidade, o aminoácido alanina pode ser convertido em glicose no fígado.

Existem três principais vias metabólicas que sintetizam ATP, descritas como anaeróbica (não requer oxigênio) ou aeróbica (requer oxigênio).

1. A *reação de fosfocreatina* (PCr) anaeróbica é a maneira mais simples e rápida de ressintetizar ATP. Ela é catalisada pela enzima creatinoquinase e pode ser vista como uma reação que retira um fosfato de uma ligação creatina-fosfato de alta energia e o transfere ao ADP, resultando em uma molécula de creatina livre e ATP:

$$ADP + PCr \rightarrow ATP + Cr$$

2. A *glicólise* anaeróbica é a conversão da glicose em 2 piruvato +2 ATP. O piruvato pode entrar nas mitocôndrias para ser usado na produção aeróbica de ATP durante as contrações musculares estáveis ou, quando as demandas de energia são muito altas, o piruvato aceita íons de hidrogênio para formar o lactato. O aparecimento de lactato no sangue é comumente utilizado como um marcador de alta taxa metabólica e fadiga.

3. A produção aeróbica de ATP ocorre em organelas especializadas chamadas de *mitocôndrias*, as quais convertem o piruvato (o produto da glicólise) e os ácidos graxos no ATP necessário para atividades prolongadas de intensidades baixa ou moderada. Embora não sejam uma fonte de energia primária em humanos saudáveis, alguns aminoácidos (as partes

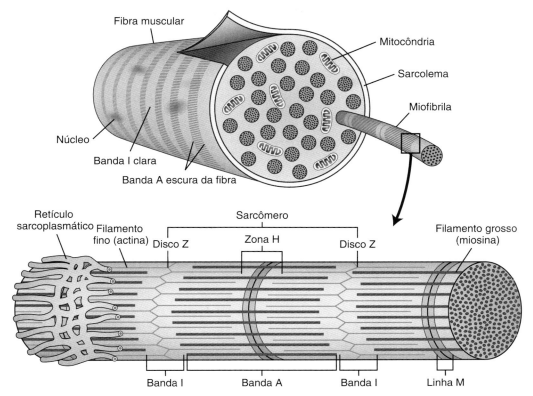

Figura 1.1 Microestrutura do músculo esquelético humano. *(Esta figura se encontra reproduzida em cores no Encarte.)*

constituintes das proteínas) também podem ser usados pelas mitocôndrias para produzir ATP. O processo aeróbico envolve duas vias químicas, o ciclo do ácido cítrico (também chamado de ciclo de Krebs) e a cadeia transportadora de elétrons. Quando o piruvato passa pela respiração aeróbica, o ganho líquido de ATP é de 32 ou 33, dependendo de a glicose ser formada como glicogênio na primeira instância. Quando um ácido graxo típico, como o palmitato, passa pela respiração aeróbica, o rendimento líquido de ATP é 129.

Propriedades contráteis do músculo

A existência de diferentes tipos de fibras no músculo esquelético é reconhecida há muito tempo. A base original para a classificação dos tipos de fibra em vermelha, branca ou intermediária surgiu da inspeção visual do tecido muscular animal. Desde a década de 1960, quando o procedimento de biopsia muscular percutânea foi reintroduzido, tornou-se possível obter amostras musculares de voluntários e estudos revelaram diferenças na composição e nas propriedades bioquímicas das fibras musculares que podem ser distinguidas por eletroforese em gel ou por diferentes técnicas histoquímicas de coloração. Ao incubar amostras de músculo em diferentes níveis de pH, a composição do tipo de fibra pode ser determinada enzimaticamente de acordo com a atividade ATPásica da miosina. Alternativamente, os tipos de fibra muscular podem ser determinados colorindo-os com anticorpos específicos contra as isoformas lenta ou rápida da cadeia pesada da miosina.

Existem três tipos principais de fibras encontradas no músculo esquelético, geralmente conhecidos como tipo 1, tipo 2A e tipo 2X. A maioria dos músculos esqueléticos contém esses três tipos de fibras puras; porém, as chamadas fibras "híbridas", com características mistas, também estão presentes. Todas as fibras musculares de uma única unidade motora compartilham as mesmas características fenotípicas (ou seja, lentas ou rápidas) e se contraem ou relaxam ao mesmo tempo de maneira "tudo ou nada".

A principal diferença funcional entre os tipos de fibra é a velocidade de contração e relaxamento. As fibras lentas do tipo 1 têm um longo tempo para alcançar o pico de força, e o tempo de relaxamento também é correspondentemente longo. As fibras de contração rápida, em contrapartida, se contraem rapidamente e o tempo de relaxamento é menor. Por exemplo, as fibras mais rápidas têm velocidade máxima de encurtamento que é cerca de 4 vezes maior do que a das fibras do tipo 1 (Bottinelli et al., 1996). Como a potência é o produto da força e da velocidade, as diferenças na potência de pico entre os tipos de fibra são maiores do que apenas para força e velocidade. As características típicas dos diferentes tipos de fibra são descritas mais detalhadamente na Tabela 1.1. As fibras lentas também possuem maior quantidade de mitocôndrias e alta proporção capilar/fibra do que as fibras rápidas e essas características fornecem uma maior capacidade de produção aeróbica de ATP e resistência à fadiga. As fibras 2X mais rápidas são – geralmente, mas nem sempre – maiores do que as fibras do tipo 1 e, além da composição da cadeia pesada de miosina diferente e da velocidade de contração mais rápida, apresentam atividade ATPásica de miosina com ação mais rápida (enzimas responsáveis por dividir as ligações de alta energia em ATP) e maior capacidade glicolítica do que as fibras lentas. As fibras do tipo 2A são geralmente vistas como fibras intermediárias com taxas mais rápidas de contração do que as fibras do tipo 1, as mitocôndrias e as densidades capilares intermediárias, e são menos fatigáveis do que as fibras do tipo 2X, embora apresentem mais fadiga do que as do tipo 1 (Tabela 1.1).

Tabela 1.1 Características dos diferentes tipos de fibra muscular.

	Tipo 1	Tipo 2A	Tipo 2X
Velocidade de encurtamento	Lenta	Rápida	Muito rápida
Produção de potência	Baixa	Alta	A mais alta
Limiar de recrutamento	Baixo	Mais alto	O mais alto
Unidades motoras	Pequenas	Maiores	As maiores
Conteúdo mitocondrial	Alto	Menor	O menor
Capacidade glicolítica	Moderada	Alta	Alta
Resistência à fadiga	Muito alta	Moderada	Baixa

Mecânica muscular e sua aplicação para força, velocidade e potência

Acoplamento excitação-contração

Os sinais que instruem o recrutamento muscular são retransmitidos ao longo dos neurônios motores como *potenciais de ação* a mais de 50 m/s e podem disparar de 5 a 30 vezes por segundo (Enoka e Fuglevand, 2001). Um potencial de ação que chega ao terminal do nervo motor desencadeia a liberação do neurotransmissor especializado *acetilcolina*, o qual se liga a seus receptores na membrana da fibra muscular e estimula um potencial de ação ao longo da fibra muscular e a liberação de Ca^{2+} no sarcolema, que é necessário para a função das pontes cruzadas que sustentam a contração muscular. Assim, a chegada de potenciais de ação do neurônio motor para a fibra muscular dita as contrações musculares. Esse processo é conhecido como *acoplamento excitação-contração*.

Ciclo de alongamento-encurtamento

Além do controle neural, também existem vários fatores mecânicos que afetam a capacidade de produção de força do músculo. Um dos mais importantes desses fatores é o tipo de ação muscular utilizada. As ações musculares podem ser divididas em ações isométricas e ações dinâmicas. Em ações isométricas, o músculo permanece no mesmo comprimento enquanto está sob tensão. Por exemplo, os flexores do cotovelo executam contrações isométricas ao segurar um peso na mão com o cotovelo flexionado a 90° e permanecendo no mesmo ângulo. As ações dinâmicas podem ser divididas em ações musculares concêntricas e excêntricas. Nas ações concêntricas, os músculos encurtam enquanto produzem tensão, fazendo com que o ângulo da articulação mude (lembre-se de que os extensores aumentam os ângulos das articulações e os flexores os diminuem). Por exemplo, as contrações concêntricas dos flexores do cotovelo diminuem progressivamente o ângulo da articulação ao levantar um peso. Em contrapartida, o músculo se alonga sob tensão durante as contrações excêntricas, como abaixar o peso usando contrações excêntricas dos flexores do cotovelo. A maioria das atividades cotidianas envolve combinações sucessivas de ações musculares excêntricas e concêntricas, como caminhar, correr, pular ou levantar/abaixar objetos, e isso é denominado *ciclo de alongamento-encurtamento*.

A força muscular é maior nas ações musculares isométricas e excêntricas do que nas concêntricas. Isso porque, a qualquer momento, mais pontes cruzadas de actina e miosina estão na posição fixada durante uma ação isométrica e excêntrica em comparação a uma ação concêntrica em que mais tempo do ciclo da ponte cruzada é gasto no estado solto. Também há consenso sobre a força e a potência musculares aumentarem em movimentos que envolvem o ciclo de alongamento-encurtamento. Embora os mecanismos precisos para esse efeito ainda estejam em debate, ele parece ser devido à *potenciação*, termo usado para descrever um processo pelo qual a ativação muscular inicial "prepara" os músculos para novas contrações, tanto de elementos contráteis quanto elásticos.

Relações comprimento-tensão e força-velocidade

Existe um comprimento ideal de cada fibra muscular em relação à sua capacidade de gerar força. Isso é denominado *relação comprimento-tensão* (Figura 1.2). O comprimento ideal do sarcômero é onde há sobreposição ótima de filamentos grossos e finos (Gordon et al., 1966). A produção de força é prejudicada quando os comprimentos do sarcômero são muito curtos, pois há sobreposição dos filamentos de actina das extremidades opostas do sarcômero. Há também uma capacidade de força reduzida quando o sarcômero é alongado além do comprimento ideal, uma vez que isso também reduz a sobreposição entre os filamentos de actina e miosina. O comprimento ideal do sarcômero ocorre quando os músculos são ligeiramente alongados além de seu comprimento natural de repouso. Por exemplo, nos extensores de joelho e flexores de cotovelo, o ângulo ideal ocorre em ângulos articulares de cerca de 80° (considerando a extensão total como 0 grau).

A chamada *relação força-velocidade* também determina a capacidade do músculo de produzir força e potência. À medida que a velocidade de ação muscular aumenta, menos força pode ser gerada durante a contração (Hill, 1938). Em palavras simples, a força máxima que pode ser produzida por um músculo é menor durante movimentos rápidos do que em movimentos mais lentos. Isso é explicado no nível do miofilamento pelo tempo que as pontes cruzadas levam para se anexar e se desprender. Especificamente, a quantidade total de pontes cruzadas formadas a qualquer momento diminui com o aumento da velocidade de encurtamento do músculo e, uma vez que a quantidade de força produzida pelo músculo está relacionada com a quantidade de pontes cruzadas formadas, a produção de força diminui com o aumento da velocidade.

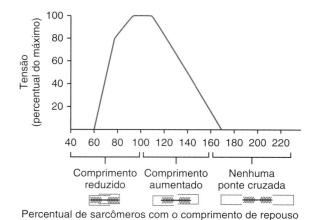

Figura 1.2 Relação comprimento-tensão do músculo esquelético. Observe que a força máxima é alcançada durante o comprimento ideal do sarcômero.

A potência muscular é diferente da força muscular. A potência é determinada pela interação entre força e velocidade de contração e é calculada simplesmente como força × velocidade (também pode ser expressa como trabalho dividido pelo tempo). Consequentemente, a produção do pico de potência muscular ocorre onde o produto da força e da velocidade é maior. Fibras individuais dissecadas em uma biopsia muscular tendem a atingir seu pico de potência quando a fibra gera apenas cerca de 20% do pico de força. Em movimentos isolados, como extensões de joelho estando sentado, o pico de potência é tipicamente alcançado em velocidades correspondentes a cerca de um terço da velocidade máxima de contração. No entanto, conforme o tipo de exercício ou estratégia de carga usada, a velocidade em que ocorre o pico de potência será muito diferente.

O braço do momento influencia a biomecânica articular

A capacidade de um músculo de produzir força também varia dependendo das características anatômicas da articulação que está sendo movida. O *braço do momento* é a distância perpendicular do ponto de aplicação da força muscular (geralmente, o tendão passando sobre uma articulação) até o ponto de rotação da articulação (geralmente, próximo ao centro da articulação). Tomando a articulação do joelho como exemplo durante a extensão do joelho, o tendão da patela na face anterior da articulação é a aplicação de força muscular, enquanto o centro de rotação da articulação ocorre profundamente em direção ao centro da articulação do joelho: a distância entre o centro de rotação e o tendão patelar é o braço do momento. Quanto maior o braço do momento, maior a força de momento máxima possível (ou torque, força que causa a rotação e a velocidade angular). Assim, um músculo posicionado com um braço do momento grande tem uma vantagem biomecânica em comparação a um músculo com força contrátil semelhante, mas com um braço do momento menor (Narici et al., 2016).

Contrações musculares, somação e tetania

Se apenas um único potencial de ação desencadear a liberação de Ca^{2+} no sarcoplasma para iniciar a função da ponte cruzada, então, ocorrerá apenas uma única *contração muscular*. Essa contração tem um período de latência muito breve, durando apenas alguns milissegundos, seguido de um período de contração que, geralmente, dura cerca de 40 ms e, depois, de um relaxamento que dura, normalmente, cerca de 50 ms. Os tempos dessas fases dependem dos tipos de fibra, já que as fibras lentas do tipo 1 se contraem e relaxam lentamente e as fibras rápidas do tipo 2 têm taxas rápidas de contração e relaxamento devido à liberação mais rápida de Ca^{2+} e à atividade ATPásica da miosina.

Se um segundo potencial de ação chega antes que o músculo esteja totalmente relaxado, mais Ca^{2+} é liberado e a força resultante se acumula sobre o primeiro, em um processo conhecido como *somação*. A somação continua progressivamente com taxas crescentes de chegada do potencial de ação (taxas de disparo da unidade motora) até um ponto em que nenhuma somação adicional é possível (geralmente, em torno de 30 a 50 Hz em músculos inteiros), o qual é conhecido como *tetania*. As ações musculares durante os movimentos de todo o corpo resultam desse processo de somação e o princípio geral é que taxas de disparo mais altas da unidade motora produzem forças musculares mais altas (Enoka e Fuglevand, 2001).

Referências bibliográficas

Al-Gindan, Y.Y., Hankey, C., Govan, L., Gallagher, D., Heymsfield, S.B., Lean, M.E., 2014. Derivation and validation of simple equations to predict total muscle mass from simple anthropometric and demographic data. The American Journal of Clinical Nutrition 100, 1041-1051.

Bottinelli, R., Canepari, M., Pellegrino, M.A., Reggiani, C., 1996. Force-velocity properties of human skeletal muscle fibres: myosin heavy chain isoform and temperature dependence. The Journal of Physiology 1 (495), 573-586.

Buchthal, F., Erminio, F., Rosenfalck, P., 1959. Motor unit territory in different human muscles. Acta physiologica Scandinavica 45, 72-87.

Enoka, R.M., Fuglevand, A.J., 2001. Motor unit physiology: some unresolved issues. Muscle & Nerve 24, 4-17.

Gordon, A.M., Huxley, A.F., Julian, F.J., 1966. The variation in isometric tension with sarcomere length in vertebrate muscle fibres. The Journal of Physiology 184, 170-192.

Henneman, E., Somjen, G., Carpenter, D.O., 1965. Functional significance of cell size in spinal motoneurons. Journal of Neurophysiology 28, 560-580.

Hill, A.V., 1938. The heat of shortening and the dynamic constants of muscle. Proceedings Biological Sciences 126 (843), 136-195.

Lüthi, J.M., Howald, H., Claassen, H., Rösler, K., Vock, P., Hoppeler, H., 1986. Structural changes in skeletal muscle tissue with heavy-resistance exercise. International Journal of Sports Medicine 7 (3), 123-127.

Narici, M., Franchi, M., Maganaris, C., 2016. Muscle structural assembly and functional consequences. The Journal of Experimental Biology 219, 276-284.

Pallafacchina, G., Blaauw, B., Schiaffino, S., 2013. Role of satellite cells in muscle growth and maintenance of muscle mass. Nutrition, Metabolism, and Cardiovascular Diseases: NMCD 23 (Suppl. 1), S12-S18.

Leitura adicional

Jones, D.A., Round, J., de Haan, A., 2004. Skeletal Muscle from Molecules to Movement: A textbook of Muscle Physiology for Sport, Exercise, Physiotherapy and Medicine. Churchill Livingstone/Elsevier Ltd, London.

Scott Powers, Edward Howley, 2017. Exercise Physiology: Theory and application of fitness and performance, Tenth ed. McGraw-Hill Education, New York.

Roger Enoka, 2015. Neuromechanics of Human Movement, fifth ed. Human Kinetics, Leeds, UK.

Capítulo | 2 |

Adaptações Musculares e Fadiga

Tommy Lundberg e Jamie McPhee

Introdução

O corpo se adapta rapidamente a novos padrões de uso ou desuso. Este capítulo apresenta adaptações típicas que ocorrem com o treinamento aeróbico regular e o treinamento de resistência regular, com foco principalmente nos músculos esqueléticos estriados. No entanto, também queremos apontar que existe uma considerável variação interindividual nas adaptações ao treinamento, ou seja, duas pessoas que executam o mesmo tipo e intensidade relativa de treinamento podem não experimentar as mesmas adaptações fisiológicas, especialmente no mesmo período de tempo. A variação na capacidade de exercício e nas respostas de adaptação tem um grande componente genético hereditário, mas nós ainda não sabemos quais combinações de genes interagem para criar o potencial de alcançar o status de atleta de elite.

Adaptações musculares ao treinamento de resistência

Conceitos importantes relacionados com o exercício de resistência

A taxa máxima de consumo de oxigênio ($\dot{V}O_{2máx}$) é importante para o desempenho de resistência, porque representa a capacidade máxima de uso de oxigênio para produzir energia durante exercícios de corpo inteiro, como corrida ou ciclismo (Bassettand Howley, 2000). A carga de trabalho ou intensidade do exercício, na qual ocorre o $\dot{V}O_{2máx}$, também é conhecida como o pico de potência aeróbica. Essa potência aeróbica é substancialmente menor do que a potência máxima que os músculos podem produzir em esforços de prazo muito curto (Zoladz et al., 2000). Por exemplo, um ciclista treinado pode atingir o $\dot{V}O_{2máx}$ a 450 W em uma bicicleta ergométrica, mas se solicitado a produzir um esforço máximo com duração de apenas 5 segundos, o mesmo ciclista pode atingir > 1.600 W; entretanto, o desempenho declina abruptamente devido à fadiga. Curiosamente, mesmo os atletas mais motivados só podem trabalhar no $\dot{V}O_{2máx}$ por períodos curtos antes que a fadiga os force a desacelerar, porque, embora a taxa de respiração aeróbica seja alta no $\dot{V}O_{2máx}$, o fluxo através da glicólise também é muito alto e os metabólitos se acumulam para causar fadiga (ver seção sobre fadiga muscular).

Portanto, esportes de resistência, como corrida de longa distância, ciclismo de estrada e esqui *cross-country*, são realizados em intensidades inferiores ao $\dot{V}O_{2máx}$ e dependem, principalmente, da produção aeróbica de trifosfato de adenosina (ATP) (Coyle, 1995; Faria et al., 2005).

Duas outras características notáveis também influenciam o desempenho de resistência: o limiar de lactato e o pico da taxa de oxidação de gordura. O limiar de lactato representa a carga de trabalho em que as concentrações de lactato acima de um certo limiar (geralmente 4 mmol/ℓ) aparecem no sangue. Esse aparecimento significa altas taxas de glicólise além da capacidade do piruvato (um produto da glicólise) de entrar na mitocôndria. O piruvato é transformado em lactato ao aceitar hidrogênio (outro produto da glicólise) e é liberado pelo músculo. Em indivíduos não treinados, o limiar de lactato pode estar entre 50 e 60% $\dot{V}O_{2máx}$, mas em indivíduos treinados pode ser tão alto quanto 80% $\dot{V}O_{2máx}$. O pico da taxa de oxidação de gordura é a carga de trabalho em que a clivagem aeróbica dos ácidos graxos para a produção de energia alcança seu pico e a partir desse ponto quaisquer requisitos adicionais de ATP devem ser atendidos pela glicose (Lundsgaard et al., 2018). Ele ocorre em intensidades menores do que o limiar de lactato, geralmente, entre 50 e 60% do $\dot{V}O_{2máx}$, e é maior em atletas treinados do que em não atletas (Venables et al., 2005).

Estímulo do treinamento de resistência

O exercício no pico da taxa de oxidação de gordura ou abaixo dele incorrerá em pouquíssima fadiga e pode ser mantido por horas ou dias, se houver motivação. O exercício no limiar de lactato pode ser sustentado por horas em pessoas treinadas e é a intensidade com que uma corrida de longa distância é geralmente concluída. O exercício acima do limiar de lactato, mas abaixo do $\dot{V}O_{2máx}$, pode ser mantido por períodos relativamente longos de tempo. O corredor recreativo médio mantém um ritmo logo abaixo do limiar de lactato, mas atletas profissionais em treinamento intenso incluem deliberadamente intervalos acima do limiar de lactato e até acima do $\dot{V}O_{2máx}$ para causar um estímulo de treinamento maior. O treinamento apresenta uma variedade de desafios fisiológicos, como a necessidade de repor o ATP e os estoques de fontes energéticas, eliminar metabólitos como CO_2 e lactato, dissipar o calor, manter o fluxo sanguíneo pelo corpo e lidar com o *feedback* sensorial que pode ser interpretado como desagradável ou doloroso.

Respostas adaptativas

O estímulo adequado do treinamento leva a adaptações fisiológicas que aumentam o suprimento de oxigênio para os músculos esqueléticos em atividade e o metabolismo aeróbico máximo dos músculos ativos. Essas adaptações aumentam o $\dot{V}O_{2máx}$, o limiar de lactato e o pico da taxa de oxidação de gordura (Jones e Carter, 2000). É importante ter em mente que o exercício agudo é o estímulo, mas os processos bioquímicos que sustentam a adaptação a longo prazo ocorrem por várias horas no período de recuperação após a interrupção do exercício. Portanto, as adaptações a longo prazo são desencadeadas pela soma das respostas fisiológicas às sessões de treinamento individuais e as adaptações ocorrem nos músculos que estavam ativos durante o exercício (Atherton et al., 2015).

O $\dot{V}O_{2máx}$ melhora, principalmente, por meio do aumento da capacidade de transportar oxigênio através do sistema cardiovascular para os músculos em atividade, não apenas nos membros ativos, mas também nos músculos respiratórios e posturais. Isso, por sua vez, está relacionado com os volumes mais elevados de plasma e sangue total, o maior conteúdo de hemoglobina (células sanguíneas da série vermelha responsáveis pelo transporte de oxigênio no sangue) e a maior contratilidade dos músculos cardíacos, especialmente do ventrículo esquerdo. Juntas, essas adaptações aumentam o volume sistólico (a quantidade de sangue bombeada para fora do coração) e, portanto, o débito cardíaco (o produto do volume sistólico × frequência cardíaca) (Bassett e Howley, 2000). A frequência cardíaca máxima muda pouco com o treinamento e, em alguns casos, pode até diminuir.

As adaptações musculares periféricas incluem aumento de atividade das enzimas mitocondriais musculares, densidades mitocondrial e capilar e estoques intracelulares de lipídios e glicogênio (Gollnick et al., 1973; Hoppeler et al., 1985). Curiosamente, os mesmos estímulos responsáveis por iniciar as contrações musculares ou aqueles que se acumulam como consequência dessas contrações, incluindo cálcio, compostos de alta energia – difosfato de adenosina (ADP) e monofosfato de adenosina (AMP) – e intermediários de ácidos graxos, juntamente com hormônios e fatores de crescimento que circulam no sangue, também desencadeiam processos de sinalização celular. Eles ativam mensageiros de proteínas secundárias e moléculas de sinalização, como a proteinoquinase ativada por mitógeno (MAPK) e a proteinoquinase ativada por AMP (AMPK), as quais, por sua vez, aumentam a expressão de genes que codificam as proteínas precisas necessárias para se adaptar (Hoppeler, 2016).

Biogênese mitocondrial

As mitocôndrias aumentam em tamanho e quantidade em todos os três tipos de fibras no período de apenas algumas semanas de treinamento de resistência. As enzimas que coordenam a produção de ATP dentro das mitocôndrias também aumentam sua atividade, de modo que cada mitocôndria melhora a utilização de todo o oxigênio disponível e de ácidos graxos como fonte de energia, o que tem a vantagem de poupar glicose (Hoppeler e Fluck, 2003). Consequentemente, o aumento no volume mitocondrial está linearmente relacionado com o potencial aeróbico muscular aumentado e com o desempenho de resistência. Uma molécula de sinalização chave que regula as melhorias mitocondriais é o receptor 1-alfa coativador do receptor gama ativado pelo proliferador de peroxissomos (PGC-1α). O PGC-1α ativa várias outras moléculas de sinalização que regulam positivamente a expressão de genes mitocondriais (as mitocôndrias contêm 37 genes mantidos separados do núcleo) e de genes nucleares. As sessões de exercício único regulam positivamente os níveis de PGC-1α, preparando os músculos para responder ainda mais rápido à sessão de exercício seguinte. Assim, PGC-1α pode ser pensado como um regulador mestre da biogênese mitocondrial em resposta ao treinamento aeróbico (Lin et al., 2005).

Angiogênese

O treinamento de resistência leva a um aumento na quantidade de capilares ao redor de cada fibra muscular. Esse processo é conhecido como angiogênese (formação de novos vasos) e serve para aumentar o suprimento de oxigênio para as fibras musculares individuais que mais precisam dele, bem como para retardar o tempo de trânsito do sangue pelo músculo para dar mais tempo para que o oxigênio seja extraído dos eritrócitos e levado para as fibras musculares. A expansão da rede capilar ocorre em paralelo com o aumento da mitocôndria e do consumo máximo de oxigênio (Klausen et al., 1981). O aumento da capilaridade é realizado, principalmente, por "brotamento" de novos capilares a partir das redes capilares existentes. Os principais estímulos que impulsionam a angiogênese são o aumento do fluxo sanguíneo, o estresse de cisalhamento à medida que o sangue empurra as paredes capilares e o aumento dos metabólitos das contrações musculares. O fator de crescimento endotelial vascular (VEGF) é o principal regulador da angiogênese. Os níveis do VEGF aumentam em resposta ao exercício agudo e sinalizam para aumentar a expressão local de genes envolvidos no crescimento capilar.

Adaptações musculares ao treinamento de resistência

O principal objetivo do treinamento de resistência é promover o aumento da força voluntária máxima. Isso é mediado, principalmente, por aumentos no tamanho do músculo (hipertrofia) e por adaptações neurais que favorecem um maior uso muscular (Folland e Williams, 2007). Fatores neurais, como impulso neural e coordenação intermuscular aprimorados associados ao controle motor, contribuem para o rápido aumento da força durante as primeiras semanas a meses de um programa de treinamento de resistência. Posteriormente, o tamanho e a força muscular parecem aumentar de modo paralelo, embora não haja necessariamente uma correlação entre o grau de crescimento muscular (hipertrofia) e o grau de ganho de força. Atletas expostos a treinamento de resistência vigorosa a longo prazo apresentam hipertrofia muscular extraordinária, o que pode refletir tanto a seleção genética quanto a resposta adaptativa ao treinamento a longo prazo, mas muito provavelmente uma combinação de ambas. Ainda há um debate considerável sobre o programa de treinamento mais eficaz para melhorar a força. O Colégio Americano de Medicina Esportiva defende a carga pesada (85 a 100% de uma repetição máxima (1RM)) e várias séries para promover o aumento da força; no entanto, essas recomendações foram legitimamente desafiadas, pois estudos recentes mostram aumentos substanciais no tamanho e na força muscular quando cargas baixas são elevadas até a falha voluntária (Schoenfeld et al., 2017).

Adaptações neurais

Exemplos indiretos de adaptações neurais são a grande discrepância na magnitude entre ganhos de força e hipertrofia muscular, notada no início de um programa de exercícios, e a observação comum de que o aumento na força é muito específico para o exercício particular realizado (princípio da especificidade) (Folland e Williams, 2007). Um exemplo disso é o fato de que o aumento da força dinâmica (1RM) é significativamente maior do que o aumento da força isométrica se o treinamento for realizado de modo dinâmico. Outro exemplo é o chamado efeito *"crossover"*, ou educação cruzada – significa que os ganhos de força podem ser observados no braço ou na perna contralateral à extremidade que estava envolvida no treinamento real (Carroll et al., 2006).

A evidência mais concreta de adaptação neural é o aumento do sinal eletromiográfico (EMG) (eletromiografia de superfície), que pode ser medido apenas após uma ou algumas semanas de treinamento de força. Um aumento no sinal elétrico através do músculo simplesmente mostra que ele é mais ativado pelo sistema nervoso. No entanto, é importante enfatizar que as medições EMG padrão não podem determinar se o sinal aumentado é devido ao recrutamento elevado de mais unidades motoras, à frequência de disparo aumentada (ou seja, codificação de taxa aumentada) ou mesmo devido à hipertrofia muscular, uma vez que o potencial elétrico está relacionado com a área da seção transversal da fibra. No entanto, o objetivo principal da adaptação neural é aumentar a ativação dos agonistas (os músculos que realizam principalmente o movimento). Outro desafio é ativar os sinergistas de modo adequado enquanto os antagonistas devem ser minimamente ativos. Ao mesmo tempo, o sistema deve aprender a lidar com o *feedback* sensorial que ocorre nos músculos e nas articulações (propriocepção e cinestesia). Embora seja um pouco difícil medir o recrutamento de unidades motoras de forma confiável, o corpo coletivo de evidências indica que o treinamento de resistência é capaz de aumentar a capacidade de recrutar de forma mais eficiente as unidades motoras de limiar mais alto (ou seja, recrutamento e taxas de disparo aumentadas).

Hipertrofia muscular

Em teoria, qualquer aumento na área de seção transversal muscular (AST) pode ser devido aos aumentos no tamanho da fibra e/ou na quantidade de fibras (hiperplasia). Geralmente, é aceito que a hipertrofia muscular do adulto ocorre predominantemente por meio de um aumento da AST das fibras individuais (Tesch, 1988). Em particular, o treinamento de resistência aumenta a área das fibras de contração rápida do tipo 2. A hipertrofia das fibras ocorre por meio da síntese e do acúmulo de novos miofilamentos, com expansão concomitante do volume da fibra. Mesmo que o processo de hipertrofia muscular comece imediatamente após a primeira sessão de treinamento, refletido como um aumento da renovação da proteína muscular líquida, leva pelo menos algumas semanas antes que a hipertrofia muscular possa ser medida de forma confiável e não invasiva por técnicas de imagem modernas (p. ex., ressonância magnética) ou invasivamente por meio da avaliação da área de fibra a partir de biopsias musculares (procedimento desconfortável).

Outras adaptações morfológicas

Embora o tipo de fibra muscular seja de maneira ampla determinado geneticamente, as fibras se adaptam metabólica e funcionalmente de forma rápida a estímulos específicos de sub ou sobrecarga, como programas de treinamento específicos. A composição das fibras musculares de diferentes atletas de elite tem sido explorada e, em geral, parece que os atletas que dependem da capacidade de resistência têm uma alta proporção de fibras do tipo 1, enquanto os atletas de potência, como corredores de *sprint*, têm uma alta proporção de fibras do tipo 2 (Costill et al., 1976). A razão para essa diferença marcante é provavelmente decorrente do viés de seleção para um esporte que se encaixa na composição genética de um indivíduo, em vez do efeito dos regimes de treinamento específicos realizados.

Se, ou não, e em que medida, as transformações do tipo de fibra ocorrem devido ao treinamento têm sido questões de debate por muitos anos (Pette e Staron, 1997; Schiaffino e Reggiani, 2011). O consenso é que o treinamento com exercícios a longo prazo em seres humanos leva a uma redução nas fibras híbridas e na isoforma do tipo 2X e a um aumento na proporção das fibras do tipo 2A (Klitgaard et al., 1990; Schiaffino e Reggiani, 2011). Embora a princípio isso possa parecer contraditório com o objetivo geral de aumentar a produção de força no que diz respeito aos atletas de treinamento de força, essa mudança é compensada por adaptações neurais, mudanças arquitetônicas e hipertrofia preferencial das fibras do tipo 2.

Outras mudanças morfológicas que podem ocorrer em resposta ao treinamento de resistência incluem um aumento no ângulo de penação da fibra, aumento do comprimento dos fascículos e remodelamento do tecido conjuntivo (Folland e Williams, 2007). Um aumento no ângulo de penação do fascículo significa aumento da AST da fibra muscular devido à adição de sarcômeros em paralelo (e, portanto, proteínas contráteis) e isso aumenta a força muscular. Se o comprimento do fascículo aumentar, isso indica que ocorreu adição em série de sarcômeros, o que, geralmente, é benéfico para a velocidade de encurtamento muscular. O treinamento de resistência também leva a adaptações no complemento músculo-tendão, aumentando a rigidez do tendão e a taxa de desenvolvimento da força. Juntos, esses fatores morfológicos contribuem para o aumento na produção de força muscular observada com o treinamento de resistência crônica.

Regulação do *turnover* (renovação) da proteína muscular

A proporção de síntese e degradação de proteínas determina o equilíbrio geral de proteínas musculares. Quando a síntese da proteína muscular excede a degradação, o *turnover* (renovação) líquido da proteína é positivo e ocorre o acúmulo de proteínas musculares. Durante o exercício agudo de resistência, tanto a síntese quanto a degradação de proteínas são estimuladas de forma que o saldo líquido seja negativo (Kumar et al., 2009). No entanto, quando os aminoácidos essenciais são consumidos após o exercício, o saldo líquido de proteínas torna-se positivo. Assim, a quantidade de proteínas contráteis atinge um novo nível de estado estacionário por meio do efeito cumulativo de sessões de exercícios repetidas e alimentação. Quando isso se repete por um período estendido, culmina em hipertrofia muscular.

Mecanotransdução

É claro que o músculo esquelético deve ter sensores que transduzem a tensão ativa ou passiva em um evento celular que favorece o aumento da síntese proteica, denominado *mecanotransdução*. Embora a compreensão desses mecanismos seja limitada até o momento, foi demonstrado que a carga aguda perturba a integridade do sarcolema e produz o ácido fosfatídico, o qual leva à ativação de cascatas de sinalização que regulam a síntese de proteínas (You et al., 2014). Além disso, uma molécula de sinalização importante, chamada de quinase de adesão focal (FAK), aumenta em resposta às contrações de alta força e diminui após a descarga, sugerindo que a FAK detecte carga mecânica (Crossland et al., 2013). Coletivamente, parece que o ácido fosfatídico e a FAK convertem a tensão mecânica em uma resposta intracelular apropriada, iniciando a síntese de proteínas e o crescimento muscular.

Regulação transcricional

Está bem estabelecido que o exercício de resistência altera a expressão de genes envolvidos em diversas funções, como crescimento de células, diferenciação, inflamação e proteólise. Embora o aumento da tradução do RNA mensageiro (mRNA) seja o principal passo regulatório para aumentar a síntese de proteínas, a resposta da expressão gênica (incluindo correguladores transcricionais) também está implicada no controle da renovação da proteína muscular. Notavelmente, a transcrição de várias centenas de genes é alterada por exercícios de resistência aguda, tanto em estados destreinados quanto habituados ao treinamento (Raue et al., 2012).

Entre os marcadores que exercem controle transcricional está a miostatina, um membro da família do fator de crescimento β-transformador que funciona como um regulador negativo do tamanho do músculo. O exercício agudo de resistência diminui a expressão da miostatina e auxilia na promoção da hipertrofia muscular, revertendo seu efeito inibitório na síntese de proteínas musculares e na atividade das células-satélite (Coffey e Hawley, 2007). Outro exemplo são as proteínas ubiquitina ligase atrogina-1 e MuRF-1, reguladas por meio de fatores de transcrição FOXO. Enquanto MuRF-1 e atrogina-1 estão relacionadas com a atrofia muscular em resposta ao desuso por direcionar proteínas contráteis para a degradação, parece que esses marcadores facilitam o remodelamento do tecido em favor do crescimento muscular no músculo esquelético saudável (Hwee et al., 2014).

Novas pesquisas têm demonstrado papéis importantes dos microRNA (miRNA) para a resposta adaptativa muscular ao exercício de resistência. Essas sequências não codificantes de RNA degradam transcritos-alvos pela ligação a sequências complementares. Vários miRNA aumentam em resposta ao exercício de resistência e podem participar da regulação das alterações induzidas pelo treinamento no músculo (Hitachi e Tsuchida, 2013).

Respostas de sinalização intracelular

A tradução do mRNA em proteína inclui os processos de iniciação, alongamento e término. A etapa de iniciação é de particular importância para esse processo, coordenada pelo complexo mecanístico do alvo da rapamicina (mTOR). O mTOR integra sinais de estímulos mecânicos, status de energia e nutrientes para coordenar eventos de sinalização a jusante. De fato, a ativação de mTOR induz aumento da síntese proteica após exercícios agudos de resistência e é crucial para a resposta hipertrófica muscular (Coffey e Hawley, 2007). Os alvos efetores a jusante de mTOR incluem p70S6 quinase (p70S6 K) e proteína 1 de ligação ao fator de iniciação eucariótico 4E (4E-BP1). Geralmente, o controle traducional da síntese de proteínas é considerado um evento molecular crucial que regula o tamanho do músculo.

A hipertrofia, impulsionada pelo saldo positivo de síntese proteica, também requer função ribossômica aumentada (Bamman et al., 2017). Os ribossomos são a organela onde os aminoácidos são ligados entre si para formar a proteína recém-construída a partir do rascunho de mRNA. Além do aumento da eficiência ribossômica, ou seja, maior tradução de mRNA por ribossomo, a tradução aumentada de proteínas também pode ocorrer por meio da capacidade ribossômica elevada – biogênese do ribossomo. De modo curioso, esse processo energeticamente caro também parece ser amplamente regulado pela atividade do mTOR.

Células-satélite e adição de mionúcleos

Durante a hipertrofia, a adição de mionúcleos poderia auxiliar na manutenção da razão mionúcleo/citoplasma estável e, portanto, proteger a capacidade de transcrição. A adição de novos núcleos às fibras existentes é mediada pela proliferação de células-satélite, que se localizam entre a lâmina basal e o sarcolema da fibra. A importância da atividade das células-satélite e da adição de mionúcleos no processo hipertrófico não é bem compreendida (Bamman et al., 2017). No entanto, em apoio a seu papel, o conteúdo de mionúcleos mostrou ser maior em levantadores de peso do que em controles não treinados e a hipertrofia de fibra induzida por treinamento de resistência foi, em alguns estudos, acompanhada por conteúdo de mionúcleos e quantidade de células-satélite aumentados.

Fadiga muscular

A fadiga muscular é a falha em manter uma determinada ação muscular ao longo do tempo e/ou ao longo de contrações sucessivas. É caracterizada por perda de força, desaceleração da velocidade de contração e da taxa de relaxamento, o que leva à perda substancial de potência (lembre-se que a potência é o produto da força × velocidade de contração) e à precisão reduzida de movimento (Enoka e Duchateau, 2008). A ação muscular é recuperada após um período de descanso, de poucos segundos a algumas horas, dependendo das circunstâncias, e qualquer perda residual de força ou potência será resultado de dano ou lesão e não fadiga.

Os mecanismos da fadiga são complexos e não totalmente compreendidos. Eles dependem do tipo e intensidade do exercício, mas podem ser classificados como tendo origem "central" ou "periférica". A *fadiga central* descreve todos os aspectos do comando motor que determinam o recrutamento da unidade motora, desde o cérebro até o terminal do axônio do neurônio motor. A *fadiga periférica* descreve todos os aspectos que ocorrem entre a troca de acetilcolina na junção neuromuscular e a cinética da ponte cruzada de actina-miosina. Os mecanismos centrais e periféricos da fadiga ocorrem durante o exercício, mas a sua importância relativa difere dependendo das características intrínsecas das unidades motoras e do período de relaxamento entre as contrações, permitindo a recuperação metabólica, bem como a intensidade e a duração do exercício (Enoka e Duchateau, 2008; Hunter, 2009). A fadiga é fortemente influenciada pelos níveis de condicionamento físico da pessoa e fatores externos, incluindo temperatura e umidade ambientais.

Fadiga durante exercícios muito intensos

Exercícios de intensidade muito alta, como corrida ou levantamento de peso, recrutam as unidades motoras maiores e mais rápidas e dependem muito de processos anaeróbicos para fornecer ATP. Há um componente central de fadiga relacionado com a "excitação" do sistema nervoso central (SNC), a evidência para isso vem de estudos em que o fornecimento de forte incentivo verbal ou outro estímulo pode aumentar o recrutamento de unidades motoras e a produção muscular (Ikai e Steinhaus, 1961). No entanto, isso normalmente é responsável por apenas cerca de 10% da fadiga geral em indivíduos muito bem-motivados e, em vez disso, o principal componente da fadiga é devido aos fatores periféricos.

Os principais locais de fadiga periférica são a propagação dos potenciais de ação ao longo do sarcolema; a liberação de Ca^{2+} do retículo sarcoplasmático; e a função das pontes cruzadas (Allen et al., 2008). Normalmente, há um influxo de Na^+ e um fluxo de saída de K^+ ao longo do sarcolema à medida que o potencial de ação se propaga. Durante a atividade muscular intensa e sustentada, o K^+ pode acumular-se nos túbulos t, restringir a recuperação do potencial da membrana e, assim, limitar qualquer ativação posterior das fibras musculares. Outro mecanismo de fadiga é que o Pi liberado do ATP durante os ciclos de ponte cruzada entra no retículo sarcoplasmático e se liga ao Ca^{2+} (formando fosfato de cálcio), o que diminui o cálcio livre disponível para liberação no sarcoplasma e, desse modo, reduz a quantidade de

Adaptações Musculares e Fadiga **Capítulo** | 2 |

pontes cruzadas que podem se formar. O Pi também pode interferir diretamente na função da ponte cruzada para diminuir sua cinética. Outros subprodutos metabólicos de intensa atividade de contração, incluindo lactato, íons de hidrogênio e ADP, também podem inibir as contrações das fibras musculares e existe a possibilidade de depleção localizada de ATP que restringiria a atividade ATPásica transportadora de íons pelo sarcolema ou ainda a atividade ATPásica da miosina ao longo dos sarcômeros. O acúmulo desses metabólitos dentro dos músculos pode estimular adicionalmente os quimiorreceptores musculares, desencadeando o *feedback* dos proprioceptores ao longo dos nervos aferentes tipo III/IV (sensoriais) que fazem sinapse com neurônios alfamotores no SNC para inibir o recrutamento da unidade motora (Garland e Kaufman, 1995; Taylor e Gandevia, 2008).

Fadiga durante exercício prolongado de resistência

O ATP necessário para alimentar o exercício intenso com duração de 2 ou 3 minutos vem igualmente de fontes aeróbicas e anaeróbicas e a intensidade é tipicamente > 90% $\dot{V}O_{2máx}$, mas exercícios prolongados que duram 20 minutos ou mais são realizados em intensidade "submáxima" < 80% $\dot{V}O_{2máx}$ e é progressivamente menor conforme a duração aumenta em até algumas horas. O ATP derivado quase inteiramente da respiração aeróbica mitocondrial fornece energia para essas atividades de duração mais longa. Os mecanismos de fadiga durante o exercício prolongado são diferentes daqueles que ocorrem durante o exercício de alta intensidade devido às claras diferenças no recrutamento da unidade motora, no metabolismo das fibras, na soma do proprioceptor e em outras informações sensoriais. Há evidências que mostram um papel importante para a fadiga central, bem como para fatores periféricos relacionados com os substratos energéticos.

A fadiga central leva a uma redução na quantidade de unidades motoras recrutadas e/ou nas taxas de disparo das unidades motoras. Essas diminuições são decorrentes do *feedback* aferente dos proprioceptores, de modo que causam inibição do recrutamento da unidade motora, bem como diminuição do impulso motor do cérebro e do SNC (Carroll et al., 2017). O SNC recebe continuamente estímulos sensoriais e, durante exercícios prolongados de resistência, fatores como temperatura corporal central, desidratação, tensão muscular, dor e lesões estão associados aos níveis aumentados de serotonina no cérebro e à redução do impulso motor. Aplicar um estímulo frio, como água, na testa e nos antebraços, ou derramar uma solução de glicose ao redor da boca, ou fornecer um forte incentivo verbal ou visual, pode superar temporariamente a fadiga central para permitir maior recrutamento da unidade motora e produção muscular, mas esses efeitos duram apenas alguns minutos e são melhoras marginais (embora importantes para atletas de elite) no desempenho (Carter et al., 2004; Jensen et al., 2018).

Os estoques de glicogênio muscular e hepático, bem como os ácidos graxos, fornecem a maior parte do combustível para a respiração aeróbica. No entanto, as reservas de glicogênio são limitadas e há relatos de depleção de glicogênio muscular durante a corrida de resistênica de longa distância (Bergstrom e Hultman, 1967). Isso pode corresponder a "bater na parede", termo usado para descrever a diminuição acentuada na intensidade do exercício e sentimentos muito fortes de fadiga e exaustão na maratona e em outros eventos de distância. No entanto, ressaltamos que as evidências científicas para a depleção de glicogênio são muito variadas e alguns estudos demonstraram reservas substanciais de glicogênio em atletas com sinais típicos de fadiga (Costill et al., 1971; Madsen et al., 1990). A depleção de glicogênio ou qualquer outro fator que reduza o uso de glicose sem qualquer ingestão adicional dessa substância retardaria a ressíntese de ATP, aumentando a dependência da oxidação beta (uso de ácidos graxos nas mitocôndrias para produzir energia). A oxidação da gordura é um processo relativamente lento e o pico da taxa ocorre em cerca de 50 a 60% do $\dot{V}O_{2máx}$ (Venables et al., 2005). As intensidades de exercício superiores a 60% do $\dot{V}O_{2máx}$ devem usar glicose e podem, de fato, inibir a oxidação de gordura (Lundsgaard et al., 2018). Uma adaptação importante do treinamento de resistência é aumentar o uso de ácidos graxos e aumentar a intensidade com que as gorduras continuam a fornecer energia para que o glicogênio possa ser poupado e melhorar o desempenho. Tomar medidas práticas para aumentar a ingestão de carboidratos nos dias anteriores a um evento de longa distância e consumir carboidratos e líquidos durante os eventos ajudam a prolongar os estoques de glicose e retardar a fadiga.

Referências bibliográficas

Allen, D.G., Lamb, G.D., Westerblad, H., 2008. Skeletal muscle fatigue: cellular mechanisms. Physiological Reviews 88, 287-332.

Atherton, P.J., Phillips, B.E., Wilkinson, D.J., 2015. Exercise and regulation of protein metabolism. Progress in Molecular Biology and Translational Science 135, 75-98.

Bamman, M.M., Roberts, B.M., Adams, G.R., 2017. Molecular regulation of exercise-induced muscle fiber hypertrophy. Cold Spring Harbor Perspectives in Medicine.

Bassett Jr., D.R., Howley, E.T., 2000. Limiting factors for maximum oxygen uptake and determinants of endurance performance. Medicine & Science in Sports & Exercise 32, 70-84.

Bergstrom, J., Hultman, E., 1967. A study of the glycogen metabolism during exercise in man. Scandinavian Journal of Clinical and Laboratory Investigation 19, 218-228.

Carroll, T.J., Herbert, R.D., Munn, J., Lee, M., Gandevia, S.C., 2006. Contralateral effects of unilateral strength training: evidence and possible mechanisms. Journal of Applied Physiology 101, 1514-1522.

Carroll, T.J., Taylor, J.L., Gandevia, S.C., 2017. Recovery of central and peripheral neuromuscular fatigue after exercise. Journal of Applied Physiology 122, 1068-1076.

Carter, J.M., Jeukendrup, A.E., Jones, D.A., 2004. The effect of carbohydrate mouth rinse on 1-h cycle time trial performance. Medicine & Science in Sports & Exercise 36, 2107-2111.

Coffey, V.G., Hawley, J.A., 2007. The molecular bases of training adaptation. Sports Medicine 37, 737-763.

Costill, D.L., Daniels, J., Evans, W., Fink, W., Krahenbuhl, G., Saltin, B., 1976. Skeletal muscle enzymes and fiber composition in male and female track athletes. Journal of Applied Physiology 40, 149-154.

Costill, D.L., Sparks, K., Gregor, R., Turner, C., 1971. Muscle glycogen utilization during exhaustive running. Journal of Applied Physiology 31, 353-356.

Coyle, E.F., 1995. Integration of the physiological factors determining endurance performance ability. Exercise and Sport Sciences Reviews 23, 25-63.

Crossland, H., Kazi, A.A., Lang, C.H., Timmons, J.A., Pierre, P., Wilkinson, D.J., et al., 2013. Focal adhesion kinase is required for IGF-I-mediated growth of skeletal muscle cells via a TSC2/mTOR/S6K1-associated pathway. American Journal of Physiology. Endocrinology and Metabolism 305, E183-E193.

Enoka, R.M., Duchateau, J., 2008. Muscle fatigue: what, why and how it influences muscle function. Journal of Physiology 586, 11-23.

Faria, E.W., Parker, D.L., Faria, I.E., 2005. The science of cycling: physiology and training – part 1. Sports Medicine 35, 285-312.

Folland, J.P., Williams, A.G., 2007. The adaptations to strength training: morphological and neurological contributions to increased strength. Sports Medicine 37, 145-168.

Garland, S.J., Kaufman, M.P., 1995. Role of muscle afferents in the inhibition of motoneurons during fatigue. Advances in Experimental Medicine and Biology 384, 271-278.

Gollnick, P.D., Armstrong, R.B., Saltin, B., Saubert, C.W., Sembrowich, W.L., Shepherd, R.E., 1973. Effect of training on enzyme activity and fiber composition of human skeletal muscle. Journal of Applied Physiology 34, 107-111.

Hitachi, K., Tsuchida, K., 2013. Role of microRNAs in skeletal muscle hypertrophy. Frontiers in Physiology 4, 408.

Hoppeler, H., Fluck, M., 2003. Plasticity of skeletal muscle mitochondria: structure and function. Medicine & Science in Sports & Exercise 35, 95-104.

Hoppeler, H., Howald, H., Conley, K., Lindstedt, S.L., Claassen, H., Vock, P., et al., 1985. Endurance training in humans: aerobic capacity and structure of skeletal muscle. Journal of Applied Physiology 59, 320-327.

Hoppeler, H., 2016. Molecular networks in skeletal muscle plasticity. Journal of Experimental Biology 219, 205-213.

Hunter, S.K., 2009. Sex differences and mechanisms of task-specific muscle fatigue. Exercise and Sport Sciences Reviews 37, 113-122.

Hwee, D.T., Baehr, L.M., Philp, A., Baar, K., Bodine, S.C., 2014. Maintenance of muscle mass and load-induced growth in Muscle RING Finger 1 null mice with age. Aging Cell 13, 92-101.

Ikai, M., Steinhaus, A.H., 1961. Some factors modifying the expression of human strength. Journal of Applied Physiology 16, 157-163.

Jensen, M., Klimstra, M., Sporer, B., Stellingwerff, T., 2018. Effect of carbohydrate mouth rinse on performance after prolonged submaximal cycling. Medicine & Science in Sports & Exercise 50, 1031 -1038.

Jones, A.M., Carter, H., 2000. The effect of endurance training on parameters of aerobic fitness. Sports Medicine 29, 373-386.

Klausen, K., Andersen, L.B., Pelle, I., 1981. Adaptive changes in work capacity, skeletal muscle capillarization and enzyme levels during training and detraining. Acta Physiologica Scandinavica 113, 9-16.

Klitgaard, H., Bergman, O., Betto, R., Salviati, G., Schiaffino, S., Clausen, T., et al., 1990. Co-existence of myosin heavy chain I and IIa isoforms in human skeletal muscle fibres with endurance training. Pflügers Archiv 416, 470-472.

Kumar, V., Atherton, P., Smith, K., Rennie, M.J., 2009. Human muscle protein synthesis and breakdown during and after exercise. Journal of Applied Physiology 106, 2026-2039.

Lin, J., Handschin, C., Spiegelman, B.M., 2005. Metabolic control through the PGC-1 family of transcription coactivators. Cell Metabolism 1, 361-370.

Lundsgaard, A.M., Fritzen, A.M., Kiens, B., 2018. Molecular regulation of fatty acid oxidation in skeletal muscle during aerobic exercise. Trends in Endocrinology and Metabolism 29, 18-30.

Madsen, K., Pedersen, P.K., Rose, P., Richter, E.A., 1990. Carbohydrate supercompensation and muscle glycogen utilization during exhaustive running in highly trained athletes. European Journal of Applied Physiology and Occupational Physiology 61, 467-472.

Pette, D., Staron, R.S., 1997. Mammalian skeletal muscle fiber type transitions. International Review of Cytology 170, 143-223.

Raue, U., Trappe, T.A., Estrem, S.T., Qian, H.R., Helvering, L.M., Smith, R.C., et al., 2012. Transcriptome signature of resistance exercise adaptations: mixed muscle and fiber type specific profiles in young and old adults. Journal of Applied Physiology 112, 1625-1636.

Schiaffino, S., Reggiani, C., 2011. Fiber types in mammalian skeletal muscles. Physiological Reviews 91, 1447-1531.

Schoenfeld, B.J., Grgic, J., Ogborn, D., Krieger, J.W., 2017. Strength and hypertrophy adaptations between low- vs. high-load resistance training: a systematic review and meta-analysis. Journal of Strength and Conditioning Research 31, 3508-3523.

Taylor, J.L., Gandevia, S.C., 2008. A comparison of central aspects of fatigue in submaximal and maximal voluntary contractions. Journal of Applied Physiology 104, 542-550.

Tesch, P.A., 1988. Skeletal muscle adaptations consequent to long-term heavy resistance exercise. Medicine & Science in Sports & Exercise 20, S132-S134.

Venables, M.C., Achten, J., Jeukendrup, A.E., 2005. Determinants of fat oxidation during exercise in healthy men and women: a cross-sectional study. Journal of Applied Physiology 98, 160-167.

You, J.S., Lincoln, H.C., Kim, C.R., Frey, J.W., Goodman, C.A., Zhong, X.P., et al., 2014. The role of diacylglycerol kinase zeta and phosphatidic acid in the mechanical activation of mammalian target of rapamycin (mTOR) signaling and skeletal muscle hypertrophy. Journal of Biological Chemistry 289, 1551-1563.

Zoladz, J.A., Rademaker, A.C., Sargeant, A.J., 2000. Human muscle power generating capability during cycling at different pedalling rates. Experimental Physiology 85, 117-124.

Capítulo | 3 |

Fisiologia do Desuso, da Imobilização e de Ambientes de Baixa Carga

Nicholas C. Clark, Mark Glaister, Lyndsey M. Cannon e Nic Perrem

Introdução

Lesões esportivas ocorrem em todas as partes do corpo (Boyce e Quigley, 2004; Tirabassi et al., 2016), com lesões articulares periféricas sendo consistentemente mais frequentes (Hootman et al., 2007; Tirabassi et al., 2016). Lesões articulares periféricas traumáticas, em particular, costumam apresentar-se com dano tecidual (Atef et al., 2016; Olsson et al., 2016; Roemer et al., 2014) e disfunções associadas a sinais e sintomas, como dor (Aarnio et al., 2017; Alaia et al., 2015), derrame (Luhmann, 2003; Man et al., 2007) e fraqueza muscular (Hohmann et al., 2016; Punt et al., 2015). Portanto, as lesões esportivas frequentemente resultam em limitações de atividade física (AF) a curto prazo e redução do tempo de participação em esportes, a fim de facilitar o processo de cicatrização e realizar a reabilitação (Hootman et al., 2007), respeitando o processo inflamatório agudo. As limitações de AF que se manifestam como resultado de lesões esportivas fazem parte de um "espectro de desuso" (Figura 3.1). Para este capítulo, o termo "desuso" refere-se à diminuição do uso de uma parte do corpo com relação aos níveis habituais de AF de um indivíduo devido às lesões traumáticas ou ao uso excessivo. O termo "imobilizar" significa evitar todo o movimento de uma parte do corpo devido a uma lesão. O termo "carga" é definido como a aplicação de força a uma parte do corpo (Whiting e Zernicke, 2008); "ambientes de baixa carga" (ABC), portanto, são definidos aqui como quando cargas inferiores às habitualmente aplicadas à parte do corpo de um indivíduo existem devido ao desuso pós-lesão. Como a lesão resulta em algum nível de desuso, vários tecidos e sistemas corporais são afetados pela diminuição dos níveis de AF (Bloomfield, 1997; Convertino, 1997).

Para desenvolver intervenções clínicas eficazes que limitem as sequelas do desuso, é necessário que os profissionais da saúde compreendam os efeitos secundários da lesão nos tecidos e sistemas corporais e como esses efeitos influenciam na prática de reabilitação (Clark, 2015). O objetivo deste capítulo, portanto, é revisar os efeitos fisiológicos do desuso, da imobilização e do ABC. Nosso grupo de pesquisa opera usando a analogia de um automóvel: você não pode condicionar o motor (sistema cardiorrespiratório) se o chassi (sistema musculoesquelético [SME]) quebrar primeiro (Clark, 2008). Essa é uma analogia importante, pois a observação clínica comum revela quantos atletas não podem realizar, por exemplo, corridas longas e lentas até que a dor pós-lesão no joelho seja resolvida. Além disso, os distúrbios do SME estão associados ao início e à progressão da doença mitigada pela AF do tipo resistência (Hawker et al., 2014; Toomey et al., 2017). Consequentemente, faremos uma revisão dos efeitos fisiológicos do desuso, da imobilização e do ABC com ênfase nos sistemas esquelético, muscular e cardiorrespiratório. Devido às limitações atuais no conhecimento e na ciência, não é ético ou tecnologicamente possível estudar alguns efeitos do desuso com paradigmas humanos *in vivo* devido à probabilidade de prejudicar os participantes do estudo. Portanto, a pesquisa empregou uma variedade de paradigmas científicos para ajudar a responder a questões clínicas; por exemplo, paradigmas animais *in vitro* e *in vivo*, humano *in vitro* e *in silico* (Huang e Wikswo, 2006; Maglio e Mabry, 2011). Uma abordagem integrativa da prática clínica baseada em evidências envolve a integração de diferentes modelos de pesquisa para responder a questões clínicas complexas (Drolet e Lorenzi, 2011; Mabry et al., 2008) e resulta em uma rica tradução da pesquisa para o contexto clínico (Drolet e Lorenzi, 2011; Rubio et al., 2010). Vamos, posteriormente, empregar múltiplos paradigmas de pesquisa em mamíferos (p. ex., humano, primata,

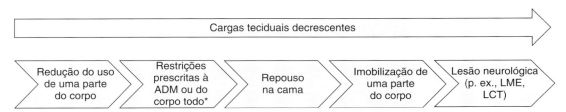

Figura 3.1 Espectro de desuso após lesão esportiva. *Normalmente aplicado com o uso de cinta e/ou muletas. ADM, amplitude de movimento; LME, lesão da medula espinal; LCT, lesão cerebral traumática. (Adaptada de Bloomfield, S., 1997. Changes in musculoskeletal structure and function with prolonged bed rest. *Medicine and Science in Sports and Exercise*, 29 (2), 197-206.)

Ossos

Os ossos formam o esqueleto que funciona para fornecer suporte e proteção para outros tecidos do corpo, um sistema de alavanca para facilitar o movimento, um reservatório de minerais e um depósito de células hematopoéticas (Weiner e Wagner, 1998; Whiting e Zernicke, 2008), contribuindo para o aparelho locomotor. Os constituintes celulares do osso são os osteoblastos e os osteoclastos, os quais são responsáveis pelo remodelamento contínuo do osso por meio da secreção da nova matriz extracelular (MEC) do osso e da erosão da MEC antiga do osso, respectivamente (Crockett et al., 2011; Feng e McDonald, 2011; Weiner e Wagner, 1998). A MEC do osso inclui componentes fibrosos (colágeno tipo I), substância fundamental (amorfa) (hidroxiapatita, cálcio, proteínas não estruturais) e água (Crockett et al., 2011; Feng e McDonald, 2011; Weiner e Wagner, 1998). A homeostase e a saúde ósseas são controladas por ações coordenadas de hormônios (Harada e Rodan, 2003) do sistema nervoso simpático (Elefteriou et al., 2014) e da mecanotransdução (Ehrlich e Lanyon, 2002; Liedert et al., 2006; Oftadeh et al., 2015; Pavalko et al., 2003; Rosa et al., 2015). Tensão intermitente e cargas de compressão são particularmente importantes para influenciar a homeostase óssea por meio de várias vias de estimulação celular, incluindo deformação física da MEC óssea, indução de fluxo de fluido canalicular e geração de fluxo elétrico lacunocanalicular (Bonewald, 2006; Oftadeh et al., 2015; Turner e Pavalko, 1998).

Redução da atividade dos osteoblastos e aumento da atividade dos osteoclastos podem ser observados logo após o desuso do membro ou a imobilização, resultando em uma diminuição líquida no volume ósseo (Weinreb et al., 1989; Wronski e Morey, 1983; Young et al., 1986). A evidência de ruptura do colágeno ósseo foi relatada após períodos prolongados de desuso (Fiore et al., 1999; Uebelhart et al., 2000) e o desuso pós-lesão e pós-cirurgia pode resultar em osteopenia tanto local quanto proximal ou distal do local da lesão primária (Ceroni et al., 2012; Ejerhed et al., 2004; Leppälä et al., 1999; Reiman et al., 2006; Smith et al., 1992). Na ressonância magnética (RM), anormalidades do sinal da medula óssea também foram relatadas após períodos de desuso e imobilização do membro (Elias et al., 2007; Nardo et al., 2013).

O desuso e a imobilização dos membros são consistentemente observados resultando em mudanças na fisiologia e estrutura ósseas, tanto locais quanto distantes do local da lesão primária ou do local de imobilização. Com a diminuição da densidade mineral óssea volumétrica e/ou mudança na estrutura óssea (geometria), vem uma diminuição na força óssea em direções específicas e um limiar mais baixo para fratura óssea (Bach-Gansmo et al., 2016; Guo e Kim, 2002; Lepola et al., 1993; Mosekilde et al., 2000; Peng et al., 1994). Após os períodos de desuso e imobilização do membro, os profissionais da saúde devem estar cientes das possíveis mudanças negativas na resistência óssea local e remota e de como isso pode influenciar a reabilitação de curto e longo prazo da lesão esportiva primária anterior.

Cartilagem articular

A cartilagem articular (CA) cobre as extremidades dos ossos formando as articulações sinoviais e facilita a transmissão de cargas por meio das superfícies articulares, permitindo o movimento quase sem fricção e minimizando a pressão no osso subcondral subjacente (Bhosale e Richardson, 2008). Os condrócitos são as células ativas na CA, sendo responsáveis pela secreção da MEC do tecido que contém uma rede de colágeno (predominantemente, tipo II) e proteínas não colágenas em uma substância viscosa semelhante à água (Lafont, 2010; Poole et al., 2001). A MEC também é composta de grandes proteoglicanos com a proteína central, agrecana, predominando (Fox et al., 2009). A cartilagem articular é avascular e, portanto, a carga intermitente é importante para alterar a pressão hidrostática intra-articular e facilitar a difusão de oxigênio e nutrientes do líquido sinovial para a CA (Bhosale e Richardson, 2008; Carter et al., 1987; Fermor et al., 2007; Vanwanseele et al., 2002b), mantendo assim a saúde dos condrócitos e a morfologia e a função da CA (Milner et al., 2012; Vanwanseele et al., 2002b).

A imobilização da articulação periférica pode resultar em mudanças no tamanho, no formato e na atividade metabólica dos condrócitos (Palmoski e Brandt, 1981; Roy, 1970). Um ambiente hipóxico pode resultar da imobilização e, por sua vez, diminuir a difusão de oxigênio do líquido sinovial (Sakamoto et al., 2009). Ambientes hipóxicos resultantes de imobilização apresentaram aumento da expressão de fator de crescimento endotelial vascular (VEGF) dentro da CA, o que pode levar à angiogênese e ao crescimento vascular para dentro do osso subcondral (Garcia-Ramirez et al., 2000; Sakamoto et al., 2009). A imobilização articular também pode desencadear apoptose de condrócitos (Mutsuzaki et al., 2017), uma quantidade reduzida de condrócitos na CA (Hagiwara et al., 2009; Iqbal et al., 2012; Palmoski e Brandt, 1981) e uma redução na concentração de proteoglicanos (Jortikka et al., 1997). As respostas celulares ao desuso e à imobilização podem ser diferentes nas zonas de CA, com as zonas profundas e calcificadas sendo menos afetadas do que a zona superficial (Sood, 1971). Uma diminuição ou ausência de mudanças intermitentes de pressão hidrostática devido ao desuso ou à imobilização está associada ao avanço da frente de ossificação para as zonas da CA (Carter et al., 1987). O afinamento da CA consistente com o da osteoartrite (OA) primária pode ser observado após a imobilização da articulação (Nomura et al., 2017; Vanwanseele et al., 2002b). Além dos efeitos locais da imobilização articular na CA, o desuso de uma parte do corpo devido a lesões em outras partes do corpo pode afetar a CA. A descarga parcial de peso devido à fratura do tornozelo pode induzir uma redução na espessura da CA em todos os compartimentos da articulação do joelho (Hinterwimmer et al., 2004). Foi relatado que a paralisia devido a lesão da medula espinal demonstra afinamento da CA nas articulações patelofemoral e tibiofemoral (Vanwanseele et al., 2002a).

Os efeitos totais do desuso, da imobilização e do ABC na CA não são bem compreendidos atualmente. A remoção da carga intermitente parece ter um impacto negativo no funcionamento fisiológico da CA (Carter et al., 1987; Milner et al., 2012; Smith et al., 1992; Vanwanseele et al., 2002b). Uma consideração importante para a prática clínica pode ser que as mudanças observadas na CA após períodos de desuso podem prejudicar a capacidade futura do tecido de tolerar a carga, tornando-o mais propenso à "sobrecarga" e, consequentemente, a uma resposta anormal ao estresse e às novas lesões após um retorno para a AF.

Ligamento

Ligamentos são faixas de tecido colagenoso que cruzam as articulações, fixando-se diretamente na região periarticular dos ossos que formam a articulação (Frank, 2004). As funções mecânicas dos ligamentos incluem aumentar a estabilidade mecânica da articulação, orientar o movimento articular e restringir o movimento articular excessivo (Bray et al., 2005). Os fibroblastos são as células predominantes encontradas no tecido ligamentar, sintetizando a MEC que inclui colágeno (predominantemente, tipo I), proteoglicanos, elastina e outras proteínas e glicoproteínas, incluindo lectina e laminina (Frank, 2004). A proliferação e a ativação de fibroblastos ocorrem especificamente em resposta às cargas de tração controladas (Gehlsen et al., 1999; Neidlinger-Wilke et al., 2001); então, os fibroblastos ativados se alinham para depositar o colágeno ao longo das linhas de tensão de tração (Eastwood et al., 1998; Mudera et al., 2000; Neidlinger-Wilke et al., 2001).

Foi relatado que a imobilização resulta na ruptura da fixação normal dos ligamentos ao osso, com aumento do local de fixação e de atividade osteoclástica periarticular e de reabsorção óssea (Klein et al., 1982; Noyes, 1977; Woo et al., 1987). Dentro dos ligamentos, a imobilização pode resultar em mudanças na quantidade, no tamanho e na forma dos fibroblastos (Chen et al., 2007; Kanda et al., 1998; Newton et al., 1995; Newton et al., 1990). As mudanças na atividade da enzima ligamentar em favor da degradação do colágeno são evidentes após a imobilização da articulação (Gamble et al., 1984). A renovação ligamentar é representada pela taxa e pelo equilíbrio entre a síntese e a degradação do colágeno, ambas alteradas após a imobilização (Amiel et al., 1982; 1983; Harwood e Amiel, 1992). Posteriormente, a composição e a estrutura do ligamento podem se alterar, com uma mudança de fibrilas de colágeno de menor para maior diâmetro sendo observada (Binkley e Peat, 1986), juntamente com padrões e alinhamento de fibras de colágeno irregulares (Chen et al., 2007). Mudanças na taxa de renovação do colágeno não parecem estar associadas a uma mudança na massa de colágeno total, embora haja uma mudança em direção a um colágeno mais imaturo e a uma densidade reduzida de fibrilas de colágeno (Amiel et al., 1982; Binkley e Peat, 1986).

As respostas celulares à imobilização estão consistentemente associadas às mudanças nas propriedades mecânicas do tecido ligamentar (Amiel et al., 1982; Newton et al., 1990; 1995; Noyes, 1977). Reduções nas cargas de tração habituais ou completas do ligamento resultam consistentemente em adaptações negativas nas características mecânicas do ligamento e da articulação (Amiel et al., 1982; Larsen et al., 1987; Newton et al., 1995; Noyes, 1977). Foi relatado que a imobilização resulta em uma diminuição na rigidez do ligamento (Amiel et al., 1982; Larsen et al., 1987; Woo et al., 1987), o que significa que uma maior tensão ou deformação do tecido ligamentar é observada após a aplicação de uma carga fixa. Períodos de desuso ou imobilização também podem resultar em uma redução na resistência final dos ligamentos (Binkley e Peat, 1986; Larsen et al., 1987; Noyes, 1977; Woo et al., 1987), o que significa que a falha do tecido pode ocorrer quando níveis mais baixos de carga externa são experimentados. Uma variedade de resultados de pesquisas relata que os períodos de imobilização levam a alterações negativas na fisiologia do ligamento e no comportamento mecânico. Após períodos de desuso e imobilização, uma consideração cuidadosa deve ser dada sobre as propriedades mecânicas inferiores dos ligamentos e sobre como isso pode impactar as intervenções clínicas direcionadas a um retorno seguro e eficaz à AF, o que demonstra ainda a necessidade de um retorno gradual e progressivo aos treinos.

Cápsula articular

As cápsulas articulares são protuberâncias de tecido conjuntivo que envolvem as articulações sinoviais, fixando-se adjacentes às margens das superfícies articulares por meio de zonas de fixação fibrocartilaginosas (Neumann, 2002; Ralphs e Benjamin, 1994). A cápsula articular é composta de duas camadas histologicamente distintas de tecido: uma camada fibrosa superficial densa ("cápsula") e uma camada membranosa profunda relativamente fina ("sinóvia") (Neumann, 2002; Ralphs e Benjamin, 1994). As funções mecânicas da cápsula incluem aumentar a estabilidade da articulação mecânica e conter o conteúdo do espaço articular (Neumann, 2002; Ralphs e Benjamin, 1994). A sinóvia é uma membrana fina que tem função mecânica desprezível na estabilidade articular, mas fornece uma barreira estéril contra o espaço extrassinovial e secreta fluido sinovial para lubrificar e nutrir o ambiente intrassinovial (Neumann, 2002; Ralphs e Benjamin, 1994; Simkin, 1991). Quanto aos ligamentos, os fibroblastos são as células predominantes encontradas no tecido capsular, sintetizando a MEC que inclui, majoritariamente, colágeno tipo I, embora colágeno tipos II e III também possam ser evidentes (Amiel et al., 1980; Gay et al., 1980; Matsumoto et al., 2002; Ralphs e Benjamin, 1994). A cápsula é composta de fibras de colágeno irregularmente organizadas, com espessamentos ou expansões específicas evidentes em torno de algumas articulações que funcionam como "ligamentos capsulares" (Neumann, 2002; Ralphs e Benjamin, 1994). A sinóvia contém dois tipos de células predominantes: sinoviócitos tipo A e tipo B (Ando et al., 2010). Por natureza, os sinoviócitos do tipo A são semelhantes aos macrófagos, enquanto os sinoviócitos do tipo B apresentam características semelhantes às dos fibroblastos (Ando et al., 2010). Os sinoviócitos do tipo A estão localizados, principalmente, na camada superficial da sinóvia, enquanto os sinoviócitos do tipo B são encontrados predominantemente na camada profunda da membrana sinovial, produzindo ácido hialurônico e fibras de colágeno (Ando et al., 2010). As fibras de colágeno na sinóvia são tipicamente dos tipos I, III, IV e V (Gay et al., 1980; Ralphs e Benjamin, 1994). Cargas de tração são importantes para estimular a atividade adequada de fibroblastos e a síntese de colágeno ao longo das linhas de estresse mecânico (Eastwood et al., 1998; Gehlsen et al., 1999; Mudera et al., 2000; Neidlinger-Wilke et al., 2001), enquanto o movimento articular fisiológico normal é crítico para garantir a homeostase celular e a saúde capsular (Kaneguchi et al., 2017; Lee et al., 2010; Yabe et al., 2013).

Os períodos de imobilização parecem estar associados a uma diminuição progressiva da densidade celular ao longo do tempo, tanto na cápsula quanto na sinóvia (Lee et al., 2010). A imobilização da articulação periférica demonstrou uma diminuição na densidade dos vasos sanguíneos capsulares, hipoxia progressiva e um aumento da presença de mediadores inflamatórios (Kaneguchi et al., 2017; Yabe et al., 2013). Em alguns trabalhos de pesquisa, proliferação de fibroblastos e aumento da síntese de colágeno foram observados (Kaneguchi et al., 2017), com outros trabalhos relatando aumento da desorganização das fibrilas de colágeno capsular, aumento relativo no colágeno tipo I e diminuição no colágeno tipo III após desuso e imobilização (Lee et al., 2010; Matsumoto et al., 2002; Yabe et al., 2013). As adesões entre as vilosidades sinoviais e o encurtamento resultante da sinóvia podem ocorrer após a imobilização (Trudel et al., 2000). Depois da imobilização da articulação periférica, a adesão da sinóvia à CA também foi relatada (Ando et al., 2010; Evans et al., 1960), assim como a proliferação de tecido intra-articular fibrogorduroso que demonstra infiltração subsequente do espaço articular (Schollmeier et al., 1994).

Quanto aos ligamentos, as respostas celulares e as adaptações do tecido à imobilização estão consistentemente associadas às mudanças no comportamento mecânico do tecido capsular e das articulações (Ando et al., 2012; Lee et al., 2010; Trudel et al., 2000; 2014). Hipomobilidade articular devido ao enrijecimento capsular ou à contratura é uma observação consistente após desuso e imobilização: quanto maior a duração do desuso e da imobilização, com menos frequência a mobilidade articular original é recuperada (Ando et al., 2012; Lee et al., 2010; Trudel et al., 2000; 2014). A localização das aderências e do enrijecimento capsular está associada à direção da restrição da mobilidade articular (Ando et al., 2010; Lobenhoffer et al., 1996; Mariani et al., 1997). Quanto aos ligamentos, uma série de resultados de pesquisas relatam que períodos de desuso e imobilização levam a alterações negativas da fisiologia capsular e do comportamento mecânico. Para cápsulas articulares, a principal preocupação clínica é como limitar o enrijecimento capsular e a contratura em situações de desuso e imobilização, podendo influenciar diretamente na amplitude de movimento (ADM) total.

Músculo esquelético

O tecido mais abundante no corpo humano é o músculo esquelético (Neumann, 2002). O músculo esquelético funciona para estabilizar e mover ossos, proteger os tecidos não contráteis de forças excessivas, absorver choques e gerar calor (termorregulação secundária) (Clark e Lephart, 2015; MacIntosh et al., 2006; Neumann, 2002). Os músculos estriados esqueléticos podem ser encontrados em muitas formas e tamanhos diferentes, sendo as células principais de um único músculo as próprias fibras musculares e as células-satélite circundantes (MacIntosh et al., 2006). O tecido conjuntivo (MEC) do músculo esquelético é identificado como epimísio, perimísio e endomísio, todos compostos, principalmente, de colágeno (tipos I-V), com alguma elastina também presente (MacIntosh et al., 2006). Uma fibra muscular é composta de muitas miofibrilas, cada miofibrila contendo proteínas contráteis (actina, miosina) e proteínas estabilizadoras (titina, nebulina) (MacIntosh et al., 2006). A estimulação das fibras musculares pelo sistema nervoso inicia o ciclo da ponte cruzada actina-miosina e a geração de força; a força é, em última análise, transmitida por meio das proteínas estabilizadoras e do tecido conjuntivo do músculo aos tendões do músculo e aos ossos nos quais os tendões se fixam (MacIntosh et al., 2006). A estimulação repetida das fibras musculares e das células-satélite é importante para manter a saúde das fibras musculares e a capacidade de geração de força (MacIntosh et al., 2006).

Após a lesão da articulação periférica e o desuso resultante, a área da seção transversal (AST) das fibras musculares individuais pode reduzir, o fenótipo das fibras musculares pode mudar, a quantidade de células-satélite pode diminuir e a quantidade de fibroblastos musculares pode aumentar (Fry et al., 2014; 2017; Noehren et al., 2016). Como a quantidade de células-satélite pode diminuir e a quantidade de fibroblastos musculares pode aumentar após o desuso do membro, uma expansão da MEC pode ocorrer dentro do músculo esquelético com desuso pós-lesão (Fry et al., 2014; 2017; Noehren et al., 2016); isso significa que há uma diminuição relativa no espaço disponível para a ocupação dos elementos contráteis do músculo esquelético em regeneração. Assim como as alterações do tecido intramuscular, o espaço intermuscular se enche com tecido adiposo com desuso e imobilização do membro (Clark, 2009). Como a AST das fibras musculares individuais reduz com o desuso pós-lesão, a AST de um músculo inteiro também pode ser vista com uma redução significativa na forma de atrofia muscular (Norte et al., 2019; Perry et al., 2015; Stevens et al., 2006). Com a imobilização

do membro, perdas significativas de AST e volume do músculo esquelético podem ser aparentes apenas após 5 dias (Wall et al., 2014). A taxa e a magnitude da atrofia muscular são maiores nos músculos antigravitacionais dos membros inferiores e da coluna lombar quando comparados aos músculos dos membros superiores (Clark, 2009).

Mudanças fisiológicas e estruturais ocorrem rapidamente no músculo esquelético após desuso ou imobilização. As alterações estruturais do músculo esquelético ocorrem de tal forma que há proliferação do tecido conjuntivo e atrofia do tecido contrátil, sendo a coluna lombar e os músculos esqueléticos dos membros inferiores os mais acometidos. Após o desuso ou a imobilização por lesões esportivas de tecidos não contráteis, é necessária uma consideração cuidadosa sobre como minimizar os períodos de desuso ou imobilização de partes do corpo e garantir a ativação frequente e intermitente das fibras musculares esqueléticas.

Sistema cardiorrespiratório

O sistema cardiorrespiratório contribui para o transporte de oxigênio, nutrientes e hormônios pelo corpo e para a remoção de subprodutos metabólicos (Wilmore et al., 2015). As adaptações cardiorrespiratórias ao exercício estão bem estabelecidas, levando a melhorias na integração de vários mecanismos centrais e periféricos de transporte de oxigênio (Wilmore et al., 2015). Em contraste, a remoção do estímulo de treinamento leva a uma reversão dessas adaptações, cuja extensão depende da extensão e duração do desuso, da imobilização e da redução da AF geral (Convertino, 1997). Os efeitos da redução da AF na principal medida de aptidão aeróbica, chamada de consumo máximo de oxigênio ($\dot{V}O_{2máx}$), são relatados como dependentes da duração da imobilização e do estado de treinamento do indivíduo. Em uma meta-análise recente, Ried-Larsen et al. (2017) relataram que o $\dot{V}O_{2máx}$ diminuiu linearmente durante o repouso no leito a uma taxa média de 0,43% ao dia quando expresso em relação à massa corporal. Além disso, a taxa de declínio no $\dot{V}O_{2máx}$ foi inversamente relacionada com o *status* de treinamento, de forma que indivíduos bem treinados experimentaram as taxas de declínio mais rápidas (Ried-Larsen et al., 2017). Os principais motivos para o declínio inicial (nas primeiras 2 semanas) no $\dot{V}O_{2máx}$ são em grande parte devido às mudanças nos mecanismos centrais de transporte de oxigênio resultantes de reduções no volume sanguíneo (hipovolemia) e de débito cardíaco (Ade et al., 2015; Convertino, 1997; 2007). No caso do primeiro, a redução da carga está associada a um aumento na excreção renal de sódio, levando a um aumento da diurese e uma redução concomitante da pressão venosa central (Convertino, 2007). De fato, o repouso na cama mostrou induzir uma redução de 10 a 30% no volume sanguíneo, a maioria das quais ocorre nas primeiras 72 horas (Convertino, 1997; 2007). Embora a diminuição do volume sanguíneo seja responsável pela maior parte do declínio do débito cardíaco, a inatividade também resulta em redução (aproximadamente, 1% por semana) na massa cardíaca; apesar de não, na maioria dos casos, a um ponto em que pareça ter qualquer influência mensurável na contratilidade miocárdica (Ade et al., 2015). Embora as adaptações centrais à AF reduzida sejam dominantes nos estágios iniciais do processo, as limitações periféricas ao $\dot{V}O_{2máx}$ elevam com o aumento da duração da inatividade; sendo responsável por aproximadamente 27% do declínio após 42 dias e 40% do declínio após 90 dias (Ade et al., 2015). Os principais motivos para as alterações periféricas no $\dot{V}O_{2máx}$ são uma diminuição no metabolismo oxidativo intracelular, devido à redução no conteúdo mitocondrial e na atividade enzimática oxidativa (Mujika e Padilla, 2001; Ringholm et al., 2011), e uma redução no volume capilar levando a um declínio no fornecimento de oxigênio periférico e uma capacidade de difusão de oxigênio reduzida (Ade et al., 2015). Essas mudanças são concomitantes com uma redução nas isoformas das fibras musculares de contração lenta e são relatadas como levando a um aumento da dependência da energia do metabolismo de carboidratos (Mujika e Padilla, 2001).

Após o desuso e a imobilização, a função cardiorrespiratória está claramente comprometida em relação aos níveis pré-lesão por causa do uso reduzido do sistema músculo-esquelético (Convertino, 2007; Frangolias et al., 1997; Widman et al., 2007). A consideração clínica é sobre como a função do sistema cardiorrespiratório pode ser otimizada durante o processo de reabilitação e quando o volume de treinamento direcionado especificamente para melhorar o desempenho cardiorrespiratório pode ser aumentado com segurança após um período inicial de reabilitação de lesões.

Resumo

As lesões traumáticas das articulações periféricas são consistentemente o tipo de lesão mais frequente em vários esportes. Os danos aos tecidos e as deficiências pós-lesão que seguem as lesões traumáticas das articulações periféricas, frequentemente, resultam em limitações de AF e restrições temporárias à participação em esportes. As limitações de AF que se manifestam como resultado de lesões esportivas são parte de um "espectro de desuso" (ver Figura 3.1).

Ossos, CA, ligamentos, cápsulas articulares e músculos esqueléticos são todos tecidos complexos com componentes celulares, MEC e fluidos. O movimento frequente e intermitente e a carga dos tecidos são importantes para nutrir uma boa fisiologia e mecânica dos tecidos. O desuso e a imobilização de partes do corpo demonstram consistentemente alterações negativas na fisiologia dos ossos, das CA, das cápsulas articulares e dos músculos esqueléticos; as alterações na fisiologia, então, parecem afetar de forma consistente e negativa a mecânica e a função dos tecidos. As alterações na fisiologia e na mecânica do tecido podem ser evidentes tanto no local quanto distantes da lesão primária (Figura 3.2). A função cardiorrespiratória e a aptidão

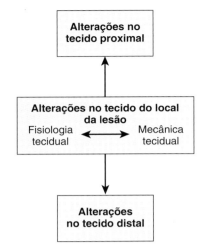

Figura 3.2 Localizações de potenciais alterações nos tecidos após o desuso.

aeróbica também são alteradas negativamente como resultado do desuso e da imobilização de partes do corpo. Embora o desuso e a imobilização alterem negativamente a fisiologia e a função do tecido muscular e esquelético, bem como a fisiologia e a função do sistema cardiorrespiratório, as intervenções subsequentes de exercícios foram relatadas como potencialmente capazes de mitigar as alterações fisiológicas e mecânicas negativas nos tecidos decorrentes do desuso (Bloomfield, 1997; Convertino, 1997; Iqbal et al., 2012; Kaneguchi et al., 2017; Noyes, 1977; Perry et al., 2015; Vanwanseele et al., 2002b; Woo et al., 1987). Os profissionais da saúde devem, portanto, considerar os efeitos locais e periféricos do desuso de parte do corpo, da imobilização e do ABC após uma lesão primária, além de quais intervenções são mais adequadas para alterar positivamente a fisiologia de um determinado tecido e sua função mecânica dentro de um processo de reabilitação clinicamente fundamentado.

Referências bibliográficas

Aarnio, M., Appel, L., Fredrikson, M., Gordh, T., Wolf, O., Sörensen, J., et al., 2017. Visualization of painful inflammation in patients with pain after traumatic ankle sprain using [11C]-D-deprenyl PET/CT. Scandinavian Journal of Pain 17, 418-424.

Ade, C.J., Broxterman, R.M., Barstow, T.J., 2015. $\dot{V}O_{2max}$ and microgravity exposure: convective versus diffusive O_2 transport. Medicine and Science in Sports and Exercise 47 (7), 1351-1361.

Alaia, M.J., Khatib, O., Shah, M., Bosco, J.A., Jazrawi, L.M., Strauss, E.J., et al., 2015. The utility of plain radiographs in the initial evaluation of knee pain amongst sports medicine patients. Knee Surgery, Sports Traumatology, Arthroscopy 23 (8), 2213-2217.

Amiel, D., Akeson, W., Harwood, F., Mechanic, G., 1980. The effect of immobilization on the types of collagen synthesized in periarticular connective tissue. Connective Tissue Research 8 (1), 27-32.

Amiel, D., Akeson, W.H., Harwood, F.L., Frank, C.B., 1983. Stress deprivation effect on metabolic turnover of the medial collateral ligament collagen. A comparison between nine-and 12-week immobilization. Clinical Orthopaedics and Related Research (172), 265-270.

Amiel, D., Woo, S.L., Harwood, F.L., Akeson, W.H., 1982. The effect of immobilization on collagen turnover in connective tissue: a biochemical–biomechanical correlation. Acta Orthopaedica Scandinavica 53 (3), 325-332.

Ando, A., Hagiwara, Y., Onoda, Y., Hatori, K., Suda, H., Chimoto, E., et al., 2010. Distribution of type A and B synoviocytes in the adhesive and shortened synovial membrane during immobilization of the knee joint in rats. The Tohoku Journal of Experimental Medicine 221 (2), 161-168.

Ando, A., Suda, H., Hagiwara, Y., Onoda, Y., Chimoto, E., Itoi, E., et al., 2012. Remobilization does not restore immobilization-induced adhesion of capsule and restricted joint motion in rat knee joints. The Tohoku Journal of Experimental Medicine 227 (1), 13-22.

Atef, A., EL-Tantawy, A., Gad, H., Hefeda, M., 2016. Prevalence of associated injuries after anterior shoulder dislocation: a prospective study. International Orthopaedics 40 (3), 519-524.

Bach-Gansmo, F.L., Wittig, N.K., Brüel, A., Thomsen, J.S., Birkedal, H., 2016. Immobilization and long-term recovery results in large changes in bone structure and strength but no corresponding alterations of osteocyte lacunar properties. Bone 91, 139-147.

Bhosale, A.M., Richardson, J.B., 2008. Articular cartilage: structure, injuries and review of management. British Medical Bulletin 87, 77-95.

Binkley, J.M., Peat, M., 1986. The effects of immobilization on the ultrastructure and mechanical properties of the medial collateral ligament of rats. Clinical Orthopaedics and Related Research 203, 301-308.

Bloomfield, S., 1997. Changes in musculoskeletal structure and function with prolonged bed rest. Medicine and Science in Sports and Exercise 29 (2), 197-206.

Bonewald, L.F., 2006. Mechanosensation and transduction in osteocytes. Bonekey Osteovision 3 (10), 7-15.

Boyce, S., Quigley, M., 2004. Review of sports injuries presenting to an accident and emergency department. Emergency Medicine Journal 21 (6), 704-706.

Bray, R.C., Salo, P.T., Lo, I.K., Ackermann, P., Rattner, J., Hart, D.A., et al., 2005. Normal ligament structure, physiology and function. Sports Medicine and Arthroscopy Review 13 (3), 127-135.

Carter, D., Orr, T., Fyhrie, D., Schurman, D., 1987. Influences of mechanical stress on prenatal and postnatal skeletal development. Clinical Orthopaedics and Related Research 219, 237-250.

Ceroni, D., Martin, X., Delhumeau, C., Rizzoli, R., Kaelin, A., Farpour-Lambert, N., et al., 2012. Effects of cast-mediated immobilization on bone mineral mass at various sites in adolescents with lower-extremity fracture. Journal of Bone and Joint Surgery America 94 (3), 208-216.

Chen, C.-H., Liu, X., Yeh, M.-L., Huang, M.-H., Zhai, Q., Lowe, W.R., et al., 2007. Pathological changes of human ligament after complete mechanical unloading. American Journal of Physical Medicine and Rehabilitation 86 (4), 282-289.

Clark, B.C., 2009. In vivo alterations in skeletal muscle form and function after disuse atrophy. Medicine and Science in Sports and Exercise 41 (10), 1869-1875.

Clark, N., Lephart, S., 2015. Management of the sensorimotor system: the lower limb. In: Jull, G., Moore, A., Falla, D., Lewis, J., McCarthy, C., Sterling, M. (Eds.), Grieve's Modern Musculoskeletal Physiotherapy. Elsevier, Edinburgh.

Clark, N.C., 2008. Strength training programme design in physiotherapy practice: what you need to know. Association of Chartered Physiotherapists in Exercise Therapy (ACPET) Study Day. University of Hertfordshire.

Clark, N.C., 2015. (vii) The role of physiotherapy in rehabilitation of soft tissue injuries of the knee. Orthopaedics and Trauma 29 (1), 48-56.

Convertino, V., 1997. Cardiovascular consequences of bed rest: effect on maximal oxygen uptake. Medicine and Science in Sports and Exercise 29 (2), 191-196.

Convertino, V.A., 2007. Blood volume response to physical activity and inactivity. The American Journal of the Medical Sciences 334 (1), 72-79.

Crockett, J.C., Rogers, M.J., Coxon, F.P., Hocking, L.J., Helfrich, M.H., 2011. Bone remodelling at a glance. Journal of Cell Science 124 (Pt 7), 991-998.

Drolet, B.C., Lorenzi, N.M., 2011. Translational research: understanding the continuum from bench to bedside. Translational Research 157 (1), 1-5.

Eastwood, M., Mudera, V., McGrouther, D., Brown, R., 1998. Effect of precise mechanical loading on fibroblast populated collagen lattices: morphological changes. Cell Motility and the Cytoskeleton 40 (1), 13-21.

Ehrlich, P., Lanyon, L., 2002. Mechanical strain and bone cell function: a review. Osteoporosis International 13 (9), 688-700.

Ejerhed, L., Kartus, J., Nilsén, R., Nilsson, U., Kullenberg, R., Karlsson, J., et al., 2004. The effect of anterior cruciate ligament surgery on bone mineral in the calcaneus: a prospective study with a 2-year follow-up evaluation. Arthroscopy 20 (4), 352-359.

Elefteriou, F., Campbell, P., Ma, Y., 2014. Control of bone remodeling by the peripheral sympathetic nervous system. Calcified Tissue International 94 (1), 140-151.

Elias, I., Zoga, A.C., Schweitzer, M.E., Ballehr, L., Morrison, W.B., Raikin, S.M., et al., 2007. A specific bone marrow edema around the foot and ankle following trauma and immobilization therapy: pattern description and potential clinical relevance. Foot and Ankle International 28 (4), 463-471.

Evans, E.B., Eggers, G., Butler, J.K., Blumel, J., 1960. Experimental immobilization and remobilization of rat knee joints. Journal of Bone and Joint Surgery America 42 (5), 737-758.

Feng, X., McDonald, J.M., 2011. Disorders of bone remodeling. Annual Review of Pathology: Mechanisms of Disease 6, 121-145.

Fermor, B., Christensen, S., Youn, I., Cernanec, J., Davies, C., Weinberg, J., et al., 2007. Oxygen, nitric oxide and articular cartilage. European Cells and Materials 13, 56-65.

Fiore, C., Pennisi, P., Ciffo, F., Scebba, C., Amico, A., Di Fazzio, S., et al., 1999. Immobilization-dependent bone collagen breakdown appears to increase with time: evidence for a lack of a new bone equilibrium in response to reduced load during prolonged bed rest. Hormone and Metabolic Research 31 (1), 31-36.

Fox, A., Bedi, A., Rodeo, S., 2009. The basic science of articular cartilage: structure, composition, and function. Sports Health 1 (6), 461-468.

Frangolias, D., Taunton, J., Rhodes, E., McConkey, J., Moon, M., 1997. Maintenance of aerobic capacity during recovery from right foot Jones fracture: a case report. Clinical Journal of Sport Medicine 7 (1), 54-57.

Frank, C., 2004. Ligament structure, physiology and function. Journal of Musculoskeletal and Neuronal Interactions 4 (2), 199-201.

Fry, C.S., Johnson, D.L., Ireland, M.L., Noehren, B., 2017. Acl injury reduces satellite cell abundance and promotes fibrogenic cell expansion within skeletal muscle. Journal of Orthopaedic Research 35 (9), 1876-1885.

Fry, C.S., Lee, J.D., Jackson, J.R., Kirby, T.J., Stasko, S.A., Liu, H., et al., 2014. Regulation of the muscle fiber microenvironment by activated satellite cells during hypertrophy. The Faseb Journal 28 (4), 1654-1665.

Gamble, J., Edwards, C., Max, S., 1984. Enzymatic adaptation in ligaments during immobilization. American Journal of Sports Medicine 12 (3), 221-228.

Garcia-Ramirez, M., Toran, N., Andaluz, P., Carrascosa, A., Audi, L., 2000. Vascular endothelial growth factor is expressed in human fetal growth cartilage. Journal of Bone and Mineral Research 15 (3), 534-540.

Gay, S., Gay, R.E., Miller, E.J., 1980. The collagens of the joint. Arthritis and Rheumatism 23 (8), 937-941.

Gehlsen, G.M., Ganion, L.R., Helfst, R., 1999. Fibroblast responses to variation in soft tissue mobilization pressure. Medicine and Science in Sports and Exercise 31 (4), 531-535.

Guo, X., Kim, C., 2002. Mechanical consequence of trabecular bone loss and its treatment: a three-dimensional model simulation. Bone 30 (2), 404-411.

Hagiwara, Y., Ando, A., Chimoto, E., Saijo, Y., Ohmori-Matsuda, K., Itoi, E., et al., 2009. Changes of articular cartilage after immobilization in a rat knee contracture model. Journal of Orthopaedic Research 27 (2), 236-242.

Harada, S.-I., Rodan, G.A., 2003. Control of osteoblast function and regulation of bone mass. Nature 423 (6937), 349-355.

Harwood, F., Amiel, D., 1992. Differential metabolic responses of periarticular ligaments and tendon to joint immobilization. Journal of Applied Physiology 72 (5), 1687-1691.

Hawker, G.A., Croxford, R., Bierman, A.S., Harvey, P.J., Ravi, B., Stanaitis, I., et al., 2014. All-cause mortality and serious cardiovascular events in people with hip and knee osteoarthritis: a population based cohort study. Plos One 9 (3), e91286.

Hinterwimmer, S., Krammer, M., Krötz, M., Glaser, C., Baumgart, R., Reiser, M., et al., 2004. Cartilage atrophy in the knees of patients after seven weeks of partial load bearing. Arthritis and Rheumatism 50 (8), 2516-2520.

Hohmann, E., Bryant, A., Tetsworth, K., 2016. Strength does not influence knee function in the ACL-deficient knee but is a correlate of knee function in the and ACL-reconstructed knee. Archives of Orthopaedic and Trauma Surgery 136 (4), 477-483.

Hootman, J.M., Dick, R., Agel, J., 2007. Epidemiology of collegiate injuries for 15 sports: summary and recommendations for injury prevention initiatives. Journal of Athletic Training 42 (2), 311-319.

Huang, S., Wikswo, J., 2006. Dimensions of systems biology. Reviews of Physiology, Biochemistry and Pharmacology 157, 81-104.

Iqbal, K., Khan, M., Minhas, L., 2012. Effects of immobilisation and remobilisation on superficial zone of articular cartilage of patella in rats. Journal of the Pakistan Medical Association 62 (6), 531-535.

Jortikka, M.O., Inkinen, R.I., Tammi, M.I., Parkkinen, J.J., Haapala, J., Kiviranta, I., et al., 1997. Immobilisation causes longlasting matrix changes both in the immobilised and contralateral joint cartilage. Annals of the Rheumatic Diseases 56 (4), 255-261.

Kanda, T., Ochi, M., Ikuta, Y., 1998. Adverse effects on rabbit anterior cruciate ligament after knee immobilization: changes in permeability of horseradish peroxidase. Archives of Orthopaedic and Trauma Surgery 117 (6-7), 307-311.

Kaneguchi, A., Ozawa, J., Kawamata, S., Yamaoka, K., 2017. Development of arthrogenic joint contracture as a result of pathological changes in remobilized rat knees. Journal of Orthopaedic Research 35 (7), 1414-1423.

Klein, L., Player, J., Heiple, K., Bahniuk, E., Goldberg, V., 1982. Isotopic evidence for resorption of soft tissues and bone in immobilized dogs. Journal of Bone and Joint Surgery America 64 (2), 225-230.

Lafont, J.E., 2010. Lack of oxygen in articular cartilage: consequences for chondrocyte biology. International Journal of Experimental Pathology 91 (2), 99-106.

Larsen, N.P., Forwood, M.R., Parker, A.W., 1987. Immobilization and retraining of cruciate ligaments in the rat. Acta Orthopaedica Scandinavica 58 (3), 260-264.

Lee, S., Sakurai, T., Ohsako, M., Saura, R., Hatta, H., Atomi, Y., et al., 2010. Tissue stiffness induced by prolonged immobilization of the rat knee joint and relevance of AGEs (pentosidine). Connective Tissue Research 51 (6), 467-477.

Lepola, V., Väänänen, K., Jalovaara, P., 1993. The effect of immobilization on the torsional strength of the rat tibia. Clinical Orthopaedics and Related Research (297), 55-61.

Leppälä, J., Kannus, P., Natri, A., Pasanen, M., Sievänen, H., Vuori, I., et al., 1999. Effect of anterior cruciate ligament injury of the knee on bone mineral density of the spine and affected lower extremity: a prospective one-year follow-up study. Calcified Tissue International 64 (4), 357-363.

Liedert, A., Kaspar, D., Blakytny, R., Claes, L., Ignatius, A., 2006. Signal transduction pathways involved in mechanotransduction in bone cells. Biochemical and Biophysical Research Communications 349 (1), 1-5.

Lobenhoffer, H., Bosch, U., Gerich, T., 1996. Role of posterior capsulotomy for the treatment of extension deficits of the knee. Knee Surgery, Sports Traumatology, Arthroscopy 4 (4), 237-241.

Luhmann, S., 2003. Acute traumatic knee effusions in children and adolescents. Journal of Pediatric Orthopedics 23 (2), 199-202.

Mabry, P.L., Olster, D.H., Morgan, G.D., Abrams, D.B., 2008. Interdisciplinarity and systems science to improve population health: a view from the nih office of behavioral and social sciences research. American Journal of Preventive Medicine 35 (Suppl. 2), S211-S224.

MacIntosh, B., Gardiner, P., McComas, A., 2006. Skeletal Muscle. Form and Function, second ed. Human Kinetics, Illinois.

Maglio, P.P., Mabry, P.L., 2011. Agent-based models and systems science approaches to public health. American Journal of Preventive Medicine 40 (3), 392-394.

Man, I., Morrissey, M., Cywinski, J., 2007. Effect of neuromuscular electrical stimulation on ankle swelling in the early period after ankle sprain. Physical Therapy 87 (1), 53-65.

Mariani, P.P., Santori, N., Rovere, P., Della Rocca, C., Adriani, E., 1997. Histological and structural study of the adhesive tissue in knee fibroarthrosis: a clinical–pathological correlation. Arthroscopy 13 (3), 313-318.

Matsumoto, F., Trudel, G., Uhthoff, H.K., 2002. High collagen type I and low collagen type Iii levels in knee joint contracture. Acta Orthopaedica Scandinavica 73 (3), 335-343.

Milner, P., Wilkins, R., Gibson, J., 2012. Cellular physiology of articular cartilage in health and disease. In: Rothschild, B. (Ed.), Principles of Osteoarthritis – Its Definition, Character, Derivation, and Modality-Related Recognition. InTech, London.

Mosekilde, L., Thomsen, J.S., Mackey, M., Phipps, R.J., 2000. Treatment with risedronate or alendronate prevents hind-limb immobilization-induced loss of bone density and strength in adult female rats. Bone 27 (5), 639-645.

Mudera, V., Pleass, R., Eastwood, M., Tarnuzzer, R., Schultz, G., Khaw, P., et al., 2000. Molecular responses of human dermal fibroblasts to dual cues: contact guidance and mechanical load. Cell Motility and the Cytoskeleton 45 (1), 1-9.

Mujika, I., Padilla, S., 2001. Cardiorespiratory and metabolic characteristics of detraining in humans. Medicine and Science in Sports and Exercise 33, 413-421.

Mutsuzaki, H., Nakajima, H., Wadano, Y., Furuhata, S., Sakane, M., 2017. Influence of knee immobilization on chondrocyte apoptosis and histological features of the anterior cruciate ligament insertion and articular cartilage in rabbits. International Journal of Molecular Sciences 18 (2), 253.

Nardo, L., Sandman, D.N., Virayavanich, W., Zhang, L., Souza, R.B., Steinbach, L., et al., 2013. Bone marrow changes related to disuse. European Radiology 23 (12), 3422-3431.

Neidlinger-Wilke, C., Grood, E., Wang, J.C., Brand, R., Claes, L., 2001. Cell alignment is induced by cyclic changes in cell length: studies of cells grown in cyclically stretched substrates. Journal of Orthopaedic Research 19 (2), 286-293.

Neumann, D., 2002. Kinesiology of the Musculoskeletal System. Mosby, St Louis.

Newton, P., Woo, S.-Y., Kitabayashi, L., Lyon, R., Anderson, D., Akeson, W., et al., 1990. Ultrastructural changes in knee ligaments following immobilization. Matrix 10 (5), 314-319.

Newton, P., Woo, S., MacKenna, D., Akeson, W., 1995. Immobilization of the knee joint alters the mechanical and ultrastructural properties of the rabbit anterior cruciate ligament. Journal of Orthopaedic Research 13 (2), 191-200.

Noehren, B., Andersen, A., Hardy, P., Johnson, D.L., Ireland, M.L., Thompson, K.L., et al., 2016. Cellular and morphological alterations in the vastus lateralis muscle as the result of ACL injury and reconstruction. Journal of Bone and Joint Surgery America 98 (18), 1541-1547.

Nomura, M., Sakitani, N., Iwasawa, H., Kohara, Y., Takano, S., Wakimoto, Y., et al., 2017. Thinning of articular cartilage after joint unloading or immobilization. An experimental investigation of the pathogenesis in mice. Osteoarthritis and Cartilage 25 (5), 727-736.

Norte, G.E., Knaus, K.R., Kuenze, C., Handsfield, G.G., Meyer, C.H., Blemker, S.S., et al., 2018. MRI-based assessment of lower extremity muscle volumes in patients before and after Acl reconstruction. Journal of Sport Rehabilitation 27 (3), 201-212.

Noyes, F.R., 1977. Functional properties of knee ligaments and alterations induced by immobilization: a correlative biomechanical and histological study in primates. Clinical Orthopaedics and Related Research (123), 210-242.

Oftadeh, R., Perez-Viloria, M., Villa-Camacho, J.C., Vaziri, A., Nazarian, A., 2015. Biomechanics and mechanobiology of trabecular bone: a review. Journal of Biomechanical Engineering 137 (1), 0108021-01080215.

Olsson, O., Isacsson, A., Englund, M., Frobell, R., 2016. Epidemiology of intra and peri-articular structural injuries in traumatic knee joint hemarthrosis – data from 1145 consecutive knees with subacute MRI. Osteoarthritis and Cartilage 24 (11), 1890-1897.

Palmoski, M., Brandt, K., 1981. Running inhibits the reversal of atrophic changes in canine knee cartilage after removal of a leg cast. Arthritis and Rheumatism 24 (11), 1329-1337.

Pavalko, F.M., Norvell, S.M., Burr, D.B., Turner, C.H., Duncan, R.L., Bidwell, J.P., et al., 2003. A model for mechanotransduction in bone cells: the load-bearing mechanosomes. Journal of Cellular Biochemistry 88 (1), 104-112.

Peng, Z., Tuukkanen, J., Zhang, H., Jämsä, T., Väänänen, H., 1994. The mechanical strength of bone in different rat models of experimental osteoporosis. Bone 15 (5), 523-532.

Perry, B.D., Levinger, P., Morris, H.G., Petersen, A.C., Garnham, A.P., Levinger, I., et al., 2015. The effects of knee injury on skeletal muscle function, Na$^+$, K$^+$-ATPase content, and isoform abundance. Physiological Reports 3 (2), e12294.

Poole, A., Kojima, T., Yasuda, T., Mwale, F., Kobayashi, M., Laverty, S., et al., 2001. Composition and structure of articular cartilage: a template for tissue repair. Clinical Orthopaedics and Related Research (Suppl. 391), S26-33.

Punt, I., Ziltener, J., Laidet, M., Armand, S., Allet, L., 2015. Gait and physical impairments in patients with acute ankle sprains who did not receive physical therapy. PM R. 7 (1), 34-41.

Ralphs, J., Benjamin, M., 1994. The joint capsule: structure, composition, ageing and disease. Journal of Anatomy 184 (Pt 3), 503-509.

Reiman, M.P., Rogers, M.E., Manske, R.C., 2006. Interlimb differences in lower extremity bone mineral density following anterior cruciate ligament reconstruction. Journal of Orthopaedic and Sports Physical Therapy 36 (11), 837-844.

Ried-Larsen, M., Aarts, H.M., Joyner, M.J., 2017. Effects of strict prolonged bed rest on cardiorespiratory fitness: systematic review and meta-analysis. Journal of Applied Physiology 123 (4), 790-799.

Ringholm, S., Biensø, R.S., Kiilerich, K., Guadalupe-Grau, A., Aachman-n-Andersen, N.J., Saltin, B., et al., 2011. Bed rest reduces metabolic protein content and abolishes exercise-induced mrna responses in human skeletal muscle. American Journal of Physiology-Endocrinology and Metabolism 301 (4), E649-E658.

Roemer, F.W., Jomaah, N., Niu, J., Almusa, E., Roger, B., D'hooghe, P., et al., 2014. Ligamentous injuries and the risk of associated tissue damage in acute ankle sprains in athletes: a cross-sectional MRI study. American Journal of Sports Medicine 42 (7), 1549-1557.

Rosa, N., Simoes, R., Magalhães, F.D., Marques, A.T., 2015. From mechanical stimulus to bone formation: a review. Medical Engineering and Physics 37 (8), 719-728.

Roy, S., 1970. Ultrastructure of articular cartilage in experimental immobilization. Annals of the Rheumatic Diseases 29 (6), 634-642.

Rubio, D.M., Schoenbaum, E.E., Lee, L.S., Schteingart, D.E., Marantz, P.R., Anderson, K.E., et al., 2010. Defining translational research: implications for training. Academic Medicine 85 (3), 470-475.

Sakamoto, J., Origuchi, T., Okita, M., Nakano, J., Kato, K., Yoshimura, T., et al., 2009. Immobilization-induced cartilage degeneration mediated through expression of hypoxia-inducible factor-1alpha, vascular endothelial growth factor, and chondromodulin-I. Connective Tissue Research 50 (1), 37-45.

Schollmeier, G., Uhthoff, H.K., Sarkar, K., Fukuhara, K., 1994. Effects of immobilization on the capsule of the canine glenohumeral joint. A structural functional study. Clinical Orthopaedics and Related Research (304), 37-42.

Simkin, P.A., 1991. Physiology of normal and abnormal synovium. Seminars in Arthritis and Rheumatism 21 (3), 179-183.

Smith, R., Thomas, K., Schurman, D., Carter, D., Wong, M., Van Der Meulen, M., et al., 1992. Rabbit knee immobilization: bone remodeling precedes cartilage degradation. Journal of Orthopaedic Research 10 (1), 88-95.

Sood, S., 1971. A study of the effects of experimental immobilisation on rabbit articular cartilage. Journal of Anatomy 108 (Pt 3), 497-507.

Stevens, J.E., Pathare, N.C., Tillman, S.M., Scarborough, M.T., Gibbs, C.P., Shah, P., et al., 2006. Relative contributions of muscle activation and muscle size to plantarflexor torque during rehabilitation after immobilization. Journal of Orthopaedic Research 24 (8), 1729-1736.

Tirabassi, J., Brou, L., Khodaee, M., Lefort, R., Fields, S., Comstock, R., et al., 2016. Epidemiology of high school sports-related injuries resulting in medical disqualification: 2005–2006 through 2013–2014 academic years. American Journal of Sports Medicine 44 (11), 2925-2932.

Toomey, C., Whittaker, J., Nettel-Aguirre, A., Reimer, R., Woodhouse, L., Ghali, B., et al., 2017. Higher fat mass is associated with a history of knee injury in youth sport. Journal of Orthopaedic and Sports Physical Therapy 47 (2), 80-87.

Trudel, G., Laneuville, O., Coletta, E., Goudreau, L., Uhthoff, H.K., 2014. Quantitative and temporal differential recovery of articular and muscular limitations of knee joint contractures; results in a rat model. Journal of Applied Physiology 117 (7), 730-737.

Trudel, G., Seki, M., Uhthoff, H., 2000. Synovial adhesions are more important than pannus proliferation in the pathogenesis of knee joint contracture after immobilization: an experimental investigation in the rat. Journal of Rheumatology 27 (2), 351-357.

Turner, C.H., Pavalko, F.M., 1998. Mechanotransduction and functional response of the skeleton to physical stress: the mechanisms and mechanics of bone adaptation. Journal of Orthopaedic Science 3 (6), 346-355.

Uebelhart, D., Bernard, J., Hartmann, D., Moro, L., Roth, M., Uebelhart, B., et al., 2000. Modifications of bone and connective tissue after orthostatic bedrest. Osteoporosis International 11 (1), 59-67.

Vanwanseele, B., Eckstein, F., Knecht, H., Stüssi, E., Spaepen, A., 2002a. Knee cartilage of spinal cord–injured patients displays progressive thinning in the absence of normal joint loading and movement. Arthritis and Rheumatism 46 (8), 2073-2078.

Vanwanseele, B., Lucchinetti, E., Stüssi, E., 2002b. The effects of immobilization on the characteristics of articular cartilage: current concepts and future directions. Osteoarthritis and Cartilage 10 (5), 408-419.

Wall, B.T., Dirks, M.L., Snijders, T., Senden, J.M., Dolmans, J., Loon, L.V., et al., 2014. Substantial skeletal muscle loss occurs during only 5 days of disuse. Acta Physiologica 210 (3), 600-611.

Weiner, S., Wagner, H.D., 1998. The material bone: structure–mechanical function relations. Annual Review of Materials Science 28, 271-298.

Weinreb, M., Rodan, G., Thompson, D., 1989. Osteopenia in the immobilized rat hind limb is associated with increased bone resorption and decreased bone formation. Bone 10 (3), 187-194.

Whiting, C., Zernicke, F., 2008. Biomechanics of Musculoskeletal Injury. Human Kinetics, Illinois.

Widman, L., Abresch, R., Styne, D., McDonald, C., 2007. Aerobic fitness and upper extremity strength in patients aged 11 to 21 years with spinal cord dysfunction as compared to ideal weight and overweight controls. Journal of Spinal Cord Medicine 30 (Suppl. 1), S88-96.

Wilmore, J., Costill, D., Kenney, W., 2015. Physiology of Sport and Exercise. Human Kinetics, Illinois.

Woo, S., Gomez, M., Sites, T., Newton, P., Orlando, C., Akeson, W., et al., 1987. The biomechanical and morphological changes in the medial collateral ligament of the rabbit after immobilization and remobilization. Journal of Bone and Joint Surgery America 69 (8), 1200-1211.

Wronski, T., Morey, E., 1983. Inhibition of cortical and trabecular bone formation in the long bones of immobilized monkeys. Clinical Orthopaedics and Related Research (181), 269-276.

Yabe, Y., Hagiwara, Y., Suda, H., Ando, A., Onoda, Y., Tsuchiya, M., et al., 2013. Joint immobilization induced hypoxic and inflammatory conditions in rat knee joints. Connective Tissue Research 54 (3), 210–217.

Young, D., Niklowitz, W., Brown, R., Jee, W., 1986. Immobilization-associated osteoporosis in primates. Bone 7 (2), 109–117.

Capítulo | 4 |

Força e Condicionamento: Aspectos Científicos, Incluindo Princípios de Reabilitação

Paul Jones e Paul Comfort

Introdução

O treinamento de força, assim como outros métodos de condicionamento, prepara o atleta fisicamente para todos aspectos do desempenho esportivo. A preparação física eficaz dos atletas deve manter seu estado de saúde e reduzir o risco de lesões esportivas sem contato, enquanto melhora seu desempenho esportivo.

Embora o papel de um treinador de força e condicionamento seja utilizar informações de todos os membros da equipe de saúde e ciência esportiva no desenvolvimento de tais programas, os fisioterapeutas devem utilizar os princípios de força e condicionamento para projetar programas de reabilitação mais eficazes para melhor preparar os atletas para o retorno ao pleno treinamento e competição. Para isso, deve ser implementado um programa de treino progressivo que siga os princípios da sobrecarga progressiva, por intermédio da manipulação eficaz do volume e da intensidade do treino/reabilitação, de modo a resultar nas adaptações adequadas aos tecidos e à estrutura fisiológica pretendidos, ao mesmo tempo que restaura a função. Este capítulo descreve os princípios científicos básicos de força e condicionamento que devem ser considerados na concepção de programas eficazes de treinamento ou reabilitação. Embora força e condicionamento possam envolver uma variedade de modalidades de treinamento para preparar os atletas para a competição, como treinamento de resistência, treinamento pliométrico, treinamento de flexibilidade e velocidade, mudança de direção e métodos de treinamento de agilidade, está além do escopo deste capítulo cobrir todos os métodos de condicionamento. Portanto, este capítulo tem o foco na importância da força e dos fatores que influenciam a expressão da força, nos princípios básicos para o desenvolvimento da força, no desenvolvimento de qualidades de força específicas, e também fornece uma visão geral com exemplos trabalhados de como projetar exercícios de "força" e a periodicidade do treinamento usando o conceito de potenciação de fase.

Importância da força muscular

A força muscular é definida como a capacidade de exercer força sobre uma resistência externa. Nos esportes, um atleta pode ser obrigado a manipular sua própria massa corporal contra a gravidade (p. ex., correr, pular), sua massa corporal e a massa corporal de um oponente (p. ex., rúgbi) ou um objeto externo (p. ex., arremesso de peso, levantamento de peso). Em última análise, a força exercida mudará ou tenderá a mudar o movimento de um corpo no espaço. Isso é baseado na segunda lei de Newton, da aceleração, em que a força (f) é igual ao produto da massa (m) e da aceleração (a). Com base nesse princípio, a aceleração de uma determinada massa é diretamente proporcional e ocorre na mesma direção da força aplicada. Portanto, a força muscular é o principal fator para produzir um movimento eficaz e eficiente do corpo de um atleta ou de um objeto externo. Esse conceito é apoiado por vários estudos científicos que encontraram uma relação entre força muscular e desempenho em uma variedade de habilidades motoras, como na corrida (Comfort et al., 2014; Kirkpatrick e Comfort, 2012; Styles et al., 2015; Seitz et al., 2014a; Wisloff et al., 2004), no salto (Hori et al., 2008; Wisloff et al., 2004) e na mudança de direção (Hori et al., 2008; Nimphius et al., 2010).

A literatura anterior indicou que tanto a taxa de desenvolvimento de força (TDF; mudança na força dividida pela mudança no tempo) quanto a potência (taxa de trabalho realizado) são duas das características mais importantes para o desempenho de um atleta (Baker et al., 2001; Morrissey et al., 1995; Stone et al., 2002). Considerando as limitações de tempo de várias tarefas esportivas, a TDF é fundamental. Por exemplo, as evidências sugerem que os indivíduos levam um período de tempo mais longo (> 300 ms) para produzir sua força máxima (Aagaard et al., 2002; Aagaard, 2003) em comparação à duração do salto e ao tempo de contato com o solo durante a corrida (Andersen e Aagaard, 2006). Além disso, os atletas têm tempo limitado para realizar o trabalho mecânico envolvido em tarefas esportivas típicas e, portanto, parece benéfico concluir o trabalho o mais rapidamente possível. Por exemplo, um atleta que conclui o trabalho exigido de uma determinada tarefa mais rapidamente pode receber uma vantagem competitiva em comparação ao seu oponente (p. ex., vencer um adversário em uma corrida até a bola no futebol). Dado que a força muscular serve como a base sobre a qual outras habilidades podem ser aprimoradas, melhorias na TDF e na produção de potência (produção de grande força em um curto período de tempo) podem resultar de aumentos na força (Suchomel e Comfort, 2017). Além disso, a menos que os atletas sejam fortes (peso máximo no agachamento com barra $\geq 1,9 \times$ massa corporal), aumentar a força parece resultar em maiores melhorias no desempenho do que o treinamento balístico ou pliométrico usando cargas mais leves, mas com foco na velocidade do movimento (Cormie et al., 2007; 2010a; 2010b; 2011).

Fatores que afetam a força muscular

Existem três tipos básicos de ações musculares: as concêntricas, as excêntricas e as isométricas (Tabela 4.1). Durante cada tipo de ação muscular, são geradas forças dentro do músculo que puxam suas extremidades uma em direção à outra, dependendo da magnitude da resistência externa. Além disso, frequentemente durante os movimentos esportivos, uma ação excêntrica é precedida por uma ação concêntrica, a qual intensifica a ação concêntrica resultante, conhecida como ciclo de alongamento-encurtamento (CAE) (Tabela 4.1). Vários fatores estão envolvidos na expressão da força humana durante tais ações, incluindo aspectos de controle neuromuscular, fatores morfológicos, comprimento muscular e velocidade de contração.

Recrutamento da unidade motora

O recrutamento de fibras musculares está diretamente relacionado com o tamanho do neurônio motor (Milner-Brown et al., 1973). Inicialmente, pequenos neurônios motores são recrutados, seguidos de grandes neurônios motores, à medida que mais força se faz necessária (Henneman et al., 1965; Henneman e Olson, 1965), comumente da região interna para externa do musculo. Isso tem sido referido como o princípio do tamanho de Henneman, em que pequenas unidades motoras (tipo I) são recrutadas primeiro e, em seguida, grandes unidades motoras (tipo II). Quanto maior o estímulo, maior a quantidade de fibras musculares estimuladas e maior a força de ação muscular. O fato de que todos os músculos contêm fibras musculares tanto do tipo I quanto do II permite que níveis graduais de contração muscular ocorram. Para que uma unidade motora seja treinada, ela deve ser recrutada; portanto, para recrutar unidades motoras de alto limiar, cargas pesadas são necessárias, juntamente com a "intenção" de acelerá-las rapidamente. Além disso, para treinar a TDF e a potência preferencial, é necessário o recrutamento de unidades motoras de alto limiar. No entanto, enquanto o recrutamento ordenado de unidades motoras existe após o treinamento do tipo balístico, as unidades motoras são recrutadas em limiares de força mais baixos (van Cutsem et al., 1998). Portanto, parece que as modalidades de treinamento que são de natureza balística (levantamento de peso, agachamento com salto etc.) permitirão o recrutamento de unidades motoras maiores do tipo II em limiares mais baixos, usando cargas externas mais baixas, permitindo, assim, a ocorrência de adaptações positivas de força e potência, sendo um possível norteador para o treinamento.

Frequência de disparo

A frequência da estimulação neural afeta a força da ação muscular. Um único estímulo neural resultará em uma contração muscular. Uma contração muscular consiste em um breve período latente seguido de uma contração muscular e, logo após, de um período de relaxamento. A força da ação e o tempo total dependerão do tipo de fibra muscular, com fibras de contração rápida se contraindo mais rapidamente e com mais força do que as fibras de contração lenta. Se uma série de estímulos neurais é usada (com 1 a 3 ms de intervalo) (Ghez, 1991), o músculo não tem tempo para relaxar e, portanto, um aumento na tensão muscular é produzido devido à soma de cada contração. Se a frequência dos estímulos neurais aumenta ainda mais, as contrações individuais são combinadas em uma única grande contração sustentada, conhecida como tetania (Ghez, 1991). Essa ação continuará até que o estímulo neural seja interrompido ou o músculo canse. As pesquisas demonstraram que, novamente, o treinamento do tipo balístico pode aumentar a frequência de disparo da unidade motora (van Cutsem et al., 1998), levando a um melhor desempenho de força-potência.

Tabela 4.1 Resumo das ações musculares comuns.

Ação muscular	Descrição
Isométrica	Uma ação muscular isométrica ocorre quando o momento gerado por um músculo ou grupo de músculos é igual ao momento resistivo. Nenhum movimento ocorre Força equivale a resistência Contração sem movimento
Concêntrica	Uma ação concêntrica ocorre quando o momento gerado pelo músculo ou grupo de músculos é maior que o momento resistivo. Isso leva ao encurtamento do complexo músculo-tendão Força maior que resistência Movimento a favor da contração
Excêntrica	Uma ação excêntrica ocorre quando o momento gerado pelo músculo ou grupo de músculos é menor que o momento resistivo. Isso leva ao alongamento do complexo músculo-tendão Força menor que resistência Movimento em direção oposta à contração
Ciclo de alongamento-encurtamento (CAE)	O CAE é quando a força de uma ação concêntrica é aumentada por uma ação muscular excêntrica precedente devido (a) ao reflexo de estiramento por meio da estimulação do fuso muscular durante a fase excêntrica e (b) ao armazenamento e à liberação de energia elástica. Ambas as ações são separadas por uma breve fase de amortização, com fases de amortização mais curtas aproveitando ambos os mecanismos, levando a uma maior potenciação na fase concêntrica. Os movimentos do CAE podem, portanto, ser subdivididos em CAE de resposta curta (< 250 ms) e longa (> 250 ms)

Modificação pelos receptores musculares e tendíneos

O sistema nervoso tem muitos mecanismos para fornecer retroalimentação na forma de informações sobre as forças aplicadas, a posição da articulação e as mudanças no comprimento do músculo. Isso permite que o movimento seja monitorado e controlado e evite lesões, limitando a força de contração dos músculos. O reflexo de alongamento é mediado por receptores no músculo (fuso muscular), o que permite que o músculo produza mais força quando é alongado repentinamente por meio de uma ação muscular excêntrica. Esse é um mecanismo do CAE, por meio do qual a força muscular concêntrica é aumentada após uma ação muscular excêntrica anterior (desde que ocorra apenas um pequeno retardo entre cada ação muscular). O treinamento pliométrico é um método para potencializar esse fenômeno muscular (Tabela 4.2).

Força e Condicionamento: Aspectos Científicos, Incluindo Princípios de Reabilitação **Capítulo** | 4 |

Tabela 4.2 **Visão geral dos diferentes métodos de treinamento de força-potência.**

Modalidade	Justificativa e benefícios	Desvantagens
Exercício utilizando o peso corporal	O exercício com peso corporal é um dos tipos mais básicos de treinamento de resistência e tem várias vantagens, incluindo o foco na melhoria da força relativa e a maior acessibilidade e versatilidade em comparação aos outros métodos de treinamento (Harrison, 2010)	A limitação mais óbvia dos exercícios com peso corporal é a incapacidade de continuar a fornecer um estímulo de sobrecarga ao atleta, impedindo o desenvolvimento significativo da força absoluta (Harrison, 2010). Os praticantes podem prescrever uma maior quantidade de repetições ou modificar o movimento (*i. e.*, variações de flexão) para progredir cada exercício. No entanto, um aumento contínuo nas repetições leva ao desenvolvimento de força-resistência em vez de força-potência necessária para melhorar o desempenho esportivo
Treinamento com peso em aparelho	Exercícios baseados em aparelhos permitem o isolamento de grupos musculares específicos, o que pode ser útil para a reabilitação de lesões	O exercício baseado em aparelhos pode não ter especificidade de movimento. Por exemplo, os movimentos atléticos raramente incluem ações musculares isoladas (Behm e Anderson, 2006). Portanto, a transferência de exercícios de isolamento para o desempenho atlético pode ser um tanto limitada (Augustsson et al., 1998; Blackburn e Morrissey, 1998)
Treinamento com pesos livres	O treinamento com pesos livres incorpora vários grupos musculares e fornece estímulo de treinamento superior ao dos exercícios isolados realizados em uma máquina (Anderson e Behm, 2005). Os exercícios com pesos livres podem recrutar estabilizadores musculares em maior extensão do que os exercícios baseados em máquinas (Haff, 2000) e, portanto, maiores adaptações de força-potência no que se refere ao desempenho esportivo	Os exercícios com pesos livres requerem maior nível de desenvolvimento da técnica em comparação aos exercícios com pesos da máquina. A utilização de exercícios com pesos livres para desenvolver a potência é limitada sem modificar o exercício, pois exercícios como o supino e o agachamento resultam em desaceleração durante os estágios posteriores da fase concêntrica (Lake et al., 2012; Newton et al., 1996). Esses exercícios podem ser modificados (balísticos) para garantir a aceleração ao longo da fase concêntrica, como supino arremessado ou agachamentos com salto (Newton et al., 1996)
Levantamento de peso	Os exercícios de levantamento de peso produzem as maiores saídas de força em comparação aos outros tipos de exercício. Os movimentos de levantamento de peso são únicos, pois exploram os aspectos de força e velocidade da produção de potência, movendo cargas moderadas a pesadas com intenção balística (Suchomel e Comfort, 2017). Uma grande vantagem do levantamento de peso é que o atleta tem como objetivo acelerar ao longo da fase concêntrica, ao contrário dos exercícios tradicionais de peso livre (*i. e.*, supino e agachamento)	Os exercícios de levantamento de peso requerem tempo gasto no desenvolvimento da competência técnica de levantamento. No entanto, derivados de levantamento de peso mais simples (*i. e.*, ações de puxar – levantamento de barra entre o meio da coxa e o quadril, levantamento de barra (*clean*) a partir do joelho) requerem menos competência técnica do que os movimentos completos de levantamento (terminando com a barra nos ombros ou acima da cabeça) e, portanto, são abordagens úteis para a taxa de desenvolvimento de força e desenvolvimento de potência (Suchomel et al., 2015)
Treinamento pliométrico	Os movimentos pliométricos podem ser definidos como movimentos rápidos de potência que usam um pré-alongamento resultando na utilização do ciclo de alongamento-encurtamento (ver Tabela 4.1). Várias meta-análises mostraram que o treinamento pliométrico pode melhorar a habilidade de salto vertical (Sáez de Villarreal et al., 2009), desempenho	A maioria dos exercícios pliométricos são implementados usando a massa corporal do atleta como resistência. No entanto, usar apenas a massa corporal do atleta como resistência pode ser limitado em termos de desenvolvimento de força-potência. Os praticantes são capazes de prescrever pequenas cargas adicionais para aumentar o estímulo de carga no atleta;

(continua)

23

Parte **| 1 |** Conceitos Básicos Importantes em Esportes

Tabela 4.2 **Visão geral dos diferentes métodos de treinamento de força-potência. (*Continuação*)**

Modalidade	Justificativa e benefícios	Desvantagens
	de *sprint* (Sáez de Villarreal et al., 2012) e habilidade de mudança de direção (Asadi et al., 2016). Além disso, o treinamento pliométrico demonstrou melhorar a economia de corrida (Spurrs et al., 2002; Turner et al., 2003) e lidar com a mecânica de pouso deficiente (Hewett et al., 1996)	porém, uma abordagem mais sensata seria aumentar a intensidade do exercício pliométrico por meio da alteração do exercício, alterando a altura da queda ou a instrução de treinamento, enquanto, simultaneamente, ajusta o volume para atender às necessidades de cada atleta
Treinamento excêntrico	As ações musculares excêntricas são aquelas que alongam o músculo como resultado de uma força aplicada a um músculo, a qual é maior do que ele mesmo pode produzir. Embora não sejam bem compreendidas, as ações musculares excêntricas possuem características moleculares e neurais únicas que podem produzir adaptações semelhantes ou maiores na função muscular, adaptações morfológicas e neuromusculares e desempenho em comparação aos treinamentos concêntrico, isométrico e tradicional (excêntrico/concêntrico) (Douglas et al., 2016a; 2016b). No entanto, pouco se sabe sobre a melhor forma de implementar o treinamento excêntrico. O treinamento excêntrico acentuado envolve a realização da fase excêntrica de um levantamento com uma carga mais pesada do que a fase concêntrica, removendo uma parte da carga, e isso tem alguns suportes na literatura. Os métodos incluem o uso de um sistema de liberação de peso (Ojasto e Häkkinen, 2009), presença de observadores (*spotters*) (Brandenburg e Docherty, 2002), o atleta deixar cair o peso (Sheppard et al., 2008) ou uso de volante (de Hoyo et al., 2015) no fim da fase excêntrica	Inicialmente, o treinamento excêntrico pode levar a altos níveis de DMIR, também chamada de dor muscular tardia, mas após algumas sessões de treinamento excêntrico, o músculo deve atingir um efeito protetor contra mais DMIR
Treinamento complexo/contraste (TC)	O TC é uma modalidade de treinamento que envolve concluir um exercício de treinamento de resistência antes de realizar um exercício balístico biomecanicamente semelhante. Por exemplo, o agachamento de costas pode ser combinado com saltos de contra movimento. O TC parece tirar vantagem da potenciação pós-ativação (PPA), que é um aumento agudo no desempenho muscular como resultado da história contrátil do músculo (Robbins, 2005). Numerosos estudos demonstraram essa melhoria de desempenho em um contexto de treinamento (ver Jones et al., 2013a; 2013b para uma revisão)	Embora a implementação de TC para aproveitar as vantagens da PPA no treinamento seja atraente, há poucas pesquisas sobre os efeitos longitudinais. Além disso, a tentativa de eliciar PPA com indivíduos mais fracos pode ser limitada, pois uma maior força muscular pode levar a uma potenciação mais rápida e maior (Seitz et al., 2014b; Suchomel et al., 2016). Dado que a pesquisa mostrou que uma recuperação > 8 min entre os exercícios pode ser necessária para tirar proveito da PPA, isso pode levar a problemas logísticos, pois muito mais tempo de treinamento é gasto na recuperação (Jones et al., 2013b)
Treinamento de resistência variável	O treinamento de resistência variável refere-se a um método de treinamento que altera a resistência externa por meio do uso de correntes ou faixas elásticas durante o exercício, a fim de maximizar a força muscular em toda a amplitude de movimento (Fleck e Kraemer, 2014). A adição de correntes ou faixas elásticas altera o perfil de carga de um exercício (Israetel et al., 2010), permitindo que	Determinar e ajustar a quantidade de carga compensada por faixas e correntes durante os exercícios de peso livre requer tempo de preparação

(continua)

Tabela 4.2 Visão geral dos diferentes métodos de treinamento de força-potência. *(Continuação)*

Modalidade	Justificativa e benefícios	Desvantagens
	o atleta corresponda às mudanças na alavancagem articular (Zatsiorsky e Kraemer, 2006) e supere as desvantagens mecânicas em vários ângulos articulares (Ebben e Jensen, 2002; Wallace et al., 2006). Parece ser uma ferramenta de treinamento eficaz para desenvolver força e potência musculares	
Treinamento com *Kettlebell*	*Kettlebells* são implementos que consistem em uma bola com peso e uma alça. Uma série de exercícios pode ser realizada com *kettlebells*, incluindo balanços, agachamentos do tipo *goblet*, balanços acelerados e exercícios de levantamento de peso modificados (*i. e.*, arrancar) com o objetivo de desenvolver força e potência. Pesquisas anteriores indicaram que o treinamento com *kettlebell* pode melhorar várias medidas de força muscular e desempenho explosivo (Lake e Lauder, 2012; Otto III et al., 2012)	Embora a pesquisa sugira que o treinamento com *kettlebell* pode fornecer um estímulo de treinamento de força eficaz, métodos tradicionais, como levantamento de peso, podem fornecer adaptações superiores quando se trata de desenvolver força máxima e explosão (Otto III et al., 2012), talvez devido à dificuldade em gerar sobrecarga progressiva (*i. e.*, tamanho do *kettlebell* vs. uma barra com peso)

DMIR, dor muscular de início retardado; *PPA*, potenciação pós-ativação.

Em contraste, o órgão tendinoso de Golgi tem um papel na inibição da força produzida pelo músculo para evitar que sejam produzidas forças que possam romper o músculo e o tendão. No entanto, o treinamento pesado de força pode diminuir a retroalimentação aferente de Ib para o conjunto de neurônios motores espinais, reduzindo a inibição neuromuscular e aumentando a produção de força (Aagaard et al., 2000). Assim, o treinamento de resistência pesado pode levar à diminuição da inibição neuromuscular, levando a um potencial maior de força e potência dos atletas.

Área transversal

Uma maior área da seção transversal (AST) de fibra muscular resulta em um tamanho maior do músculo como um todo. De uma perspectiva fisiológica, uma maior AST muscular aumenta a produção de força devido a uma maior quantidade de sarcômeros em paralelo (maior soma espacial). Um aumento na quantidade de sarcômeros (*i. e.*, a menor unidade contrátil dentro de uma célula muscular) eleva a quantidade de interações potenciais entre microfilamentos de actina e miosina (*i. e.*, pontes cruzadas), o que, em última análise, aumenta a força que um músculo pode produzir.

Arquitetura muscular

As propriedades arquitetônicas do músculo esquelético também mostraram afetar a força e a velocidade das ações musculares. Uma diminuição no ângulo de penação ou um aumento no comprimento do fascículo resulta em elevação na velocidade de contração devido ao aumento do comprimento do componente contrátil (Blazevich, 2006; Earp et al., 2010). Em contraste, uma ampliação no ângulo de penação resulta em um aumento na quantidade de fibras para uma determinada AST, o que eleva a capacidade de geração de força (Blazevich, 2006; Manal et al., 2006; Earp et al., 2010).

Comprimento do músculo e o modelo mecânico do músculo

Quando um músculo está em seu comprimento de repouso, os filamentos de actina e miosina ficam próximos uns dos outros, de modo que uma quantidade máxima de locais de pontes cruzadas potenciais estão disponíveis. Isso permite que um maior nível de força seja gerado no comprimento de repouso. Quando um músculo encurta, os filamentos de actina se sobrepõem e o resultado é que a quantidade de pontos de pontes cruzadas é reduzida, diminuindo o potencial de geração de força. Quando o músculo é alongado, uma proporção reduzida de filamentos de actina e miosina fica uma ao lado da outra, novamente reduzindo o potencial de geração de força. Esse fenômeno descreve a relação comprimento-tensão do músculo (Figura 4.1). Devido à natureza de muitos esportes, é essencial treinar os músculos em toda a sua extensão, sempre que possível.

A Figura 4.2 ilustra o modelo mecânico do músculo, composto do componente contrátil e dos componentes elásticos em paralelo e em série. Quando o complexo músculo-tendão é alongado durante uma ação muscular excêntrica, a tensão "passivamente" aumenta no complexo músculo-tendão, devido às propriedades elásticas do tendão e dos tecidos ao redor das fibras musculares (ver Figura 4.1), particularmente com a elevação da velocidade. Durante os movimentos de CAE, a energia elástica armazenada, principalmente no tendão, é utilizada durante a fase concêntrica subsequente, levando a uma maior produção de força e proporcionando um pequeno retardo entre as ações musculares excêntricas e concêntricas (além do reflexo de estiramento mencionado anteriormente). Além disso, a relação comprimento-tensão do músculo (ver Figura 4.1) tem implicações no treinamento excêntrico em que cargas maiores (*i. e.*, 110% de uma repetição máxima (1RM) para treinadores novatos) são necessárias (apenas em comparação às ações concêntricas) durante as fases excêntricas dos exercícios (p. ex., descida de um agachamento com barra).

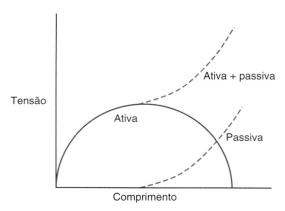

Figura 4.1 Relação comprimento-tensão do músculo.

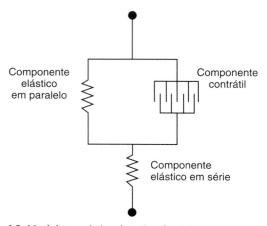

Figura 4.2 Modelo mecânico de músculo. O "componente contrátil" refere-se aos filamentos de actina-miosina, a principal fonte de geração de força muscular durante ações concêntricas. O "componente elástico em série" (*i. e.*, tendão) armazena energia elástica quando esticado, aumentando a produção de força. O "componente elástico em paralelo" (*i. e.*, epimísio, perimísio, endomísio e sarcolema) exerce tensão "passiva" quando o músculo é alongado. (Adaptada de Hill, A.V. (1970). *First and Last Experiments in Muscle Mechanics*. London: Cambridge University Press.)

Velocidade de contração

Com base no trabalho clássico sobre músculo animal isolado de Hill (1970), a capacidade de força do músculo diminui à medida que a velocidade de contração aumenta, talvez devido a um declínio nas pontes cruzadas formadas à medida que a velocidade de encurtamento aumenta. A relação é curvilínea, com o declínio na capacidade de força mais acentuado na faixa inferior de velocidades de movimento (Figura 4.3). Como mencionado acima, os atletas são obrigados a trabalhar contra uma variedade de resistências no esporte (*i. e.*, seu próprio corpo, um oponente ou objeto esportivo) e, portanto, dependendo das demandas esportivas específicas, os atletas podem ser obrigados a desenvolver diferentes partes da curva força-velocidade (a extremidade de alta ou baixa velocidade, ou ambas). Isso requer manipulação de carga e seleção de exercício (Suchomel et al., 2017).

Princípios básicos para aumentar a força e a potência musculares

Existe uma variedade de regimes de exercícios para aumentar a força e a potência musculares. Um resumo é fornecido na Tabela 4.2.

Os princípios importantes para o desenvolvimento de força e potência são sobrecarga, especificidade, individualidade, reversibilidade e rendimentos decrescentes.

Sobrecarga

Para que qualquer um dos sistemas do corpo se adapte, os estímulos devem ser suficientes para criar sobrecarga, ou seja, é necessário expor o tecido a uma carga maior do que aquela a que foi submetido recentemente. Para melhorar a força (ou outras qualidades de aptidão) de um músculo, ele deve ser *progressivamente* e apropriadamente sobrecarregado (Bruton, 2002). Para criar sobrecarga ao fortalecer um músculo, a resistência (carga) deve ser maior do que os músculos estão acostumados durante as atividades diárias; e, à medida que o músculo ganha força, a resistência deve ser aumentada progressivamente. A sobrecarga, neste caso, pode ser alcançada, inicialmente, por meio de um ligeiro aumento nas repetições (2 a 6) ou séries (3 a 6); no entanto, uma vez que a quantidade máxima de repetições seja alcançada em dada resistência, esta (carga externa) deverá ser aumentada (geralmente ≥ 85% do máximo). Aumentar ainda mais as repetições altera o foco da força muscular para a resistência muscular. Ao aumentar a resistência muscular, deve haver ampliação progressiva no volume do exercício, novamente por meio de um aumento nas repetições (10 a 20) das séries (2 a 3), embora, assim como ocorre com a força, se a quantidade máxima de repetições pode ser alcançada com uma dada resistência, a resistência deve ser aumentada. É essa natureza progressiva que garante que a sobrecarga continue durante as sessões de reabilitação/treinamento.

Especificidade

Este princípio diz respeito à adaptação específica do músculo às demandas impostas (princípio SAID, do inglês *specific adaptation to imposed demands*) (DiNubile, 1991). O efeito no músculo é específico à natureza do exercício (ver seção *Desenvolvimento de qualidades específicas*). A implicação na especificidade é que o exercício prescrito não precisa espelhar o padrão de movimento da atividade funcional que visa melhorar (*i. e.*, copiar diretamente os padrões de movimento da ação esportiva). A atividade precisa ter como alvo a musculatura apropriada e a carga e/ou velocidade do movimento precisa ser específica para que a sobrecarga apropriada, em relação com o objetivo, seja alcançada. Por exemplo, o fortalecimento do quadríceps deve envolver alta resistência e baixa repetição, mas o exercício pode ser um agachamento (p. ex., agachamento frontal,

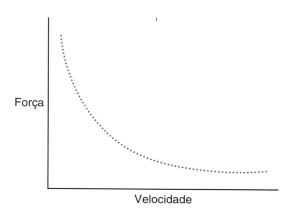

Figura 4.3 Relação força-velocidade do músculo.

agachamento com barra, *box squat*), uma variação de afundo (p. ex., para frente, reverso, com halter e perna de trás elevada) ou um simples exercício de extensão do joelho. No entanto, a transferência da extensão do joelho para, por exemplo, um típico sentar e ficar em pé será muito menos eficaz do que partir de uma variação de agachamento ou afundo (Augustsson et al., 1998; Blackburn e Morrissey, 1998).

Individualidade

Os indivíduos responderão de maneira diferente ao mesmo exercício; essa resposta é determinada pela genética, pelas taxas de crescimento celular, pelo metabolismo e pelas regulações neural e endócrina. Por exemplo, um exercício aplicado a uma pessoa de 80 anos e a uma de 26 anos de idade terá efeitos diferentes, pois aos 60 anos a quantidade de fibras de contração rápida diminui. As diferenças nos níveis de força entre homens de meia-idade e homens mais velhos são parcialmente explicadas pela diminuição dos hormônios anabólicos associados ao envelhecimento (Izquierdo et al., 2001), embora essas diminuições na força sejam um tanto reversíveis com o treinamento de força apropriado (Suetta et al., 2004). O *status* do treinamento com base nos níveis de força também determina a resposta ao treinamento subsequente, com indivíduos que já são fortes progredindo em um ritmo mais lento (Cormie et al., 2010a) devido à lei dos rendimentos decrescentes.

Rendimentos decrescentes

Um regime de exercícios produzirá uma melhora maior nas pessoas em más condições físicas do que naquelas que já estão em boas condições físicas (Figura 4.4). É importante notar, entretanto, que poucos atletas estão realmente próximos de seu teto genético para força ou capacidade aeróbica, especialmente em esportes de equipe.

Reversibilidade

Quando o treinamento é interrompido, qualquer ganho de força (ou outra qualidade) será perdido progressivamente (Bruton, 2002), por exemplo, quando um membro é imobilizado, a força e o tamanho dos músculos do membro diminuem. A taxa de declínio é mais lenta em atletas bem treinados e mais experientes.

Desenvolvimento de qualidades específicas

Os princípios acima precisam ser levados em consideração ao se almejar o desenvolvimento da força de um indivíduo. A resistência necessária para desenvolver força pode ser fornecida por vários métodos (ver Tabela 4.2). Durante as primeiras 6 a 8 semanas de treinamento de força, as adaptações são amplamente neurais com aumentos na produção de força observados (Enoka, 1988). Essas mudanças incluem aumento da ativação neural do músculo (p. ex., aumento do recrutamento e sincronização de unidades motoras) (Sale et al., 1983; Komi, 1986), o qual é paralelo ao aumento da força muscular, ao aumento da ativação dos motores primários (Sale, 1988), à melhora da coordenação intermuscular (Sale, 1988) e à diminuição da ativação de antagonistas.

Após as adaptações neurológicas iniciais, aumentos subsequentes na força são atribuíveis às adaptações arquitetônicas

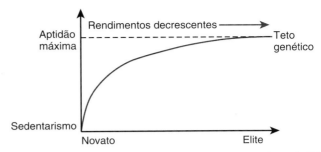

Figura 4.4 Conceito de rendimentos decrescentes. Todos os indivíduos têm um limite genético no que diz respeito ao desenvolvimento de uma qualidade de aptidão específica. O impacto de um regime de exercícios será reduzido com o ganho de aptidão.

do músculo e às ampliações na AST (hipertrofia). As mudanças incluem um aumento na AST do músculo (Housh et al., 1992; Narici et al., 1996) e nas fibras musculares (Andersen e Aagaard, 2000; Melissa et al., 1997); um aumento na proporção de fibras do tipo IIa e uma diminuição nas fibras do tipo IIx (Andersen e Aagaard, 2000; Hortobagyi et al., 1996); alteração nos ângulos de penação (Kawakami et al., 1993; 1995); alteração na capacidade metabólica do músculo (Simoneau et al., 1986); alteração nas isoformas da cadeia pesada da miosina (MHC) (Andersen e Aagaard, 2000; Gea, 1997); e aumento do tecido conjuntivo encontrado nas estruturas musculares proporcionais à hipertrofia muscular.

A *resistência muscular* se refere à capacidade de um músculo de produzir uma força específica repetidamente ou de sustentar uma ação isométrica por um período de tempo (Bruton, 2002). Para aumentar a resistência muscular, cargas baixas são usadas para várias repetições (2 a 3 séries de 10 a 20 repetições). Esses intervalos de intensidade e repetição ajudam a aumentar a capacidade de trabalho dos músculos, mas, devido ao alto volume (séries × repetições × carga levantada) associado a esse treinamento, é provável que haja uma resposta hipertrófica. Além disso, o aumento inicial da força deve aumentar a resistência muscular, pois as atividades realizadas pelo indivíduo não estão mais próximas da intensidade máxima.

Uma grande quantidade de repetições de ações musculares contra uma resistência moderada aumenta a resistência muscular, efetuando uma mudança no músculo (p. ex., ampliação da AST, aumento das enzimas glicolíticas e do armazenamento de glicogênio). O estímulo é a demanda metabólica e o estresse de tração no músculo, e isso reflete sobre a natureza das mudanças, incluindo aumentos na quantidade de fibras dos tipos I e IIa (Demirel et al., 1999; Ingjer, 1979), na AST de fibras dos tipos I e IIx (Ingjer, 1979), na quantidade de capilares em torno de cada fibra muscular (Ingjer, 1979), no fluxo sanguíneo no músculo (Rohter et al., 1963; Vanderhoof et al., 1961), no conteúdo de mioglobina (Holloszy, 1976); e uma diminuição nas fibras do tipo IIx (Demirel et al., 1999; Ingjer, 1979).

A *potência muscular* é uma função da força e da velocidade musculares; a melhora em um ou ambos os aspectos resulta em aumento na potência muscular. Além disso, acredita-se que a prática repetida do movimento ou de um componente do movimento, na velocidade, produz melhora na força muscular, provavelmente devido à maior eficiência do movimento e à diminuição da ativação antagonista (deVries e Housh, 1994).

A produção de força é o principal determinante da potência; como mencionado anteriormente, o aumento da produção de força resulta em um aumento da capacidade de acelerar um

Parte | 1 | Conceitos Básicos Importantes em Esportes

objeto (segunda lei de Newton). Se a aceleração de um objeto aumenta a partir de elevação na produção de força, há um aumento resultante na velocidade do movimento. Portanto, o aumento da força e da velocidade resulta em maior melhoria na potência (potência = força × velocidade).

Foi sugerido que o movimento deve ser realizado o mais rápido possível contra uma resistência de 30% da força *isométrica* máxima, embora os exercícios realizados com cargas baixas resultem apenas na melhora da potência com cargas baixas, enquanto os exercícios com cargas moderadas ou pesadas aumentam a potência em todos cargas (Kaneko et al., 1983; Toji e Kaneko, 2004). Em linha com o princípio da especificidade, a carga e a velocidade resultante geram os maiores aumentos de potência nessas cargas e velocidades. No entanto, o treinamento de carga pesada resulta em maiores melhorias na potência em uma gama de cargas (Harris et al., 2008; Kaneko et al., 1983; Toji et al., 1997; Toji e Kaneko, 2004). O fator chave no desenvolvimento de potência parece ser a habilidade de produzir força rapidamente, esse é o melhor treinamento com foco maior no desenvolvimento de força do que de potência, a menos que o indivíduo já seja forte (Cormie et al., 2010b).

Projetando um treino de "força"

Análise das necessidades

Um primeiro passo importante para o desenvolvimento de um programa de "força" é realizar uma "análise das necessidades". A análise de necessidades deve avaliar as demandas do esporte, as lesões comuns e as suas causas e o atleta em relação com um perfil acordado do esporte. Ao avaliar as demandas do esporte, o seguinte deve ser considerado:

1. É necessária uma *análise biomecânica/de movimento*. A fim de selecionar exercícios com algum grau de "transferência" de movimento, as ações de movimento importantes (corrida, salto etc.) do esporte precisam ser identificadas primeiro. Uma vez que esses movimentos tenham sido identificados, as características biomecânicas dessas ações precisam ser compreendidas. Por exemplo: quais forças são geradas e absorvidas e em que duração? Quais são as velocidades, amplitudes de movimento e ações musculares dos segmentos corporais envolvidos no movimento? A literatura biomecânica deve ser considerada para identificar essas características. No entanto, se esses dados não estiverem disponíveis na literatura, uma avaliação "qualitativa" dos movimentos esportivos comuns deve ser realizada para compreender essas características.

2. A *análise fisiológica* é necessária para identificar as qualidades físicas importantes exigidas para o sucesso naquele esporte. Geralmente, isso forma o objetivo principal do treinamento (*i. e.*, desenvolvimento de potência para um arremessador de peso). Aqui, o praticante precisa considerar quaisquer dados fisiológicos (p. ex., frequência cardíaca média e de pico), movimentos temporais ou sistemas de posicionamento global (GPS) da competição, a fim de identificar distâncias típicas percorridas em diferentes velocidades de locomoção, quantidade de mudanças de direção, trabalho típico: repouso, por exemplo. Além disso, os dados normativos de atletas de alto nível devem ser considerados para decidir quais fatores físicos são importantes para o sucesso e para discriminar entre os níveis de elite e subelite de desempenho.

3. A *análise de lesões* é necessária para identificar os locais comuns para lesões articulares e musculares pertencentes ao esporte. A literatura epidemiológica deve ser consultada para identificar as lesões comuns associadas ao esporte. Além disso, é importante entender os mecanismos subjacentes dessas lesões e se eles são modificáveis por intervenção de treinamento. Estudos prospectivos/de rastreamento e biomecânicos dos mecanismos de lesão devem ser consultados aqui.

A avaliação do atleta deve considerar o seguinte: estado de treinamento e experiência, análise retrospectiva da(s) temporada(s) anterior(es), histórico de lesões do atleta e resultados de testes de desempenho/pré-seleção *objetivos* (*i. e.*, quaisquer testes realizados são baseados nas demandas do esporte).

A análise das necessidades permite que metas de treinamento adequadas sejam definidas em relação ao programa de treinamento de força. Por exemplo, o objetivo principal de treinamento de um velocista (Boxe 4.1) pode ser o desenvolvimento de potência; entretanto, como já foi mencionado, o desenvolvimento de uma base de força é necessário, pois a capacidade de produzir força sustenta a potência. Portanto, o treinamento precisa ser periodizado (ver *Periodização do treinamento*), a fim de permitir a "potenciação de fase" (*i. e.*, o desenvolvimento da força em um bloco de treinamento anterior permite um maior desenvolvimento de força no bloco subsequente devido ao aumento da capacidade de produzir força). Consulte a Tabela 4.3 para obter um exemplo.

Frequência de treinamento

A frequência de treinamento se refere à quantidade de sessões de treinamento realizadas em um determinado período de tempo, normalmente 1 semana. Ao determinar a frequência de treinamento, o *status* de treinamento do atleta, a temporada esportiva, as cargas de exercício projetadas, os tipos de exercícios e os outros treinamentos ou atividades simultâneas devem ser considerados.

Normalmente, três sessões de "força" por semana são recomendadas, o que permite aos atletas uma recuperação de no mínimo 1 dia entre os treinos (uma regra geral é permitir 1 dia de descanso entre os treinos, porém não mais do que três entre as sessões que estressam a mesma parte do corpo). Conforme o atleta se adapta ao treinamento, outros exercícios podem ser realizados. Os atletas podem aumentar seu treinamento usando *rotinas divididas*, nas quais diferentes grupos de músculos são treinados em dias diferentes. Observe que o uso de cargas máximas ou quase máximas pode exigir mais recuperação entre os treinos, impactando, assim, a frequência do treinamento. No entanto, isso pode ser gerenciado alternando cargas pesadas e leves durante a semana de treinamento. O uso dos termos "pesado" e "leve" na literatura é um tanto enganoso, pois a manipulação adequada das sessões de treinamento em 1 semana deve manter a intensidade e alterar o volume total de trabalho realizado, geralmente por meio de alterações nas séries e faixas de repetição realizadas dentro de uma sessão de treinamento.

A temporada esportiva do atleta também influencia a frequência de treinamento. Por exemplo, na temporada, há demandas crescentes de jogos e práticas específicas de esportes, o que leva a uma diminuição no tempo disponível para atividades de "condicionamento". Além disso, a frequência do treinamento é influenciada pela quantidade geral de estresse físico. Assim, se o programa de força de um atleta é executado simultaneamente com outro treinamento (*i. e.*, aeróbico ou anaeróbico) e outra prática esportiva específica, os efeitos de outros tipos de

Boxe 4.1 Aplicação dos princípios de prescrição de exercícios no projeto de sessões de treinamento de força-potência para um velocista (100 e 200 m)

Análise das necessidades

A duração dos eventos de 100 e 200 m para velocistas de alto nível varia de aproximadamente 10 segundos (100 m) a 21 segundos (200 m). Portanto, para esses atletas, há maior ênfase no condicionamento "anaeróbico" e uma necessidade de produzir rapidamente altas forças em condições de alta velocidade (i. e., potência). Os programas de treinamento de resistência para velocistas devem se concentrar, principalmente, no objetivo de desenvolver potência; no entanto, isso deve ser depois de desenvolver uma base de força (Tabela 4.3), pois a força máxima sustenta a potência. O sprint de 100 m pode ser subdividido em uma fase de aceleração (0 a 40 m), uma fase de velocidade máxima (40 a 70 m), com o restante do sprint focado na manutenção da velocidade (i. e., endurance de velocidade). Ambas as fases de aceleração e velocidade máxima envolvem biomecânica distintamente diferente, o que tem implicações na seleção de exercícios de treinamento. A fase de aceleração envolve contatos curtos (0,12 a 0,2 segundo) com o solo (Atwater, 1982; Salo et al., 2005), com ênfase na geração de força de propulsão horizontal e impulso (Hunter et al., 2005), enquanto minimiza as forças de frenagem. As articulações dos membros inferiores se estendem durante o contato com o solo, com ênfase na geração de força concêntrica no tornozelo e joelho (Buckley et al., 2001). É necessária uma inclinação maior do tronco (aproximadamente 45°) para ajudar a gerar a força propulsora horizontal (Kugler e Janssen, 2010). Portanto, exercícios com maior ênfase na geração de força concêntrica horizontal (ou pliometria de resposta longa) devem ser incorporados (i. e., saltos longos em pé; ver Tabela 4.3). A fase de velocidade máxima é caracterizada por contatos mais curtos com o solo (0,09 a 0,12 segundo) (Atwater, 1982; Kuitenen et al., 2002; Mann e Herman, 1985), novamente destacando a importância da taxa de desenvolvimento de força para o desempenho de sprint. No entanto, a produção ideal de força vertical é necessária para preservar a fase de voo (Weyland et al., 2000), ao mesmo tempo que visa minimizar o tempo de contato e as forças de frenagem. Durante o contato com o solo na fase de velocidade máxima, maior ênfase é colocada na absorção de potência excêntrica (Bezodis et al., 2008) no tornozelo e no joelho, pois um velocista faz maior uso do CAE (resposta rápida/curta) durante essa fase, daí a necessidade de exercícios pliométricos no programa (drop jumps [queda de altura predeterminada, seguida de salto máximo] simples e bilaterais, obstáculos etc.; ver Tabela 4.3). As articulações dos membros inferiores se estendem durante a fase posterior do contato com o solo, daí a necessidade de movimentos semelhantes serem incorporados ao programa (i. e., agachamentos, levantamento de peso, puxadas). No entanto, um nível ideal de extensão do quadril é necessário para evitar o aumento do tempo de contato com o solo e, assim, reduzir a frequência do passo (Mann e

Herman, 1985). A natureza unilateral da corrida de velocidade sugere que os exercícios unilaterais devem ser incorporados ao programa, uma vez que o atleta esteja adequadamente condicionado para executá-los com segurança e eficácia. Finalmente, as lesões por distensão dos isquiotibiais são comuns em velocistas (Lynsholm e Wiklander, 1987), o que pode ser resultado de uma fraqueza excêntrica dos isquiotibiais, tornando o grupo muscular mais suscetível a lesões por distensão durante o balanço tardio (Schache et al., 2012). Portanto, os exercícios dedicados ao desenvolvimento da força excêntrica dos isquiotibiais (i. e., exercícios nórdicos para isquiotibiais [Nordic Hamstrings]) devem ser incluídos no programa.

Exemplo de sessões focadas em "potência" assumindo um status de treinamento avançado

Exemplo de sessão 1				*Exemplo de sessão 2*			
Exercício	Carga (% 1RM)	Repetições	Séries	Exercício	Carga (% 1RM)	Repetições	Séries
Levantamento de peso entre a coxa e o quadril (mid thigh clean)	70%[c]	3	3	Puxada do tipo mid thigh clean	60[c]	3	3
Agachamento com barra[a]	90%	4	3	Jerk dividido (Split jerk)	80%	3	4
Afundo para frente[a]	85%	6	2	Agachamento frontal[a]	90%	4	3
Exercícios nórdicos para isquiotibiais (Nordic Hamstrings)[b]	PC	4	3	Levantamento terra romeno[b]	87%	5	2

[a]Incluído para preservar a força máxima, enquanto o programa se concentra na potência; [b]Incluído para prevenção de lesões; [c]% 1RM power clean; PC, peso corporal; RM, repetição máxima.

Atwater, A., 1982. Kinematic analyses of sprinting. Track and Field Quarterly Review 82, 12-16.

Bezodis, I., Kerwin, D., Salo, A., 2008. Lower-limb mechanics during support phases of maximum-velocity sprint running. Med. Sci. Sports Exerc. 40, 707-715.

Hunter, J., Marshall, R., Mcnair, P., 2005. Relationships between ground reaction force impulse and kinematics of sprint-running accleration. J. Appl. Biomech. 21, 31-43.

Johnson, M., Buckley, J., 2001. Muscle power patterns in the mid-acceleration phase of sprinting. J. Sports Sci. 19, 263-272.

Kugler, F., Janshen, L., 2010. Body position determines propulsive forces in accelerated running. J. Biomech. 43, 343-348.

Kuitenen, S., Komi, P., Kyrolainen, H., 2002. Knee and ankle joint stiffness in sprint running. Med. Sci. Sports Exerc. 34, 166-173.

Lysholm, J., Wiklander, J., 1987. Injuries in runners. American Journal of Sports Medicine 15, 168-171.

Mann, R., Herman, J., 1985. Kinematic analysis of olympic sprint performance: men's 200 meters. Int. J. Sport Biomech. 1, 151-162.

Salo, A., Keranen, T., Viitasalo, J., 2005. Force production in the first four steps of sprint running. In: Wang, Q. (Ed.), XXIII International Symposium on Biomechanics on Sport. The China Institute of Sports Science, Beijing, pp. 313-317.

Schache, A.G., Dorn, T.W., Blanch, P.D., Brown, N.A.T., Pandy., M.G., 2012. Mechanics of the human hamstring muscles during sprinting. Medicine and Science in Sports and Exercise 44 (4), 647-658.

Weyand, P.G., Sternlight, D.B., Bellizzi, M.J., Wright, S., 2000. Faster top running speeds are achieved with greater ground forces not more rapid leg movements. Journal of Applied Physiology 89, 1991-1999.

Tabela 4.3 **Exemplo de periodização para um velocista de pista (100 e 200 m).**

MACROCICLO	PREPARAÇÃO			COMPETIÇÃO	
Fase de treinamento	**Preparação geral**		**Preparação específica**	**Pré-competição**	**Competição**
Mesociclos	**Adaptação anatômica[a] (EM/técnica)**	**Força geral (hip./força)[a]**	**Força máxima[a,b]** ... **Potência[b]**	**Velocidade**	**Pico**
Exemplos de sessão 1	Primeira puxada do *clean* (*clean pull*) (60 a 70% 1RM[d] × 10 × 3)[c] Agachamento com peso (65 a 70% 1RM × 10 a 15 × 3) Agachamento dividido (67% 1RM × 12 (6 em cada perna) × 3) LTR (75% 1RM × 10 × 3)	Primeira puxada do (*clean pull*) (70 a 80% 1RM[d] × 10 × 3)[c] Agachamento com peso (67 a 80% 1RM × 8 a 12 × 3) Afundo para frente (*forward lunge*) (80% 1RM × 8 × 4) LTR (80% 1RM × 8 × 4)	*Power clean* (80% 1RM[d] × 2 a 4 × 4) Agachamento com peso (85 a 87% 1RM × 5 a 6 × 3) Avanço (*walking lunge*) (80 a 85% 1RM × 6 a 8 × 3 a 4 por perna) LTR (87 a 90% 1RM × 4 a 5 × 3) ‖ *Hang clean* (60% 1RM[d] × 5 × 4) Agachamento com salto (20 a 40% 1RM[e] × 5 × 3) Avanço (*walking lunge*) (87% 1RM × 5 × 2 por perna)/alternando com uma perna única 5 a 6 × 2 cada perna LTR (87 a 90% 1RM × 4 a 5 × 3)	Levantamento de peso entre a coxa e o quadril (*mid-thigh clean*) (40% 1RM[d] × 5 × 3) Agachamento com salto (0% 1RM[e] × 5 × 3) *Drop jump* horizontal de perna única (PC × 4 × 4) LTR (87% 1RM × 5 × 2)	Levantamento de peso entre a coxa e o quadril (*mid-thigh clean*) (60% 1RM[d] × 3 × 3) *Split jerk* (60% 1RM × 3 × 2) A manutenção antes do pico pode incorporar exercício de força (*i. e.*, agachamento) com alta carga/baixo volume (*i. e.*, 90% 1RM × 3 a 4 × 2)
Exemplos de sessão 2	Levantamento terra (65 a 70% 1RM × 10 a 15 × 3) Agachamento dividido (65 a 75% 1RM × 8 a 12 × 3) Exercício nórdico para isquiotibiais (*Nordic hamstring*) (PC × 3 × 3) Elevação da panturrilha (65% 1RM × 15 × 3)	Levantamento terra (80% 1RM × 8 × 3) Agachamento búlgaro/ agachamento dividido (80% 1RM × 8 × 4) Exercício nórdico para isquiotibiais (*Nordic hamstring*) (PC × 4 a 6 × 3 a 4) Elevação da panturrilha (67 a 80% 1RM × 12 a 8 × 3)	Levantamento terra (90% 1RM × 4 × 3) Agachamento unilateral (85% 1RM × 6 × 2 [cada perna]) Exercício nórdico para isquiotibiais (*Nordic hamstring*) (PC + colete de peso × 5 a 6 × 3 a 4) Elevação da panturrilha (85% 1RM × 6 × 3) ‖ *Clean* a partir do joelho (80 a 90% 1RM[d] × 2 a 4 × 2 a 4) Saltos em uma única perna (PC + 6 × 2 (cada perna)) Exercício nórdico para isquiotibiais (*Nordic hamstring*) (PC + colete de peso × 5 a 6 × 3 a 4) Elevação da panturrilha (90% 1RM × 4 × 2)	*Mid-thigh clean pull* (60% 1RM[d] × 5 × 3) *Split jerk* (60% 1RM × 4 × 3) Salto em distância em pé (PC × 5 × 4) Exercício nórdico para isquiotibiais inferiores (PC × 3 × 3) (manutenção)	*Mid-thigh pull* (40% 1RM[d] × 3 × 2) *Split jerk* (60% 1RM × 3 × 2) A manutenção antes do pico pode incorporar exercício de força (*i. e.*, agachamento com barra) com alta carga/baixo volume (*i. e.*, 90% 1RM × 3 a 4 × 2)

[a]Exercícios para a parte superior do corpo utilizados para o condicionamento de todo o corpo (*i. e.*, remada unilateral, *shoulder press*) nessas fases; [b]As fases podem ser repetidas: força máxima – potência – força máxima – potência para proporcionar maior variação de treinamento ao longo dessa fase de treinamento; [c]Conjuntos usados para manter a técnica e a velocidade (p. ex., 15 repetições divididas em 3 grupos de 5 repetições com um descanso intraconjunto de 20 a 30 segundos); [d]% 1RM *power clean*; [e]% 1RM agachamento com barra. *PC*, peso corporal; *Hip.*, hipertrofia; *EM*, endurance muscular; *LTR*, levantamento terra romeno; *RM*, repetição máxima.

Força e Condicionamento: Aspectos Científicos, Incluindo Princípios de Reabilitação **Capítulo** | **4** |

treinamentos devem ser considerados para evitar efeitos negativos nos exercícios de força. Dessa maneira, a organização da frequência de treinamento pode ser usada para reduzir o volume geral de treinamento semanal.

Seleção de exercícios

A fim de selecionar os exercícios mais adequados para o programa do atleta, o praticante deve compreender as características biomecânicas dos vários tipos de exercícios de treinamento, os movimentos e os requisitos musculares do esporte e a experiência técnica de exercício do atleta. Além disso, os recursos de treinamento e o tempo disponível podem ser aspectos adicionais a serem considerados antes de projetar o programa. O exercício pode ser classificado como "*core*", "assistência" ou "potência". Os *exercícios de core* são essencialmente exercícios multiarticulares (p. ex., agachamento, levantamento terra, *power cleans*) que recrutam uma ou mais áreas musculares, envolvem um mínimo de duas articulações primárias e demonstram semelhança aos padrões de movimento esportivo do atleta. Os *exercícios de assistência* são essencialmente exercícios uniarticulares (p. ex., flexão do joelho, extensão do joelho), que visam a um grupo de músculos e podem ser incluídos no programa para fins de "assistência" ou prevenção de lesões. Os *exercícios de potência* são exercícios estruturais (*i. e.*, exercícios que carregam a coluna diretamente) realizados rapidamente com ênfase no desenvolvimento de potência. Os exercícios de levantamento de peso e seus derivados se enquadram nessa categoria, junto com os exercícios balísticos (*i. e.*, saltos, agachamentos, supino, arremessos).

Com base no princípio da especificidade declarado anteriormente, os exercícios selecionados dentro de um programa precisam ter relevância para as atividades associadas ao esporte no que diz respeito aos músculos e às ações musculares envolvidas, às cargas (intensidade), à velocidade e à amplitude de movimento. Por exemplo, no Boxe 4.1, um velocista pode adotar puxadas do tipo *mid-thigh clean* durante uma fase de potência de seu treinamento. Embora o exercício possa não replicar o padrão de movimento exato da corrida, ele satisfaz o princípio da especificidade. Isso ocorre porque a tração limpa no meio da coxa (*mid-thigh clean pull*) (a) usa os mesmos músculos dos membros inferiores, (b) envolve a extensão tripla das articulações dos membros inferiores a partir de um ângulo de joelho semelhante ao da fase de postura média do ciclo de marcha, (c) envolve uma alta velocidade de movimento (dependente da carga usada) e (d) envolve a produção rápida de força.

Os exercícios também devem ser incluídos no programa para lidar com quaisquer desequilíbrios musculares indesejados decorrentes do desenvolvimento. Por exemplo, no Boxe 4.1 e na Tabela 4.3, o velocista precisa incluir exercícios para atingir o desenvolvimento da força dos isquiotibiais (*i. e.*, exercícios nórdicos para isquiotibiais, levantamento terra romeno), já que outros exercícios no programa junto com o programa de corrida podem ter muito foco no quadríceps e, portanto, levam a desequilíbrios musculares e a lesões potenciais. Exercícios focados nos isquiotibiais são necessários para evitar o desenvolvimento desses desequilíbrios, enquanto exercícios como o levantamento terra romeno podem ajudar na extensão forçada do quadril, essencial para a corrida.

Prescrição de exercícios

Ordem do exercício

Uma vez que a meta de treinamento do atleta para uma sessão é decidida, o praticante precisa determinar a ordem correta dos exercícios, a sua carga e faixa de repetição, a quantidade de séries e a recuperação. No que diz respeito à ordem dos exercícios, de um modo geral, a sessão deve ser concebida da seguinte forma: exercícios de potência primeiro (*i. e.*, *power clean* – variação da primeira fase do arremesso de peso em que o atleta não se abaixa completamente), seguidos de outros exercícios de força multiarticulares (*i. e.*, agachamento com barra) e, posteriormente, exercícios de "assistência" uniarticulares. A justificativa para essa ordem é que os exercícios de potência requerem o mais alto nível de habilidade e concentração de todos os exercícios e podem ser afetados pela fadiga, aumentando o risco de lesões (Fleck e Kraemer, 2014). Além disso, os movimentos de levantamento de peso que muitas vezes são realizados como exercícios de potência resultam no maior gasto de energia e são tecnicamente os mais exigentes em comparação aos outros exercícios (Stone et al., 2006). Portanto, esses exercícios são realizados primeiro na sessão, quando o atleta está "fresco". Se os exercícios de potência não forem realizados, então, exercícios multiarticulares de "*core*" são realizados seguidos de exercícios de "assistência".

Um método para facilitar a recuperação do atleta durante uma sessão de treinamento e fazer uso mais eficiente do tempo de treinamento é alternar exercícios para a parte inferior e superior do corpo durante a sessão (Sheppard e Triplett, 2016). Outro método consiste em alternar entre exercícios de empurrar (*i. e.*, supino) e puxar (*i. e.*, remada unilateral); isso garante que o mesmo grupo muscular não seja usado em exercícios sucessivos e facilita a recuperação durante a sessão (Sheppard e Triplett, 2016).

Carga de treinamento e repetições

Carga simplesmente se refere à quantidade de carga atribuída a um conjunto de exercícios e é o aspecto mais crítico de um programa de treinamento de resistência. A quantidade de repetições realizadas está inversamente relacionada com a carga levantada (*i. e.*, quanto mais pesada a carga, menor a quantidade de repetições realizadas). O objetivo do treinamento influencia diretamente a seleção da carga e as repetições que a acompanham:

Força máxima

Alta resistência e baixa repetição (geralmente 2 a 6 repetições) resultam em um aumento na força muscular (Hakkinen et al., 1998; Staron et al., 1994). O treinamento até o ponto de falha muscular momentânea (*i. e.*, nenhuma repetição adicional pode ser realizada dentro da série) não é necessário (Izquierdo et al., 2006), desde que o exercício seja realizado com carga suficiente (geralmente, $\geq 80\%$ 1RM). Normalmente, 2 a 6 séries podem ser realizadas.

Hipertrofia

Normalmente, isso é alcançado por meio de um alto volume de trabalho (quantidade moderada a alta de repetições por série, com uma alta quantidade de séries realizadas [3 a 6]) e concluídas com intensidades moderadas a moderadamente altas (60 a 80% 1RM) (Suchomel e Comfort, 2017).

31

Resistência muscular

Baixa resistência (60 a 75% 1RM) e alta repetição (10 a 20 repetições) resultarão em um aumento na resistência muscular. Apenas pequenos aumentos na força estão associados à resposta hipertrófica ao treinamento de endurance muscular, resultando em um aumento da AST de um músculo. O treinamento até a falha muscular momentânea parece ser vantajoso (Izquierdo et al., 2006). Normalmente, 2 a 3 séries são realizadas para evitar inflar excessivamente a carga de volume geral.

Potência

Baixas resistências (≤ 40% 1RM) movidas em alta velocidade irão aumentar a potência muscular, ou seja, uma elevação na velocidade de encurtamento do fascículo. A potência também pode ser aumentada com cargas maiores (≥ 60% 1RM), desde que a intenção seja mover-se rapidamente, mesmo que o nível de resistência resulte em uma velocidade de movimento relativamente baixa (Behm e Sale, 1993); embora, normalmente, essas cargas sejam utilizadas durante exercícios de levantamento de peso e seus derivados (Suchomel et al., 2017). Para maximizar a qualidade do exercício, normalmente, são realizadas de 3 a 5 séries. A fadiga também pode ser gerenciada pela utilização de séries de *cluster* (recuperações curtas de < 30 s entre as repetições dentro de uma série) (Haff et al., 2003; 2008; Lawton et al., 2006).

Antes de atribuir as cargas de treinamento, o praticante precisa avaliar o nível de força do atleta para o(s) exercício(s) realizado(s) no programa. Isso é comumente alcançado avaliando 1RM do atleta para o exercício. No entanto, isso pode não ser seguro para indivíduos menos experientes e pode não ser prático usar esse método para todos os exercícios. Estratégias alternativas podem ser usadas para atribuir cargas de treinamento (Tabela 4.4).

Recuperação

Repetições máximas ou quase máximas envolvidas com exercícios de força e potência, geralmente, requerem longos intervalos de descanso entre séries para permitir a recuperação do sistema de fosfocreatina. Ao treinar para hipertrofia muscular, recuperações entre séries curtas a moderadas são usadas (30 a

Tabela 4.4 Métodos para determinar a carga de treinamento.

Teste de 1RM	Múltiplos RM	
Medir diretamente 1RM	Estimar 1RM a partir de um teste de RM múltiplos (*i. e.*, 5RM)	Múltiplos RM com base no número de repetições planejadas para esse exercício durante o bloco de treinamento (*i. e.*, 5 repetições por série)
Aquecimento com resistência leve. Calcule uma carga de aquecimento para permitir que o atleta complete 3 a 5 repetições 2 min de recuperação Estime uma carga conservadora quase máxima para permitir que o atleta execute 2 a 3 repetições 2 a 4 min de descanso Tente 1RM e repita até que seja alcançada 1RM (isso deve ocorrer em 2 ou 3 tentativas). Permita 2 a 4 min entre as tentativas Nota: se o atleta falhar na primeira tentativa, forneça 2 a 4 min de recuperação e, em seguida, trate a tentativa com uma carga mais leve (*i. e.*, 2,5 a 5% inferior [parte superior do corpo] a 5 a 10% [parte inferior do corpo])	Selecione as repetições-alvo (*i. e.*, 10RM) Aquecimento com resistência leve. Estime uma carga de aquecimento para permitir que o atleta complete o número desejado de repetições 2 min de recuperação Estime uma carga conservadora quase máxima para permitir que o atleta execute o número desejado de repetições Tente RM e repita até que RM seja alcançada (isso deve ocorrer em 2 ou 3 tentativas) Uma vez que a carga de RM é alcançada, 1RM pode ser estimada por meio de equações de regressão ou tabelas de conversão (ver Sheppard e Triplett, 2016)	Selecione as repetições-alvo (*i. e.*, 5RM) Aquecimento com resistência leve; estimar uma carga de aquecimento para permitir que o atleta complete o número desejado de repetições 2 min de recuperação Estime uma carga conservadora quase máxima para permitir que o atleta execute o número desejado de repetições 2 a 4 min de descanso Tente RM e repita até que RM seja alcançada (isso deve ocorrer em 2 ou 3 tentativas) Uma vez que a carga de RM seja atingida, pode ser usada no bloco de treinamento subsequente para esse exercício. A carga deve ser progredida de acordo com o bloco de treinamento (sobrecarga progressiva)
Adequado apenas para treinadores experientes	Apropriado para treinadores experientes e menos experientes	Apropriado para treinadores experientes e menos experientes Pode ser usado para estimar a carga de treinamento em todos os exercícios usados no bloco de treinamento subsequente – a avaliação ocorre na semana de descarga
Logisticamente difícil de realizar em todos os exercícios dentro de um programa Apenas exercícios básicos (*i. e.*, agachamento de costas, supino, levantamento terra, *power clean*) devem ser usados por segurança	Logisticamente difícil de realizar em todos os exercícios dentro de um programa Precisão de previsão de 1RM reduzida com o aumento da quantidade de repetições no teste Talvez não seja apropriado para exercícios de potência, como o *power clean*	É preciso ter cuidado ao usar exercícios que são mais desafiadores do ponto de vista metabólico (*i. e.*, *power clean*)

RM, repetição máxima.

Força e Condicionamento: Aspectos Científicos, Incluindo Princípios de Reabilitação **Capítulo** | **4** |

90 segundos), pois é recomendado que o atleta comece a série subsequente antes que a recuperação completa seja alcançada. A fim de satisfazer o princípio da especificidade, períodos curtos de recuperação (30 segundos) são frequentemente utilizados para almejar a resistência muscular (Sheppard e Triplett, 2016).

A Tabela 4.5 resume as diretrizes para a prescrição de exercícios de resistência com base na meta do treinamento, com um exemplo prático que ilustra sua aplicação no Boxe 4.1.

Periodização do treinamento

A periodização pode ser definida como "distribuição planejada ou variação nos métodos de treinamento" e significa uma "base cíclica ou periódica" (Plisk e Stone, 2003). Os objetivos da periodização são (1) explorar os efeitos do treinamento complementar em momentos ótimos, (2) controlar a fadiga e (3) prevenir a estagnação ou o supertreinamento. Uma abundância de modelos de periodização existe dentro do campo de força e condicionamento, como o tradicional (muitas vezes erroneamente denominado "linear"), o ondulante e o conjugado (Plisk e Stone, 2003). Grande parte da literatura existente apoia a noção de que a periodização de blocos pode fornecer resultados superiores em comparação aos outros modelos (DeWeese et al., 2015a; 2015b; Insurrin, 2008; 2010). A periodização do bloco é baseada na ideia de que uma carga concentrada pode ser usada para treinar uma característica específica durante cada fase de treinamento, mantendo as características previamente desenvolvidas, em vez de desenvolver múltiplas características fisiológicas ou habilidades motoras simultaneamente, o que pode ser contraproducente.

Como mencionado acima, a *sobrecarga progressiva* é vital em todos os aspectos do treinamento físico, seja o objetivo melhorar o desempenho esportivo ou reabilitar um atleta. Durante um modelo periodizado, o atleta progride por meio de fases (blocos), com cada uma visando à qualidade de condicionamento físico específico, culminando com o atleta atingindo o pico de condicionamento físico específico no momento exato da competição principal. Por exemplo, o treinamento pode começar com um foco básico geral antes de mudar para o condicionamento específico para esportes. Essa mudança de ênfase requer alterações no volume e na intensidade do treinamento (geralmente, para um atleta de potência de alto volume/baixa intensidade para baixo volume/alta intensidade) e na especificidade do treinamento (i. e., o treinamento se torna mais específico em relação às demandas mecânicas e metabólicas do esporte; ver Tabela 4.3).

Um aspecto importante da periodização do treinamento de força é controlar a fadiga. A Figura 4.5 ilustra o modelo de condicionamento físico-fadiga, segundo o qual, após um treino, o efeito da fadiga é grande, mas de curta duração, enquanto qualquer ganho de condicionamento físico é pequeno, porém de maior durabilidade. Assim, após um período de recuperação, quando a fadiga diminui, a qualidade de aptidão específica supercompensa. A implicação nisso é que o treinamento precisa ser cuidadosamente estruturado em microciclos (1 semana de treinamento) e mesociclos (bloco de treinamento), uma vez que os ganhos de condicionamento físico não são realizados até depois de um período de recuperação. Com relação aos mesociclos, a maioria dos treinadores planeja o treinamento em blocos de 4 semanas (Figura 4.6), nas quais o treinamento aumenta ao longo de um período de 3 semanas e é seguido de 1 semana de descarga para permitir a recuperação completa; geralmente, isso é obtido por meio da redução do volume, mantendo a intensidade. Observe que os blocos de 3 semanas podem ser usados para atletas jovens ou novatos, pois eles podem não possuir o histórico de treinamento necessário para tolerar um aumento de 3 semanas na carga de volume; dessa forma, um paradigma 2:1 é usado, em que o treinamento é progredido por 2 semanas e seguido de 1 semana de descarga.

O ano geral de treinamento é frequentemente referido como macrociclo (Bompa e Haff, 2009), que consiste em micro e mesociclos separados. O ano de treinamento pode ser dividido em fases de preparação e competição separadas por uma fase de transição, geralmente pré-competição (final da preparação) e recuperação ativa (final da temporada competitiva). Conforme mencionado acima, as fases de preparação podem ser divididas em preparação geral e específica (ver Tabela 4.3). Normalmente, a fase de condicionamento geral é mais focada na hipertrofia/resistência muscular e na força básica, enquanto a preparação específica pode se

Tabela 4.5 Resumo das diretrizes de prescrição de exercícios.

	Força	**Resistência muscular**	**Hipertrofia**	**Potência**
Ordem do exercício	• Mais elevações técnicas primeiro • Essencial • Assistência	• Essencial • Assistência	• Essencial • Assistência	• Potência • Outro essencial • Assistência
Carga	Alta: ≥ 85% 1RM	Baixa: ≤ 67% 1RM	Moderada: 67 a 85% 1RM	0 a 80% 1RM[a]
Repetições	≤ 6	12 a 20	6 a 12	1 a 6[b]
Séries	2 a 6	2 a 3	3 a 6	3 a 5
Recuperação	2 a 5 min	≥ 30 s	30 a 90 s	2 a 5 min

[a]Depende de objetivos de treinamento específicos (i. e., velocidade baixa *versus* alta) e de exercício de treinamento (ver Suchomel et al., 2017); [b]A produção de potência pode se deteriorar durante um conjunto de 3 a 6 repetições, mas pode ser minimizada, e a sobrecarga maximizada usando conjuntos de *cluster* (Haff et al., 2003; 2008; Lawton et al., 2006). Por exemplo, 6 repetições realizadas como 3 grupos de 2 repetições, com repouso intrarrepetição de 15 s entre cada uma das 2 repetições. RM, repetição máxima. (Adaptada de Sheppard, J.M., Triplett, N.T., 2016. Program design for resistance training. In: Haff, G.G., Triplett N.T. (Eds.) Essentials of Strength Training and Conditioning, fourth ed. Human Kinetics, Champaign, IL. pp. 439-469.)

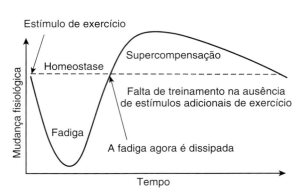

Figura 4.5 Paradigma de fadiga-aptidão no qual a periodização se baseia.

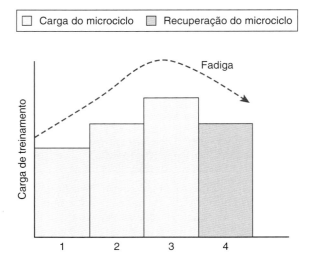

Figura 4.6 Exemplo de mesociclo de paradigma 3:1.

concentrar em força e potência máximas para um atleta típico de força-potência.

O exemplo mostrado na Tabela 4.3 ilustra uma abordagem de periodização bloqueada para um velocista seguindo o exemplo do Boxe 4.1. Aqui, o atleta começa o ano de treinamento com treinamento de resistência de alto volume e baixa intensidade (condicionamento geral). Isso fornece uma base para as fases posteriores de força e potência máximas (condicionamento específico). Cada bloco de treinamento seguiria um paradigma 3:1 (*i. e.*, 3 semanas de treinamento com carga de volume crescente e, em seguida, 1 semana de descarga, quando o volume do atleta diminui para facilitar a adaptação). Aqui, os exercícios são bem gerais e se tornam mais "específicos do esporte" à medida que o ano de treinamento se desenvolve em direção a uma grande competição. A pré-temporada para esse tipo de atleta é geralmente longa e, portanto, para evitar a monotonia e a estagnação, uma vez que uma base de força é estabelecida, os ciclos do atleta "bloqueiam" com foco na força máxima (70% da força/30% da potência) ou potência máxima (70% da potência/30% da força) para desenvolver ainda mais cada qualidade, enquanto permitem a manutenção da qualidade física previamente adquirida. Uma vez que o atleta chega à temporada competitiva, ele mantém ambas as qualidades antes de atingir o pico de potência antes da competição. O Boxe 4.2 ilustra o uso de uma abordagem de periodização para a reabilitação de um jogador de futebol devido a uma lesão por distensão da coxa.

A abordagem de periodização de bloco é altamente apropriada para atletas em esportes em que um único pico de competição é necessário. As dificuldades residem nos esportes em que há longas temporadas competitivas que exigem a manutenção das qualidades físicas ao longo das temporadas. Aqui, uma abordagem de periodização bloqueada pode ser usada na pré-temporada, anteriormente à temporada competitiva, para desenvolver qualidades físicas importantes, antes de mudar para uma abordagem de microciclos somados (Baker, 1998; 2001) durante a temporada, a fim de preservar as qualidades físicas desenvolvidas. Está além do escopo deste capítulo fornecer um exame aprofundado das diferentes abordagens de periodização disponíveis aos profissionais ou discutir outras questões, como treinamento simultâneo e redução gradual. O leitor interessado pode dirigir-se a Bompa e Haff (2009) para mais informações sobre periodização.

Resumo

Força e condicionamento são a aplicação do treinamento de força e os outros métodos de condicionamento para preparar fisicamente os atletas para o desempenho esportivo. Os terapeutas devem utilizar os princípios de força e condicionamento a fim de projetar programas de reabilitação eficazes que preparem melhor os atletas para o retorno ao jogo/competição. A força muscular é a capacidade de exercer força e é a base de TDF (taxa de desenvolvimento de força), potência, desempenho atlético e prevenção de lesões. A capacidade de expressar força depende de fatores neurais e morfológicos modificáveis. Para evocar essas adaptações, os programas de treinamento de força devem buscar proporcionar sobrecarga e levar em consideração a especificidade do estímulo, bem como a individualidade e o estado de treinamento do atleta. O modelo de periodização, a modalidade de treinamento de resistência e a prescrição de exercícios podem afetar ainda mais a força muscular, as adaptações de potência e a ênfase do treinamento. Os programas de treinamento de indivíduos mais fracos devem se concentrar em melhorar a força muscular antes de focar especificamente na potência. Em contraste, atletas mais fortes podem usar estratégias de treinamento avançadas para aumentar a potência enquanto mantêm ou melhoram seu nível de força.

Boxe 4.2 Exemplo de programa de recondicionamento periódico de isquiotibiais para um jogador de futebol

Lesões por estiramento dos isquiotibiais (LEI) são comuns no futebol (Ekstrand et al., 2011; 2013; Hawkins et al., 2001). Uma ampla gama de fatores de risco extrínsecos (p. ex., intervalo curto entre partidas, aumentos bruscos no volume da corrida de alta velocidade [CAV]) e intrínsecos (p. ex., comprimento do fascículo reduzido) está associada às LEI (Bengtsson et al., 2013; Duhig et al., 2016; Timmins et al., 2015). Lesão prévia é o fator mais comumente implicado devido às perdas de força e às mudanças morfológicas. A LEI resulta em carga excêntrica de alta velocidade (Schache et al., 2012), pois, durante a fase final de balanço do ciclo da marcha, os isquiotibiais trabalham excentricamente para desacelerar a coxa e a perna em preparação para o contato com o solo; as LEI foram associadas a essa fase (Heidercheit et al., 2005; Schache et al., 2012; Thelen et al., 2005). Assim, as características da força dos músculos isquiotibiais, particularmente a força excêntrica baixa (Jonhagen et al., 1994; Opar et al., 2015), também foram associadas à LEI. Uma compreensão da *periodização* é essencial para concluir uma reabilitação eficaz da LEI. No exemplo a seguir, o jogador sofreu uma ruptura de grau 2 no isquiotibial e está embarcando em um programa de reabilitação de 12 semanas antes de ser considerado para a seleção do time. Anteriormente a esse exemplo, o jogador foi submetido a tratamento inicial (repouso, gelo, compressão e elevação), seguido de alguma restauração da amplitude de movimento (alongamentos, 30 a 45 segundos por alongamento, realizados de 3 a 4 vezes/dia, juntamente com exercícios isométricos e de sustentação de peso sem dor).

Exemplo de programa de reabilitação para lesão do isquiotibial.

Preparação geral		*Preparação específica*	
Mesociclo 1	**Mesociclo 2**	**Mesociclo 3**	**Mesociclo 4**
3 semanas (paradigma 2:1)	**3 semanas (paradigma 2:1)**	**3 semanas (paradigma 2:1)**	**3 semanas (paradigma 2:1)**
Fortalecimento inicial	**Força geral (excêntrico de baixa velocidade)**	**Força/potência específica (excêntrico de alta velocidade)**	**Pré-competição**
Fortalecimento com foco em exercícios específicos para isquiotibiais (*i. e.*, flexão de perna; levantamento terra romeno). Aumentos graduais na amplitude de movimento (ADM). Os exercícios lombopélvicos (*i. e.*, pranchas, pontes de joelho dobradas e retas unilaterais e bilaterais, elevação dos glúteos) devem ser realizados em sessões separadas	Comece atividades excêntricas de baixa velocidade: levantamento terra romeno modificado, exercício nórdico para isquiotibiais, agachamentos/afundos divididos. Os exercícios lombopélvicos (*i. e.*, pranchas, pontes de joelho dobradas e retas unilaterais e bilaterais, elevação dos glúteos) devem ser realizados em sessões separadas	Exercícios excêntricos de alta velocidade (*i. e.*, pliometria) incorporados para desenvolver força excêntrica de alta velocidade. Os exercícios lombopélvicos (*i. e.*, pranchas, pontes de joelho dobradas e retas unilaterais e bilaterais, elevação dos glúteos) devem ser realizados em sessões separadas	Progresso para *sprint* específico para esportes, exercícios de mudança de direção. Exercícios pliométricos e exercícios de levantamento de peso enfatizando posições de "pegada" mais profundas, para aumentar a carga excêntrica dos isquiotibiais, formam a base das sessões de ginástica (detalhadas abaixo). Força e ADM devem ser mantidas. Os exercícios lombopélvicos (*i. e.*, pranchas, pontes de joelho dobradas e retas unilaterais e bilaterais, elevação dos glúteos) devem ser realizados em sessões separadas
Sessão 1			
Agachamento com peso (70 a 75% 1RM × 10 × 3) Levantamento terra romeno (70 a 75% 1RM × 10 × 3)	Agachamento dividido (85% 1RM × 6 × 3) Levantamento terra romeno excêntrico (LTR)/ levantamento terra concêntrico (110% 1RM LTR × 3 a 4 × 2 a 3)	*Hang clean* (40 a 60% 1RM *clean* × 5 × 3) Afundo excêntrico (3 × 5 em cada perna) LTR de perna única (50% LTR 1RM × 6 × 3)	Arremesso em suspensão (*hang squat clean*) (80% 1RM *clean* × 3 × 3) Saltos de barreira frontal e lateral bilateral ou unipodal (4 × 10)

(continua)

Boxe 4.2 Exemplo de programa de recondicionamento periódico de isquiotibiais para um jogador de futebol *(Continuação)*			
Preparação geral		*Preparação específica*	
Mesociclo 1	**Mesociclo 2**	**Mesociclo 3**	**Mesociclo 4**
3 semanas (paradigma 2:1)	**3 semanas (paradigma 2:1)**	**3 semanas (paradigma 2:1)**	**3 semanas (paradigma 2:1)**
Fortalecimento inicial	**Força geral (excêntrico de baixa velocidade)**	**Força/potência específica (excêntrico de alta velocidade)**	**Pré-competição**
Sessão 2			
Agachamento frontal (70 a 75% 1RM × 10 × 3) Flexão de perna em bola suíça (10 a 12 × 3)	Afundo para frente (85% 1RM × 6 × 3) Exercício nórdico para isquiotibiais (PC × 3 × 2 a 4)	*Hang snatch pulls* (40 a 60% 1RM *snatch* × 5 × 3) Avanço (85% 1RM × 5 × 2 cada perna) *Box drop* do tipo excêntrica (3 × 6)	*Hang squat snatch* (70% 1RM *snatch* × 3 × 3) Saltos em profundidade (3 × 6)

ADM, amplitude de movimento; *RM*, repetição máxima; *LTR*, levantamento terra romeno; *PC*, peso corporal. (Adaptado de Bengtsson, H., Ekstrand, J., & Hägglund, M., 2013. Muscle injury rates in professional football increase with fixture congestion: an 11-year follow-up of the UEFA Champions League injury study. Brit. J. Sports Med. 47, 743–747.

Duhig, S., Shield, A.J., Opar, D., Gabbett, T.J., Ferguson, C., Williams, M., 2016. Effect of high-speed running on hamstring strain injury risk. British Journal of Sports Medicine 50, 1536–1540.
Ekstrand, J., Hägglund, M., Waldén, M., 2011. Epidemiology of muscle injuries in professional football (soccer). The American Journal of Sports Medicine 39, 1226–1232.
Ekstrand, J., Hägglund, M., Kristenson, K., Magnusson, H., Waldén, M., 2013. Fewer ligament injuries but no preventive effect on muscle injuries and severe injuries: an 11-year follow-up of the UEFA champions league injury study. British Journal of Sports Medicine 47, 732–737.
Hawkins, R.D., Hulse, M.A., Wilkinson, C., Hodson, A., Gibson, M., 2001. The association football medical research programme: an audit of injuries in professional football. British Journal of Sports Medicine 35, 43–47.
Heiderscheit, B.C., Hoerth, D.M., Chumanov, E.S., Swanson, S.C., Thelen, B.J., Thelen, D.G., 2005. Identifying the time of occurrence of a hamstring strain injury during treadmill running: a case study. Clinical Biomechanics 20, 1072–1078.
Jonhagen, S., Nemeth, G., Eriksson, E., 1994. Hamstring injuries in sprinters. the role of concentric and eccentric hamstring muscle strength and flexibility. The American Journal of Sports Medicine 22, 262–266.
Opar, D.A., Williams, M.D., Timmins, R.G., Hickey, J., Duhig, S.J., Shield, A.J., 2015. Eccentric hamstring strength and hamstring injury risk in Australian footballers. Medicine and Science in Sports and Exercise 47 (4), 857–865.
Schache, A.G., Dorn, T.W., Blanch, P.D., Brown, N.A.T., Pandy., M.G., 2012. Mechanics of the human hamstring muscles during sprinting. Medicine and Science in Sports and Exercise 44 (4), 647–658.
Thelen, D.G., Chumanov, E.S., Best, T.M., Swanson, S.C., Heiderscheit, B.C., 2005. Simulation of biceps femoris musculo-tendon mechanics during the swing phase of sprinting. Medicine and Science in Sports and Exercise 37, 1931–1938.
Timmins, R.G., Bourne, M.N., Shield, A.J., Williams, M.D., Lorenzen, C., Opar, D.A., 2015. A short biceps femoris long head fascicle length and eccentric knee flexor weakness increase risk of hamstring injury: a prospective cohort study in 152 elite professional football players. British Journal of Sports Medicine 50 (24), 1524–1535.)

Parte | 1 | Conceitos Básicos Importantes em Esportes

Referências bibliográficas

Aagaard, P., Simonsen, E.B., Andersen, J.L., Magnusson, P., Dyhre-Poulsen, P., 2002. Increased rate of force development and neural drive of human skeletal muscle following resistance training. Journal of Applied Physiology 93, 1318-1326.

Aagaard, P., 2003. Training-induced changes in neural function. Exercise and Sport Sciences Reviews 31, 61-67.

Aagaard, P., Simonsen, E.B., Andersen, J.L., Magnusson, S.P., Halkjaer-Kristensen, J., Dyhre-Poulsen, P., 2000. Neural inhibition during maximal eccentric and concentric quadriceps contraction: effects of resistance training. Journal of Applied Physiology 89, 2249-2257.

Andersen, L.L., Aagaard, P., 2006. Influence of maximal muscle strength and intrinsic muscle contractile properties on contractile rate of force development. European Journal of Applied Physiology 96, 46-52.

Anderson, K., Behm, D.G., 2005. Trunk muscle activity increases with unstable squat movements. Canadian Journal of Applied Physiology 30, 33-45.

Asadi, A., Arazi, H., Young, W.B., Sáez de Villarreal, E., 2016. The effects of plyometric training on change of direction ability: A meta-analysis. International Journal of Sports Physiology and Performance 11, 563-573.

Augustsson, J., Esko, A., Thomee, R., Sventesson, U., 1998. Weight training of the thigh muscles using closed vs. open kinetic chain exercises: a comparison of performance enhancement. Journal of Orthopaedic Sports Physical Therapy 27, 3-8.

Baker, D., 1998. Applying the in-season periodisation of strength and power training to football. Strength & Conditioning 20 (2), 18-27.

Baker, D., 2001. The effects of an in-season of concurrent training on the maintenance of maximal strength and power in professional and college-aged rugby league players. Journal of Strength and Conditioning Research 15 (2), 172-177.

Baker, D., 2001. Comparison of upper-body strength and power between professional and college-aged rugby league players. Journal of Strength and Conditioning Research 15, 30-35.

Blazevich, A.J., 2006. Effects of physical training and detraining, immobilisation, growth and aging on human fascicle geometry. Sports Medicine 36, 1003-1017.

Bruton, A., 2002. Muscle plasticity: response to training and detraining. Physiotherapy 88 (7), 398-408.

Behm, D.G., Anderson, K.G., 2006. The role of instability with resistance training. Journal of Strength and Conditioning Research 20, 716-722.

Behm, D.G., Sale, D.G., 1993. Intended rather than actual movement velocity determines velocity-specific training response. Journal of Applied Physiology 74, 359-368.

Blackburn, J.R., Morrissey, M.C., 1998. The relationship between open and closed kinetic chain strength of the lower limb and jumping performance. Journal of Orthopaedic Sports Physical Therapy 27 (6), 430-435.

Bompa, T.O., Haff, G., 2009. Periodization: Theory and Methodology of Training. Human Kinetics, Champaign, IL.

Brandenburg, J.E., Docherty, D., 2002. The effects of accentuated eccentric loading on strength, muscle hypertrophy, and neural adaptations in trained individuals. Journal of Strength and Conditioning Research 16, 25-32.

Comfort, P., Stewart, A., Bloom, L., Clarkson, B., 2014. Relationships between strength, sprint, and jump performance in well-trained youth soccer players. Journal of Strength & Conditioning Research 28 (1), 173-177.

Cormie, P., McCaulley, G.O., McBride, J.M., 2007. Power versus strength–power jump squat training: influence on the load–power relationship. Medicine and Science in Sports and Exercise 39 (6), 996-1003.

Cormie, P., McGuigan, M.R., Newton, R.U., 2010a. Influence of strength on magnitude and mechanisms of adaptation to power training. Medicine and Science in Sports and Exercise 42 1566-158.

Cormie, P., McGuigan, M.R., Newton, R.U., 2010b. Adaptations in athletic performance after ballistic power versus strength training. Medicine and Science in Sports and Exercise 42 (8), 1582-1598.

Cormie, P., McGuigan, M.R., Newton, R.U., 2011. Developing maximal neuromuscular power: Part 2 – training considerations for improving maximal power production. Sports Medicine 41 (2), 125-146.

De Hoyo, M., Pozzo, M., Sañudo, B., Carrasco, L., Gonzalo-Skok, O., Domínguez-Cobo, S., et al., 2015. Effects of a 10-week in-season eccentric-overload training program on muscle-injury prevention and performance in junior elite soccer players. International Journal of Sports Physiology and Performance 10, 46-52.

Demirel, H.A., Powers, S.K., Naito, H., Hughes, M., Coombes, J.S., 1999. Exercise-induced alterations in skeletal muscle myosin heavy chain phenotype: dose–response relationship. Journal of Applied Physiology (1985) 86 (3), 1002-1008.

Devries, H.A., Housh, T.J., 1994. Physiology of Exercise for Physical Education, Athletics and Exercise Science, fifth ed. Brown & Benchmark, Madison, WI.

Deweese, B.H., Hornsby, G., Stone, M., Stone, M.H., 2015a. The training process: planning for strength–power training in track and field. Part 1: theoretical aspects. The Journal of Sport and Health Science 4, 308-317.

Deweese, B.H., Hornsby, G., Stone, M., Stone, M.H., 2015b. The training process: planning for strength–power training in track and field. Part 2: practical and applied aspects. The Journal of Sport and Health Science 4, 318-324.

Dinubile, N.A., 1991. Strength training. Clinics in Sports Medicine 10 (1), 33-62.

Douglas, J., Pearson, S., Ross, A., McGuigan, M.R., 2016a. Chronic adaptations to eccentric training: a systematic review. Sports Medicine 47 (5), 917-941.

Douglas, J., Pearson, S., Ross, A., McGuigan, M.R., 2016b. Eccentric exercise: physiological characteristics and acute responses. Sports Medicine 47 (4), 663-675.

Earp, J.E., Kraemer, W.J., Newton, R.U., Comstock, B.A., Fragala, M.S., Dunn-Lewis, C., et al., 2010. Lower-body muscle structure and its role in jump performance during squat, countermovement, and depth drop jumps. Journal of Strength and Conditioning Research 24, 722-729.

Ebben, W.P., Jensen, R.L., 2002. Electromyographic and kinetic analysis of traditional, chain, and elastic band squats. Journal of Strength and Conditioning Research 16, 547-550.

Enoka, R.M., 1988. Muscle strength and its development: new perspectives. Sports Medicine 6, 146-168.

Fleck, S.J., Kraemer, W.J., 2014. Designing Resistance Training Programs, fouth ed. Human Kinetics, Champaign, IL.

Gea, J.G., 1997. Myosin gene expression in the respiratory muscles. The European Respiratory Journal 10, 2404-2410.

Ghez, C., 1991. Muscles: effectors of the motor systems. In: Kandel, E.R., Schwartz, J.H., Jessell, T.M. (Eds.), Principles of Neural Science, third ed. Elsevier, New York, pp. 548-563.

Haff, G.G., 2000. Roundtable discussion: machines versus free weights. Strength and Conditioning Journal 22, 18-30.

Haff, G.G., Whitley, L.B., McCoy, H.S., O'Bryant, J.L., Kilgore, E., Haff, E.,K., et al., 2003. Effects of different set configurations on barbell velocity and displacement during a clean pull. Journal of Strength and Conditioning Research 17, 95-103.

Haff, G.G., Hobbs, R.T., Haff, E., Sands, W.A., Pierce, K.C., Stone, M.H., 2008. Cluster training: a novel method for introduction training program variation. Strength and Conditioning Journal 30, 67-76.

Hakkinen, K., Newton, R.U., Gordon, S.E., McCormick, M., Volek, J.S., Nindl, B.C., et al., 1998. Changes in muscle morphology, electromyographic activity, and force production characteristics during progressive strength training in young and older men. The Journals of Gerontology 53A (6), B415-B423.

Harris, N.K., Cronin, J.B., Hopkins, W.G., Hansen, K.T., 2008. Squat jump training at maximal power loads vs. heavy loads: effect on sprint ability. Journal of Strength and Conditioning Research 22, 1742-1749.

Harrison, J.S., 2010. Bodyweight training: a return to basics. Strength and Conditioning Journal 32, 52-55.

Henneman, E., Olson, C.B., 1965. Relations between structure and function in the design of skeletal muscles. Journal of Neurophysiology 28, 581-598.

Henneman, E., Somjen, G., Carpenter, D.O., 1965. Functional significance of cell size in spinal motoneurons. Journal of Neurophysiology 28, 560-580.

Hewett, T.E., Stroupe, A.L., Nance, T.A., Noyes, F.R., 1996. Plyometric training in female athletes. decreased impact forces and increased hamstring torques. The American Journal of Sports Medicine 24 (6), 765-773.

Hill, A.V., 1970. First and Last Experiments in Muscle Mechanics. Cambridge University Press, London.

Holloszy, J.O., 1976. Adaptations of muscular tissue to training. Prog. Cardiovasc. Dis. 18 (6), 445-458.

Hori, N., Newton, R.U., Andres, W.A., Kawamori, N., McGuigan, M.R., Nosaka, K., 2008. Does performance of hang power clean differentiate performance of jumping, sprinting, and changing of direction? Journal of Strength & Conditioning Research 22 (2), 412-418.

Hortobagyi, T., Hill, J.P., Houmard, J.A., Fraser, D.D., Lambert, N.J., Israel, R.G., 1996. Adaptive responses to muscle lengthening and shortening in humans. Journal of Applied Physiology (1985) 80 (3), 765-772.

Housh, D.J., Housh, T.J., Johnson, G.O., Chu, W.K., 1992. Hypertrophic response to unilateral concentric isokinetic resistance training. Journal of Applied Physiology (1985) 73 (1), 65-70.

Jones, P.A., Bampouras, T., Comfort, P., 2013a. A review of complex and contrast training: implications for practice. Part 1. Professional Strength & Conditioning 29, 11-20.

Jones, P.A., Bampouras, T., Comfort, P., 2013b. A review of complex and contrast training: implications for practice. Part 2. Professional Strength & Conditioning 30, 27-30.

Ingjer, F., 1979. Capillary supply and mitochondrial content of different skeletal muscle fiber types in untrained and endurance-trained men. A histochemical and ultrastructural study. European Journal of Applied Physiology and Occupational Physiology 40, 197-209.

Israetel, M.A., McBride, J.M., Nuzzo, J.L., Skinner, J.W., Dayne, A.M., 2010. Kinetic and kinematic differences between squats performed with and without elastic bands. Journal of Strength and Conditioning Research 24, 190-194.

Issurin, V.B., 2008. Block periodization versus traditional training theory: a review. The Journal of Sports Medicine and Physical Fitness 48, 65-75.

Issurin, V.B., 2010. New horizons for the methodology and physiology of training periodization. Sports Medicine 40, 189-206.

Izquierdo, M., Hakkinen, K., Anton, A., Garrues, M., Ibanez, J., Ruesta, M., et al., 2001. Maximal strength and power, endurance performance, and serum hormones in middle-aged and elderly men. Medicine and Science in Sports and Exercise 33, 1577-1587.

Izquierdo, M., Ibanez, J., Gonzalez-Badillo, J.J., Hakkinen, K., Ratamess, N.A., Kraemer, W.J., et al., 2006. Differential effects of strength training leading to failure versus not to failure on hormonal responses, strength, and muscle power gains. Journal of Applied Physiology (1985) 100, 1647-1656.

Kaneko, M., Fuchimoto, T., Toji, H., Suei, K., 1983. Training effect of different loads on the force–velocity relationship and mechanical power output in human muscle. Scandinavian Journal of Medicine & Science in Sports 5, 50-55.

Kawakami, Y., Abe, T., Fukunaga, T., 1993. Muscle-fiber pennation angles are greater in hypertrophied than in normal muscles. Journal of Applied Physiology 74 (6), 2740-2744.

Kawakami, Y., Abe, T., Kuno, S.-Y., Fukunaga, T., 1995. Training-induced changes in muscle architecture and specific tension. European Journal of Applied Physiology 72 (1-2), 37-43.

Kirkpatrick, J., Comfort, P., 2012. Strength, power, and speed qualities in English junior elite rugby league players. Journal of Strength and Conditioning Research 27 (9), 2414-2419.

Komi, P.V., 1986. Training of muscle strength and power: interaction of neuromotoric, hypertrophic, and mechanical factors. Journal of Strength and Conditioning Research 7 (Suppl.), 10-15.

Lake, J.P., Lauder, M.A., 2012. Kettlebell swing training improves maximal and explosive strength. Journal of Strength and Conditioning Research 26, 2228-2233.

Lake, J.P., Lauder, M.A., Smith, N.A., Shorter, K.A., 2012. A comparison of ballistic and non-ballistic lower-body resistance exercise and the methods used to identify their positive lifting phases. Journal of Applied Biomechanics 28, 431-437.

Lawton, T.W., Croin, J.B., Lindsell, R.P., 2006. Effect of inter-repetition rest intervals on weight training repetition power output. Journal of Strength and Conditioning Research 20, 172-176.

Manal, K., Roberts, D.P., Buchanan, T.S., 2006. Optimal pennation angle of the primary ankle plantar and dorsiflexors: variations with sex, contraction intensity, and limb. Journal of Applied Biomechanics 22, 255-263.

Melissa, L., MacDougall, J.D., Tarnopolsky, M.A., Cipriano, N., Green, H.J., 1997. Skeletal muscle adaptations to training under normobaric hypoxic versus normoxic conditions. Medicine and Science in Sports and Exercise 29 (2), 238-243.

Milner-Brown, H.S., Stein, R.B., Yemm, R., 1973. The orderly recruitment of human motor units during voluntary isometric contractions. Journal of Physiology (London) 230, 359-370.

Morrissey, M.C., Harman, E.A., Johnson, M.J., 1995. Resistance training modes: specificity and effectiveness. Medicine and Science in Sports and Exercise 27, 648-660.

Narici, M.V., Hoppeler, H., Kayser, B., Landoni, L., Claassen, H., Gavardi, C., et al., 1996. Human quadriceps cross-sectional area, torque and neural activation during 6 months strength training. Acta Physiologica Scandinavica 157 (2), 175-186.

Newton, R.U., Kraemer, W.J., Häkkinen, K., Humphries, B., Murphy, A.J., 1996. Kinematics, kinetics, and muscle activation during explosive upper body movements. Journal of Applied Biomechanics 12, 31-43.

Nimphius, S., McGuigan, M.R., Newton, R.U., 2010. Relationship between strength, power, speed, and change of direction performance of female softball players. Journal of Strength and Conditioning Research 24 (4), 885-895.

Ojasto, T., Häkkinen, K., 2009. Effects of different accentuated eccentric load levels in eccentric-concentric actions on acute neuromuscular, maximal force, and power responses. Journal of Strength and Conditioning Research 23, 996-1004.

Otto III, W.H., Coburn, J.W., Brown, L.E., Spiering, B.A., 2012. Effects of weightlifting vs. kettlebell training on vertical jump, strength, and body composition. Journal of Strength and Conditioning Research 26, 1199-1202.

Plisk, S.S., Stone, M.H., 2003. Periodization strategies. Strength & Conditioning Journal 25 (6), 19-37.

Robbins, D.W., 2005. Postactivation potentiation and its practical applicability: a brief review. Journal of Strength and Conditioning Research 19, 453-458.

Rohter, F.D., Rochelle, R.H., Hyman, C., 1963. Exercise blood flow changes in the human forearm during physical training. Journal of Applied Physiology 18 (4), 789-793.

Sáez de Villarreal, E., Kellis, E., Kraemer, W.J., Izquierdo, M., 2009. Determining variables of plyometric training for improving vertical jump height performance: a meta-analysis. Journal of Strength and Conditioning Research 23 (2), 495-506.

Sáez de Villarreal, E., Requena, B., Cronin, J.B., 2012. The effects of plyometric training on sprint performance: a meta-analysis. Journal of Strength and Conditioning Research 26 (2), 575-584 2012.

Sale, D.G., 1988. Neural adaptation to resistance training. Medicine and Science in Sports and Exercise 20 (5), S135-S145.

Sale, D.G., MacDougall, J.D., Upton, A.R.M., McComas, A.J., 1983. Effect of strength training upon motor neurone excitability in man. Medicine and Science in Sports and Exercise 15 (1), 57-62.

Seitz, L.B., Reyes, A., Tran, T.T., Sáez de Villarreal, E., Haff, G.G., 2014a. Increases in lower-body strength transfer positively to sprint performance: a systematic review with meta-analysis. Sports Medicine 44 (12), 1693-1702.

Seitz, L.B., Sáez de Villarreal, E., Haff, G.G., 2014b. The temporal profile of postactivation potentiation is related to strength level. Journal of Strength and Conditioning Research 28, 706-715.

Sheppard, J., Hobson, S., Barker, M., Taylor, K., Chapman, D., McGuigan, M., et al., 2008. The effect of training with accentuated eccentric load counter-movement jumps on strength and power characteristics of high-performance volleyball players. The International Journal of Sports Science & Coaching 3, 355-363.

Sheppard, J.M., Triplett , N.T., 2016. Program design for resistance training. In: Haff, G.G., Triplett, N.T. (Eds.), Essentials of Strength Training and Conditioning, fourth ed. Human Kinetics, Champaign, IL, pp. 439-469.

Simoneau, J.A., Lortie, G., Boulay, M.R., Marcotte, M., Thibault, M.C., Bouchard, C., 1986. Inheritance of human skeletal muscle and anaerobic capacity adaptation to high-intensity intermittent training. International Journal of Sports Medicine 7 (3), 167-171.

Spurrs, R.W., Murphy, A.J., Watsford, M.L., 2002. The effect of plyometric training on distance running performance. European Journal of Applied Physiology 89, 1-7.

Staron, R.S., Karapondo, D.L., Kraemer, W.J., Fry, A.C., Gordon, S.E., Falkel, J.E., et al., 1994. Skeletal muscle adaptations during early phase of heavy-resistance training in men and women. Journal of Applied Physiology 76 (3), 1247-1255.

Stone, M.H., Moir, G., Glaister, M., Sanders, R., 2002. How much strength is necessary? Physical Therapy in Sport 3, 88-96.

Stone, M.H., Pierce, K.C., Sands, W.A., Stone, M.E., 2006. Weightlifting: a brief review. Strength and Conditioning Journal 28 (1), 50-66.

Styles, W.J., Matthews, M.J., Comfort, P., 2015. Effects of strength training on squat and sprint performance in soccer players. Journal of Strength & Conditioning Research 30 (6), 1534-1539.

Suchomel, T.J., Comfort, P., 2017. Developing strength and power. In: Tuner, A., Comfort, P. (Eds.), Advanced Strength and Conditioning. Routledge, Oxon, pp. 13-38.

Suchomel, T.J., Comfort, P., Lake, J.P., 2017. Enhancing the force–velocity profile of athletes using weightlifting derivatives. Strength & Conditioning Journal 39 (1), 10-20.

Suchomel, T.J., Comfort, P., Stone, M.H., 2015. Weightlifting pulling derivatives: rationale for implementation and application. Sports Medicine 45 (6), 823-839.

Suchomel, T.J., Sato, K., Deweese, B.H., Ebben, W.P., Stone, M.H., 2016. Potentiation following ballistic and non-ballistic complexes: the effect of strength level. Journal of Strength and Conditioning Research 30, 1825-1833.

Suetta, C., Aagaard, P., Rosted, A., Jakobsen, A.K., Duus, B., Kjaer, M., et al., 2004. Training-induced changes in muscle CSA, muscle strength, EMG, and rate of force development in elderly subjects after long-term unilateral disuse. Journal of Applied Physiology (1985) 97, 1954-1961.

Toji, H., Suei, K., Kaneko, M., 1997. Effects of combined training loads on relations among force, velocity, and power development. Canadian Journal of Applied Physiology 22, 328-336.

Toji, H., Kaneko, M., 2004. Effect of multiple-load training on the force–velocity relationship. Journal of Strength and Conditioning Research 18, 792-795.

Turner, A.M., Owings, M., Schwane, J.A., 2003. Improvements in running economy after 6 weeks of plyometric training. Journal of Strength and Conditioning Research 17, 60-67.

Van Cutsem, M., Duchateau, J., Hainaut, K., 1998. Changes in single motor unit behaviour contribute to the increase in contraction speed after dynamic training in humans. The Journal of Physiology 513, 295-305.

Vanderhoof, E.R., Imig, C.J., Hines, H.M., 1961. Effect of muscle strength and endurance development on blood flow. Journal of Applied Physiology 16 (5), 873-877.

Wallace, B.J., Winchester, J.B., McGuigan, M.R., 2006. Effects of elastic bands on force and power characteristics during the back squat exercise. Journal of Strength and Conditioning Research 20, 268-272.

Wisloff, U., Castagna, C., Helgerud, J., Jones, R., Hoff, J., 2004. Strong correlation of maximal squat strength with sprint performance and vertical jump height in elite soccer players. British Journal of Sports Medicine 38 (3), 285-288.

Zatsiorsky, V.M., Kraemer, W.J., 2006. Science and Practice of Strength Training, second ed. Human Kinetics, Champaign, IL.

Capítulo | 5 |

Biomecânica das Lesões Esportivas, Manejo e Considerações Clínicas

Jim Richards, Carrie Docherty, Brent Arnold, Kim Hébert-Losier, Charlotte Häger, Bruno Mazuquin e Puneet Monga

Introdução

Este capítulo focará nos fatores biomecânicos associados a diferentes lesões esportivas e nas considerações clínicas em seu tratamento, além de concentrar-se em três dos locais de lesão mais comuns: tornozelo lateral e ligamento cruzado anterior no joelho e no ombro.

Lesões no tornozelo

Carrie Docherty, Brent Arnold

Epidemiologia

A entorse lateral do tornozelo é a lesão mais comum que ocorre durante a atividade física (Hootman et al., 2007). Nos EUA, a incidência de entorses de tornozelo em indivíduos fisicamente ativos é de 0,68 a 3,85 entorses de tornozelo por mil pessoas/dia ou 5 a 7 entorses por mil pessoas/ano. Isso equivale a aproximadamente 2 milhões de entorses de tornozelo agudas a cada ano apenas nos EUA (Waterman et al., 2010). Existem disparidades entre a incidência de entorses de tornozelo entre homens e mulheres, com as mulheres sofrendo entorses de tornozelo a uma taxa mais elevada de 13,6 por mil em comparação a 6,9 por mil para os homens (Doherty et al., 2014).

Mecanismo e apresentação clínica

As entorses laterais de tornozelo podem ser causadas por mecanismos de contato e sem contato. Lesões sem contato são normalmente o resultado de inversão descontrolada e rotação interna após o contato inicial do pé (Gehring et al., 2013). Ao que parece, esse mecanismo pode ocorrer com ou sem a presença de flexão plantar. Em contrapartida, as lesões por contato são mais frequentemente o resultado de (1) contato jogador contra jogador no aspecto medial da perna um pouco antes ou no golpe do pé causando um mecanismo de inversão ou (2) flexão plantar forçada, em que o jogador lesionado bateu no pé do adversário ao tentar arremessar ou chutar a bola. Essas lesões são mais comumente vistas em esportes de campo e de quadra, com a entorse de tornozelo sendo responsável por 15% de todas as lesões no atletismo escolar organizado (Hootman et al., 2007).

Ao avaliar a anatomia do tornozelo, é fundamental perceber o importante papel que a tíbia e a fíbula desempenham na ocorrência de lesões no tornozelo. O lado medial do tornozelo não é comumente lesionado, porque a fíbula cria um bloqueio ósseo que reduz a amplitude de movimento durante os movimentos de eversão. No entanto, a parte lateral do tornozelo carece dessa infraestrutura óssea; assim, as estruturas laterais são mais facilmente danificadas. Quando ocorre uma entorse de tornozelo por inversão, ela tem o potencial de causar danos aos ligamentos, bem como aos músculos e aos nervos que cruzam a articulação do tornozelo. Portanto, todas essas estruturas devem ser consideradas no manejo dessa lesão, sendo necessária uma avaliação direcionada.

Não apenas a lesão inicial é uma área de preocupação, mas a incidência de nova lesão, instabilidade recorrente e consequências a longo prazo de uma entorse lateral de tornozelo são reconhecidas como um grande fardo para a saúde. Estudos epidemiológicos descobriram que as taxas de recorrência de entorse de tornozelo entre atletas nacionais, competitivos e recreativos chegam a 73%, com 22% sofrendo cinco ou mais lesões no mesmo tornozelo ao longo da vida (Yeung et al., 1994). Muitos indivíduos continuarão a descrever sensações recorrentes de instabilidade por meses e até anos após a lesão inicial. Esse fenômeno é conhecido como instabilidade crônica do tornozelo. Esses problemas recorrentes estão criando um fardo financeiro por meio do aumento dos custos de saúde, bem como fardos para a saúde. Indivíduos com histórico de lesões no tornozelo são menos ativos fisicamente à medida que envelhecem e podem apresentar o aparecimento precoce de osteoartrose do tornozelo. Foi relatado que quase 90% dos pacientes de 19 anos ou mais com entorse lateral aguda do tornozelo têm lesões osteocondrais (Taga et al., 1993). Uma possível explicação para essas consequências a longo prazo é o rápido retorno ao jogo após uma lesão.

A maioria dos indivíduos retorna à prática esportiva após uma entorse de tornozelo pela primeira vez depois de 3 dias, enquanto os indivíduos que sofrem de entorse de tornozelo recorrente retornam em apenas 1 dia (McKeon et al., 2014). Esse rápido retorno ao jogo ocorre mesmo que os indivíduos experimentem frouxidão mecânica por até 1 ano após a lesão inicial (Hubbard e Hicks-Little, 2008). Portanto, o tratamento de entorses de tornozelo deve incorporar a reabilitação a longo prazo, a qual pode diminuir as chances de uma nova lesão.

Protocolos de reabilitação do tornozelo

Os protocolos de reabilitação do tornozelo podem ser divididos em três grandes áreas: treinamento de equilíbrio como a única intervenção (Lee e Lin, 2008; Matsusaka et al., 2001), treinamento de força (Docherty et al., 1998; Sekir et al., 2007) e treinamento neuromuscular (Coughlan e Caulfield, 2007; Ross et al., 2007). Os estudos de reabilitação usaram uma variedade de medidas que abrange um contínuo para avaliar a eficácia, incluindo a fisiologia, os prejuízos, a limitação funcional (muitas vezes ignorada em avaliações rápidas) e a deficiência.

As medidas fisiológicas do desempenho neuromuscular na reabilitação incluem latências reflexas e propriocepção. O prejuízo pode ser representado por mudanças no nível do órgão (McLeod et al., 2008; Snyder et al., 2008). Isso inclui medidas associadas ao desempenho da extremidade inferior e são representadas como medidas de equilíbrio e testes de desempenho físico, como salto. A função autorrelatada inclui a avaliação das atividades da vida diária, englobando as esportivas. Estas podem ser medidas pelo Índice de Incapacidade de Pé e Tornozelo (FADI, *Foot and Ankle Disability Index*); pelo FADI *Sport*; pela medida de habilidade do pé e tornozelo (FAAM, *Foot and Ankle Ability Measure*) e pela ferramenta de avaliação funcional da articulação do tornozelo (AJFAT, *Ankle Joint Functional Assessment Tool*), enquanto a deficiência é frequentemente medida como qualidade de vida relacionada com a saúde geral (QVRS).

Protocolos de treinamento de força

Um dos métodos mais comuns de treinamento de força do tornozelo é o exercício com uso de faixa elástica. Docherty et al. (1998) descobriram que os exercícios de faixa elástica melhoram a força do dorsiflexor e do eversor, além de também melhorarem a sensação de reposição articular ativa nas direções de inversão e flexão plantar. Do mesmo modo, Hall et al. (2015) concluíram que o treinamento com faixa elástica melhora a força dos inversores, eversores, flexores plantares e dorsiflexores. No entanto, em contrapartida, Wright et al., 2016 descobriram que o treinamento com faixa elástica falhou em melhorar a força. Essas discrepâncias podem ser explicadas pelo fato de que diferentes níveis de resistência foram utilizados durante os protocolos de treinamento.

Como alternativa ao exercício com faixa elástica, Sekir et al. (2007) demonstraram que o exercício isocinético melhorou a força em tornozelos instáveis. Os picos de torque concêntrico de inversão e de eversão foram significativamente maiores após o treinamento. Esse déficit funcional é apoiado sobre uma metanálise da força do tornozelo em tornozelos instáveis e é discutido por Arnold et al. (2009), que descobriram que tornozelos instáveis eram mais fracos do que tornozelos não lesionados, e Feger et al. (2016), que identificaram uma diminuição do volume muscular com instabilidade crônica. Isso sugere que os tornozelos lesionados são realmente mais fracos, mas talvez as medidas de força do tornozelo tenham uma capacidade de resposta limitada às mudanças induzidas pela reabilitação.

Treino de equilíbrio

Alterações na fisiopatologia

O treinamento de equilíbrio é um tratamento comum usado para a instabilidade do tornozelo e, geralmente, é combinado com outras terapias. Vários estudos relataram os efeitos do treinamento de equilíbrio (Lee e Lin, 2008; Wright et al., 2016).

O uso de dispositivos de alçapão para medir as latências do fibular longo e do tibial anterior mostrou que o treinamento de equilíbrio diminui os tempos de latência em ambos os músculos em até 30% em comparação aos controles. Isso indica que a resposta à perturbação inesperada é mais rápida após o treinamento. No entanto, não se sabe como isso se traduz em melhora do paciente.

Também foi demonstrado que a sensação de reposição articular ativa e passiva é melhorada após o treinamento de equilíbrio. Novamente, não se sabe se essas mudanças estão relacionadas com a melhora do paciente. No entanto, há algumas evidências de que o treinamento de equilíbrio melhora as deficiências fisiopatológicas do tornozelo.

Efeitos nas medidas de deficiência

As medidas de comprometimento do tornozelo incluem medidas de equilíbrio e medidas baseadas no desempenho, como salto. Essas medidas podem ser subdivididas em medidas laboratoriais e clínicas.[1]

Conforme os definimos, os métodos baseados em equipamentos laboratoriais incluem aqueles procedimentos que requerem equipamentos normalmente encontrados no ambiente do laboratório. Isso não quer dizer que esses equipamentos não possam estar disponíveis para os profissionais de saúde; no entanto, em geral, normalmente não estão disponíveis para o clínico.[2] Para a pesquisa de reabilitação do tornozelo, isso foi limitado a medidas de equilíbrio instrumentadas de plataformas de força ou o uso de sistemas de estabilidade como o Biodex. Em ambos os casos, foram encontradas melhorias nessas medidas após o treinamento de equilíbrio. Para medidas de plataforma de força, uma variedade de medidas dependentes foi considerada responsiva ao treinamento de equilíbrio, incluindo: velocidade do centro de pressão, comprimento do caminho de oscilação medial/lateral, raio do centro de pressão, tempo até o limite e área do centro de pressão. As medidas coletadas com o Sistema de Estabilidade Biodex também produziram um efeito substancial, o que indica claramente que o treinamento de equilíbrio tem um efeito potente sobre essas medidas. No entanto, atualmente, não se sabe se essas mudanças se traduzem em melhorias significativas para o paciente.

Os métodos clínicos incluem as avaliações que requerem uma quantidade mínima de equipamentos e são facilmente utilizados no ambiente clínico. Dependendo da medida, essas medidas clínicas simples mostraram melhorar com a reabilitação. O teste de equilíbrio de excursão em estrela (SEBT, *star excursion balance test*)[3] é uma das medidas com base na clínica mais frequentemente usadas, com melhora no equilíbrio após a reabilitação do tornozelo relatada (Linens et al., 2016; Wright et al., 2016). Outras medidas igualmente simples com base na clínica também mostraram responder à reabilitação do tornozelo. Isso inclui o teste de levantamento do pé, o teste de equilíbrio do tempo, o salto em forma de oito e o salto lateral.

Em resumo, medidas laboratoriais de deficiência são aprimoradas após o treinamento de equilíbrio e podem ser úteis quando o equipamento estiver disponível. Pesquisas mais recentes demonstraram que medidas com base na clínica podem ser tão responsivas quanto testes laboratoriais e têm o benefício de necessitar de equipamento mínimo.

Efeito nas medidas de função autorrelatada

As medidas de função autorrelatada incluem aquelas com base em questionários que avaliam a capacidade do paciente de realizar atividades da vida diária e atividades relacionadas com o esporte,

---

[1] N.R.T.: são fundamentais, em caso de atletas, medidas prévias para comparação pós-lesão e durante a reabilitação.

[2] N.R.T.: é mais facilmente encontrada em universidades ou clubes esportivos.

[3] N.R.T.: adaptado para Y teste em uma versão específica.

por exemplo, FADI e FADI *Sport*. Embora as medidas anteriores possam ser conceitualmente vinculadas por médicos e pacientes às medidas de fisiopatologia e ao comprometimento, elas avaliam mais diretamente aquelas tarefas funcionais que são importantes para os pacientes. Vários estudos mostraram melhorias significativas com essas medidas após o treinamento de equilíbrio (Cruz-Diaz et al., 2015; Linens et al., 2016; Wright et al., 2016). Isso fornece evidências claras de que o treinamento de equilíbrio melhora a função que é mais importante para o paciente. Não está claro qual medida é a mais adequada, uma vez que não foram feitas comparações diretas.

Tratamentos e protocolos de treinamento

Estudos que usam múltiplas terapias são aqueles estudos que combinam diferentes modos de tratamento em um único plano de tratamento geral. Por exemplo, essas terapias incluíram vários exercícios de chute com faixa elástica (Han et al., 2009), várias tarefas de salto combinadas com tarefas de equilíbrio (McKeon et al., 2008) e tarefas de equilíbrio combinadas com amplitude de movimento padrão e exercícios de força (Hale et al., 2007). Do ponto de vista científico, a variedade de medidas, exercícios e sua dosagem (diária e semanal) dentro dos protocolos e a variação na duração da reabilitação, a qual inclui 4, 6, 8 e 36 semanas, dificultam as comparações entre os estudos, sendo limitadoras da evidência. No entanto, os planos de tratamento têm se mostrado eficazes em pelo menos uma das variáveis dependentes medidas (Hale et al., 2007; McKeon et al., 2009; Ross et al., 2007).

Efeitos nas medidas de deficiência

Semelhante aos protocolos de treinamento de equilíbrio, o desempenho no SEBT demonstrou melhorar os seguintes protocolos de tratamento que incluíam equilíbrio, testes funcionais, exercícios de força e exercícios de amplitude de movimento (Hale et al., 2007). Do mesmo modo, a reabilitação que consiste em tarefas de salto e equilíbrio também mostrou melhoras na distância de alcance do SEBT (McKeon et al., 2008). No entanto, a dificuldade desses estudos é que não é possível saber se esses efeitos foram potencializados pelo uso de múltiplos tratamentos ou se foram o único produto do treinamento de equilíbrio, sendo os demais componentes supérfluos.

Efeitos nas medidas de limitação funcional

Dois ensaios clínicos randomizados avaliaram vários protocolos de tratamento em termos de medidas de limitações funcionais. Hale et al. (2007) usaram equilíbrio, testes funcionais, exercícios de força e de amplitude de movimento e demonstraram melhorias significativas nos escores FADI e FADI *Sport*. Do mesmo modo, usando saltos e tarefas de equilíbrio McKeon et al. (2008) também demonstraram melhorias na FADI e FADI *Sport*. Claramente, com base nesses estudos e naqueles descritos anteriormente, os protocolos de reabilitação do tornozelo podem melhorar as limitações funcionais dos pacientes, talvez independentemente do modo de treinamento.

Resumo

Em resumo, esses protocolos são eficazes, porém complexos. Normalmente, eles envolvem muitos exercícios e, frequentemente, combinam diferentes modos de exercício ou tratamento. A frequência e a duração do tratamento também variam significativamente, dificultando a comparação entre os estudos. Por fim, a complexidade dos protocolos de tratamento e o tempo necessário por sessão para concluir o tratamento podem representar uma sobrecarga de tempo impraticável para o paciente e o médico.

Incapacidade do paciente resultante de doença do tornozelo

O *Short Form* (36) *Health Survey* (SF-36) foi usado para avaliar a QVRS em pacientes com patologias do tornozelo, como artrose do tornozelo, osteoartrite, fraturas e entorses (Bhandari et al., 2004; Ponzer et al., 1999; Saltzman et al., 2006). Em entorses de tornozelo, foi relatado que, em comparação aos indivíduos ilesos, os indivíduos com lesão no tornozelo tiveram pontuações mais baixas na escala de "Saúde Geral" e "Resumo do Componente Físico" (RCF) do SF-36. Um estudo de reabilitação mais recente demonstrou que o treinamento em prancha de equilíbrio, mas não o treinamento de força, pode produzir melhorias no RCF em níveis que estão associados a uma melhor capacidade de trabalho e a menor risco de perda de emprego (Wright et al., 2016). Esses estudos indicam que as entorses de tornozelo levam a uma redução da QVRS e que o treinamento na prancha de equilíbrio pode ser eficaz na melhora da QVRS.

Efeitos da reabilitação na incidência e recorrência

Além das medidas descritas anteriormente, alguns estudos (Emery et al., 2007; Mohammadi, 2007) relataram medidas epidemiológicas de incidência/recorrência. Todos, exceto um desses estudos, mostraram que o treinamento de equilíbrio diminui o risco de entorse de tornozelo em 2 a 8 vezes, com o estudo de Mohammadi (2007) também apontando que o treinamento de força pode reduzir o risco em duas vezes e demonstrando que o treinamento de equilíbrio foi superior ao treinamento de força.

Mensagem para levar para casa

Com base na pesquisa disponível, o treinamento de equilíbrio melhora a função do tornozelo em todo o espectro de deficiência e reduz a recorrência de entorse. Combinar o treinamento de equilíbrio com outras formas de reabilitação também é eficaz, mas não está claro se essa abordagem combinada é melhor do que apenas o treinamento de equilíbrio. A eficácia do treinamento de força ainda não está clara.

Lesões do ligamento cruzado anterior

Kim Hébert-Losier, Charlotte Häger

Introdução

As rupturas do ligamento cruzado anterior (LCA) são uma das lesões mais comuns do joelho, com taxas de incidência anuais de 0,05 a 0,08% (Moses e Orchard, 2012). Só nos EUA, há aproximadamente um quarto de milhão de novas lesões do LCA por ano (Silvers e Mandelbaum, 2011). Com base em uma análise de custo-utilidade do banco de dados multicêntricos (Mather et al., 2013), evitar uma lesão do LCA em alguém com menos de 25 anos resulta em uma economia social e financeira ao longo da vida de US$ 50.000 a US$ 95.000. A maioria das lesões do LCA ocorre durante atividades esportivas, que não afetam apenas a função dos indivíduos a curto prazo, mas também podem afetar várias décadas após a lesão (Hébert-Losier et al., 2015).

Anatomia

O LCA é um ligamento extrassinovial intra-articular orientado obliquamente desde a face posteromedial da incisura do côndilo femoral intercondilar até um espaço triangular na tíbia, entre a eminência intercondilar medial e os cornos anteriores dos meniscos (Figura 5.1). A inserção óssea femoral do LCA está em continuidade com a cortical posterior do fêmur. A inserção tibial do LCA é em forma de C e se mistura com as inserções do menisco lateral. Frequentemente, o LCA é descrito como contendo dois feixes (anteromedial e posterolateral), nomeados de acordo com seus locais de inserção tibial na área intercondilar anterior. O principal papel do LCA é prevenir a translação anterior da tíbia em relação com o fêmur. O LCA também restringe rotação tibial interna excessiva, hiperextensão do joelho e valgo e varo do joelho, especialmente na sustentação de peso.

Mecanismos de lesão e fatores de risco

Compreender os mecanismos de lesão é um componente chave na prevenção de lesões. A maioria das lesões do LCA ocorre em esportes de pivô, especialmente no futebol, com até 85% das lesões acontecendo durante situações de contato indireto ou até mesmo sem contato. Em particular, essas lesões ocorrem durante as manobras de desaceleração, corte lateral, pouso e equilíbrio (Waldén et al., 2015). Embora a incidência absoluta de lesões e cirurgias do LCA seja maior em homens (Gornitzky et al., 2016), o risco relativo de sofrer uma lesão do LCA é, em geral, 3 vezes maior em mulheres (Agel et al., 2005; Prodromos et al., 2007). Além do futebol, do futebol americano, da ginástica, do basquete, do *lacrosse* e da luta livre, há taxas relativamente altas de lesões do LCA (Hootman et al., 2007) em esportes como rúgbi, handebol, *floorball* e esqui. Lesões e cirurgias do LCA são menos comuns na pré-puberdade. Tem sido sugerido que o pico ocorre entre 14 e 19 anos de idade em mulheres e 15 a 34 anos em homens (Sanders et al., 2016).

As lesões do LCA ocorrem quando a carga excede a capacidade do tecido biológico. Suspeita-se que as lesões ocorram entre 20 e 50 ms após a distensão inicial (Koga et al., 2010), com a carga em múltiplos planos no joelho sustentando peso sendo o modo mais comum de lesão sem contato do LCA. O joelho está frequentemente em hiperextensão ou leve flexão e sofre um movimento em valgo com rotação interna ou externa (Shimokochi e Shultz, 2008), em posição de "joelho para dentro e dedos para fora" (Figura 5.2). Os termos *valgo dinâmico* e *valgo dinâmico da extremidade inferior* são comumente usados na literatura para descrever os movimentos multiplano e multiarticular que caracterizam o mecanismo de lesão do LCA, envolvendo adução e rotação interna do quadril, abdução do joelho, rotação externa da tíbia e translação anterior, além de eversão do tornozelo (Hewett et al., 2006). Na verdade, as explicações para os mecanismos de lesão do LCA devem considerar toda a cadeia cinemática. Por exemplo, baixo grau de flexão plantar do tornozelo, grande flexão do quadril (Carlson et al., 2016), baixo grau de flexão do joelho, flexão lateral do tronco e pouca flexão do tronco são todos os movimentos que foram observados durante as rupturas do LCA (Hewett et al., 2009; Hewett et al., 2011).

Além da participação em esportes de pivô e dos padrões de movimento *dinâmico em valgo* (Hewett et al., 2006), os fatores predisponentes a lesões do LCA sem contato comuns a ambos os sexos incluem: frouxidão generalizada e/ou articular do joelho (Vacek et al., 2016), lesão prévia do LCA (Arden et al., 2014), rotação de quadril restrita (VandenBerg et al., 2017), histórico familiar de lesões do LCA (Vacek et al., 2016) e fatores anatômicos, como uma incisura intercondilar estreita (Zeng et al., 2013) e/ou declive tibial íngreme (Hashemi et al., 2010). Evidências emergentes na última década sugerem o envolvimento de fatores hereditários, em que a genética pode desempenhar um papel nos fatores de risco anatômicos, como geometria óssea e estrutura de colágeno (O'Connell et al., 2015), incluindo comportamentos de risco. Outros fatores de risco propostos como sendo mais específicos para os homens incluem diminuição da dorsiflexão do tornozelo, diminuição da rotação interna do quadril e aumento da anteversão do quadril. Aqueles específicos para mulheres incluem diminuição das capacidades musculares dos isquiotibiais aos quadríceps (Myer et al., 2009), aumento do índice de massa corporal (Uhorchak et al., 2003) e estar na primeira metade do ciclo menstrual (fases pré-ovulatória e ovulatória) (Herzberg et al., 2017) devido às variações inter-relacionadas com a frouxidão do LCA (Zazulak et al., 2006). Não está claro se as lesões do LCA são mais frequentes no lado dominante ou não dominante, o que depende das diferenças entre os sexos, os esportes, os mecanismos de lesão e a definição de dominância lateral entre os estudos (Ruedl et al., 2012).

Triagem e prevenção

Os testes de triagem visam identificar os atletas com alto risco de sofrer uma lesão e justificar a implementação de estratégias direcionadas de prevenção de lesões. Os testes de triagem devem ser sensíveis (*i. e.*, identificar corretamente os indivíduos de alto risco) e específicos (*i. e.*, identificar corretamente os indivíduos de baixo risco), além de serem custo-efetivos. A triagem com relação a padrões de movimento potencialmente prejudiciais durante *drop jumps* verticais e saltos do tipo *wall jump* ou *tuck jumps* (Padua et al., 2015), bem como a estabilidade postural prejudicada (Dingeman et al., 2016), tem recebido alguma atenção ao longo dos anos com relação à previsão de lesões do LCA. No entanto, há algumas preocupações envolvendo a confiabilidade, validade, praticidade, eficiência e especificidade esportiva desses métodos de triagem, com apenas um estudo demonstrando uma capacidade de medidas baseadas em campo para identificar prospectivamente atletas de futebol juvenil que sofreram uma lesão do LCA por meio de *drop jump* verticais (Padua et al., 2015). Há necessidade de maior desenvolvimento e validação de testes de triagem que possam ser usados na prevenção primária e secundária de lesões do LCA, que considerem o sistema sensorimotor e a qualidade do movimento (van Melick et al., 2016; Dingenen e Gokeler, 2017).

Dados os desafios associados à previsão do risco de lesões por meio de iniciativas de triagem em massa, a implementação sistemática de programas de prevenção de lesões do LCA tem sido recomendada, especialmente para indivíduos que são jovens, do sexo feminino, que participam de esportes de alto risco e que apresentam histórico pessoal ou familiar de lesão do LCA. Vários programas de prevenção estão disponíveis e têm como alvo fatores de risco modificáveis para lesões do LCA sem contato. Normalmente, esses programas incluem um ou vários dos seguintes componentes, organizados de maneira sistemática: pliometria, equilíbrio, propriocepção, fortalecimento, controle do núcleo e do tronco, agilidade, correção de técnica com *feedback*, consciência corporal, educação e alongamento (Alentorn-Geli et al., 2009; Bien et al., 2011). Programas direcionados a vários componentes parecem ser os mais eficazes na prevenção de lesões do LCA, particularmente ao integrar exercícios de fortalecimento, controle proximal, pliometria e *feedback*. Os programas também são mais eficazes quando realizados na temporada do que quando na pré-temporada (Michaelidis e Koumantakis, 2014), com conformidade e dosagem sendo fatores-chave para a redução bem-sucedida da incidência de lesões do LCA. A recomendação atual é de três sessões por semana na pré-temporada e duas sessões

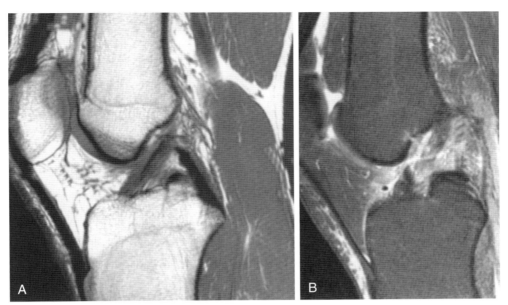

Figura 5.1 Ressonância magnética de ligamento cruzado anterior intacto (A) e ruptura do ligamento cruzado anterior do joelho (B).

por semana na temporada, com cada sessão durando pelo menos 20 minutos (Sugimoto et al., 2014). Semelhantemente às iniciativas de triagem, existe uma preocupação com o custo-benefício dos programas de prevenção de lesões – aproximadamente 100 a 120 atletas precisam seguir um programa eficaz para prevenir uma lesão do LCA sem contato (Noyes et al., 2014). Outras estratégias preconizadas na prevenção primária e secundária de lesões do LCA incluem o uso de joelheiras (Ewing et al., 2016), bandagem (Harput et al., 2016) ou órteses para os pés (Jenkins et al., 2008), embora mais evidências sejam necessárias para apoiar a eficácia dessas intervenções.

Tratamento

As rupturas do LCA são tratadas de forma conservadora, usando uma abordagem de reabilitação baseada em fisioterapia, muitas vezes com modificações da atividade como um conceito principal, ou são tratadas cirurgicamente em conjunto com a fisioterapia pré e pós-operatória. Os autoenxertos osso-tendão patelar-osso e isquiotibial-tendão são os tecidos autólogos mais comumente colhidos e usados em reconstruções cirúrgicas, com o tendão do quadríceps também mostrando resultados promissores. Outras opções de enxerto incluem aloenxertos e enxertos sintéticos (Kay et al., 2017).

A escolha do manejo não operatório *versus* operatório é uma decisão complexa, com um limite inferior para oferecer cirurgia na presença de lesões do LCA com lesões meniscais associadas ou lesões multiligamentares em comparação às rupturas ou às rupturas isoladas do LCA.

Ainda há uma falta de evidências conclusivas sobre qual abordagem de tratamento é a melhor (i. e., não cirúrgico *versus* cirúrgico) em um nível individual. A pesquisa indica resultados comparáveis quanto a retorno ao esporte, necessidade de cirurgia secundária, desenvolvimento de osteoartrite, simetria dos membros, resultados relatados pelo paciente e satisfação (Frobell et al., 2013; Grindhem et al., 2014; Smith et al., 2014; Tengman et al., 2014). Além disso, há evidências de que seguir um programa de reabilitação estruturado pode levar à recuperação do desempenho físico e da força muscular com ou sem intervenção cirúrgica em adultos jovens ativos (Ericsson et al., 2013).

Comparar resultados diretamente entre as abordagens não operatórias e operatórias é um desafio, dada a dificuldade de conduzir e a falta de ensaios clínicos randomizados nesta área, bem como a evolução contínua das abordagens conservadoras e cirúrgicas. Independentemente da abordagem de tratamento, estudos transversais sobre o tema indicam a presença e a persistência de mecanismos compensatórios e as estratégias biomecânicas alteradas (Roos et al., 2014; Tengman et al., 2015), com nem todos os indivíduos retornando com sucesso aos níveis de atividade física pré-lesão.

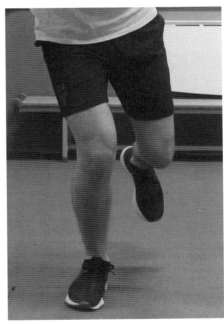

Figura 5.2 Foto de uma posição de risco potencial da extremidade inferior em relação à lesão do ligamento cruzado anterior, em que o joelho está em movimento valgo e o pé está girado externamente, configuração chamada de "joelho para dentro e pé para fora".

Parte | 1 | Conceitos Básicos Importantes em Esportes

Independentemente da escolha do manejo primário, a realização de um programa estruturado de fisioterapia e reabilitação é recomendada e deve durar no mínimo 24 semanas se não operatório (Frobell et al., 2010) e entre 9 e 12 meses após a cirurgia (van Melick et al., 2016). Vários fatores devem ser considerados durante o processo de reabilitação, incluindo o tipo e o nível ideal de atividade física, os estágios de cicatrização do tecido, a capacidade de tolerar carga, a dor e a efusão, a função autoavaliada e a prontidão psicológica (Arden et al., 2011). Geralmente, os programas de reabilitação se concentram em manejo dos sintomas (dor, inchaço, episódios de fraqueza), amplitude de movimento, força muscular, marcha, equilíbrio, propriocepção, controle neuromuscular, estabilidade dinâmica do joelho, qualidade do movimento, exercícios específicos do esporte e retorno gradual ao jogo. O uso de joelheiras funcionais durante a reabilitação oferece resistência contra a translação anterior da tíbia e proteção contra a extensão total, e o uso participando em atividades de alto risco (p. ex., esqui alpino e esportes de pivô) é prevalente no manejo tanto operatório quanto não operatório de rupturas do LCA. No entanto, atualmente, não há evidências definitivas de melhores resultados de tratamento e a prescrição de órtese funcional no tratamento da ruptura do LCA não é rotina (Lowe et al., 2017). A bandagem elástica nas fases iniciais da reabilitação também foi examinada (Balki et al., 2016), mas não foi consistentemente associada a resultados superiores.

Medidas de resultado

Não existe um padrão ouro atual em termos de avaliação dos resultados do tratamento do LCA (Ahmad et al., 2017) ou de estabelecimento de quando um atleta está pronto para retornar ao esporte (Dingeman e Gokeler, 2017). Ensaios clínicos de lesão de LCA nível I altamente citados comumente relatam frouxidão da articulação do joelho, pontuações subjetivas relatadas pelo paciente, falha do enxerto e dados de amplitude de movimento (Ahmad et al., 2017). Mais raramente, as medidas diretas da função sensorimotora ou da qualidade do movimento são incluídas em estudos clínicos, o que é uma lacuna na literatura empírica dada a persistência de déficits observados a longo prazo. De modo a avaliar a prontidão para voltar a jogar, as principais diretrizes utilizadas são tempo pós-cirurgia, medidas clínicas relacionadas com a mobilidade e com a força, testes de desempenho funcional e resultados relatados pelo paciente (Gokeler et al., 2017).

As medidas clínicas usadas para quantificar objetivamente os resultados incluem testes de amplitude de movimento, força e integridade ligamentar (teste *pivot shift* e teste de Lachman). Alguns dos principais resultados disponíveis relatados pelo paciente são escore de Lysholm, escala de atividade de Tegner, atividades da vida diária, *"International Knee Documentation Scores"* (traduzida e adaptada transculturalmente para a língua portuguesa), *"Knee Injury and Osteoarthritis Outcome Score"* (KOOS), questionário *"ACL Return to Sports after Injury"* (ACL-RSI) (adaptado e traduzido para língua portuguesa) e escala *"Injury Psychological Readiness to Return to Sport"*. Evidências crescentes indicam que fatores psicológicos (p. ex., motivação, medo de movimento) desempenham um papel na reabilitação, na satisfação do paciente e no retorno aos níveis de atividade física pré-lesão (Arden et al., 2011). As escalas que abordam o medo do movimento (p. ex., *"Tampa Scale for Kinesiophobia"*, escala de Tampa, traduzida e validada para a língua portuguesa) estão sendo cada vez mais usadas na prática e na pesquisa.

Em termos de desempenho funcional, os testes de salto (p. ex., para saltos em distância, altura ou laterais, *crossover*, salto triplo e cronometrado de 6 m) são os mais frequentemente usados. Um dos critérios mais usados para avaliar o retorno à função "normal" ou "anormal" tem sido o índice de simetria do membro (LSI, *limb symmetry index*; membro envolvido/membro não envolvido × 100%), em que um LSI > 90% é considerado satisfatório (Thomeé et al., 2011). No entanto, existem várias preocupações com relação ao uso do LSI como uma medida de resultado ou único critério de retorno ao jogo. O LSI pode mascarar a presença de déficits bilaterais, ocultar resultados individuais, deixar de considerar o desempenho absoluto e superestimar a função do joelho após uma lesão do LCA (Wellsandt et al., 2017). Os testes de desempenho funcional não devem ser usados como critérios únicos de retorno ao esporte e uma bateria de testes abrangente deve ser empregada (van Melick et al., 2016) em combinação com escalas de prontidão psicológica (Arden et al., 2016), tempo pós-cirurgia e nível de retorno ao esporte (Grindem et al., 2020).

Consequências

Não há uma definição clara de qual período de tempo constitui um resultado de curto, médio ou longo prazo na literatura do LCA, com 6, 9, 12, 18 e 24 meses sendo os períodos de acompanhamento de referência. Há um número crescente de estudos com acompanhamentos de 2 a 10 anos, 10 a 20 anos e além de 20 anos. Todos esses estudos fornecem informações sobre as consequências potenciais de lesões do LCA, que incluem alterações de curto, médio e longo prazo em marcha (*i. e.*, caminhada, corrida e uso de escada), equilíbrio, propriocepção, sentido da posição da articulação do joelho, consciência articular, padrões de carga nas extremidades inferiores, estratégias de movimento, risco de lesões, participação em esportes e níveis de atividade física e o risco aumentado de desenvolver osteoartrite.

Ao sintetizar a literatura, Ardern et al. (2014) determinaram que 81% dos indivíduos retornaram a alguma forma de esporte após a reconstrução do LCA, mas apenas 65% retornaram aos níveis pré-lesão e 55% ao esporte competitivo. Parece não haver diferença clara nas taxas de retorno ao esporte entre as abordagens de tratamento operatório e não operatório (Kessler et al., 2008), exceto em crianças e adolescentes, entre os quais o tratamento operatório tem sido associado a maiores taxas de retorno ao esporte e a melhores resultados funcionais (Fabricant et al., 2016), pelo menos a curto prazo.

A combinação de informações de várias fontes coloca as taxas secundárias de lesão do LCA nos 5 anos após uma reconstrução do LCA em 17,6%, 5,8% no lado ipsilateral e 11,8% no lado contralateral (Wright et al., 2011), com taxas chegando a 32% nos 15 anos pós-cirurgia reconstrutiva (Leys et al., 2012). O risco relativo de sofrer uma nova lesão no joelho é mais de três vezes maior em atletas com um joelho com reconstrução do LCA do que naqueles sem (Waldén et al., 2006). O risco de nova ruptura parece ser maior em indivíduos mais jovens e nos primeiros 2 anos após a reconstrução (Schlumberger et al., 2017). Menos informações estão disponíveis para indivíduos não operados, com estudos indicando que a cirurgia do joelho é necessária em aproximadamente 25% dos casos em acompanhamentos de 14 anos (Chalmers et al., 2014).

Em prazo muito longo (> 20 anos), indivíduos com lesão do LCA tendem a relatar níveis mais baixos de atividade física específica do joelho com base nos escores de Tegner e Lysholm quando comparados aos controles pareados, especialmente na presença de osteoartrite do joelho. A osteoartrite é observada em 50 a 90% dos indivíduos com lesão do LCA (Tengman et al., 2014), um risco relativo três a quatro vezes maior em comparação aos indivíduos não lesionados (Suter et al., 2017), independentemente da abordagem de tratamento. Além disso, a pesquisa fornece evidências de alteração de estabilidade dinâmica da articulação do joelho durante tarefas funcionais, capacidade de salto,

Biomecânica das Lesões Esportivas, Manejo e Considerações Clínicas **Capítulo** | 5 |

equilíbrio e força em comparação aos controles, não apenas na perna lesionada, mas também na perna não lesionada (Grip et al., 2015; Hébert-Losier et al., 2015; Tengman et al., 2014; 2015). Esses achados indicam que pode ser aconselhável continuar realizando alguma forma de reabilitação ao longo da vida para limitar as sequelas a longo prazo resultantes das lesões do LCA.

Mensagem para levar para casa

Lesões do LCA são uma grande preocupação em esportes e medicina ortopédica. A biomecânica desempenha um papel central na compreensão e abordagem das lesões do LCA e do seu tratamento. Não há, no entanto, nenhum padrão ouro atual para detectar indivíduos com alto risco de lesões, prescrever programas de prevenção de lesões, selecionar tratamento operatório *versus* não operatório, avaliar os resultados do tratamento do LCA, retornar os indivíduos ao esporte, reduzir as taxas de novas lesões e osteoartrite e abordar a longo prazo déficits funcionais. A ausência de diretrizes definitivas se deve à natureza multifatorial e multidimensional das lesões do LCA e à falta de consenso, apesar de ser um campo de pesquisa em constante crescimento. Portanto, as lesões do LCA devem ser tratadas caso a caso, usando as informações disponíveis mais atualizadas para garantir o gerenciamento das melhores práticas.

Lesões no ombro

Bruno Mazuquin, Puneet Monga

Introdução

O ombro possui características inerentes integrando estruturas anatômicas para permitir a maior amplitude de movimento entre todas as articulações do corpo humano. Sua mobilidade é responsável por suportar o deslocamento espacial dos braços, permitindo um amplo escopo de atividades dos membros superiores. No entanto, a forma anatômica da articulação glenoumeral, com cabeça umeral muito maior do que a fossa glenoide, aumenta o risco de instabilidade. Para realizar um movimento suave e controlado, os músculos ao redor do ombro precisam fornecer forças equilibradas; isso se baseia em informações de mecanorreceptores dentro dos próprios músculos e de outras estruturas adjacentes, como ligamentos e cápsula. Essas informações importantes garantem a segurança das estruturas, principalmente quando a junta atinge os limites de um movimento. Quando partes das estruturas do ombro não funcionam corretamente, ou quando os estabilizadores dinâmicos, ou seja, os músculos do manguito rotador (supraespinal, infraespinal, redondo menor e subescapular), não são capazes de controlar a cabeça do úmero, podem ocorrer danos e interromper a biomecânica inerente da junta. Por sua vez, isso pode prejudicar o desempenho esportivo e causar sintomas incapacitantes, como dor. Nesta seção, revisamos as três lesões esportivas mais comumente observadas que afetam o ombro: impacto interno, rupturas e instabilidade do manguito rotador.

Impacto interno

O impacto interno é uma condição comumente observada em atletas arremessadores, especialmente no futebol americano. O cenário clássico dessa ocorrência acontece quando uma bola é arremessada – a elevação e rotação do ombro são necessárias. O choque interno acontece, principalmente, durante a fase de armar, momento em que o úmero está acima de 90° de abdução combinado com mais de 90° de rotação externa. Nessa posição, o lado articular do supraespinal pode ser comprimido entre a cabeça do úmero e o labrum posterossuperior. Esse contato em si não é uma grande preocupação, pois é um evento relativamente normal quando o braço está posicionado a 90° de abdução e 90° de rotação externa. No entanto, devido à natureza repetitiva das atividades esportivas, a sobrecarga contínua e cumulativa dos músculos do manguito rotador pode levar a lesões no labrum e no tendão (Burkhart et al., 2003).

Os principais sintomas relacionados com o impacto interno são dor durante a abdução máxima e rotação externa, diminuição progressiva da velocidade de movimento, perda de controle e deterioração do desempenho esportivo. Geralmente, o atleta mostra sinais de sensibilidade na linha articular glenoumeral posterior, perda de rotação interna e rotação externa excessiva. Além disso, exames de imagem complementares podem revelar outros problemas estruturais em potencial, como rupturas do manguito rotador e dos labiais.

Rupturas do manguito rotador

Por definição, rupturas do manguito rotador são as rupturas de um ou mais tendões dos músculos do manguito rotador devido a trauma ou a um processo degenerativo (Opsha et al., 2008). Essa é uma das principais causas de dor no ombro e é um distúrbio comum que afeta aproximadamente 30% das pessoas com mais de 60 anos, tendo uma taxa crescente associada ao envelhecimento (Yamaguchi et al., 2006; Yamamoto et al., 2010). Na população esportiva, as rupturas do manguito rotador são comuns em atletas arremessadores; rupturas parciais foram observadas em 48% e rupturas de espessura total em 21% (McMahon et al., 2014). Como resultado, as rupturas do manguito rotador são responsáveis por aproximadamente 450 mil operações por ano apenas nos EUA (Thigpen et al., 2016).

Considerando o papel estabilizador do manguito rotador, a presença de uma ruptura em um dos quatro tendões pode potencialmente perturbar a biomecânica do ombro e o controle do movimento. Por exemplo, se o subescapular ou supraespinal estiver prejudicado, a força que puxa a cabeça do úmero para baixo durante a elevação será deficiente. Portanto, a cabeça do úmero migrará em direção ao acrômio devido à tração sem oposição do deltoide, o qual comprimirá as estruturas sob o espaço subacromial e, consequentemente, poderá provocar dor e desconforto.

Mecanismo de lesão

Os mecanismos que levam à falha dos tendões do manguito rotador em atletas estão relacionados com trauma ou uso excessivo. Eventos traumáticos de ruptura do manguito rotador em esportes são mais prováveis de acontecer em uma queda ou com tração; em contraste, os processos crônicos são comuns em atletas arremessadores, como arremessadores de beisebol e jogadores de tênis. Nesses esportes, a repetição do movimento é necessária, o que exige o uso prolongado dos músculos do manguito rotador como um estabilizador dinâmico em posições de alta carga. O estresse contínuo aplicado sobre os tendões do manguito pode causar microtrauma, que com o tempo pode resultar em falha do tecido.

Manejo do impacto interno e rupturas do manguito rotador

A primeira opção de tratamento para impacto interno e rupturas crônicas do manguito rotador costuma ser a fisioterapia. A realização de exercícios com o objetivo de melhorar o controle motor

47

e o recrutamento do manguito rotador tem se mostrado eficaz na resolução dos sintomas de dor e na melhora da função (Kuhn et al., 2013). Além disso, focar em exercícios que envolvem toda a cadeia cinética também é fortemente recomendado. Esse tipo de exercício consiste em treinar a potência e a energia geradas a partir dos membros inferiores para que sejam transferidas de forma mais eficiente pelo tronco até atingir os membros superiores, reduzindo, assim, o estresse imposto ao ombro na realização de movimentos esportivos (McMullen e Uhl, 2000). A maioria dos pacientes mostra uma resposta positiva na redução dos sintomas quando essa fisioterapia é realizada por cerca de 12 semanas (Kuhn et al., 2013). Outra opção conservadora são as injeções de corticosteroides, que são usadas para reduzir a inflamação. No entanto, a evidência mostra que esse tratamento tem bons efeitos a curto prazo, mas não tem benefícios de longa duração. Além disso, existem preocupações de que o uso de corticosteroides pode comprometer os tecidos do tendão e da cartilagem por impactar negativamente a expressão do colágeno (Abdul-Wahab Taiceer et al., 2016).

Quando as abordagens conservadoras não alcançam um resultado satisfatório, a cirurgia é considerada. Para rupturas do manguito rotador, a cirurgia envolve a reparação dos tendões danificados, reinserindo-os em sua fixação no úmero. Dependendo do tamanho da ruptura e da qualidade do tecido, diferentes técnicas podem ser usadas para fornecer maior estabilidade à pegada. No entanto, os estudos não mostraram diferenças estatisticamente significativas nas medidas de resultados relatados pelo paciente comparando métodos de linha única ou dupla (McCormick et al., 2014; Trappey e Gartsman, 2011).

Em contraste com as rupturas crônicas do manguito rotador, a cirurgia é considerada a primeira opção de tratamento para as rupturas agudas. A cirurgia precoce, até 3 meses após o evento, demonstrou melhorar significativamente os resultados dos pacientes e aumentar a probabilidade de retorno ao jogo. Klouche et al. (2016) realizaram uma revisão sistemática com metanálise para determinar a taxa de retorno ao esporte após reparos do manguito rotador. Os autores encontraram uma taxa geral de retorno de 84,7% para atletas recreativos, dos quais 65,4% retornaram a um nível semelhante de jogo, enquanto 49,9% dos profissionais e indivíduos competitivos retornaram ao esporte em nível semelhante ao de antes da cirurgia. Além disso, Antoni et al. (2016) relataram bons resultados para atletas recreativos; isso incluiu indivíduos que tiveram um reparo do manguito rotador e um acompanhamento mínimo de 2 anos. Destes, 88,2% dos atletas retornaram às atividades esportivas com tempo médio de 6 meses (DP = 4,9 meses).

Atualmente, a fisioterapia após o reparo do manguito rotador é uma área de debate considerável, particularmente com relação ao tempo de uso da tipoia após a cirurgia. Antes, um período de imobilização de 6 semanas após a cirurgia era recomendado para evitar episódios de novas rupturas. No entanto, o uso de uma tipoia por longos períodos de tempo pode causar rigidez e mostrou alterar a atividade nos córtices motor e somatossensorial (Berth et al., 2009; Huber et al., 2006). Uma visão geral das revisões sistemáticas demonstrou que o uso de uma tipoia por menos de 6 semanas não é a principal causa de taxas de rerruptura mais altas (Mazuquin et al., 2018). O tendão e o tecido muscular são geralmente de boa qualidade na população jovem, o que possibilita um bom reparo com maior chance de boa estabilidade e potencialmente menor tensão em rupturas agudas nessa faixa etária. Para esses reparos, iniciar a mobilização antes do período de 6 semanas pode trazer maiores benefícios e reduzir o tempo de retorno ao esporte, embora seja importante uma abordagem individualizada e um consenso entre o cirurgião e o terapeuta.

Instabilidade

A instabilidade do ombro é um movimento sintomático anormal do úmero na fossa glenoide que pode causar dor, subluxação ou luxação (Lewis et al., 2004). Existem vários métodos para classificar a instabilidade do ombro. Um dos mais comuns é o sistema de classificação de Stanmore, que classifica os pacientes em três grupos polares principais que diferem de acordo com a causa da instabilidade (Lewis et al., 2004) (Figura 5.3). Embora sejam definidos três grupos distintos, alguns pacientes também podem apresentar características mútuas de mais de um tipo polar e, portanto, estar posicionados entre dois polos do triângulo.

- Polar I: provocado por um evento traumático que lesiona as estruturas anatômicas responsáveis pela estabilidade do ombro, principalmente os estabilizadores estáticos (labrum, cápsula, ligamentos)
- Polar II: causado por defeitos estruturais que podem não ser consequência de traumas
- Polar III: não estrutural e causado principalmente por atividade muscular anormal.

Os principais sintomas dos pacientes que estão sob a classificação de instabilidade polar I serão apreensão de luxação ao testar a instabilidade anterior com o teste de apreensão. Geralmente, há histórico de lesão e, além disso, podem apresentar fraqueza na rotação interna se o subescapular for afetado. Para fraqueza do subescapular, o teste de Gerber pode ser usado (Monga e Funk, 2017). O paciente polar tipo II também apresentará apreensão, a qual pode estar associada a déficit de rotação interna e aumento da rotação externa. Isso, por sua vez, pode estar associado à hiperfrouxidão articular. O polar tipo III, geralmente, mostrará menos apreensão; em vez disso, observa-se um controle muscular deficiente, especialmente para o manguito rotador ao realizar vários movimentos do ombro.

Para aqueles pacientes que apresentam instabilidade por envolvimento estrutural, exames de imagem como a ressonância magnética (RM) e a radiografia são benéficos para observar quais estruturas estão comprometidas e para planejar a intervenção cirúrgica.

Mecanismo de lesão

Em esportes como rúgbi e futebol americano, a grande maioria da instabilidade do ombro é causada por eventos traumáticos que, consequentemente, comprometem a integridade da estrutura anatômica do ombro (Crichton et al., 2012; Gibbs et al., 2015). A situação de jogo mais comum que expõe os atletas a

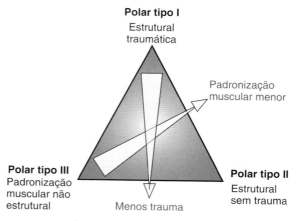

Figura 5.3 Triângulo Stanmore.

Biomecânica das Lesões Esportivas, Manejo e Considerações Clínicas — Capítulo | 5 |

lesões por instabilidade do ombro é quando vai para um *tackle* (ombro abduzido) ou quando tenta alcançar a bola e pousar com o braço flexionado a mais de 90°. Em ambas as situações, um impacto de alta energia gera forças na direção anterior ou posterior que são aplicadas na extremidade distal do membro; consequentemente, essas forças produzem um efeito de alavanca na articulação glenoumeral movendo a cabeça do úmero anterior ou posteriormente, respectivamente (Crichton et al., 2012). As lesões mais comuns e as respectivas estruturas do ombro afetadas em cada uma estão descritas na Tabela 5.1.

Manejo de instabilidade

O manejo vai depender do tipo de instabilidade que o paciente apresenta. Aqueles com polar tipo I, menos de 20 anos e que pretendem retornar ao esporte têm maior benefício com a cirurgia (Jaggi e Lambert, 2010). Nesse cenário, a cirurgia demonstrou evitar a recorrência e uma alta porcentagem de pacientes retorna ao esporte no mesmo nível e, muitas vezes, em cerca de 4 meses (Gibson et al., 2016; Kim et al., 2003).

Em contraste, os pacientes com instabilidade de origem não traumática podem se beneficiar do tratamento conservador, como fisioterapia, primeiro. Nesses casos, a fisioterapia tem se mostrado eficaz em evitar a cirurgia em até 80% dos indivíduos (Jaggi e Lambert, 2010). Os programas de reabilitação devem priorizar exercícios com o objetivo de melhorar seus déficits de atividade muscular inter-relacionados do manguito rotador. Além disso, exercícios com o objetivo de fortalecer outros músculos do ombro devem ser considerados. Semelhantemente ao programa de reabilitação para lesão interna e rupturas do manguito rotador, esses pacientes também se beneficiam de exercícios que incorporam a cadeia cinética para desenvolver a eficiência do movimento. Para pacientes classificados como polar tipo II, a cirurgia seria recomendada após um período de 6 meses de tentativa de fisioterapia (Jaggi e Lambert, 2010).

O primeiro estágio após a cirurgia requer cautela para permitir uma boa cicatrização das estruturas reparadas. Nesse estágio, a fisioterapia precisa encontrar o equilíbrio, mobilizando a articulação para evitar a rigidez sem ultrapassar os limites que podem causar danos aos tecidos reparados. Portanto, exercícios em cadeia fechada são uma boa opção na fase inicial de reabilitação, pois a amplitude de movimento pode ser controlada e, ao mesmo tempo, os músculos já começam a ser estimulados e recrutados. À medida que os pacientes progridem e os níveis de dor melhoram, os exercícios podem avançar para melhorar a força, o treino de resistência e a amplitude de movimento, passando de cadeia fechada para cadeia aberta e ajustando adequadamente os braços de alavanca e a resistência.

As taxas de retorno ao jogo após a cirurgia de instabilidade são altas. Elsenbeck e Dickens (2017) demonstraram em sua revisão que a taxa de retorno ao esporte varia de 63 a 100%, com a maioria dos estudos mostrando uma taxa acima de 80%, o que foi confirmado por Robins et al. (2017).

Mensagem para levar para casa

Devido a sua grande mobilidade, o ombro fica exposto a lesões e conta com a integridade de estabilizadores estáticos e dinâmicos que atuam em sinergia para manter a fluidez biomecânica articular. Atletas com sobrecarga são mais propensos a lesões internas e rupturas do manguito rotador, enquanto os atletas que participam de esportes de contato podem ser mais suscetíveis à instabilidade. As intervenções cirúrgicas têm demonstrado resultados positivos com relação ao retorno ao jogo e a fisioterapia desempenha um papel importante na recuperação dos atletas, seja como primeira opção de tratamento ou após procedimentos cirúrgicos.

Tabela 5.1 Estruturas comuns afetadas na instabilidade do ombro.

Lesão	Estrutura
LSAP	Labrum superior
Bankart	Labrum anteroinferior
Hill–Sachs	Perda óssea sobre a cabeça do úmero
AULG	Avulsão da inserção umeral do ligamento glenoumeral

AULG, avulsão umeral do ligamento glenoumeral; *LSAP*, labrum superior anteroposterior.

Referências bibliográficas

Lesões do tornozelo

Arnold, B.L., Linens, S.W., de la Motte, S.J., Ross, S.E., 2009. Concentric evertor strength differences and functional ankle instability: A meta-analysis. Journal of Athletic Training 44 (6), 653-662.

Bhandari, M., Sprague, S., Hanson, B., Busse, J.W., Dawe, D.E., Moro, J.K., et al., 2004. Health-related quality of life following operative treatment of unstable ankle fractures: A prospective observational study. Journal of Orthopaedic Trauma 18 (6), 338-345.

Coughlan, G., Caulfield, B., 2007. A 4-week neuromuscular training program and gait patterns at the ankle joint. Journal of Athletic Training 42 (1), 51-59.

Cruz-Diaz, D., Lomas-Vega, R., Osuna-Perez, M.C., Contreras, F.H., Martinez-Amat, A., 2015. Effects of 6 weeks of balance training on chronic ankle instability in athletes: A randomized controlled trial. International Journal of Sports Medicine 36 (9), 754-760.

Docherty, C.L., Moore, J.H., Arnold, B.L., 1998. Effects of strength training on strength development and joint position sense in functionally unstable ankles. Journal of Athletic Training 33 (4), 310-314.

Doherty, C., Delahunt, E., Caulfield, B., Hertel, J., Ryan, J., Bleakley, C., et al., 2014. The incidence and prevalence of ankle sprain injury: a systematic review and meta-analysis of prospective epidemiological studies. Journal of Sports Medicine 44, 123-140.

Emery, C.A., Rose, M.S., McAllister, J.R., Meeuwisse, W.H., 2007. A prevention strategy to reduce the incidence of injury in high school basketball: A cluster randomized controlled trial. Clinical Journal of Sport Medicine 17 (1), 17-24.

Feger, M.A., Snell, S., Handsfield, G.G., Blemker, S.S., Wombacher, E., Fry, R., et al., 2016. Diminished foot and ankle muscle volumes in young adults with chronic ankle instability. Orthopaedic Journal of Sports Medicine 4 (6), 2325967116653719.

Gehring, D., Wissler, S., Mornieux, G., Gollhofer, A., 2013. How to sprain your ankle – a biomechanical case report of an inversion trauma. Journal of Biomechanics 46 (1), 175-178.

Hale, S.A., Hertel, J., Olmsted-Kramer, L.C., 2007. The effect of a 4-week comprehensive rehabilitation program on postural control and lower extremity function in individuals with chronic ankle instability. Journal of Orthopaedic & Sports Physical Therapy 37 (6), 303-311.

Hall, E.A., Docherty, C.L., Simon, J., Kingma, J.J., Klossner, J.C., 2015. Strength-training protocols to improve deficits in participants with chronic ankle instability: A randomized controlled trial. Journal of Athletic Training 50 (1), 36-44.

Han, K., Ricard, M.D., Fellingham, G.W., 2009. Effects of a 4-week exercise program on balance using elastic tubing as a perturbation force for individuals with a history of ankle sprains. Journal of Orthopaedic & Sports Physical Therapy 39 (4), 246-255.

Hootman, J., Dick, R., Agel, J., 2007. Epidemiology of collegiate injuries for 15 sports: summary and recommendations for injury prevention initiatives. Journal of Athletic Training 42, 311-319.

Hubbard, T.J., Hicks-Little, C.A., 2008. Ankle ligament healing after an acute ankle sprain: an evidence-based approach. Journal of Athletic Training 43 (5), 523-529.

Lee, A.J.Y., Lin, W., 2008. Twelve-week biomechanical ankle platform system training on postural stability and ankle proprioception in subjects with unilateral functional ankle instability. Clinical Biomechanics 23, 1065-1072.

Linens, S.W., Ross, S.E., Arnold, B.L., 2016. Wobble board rehabilitation for improving balance in ankles with chronic instability. Clinical Journal of Sport Medicine 26 (1), 76-82.

Matsusaka, N., Yokoyama, S., Tsurusaki, T., Inokuchi, S., Okita, M., 2001. Effect of ankle disk training combined with tactile stimulation to the leg and foot on functional instability of the ankle. American Journal of Sports Medicine 29 (1), 25-30.

McKeon, J.M., Bush, H.M., Reed, A., Whittington, A., Uhl, T.L., McKeon, P.O., 2014. Return-to-play probabilities following new versus recurrent ankle sprains in high school athletes. Journal of Science and Medicine in Sport 17 (1), 23-28.

McKeon, P.O., Ingersoll, C.D., Kerrigan, D.C., Saliba, E., Bennett, B.C., Hertel, J., et al., 2008. Balance training improves function and postural control in those with chronic ankle instability. Medicine and Science in Sports and Exercise 40 (10), 1810-1819.

McKeon, P.O., Paolini, G., Ingersoll, C.D., Kerrigan, D.C., Saliba, E.N., Bennett, B.C., et al., 2009. Effects of balance training on gait parameters in patients with chronic ankle instability: A randomized controlled trial. Clinical Rehabilitation 23 (7), 609-621.

McLeod, T.C.V., Snyder, A.R., Parsons, J.T., Bay, R.C., Michener, L.A., Sauers, E.L., et al., 2008. Using disablement models and clinical outcomes assessment to enable evidence-based athletic training practice, part II: Clinical outcomes assessment. Journal of Athletic Training 43 (4), 437-445.

Mohammadi, F., 2007. Comparison of 3 preventive methods to reduce the recurrence of ankle inversion sprains in male soccer players. American Journal of Sports Medicine 35 (6), 922-926.

Ponzer, S., Nasell, H., Bergman, B., Tornkvist, H., 1999. Functional outcome and quality of life in patients with type B ankle fractures: A two-year follow-up study. Journal of Orthopaedic Trauma 13 (5), 363-368.

Ross, S.E., Arnold, B.L., Blackburn, J.T., Brown, C.N., Guskiewicz, K.M., 2007. Enhanced balance associated with coordination training with stochastic resonance stimulation in subjects with functional ankle instability: An experimental trial. Journal of Neuroengineering and Rehabilitation 4, 47.

Saltzman, C.L., Zimmerman, M.B., O'Rourke, M., Brown, T.D., Buckwalter, J.A., Johnston, R., et al., 2006. Impact of comorbidities on the measurement of health in patients with ankle osteoarthritis. Journal of Bone and Joint Surgery. American Volume 88 (11), 2366-2372.

Sekir, U., Yildiz, Y., Hazneci, B., Ors, F., Aydin, T., 2007. Effect of isokinetic training on strength, functionality and proprioception in athletes with functional ankle instability. Knee Surgery, Sports Traumatology, Arthroscopy 15 (5), 654-664.

Snyder, A.R., Parsons, J.T., McLeod, T.C.V., Bay, R.C., Michener, L.A., Sauers, E.L., et al., 2008. Using disablement models and clinical outcomes assessment to enable evidence-based athletic training practice, part I: Disablement models. Journal of Athletic Training 43 (4), 428-436.

Taga, I., Shoni, K., Inoue, M., Nakata, K., Maeda, J., 1993. Articular cartilage lesions in ankles with lateral ligament injury. An arthrocospic study. The American Journal of Sports Medicine 21 (1), 120-126.

Waterman, B.R., Belmont, P.J., Cameron, K.L., DeBerardino, T.M., Owens, B.D., 2010. Epidemiology of ankle sprain at the United States Military Academy. The American Journal of Sports Medicine 38, 797-803.

Wright, C.J., Linens, S.W., Cain, M.S., 2016. A randomized controlled trial comparing rehabilitation efficacy in chronic ankle instability. Journal of Sport Rehabilitation 26 (4), 238-249.

Yeung, M., Chang, K., So, C., 1994. An epidemiological survey on ankle sprain. British Journal of Sports Medicine 28, 112-116.

Anterior cruciate ligament injuries

Agel, J., Arendt, E.A., Bershadsky, B., 2005. Anterior cruciate ligament injury in national collegiate athletic association basketball and soccer. The American Journal of Sports Medicine 33 (4), 524-531.

Ahmad, S.S., Meyer, J.C., Krismer, A.M., Ahmad, S.S., Evangelopoulos, D.S., Hoppe, S., et al., 2017. Outcome measures in clinical ACL studies: An analysis of highly cited level I trials. Knee Surgery, Sports Traumatology, Arthroscopy 25 (5), 1517-1527.

Alentorn-Geli, E., Myer, G.D., Silvers, H.J., Samitier, G., Romero, D., Lázaro-Haro, C., et al., 2009. Prevention of non-contact anterior cruciate ligament injuries in soccer players. Part 2: A review of prevention programs aimed to modify risk factors and to reduce injury rates. Knee Surgery, Sports Traumatology, Arthroscopy 17 (8), 859-879.

Ardern, C.L., Glasgow, P., Schneiders, A., Witvrouw, E., Clarsen, B., Cools, A., et al., 2016. Consensus statement on return to sport from the first world congress in sports physical therapy, Bern. British Journal of Sports Medicine 50 (14), 853-864.

Ardern, C.L., Taylor, N.F., Feller, J.A., Webster, K.E., 2014. Fifty-five per cent return to competitive sport following anterior cruciate ligament reconstruction surgery: an updated systematic review and meta-analysis including aspects of physical functioning and contextual factors. British Journal of Sports Medicine 48 (21), 1543-1552.

Ardern, C.L., Webster, K.E., Taylor, N.F., Feller, J.A., 2011. Return to sport following anterior cruciate ligament reconstruction surgery: A systematic review and meta-analysis of the state of play. British Journal of Sports Medicine 45 (7), 596-606.

Balki, S., Göktaş, H., Öztemur, Z., 2016. Kinesio taping as a treatment method in the acute phase of ACL reconstruction: A double-blind, placebo-controlled study. Acta Orthopaedica et Traumatologica Turcica 50 (6), 628-634.

Bien, D.P., 2011. Rationale and implementation of anterior cruciate ligament injury prevention warm-up programs in female athletes. Journal of Strength and Conditioning Research 25 (1), 271-285.

Carlson, V.R., Sheehan, F.T., Boden, B.P., 2016. Video analysis of anterior cruciate ligament (ACL) injuries: A systematic review. JBJS Rev. 4 (11).

Chalmers, P.N., Mall, N.A., Moric, M., Sherman, S.L., Paletta, G.P., Cole, B.J., et al., 2014. Does ACL reconstruction alter natural history? A systematic literature review of long-term outcomes. The Journal of Bone and Joint Surgery. American volume 96 (4), 292-300.

Dingenen, B., Gokeler, A., 2017. Optimization of the return-to-sport paradigm after anterior cruciate ligament reconstruction: A critical step back to move forward. Journal of Sports Medicine 47 (8), 1487-1500.

Dingenen, B., Malfait, B., Nijs, S., Peers, K.H., Vereecken, S., Verschueren, S.M., et al., 2016. Postural stability during single-leg stance: A preliminary evaluation of noncontact lower extremity injury risk. The Journal of Orthopaedic and Sports Physical Therapy 46 (8), 650-657.

Ericsson, Y.B., Roos, E.M., Frobell, R.B., 2013. Lower extremity performance following ACL rehabilitation in the KANON-trial: Impact of reconstruction and predictive value at 2 and 5 years. British Journal of Sports Medicine 47 (15), 980-985.

Ewing, K.A., Fernandez, J.W., Begg, R.K., Galea, M.P., Lee, P.V., 2016. Prophylactic knee bracing alters lower-limb muscle forces during a double-leg drop landing. Journal of Biomechanics 49 (14), 3347-3354.

Fabricant, P.D., Lakomkin, N., Cruz, A.I., Spitzer, E., Marx, R.G., 2016. ACL reconstruction in youth athletes results in an improved rate of return to athletic activity when compared with non-operative treatment: a systematic review of the literature. Journal of ISAKOS: Joint Disorders & Orthopaedic Sports Medicine 1, 62-69.

Frobell, R.B., Roos, E.M., Roos, H.P., Ranstam, J., Lohmander, L.S., 2010. A randomized trial of treatment for acute anterior cruciate ligament tears. The New England Journal of Medicine 363 (4), 331-342.

Frobell, R.B., Roos, H.P., Roos, E.M., Roemer, F.W., Ranstam, J., Lohmander, L.S., 2013. Treatment for acute anterior cruciate ligament tear: five year outcome of randomised trial. British Medical Journal 346:f232.

Gokeler, A., Welling, W., Benjaminse, A., Lemmink, K., Seil, R., Zaffagnini, S., et al., 2017. A critical analysis of limb symmetry indices of hop tests in athletes after anterior cruciate ligament reconstruction: A case control study. Orthopaedics and Traumatology, Surgery and Research 103 (6), 947-951.

Gornitzky, A.L., Lott, A., Yellin, J.L., Fabricant, P.D., Lawrence, J.T., Ganley, T.J., et al., 2016. Sport-specific yearly risk and incidence of anterior cruciate ligament tears in high school athletes: A systematic review and meta-analysis. The American Journal of Sports Medicine 44 (10), 2716-2723.

Grindem, H., Eitzen, I., Engebretsen, L., Snyder-Mackler, L., Risberg, M.A., 2014. Nonsurgical or surgical treatment of ACL injuries: Knee function, sports participation, and knee reinjury: The Delaware–Oslo ACL Cohort Study. The Journal of Bone and Joint Surgery. American volume 96 (15), 1233-1241.

Grindem, H., Engebretsen, L., Axe, M., Snyder-Mackler, L., Risberg, M.A., 2020. Activity and functional readiness, not age, are the critical factors for second anterior cruciate ligament injury - the Delaware-Oslo ACL cohort study. British Journal of Sports Medicine 54, 1099-1102.

Grip, H., Tengman, E., Hager, C.K., 2015. Dynamic knee stability estimated by finite helical axis methods during functional performance approximately twenty years after anterior cruciate ligament injury. Journal of Biomechanics 48 (10), 1906-1914.

Harput, G., Ulusoy, B., Ozer, H., Baltaci, G., Richards, J., 2016. External supports improve knee performance in anterior cruciate ligament reconstructed individuals with higher kinesiophobia levels. Knee 23 (5), 807-812.

Hashemi, J., Chandrashekar, N., Mansouri, H., Gill, B., Slauterbeck, J.R., Schutt Jr., R.C., et al., 2010. Shallow medial tibial plateau and steep medial and lateral tibial slopes: New risk factors for anterior cruciate ligament injuries. The American Journal of Sports Medicine 38 (1), 54-62.

Hébert-Losier, K., Pini, A., Vantini, S., Strandberg, J., Abramowicz, K., Schelin, L., et al., 2015. One-leg hop kinematics 20 years following anterior cruciate ligament rupture: Data revisited using functional data analysis. Clinical Biomechanics (Bristol, Avon) 30 (10), 1153-1161.

Herzberg, S.D., Motu'apuaka, M.L., Lambert, W., Fu, R., Brady, J., Guise, J.M., et al., 2017. The effect of menstrual cycle and contraceptives on ACL injuries and laxity: A systematic review and meta-analysis. Orthopaedic Journal of Sports Medicine 5 (7), 2325967117718781.

Hewett, T.E., Myer, G.D., Ford, K.R., 2006. Anterior cruciate ligament injuries in female athletes: Part 1, mechanisms and risk factors. The American Journal of Sports Medicine 34 (2), 299-311.

Hewett, T.E., Myer, G.D., 2011. The mechanistic connection between the trunk, hip, knee, and anterior cruciate ligament injury. Exercise and Sport Sciences Reviews 39 (4), 161-166.

Hewett, T.E., Torg, J.S., Boden, B.P., 2009. Video analysis of trunk and knee motion during non-contact anterior cruciate ligament injury in female athletes: Lateral trunk and knee abduction motion are combined components of the injury mechanism. British Journal of Sports Medicine 43 (6), 417-422.

Jenkins, W.L, Raedeke, S.G., Williams 3rd, D.S.B., 2008. The relationship between the use of foot orthoses and knee ligament injury in female collegiate basketball players. Journal of the American Podiatric Medical Association 98 (3), 207-211.

Kay, J., Naji, L., de SA, D., et al., 2017. Graft choice has no significant influence on the rate of return to sport at the preinjury level after revision anterior cruciate ligament reconstruction: A systematic review and meta-analysis. Journal of ISAKOS: Joint Disorders & Orthopaedic Sports Medicine 2 (1), 21-30.

Kessler, M.A., Behrend, H., Henz, S., Stutz, G., Rukavina, A., Kuster, M.S., et al., 2008. Function, osteoarthritis and activity after ACL-rupture: 11 years follow-up results of conservative versus reconstructive treatment. Knee Surgery, Sports Traumatology, Arthroscopy 16 (5), 442-448.

Kiadaliri, A.A., Englund, M., Lohmander, L.S., Carlsson, K.S., Frobell, R.B., 2016. No economic benefit of early knee reconstruction over optional delayed reconstruction for ACL tears: Registry enriched randomised controlled trial data. British Journal of Sports Medicine 50 (9), 558-563.

Koga, H., Nakamae, A., Shima, Y., Iwasa, J., Myklebust, G., Engebretsen, L., et al., 2010. Mechanisms for noncontact anterior cruciate ligament injuries: Knee joint kinematics in 10 injury situations from female team handball and basketball. The American Journal of Sports Medicine 38 (11), 2218-2225.

Leys, T., Salmon, L., Waller, A., Linklater, J., Pinczewski, L., 2012. Clinical results and risk factors for reinjury 15 years after anterior cruciate ligament reconstruction: A prospective study of hamstring and patellar tendon grafts. The American Journal of Sports Medicine 40 (3), 592-605.

Lowe, W.R., Warth, R.J., Davis, E.P., Bailey, L., 2017. Functional bracing after anterior cruciate ligament reconstruction: A systematic review. The Journal of the American Academy of Orthopaedic Surgeons 25 (3), 239-249.

Mather 3rd, R.C., Koenig, L., Kocher, M.S., Dall, T.M., et al., 2013. Societal and economic impact of anterior cruciate ligament tears. The Journal of Bone and Joint Surgery. American volume 95 (19), 1751.

Michaelidis, M., Koumantakis, G.A., 2014. Effects of knee injury primary prevention programs on anterior cruciate ligament injury rates in female athletes in different sports: A systematic review. Physical Therapy in Sport 15 (3), 200-210.

Moses, B., Orchard, J., 2012. Systematic review: Annual incidence of ACL injury and surgery in various populations. Research in Sports Medicine 20 (3-4), 157-179.

Myer, G.D., Ford, K.R., Barber Foss, K.D., Liu, C., Nick, T.G., Hewett, T.E., et al., 2009. The relationship of hamstrings and quadriceps strength to anterior cruciate ligament injury in female athletes. Clinical Journal of Sport Medicine 19 (1), 3-8.

Noyes, F.R., Barber-Westin, S.D., 2014. Neuromuscular retraining intervention programs: Do they reduce noncontact anterior cruciate

ligament injury rates in adolescent female athletes? Arthroscopy 30 (2), 245-255.

O'Connell, K., Knight, H., Ficek, K., Leonska-Duniec, A., Maciejewska-Karlowska, A., Sawczuk, M., et al., 2015. Interactions between collagen gene variants and risk of anterior cruciate ligament rupture. European Journal of Sport Science 15 (4), 341-350.

Padua, D.A., DiStefano, L.J., Beutler, A.I., de la Motte, S.J., DiStefano, M.J., Marshall, S.W., et al., 2015. The Landing Error Scoring System as a screening tool for an anterior cruciate ligament injury-prevention program in elite-youth soccer athletes. Journal of Athletic Training 50 (6), 589-595.

Prodromos, C.C., Han, Y., Rogowski, J., Joyce, B., Shi, K., 2007. A meta-analysis of the incidence of anterior cruciate ligament tears as a function of gender, sport, and a knee injury-reduction regimen. Arthroscopy 23 (12), 1320-1325.e1326.

Roos, P.E., Button, K., Sparkes, V., van Deursen, R.W., 2014. Altered biomechanical strategies and medio-lateral control of the knee represent incomplete recovery of individuals with injury during single leg hop. Journal of Biomechanics 47 (3), 675-680.

Ruedl, G., Webhofer, M., Helle, K., Strobl, M., Schranz, A., Fink, C., et al., 2012. Leg dominance is a risk factor for noncontact anterior cruciate ligament injuries in female recreational skiers. The American Journal of Sports Medicine 40 (6), 1269-1273.

Sanders, T.L., Maradit Kremers, H., Bryan, A.J., Larson, D.R., Dahm, D.L., Levy, B.A., et al., 2016. Incidence of anterior cruciate ligament tears and reconstruction: A 21-year population-based study. The American Journal of Sports Medicine 44 (6), 1502-1507.

Schlumberger, M., Schuster, P., Schulz, M., Immendörfer, M., Mayer, P., Bartholomä, J., et al., 2017. Traumatic graft rupture after primary and revision anterior cruciate ligament reconstruction: retrospective analysis of incidence and risk factors in 2915 cases. Knee Surgery, Sports Traumatology, Arthroscopy 25 (5), 1535-1541.

Shimokochi, Y., Shultz, S.J., 2008. Mechanisms of noncontact anterior cruciate ligament injury. Journal of Athletic Training 43 (4), 396-408.

Silvers, H.J., Mandelbaum, B.R., 2011. ACL injury prevention in the athlete. Sports Orthopaedics and Traumatology 27 (1), 18-26.

Smith, T.O., Postle, K., Penny, F., McNamara, I., Mann, C.J.V., 2014. Is reconstruction the best management strategy for anterior cruciate ligament rupture? A systematic review and meta-analysis comparing anterior cruciate ligament reconstruction versus non-operative treatment. Knee 21 (2), 462-470.

Sugimoto, D., Myer, G.D., Foss, K.D., Hewett, T.E., 2014. Dosage effects of neuromuscular training intervention to reduce anterior cruciate ligament injuries in female athletes: Meta- and sub-group analyses. Journal of Sports Medicine 44 (4), 551-562.

Suter, L.G., Smith, S.R., Katz, J.N., Englund, M., Hunter, D.J., Frobell, R., et al., 2017. Projecting lifetime risk of symptomatic knee osteoarthritis and total knee replacement in individuals sustaining a complete anterior cruciate ligament tear in early adulthood. Arthritis Care & Research 69 (2), 201-208.

Tengman, E., Brax Olofsson, L., Stensdotter, A.K., Nilsson, K.G., Häger, C.K., 2014. Anterior cruciate ligament injury after more than 20 years. II. Concentric and eccentric knee muscle strength. Scandinavian Journal of Medicine & Science in Sports 24 (6), e501-e509.

Tengman, E., Grip, H., Stensdotter, A.K., Hager, C.K., 2015. Anterior cruciate ligament injury about 20 years post-treatment: A kinematic analysis of one-leg hop. Scandinavian Journal of Medicine & Science in Sports 25 (6), 818-827.

Tengman, E., Olofsson, L.B., Nilsson, K.G., Tegner, Y., Lundgren, L., Hager, C.K., et al., 2014. Anterior cruciate ligament injury after more than 20 years: I. Physical activity level and knee function. Scandinavian Journal of Medicine & Science in Sports 24 (6), e491-e500.

Thomeé, R., Kaplan, Y., Kvist, J., Myklebust, G., Risberg, M.A., Theisen, D., et al., 2011. Muscle strength and hop performance criteria prior to return to sports after ACL reconstruction. Knee Surgery, Sports Traumatology, Arthroscopy 19 (11), 1798-1805.

Uhorchak, J.M., Scoville, C.R., Williams, G.N., Arciero, R.A., St Pierre, P., Taylor, D.C., et al., 2003. Risk factors associated with noncontact injury of the anterior cruciate ligament: a prospective four-year evaluation of 859 West Point cadets. The American Journal of Sports Medicine 31 (6), 831-842.

Vacek, P.M., Slauterbeck, J.R., Tourville, T.W., Sturnick, D.R., Holterman, L.A., Smith, H.C., et al., 2016. Multivariate analysis of the risk factors for first-time noncontact ACL injury in high school and college athletes. The American Journal of Sports Medicine 44 (6), 1492-1501.

van Melick, N., van Cingel, R.E., Brooijmans, F., Neeter, C., van Tienen, T., Hullegie, W., et al., 2016. Evidence-based clinical practice update: Practice guidelines for anterior cruciate ligament rehabilitation based on a systematic review and multidisciplinary consensus. British Journal of Sports Medicine 50 (24), 1506-1515.

VandenBerg, C., Crawford, E.A., Sibilsky Enselman, E., Robbins, C.B., Wojtys, E.M., Bedi, A., et al., 2017. Restricted hip rotation is correlated with an increased risk for anterior cruciate ligament injury. Arthroscopy 33 (2), 317-325.

Waldén, M., Hägglund, M., Ekstrand, J., 2006. High risk of new knee injury in elite footballers with previous anterior cruciate ligament injury. British Journal of Sports Medicine 40 (2), 158-162.

Waldén, M., Krosshaug, T., Bjørneboe, J., Andersen, T.E., Faul, O., Hägglund, M., et al., 2015. Three distinct mechanisms predominate in non-contact anterior cruciate ligament injuries in male professional football players: A systematic video analysis of 39 cases. British Journal of Sports Medicine 49 (22), 1452-1460.

Wellsandt, E., Failla, M.J., Snyder-Mackler, L., 2017. Limb symmetry indexes can overestimate knee function after anterior cruciate ligament injury. The Journal of Orthopaedic and Sports Physical Therapy 47 (5), 334-338.

Wright, R.W., Magnussen, R.A., Dunn, W.R., Spindler, K.P., 2011. Ipsilateral graft and contralateral ACL rupture at five years or more following ACL reconstruction: A systematic review. The Journal of Bone and Joint Surgery. American volume 93 (12), 1159-1165.

Zeng, C., Gao, S.G., Wei, J., Yang, T.B., Cheng, L., Luo, W., et al., 2013. The influence of the intercondylar notch dimensions on injury of the anterior cruciate ligament: a meta-analysis. Knee Surgery, Sports Traumatology, Arthroscopy 21 (4), 804-815.

Lesões do ombro

Abdul-Wahab, T.A., Betancourt, J.P., Hassan, F., Thani, S.A., Choueiri, H., Jain, N.B., et al., 2016. Initial treatment of complete rotator cuff tear and transition to surgical treatment: systematic review of the evidence. Muscles, Ligaments and Tendons Journal 6 (1), 35-47.

Antoni, M., Klouche, S., Mas, V., Ferrand, M., Bauer, T., Hardy, P., et al., 2016. Return to recreational sport and clinical outcomes with at least 2 years follow-up after arthroscopic repair of rotator cuff tears. Orthopaedics & Traumatology: Surgery & Research 102 (5), 563-567.

Berth, A., Pap, G., Awiszus, F., Neumann, W., 2009. Central motor deficits of the deltoid muscle in patients with chronic rotator cuff tears. Acta Chirurgiae Orthopaedicae et Traumatologiae Cechoslovaca 76 (6), 456-461.

Burkhart, S.S., Morgan, C.D., Kibler, W.B., 2003. The disabled throwing shoulder: Spectrum of pathology part I: Pathoanatomy and biomechanics. Arthroscopy 19 (4), 404-420.

Crichton, J., Jones, D.R., Funk, L., 2012. Mechanisms of traumatic shoulder injury in elite rugby players. British Journal of Sports Medicine 46 (7), 538-542.

Elsenbeck, M.J., Dickens, J.F., 2017. Return to sports after shoulder stabilization surgery for anterior shoulder instability. Current Reviews in Musculoskeletal Medicine 10 (4), 491-498.

Gibbs, D.B., Lynch, T.S., Nuber, E.D., Nuber, G.W., 2015. Common shoulder injuries in american football athletes. Current Sports Medicine Reports 14 (5), 413-419.

Gibson, J., Kerss, J., Morgan, C., Brownson, P., 2016. Accelerated rehabilitation after arthroscopic Bankart repair in professional footballers. Shoulder & Elbow 8 (4), 279-286.

Huber, R., Ghilardi, M.F., Massimini, M., Ferrarelli, F., Riedner, B.A., Peterson, M.J., et al., 2006. Arm immobilization causes cortical plastic changes and locally decreases sleep slow wave activity. Nature Neuroscience 9 (9), 1169-1176.

Jaggi, A., Lambert, S., 2010. Rehabilitation for shoulder instability. British Journal of Sports Medicine 44 (5), 333-340.

Kim, S.H., Ha, K.I., Jung, M.W., Lim, M.S., Kim, Y.M., Park, J.H., et al., 2003. Accelerated rehabilitation after arthroscopic Bankart repair for selected cases: a prospective randomized clinical study. Arthroscopy 19 (7), 722-731.

Klouche, S., Lefevre, N., Herman, S., Gerometta, A., Bohu, Y., 2016. Return to sport after rotator cuff tear repair. The American Journal of Sports Medicine 44 (7), 1877-1887.

Kuhn, J.E., Dunn, W.R., Sanders, R., An, Q., Baumgarten, K.M., Bishop, J.Y., et al., 2013. Effectiveness of physical therapy in treating atraumatic full-thickness rotator cuff tears: a multicenter prospective cohort study. Journal of Shoulder and Elbow Surgery 22 (10), 1371-1379.

Lewis, A., Kitamura, T., Bayley, J.I., 2004. (ii) The classification of shoulder instability: new light through old windows! Current Orthopaedics 18 (2), 97-108.

Mazuquin, B.F., Wright, A.C., Russell, S., Monga, P., Selfe, J., Richards, J., et al., 2018. Effectiveness of early compared with conservative rehabilitation for patients having rotator cuff repair surgery: An overview of systematic reviews. British Journal of Sports Medicine 52 (2), 111-121.

McCormick, F., Gupta, A., Bruce, B., Harris, J., Abrams, G., Wilson, H., et al., 2014. Single-row, double-row, and transosseous equivalent techniques for isolated supraspinatus tendon tears with minimal atrophy: A retrospective comparative outcome and radiographic analysis at minimum 2-year follow-up. International Journal of Shoulder Surgery 8 (1), 15-20.

McMahon, P.J., Prasad, A., Francis, K.A., 2014. What is the prevalence of senior-athlete rotator cuff injuries and are they associated with pain and dysfunction? Clinical Orthopaedics and Related Research 472 (8), 2427-2432.

McMullen, J., Uhl, T.L., 2000. A kinetic chain approach for shoulder rehabilitation. Journal of Athletic Training 35 (3), 329-337.

Monga, P., Funk, L., 2017. Diagnostic Clusters in Shoulder Conditions. Springer International Publishing, New York.

Opsha, O., Malik, A., Baltazar, R., Primakov, D., Beltran, S., Miller, T.T., et al., 2008. MRI of the rotator cuff and internal derangement. European Journal of Radiology 68 (1), 36-56.

Robins, R.J., Daruwalla, J.H., Gamradt, S.C., McCarty, E.C., Dragoo, J.L., Hancock, R.E., et al., 2017. Return to play after shoulder instability surgery in National Collegiate Athletic Association Division I intercollegiate football athletes. The American Journal of Sports Medicine 45 (10), 2329-2335.

Thigpen, C.A., Shaffer, M.A., Gaunt, B.W., Leggin, B.G., Williams, G.R., Wilcox 3rd, R.B., et al., 2016. The American Society of Shoulder and Elbow Therapists' consensus statement on rehabilitation following arthroscopic rotator cuff repair. Journal of Shoulder and Elbow Surgery 25 (4), 521-535.

Trappey, G.J., Gartsman, G.M., 2011. A systematic review of the clinical outcomes of single row versus double row rotator cuff repairs. Journal of Shoulder and Elbow Surgery 20 (Suppl. 2), S14-S19.

Yamaguchi, K., Ditsios, K., Middleton, W.D., Hildebolt, C.F., Galatz, L.M., Teefey, S.A., et al., 2006. The demographic and morphological features of rotator cuff disease – A comparison of asymptomatic and symptomatic shoulders. The Journal of Bone and Joint Surgery. American volume 88 (8), 1699-1704 2006 Aug.

Yamamoto, A., Takagishi, K., Osawa, T., Yanagawa, T., Nakajima, D., Shitara, H., et al., 2010. Prevalence and risk factors of a rotator cuff tear in the general population. Journal of Shoulder and Elbow Surgery 19 (1), 116-120.

Capítulo | 6 |

Agentes Eletrofísicos: Fisiologia e Evidências

Tim Watson

Introdução

Há uma tendência geral de se afastar do termo "eletroterapia" em direção ao termo mais abrangente "agentes eletrofísicos" (AEF). Eletroterapia, no sentido mais estrito, só se aplica às modalidades que envolvem o fornecimento de energia elétrica e, possivelmente, também eletromagnética. Como um termo, "AEF" é mais inclusivo e é um reflexo mais preciso da ampla gama de modalidades empregadas na terapia, como ultrassom (US), *laser* e ondas de choque (Watson, 2010).

O uso moderno dos AEF deve ser baseado em evidências, e as modalidades, escolhidas criteriosamente. Quando usadas de maneira adequada, essas modalidades têm a capacidade estabelecida e demonstrável de alcançar um benefício significativo. Usadas imprudentemente, não farão nenhum bem ou, pior ainda, agravarão o quadro clínico. Além das habilidades necessárias para entregar cada modalidade, há habilidade para tomar a decisão clínica apropriada sobre qual modalidade usar e quando. Existem poucas circunstâncias, se houver, nas quais as modalidades são mais eficazes quando usadas isoladamente. Seu uso como parte de um programa de tratamento integrado e personalizado é o modo em que eles são capazes de alcançar o benefício máximo. Os AEF não são um componente essencial para todos os pacientes e só devem ser usados quando e onde forem justificados e benefícios significativos possam ser razoavelmente esperados.

O objetivo deste capítulo é permitir ao leitor identificar rapidamente as principais modalidades que são capazes de influenciar a reparação e recuperação de tecidos de uma lesão. Não tem como objetivo examinar ou explicar completamente as evidências para todas as modalidades e há muitas modalidades que foram excluídas. Isso é um reflexo da complexidade das evidências e práticas modernas dos AEF. Mais detalhes estão disponíveis em outros textos (p. ex., Bellew et al., 2016; Knight e Draper, 2012; Michlovitz et al., 2012; Watson e Nussbaum, 2020). As referências principais são fornecidas no final do capítulo e o recurso *online* (acesso aberto) www.electrotherapy.org tem detalhes sobre todas as modalidades, juntamente com um resumo objetivo da literatura principal.

Ultrassom terapêutico

A terapia de US é um dos tratamentos eletrofísicos mais comumente empregados (Shah e Farrow, 2012) e tem uma ampla gama de aplicações em tecidos moles e reparo e recuperação relacionados com os esportes (de Brito Viera et al., 2012; Watson, 2014).

O US é um tipo de energia mecânica. A faixa normal de som humano é de 16 Hz a aproximadamente 20 mil Hz. Além desse limite superior, a vibração mecânica é conhecida como US. As frequências usadas na terapia são normalmente 1 e 3 MHz (1 MHz = 1 milhão de ciclos por segundo) e, portanto, estão além do alcance auditivo humano. Alguns dispositivos de terapia oferecem frequências de aplicação em outras taxas, como 1,5 e 0,75 MHz e dispositivos de US de ondas longas que operam na faixa de quilohertz (p. ex., 48 kHz e 150 kHz). O desenvolvimento relativamente recente do US pulsado de baixa intensidade (LIPUS, do inglês *low-intensity pulsed ultrasound*) é usado principalmente em relação com as lesões ósseas, em particular no reparo de fraturas, comumente empregando uma frequência de aplicação de 1,5 MHz.

As ondas sonoras são ondas longitudinais que consistem em zonas de compressão e rarefação. Quando expostas a uma onda sonora, as partículas de um material oscilam em torno de um ponto fixo. Qualquer aumento da vibração molecular no tecido pode resultar na geração de calor e o US pode ser usado para produzir mudanças térmicas nos tecidos, embora a maioria do uso atual na terapia não se concentre nesse fenômeno (Baker et al., 2001; Nussbaum, 1997; ter Haar, 1999; Watson, 2020). A vibração dos tecidos tem efeitos considerados de natureza "não térmica", embora, como em outras modalidades, deva haver um componente térmico, por menor que seja, não suficiente para alterações clinicamente significativas. À medida que a onda dos US passa por um material (os tecidos), os níveis de energia dentro da onda diminuem conforme a energia é transferida para o material.

Um meio de acoplamento é empregado para permitir a transferência da energia sonora para os tecidos. No momento, os meios à base de gel são preferíveis aos à base de óleos e cremes. A água é um meio de transmissão eficaz e pode ser usada como alternativa. Não há diferença realista (clínica) entre os géis de uso clínico comum (Poltawski e Watson, 2007).

A absorção de energia dos US segue uma distribuição exponencial. Para que a energia tenha efeito, ela deve ser absorvida. À medida que a energia dos US penetra mais nos tecidos, uma proporção maior da energia terá sido absorvida e, portanto, haverá menos energia disponível para atingir os efeitos terapêuticos. O US pode ser clinicamente eficaz em profundidades de 5 a 6 cm.

Alguns tecidos são capazes de maior absorção de energia dos US do que outros. Tecidos com maior teor de proteína absorvem os US em maior extensão. Assim, os tecidos com alto teor de água e baixo teor de proteína absorvem pouca energia (p. ex., sangue e gordura), enquanto os tecidos com menor teor de água e maior teor de proteína irão absorver US com muito mais eficiência. Foi sugerido que os tecidos podem, portanto, ser classificados de acordo com sua absorção (Figura 6.1).

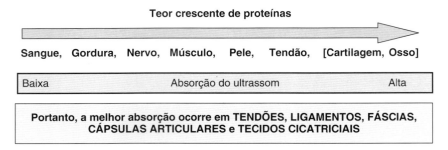

Figura 6.1 Absorção de ultrassom em diferentes tecidos.

Embora a cartilagem e o osso estejam na extremidade superior dessa escala, os problemas associados à reflexão das ondas significam que a maior parte da energia dos US que atinge a superfície de qualquer um desses tecidos, provavelmente, será refletida. Os tecidos com melhor absorção na prática clínica são aqueles com alto teor de colágeno; ligamento, tendão, fáscia, cápsula articular, tecido cicatricial (Nussbaum, 1998; ter Haar, 1999; Watson, 2000; 2008; 2020).

A maioria das máquinas oferece a facilidade de saída dos ultrassons pulsados. Os formatos de pulso típicos são 1:1 e 1:4, embora outros estejam disponíveis. No modo 1:1, a máquina oferece uma saída de 2 ms seguido de 2 ms de repouso. No modo 1:4, a saída de 2 ms é seguida de um período de descanso de 8 ms. Os efeitos do US pulsado são bem documentados (Watson, 2020; Watson e Nussbaum, 2020), e esse tipo de saída é preferível, principalmente, no tratamento de lesões mais agudas. Isso evita o acúmulo de energia suficiente para gerar calor, mantendo, no entanto, os efeitos atérmicos do US, como micromassagem e cavitação.

Usos clínicos da terapia de ultrassom

Geralmente, os efeitos terapêuticos do US são divididos nas categorias *térmica* e *não térmica*. Enquanto a aplicação de energia dos US em níveis de potência suficientes será capaz de gerar mudança térmica nos tecidos (Draper et al., 1995; Draper e Ricard, 1995; Meakins e Watson, 2006; Nussbaum, 1998), nos tecidos moles e na terapia relacionada com esportes, aplicações pulsadas de baixa dosagem com intenção não térmica dominam as evidências. Doses mais altas com potenciais térmicos têm um lugar a longo prazo e para apresentações mais crônicas.

Efeitos e usos não térmicos do ultrassom

Agora, os efeitos não térmicos do US são atribuídos, principalmente, a uma combinação de *cavitação* e *correntes acústicas* (Baker et al., 2001; ter Haar, 1999; Watson e Nussbaum, 2020). Os detalhes desses efeitos físicos primários do US são descritos em textos e artigos apropriados (Robertson et al., 2006; Watson, 2020).

O resultado dos efeitos combinados da cavitação estável e das correntes acústicas é que a membrana celular se torna "excitada" (ou seja, ela se regula positivamente), aumentando seus níveis de atividade. A energia dos US atua como um gatilho para esse processo, mas é o aumento da atividade celular que é efetivamente responsável pelos benefícios terapêuticos da modalidade (Izadifar et al., 2017; Watson, 2000; 2008; 2020). Evidências recentes identificam fortemente que a energia mecânica aplicada resulta em regulação positiva celular e, como resultado, estimula a liberação/síntese/expressão de vários mediadores químicos, fatores de crescimento e citocinas, que são responsáveis pelos efeitos fisiológicos e clínicos observados (Watson, 2016).

Aplicação de ultrassom em relação ao reparo tecidual

O processo de reparo tecidual é uma série complexa de eventos em cascata mediados quimicamente que levam à produção de tecido cicatricial, o qual constitui um material eficaz para restaurar a continuidade do tecido danificado.

Inflamação

Durante a fase inflamatória, o US tem um efeito estimulante sobre os mastócitos, as plaquetas, os glóbulos brancos com funções fagocíticas e os macrófagos (Maxwell, 1992; Nussbaum, 1997; ter Haar, 1999). A aplicação do US induz a degranulação dos mastócitos, causando a liberação de ácido araquidônico, o qual, por sua vez, é um precursor da síntese de prostaglandinas e leucotrienos – que atuam como mediadores inflamatórios (Nussbaum, 1997). Ao aumentar a atividade dessas células, a influência geral do US terapêutico é mais *pró-inflamatória* do que *anti-inflamatória*. O benefício não é "aumentar" a resposta inflamatória, mas sim atuar como um "otimizador inflamatório". A resposta inflamatória é essencial para o reparo eficaz do tecido e quanto mais eficientemente o processo puder ser concluído, mais efetivamente o tecido poderá progredir para a próxima fase (proliferação). O US é eficaz na promoção de eventos inflamatórios normais e, como tal, tem valor terapêutico na promoção de eventos gerais de reparo. Outro benefício é que os eventos inflamatórios mediados quimicamente estão associados à estimulação da fase proliferativa e, por meio dessa via, também promovem o reparo.

A evidência de efeitos de US mediados quimicamente é identificada em muitas publicações (Bajpai et al., 2018; Kim et al., 2020; Maxwell, 1992; Nakamura et al., 2010; Nussbaum, 1997; Renno et al., 2011; Sahu et al., 2020; ter Haar, 1999; Watson, 2014; 2020; Watson e Nussbaum, 2020; Zhou et al., 2008).

Empregado em uma dose de tratamento apropriada, com parâmetros de tratamento ideais (intensidade, pulsação, tempo), o benefício do US é induzir a fase de reparo inicial alcançada com mais eficiência, promovendo, assim, a cascata de cura.

Proliferação

Durante a fase proliferativa, o US também tem um efeito estimulante (regulação celular positiva) e os alvos ativos primários são fibroblastos, células endoteliais e miofibroblastos (Maxwell, 1992; Nussbaum, 1997; 1998; Ramirez et al., 1997). Normalmente, todas essas células são ativas durante a produção de reparo tecidual; portanto, o US é *pró-proliferativo*. Ele não altera a fase proliferativa normal, mas maximiza sua eficiência; produzindo o tecido cicatricial necessário de uma maneira ideal. Harvey et al. (1975) demonstraram que o US pulsado de baixa dosagem aumenta a síntese de proteínas e vários grupos de pesquisa observaram fibroplasia e síntese de colágeno aumentadas

(Enwemeka et al., 1990; Ramirez et al., 1997; Turner et al., 1989). Um trabalho recente identificou o papel crítico de vários fatores de crescimento em relação com o reparo tecidual e algumas evidências acumuladas identificaram que o US terapêutico tem um papel positivo para desempenhar nesse contexto (de Oliveira Perrucini et al., 2020; Leung et al., 2006; Lovric et al., 2013; McBrier et al., 2007; Watson, 2016).

Remodelamento

Durante a fase de remodelamento do reparo, a cicatriz genérica, que é produzida durante a proliferação, é refinada. Isso é alcançado por uma série de processos, sobretudo relacionados com a orientação das fibras de colágeno na cicatriz em desenvolvimento e com a mudança no tipo de colágeno, de predominantemente tipo III para predominantemente tipo I (Watson, 2006) – ambos determinam a qualidade e a resistência do reparo.

A aplicação de US terapêutico pode influenciar o remodelamento do tecido cicatricial, pois melhora a orientação das fibras de colágeno recém-formadas (Byl et al., 1996) e estimula a mudança de colágeno do tipo III para uma construção mais predominantemente do tipo I, aumentando a resistência à tração e a mobilidade da cicatriz (Nussbaum, 1998; Wang, 1998). O US aplicado aos tecidos também eleva a capacidade funcional dos tecidos da cicatriz (Nussbaum, 1998; Yeung et al., 2006).

A aplicação do US durante as fases inflamatória, proliferativa e de reparo não altera a sequência normal de eventos; em vez disso, tem a capacidade de estimular ou aumentar esses eventos normais e, assim, ampliar a eficiência das fases de reparo (ter Haar, 1999; Watson, 2006; 2008; 2014). Recentemente, foi proposto (Watson, 2016) que o modo de ação, de acordo com outras modalidades eletrofísicas, se dá principalmente, pelo aumento dos eventos inflamatórios, proliferativos e de remodelamento mediados quimicamente. A aplicação eficaz do US para atingir esses objetivos depende da dose. Os detalhes das aplicações de dose estão além do escopo deste texto, mas são revisados em www.electrotherapy.org.

Embora a ênfase da evidência revisada nesta seção tenha sido relacionada com o reparo tecidual, claramente, existem circunstâncias em que a inflamação está presente sem lesão evidente. A evidência publicada ilustra que o US tem um benefício demonstrável nessas lesões inflamatórias, por exemplo, alterações relacionadas com a osteoartrite (Yegin et al., 2017; Zeng et al., 2014; Zhang et al., 2016), a síndrome do túnel do carpo (Ahmed et al., 2017; Huisstede et al., 2018), a síndrome da dor miofascial (Ilter et al., 2015) e a epicondilite (Dingemanse et al., 2014).

Ultrassom pulsado de baixa intensidade e cicatrização de fraturas

Vários trabalhos de pesquisa recentes identificaram o potencial do US pulsado de baixa intensidade (LIPUS) para promover o reparo tecidual, mais fortemente evidenciado em relação a fraturas, incluindo cenários clínicos normais, tardios/não união e pós-cirúrgicos.

Uma revisão sistemática e metanálise (Busse et al., 2009) considerou as evidências para o efeito do LIPUS no tempo de consolidação da fratura. Eles concluíram a partir das evidências de dados agrupados de ensaios clínicos randomizados (ECR) (três estudos, 158 fraturas) que o tempo para a consolidação da fratura foi significativamente reduzido nos grupos tratados com US em comparação aos grupos de controle, e a diferença média no tempo de cicatrização foi de 64 dias. Uma revisão sistemática (Griffin et al., 2008) avaliando o uso de LIPUS para fraturas recentes, considerando sete ECR e duas metanálises, sugeriu que esse corpo de evidências é de suporte.

O mecanismo pelo qual o LIPUS aumenta ou estimula a sequência de reparo da fratura está resumido na Figura 6.2 e é abordado de forma útil por Claes e Willie (2007); Della Roca (2009); Jingushi (2009); Lu et al. (2009); Padilla et al. (2014); Zhang et al. (2017) e Zuo et al. (2018). O mecanismo é, principalmente, por meio de vias de mediação química aprimoradas, como é o caso do US tradicional.

As máquinas utilizadas para esses tratamentos entregam uma intensidade muito baixa (0,03 W/cm² ou 30 mW/cm²), a 1,5 MHz pulsado na proporção de 1:4 a 1 kHz, aplicado por 20 minutos diários. A intensidade dessa aplicação é consideravelmente menor do que a intensidade mais baixa que é fornecida pela maioria das máquinas de US atuais (normalmente 0,1 W/cm²). Atualmente, uma máquina de US de terapia convencional não fornecerá uma dose baixa suficientemente controlada para tornar o LIPUS uma opção. Dispositivos específicos do LIPUS são comercializados, embora seja provável futuras máquinas clínicas oferecerem uma opção do LIPUS.

Os primeiros estudos clínicos (p. ex., Heckman et al., 1994; Kristiansen et al., 1997) demonstraram uma aceleração nas taxas de consolidação de fraturas de 30 a 38%. Jensen (1998) identifica os efeitos benéficos do US no tratamento de fraturas por estresse, comum em atletas, com uma taxa de sucesso geral de 96%. Mayr et al. (2000) relatam uma série de resultados ao usar US pulsado de baixa intensidade para pacientes com união tardia (n = 951) e não união (n = 366). A taxa geral de sucesso para a união tardia foi de 91% e para não união foi de 86%.

Numerosas revisões recentes baseadas em evidências foram publicadas (Bayat et al., 2018; Harrison et al., 2016; Mehta et al., 2015; Padilla et al., 2016), todas apoiando essa intervenção. Uma sugestão recente de que os efeitos clínicos do LIPUS não são tão pronunciados como levantado originalmente (Schandelmaier et al., 2017) foi contestada por Aspenberg (2017), entre outros. O peso atual da evidência é a favor das aplicações do LIPUS como um meio de melhorar o reparo de fraturas recentes e para instigar uma resposta em apresentações clínicas tardias e não consolidadas. O uso de LIPUS na terapia, provavelmente, aumentará com base nisso.

Terapia por ondas curtas pulsadas e outras aplicações de radiofrequência

A terapia por ondas curtas pulsadas (TOCP) é uma modalidade amplamente utilizada (Al Mandeel e Watson, 2006). O termo mais antigo, "diatermia de ondas curtas pulsadas", não é realmente apropriado, pois a modalidade não é empregada principalmente como diatermia (literalmente, "por meio de aquecimento").

A saída da máquina de ondas curtas (operando a 27,12 MHz) é pulsada de modo que o tempo "ligado" seja consideravelmente mais curto do que o tempo "desligado"; assim, a potência média fornecida ao paciente é relativamente baixa, embora a potência de pico (durante os pulsos "ligados") possa ser alta (normalmente em torno de 150 a 200 W com máquinas modernas).

O usuário pode variar (a) a potência média fornecida ao paciente e (b) os parâmetros de pulsação que governam o modo de distribuição da energia. A evidência atual sugere que a *potência média* é o parâmetro mais importante (Al Mandeel e Watson, 2020; Hill et al., 2002).

Ao usar ondas curtas pulsadas no ambiente clínico, existem dois "modos" de aplicação. As informações nesta seção se referem à aplicação usando o eletrodo "monodo" ou "tambor" em vez do sistema de distribuição da placa do capacitor que carece de evidências de suporte suficientes.

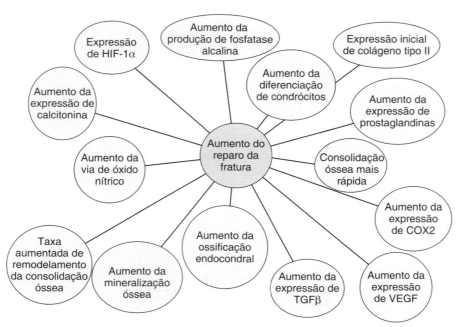

Figura 6.2 Mecanismos com evidência para a ação do ultrassom pulsado de baixa intensidade (LIPUS) em relação ao reparo de fraturas. *COX2*, ciclo-oxigenase-2; *HIF-1α*, fator-1alfa induzível por hipoxia; *TGFβ*, fator de crescimento transformador beta; *VEGF*, fator de crescimento endotelial vascular.

Parâmetros principais. A taxa de repetição do pulso (Hz ou pulsos/segundo) controla a quantidade de pulsos de energia de ondas curtas que é entregue ao paciente em um segundo. A duração do pulso (largura do pulso) refere-se à duração, em microssegundos (μs), de cada pulso individual de energia.

A combinação de frequência de pulso e gerenciamento de duração permite que o usuário influencie a potência média fornecida ao paciente, que é o parâmetro crítico do tratamento.

Normalmente, o pico de potência é em torno de 150 a 200 W em máquinas modernas. Essa é a "força" das ondas curtas enquanto o pulso está "ligado". A *potência média* leva em consideração o fato de que existem as fases "ligada" e "desligada", ou seja, o fornecimento de energia é intermitente; descreve a saída de potência média em vez da saída de potência em qualquer momento (que pode ser máxima ou zero).

As aplicações clínicas, geralmente, variam de 10 a 20 minutos em níveis de potência médios de < 5 W (lesões agudas) até 48 W (dose térmica, lesões crônicas).

A relação entre os parâmetros de pulso e os níveis de potência é ilustrada na Figura 6.3.

Aquecimento tecidual. Com relação aos efeitos da onda curta pulsada, há um elemento de aquecimento tecidual que ocorre durante o pulso "ligado", mas isso é dissipado durante a fase "desligada" prolongada. Portanto, é possível administrar o tratamento sem aumento líquido na temperatura tecidual, por isso indicado em fases inflamatórias agudas. A Figura 6.4 A não demonstra nenhum acúmulo de efeitos térmicos ou não térmicos. Na Figura 6.4 B, os pulsos estão suficientemente próximos para gerar um efeito acumulativo não térmico. Por sua vez, na Figura 6.4 C, há um acúmulo de efeitos térmicos e não térmicos. As configurações aplicadas à máquina determinarão quais efeitos serão obtidos em determinado tratamento. Em geral, os efeitos "não térmicos" da modalidade são considerados de maior significado, especialmente em tecidos moles/aplicações relacionadas com esportes. Eles parecem se acumular durante o tempo de tratamento e têm um efeito significativo após um período latente, possivelmente da ordem de 6 a 8 horas. É sugerido (Hayne, 1984) que os níveis de energia necessários para produzir esse efeito em humanos são baixos.

A pesquisa demonstrou que a TOCP tem um componente térmico e que pode ocorrer aquecimento real do tecido (Bricknell e Watson, 1995). Um efeito de aquecimento mensurável pode ser demonstrado em níveis de potência acima de 5 W; contudo, no geral, ele se torna aparente em potência média de 11 W ou mais.

Se um tratamento "não térmico" for necessário (p. ex., para o manejo de lesões agudas), o tratamento deve ser administrado em um nível abaixo de 5 W de potência média. Se for pretendido um efeito térmico, são necessários níveis de potência superiores a 5 W; porém, se realizado, o terapeuta deve garantir que sejam tomadas as precauções como em qualquer outra intervenção térmica.

Terapia por ondas curtas pulsadas: efeitos clínicos

Os efeitos clínicos da TOCP estão, principalmente, relacionados com as fases inflamatória e de reparo nos tecidos musculoesqueléticos. Goldin et al. (1981) listaram os efeitos da modalidade (seguindo pesquisas de reparo de tecidos moles após aplicação

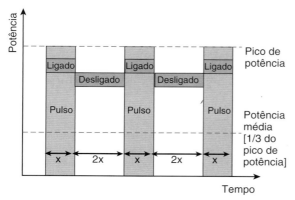

Figura 6.3 Relação entre os parâmetros de pulso e os níveis de potência com terapia por ondas curtas pulsadas.

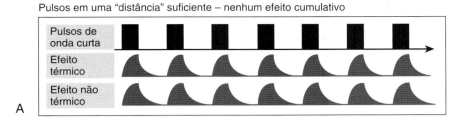
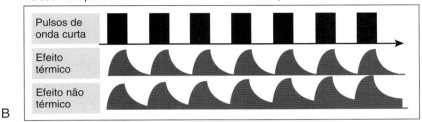
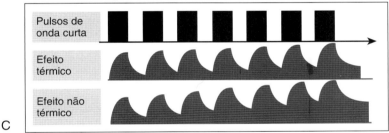

Figura 6.4 Efeito da variação dos parâmetros de pulso sobre o calor acumulado gerado nos tecidos.

de enxerto de pele). Os efeitos são abordados nos textos padrões (Al Mandeel e Watson, 2020; Robertson et al., 2006; Watson, 2006). É mais eficaz quando empregada após lesões de tecido em níveis baixos (não térmicos), enquanto aplicações de alta potência são benéficas em apresentações mais crônicas. Considerando que a terapia de US é a modalidade de escolha para o tratamento de tecido colagenoso denso (ligamento, tendão, fáscia, cápsula articular, tecido cicatricial), a onda curta pulsada é empregada de maneira ideal quando o tecido-alvo tem um alto teor de água (músculo, nervo, áreas de edema, hematoma). Os efeitos das duas modalidades de terapia são basicamente os mesmos; é o tipo de tecido no qual os efeitos são alcançados que varia entre elas. O uso de ondas curtas pulsadas foi revisado recentemente em condições agudas e crônicas (Kumaran e Watson, 2015; 2016) com evidências de suporte em ambos os grupos.

Aplicações de altas doses foram relatadas na literatura esportiva com efeito aparentemente bom para o manejo de lesões de longa duração (Draper et al., 2017). No outro extremo, unidades de uso doméstico portáteis de dose muito baixa distribuindo ondas curtas por meio de um circuito de contato com a pele têm uso potencial em lesões agudas (incluindo pós-cirurgia), sendo usadas por horas ao longo do dia em vez de dezenas de minutos (Brook et al., 2012).

Aplicações de radiofrequência de ondas não curtas (Tecar)

O fornecimento de energia de radiofrequência (RF) em frequências de ondas não curtas (normalmente, abaixo de 1 MHz) está ganhando força, inclusive na área de medicina esportiva. O tópico foi revisado recentemente (Kumaran e Watson, 2015; 2016), incluindo RF em frequências de ondas curtas e não curtas. Normalmente, o tratamento é administrado com um sistema de dois eletrodos (um eletrodo ativo menor e uma placa de retorno maior) em modo capacitivo ou resistivo. Os eletrodos estão em contato direto com os tecidos por meio de um creme condutor; assim, uma corrente fluirá pelos tecidos, ocasionando um efeito térmico significativo quando aplicada com energia suficiente.

Além das mudanças de temperatura do tecido, fisiologicamente, há um efeito altamente significativo no fluxo sanguíneo local, tanto em nível superficial quanto profundo. Essas mudanças são evidentes mesmo em doses baixas (não térmicas) (Kumaran e Watson, 2017). Além disso, esses efeitos têm uma duração significativamente mais longa do que os níveis de energia equivalentes aplicados com dispositivos de ondas curtas pulsadas (Kumaran e Watson, 2018).

O aumento do fluxo sanguíneo é uma reação tecidual essencial durante a sequência de reparo (Watson, 2006) e, portanto, é proposto que, ao aumentar essa resposta local, o processo de reparo tecidual será aprimorado. As primeiras evidências clínicas apoiam essa proposição (Kumaran e Watson, 2018).

Terapia a *laser*/fotobiomodulação

O termo *laser* é um acrônimo em inglês para *amplificação de luz por emissão estimulada de radiação* (*light amplification by stimulated emission of radiation*). Em termos simples, o *laser* pode ser considerado um tipo de amplificador de luz – ele fornece o aprimoramento de propriedades específicas da energia luminosa.

A luz do *laser* se comporta de acordo com as leis básicas da luz, no sentido de que viaja em linha reta a uma velocidade constante no espaço. Ele pode ser transmitido, refletido, refratado e absorvido. O *laser* também pode ser colocado dentro do espectro eletromagnético de acordo com seu comprimento de onda/frequência, que irá variar conforme o gerador específico considerado (Figura 6.5).

Existem vários aspectos da luz *laser* que são considerados únicos e são, frequentemente, mencionados na literatura. Estes incluem *monocromacia*, *coerência* e *polarização* (para detalhes de física e mecanismo de interação, ver Baxter e Nussbaum, 2020; Hamblin e Huang, 2013; Karu, 1998; Tuner e Hode, 2004).

Terminologia. Os termos "terapia a *laser* de baixo nível" (LLLT, do inglês *low-level laser therapy*) e "terapia a *laser* de baixa intensidade" (LILT, do inglês *low-intensity laser therapy*) são usados como equivalentes. Recentemente, os termos "fotomodulação" ou "fotobiomodulação" foram adotados como os termos preferenciais para essa terapia (Hamblin, 2016).

Os *lasers* de terapia têm várias características comuns que são resumidas brevemente a seguir.

Parâmetros. O aparelho de LLLT gera luz nas bandas do vermelho visível e próximas ao infravermelho no espectro eletromagnético, com comprimentos de onda típicos de 600 a 1000 nm. Em geral, a potência média desses dispositivos é baixa (1 a 100 mW). O dispositivo de tratamento pode ser um único emissor ou um conjunto de vários emissores. Normalmente, o feixe de sondas simples é estreito (Ø 1 a 7 mm) na fonte. Um conjunto de sondas costuma incorporar emissores de alta e baixa potências de diferentes comprimentos de onda. A saída pode ser contínua ou pulsada, com larguras de pulso estreitas (nas faixas de nano ou microssegundos) e uma ampla variedade de taxas de repetição de pulso de 2 Hz até vários milhares de Hz. É difícil identificar as evidências para o uso de pulsação na literatura científica, embora isso afete a energia aplicada e, portanto, tenha impacto nos parâmetros de dose.

A recente promoção de *lasers* de alta potência (muitas vezes descritos em virtude de sua classificação de segurança, *lasers* de classe 4) baseia-se no fato de que, com níveis de energia entregues mais elevados, a penetração da energia luminosa no tecido será maior (nenhuma evidência identificada) e os tempos de tratamento serão mais curtos (de acordo com evidências baseadas nos tempos de entrega de energia).

Geradores alternativos usando diodos emissores de luz (LED) ou diodos *laser* estão disponíveis. As evidências sugerem que essas fontes alternativas de luz serão capazes de atingir efeitos equivalentes desde que a energia aplicada esteja no mesmo nível (de Abru Chaves et al., 2014; Lima et al., 2017).

Absorção de luz pelos tecidos

A absorção de energia luminosa dentro dos tecidos é uma questão complexa, mas, geralmente, os comprimentos de onda mais curtos (ultravioleta e visível mais curto) são absorvidos, principalmente, na epiderme por pigmentos, aminoácidos e ácidos nucleicos. Os comprimentos de onda infravermelhos mais longos (> 1.300 nm) parecem ser rapidamente absorvidos pela água e, portanto, têm uma penetração limitada nos tecidos. A banda de 600 a 1.000 nm é capaz de penetração além da epiderme superficial e está disponível para absorção por tecidos mais profundos.

Embora grande parte da luz de *laser* aplicada seja absorvida nos tecidos superficiais, é proposto que efeitos mais profundos ou mais distantes podem ser alcançados como uma consequência secundária por meio de mediadores químicos ou sistemas de segundo mensageiro, embora haja evidências limitadas para apoiar totalmente essa alegação. A maior parte da energia luminosa aplicada será absorvida nos primeiros 5 mm de profundidade do tecido quando os comprimentos de onda na parte vermelha visível do espectro forem empregados. Uma porcentagem útil da energia luminosa disponível na superfície estará disponível em 10 a 15 mm nos tecidos com comprimentos de onda infravermelhos (acima de 770 nm), mas a penetração clinicamente eficaz além desse nível é discutível.

Interação *laser*-tecido

Fotobiomodulação ou *fotobioativação* são termos comumente usados em conexão com a terapia a *laser* e se referem à estimulação de vários eventos biológicos usando energia luminosa, mas sem mudanças significativas de temperatura. Eles já foram adotados como termos preferenciais para essa modalidade (Hamblin, 2016).

Os primeiros princípios da fotobioativação foram propostos por Karu (1987), que relatou e demonstrou vários fatores-chave. Ela observa em seu artigo que algumas biomoléculas mudam sua atividade em resposta à exposição à luz visível de baixa intensidade, mas que essas moléculas não parecem absorver a luz diretamente. A célula e as membranas mitocondriais são os absorvedores primários da energia que, por sua vez, geram efeitos intracelulares por meio de um segundo mensageiro/resposta em cascata. A magnitude da resposta à luz parece ser determinada

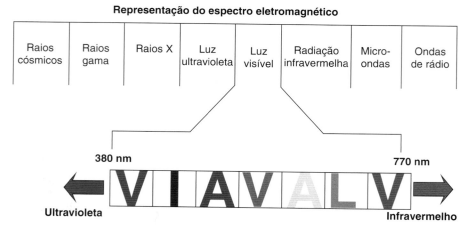

Figura 6.5 Energia luminosa como parte do espectro eletromagnético.

pelo estado dos tecidos antes da irradiação. A irradiação do *laser* nos tecidos é um gatilho para a alteração dos processos metabólicos celulares, por meio de um processo de transdução do sinal luminoso. Embora a pesquisa de Karu não seja recente, foi a primeira demonstração robusta desses efeitos, confirmados por muitos autores posteriormente. As metas de nível celular e os efeitos alcançados foram revistos de forma útil por Hamblin (2017).

A seguinte lista de efeitos de nível fisiológico e celular é compilada a partir de várias revisões e artigos de pesquisa (Baxter, 2002; 2008; Hamblin et al., 2013; Tuner e Hode, 2004):

- Proliferação celular alterada
- Motilidade celular alterada
- Ativação de fagócitos
- Estimulação de respostas imunológicas
- Aumento do metabolismo celular
- Estimulação de macrófagos
- Estimulação da degranulação dos mastócitos
- Ativação e proliferação de fibroblastos
- Alteração dos potenciais de membrana celular
- Estimulação da angiogênese
- Alteração dos potenciais de ação
- Produção alterada de prostaglandina
- Produção de opioides endógenos alterada.

Os efeitos da fotobiomodulação a *laser* na *fase inflamatória* do reparo são muito semelhantes aos alcançados pela terapia de US e quase certamente aos alcançados por meio de mediação química e ativação de sistema semelhante (Alves et al., 2013; 2014; Aras et al., 2015; Dos Santos et al., 2014; Hamblin, 2017; Hwang et al., 2015; Moura Júnior et al., 2014; Pires et al., 2011; Silva et al., 2015; Torres-Silva et al., 2015). Na *fase proliferativa*, os efeitos do *laser* refletem mais uma vez amplamente aqueles alcançados por terapias baseadas em US (Alves et al., 2013; Chen et al., 2015; Colombo et al., 2013; Cury et al., 2013; Dungel et al., 2014; Ginani et al., 2015; Halon et al., 2015; Kuryliszyn-Moskal et al., 2015; Park et al., 2015; Rhee et al., 2016; Solmaz et al., 2017; Staffoli et al., 2017). O *laser* tem efeitos menos bem demonstrados no *estágio de remodelamento* (quando comparado ao US), embora algumas evidências de eficácia e mecanismos de ação tenham sido identificadas (De Souza et al., 2011).

Doses terapêuticas

A maioria dos grupos de pesquisa recomenda que a dose administrada a um paciente durante uma sessão de tratamento deve ser baseada em *densidade energética*, e não em potência ou outra medida de dose. A densidade energética é medida em *joules* por centímetro quadrado (J/cm²). Atualmente, argumenta-se que os *joules* (i. e., *energia*) podem de fato ser o parâmetro mais crítico, em vez da densidade energética. O debate ainda não foi resolvido, e a densidade energética é usada aqui como a pesquisa publicada que o cita quase exclusivamente.

A maioria das autoridades sugere que a densidade energética por sessão de tratamento deve, geralmente, cair na faixa de 0,1 a 12 J/cm², embora haja algumas recomendações que vão até 30 J/cm². Novamente, como regra geral, doses mais baixas devem ser aplicadas às lesões mais agudas que parecem ser mais sensíveis à energia.

Aplicações clínicas

A pesquisa recente concentra-se em algumas áreas-chave. As mais dominantes entre elas são cicatrização de feridas, artropatias inflamatórias, lesões em tecidos moles e alívio da dor (que inclui acupuntura a *laser*).

Feridas abertas

Há um crescente corpo de evidências para o uso do tratamento a *laser* nesse contexto, com a maioria sendo ensaios de resultados positivos (há seções úteis em Baxter, 1994; Baxter e Nussbaum, 2020; Hamblin, 2013; Tuner e Hode, 2004). Embora as evidências para essas aplicações permaneçam fortes, elas não são amplamente utilizadas na prática da medicina esportiva.[1]

Artropatias inflamatórias

Houve vários estudos envolvendo o uso de LILT para vários problemas inflamatórios nas articulações. Os resultados são mistos, mas a tendência geral é favorável. A revisão do Painel de Ottawa (2004) apoia a terapia a *laser* na artrite reumatoide. Há um volume relativamente pequeno de literatura relacionada com a artropatia inflamatória na medicina esportiva – ela é dominada por apresentações do tipo degenerativa (osteoartrite) e inflamatória clássica (artrite reumatoide) (Rayegani et al., 2017).

Lesão de tecido mole

Há um uso generalizado de LILT em aplicações nos tecidos moles. Tuner e Hode (2004) descrevem vários exemplos de tratamentos eficazes de tecidos moles e identificam algumas das principais pesquisas nessa área. Mais materiais também estão incluídos na revisão de Baxter e Nussbaum (2020) e no texto de Hamblin (2013). Trabalhos recentes concentraram-se no efeito do *laser* como uma intervenção pré-exercício para limitar a dor muscular de início tardio (DMIT) e melhorar a recuperação, em vez de um tratamento de lesões *em si*. Os resultados foram mistos, mas, em alguns casos, a aplicação de *laser* antes do exercício demonstrou um benefício de recuperação significativo para os atletas (De Marchi et al., 2017; de Oliveira et al., 2017; Jowko et al., 2019; Pinto et al., 2016).

Dor

Tem sido amplamente assumido que o efeito da terapia a *laser* para o alívio da dor é um efeito secundário de lidar com o estado inflamatório. Embora o alívio da dor sintomática possa ser benéfico do ponto de vista do paciente (de Souza et al., 2018; Izukura et al., 2017), argumenta-se que o uso de *laser* para afetar a lesão/patologia subjacente tem o potencial de proporcionar efeitos mais duradouros. Há evidências crescentes de que a terapia a *laser* tem um efeito direto nas características de condução nervosa e pode resultar em redução da dor como efeito direto (Casale et al., 2013; Chow e Armati, 2016).

Nos últimos anos, houve vários estudos avaliando a terapia a *laser* como um meio de modificar a dor (DMIT) ou melhorar a recuperação muscular pós-exercício (Antonialli et al., 2014; de Oliveira et al., 2017). Embora essas não sejam aplicações clínicas totalmente estabelecidas, há, certamente, evidências suficientes para identificá-las como aplicações promissoras.

Resumo

Em termos de melhorar a reparação de tecidos e a recuperação de lesões, as terapias baseadas em *laser* têm uma base de evidências de suporte substancial. Os efeitos da terapia são muito semelhantes aos alcançados pela terapia de US, embora o tecido-alvo seja diferente – o *laser* é mais eficaz nos tecidos

---

[1] N.R.T.: ao usar o tratamento a *laser*, é importante sempre respeitar os métodos de prevenção de contaminação por contato direto entre a ponteira e a ferida, a qual deve estar recoberta de plástico especial.

Terapia por ondas de choque

A terapia por ondas de choque é um desenvolvimento relativamente recente para aplicações relacionadas com as lesões e os esportes.

Inicialmente, as ondas de choque foram empregadas como tratamento não invasivo para cálculos renais nas décadas de 1970 e 1980 e isso se tornou uma intervenção de primeira linha para essas condições. Os experimentos com modelos animais associados a esse trabalho identificaram que as ondas de choque podem ter um efeito (adverso) no osso. Isso levou a uma série de investigações experimentais avaliando o efeito das ondas de choque no osso, na cartilagem e nos tecidos moles (tendão, ligamento, fáscia), resultando nas aplicações atuais da terapia.

Uma história sucinta do desenvolvimento de ondas de choque para aplicações médicas pode ser encontrada em Thiel (2001). Os geradores de ondas de choque pneumáticos (balísticos) são mais comumente empregados na terapia.

Existem essencialmente dois "modos" de terapia por ondas de choque: *focada* e *radial*. A versão focada é "mais forte", ou seja, a energia aplicada atinge um ponto focal no tecido e é, geralmente, considerada a forma mais poderosa da terapia. É avaliada como eficaz até uma profundidade de tecido de aproximadamente 12 cm. O modo radial é mais comumente gerado com um mecanismo de ar comprimido, enviando um projétil ao longo de um cilindro, atingindo a placa final no aplicador. Atualmente, existem dispositivos eletromagnéticos que operam de maneira semelhante. A onda de pressão acústica é transmitida aos tecidos (normalmente, por meio de um gel condutor, que melhora a eficácia e o conforto). A energia não atinge um ponto de concentração no tecido e, portanto, nunca é mais "concentrada" do que na superfície. É sugerido que essa energia é clinicamente eficaz em profundidades de 5 a 6 cm no tecido (Eaton e Watson, 2020; Foldager et al., 2012).

Quando a onda de choque entra nos tecidos, ela é refletida, refratada, transmitida e dissipada da mesma forma que qualquer outra energia. O conteúdo de energia e a propagação da onda variam com o tipo de tecido.

As ondas de choque podem ser aplicadas em potências altas e baixas. Os tratamentos de alta potência (> 0,6 mJ/mm²) são administrados como "únicos" e geram uma quantidade significativa de dor. Frequentemente, é necessário algum tipo de anestesia local para que o paciente seja capaz de tolerar o tratamento. A abordagem mais comum é usar várias (geralmente de três a cinco) aplicações em baixa potência (até 0,08 mJ/mm²; nenhuma anestesia é necessária), em geral 1.500 a 2.000 choques administrados por sessão usando um dispositivo de onda de choque radial.

Conforme a onda de choque viaja através de um meio e chega a uma interface, parte da onda é refletida e parte é transmitida. A dissipação da energia na interface é responsável pela geração dos efeitos físicos, fisiológicos e terapêuticos.

A terapia por ondas de choque é mais eficaz quando empregada como parte de um programa de tratamento para apresentações do tipo tendinopatia crônica. Isso inclui fascite plantar; lesões no tendão calcâneo (porções média e de inserção), patelares, epicondilares medial e lateral; supraespinal (calcificada e não calcificada) e outras lesões do manguito rotador. Existem inúmeras aplicações de tratamento em desenvolvimento, incluindo síndrome da dor trocantérica maior, síndrome de estresse tibial medial, miosite ossificante, problemas musculares locais, lesões ligamentares, cicatrização óssea problemática e cerca de 20 ou 30 outros exemplos. Embora alguns deles sejam de desenvolvimento, já existem evidências de pesquisas publicadas para apoiá-los.

A literatura de tendinopatia é resumida em várias revisões importantes e documentos de compilação de evidências (Aqil et al., 2013; Császár e Schmidt, 2013; Everhart et al., 2017; Hawk et al., 2017; Ioppolo et al., 2013; Korakakis et al., 2018; Leal et al., 2015; Roehrig et al., 2005; Romeo et al., 2014; Santamato et al., 2016; Speed, 2014; Taheri et al., 2017; van der Worp et al., 2013; Verstraelen et al., 2014; Wang et al., 2012; Yin et al., 2014).

Essa é uma intervenção provocativa e não se destina a "acalmar" o tecido no qual é aplicada. Ao provocar a lesão crônica com níveis de energia relativamente elevados, uma lesão mais aguda será ativada com mecanismos pró-inflamatórios associados.

O papel da terapia por ondas de choque irá estabilizar-se com o tempo (*i. e.*, as apresentações clínicas para as quais ela é mais/menos eficaz irão tornar-se estabelecidas); no entanto, atualmente, seu uso em casos de tendinopatia crônica é reconhecido e é apoiado por pesquisas clínicas e revisões sistemáticas.

Terapia de microcorrente

A terapia de microcorrente está se tornando cada vez mais empregada no ambiente clínico como uma modalidade nova e emergente, embora fortes evidências para apoiar seu uso datem de várias décadas.

Curiosamente, parece quebrar todas as "regras" de classificação identificadas anteriormente neste capítulo. Não é entregue com a intenção de estimular os nervos, ao contrário, atua no ambiente bioelétrico dos tecidos e, portanto, tem um efeito primário em termos de reparo tecidual (Poltawski e Watson, 2009; Watson e Nussbaum, 2020). A característica geral desse tipo de terapia é utilizar uma corrente direta (pulsada ou contínua), administrada em amplitude muito baixa (na faixa de microampere [milionésimos de ampere]), que costuma ser subsensorial do ponto de vista do paciente. Esse tipo de terapia já demonstrou ser eficaz em várias áreas clínicas, principalmente no reparo de fraturas (Ciombor e Aaron, 2005; Simonis et al., 2003) e na cicatrização de feridas abertas (Evans et al., 2001; Watson, 1996; 2008). A pesquisa de reparo de tecidos moles está evoluindo e mostra um forte potencial para o futuro. O uso dessa terapia no tratamento de lesões teciduais foi revisado recentemente (Poltawski e Watson, 2009) e alguns resultados de ensaios clínicos de suporte foram publicados (Chapman-Jones e Hill, 2002; Poltawski et al., 2012).

Os dispositivos de terapia de microcorrente parecem ser empregados de modo mais eficaz quando usados por horas ao longo do dia (em vez de minutos por semana na clínica). Portanto, a terapia domiciliar com dispositivos portáteis pequenos e baratos é um provável caminho a seguir.

Conclusão

Os agentes eletrofísicos têm um papel baseado em evidências na prática fisioterapêutica. Este capítulo tentou resumir as

Agentes Eletrofísicos: Fisiologia e Evidências **Capítulo** |6|

principais modalidades em uso no ambiente clínico atual, com foco nas modalidades com o papel mais importante a desempenhar na cura e no tratamento pós-lesão. Cada modalidade tem uma gama de efeitos fisiológicos específicos, os quais podem ser empregados, por sua vez, para produzir efeitos terapêuticos.

O uso excessivo da eletroterapia no passado resultou no fim dessa área de prática. Este capítulo tentou identificar as questões-chave para modalidades relevantes, ilustrar suas aplicações clínicas potenciais com base nas evidências disponíveis e apontar fontes detalhadas para informações adicionais.

Referências bibliográficas

Ahmed, O.F., Elkharbotly, A.M., Taha, N., Bekheet, A.B., 2017. Treatment of mild to moderate carpal tunnel syndrome in patients with diabetic neuropathy using low level laser therapy versus ultrasound controlled comparative study. Biochimica et Biophysica Acta Clinical 8, 43-47.

Al-Mandeel, M., Watson, T., 2020. Pulsed and continuous shortwave and radiofrequency therapies. In: Watson, T. and Nussbaum, N. (Eds.), Electrophysical Agents: Evidence-Based Practice, thirteenth ed. Elsevier, Edinburgh, pp. 132-149.

Al-Mandeel, M., Watson, T., 2006. An audit of patient records into the nature of pulsed shortwave therapy use. International Journal of Therapy and Rehabilitation 13 (9), 414-420.

Alves, A.C., Vieira, R., Leal-Junior, E., dos Santos, S., Ligeiro, A.P., Albertini, R., et al., 2013. Effect of low-level laser therapy on the expression of inflammatory mediators and on neutrophils and macrophages in acute joint inflammation. Arthritis Research & Therapy 15 (5), R116.

Alves, A.N., Fernandes, K.P., Deana, A.M., Bussadori, S.K., Mesquita-Ferrari, R.A., 2014. Effects of low-level laser therapy on skeletal muscle repair: a systematic review. American Journal of Physical Medicine & Rehabilitation 93 (12), 1073-1085.

Antonialli, F.C., De Marchi, T., Tomazoni, S.S., Vanin, A.A., Dos Santos Grandinetti, V., de Paiva, P.R., et al., 2014. Phototherapy in skeletal muscle performance and recovery after exercise: effect of combination of super-pulsed laser and light-emitting diodes. Lasers in Medical Science 29 (6), 1967-1976.

Aqil, A., Siddiqui, M.S., Solan, M., Redfern, D., Gulati, V., Cobb, J., 2013. Extracorporeal shock wave therapy is effective in treating chronic plantar fasciitis: a meta-analysis of RCTs. Clinical Orthopaedics and Related Research 471 (11), 3645-3652.

Aras, M.H., Bozdag, Z., Demir, T., Oksayan, R., Yanik, S., Sokucu, O., 2015. Effects of low-level laser therapy on changes in inflammation and in the activity of osteoblasts in the expanded premaxillary suture in an ovariectomized rat model. Photomedicine and Laser Surgery 33 (3), 136-144.

Aspenberg, P., 2017. Comment to a BMJ Editorial: is LIPUS the baby in the bathwater? Acta Orthopaedica 88 (1), 1.

Bajpai, A., Nadkarni, S., Neidrauer, M., Weingarten, M.S., Lewin, P.A., Spiller, K.L., 2018. Effects of non-thermal, non-cavitational ultrasound exposure on human diabetic ulcer healing and inflammatory gene expression in a pilot study. Ultrasound in Medicine & Biology 44 (9), 2043-2049.

Baker, K.G., Robertson, V.J., Duck, F.A., 2001. A review of therapeutic ultrasound: biophysical effects. Physical Therapy 81 (7), 1351-1358.

Baxter, D., 1994. Therapeutic Lasers: Theory & Practice. Churchill Livingstone, Edinburgh.

Baxter, D., 2002. Low-intensity laser therapy. In: Kitchen, S. (Ed.), Electrotherapy: Evidence Based Practice, eleventh ed. Churchill Livingstone/Elsevier, Edinburgh.

Baxter, D., Nussbaum, E., 2020. Laser/photobiomodulation. In: Watson, T. and Nussbaum, N. (Eds.), Electrophysical Agents: Evidence-Based Practice, thirteenth ed. Elsevier, Edinburgh, pp. 189-207.

Bayat, M., Virdi, A., Rezaei, F., Chien, S., 2018. Comparison of the in vitro effects of low-level laser therapy and low-intensity pulsed ultrasound therapy on bony cells and stem cells. Progress in Biophysics and Molecular Biology 133, 36-48 2018.

Bellew, J.W., Michlovitz, S.L., Nolan, T., 2016. Michlovitz's Modalities for Therapeutic Intervention, sixth ed. F.A. Davis Company, Philadelphia, PA.

Bricknell, R., Watson, T., 1995. The thermal effects of pulsed shortwave therapy. British Journal of Therapy & Rehabilitation 2 (8), 430-434.

Brook, J., Dauphinee, D.M., Korpinen, J., Rawe, I.M., 2012. Pulsed radiofrequency electromagnetic field therapy: a potential novel treatment of plantar fasciitis. The Journal of Foot and Ankle Surgery 51 (3), 312-316.

Busse, J.W., Kaur, J., Mollon, B., Bhandari, M., Tornetta 3rd, P., Schunemann, H.J., et al., 2009. Low intensity pulsed ultrasonography for fractures: systematic review of randomised controlled trials. British Medical Journal 338, b351.

Byl, N.N., Hill Toulouse, L., Sitton, P., Hall, J., Stern, R., 1996. Effects of ultrasound on the orientation of fibroblasts: an in-vitro study. European Journal of Physical and Rehabilitation Medicine 6 (6), 180-184.

Casale, R., Damiani, C., Maestri, R., Wells, C.D., 2013. Pain and electrophysiological parameters are improved by combined 830-1064 high-intensity LASER in symptomatic carpal tunnel syndrome versus transcutaneous electrical nerve stimulation. A randomized controlled study. European Journal of Physical and Rehabilitation Medicine 49 (2), 205-211.

Chapman-Jones, D., Hill, D., 2002. Novel microcurrent treatment is more effective than conventional therapy for chronic Achilles tendinopathy: randomised comparative trial. Physiotherapy 88 (8), 471-480.

Chen, M.H., Huang, Y.C., Sun, J.S., Chao, Y.H., 2015. Second messengers mediating the proliferation and collagen synthesis of tenocytes induced by low-level laser irradiation. Lasers in Medical Science 30 (1), 263-272.

Chow, R.T., Armati, P.J., 2016. Photobiomodulation: implications for anesthesia and pain relief. Photomedicine and Laser Surgery 34 (12), 599-609.

Ciombor, D.M., Aaron, R.K., 2005. The role of electrical stimulation in bone repair. Foot and Ankle Clinics 10 (4), 579-593 vii.

Claes, L., Willie, B., 2007. The enhancement of bone regeneration by ultrasound. Progress in Biophysics and Molecular Biology 93 (1-3), 384-398.

Colombo, F., Neto Ade, A., Sousa, A.P., Marchionni, A.M., Pinheiro, A.L., Reis, S.R., et al., 2013. Effect of low-level laser therapy (λ660 nm) on angiogenesis in wound healing: a immunohistochemical study in a rodent model. Brazilian Dental Journal 24 (4), 308-312.

Császár, N.B., Schmitz, C., 2013. Extracorporeal shock wave therapy in musculoskeletal disorders. Journal of Orthopaedic Surgery and Research 8 (1), 22.

Cury, V., Moretti, A.I., Assis, L., Bossini, P., Crusca Jde, S., Neto, C.B., et al., 2013. Low level laser therapy increases angiogenesis in a model of ischemic skin flap in rats mediated by VEGF, HIF-1α and MMP-2. Journal of Photochemistry and Photobiology. B, Biology 125, 164-170.

de Abreu Chaves, M.E., de Araújo, A.R., Piancastelli, A.C.C., Pinotti, M., 2014. Effects of low-power light therapy on wound healing: LASER x LED. Anais Brasileiros de Dermatologia 89 (4), 616-623.

de Brito Vieira, W.H., Aguiar, K.A., da Silva, K.M., Canela, P.M., da Silva, F.S., Abreu, B.J., et al., 2012. Overview of ultrasound usage trends in orthopedic and sports physiotherapy. Critical Ultrasound Journal 4 (1), 11.

De Marchi, T., Schmitt, V.M., Danubia da Silva Fabro, C., da Silva, L.L., Sene, J., Tairova, O., et al., 2017. Phototherapy for improvement of performance and exercise recovery: comparison of 3 commercially available devices. Journal of Athletic Training 52 (5), 429-438.

de Oliveira, A.R., Vanin, A.A., Tomazoni, S.S., Miranda, E.F., Albuquerque-Pontes, G.M., De Marchi, T., et al., 2017. Pre-exercise infrared photobiomodulation therapy (810 nm) in skeletal muscle performance and postexercise recovery in humans: what is the optimal power output? Photomedicine and Laser Surgery 35 (11), 595-603.

de Oliveira Perrucini, P.D., Poli-Frederico, R.C., de Almeida Pires-Oliveira, D.A., Dragonetti Bertin, L., Beltrao Pires, F., Shimoya-Bittencourt, W., et al., 2020. Anti-inflammatory and healing effects of pulsed ultrasound therapy on fibroblasts. American Journal of Physical Medicine & Rehabilitation 99 (1), 19-25.

de Souza, R.C., de Sousa, E.T., Scudine, K.G., Meira, U.M., de Oliveira, E.S.E.M., Gomes, A.C., et al., 2018. Low-level laser therapy and anesthetic infiltration for orofacial pain in patients with fibromyalgia: a randomized clinical trial. Medicina Oral, Patologia Oral y Cirugia Bucal 23 (1), e65-e71.

de Souza, T., Mesquita, D., Ferrari, R., dos Santos Pinto, D., Correa, L., Bussadori, S., et al., 2011. Phototherapy with low-level laser affects the

61

remodeling of types I and III collagen in skeletal muscle repair. Lasers in Medical Science 26 (6), 803-814.

Della Rocca, G., 2009. The science of ultrasound therapy for fracture healing. Indian Journal of Orthopaedics 43 (2), 121-126.

Dingemanse, R., Randsdorp, M., Koes, B.W., Huisstede, B.M.A., 2014. Evidence for the effectiveness of electrophysical modalities for treatment of medial and lateral epicondylitis: a systematic review. British Journal of Sports Medicine 48 (12), 957-965.

dos Santos, S.A., Alves, A.C., Leal-Junior, E.C., Albertini, R., Vieira Rde, P., Ligeiro, A.P., et al., 2014. Comparative analysis of two low-level laser doses on the expression of inflammatory mediators and on neutrophils and macrophages in acute joint inflammation. Lasers in Medical Science 29 (3), 1051-1058.

Draper, D.O., Ricard, M.D., 1995. Rate of temperature decay in human muscle following 3 MHz ultrasound: the stretching window revealed. Journal of Athletic Training 30 (4), 304-307.

Draper, D.O., Schulthies, S., Sorvisto, P., Hautala, A.M., 1995. Temperature changes in deep muscles of humans during ice and ultrasound therapies: an in vivo study. The Journal of Orthopaedic and Sports Physical Therapy 21 (3), 153-157.

Draper, D.O., Veazey, E., 2017. Pulsed shortwave diathermy and joint mobilizations restore a twice fractured elbow with metal implants to full range of motion. Journal of Novel Physiotherapy and Rehabilitation 1, 020-026.

Dungel, P., Hartinger, J., Chaudary, S., Slezak, P., Hofmann, A., Hausner, T., et al., 2014. Low level light therapy by LED of different wavelength induces angiogenesis and improves ischemic wound healing. Lasers in Surgery and Medicine 46 (10), 773-780.

Dyson, M., Smalley, D., 1983. Effects of ultrasound on wound contraction. In: Millner, R., Rosenfeld, E., Cobet, U. (Eds.), Ultrasound Interactions in Biology & Medicine. Plenum Press, New York, pp. 151-158.

Eaton, C., Watson, T., 2020. Shockwave. In: Watson, T. and Nussbaum, N. (Eds.), Electrophysical Agents: Evidence-Based Practice, thirteenth ed. Elsevier, Edinburgh, pp. 229-246.

Enwemeka, C.S., Rodriguez, O., Mendosa, S., 1990. The miomechanical effects of low intensity ultrasound on healing tendons. Ultrasound in Medicine & Biology 16 (8), 801-807.

Evans, R.D., Foltz, D., Foltz, K., 2001. Electrical stimulation with bone and wound healing. Clinics in Podiatric Medicine and Surgery 18 (1), 79-95 vi.

Everhart, J.S., Cole, D., Sojka, J.H., Higgins, J.D., Magnussen, R.A., Schmitt, L.C., et al., 2017. Treatment options for patellar tendinopathy: a systematic review. Arthroscopy 33 (4), 861-872.

Foldager, C.B., Kearney, C., Spector, M., 2012. Clinical application of extracorporeal shock wave therapy in orthopedics: focused versus unfocused shock waves. Ultrasound in Medicine & Biology 38 (10), 1673-1680.

Ginani, F., Soares, D.M., Barreto, M.P., Barboza, C.A., 2015. Effect of low-level laser therapy on mesenchymal stem cell proliferation: a systematic review. Lasers in Medical Science 30 (8), 2189-2194.

Goldin, J.H., Broadbent, N.R.G., Nancarrow, J.D., Marshall, T., 1981. The effects of Diapulse on the healing of wounds: a double-blind randomised controlled trial in man. British Journal of Plastic Surgery 34 (3), 267-270.

Griffin, X.L., Costello, I., Costa, M.L., 2008. The role of low intensity pulsed ultrasound therapy in the management of acute fractures: a systematic review. The Journal of Trauma 65 (6), 1446-1452.

Halon, A., Donizy, P., Dziegala, M., Dobrakowski, R., Simon, K., 2015. Tissue laser biostimulation promotes post-extraction neoangiogenesis in HIV-infected patients. Lasers in Medical Science 30 (2), 701-706.

Hamblin, M.R., 2016. Photobiomodulation or low-level laser therapy. Journal of Biophotonics 9 (11-12), 1122-1124.

Hamblin, M.R., 2017. Mechanisms and applications of the anti-inflammatory effects of photobiomodulation. American Institute of Mathematical Sciences Biophysics 4 (3), 337-361.

Hamblin, M.R., Huang, Y., 2013. Handbook of Photomedicine. CRC Press, Boca Raton, FL.

Harrison, A., Lin, S., Pounder, N., Mikuni-Takagaki, Y., 2016. Mode & mechanism of low intensity pulsed ultrasound (LIPUS) in fracture repair. Ultrasonics 70, 45-52.

Harvey, W., Dyson, M., Pond, J.B., Grahame, R., 1975. The stimulation of protein synthesis in human fibroblasts by therapeutic ultrasound. Rheumatology & Rehabilitation 14 (4), 237.

Hawk, C., Minkalis, A.L., Khorsan, R., Daniels, C.J., Homack, D., Gliedt, J.A., et al., 2017. Systematic review of nondrug, nonsurgical treatment of shoulder conditions. Journal of Manipulative and Physiological Therapeutics 40 (5), 293-319.

Hayne, C.R., 1984. Pulsed high frequency energy – Its place in physiotherapy. Physiotherapy 70, 459-464.

Heckman, J.D., Ryaby, J.P., McCabe, J., Frey, J.J., Kilcoyne, R.F., 1994. Acceleration of tibial fracture-healing by non-invasive, low-intensity pulsed ultrasound. The Journal of Bone and Joint Surgery. American Volume 76 (1), 26-34.

Hill, J., Lewis, M., Mills, P., Kielty, C., 2002. Pulsed short-wave diathermy effects on human fibroblast proliferation. Archives of Physical Medicine and Rehabilitation 83 (6), 832-836.

Huisstede, B.M.A., Hoogvliet, P., Franke, T.P.C., Randsdorp, M.S., Koes, B.W., 2018. Carpal tunnel syndrome: effectiveness of physical therapy and electrophysical modalities. An updated systematic review of randomized controlled trials. Archives of Physical Medicine and Rehabilitation 99 (8), 1623-1634.e23.

Hwang, M.H., Shin, J.H., Kim, K.S., Yoo, C.M., Jo, G.E., Kim, J.H., et al., 2015. Low level light therapy modulates inflammatory mediators secreted by human annulus fibrosus cells during intervertebral disc degeneration in vitro. Photochemistry and Photobiology 91 (2), 403-410.

Ilter, L., Dilek, B., Batmaz, I., Ulu, M.A., Sariyildiz, M.A., Nas, K., et al., 2015. Efficacy of pulsed and continuous therapeutic ultrasound in myofascial pain syndrome: a randomized controlled study. American Journal of Physical Medicine & Rehabilitation 94 (7), 547-554.

Ioppolo, F., Tattoli, M., Di Sante, L., Venditto, T., Tognolo, L., Delicata, M., et al., 2013. Clinical improvement and resorption of calcifications in calcific tendinitis of the shoulder after shock wave therapy at 6 months' follow-up: a systematic review and meta-analysis. Archives of Physical Medicine and Rehabilitation 94 (9), 1699-1706.

Izadifar, Z., Babyn, P., Chapman, D., 2017. Mechanical and biological effects of ultrasound: a review of present knowledge. Ultrasound in Medicine & Biology 43 (6), 1085-1104.

Izukura, H., Miyagi, M., Harada, T., Ohshiro, T., Ebihara, S., 2017. Low Level Laser Therapy in patients with chronic foot and ankle joint pain. Laser Therapy 26 (1), 19-24.

Jensen, J.E., 1998. Stress fracture in the world class athlete: a case study. Medicine and Science in Sports and Exercise 30 (6), 783-787.

Jingushi, S., 2009. [Bone fracture and the healing mechanisms. Fracture treatment by low-intensity pulsed ultrasound]. Clinical Calcium 19 (5), 704-708.

Jowko, E., Plaszewski, M., Cieslinski, M., Sacewicz, T., Cieslinski I., Jarocka, M., 2019. The effect of low level laser irradiation on oxidative stress, muscle damage and function following neuromuscular electrical stimulation. A double blind, randomised, crossover trial. BMC Sports Science, Medicine and Rehabilitation 11, 38.

Karu, T., 1987. Photobiological fundamentals of low-power laser therapy. IEEE Journal of Quantum Electronics 23 (10), 1703-1717.

Karu, T., 1998. The Science of Low-Power Laser Therapy. Gordon & Breach Science Publishers, Amsterdam.

Kim, K.H., Im, H.W., Karmacharya, M.B., Kim, S., Min, B.H., Park, S.R., Choi, B.H., 2020. Low-intensity ultrasound attenuates paw edema formation and decreases vascular permeability induced by carrageenan injection in rats. Journal of Inflammation 17 (1), 7.

Knight, K.L., Draper, D.O., 2012. Therapeutic Modalities: The Art and Science. Lippincott Williams & Wilkins, Baltimore, MD.

Korakakis, V., Whiteley, R., Tzavara, A., Malliaropoulos, N., 2018. The effectiveness of extracorporeal shockwave therapy in common lower limb conditions: a systematic review including quantification of patient-rated pain reduction. British Journal of Sports Medicine 52 (6), 387-407.

Kristiansen, T.K., Ryaby, J.P., McCabe, J., Frey, J.J., Roe, L.R., 1997. Accelerated healing of distal radial fractures with the use of specific, low-intensity ultrasound. A multicenter, prospective, randomized, double-blind, placebo-controlled study. The Journal of Bone and Joint Surgery. American Volume 79 (7), 961-973.

Kumaran, B., Herbland, A., Watson, T., 2017. Continuous-mode 448 kHz capacitive resistive monopolar radiofrequency induces greater deep blood flow changes compared to pulsed mode shortwave: a crossover study in healthy adults. European Journal of Physiotherapy 19 (3), 137-146.

Kumaran, B., Watson, T., 2015. Radiofrequency-based treatment in therapy-related clinical practice – a narrative review. Part I: acute conditions. Physical Therapy Reviews 20 (4), 241-254.

Kumaran, B., Watson, T., 2016. Radiofrequency-based treatment in therapy-related clinical practice – a narrative review. Part II: chronic conditions. Physical Therapy Reviews 20 (5-6), 325-343.

Kumaran, B., Watson, T., 2018. Skin thermophysiological effects of 448 kHz capacitive resistive monopolar radiofrequency in healthy adults: a randomised crossover study and comparison with pulsed shortwave therapy. Electromagnetic Biology and Medicine 37 (1), 1-12.

Kuryliszyn-Moskal, A., Kita, J., Dakowicz, A., Chwiesko-Minarowska, S., Moskal, D., Kosztyla-Hojna, B., et al., 2015. The influence of Multiwave Locked System (MLS) laser therapy on clinical features, microcirculatory abnormalities and selected modulators of angiogenesis in patients with Raynaud's phenomenon. Clinical Rheumatology 34 (3), 489-496.

Leal, C., Ramon, S., Furia, J., Fernandez, A., Romero, L., Hernandez-Sierra, L., et al., 2015. Current concepts of shockwave therapy in chronic patellar tendinopathy. International Journal of Surgery 24 (Pt B), 160-164.

Leung, M.C., Ng, G.Y., Yip, K.K., 2006. Therapeutic ultrasound enhances medial collateral ligament repair in rats. Ultrasound in Medicine & Biology 32 (3), 449-452.

Lima, A.C., Fernandes, G.A., de Barros Araujo, R., Gonzaga, I.C., de Oliveira, R.A., Nicolau, R.A., et al., 2017. Photobiomodulation (laser and LED) on sternotomy healing in hyperglycemic and normoglycemic patients who underwent coronary bypass surgery with internal mammary artery grafts: a randomized, double-blind study with follow-up. Photomedicine and Laser Surgery 35 (1), 24-31.

Lovric, V., Ledger, M., Goldberg, J., Harper, W., Bertollo, N., Pelletier, M.H., et al., 2013. The effects of low-intensity pulsed ultrasound on tendon–bone healing in a transosseous-equivalent sheep rotator cuff model. Knee Surgery, Sports Traumatology, Arthroscopy 21 (2), 466-475.

Lu, H., Qin, L., Lee, K., Cheung, W., Chan, K., Leung, K., et al., 2009. Identification of genes responsive to low-intensity pulsed ultrasound stimulations. Biochemical and Biophysical Research Communications 378 (3), 569-573.

Maxwell, L., 1992. Therapeutic ultrasound: its effects on the cellular and molecular mechanisms of inflammation and repair. Physiotherapy 78 (6), 421-426.

Mayr, E., Frankel, V., Ruter, A., 2000. Ultrasound – an alternative healing method for nonunions? Archives of Orthopaedic and Trauma Surgery 120 (1-2), 1-8.

McBrier, N.M., Lekan, J.M., Druhan, L.J., Devor, S.T., Merrick, M.A., 2007. Therapeutic ultrasound decreases mechano-growth factor messenger ribonucleic acid expression after muscle contusion injury. Archives of Physical Medicine and Rehabilitation 88 (7), 936-940.

Meakins, A., Watson, T., 2006. Longwave ultrasound and conductive heating increase functional ankle mobility in asymptomatic subjects. Physical Therapy in Sport 7, 74-80.

Mehta, S., Long, K., DeKoven, M., Smith, E., Steen, R.G., 2015. Low-intensity pulsed ultrasound (LIPUS) can decrease the economic burden of fracture non-union. Journal of Medical Economics 18 (7), 542-549.

Michlovitz, S.L., Bellew, J.W., Nolan, T.P., 2012. Modalities for Therapeutic Intervention, fifth ed. F. A. Davis Company, Philadelphia, PA.

Moura Júnior, M. de J., Arisawa, E.Â., Martin, A.A., de Carvalho, J.P., da Silva, J.M., Silva, J.F., et al., 2014. Effects of low-power LED and therapeutic ultrasound in the tissue healing and inflammation in a tendinitis experimental model in rats. Lasers in Medical Science 29 (1), 301-311.

Nakamura, T., Fujihara, S., Katsura, T., Yamamoto, K., Inubushi, T., Tanimoto, K., et al., 2010. Effects of low-intensity pulsed ultrasound on the expression and activity of hyaluronan synthase and hyaluronidase in IL-1beta-stimulated synovial cells. Annals of Biomedical Engineering 38 (11), 3363-3370.

Nussbaum, E., 1997. Ultrasound: to heat or not to heat – that is the question. Physical Therapy Reviews 2 (2), 59-72.

Nussbaum, E., 1998. The influence of ultrasound on healing tissues. Journal of Hand Therapy 11 (2), 140-147.

Ottawa Panel, 2004. Ottawa Panel evidence-based clinical practice guidelines for electrotherapy and thermotherapy interventions in the management of rheumatoid arthritis in adults. Physical Therapy 84 (11), 1016-1043.

Padilla, F., Puts, R., Vico, L., Guignandon, A., Raum, K., 2016. Stimulation of Bone Repair with Ultrasound. Advances in Experimental Medicine and Biology 880, 385-427.

Padilla, F., Puts, R., Vico, L., Raum, K., 2014. Stimulation of bone repair with ultrasound: a review of the possible mechanic effects. Ultrasonics 54 (5), 1125-1145.

Park, I.S., Chung, P.S., Ahn, J.C., 2015. Adipose-derived stromal cell cluster with light therapy enhance angiogenesis and skin wound healing in mice. Biochemical and Biophysical Research Communications 462 (3), 171-177.

Pinto, H.D., Vanin, A.A., Miranda, E.F., Tomazoni, S.S., Johnson, D.S., Albuquerque-Pontes, G.M., et al., 2016. Photobiomodulation therapy improves performance and accelerates recovery of high-level rugby players in field test: a randomized, crossover, double-blind, placebo-controlled clinical study. Journal of Strength and Conditioning Research 30 (12), 3329-3338.

Pires, D., Xavier, M., Araujo, T., Silva Jr., J.A., Aimbire, F., Albertini, R., et al., 2011. Low-level laser therapy (LLLT; 780 nm) acts differently on mRNA expression of anti- and pro-inflammatory mediators in an experimental model of collagenase-induced tendinitis in rat. Lasers in Medical Science 26 (1), 85-94.

Poltawski, L., Johnson, M., Watson, T., 2012. Microcurrent therapy in the management of chronic tennis elbow: pilot studies to optimize parameters. Physiotherapy Research International 17 (3), 157-166.

Poltawski, L., Watson, T., 2007. Relative transmissivity of ultrasound coupling agents commonly used by therapists in the UK. Ultrasound in Medicine & Biology 33 (1), 120-128.

Poltawski, L., Watson, T., 2009. Bioelectricity and microcurrent therapy for tissue healing – a narrative review. Physical Therapy Reviews 14 (2), 104-114.

Ramirez, A., Schwane, J.A., McFarland, C., Starcher, B., 1997. The effect of ultrasound on collagen synthesis and fibroblast proliferation in vitro. Medicine and Science in Sports and Exercise 29 (3), 326-332.

Rayegani, S.M., Raeissadat, S.A., Heidari, S., Moradi-Joo, M., 2017. Safety and effectiveness of low-level laser therapy in patients with knee osteoarthritis: a systematic review and meta-analysis. Journal of Lasers in Medical Sciences 8 (Suppl. 1), S12-S19.

Renno, A.C., Toma, R.L., Feitosa, S.M., Fernandes, K., Bossini, P.S., de Oliveira, P., et al., 2011. Comparative effects of low-intensity pulsed ultrasound and low-level laser therapy on injured skeletal muscle. Photomedicine and Laser Surgery 29 (1), 5-10.

Rhee, Y.H., Moon, J.H., Choi, S.H., Ahn, J.C., 2016. Low-level laser therapy promoted aggressive proliferation and angiogenesis through decreasing of transforming growth factor-β1 and increasing of akt/hypoxia inducible factor-1α in anaplastic thyroid cancer. Photomedicine and Laser Surgery 34 (6), 229-235.

Robertson, V.J., Ward, A., Low, J., Reed, A., 2006. Electrotherapy Explained: Principles and Practice, fourth ed. Butterworth-Heinemann/Elsevier, Oxford.

Roehrig, G.J., Baumhauer, J., DiGiovanni, B.F., Flemister, A.S., 2005. The role of extracorporeal shock wave on plantar fasciitis. Foot Ankle Clinics 10 (4), 699-712 ix.

Romeo, P., Lavanga, V., Pagani, D., Sansone, V., 2014. Extracorporeal shock wave therapy in musculoskeletal disorders: a review. Medical Principles and Practice 23 (1), 7-13.

Sahu, N., Viljoen, H.J., Subramanian, A., 2019. Continuous low-intensity ultrasound attenuates IL-6 and TNFalpha-induced catabolic effects and repairs chondral fissures in bovine osteochondral explants. BMC Musculoskeletal Disorders 20 (1), 193.

Santamato, A., Panza, F., Notarnicola, A., Cassatella, G., Fortunato, F., de Sanctis, J.L., et al., 2016. Is extracorporeal shockwave therapy combined with isokinetic exercise more effective than extracorporeal shockwave therapy alone for subacromial impingement syndrome? A randomized clinical trial. The Journal of Orthopaedic and Sports Physical Therapy 46 (9), 714-725.

Schandelmaier, S., Kaushal, A., Lytvyn, L., Heels-Ansdell, D., Siemieniuk, R.A.C., Agoritsas, T., et al., 2017. Low intensity pulsed ultrasound for bone healing: systematic review of randomized controlled trials. British Medical Journal 356, j656.

Shah, S.G.S., Farrow, A., 2012. Trends in the availability and usage of electrophysical agents in physiotherapy practices from 1990 to 2010: a review. Physical Therapy Reviews 17 (4), 207-226.

Silva, G.B., Sacono, N.T., Othon-Leite, A.F., Mendonca, E.F., Arantes, A.M., Bariani, C., et al., 2015. Effect of low-level laser therapy on inflammatory mediator release during chemotherapy-induced oral mucositis: a randomized preliminary study. Lasers in Medical Science 30 (1), 117-126.

Simonis, R.B., Parnell, E.J., Ray, P.S., Peacock, J.L., 2003. Electrical treatment of tibial non-union: a prospective, randomised, double-blind trial. Injury 34 (5), 357-362.

Solmaz, H., Ulgen, Y., Gulsoy, M., 2017. Photobiomodulation of wound healing via visible and infrared laser irradiation. Lasers in Medical Science 32 (4), 903-910.

Speed, C., 2014. A systematic review of shockwave therapies in soft tissue conditions: focusing on the evidence. British Journal of Sports Medicine 48 (21), 1538-1542.

Staffoli, S., Romeo, U., Amorim, R.N.S., Migliau, G., Palaia, G., Resende, L., et al., 2017. The effects of low level laser irradiation on proliferation of human dental pulp: a narrative review. La Clinica Terapeutica 168 (5), e320-e326.

Taheri, P., Emadi, M., Poorghasemian, J., 2017. Comparison the effect of extra corporeal shockwave therapy with low dosage versus high dosage in treatment of the patients with lateral epicondylitis. Advanced Biomedical Research 6, 61.

ter Haar, G., 1999. Therapeutic ultrasound. European Journal of Ultrasound 9 (1), 3-9.

Thiel, M., 2001. Application of shock waves in medicine. Clinical Orthopaedics & Related Research 387, 18-21.

Torres-Silva, R., Lopes-Martins, R.A., Bjordal, J.M., Frigo, L., Rahouadj, R., Arnold, G., et al., 2015. The low level laser therapy (LLLT) operating in 660 nm reduce gene expression of inflammatory mediators in the experimental model of collagenase-induced rat tendinitis. Lasers in Medical Science 30 (7), 1985-1990.

Tuner, J., Hode, L., 2004. The Laser Therapy Handbook. Prima Books, Grangesberg, Sweden.

Turner, S., Powell, E., Ng, C., 1989. The effect of ultrasound on the healing of repaired cockerel tendon: is collagen cross-linkage a factor? The Journal of Hand Surgery 14 (4), 428-433.

van der Worp, H., van den Akker-Scheek, I., van Schie, H., Zwerver, J., 2013. ESWT for tendinopathy: technology and clinical implications. Knee Surgery, Sports Traumatology, Arthroscopy 21 (6), 1451-1458.

Verstraelen, F.U., In den Kleef, N.J., Jansen, L., Morrenhof, J.W., 2014. High-energy versus low-energy extracorporeal shock wave therapy for calcifying tendinitis of the shoulder: which is superior? A meta-analysis. Clinical Orthopaedics and Related Research 472 (9), 2816-2825.

Wang, C.J., 2012. Extracorporeal shockwave therapy in musculoskeletal disorders. Journal of Orthopaedic Surgery and Research 7 (1), 11.

Wang, E.D., 1998. Tendon repair. Journal of Hand Therapy 11 (2), 105-110.

Watson, T., 1996. Electrical stimulation for wound healing. Physical Therapy Reviews 1 (2), 89-103.

Watson, T., 2000. The role of electrotherapy in contemporary physiotherapy practice. Manual Therapy 5 (3), 132-141.

Watson, T., 2006. Electrotherapy and tissue repair. Journal of Sportex Medicine 29, 7-13.

Watson, T., 2010. Narrative review: key concepts with electrophysical agents. Physical Therapy Reviews 15 (4), 351-359.

Watson, T., 2014. Crest of a wave: effectiveness of therapeutic ultrasound in musculoskeletal injury. International Therapist (110), 18-20.

Watson, T., 2016. Expanding our Understanding of the Inflammatory Process and its Role in Pain & Tissue Healing. IFOMPT 2016, Glasgow.

Watson, T., 2020. Electrophysical Agents: Evidence-Based Practice, thirteenth ed. Elsevier, Edinburgh.

Watson, T., 2020. Ultrasound. In: Watson, T. and Nussbaum, N. (Eds.), Electrophysical Agents: Evidence-Based Practice, thirteenth ed. Elsevier, Edinburgh, pp. 164-188.

Williams, R., 1987. Production and transmission of ultrasound. Physiotherapy 73 (3), 113-116.

Yegin, T., Altan, L., Kasapoglu Aksoy, M., 2017. The effect of therapeutic ultrasound on pain and physical function in patients with knee osteoarthritis. Ultrasound in Medicine & Biology 43 (1), 187-194.

Yeung, C.K., Guo, X., Ng, Y.F., 2006. Pulsed ultrasound treatment accelerates the repair of Achilles tendon rupture in rats. Journal of Orthopaedic Research 24 (2), 193-201.

Yin, M.C., Ye, J., Yao, M., Cui, X.J., Xia, Y., Shen, Q.X., et al., 2014. Is extracorporeal shock wave therapy clinical efficacy for relief of chronic, recalcitrant plantar fasciitis? A systematic review and meta-analysis of randomized placebo or active-treatment controlled trials. Archives of Physical Medicine and Rehabilitation 95 (8), 1585-1593.

Zeng, C., Li, H., Yang, T., Deng, Z.H., Yang, Y., Zhang, Y., et al., 2014. Effectiveness of continuous and pulsed ultrasound for the management of knee osteoarthritis: a systematic review and network meta-analysis. Osteoarthritis Research Society 22 (8), 1090-1099.

Zhang, C., Xie, Y., Luo, X., Ji, Q., Lu, C., He, C., et al., 2016. Effects of therapeutic ultrasound on pain, physical functions and safety outcomes in patients with knee osteoarthritis: a systematic review and meta-analysis. Clinical Rehabilitation 30 (10), 960-971.

Zhang, N., Chow, S.K.-H., Leung, K.-S., Cheung, W.-H., 2017. Ultrasound as a stimulus for musculoskeletal disorders. Journal of Orthopaedic Translation 9, 52-59.

Zhou, S., Bachem, M.G., Seufferlein, T., Li, Y., Gross, H.J., Schmelz, A., et al., 2008. Low intensity pulsed ultrasound accelerates macrophage phagocytosis by a pathway that requires actin polymerization, Rho, and Src/MAPKs activity. Cellular Signalling 20 (4), 695-704.

Zuo, J., Zhen, J., Wang, F., Li, Y., Zhou, Z., 2018. Effect of low-intensity pulsed ultrasound on the expression of calcium ion transport-related proteins during tertiary dentin formation. Ultrasound in Medicine & Biology 44 (1), 223-233.

Capítulo | 7 |

Crioterapia: Fisiologia e Novas Abordagens

James Selfe, Cari Thorpe, Karen May e Jill Alexander

Introdução

Em um capítulo que foca a crioterapia, é irônico notar que os mecanismos homeostáticos para a termorregulação humana são, na verdade, voltados para a proteção contra o superaquecimento (Sawka e Wegner, 1988). Os humanos têm uma capacidade muito menor de se adaptar à exposição prolongada ao frio em comparação à exposição prolongada ao calor (Young, 1988). Clinicamente, a hipotermia é mais comum do que a hipertermia (Kelman, 1980).

De acordo com Fu et al. (2016), a regulação da temperatura do corpo humano ocorre em uma ordem hierárquica:
- Recepção térmica por neurônios sensíveis à temperatura
- Integração de dados térmicos por vias neurais
- Resposta termorregulatória por meio de ramos separados do sistema nervoso.

Existem dois conjuntos de receptores térmicos no corpo: aqueles localizados principalmente na pele, que monitoram a temperatura ambiente externa, e aqueles localizados principalmente no hipotálamo, que monitoram a temperatura central interna (Kelman, 1980). A maior parte do processamento e da integração dos dados sensoriais térmicos ocorre no hipotálamo, o qual fornece uma resposta termorregulatória apropriada (Boxe 7.1). O hipotálamo mantém a temperatura corporal central em uma faixa estreita em torno de 37°C (Fu et al., 2016), geralmente entre 36,1 e 37,8°C (Anderson e Hall, 1995). O hipotálamo anterior controla a perda de calor por meio da vasodilatação na pele e da sudorese quando a temperatura corporal aumenta; o hipotálamo posterior estimula a produção de calor por meio de tremores e aumento do metabolismo quando a temperatura corporal diminui (Green, 1981).

A temperatura da pele humana é inferior à temperatura central. Ao contrário da temperatura central, a temperatura da pele pode oscilar amplamente. A perda de calor para o ambiente é reduzida quando o fluxo sanguíneo na pele é baixo; inversamente, quando há alto fluxo sanguíneo na pele, a temperatura da pele aumenta, assim como a perda de calor para o ambiente (Green, 1981). Em seres humanos, geralmente, há um gradiente decrescente de temperatura da pele ao mover-se do tronco ao longo dos membros (Figura 7.1).

A principal exceção à redução geral da temperatura da pele ao longo dos membros ocorre no joelho, onde a patela atua como isolante térmico e, normalmente, é mais fria do que a perna e a panturrilha mais distais (Ammer, 2012) (Figura 7.2). Isso é importante em termos de raciocínio clínico e compreensão do que é normal

---

Boxe 7.1 Fatores principais envolvidos na homeostase térmica

O estresse térmico imposto ao corpo devido ao desafio do frio é altamente relativo e depende dos seguintes fatores (Toner et al., 1984):
- Temperatura ambiente
- Temperatura do meio de resfriamento
- Diferenças fisiológicas individuais.

Fu et al. (2016) listam as seguintes características fisiológicas importantes que influenciam a resposta de um indivíduo ao estresse térmico:
- Peso corporal total
- Área da superfície corporal
- Capacitância térmica
- Condutância de gordura
- Fluxo sanguíneo
- Absorção solar para a cor da pele
- Idade
- Sexo
- Capacidade de aclimatação.

As seguintes diferenças de sexo na reação ao estresse térmico foram observadas (Anderson e Hall, 1995; Burse, 1979; Otte et al., 2002):
- Há pouca diferença na tolerância ao calor entre os sexos
- As mulheres têm uma maior quantidade de glândulas sudoríparas ativadas pelo calor, mas suam menos
- As mulheres começam a suar em temperaturas mais altas, tanto superficial quanto central
- As mulheres dependem de mecanismos circulatórios para dissipação de calor
- Os homens contam com a evaporação para resfriamento
- As mulheres, normalmente, têm níveis maiores de tecido adiposo, portanto, demonstram uma resposta de isolamento maior ao resfriamento.

Anderson, M., Hall, S.,1995. *Sports Injury Management*. Lippincott Williams and Wilkins, Baltimore, MD.

Burse, R.L., 1979. Sex differences in human thermoregulatory response to heat and cold stress. Human Factors 21 (6), 687-699.

Fu, M., Weng, W., Chen, W., Luo, N., 2016. Review on modelling heat transfer and thermoregulatory responses in the human body. Journal of Thermal Biology 62, 189-200.

Otte, J.W., Merrick, M.A., Ingersoll, C.D., Cordova, M.L., 2002. Subcutaneous adipose tissue thickness alters cooling time during cryotherapy. Archives of Physical Medicine and Rehabilitation 83 (11), 1501-1505.

Toner, M.M., Sawka, M.N., Pandolf, K.B., 1984. Thermal responses during arm and leg and combined arm–leg exercise in water. J Appl Physiol Respir Environ Exerc Physiol 56 (5), 1355-1360.

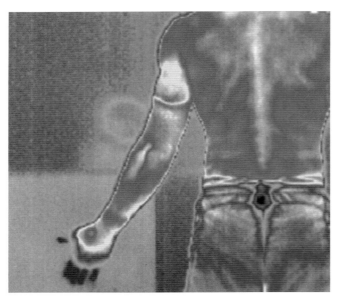

Figura 7.1 Imagem térmica infravermelha mostrando o gradiente de temperatura da pele do membro superior (*vermelho* mais quente do que *azul*) em sujeito adulto saudável do sexo masculino. (*Esta figura se encontra reproduzida em cores no Encarte.*)

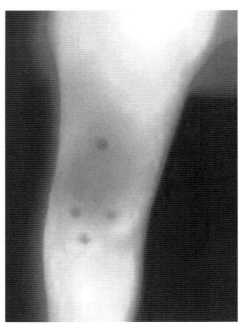

Figura 7.2 Imagem térmica infravermelha com quatro marcadores anatômicos termicamente inertes no local, mostrando uma temperatura da pele mais fria (*laranja*) sobre um joelho saudável. (*Esta figura se encontra reproduzida em cores no Encarte.*)

e o que é potencialmente um sinal de patologia e ao se aplicar a crioterapia localmente. Por exemplo, a dose/resposta pode ser diferente ao se aplicar a crioterapia em uma lesão muscular na parte inferior da perna em comparação a sua aplicação em um joelho inchado e dolorido. Em um ambiente clínico, seja aplicando crioterapia localmente ou em todo o corpo, também existem fatores psicológicos significativos que podem mediar a resposta de um indivíduo. Isso inclui a compreensão do motivo da aplicação da crioterapia e a percepção única de um indivíduo e sua reação emocional ao frio em termos de sensação e conforto térmicos.

Transferência de calor

Em uma escala microscópica, a energia cinética das moléculas está em relação direta com a energia térmica. À medida que a temperatura sobe, há um aumento molecular na energia cinética (agitação térmica) manifestado pelo aumento do movimento e da vibração. Conforme a temperatura diminui, há menos movimento e vibração moleculares. O *equilíbrio térmico* é uma condição em que duas substâncias em contato físico uma com a outra atingem a mesma temperatura – nenhum fluxo de calor ocorre entre elas e elas mantêm uma temperatura constante. A *transferência de calor* é o ato físico de troca de energia térmica entre dois sistemas em temperaturas diferentes. A transferência de calor é sempre unidirecional da mais alta para a mais baixa; portanto, regiões que contêm maior energia cinética transferem energia para regiões com menor energia cinética (Gonzales, 2015). Merrick et al. (2003) afirmam que as modalidades de crioterapia não transferem o frio para os tecidos, pois o frio (baixa energia cinética) não é transferível. São os tecidos que aquecem as modalidades frias, perdendo calor para elas. Dito de outra forma, como a transferência de calor é unidirecional, as modalidades de crioterapia funcionam absorvendo o calor da pele e do tecido superficial. Por sua vez, os tecidos mais profundos são resfriados pela perda de calor para os tecidos mais superficiais. Essa relação é negativamente quadrática por natureza (consulte a relação entre a superfície da pele e a temperatura do tecido profundo). Existem cinco métodos de transferência de calor aplicáveis a seres humanos; eles são descritos a seguir.

Convecção

Quando um fluido (gás ou líquido) é aquecido, as moléculas se expandem, tornam-se menos densas, sobem e são substituídas por moléculas mais densas e mais frias. Estas, por sua vez, aquecem, e esse processo repetitivo cria um ciclo identificável como uma corrente de convecção. Em seres humanos, esta é provavelmente a fonte mais importante de perda de calor, pois o ar quente da superfície da pele sobe e é substituído por ar mais frio, causando um resfriamento da pele. Esse processo é potencializado pelo movimento do ar, que ajuda a explicar o conceito de índice de resfriamento (Kelman, 1980). Quando a crioterapia é aplicada à pele, é criado um desequilíbrio térmico. Parte da resposta fisiológica na tentativa de restaurar o equilíbrio térmico é a circulação de sangue quente nos tecidos superficiais – isso transfere calor para a área resfriada da pele em contato com a crioterapia.

Condução

A condução transfere calor por meio de colisão molecular direta e é a forma mais comum de transferência de calor. Terapeuticamente, isso costuma ser obtido por meio da crioterapia local. Ao usar modalidades de crioterapia, o calor é transferido unidirecionalmente do paciente para a modalidade. Quanto maior a diferença de temperatura entre a crioterapia e a pele do paciente, mais rápida é a taxa de transferência de calor (Cameron, 1999). A água tem grande capacidade de calor específico (ver Tabela 7.2, mais adiante), muito maior do que a do ar; a 10°C, a condutividade do ar é de apenas 0,0151 W/mK em comparação à da água, que é de 0,5846 W/mK (Holmes e Willoughby, 2016). Portanto, o resfriamento ocorre de forma mais rápida e eficiente na água ou em um material úmido colocado contra a pele. Essa é uma das justificativas para colocar uma toalha úmida entre um saco de gelo picado e a pele durante o tratamento. LaVelle e Snyder (1985) confirmaram isso ao examinar o efeito de uma variedade de barreiras na temperatura da pele ao aplicar 500 g de gelo picado em um saco plástico por 30 minutos no tornozelo direito (Tabela 7.1).

Crioterapia: Fisiologia e Novas Abordagens **Capítulo** | **7** |

Tabela 7.1 **Efeito das diferentes barreiras entre a pele e o gelo.**

Tipo de barreira	Temperatura média da pele
Bandagem acolchoada	30,5°C
Bandagem não acolchoada	20,5°C
Pano seco	17,8°C
Sem barreira	10,8°C
Pano úmido	9,9°C

Adaptada de LaVelle, B.E., Snyder, M., 1985. Differential conduction of cold though barriers. Journal of Advanced Nursing 10 (1), 55-61.

Radiação

A radiação térmica é o resultado de movimentos aleatórios de átomos e moléculas na matéria. O movimento de prótons e elétrons carregados resulta na emissão de radiação eletromagnética. A emissividade é definida como a eficácia de um objeto em emitir energia como radiação térmica. A emissividade da radiação térmica é quantificada em torno dos extremos teóricos de um emissor perfeito (corpo negro = 1) e um refletor perfeito (= 0). Os seres humanos emitem quantidades significativas de radiação infravermelha e a emissividade da pele humana é, geralmente, relatada como 0,97 ou 0,98, semelhante à emissividade do gelo (0,97). Isso se deve ao alto teor de água da pele. Câmeras de imagem térmica infravermelha podem, portanto, ser usadas clinicamente para medir mudanças na radiação térmica da pele.

Evaporação

Em seres humanos, o suor na superfície da pele é aquecido e evapora; as partículas de água remanescentes no suor têm uma energia cinética média mais baixa, fazendo com que a pele resfrie à medida que ocorre a evaporação. Se o suor escorre da pele e não evapora, o resfriamento não ocorre. A umidade relativa é o fator mais importante que determina a eficácia da perda de calor por evaporação. Os seres humanos podem suportar temperaturas ambientais muito altas se o ar estiver seco, mas temperaturas bem abaixo da temperatura corporal podem ser desconfortáveis se a umidade for alta (Green, 1981).

Conversão

A transferência de calor também pode ocorrer quando as formas não térmicas de energia são convertidas em calor (Cameron, 1999). Os exemplos terapêuticos mais comuns são o ultrassom e a diatermia por ondas curtas, que criam calor devido ao atrito como resultado da agitação molecular. Do ponto de vista do resfriamento, algumas compressas frias funcionam por meio de reações químicas endotérmicas impulsionadas pela conversão do calor absorvido do corpo.

Calor específico

O calor específico de uma substância é a quantidade de energia necessária para alterar a temperatura de 1 g da substância em 1°C (Cameron, 1999). Tecidos com maior calor específico requerem mais energia para aquecê-los ou maior remoção de energia para resfriá-los. Esses tecidos armazenam mais energia do que os materiais com menor calor específico quando ambos estão na mesma temperatura. O corpo humano tem um calor específico

semelhante ao da água, o que não é surpreendente considerando que o conteúdo médio de água do corpo humano adulto é de aproximadamente 65% (Watson et al., 1980).

É interessante notar que, devido aos seus altos teores de água, ervilhas congeladas e gelo têm calores específicos semelhantes (Tabela 7.2). Sacos de ervilhas congeladas têm sido frequentemente sugeridos como uma forma de aplicação de crioterapia. Com base no calor específico, é, portanto, razoável substituir o gelo picado por ervilhas congeladas se o gelo picado não estiver disponível. Também é digno de nota que a composição química precisa dos pacotes de gel varia amplamente – atualmente, existem mais de 100 produtos diferentes na lista de dispositivos da Food and Drug Administration (FDA, 2017), e isso pode ter uma influência marcante em seus desempenhos como agentes de resfriamento.

Calor latente de fusão

O calor latente de fusão (entalpia) é a quantidade de calor necessária para um material sofrer mudança de fase, por exemplo, para o gelo (sólido) derreter em água (líquido). Quando um material passa por mudança de fase, uma grande quantidade de energia é necessária para quebrar as ligações que prendem os átomos no lugar, mas a temperatura do material permanece a mesma. Essa é uma das razões pelas quais o gelo é uma modalidade de crioterapia tão boa, tendo em vista que grandes quantidades de calor do corpo são necessárias para conseguir a mudança de fase de sólido para líquido.

Base científica

A crioterapia é geralmente barata, facilmente autoadministrada, não invasiva e tem poucos efeitos colaterais (Song et al., 2016). Portanto, é uma intervenção clínica muito popular e comumente usada. A crioterapia tem sido considerada o tratamento de

Tabela 7.2 **Calor específico de diferentes materiais.**

Material	Calor específico (J/g/°C)
Média para o corpo humano	3,56
Pele	3,77
Músculo	3,75
Gordura	2,30
Osso	1,59
Pacote de gel: gel de sílica	1,13
Pacote de gel: hidroxietil celulose	3,85 a 4,15
Ervilhas congeladas	1,98
Água	4,19
Gelo	2,11
Ar	1,01

Adaptada de Cameron, M., 1999. Physical Agents in Rehabilitation. From Research to Practice. W.B. Saunders Company. Philadelphia, PA; Moschiano, H., Dabney, W., Johnson, R., Placek, L., 2010. Thermal and electrical characterization of PAA and HEC gel used in MRI testing of active and passive medical implants. Proceedings of International Society for Magnetic Resonance in Medicine 18, Sweden.

Parte | 1 | Conceitos Básicos Importantes em Esportes

padrão-ouro para lesões agudas por muitos anos, principalmente, para aquelas ligadas ao esporte. O principal objetivo de muitos profissionais de reabilitação é minimizar os efeitos da inflamação e, por fim, auxiliar no retorno à função, ou seja, ao trabalho e ao esporte, o mais rápido possível (Smith, 2005). No entanto, apesar de pesquisas significativas sobre a crioterapia e em contraste com a compreensão dos princípios físicos da termodinâmica, há algumas confusões sobre quais são os efeitos precisos da crioterapia nos tecidos lesionados e quais deveriam ser os protocolos de aplicação clínica ideais para esse tratamento (MacAuley, 2001) (Boxe 7.2).

É bem conhecido que a velocidade das reações químicas depende da temperatura. Q10 é a magnitude da mudança na taxa de uma reação química quando há uma mudança de 10°C na temperatura. É frequentemente sugerido que Q10 = 2, isto é, a taxa de reação dobra a cada aumento de 10°C na temperatura e vice-versa. Apesar de ser um conceito importante ao se considerar a crioterapia, não se sabe qual é o Q10 para reações enzimáticas específicas após lesões musculoesqueléticas (Merrick, 2007).

Um dos desafios clínicos interessantes em relação à crioterapia é a escolha da temperatura. Na maioria das circunstâncias, os profissionais têm pouquíssimo controle sobre a quantidade de resfriamento produzida pela maioria das modalidades comumente disponíveis. Baranov e Malyseva (2006) apontam corretamente que a temperatura resultante é, em geral, determinada pelas propriedades de resfriamento da modalidade, não pelas do objetivo fisiológico/terapêutico.

Vários estudos compararam diferentes modalidades de crioterapia para tentar determinar a aplicação mais eficaz. O gelo consistentemente esmagado ou molhado é relatado como o mais eficaz; em contrapartida, os pacotes de gel são os menos eficazes na redução da temperatura da pele (T_{pl}) para induzir uma resposta analgésica ou para reduzir a temperatura intramuscular (T_{im}) (Dykstra et al., 2009; Hardy e Woodall, 1998; Kennet et al., 2007; Selfe et al., 2009). Herrera et al. (2010) relataram que o uso de imersão em água fria (IAF) teve o efeito mais significativo na velocidade de condução nervosa (VCN); isso, provavelmente, se deve à grande área de superfície de contato.

As diretrizes clínicas mais bem estabelecidas para a aplicação da crioterapia local seguem o protocolo definido pelo acrônimo PRICE (proteção, repouso, gelo, compressão, elevação; do inglês *protection, rest, ice, compression* e *elevation*) (Bleakley et al., 2011). No entanto, ele tem sido substituído pelo acrônimo POLICE (proteção, carga ideal, gelo, compressão e elevação; do inglês *protection, optimal loading, ice, compression* e *elevation*) (Bleakley et al., 2012c). A progressão da diretriz PRICE original para a estratégia POLICE incentiva o pensamento diverso para a prescrição adicional de carga eficaz e controlada durante o tratamento inicial de lesões de tecidos moles (Bleakley et al., 2012c). A regulação da carga ideal durante os estágios iniciais de reabilitação é vital para a recuperação; Bleakley et al. (2012c) sugerem que o carregamento ideal deve incluir intervenções como técnicas manuais e regulação do movimento por meio do uso de muletas ou suspensórios.

> **Boxe 7.2 Alguns motivos de controvérsia na base científica para a crioterapia**
>
> - Metodologias experimentais variadas
> - Diferentes propriedades termodinâmicas da crioterapia (condutividade térmica e calor específico)
> - Variação no gradiente térmico, ou seja, a diferença entre a temperatura inicial da pele (T_{pl}) e a temperatura da crioterapia (lei de Fourier)
> - Diferenças no tamanho das áreas de contato: a compressão pode fazer com que uma parte maior da modalidade de crioterapia fique em contato mais próximo com a pele, resultando em um melhor resfriamento
> - Variação da duração dos tempos de aplicação/exposição
> - Frequências diferentes de cronogramas de intervenção
> - Variedade de áreas corporais (músculos ou articulações)
> - Indivíduos saudáveis vs. lesionados, diferentes tipos de lesões e gravidade das lesões
> - Diferentes níveis de gordura subcutânea
> - Diferentes sexos
> - Tamanhos amostrais pequenos.

Dose-resposta

Não há consenso sobre o método ideal de aplicação da crioterapia para o manejo de lesões (Merrick et al., 2003; Myrer et al., 2001; White e Wells, 2013) ou, então, sobre as relações dose-resposta. As principais variáveis a serem ainda compreendidas são:
- Temperatura ideal
- Tempo ideal (*i. e.*, duração de cada exposição)
- Quantidades ideais de exposições por dia e de sessões por semana.

Além disso, há uma percepção crescente de que fatores como sexo e adiposidade têm uma influência significativa na dose-resposta à crioterapia, levando os pesquisadores a considerar esses fatores mais de perto na tentativa de "personalizar" ou direcionar a crioterapia para o indivíduo.

A dor costuma ser o sintoma mais óbvio da lesão inicial e a razão pela qual a maioria dos pacientes busca aconselhamento e tratamento. O principal objetivo da crioterapia é diminuir a temperatura do tecido, resultando em uma redução na percepção da dor, na VCN, no metabolismo celular e no edema (Algafly e George, 2007; Bugaj, 1975; Jutte et al., 2001; Topp et al., 2003). Observa-se que a VCN reduz significativamente em correlação com a T_{pl}, com diminuição sensorial média de 33% demonstrada a uma T_{pl} de 10°C (Algafly e George, 2007). Apoiando o conceito de que a redução da VCN é importante para o controle da dor, Algafly e George (2007) relataram que alterações na tolerância à dor e no limiar da dor foram encontradas em áreas remotas até a área de aplicação de gelo, desafiando o conceito de que a crioterapia influencia a dor em relação à teoria do portão da dor ou teoria das comportas.

---

fur6Bleakley, C., Costello, J.T., Glasgow, P.D., 2012. Should athletes return to sport after applying ice. A systematic review of the effect of local cooling on functional performance. Sports Medicine 42 (1), 69-87.

fur7Crystal, N.J., Townson, D.H., Cook, S.B., LaRoche, D.P., 2013. Effect of cryotherapy on muscle recovery and inflammation following a bout of damaging exercise. European Journal of Applied Physiology 113 (10), 2577-2586.

fur8Hubbard, T.J., Denegar, C.R., 2004. Does cryotherapy improve outcomes with soft tissue injury? Journal of Athletic Training 39 (3), 278-279.

fur9MacAuley, D.C., 2001. Ice therapy: how good is the evidence? International Journal of Sports Medicine 22 (5), 379-384.

fur10Merrick, M., Jutte, L., Smith, M., 2003. Cold modalities with different thermodynamic properties produce different surface and intramuscular temperatures. Journal of Athletic Training 38 (1), 28-33.

fur11Merrick, M., Knight, K., Ingersoll, C., Potteiger, J., 1993. The effects of ice and compression wraps on intramuscular temperatures at various depths. Journal of Athletic Training 28 (3), 236-245.

fur12Smith, M., 2005. A review of the initial management of soft tissue sports injuries. Journal of Orthopaedic Nursing 9 (2), 103-107.

fur13Von Nieda, K., Michlovitz, S.L., 1996. Cryotherapy. In: Michlovitz, S.L. (Ed.), Thermal Agents in Rehabilitation, third, 3rd ed. F.A. Davies Company, Philadelphia, PA.

fur14White, G.E., Wells, G.D., 2013. Cold-water immersion and other forms of cryotherapy: physiological changes potentially affecting recovery from high-intensity exercise. Extreme Physiology and Medicine 2 (1), 26.

Sugere-se que quanto mais precoce for a aplicação da crioterapia, mais benéfico será o efeito, pois a redução mais precoce da taxa metabólica minimizará o efeito do dano secundário (Merrick et al., 2003). Frequentemente, a crioterapia é aplicada com compressão. Isso tem demonstrado temperaturas mais baixas, as quais são alcançadas mais rapidamente, e maiores melhorias na dor e no edema em comparação à crioterapia isolada (Song et al., 2016). As evidências também sugerem que a aplicação intermitente de crioterapia em conjunto com exercícios permite que os pacientes retornem às funções mais cedo (Bleakley et al., 2011).

Relação entre as temperaturas da superfície da pele e do tecido profundo

Para determinar os efeitos das modalidades de crioterapia, a medição da temperatura da superfície da pele (T_{pl}) é um método eficaz (Hardaker et al., 2007; Hildebrandt et al., 2010; Kennet et al., 2007; Selfe et al., 2009). A imagem térmica usada de acordo com as diretrizes de "Imagens termográficas na medicina do esporte e do exercício" (Moreira et al., 2017) fornece análises não invasivas em tempo real, produzindo dados precisos e confiáveis (Costello et al., 2012c; Ring e Ammer, 2000; Selfe et al., 2006), com limitações entre a diferença dos músculos superficiais e profundos. Vários outros dispositivos estão disponíveis para registrar medidas clinicamente relevantes de T_{pl}, incluindo termômetros digitais portáteis infravermelhos (Figura 7.3), termistores e dispositivos de termografia de contato (Erande et al., 2016; Merrick et al., 2003). O uso da medição da temperatura timpânica é relatado como de baixa precisão ao avaliar aplicações de crioterapia em todo o corpo (Cuttell et al., 2017).

Existe uma relação entre T_{pl} e T_{im} após a aplicação da crioterapia, com transferência de calor unidirecional ocorrendo de estruturas de tecido profundas para superficiais. O efeito do fluxo sanguíneo dentro do tecido muscular e o isolamento fornecido pelo tecido adiposo reduzem o efeito do resfriamento (Hardy e Woodall, 1998; Otte et al., 2002). Há uma relação quadrática negativa entre T_{pl} e T_{im}, isto é, à medida que a T_{pl} aumenta, a T_{im} diminui (Hardaker et al., 2007) (Figura 7.4). Isso significa que as estruturas mais profundas dos tecidos moles continuam resfriando após a remoção da crioterapia, pois o calor dos tecidos mais profundos é transferido para os tecidos superficiais com o intuito de reaquecer a pele. Hardaker et al. (2007) relatam que o resfriamento do tecido profundo continua após a remoção da crioterapia no tecido subadiposo em 3 cm de profundidade

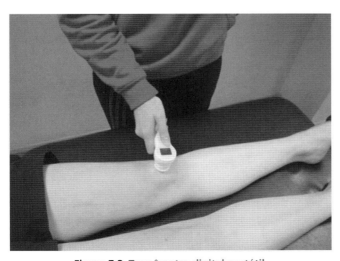

Figura 7.3 Termômetro digital portátil.

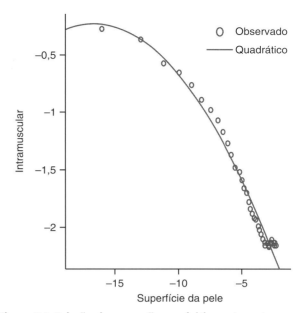

Figura 7.4 Relação de regressão quadrática entre a temperatura intramuscular e a temperatura da superfície da pele após o resfriamento do quadríceps. (Adaptada de Hardaker, N., Moss, A., Richards, J., Jarvis., S., McEwan, I., Selfe, J., 2007. The relationship between skin surface temperatures measured via non-contact thermal imaging and intra-muscular temperature of the rectus femoris muscle. Thermology International 17(1), 45-50.)

por até 30 a 40 min. Isso destaca a necessidade de considerar períodos de reaquecimento apropriados para os tecidos mais profundos após a crioterapia e o efeito que isso provavelmente terá na função muscular. Clinicamente, isso se torna relevante ao decidir retornar um atleta às tarefas funcionais de sustentação de peso ou ao campo de jogo após a crioterapia.

Efeito do resfriamento no músculo

Uma variedade de mudanças fisiológicas, como alterações na rigidez muscular (Point et al., 2017), saída de torque (Dewhurst et al., 2010), força muscular, potência (Thornley et al., 2013) e recuperação de desempenho (Poppendieck et al., 2013) após a crioterapia local, é relatada na literatura. Embora exista consenso sobre a redução da VCN mediada por crioterapia local, a qual contribui para decréscimos na força e na função musculares, alguns autores sugerem diminuições nas taxas de disparo do receptor (Knight, 1995) e na atividade do fuso muscular (Oska et al., 2000) causando déficits de força pós-crioterapia. No entanto, a magnitude da redução da força muscular relatada varia. Burgh e Ekblom (1979) relataram reduções no torque de extensão e na potência de cerca de 5% para cada diminuição de 1°C na T_{im}. Outros, entretanto, descrevem mudanças moderadas (Thornley et al., 2003) ou contraditórias com aumentos na força muscular isométrica (Sanya e Bello, 1999) no membro inferior após crioterapia local. Os efeitos agudos da crioterapia no membro superior também demonstraram resultados conflitantes. De Nardi et al. (2017) relataram que a força de preensão manual melhorou após o resfriamento parcial do corpo a -110°C em uma câmara de crioterapia. Em contraste, após a crioterapia local, reduções na força de preensão voluntária máxima depois da IAF da mão e antebraço (Pathak, 2014; Rabelo et al., 2016; Vincent e Tipton, 1988) foram relatadas. Torres et al. (2017)

Parte |1| Conceitos Básicos Importantes em Esportes

descreveram reduções na força muscular após uma aplicação local de crioterapia no ombro.

A evidência de aumento da rigidez muscular (Point et al., 2017) apoia a sugestão de que a variação do reflexo de estiramento miotático ocorre devido às reduções na atividade enzimática como resultado das temperaturas reduzidas associadas à crioterapia (Ferretti, 1992; Ranatunga et al., 1987; Rutkove, 2001). Isso, no entanto, não é universalmente aceito, e alguns pesquisadores sugerem que mudanças na ativação muscular se devem aos aumentos na excitabilidade do neurônio motor (Oksa et al., 2000; Palmieri-Smith et al., 2007) e, mais recentemente, que ocorrem mudanças viscoelásticas globais após a mudança de temperatura (Point et al., 2017). Dentro da matriz extracelular, Point et al. (2017) descrevem mudanças nos componentes elásticos ativos e passivos que são considerados causadores de aumentos nas propriedades mecânicas dos tecidos moles. Sabe-se que a rigidez músculo-tendão está relacionada com a incidência de tensões musculares (Watsford et al., 2010); portanto, uma incapacidade intrínseca de monitorar efetivamente o reflexo de estiramento dentro do músculo após a crioterapia pode aumentar o risco de lesões. Acredita-se que isso seja devido às limitações na capacidade da unidade músculo-tendão de sustentar a tensão associada aos aumentos no módulo de cisalhamento do tecido muscular.

Efeito do resfriamento no sentido da posição articular

Alterações no senso de posição articular (SPA) e propriocepção (Alexander et al., 2016; 2018; Costello e Donnelly, 2010) foram relatadas após a crioterapia. O SPA é um componente complexo do sistema sensorial somático. É uma submodalidade da propriocepção específica para a consciência de uma articulação dentro de um determinado espaço e é controlada por mecanorreceptores localizados na unidade musculotendínea, nos ligamentos e na pele (Grob et al., 2002; Lephart et al., 1997). A acuidade do SPA é importante, não apenas para o desempenho, mas também como um preditor de risco de lesão (Kaynak et al., 2019). O efeito da crioterapia no SPA é amplamente debatido. Há pouco consenso sobre como o SPA no joelho, por exemplo, é afetado pela aplicação da crioterapia; revisões sistemáticas recentes relatam conclusões variadas (Bleakley et al., 2012a; Bleakley e Costello, 2013). Estudos sobre o tornozelo (Costello e Donnelly, 2011; Hopper et al. 1997; LaRiviere e Osternig, 1994) e o ombro (Dover e Powers, 2004; Wassinger et al., 2007) também demonstraram resultados conflitantes.

Alexander et al. (2015) relataram que uma aplicação de gelo picado no membro não dominante por 20 minutos teve um efeito adverso imediato no reposicionamento da articulação do joelho com suporte de peso, em particular, a reprodução da flexão do joelho com controle reduzido durante carga excêntrica em uma pequena flexão de joelho. Isso é consistente com pesquisas publicadas anteriormente (Sürenkök et al., 2008; Uchio et al., 2003). Da mesma forma, Alexander et al. (2016) destacaram respostas adversas prolongadas no SPA de joelho com suporte de peso com reduções significativas no controle rotacional 20 minutos após a remoção do gelo. Não se sabe se esses efeitos relatados no reposicionamento e na estabilidade dinâmica ocorreram em relação ao aumento da rigidez articular ou às adaptações neuromusculares.

Embora os efeitos da crioterapia no SPA não sejam totalmente compreendidos (Alexander et al., 2015; 2016; Costello e Donnelly, 2010), os médicos e terapeutas continuam a usar a crioterapia nos ambientes clínicos e no campo (Bleakley et al., 2010) durante os intervalos intermitentes do jogo para permitir que seus atletas continuem a treinar ou a competir. Potencialmente,

isso expõe seus atletas a um risco maior de lesões devido a um déficit proprioceptivo (Bleakley et al., 2006). Os médicos da equipe, os clínicos e os terapeutas devem considerar esses achados ao decidir retornar um atleta, após a crioterapia, às tarefas funcionais de levantamento de peso ou ao campo de jogo, visto que existe potencial de aumento do risco de lesão imediatamente e em 20 minutos depois da crioterapia.

Atrapalha ou otimiza?

A inflamação é um componente natural e normal de cura. Então, por que gastamos tanto tempo e esforço usando a crioterapia para minimizá-la? Uma teoria sugere que a redução do inchaço "acelera" o processo de cicatrização, auxiliando, assim, um retorno mais rápido à função. No entanto, se considerarmos que a inflamação junto com os componentes desse processo são os blocos de construção nos estágios iniciais da cura, podemos questionar a premissa de minimizá-la. Fisiologicamente, é improvável que a cura possa ser acelerada com o uso da crioterapia. Entretanto, as condições para que ocorra a cura podem ser otimizadas. Alguns profissionais da saúde argumentam que estamos usando a crioterapia para garantir que o processo inflamatório não fique fora de controle. No entanto, como sabemos o que está "fora de controle" e se o retorno à função está atrasado? Parece lógico que qualquer coisa que reduza a inflamação, na verdade, retarde a cura. As evidências para o uso da crioterapia no controle do edema também são contraditórias. Na fase pós-lesão inicial, ocorre a morte secundária do tecido (Merrick, 2002), o que foi sugerido ser devido à natureza hipóxica do ambiente e à atividade enzimática após a lesão inicial (Knight, 1995). Merrick (2002) afirma que a habilidade de distinguir a morte celular primária e secundária é difícil, pois há uma sobreposição considerável das duas, bem como uma incapacidade de determinar a morte celular secundária a partir da extensão da lesão ou do ambiente hipóxico. Merrick (2002) também discutiu a natureza isquêmica do tecido, possivelmente, resultando em morte celular secundária.

A redução da temperatura do tecido resulta em diminuição no metabolismo celular, reduzindo assim o efeito isquêmico ou hipóxico e a morte celular secundária. A aplicação de crioterapia também é considerada para reduzir o fluxo sanguíneo por intermédio da vasoconstrição, diminuindo, dessa maneira, o edema e mais efeitos isquêmicos no tecido (Bleakley et al., 2007). No entanto, a maioria dos estudos relacionados com isso foi realizada em tecido saudável e a controvérsia sobre a perfusão do tecido após a crioterapia permanece (Merrick, 2002). A redução do edema é considerada útil na diminuição do fluxo sanguíneo em estudos com animais, resultando na minimização do inchaço e da pressão nos tecidos circundantes, o que teria, então, impacto na dor e na amplitude de movimento. Entretanto, isso ainda não foi replicado em testes em seres humanos (Bleakley et al., 2011).

Embora o resfriamento dos tecidos resulte em redução do fluxo sanguíneo e possa servir para reduzir o inchaço e a pressão, verificou-se que a aplicação prolongada de crioterapia pode causar danos aos vasos linfáticos superficiais, resultando em um aumento na circunferência do membro e no fluxo sanguíneo com aplicação de modalidades de frio superficial (McMaster e Liddle, 1980; Meeusen e Lievens, 1986). O aumento do fluxo sanguíneo durante a fase inflamatória da cura precisa ser considerado.

Modalidades e métodos de crioterapia

Existem muitas modalidades de crioterapia local, com diferenças em sua capacidade de atingir uma T_{pl} clinicamente terapêutica, variando entre 10 e 15°C (Kennet et al., 2007). Isso torna a escolha da modalidade um aspecto importante da tomada de decisão clínica (Kennet et al., 2007). As modalidades de crioterapia incluem:

- Gelo (em cubos, triturado, em flocos e umedecido)
- Imersão em água fria
- Pacotes de gel
- *Sprays* frios
- Massagem com gelo
- Ervilhas congeladas
- Dispositivos *IceMan*
- Dispositivos *CryoCuff*
- Dispositivos *Game Ready*
- Dispositivos *Swellaway*.

Gelo (triturado/em cubos/umedecido)

É consenso que as modalidades com maior calor específico e aquelas que passam pela mudança de fase são mais eficazes no resfriamento da pele e na redução da temperatura intramuscular (Dykstra et al., 2009). Tradicionalmente, o gelo picado é mais usado e relatado como a modalidade de crioterapia mais eficaz. Dykstra et al. (2009) compararam vários tipos de gelo usados clinicamente, como triturados, umedecidos e em cubos; eles relataram que o gelo úmido foi mais eficaz do que o gelo triturado ou em cubos na redução da T_{pl}. A capacidade de o gelo umedecido extrair calor dos tecidos superficiais é clara e pode ser aumentada devido à capacidade do gelo umedecido de também se moldar bem aos contornos corporais, o que aumenta a área de superfície de contato.

Imersão em água fria

A IAF permite que temperaturas mais baixas sejam alcançadas e mantidas em comparação a outras modalidades e é frequentemente usada no esporte para recuperação – comumente para redução da dor muscular de início tardio (DMIT) (Bleakley et al., 2012b; White e Wells, 2013). A DMIT é frequentemente usada como um modelo de lesão para avaliar a eficácia da IAF, mas a generalização dessa abordagem está em questão, pois uma associação entre o processo inflamatório após a lesão e o encontrado pós-exercício ainda não foi comprovada (Hawkins, 2016). A IAF é comumente usada no tratamento de lesões agudas de tecidos moles, com mais frequência, nos membros inferiores (Thain et al., 2015). Em particular, os autores relataram benefícios percebidos na fadiga e na dor muscular (Crystal et al., 2013; Hohenauer et al., 2015; White e Wells, 2013), bem como maior recuperação de função muscular, redução do inchaço, saturação venosa de O_2 e mioglobina plasmática (Roberts et al., 2014). Após a IAF, ocorre analgesia induzida pelo frio, o que facilita os primeiros exercícios de reabilitação (Bleakley et al., 2004; Knight et al., 2000).

A IAF também foi adotada como uma estratégia para reduzir os sintomas que possivelmente interfeririam no desempenho durante a competição e/ou o treinamento. No entanto, Stephens et al. (2017) apontam que há variabilidade na literatura atual sobre a eficácia da IAF para a recuperação e, recentemente, foi relatado que a aplicação regular da IAF pode atenuar as adaptações a longo prazo ao treinamento, principalmente, ganhos de força (Peake et al., 2017). Os estudos da IAF que investigam o efeito na recuperação tendem a observar marcadores sistêmicos de inflamação após exercícios excêntricos ou resistência tradicional, mas, como Roberts et al. (2014) destacaram, a pesquisa falha em observar mudanças após o exercício de resistência de 1 a 24 horas após a sessão. Roberts et al. (2014) relataram que a IAF melhorou a recuperação da função muscular submáxima,

embora em comparação à recuperação ativa, a IAF não alterou a recuperação da força máxima ou o desempenho do salto de contramovimento. Pointon et al. (2012) examinaram os efeitos da IAF após uma colisão esportiva simulada no rúgbi; eles sugeriram o uso da IAF depois que os exercícios de contato simulados reduziram a percepção de dor nos jogadores.

Allan e Mawhinney (2017) relatam que há uma falta de evidências para apoiar os efeitos da IAF nas respostas inflamatórias e de estresse celular pós-exercício. Foi sugerido que IAF usada durante o treinamento de pré-temporada para respostas hipertróficas carece de justificativa por causa das reduções nas respostas de treinamento adaptativo que essa modalidade causa. É importante ressaltar que, em geral, os estudos disponíveis apoiam o uso da IAF em ambientes de competição, mais comumente em esportes com rápida reviravolta em torneios ou que são altamente prejudiciais por natureza. O uso da IAF como uma estratégia de recuperação parece mais promissor para a recuperação a curto prazo, ou seja, durante a fase competitiva para permitir uma recuperação rápida entre eventos, mas o uso a longo prazo parece prejudicial para os ganhos de força e massa muscular (Peake et al., 2017), sendo necessário levar em consideração o momento do atleta.

Crioterapia e compressão

As diretrizes PRICE (Bleakley et al., 2011) relataram que havia pouca evidência de um nível ideal de compressão. O grau de compressão externa para manter as modalidades de crioterapia no lugar durante a aplicação varia entre os dispositivos e os profissionais de saúde; portanto, ocorrem diferenças na magnitude do resfriamento do tecido (Tomchuck et al., 2010).

Estudos que investigam compressão *versus* não compressão durante a crioterapia sugerem que o resfriamento mais profundo dos tecidos intramusculares ocorre quando a compressão é aplicada (Jutte et al., 2001; Merrick et al., 1993). Dispositivos do tipo *Flex-i-Wrap* (Cramer Products Inc., Gardner, KS) e envoltórios de filme elástico são comumente usados para manter sacos de gelo no lugar durante as aplicações ao lado do campo, enquanto produtos como *IceMan* ou *CryoCuff* aplicam um elemento de compressão ao redor do membro durante aplicação da pressão do líquido no *design* do produto. Tomchuck et al. (2010) compararam os efeitos de dois tipos comuns de compressão externa na magnitude dos resfriamentos superficial e intramuscular no membro inferior durante e após um tratamento com bolsa de gelo de 30 minutos e relataram que o envoltório elástico foi mais eficaz em reduzir a temperatura intramuscular do que o dispositivo *Flex-i-Wrap*. O envoltório elástico, provavelmente, proporciona um maior efeito isolante (Tomchuck et al., 2010).

Aplicações ao lado do campo

A aplicação de crioterapia ao lado do campo pode ser considerada como "não padronizada" em comparação ao seu uso no ambiente clínico. Há uma grande variabilidade nos tempos de exposição/duração de muitas modalidades aplicadas durante jogos competitivos em comparação às diretrizes PRICE tradicionais, as quais sugerem que uma exposição de 20 minutos é necessária para induzir mudanças fisiológicas nos tecidos, levando a um efeito analgésico após lesão aguda de tecidos moles (Bleakley et al., 2012a). Especificamente, a T_{pl} inferior a 13°C induz uma resposta analgésica ideal (Bleakley e Hopkins, 2010; Bugaj, 1975). Em uma revisão recente da prática dos fisioterapeutas esportivos, Hawkins e Hawkins (2016) relataram uma grande variabilidade na aplicação da crioterapia. A crioterapia é conhecida por ser aplicada aleatoriamente por meio de pausas nos jogos ou nos intervalos em jogos competitivos (Fullam et al., 2015), mas os tempos de aplicação ideais para obter respostas terapêuticas são desconhecidos, assim como o período seguro para os atletas retornarem ao pós-arrefecimento esportivo nessas circunstâncias. Uma série de estudos relatam preocupações com relação aos atletas que retornam ao jogo após exposições ao resfriamento do lado do campo nas articulações periféricas dos membros inferiores (Alexander et al., 2016; Costello e Donnelly, 2010; Fullam et al., 2015) devido ao risco de novas lesões. No entanto, alguns estudos de aplicação de crioterapia de curta duração sugerem que há efeitos deletérios mínimos dessas exposições (Thain et al., 2015).

Crioterapia de corpo inteiro

Embasamento

Desenvolvida no Japão na década de 1970, a crioterapia de corpo inteiro (CCI) ganhou popularidade nos últimos 15 a 30 anos na América do Norte e na Europa. Introduzida na prática clínica para o manejo de pacientes com artrite reumatoide (Yamauchi et al., 1981a; 1981b), a CCI está se tornando mais acessível e tem crescido em uso nas populações esportivas (Bleakley et al., 2014) e na medicina esportiva, apesar da falta de evidências empíricas. Sendo uma aplicação terapêutica de ar frio e seco, a CCI é creditada anedoticamente com a capacidade de reduzir o tempo de recuperação pós-exercício, prevenir lesões e reduzir as respostas inflamatórias à patologia ou ao uso excessivo (Furmanek et al., 2014) por meio de uma única exposição de temperaturas entre –110°C e –140°C (Costello et al., 2015) (Figura 7.5).

O uso de CCI é controverso e, em 2016, a FDA, dos EUA, divulgou uma declaração de informações sobre a saúde do consumidor intitulada *Crioterapia de Corpo inteiro (CCI): Uma tendência "legal" que carece de evidências apresenta riscos* (FDA, 2016). Isso alertou os consumidores sobre alegações enganosas de profissionais da saúde sobre o uso de CCI e apontou que nenhum de seus dispositivos naquela época havia recebido autorização ou aprovação da FDA para ser uma ferramenta clínica segura e eficaz. No entanto, a CCI não está estritamente limitada a apenas tratar condições de saúde; também está sendo usada no esporte para melhorar o desempenho e a recuperação. Entretanto, as preocupações expressas pela FDA sobre a falta de evidências em relação à segurança e à eficácia da CCI permanecem pertinentes para qualquer profissional envolvido na administração de CCI, seja para aplicações médicas ou esportivas.

Existem dois tipos principais de câmara criogênica: câmaras de CCI que incluem o resfriamento da cabeça (Figura 7.5) e câmaras de crioterapia localizada (CL), nas quais o desenho da câmara exclui a cabeça.

Louis et al. (2015) relataram que tanto a CCI quanto a CL estimulam o sistema nervoso autônomo (SNA), com a CCI fornecendo apenas uma estimulação ligeiramente maior do que a CL. Portanto, a exposição ao resfriamento por meio da crioestimulação de todo o corpo, incluindo a cabeça, pode não ser a principal influência das alterações do SNA (Louis et al., 2015). Algumas pesquisas de CCI indicam que ela proporciona melhora na recuperação e redução da dor muscular, com foco específico nos efeitos fisiológicos e moleculares (Russell et al., 2017; Ziemann et al., 2014). Os protocolos de CCI ideais para sessões de tratamento em ambientes esportivos e clínicos ainda são controversos, com considerações sobre a antropometria e o sexo influenciando a duração e os tempos de exposição (Cuttell et al., 2017; Hammond et al., 2014). Normalmente, os tempos de exposição são cotados entre 1 e 3 minutos por sessão única, embora existam diferenças conhecidas nos resultados fisiológicos ao comparar os tempos de exposição de sessão única. Selfe et al. (2014) relataram uma exposição ótima de 2 minutos a –135°C, em que uma exposição de 2 minutos à CCI induziu alterações fisiológicas e perceptivas potencialmente benéficas, maiores do que as alcançadas após uma exposição de 1 minuto à CCI, mas sem nenhum dos efeitos negativos demonstrados por uma exposição de 3 minutos. Em contraste, Pournot et al. (2011) observaram mudanças positivas após múltiplas exposições à CCI de 3 minutos, sugerindo reduções positivas nas respostas inflamatórias pós-exercício. Uma revisão recente da Cochrane destaca que as exposições de 2 a 4 minutos em sessão única são, geralmente, implementadas em protocolos de CCI (Costello et al., 2015).

Crioterapia de corpo inteiro e fisiologia

Parece haver reações fisiológicas significativas em resposta à CCI, incluindo reações de analgesia nos sistemas circulatório e imunológico, bem como reduções no inchaço (Lombardi et al., 2017). Alguns autores destacaram que a CCI não reduz a T_{pl} a < 13°C para induzir analgesia na região da patela (Costello et al., 2014), ao contrário das modalidades de resfriamento direto. No que diz respeito à determinação da profundidade de resfriamento alcançada pela CCI (em temperatura corporal superficial, profunda, muscular ou central), há uma quantidade muito limitada de estudos disponíveis (Holmes e Willoughby, 2016). Selfe et al. (2014) relataram mudanças na T_{pl} e na temperatura corporal central após três exposições aleatórias à CCI, observando reduções significativas na T_{pl}, mas nenhuma mudança na temperatura corporal central. Foi sugerido que isso pode ser devido ao desvio vascular para manter a função de órgãos vitais. Além disso, Costello et al. (2012b) investigaram a exposição pré e pós-CCI na T_{im} e relataram diminuições comparáveis na pele, no músculo e na temperatura central para aplicações de IAF após uma única exposição à CCI de –110°C.

Como mencionado anteriormente, a composição corporal pode afetar a eficiência de resfriamento da CCI e, potencialmente, a eficácia do tratamento, com um estudo recente de Cuttell et al. (2017) destacando as diferenças observadas na temperatura corporal média entre os sexos e as medições de T_{pl} específicas do local. Esse estudo identificou a importância de otimizar os tratamentos com CCI, levando em consideração o dimorfismo entre os sexos. Um estudo anterior de Hammond et al. (2014) observou a relação entre a porcentagem de gordura corporal e a resposta da T_{pl} após a CCI; eles descobriram que os homens que apresentavam níveis mais elevados de tecido adiposo resfriaram significativamente mais do que aqueles com menos tecido adiposo.

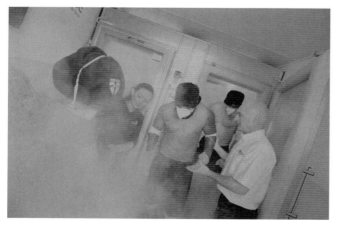

Figura 7.5 Jogadores profissionais da liga de rúgbi saindo de uma unidade móvel de crioterapia de corpo inteiro.

Crioterapia: Fisiologia e Novas Abordagens

Acredita-se que reduções nos marcadores inflamatórios (Banfi et al., 2009; 2010; Lubkowska et al., 2010; Wozniak et al., 2007) e alterações nos perfis hematológicos (Twist et al., 2012) tenham efeitos positivos sobre o dano muscular induzido pelo exercício (DMIE) e a DMIT (Pournot et al., 2011). Uma série de artigos sugere que a reabsorção óssea induzida por inflamação pode ser contrabalançada após a CCI (Lombardi et al., 2017), portanto, o uso de CCI pode apoiar a recuperação pós-fratura (Galliera et al., 2012).

A maioria dos estudos endocrinológicos sugere que ocorrem mudanças nos níveis hormonais com a exposição à CCI (Lombardi et al., 2017), as quais, particularmente, são importantes quando se considera a carga de trabalho em atletas. Na maior parte dos estudos usando populações esportivas, os níveis de hormônios como o cortisol associados ao estresse psicofísico mudaram, de modo que ou diminuíram (Wozniak et al., 2013) ou aumentaram (Ziemann et al., 2012). No entanto, alguns autores não relataram nenhuma mudança (Russell et al., 2017; Sutkowy et al., 2014). Aumentos nos níveis de testosterona também foram relatados (Grasso et al., 2014; Russell et al., 2017), mas outros estudos não demonstram nenhuma alteração pós-exposição à CCI (Sutkowy et al., 2014). Essas inconsistências nos resultados provavelmente destacam as diferenças nos níveis de estresse aplicados em diferentes esportes e nos diferentes protocolos de CCI usados.

Os marcadores inflamatórios têm sido mais comumente investigados (Lombardi et al., 2017) e são um tópico de interesse chave. Sugestões de que a CCI reduz a inflamação são comuns; no entanto, como mencionado anteriormente, a comparação entre os estudos é difícil devido à variabilidade do protocolo e à heterogeneidade dos participantes que abrange uma diversidade de populações de patologia esportiva, não esportiva, normativa e sistêmica (Bettoni et al., 2013; Lombardi et al., 2017). Apesar disso, ainda parece haver uma escassez de literatura na qual se pode formar um consenso sobre se os níveis de inflamação são reduzidos pela CCI e se isso tem algum benefício positivo no desempenho ou na recuperação.

Crioterapia de corpo inteiro e recuperação

Ziemann et al. (2012; 2014) não relataram mudanças nas taxas metabólicas de repouso ou no gasto de energia durante o exercício após tratamentos com múltiplas exposições à CCI. Costello et al. (2015) sugerem que mais estudos devem comparar a CCI às modalidades eficazes conhecidas, como a IAF, ao avaliar sua eficácia na recuperação muscular pós-exercício. Uma série de estudos investigou o papel da CCI no auxílio à recuperação muscular (Fonda e Sarabon, 2013; Markovic et al., 2014; Pournot et al., 2011; Selfe et al., 2014) e em comparação às outras modalidades de crioterapia (Abaïdia et al., 2017; Holmes e Willoughby, 2016). Bleakley et al. (2014) propõem que, embora a CCI possa atingir reduções na temperatura do tecido comparáveis às dos outros métodos de crioterapia, a percepção de recuperação pode ser diminuída pela consciência do padrão fraco de evidência; isso pode anular ou diminuir o impacto da recuperação real por meio de desempenho ou função aprimorada ao combater DMIE. Holmes e Willoughby (2016) tentaram sintetizar dados atuais da CCI, mas não foram capazes de estabelecer diretrizes gerais ou protocolos de uso em populações esportivas para benefícios de recuperação. Isso provavelmente se deve à variedade de marcadores inflamatórios usados nos estudos. Holmes e Willoughby (2016) compararam a CCI à IAF usando vários marcadores de mudança fisiológica comumente associados à recuperação esportiva (White e Wells, 2013) e relataram que a CCI foi menos eficaz do que a IAF na redução da temperatura do tecido. Eles sugerem

que isso se deve ao aumento da velocidade de reaquecimento pós-exposição à CCI.

Um dos principais biomarcadores medidos nesse campo de pesquisa é a interleucina 6 (IL-6), que é secretada pelas células T e pelos macrófagos durante a infecção e após o trauma. A IL-6 é tanto pró quanto anti-inflamatória, pois auxilia no início da resposta imune e desempenha um papel no combate à infecção. Lombardi et al. (2017) confirmam que um efeito anti-inflamatório ocorre em resposta à CCI, mas que as diferenças nos níveis relatados de IL-6 ocorrem entre os estudos devido à variação do protocolo. O consenso sugere que sessões únicas de CCI aumentam a concentração de IL-6, enquanto os níveis basais se recuperam após múltiplas exposições (Lombardi et al., 2017).

O impacto das exposições à CCI no desempenho esportivo com relação à recuperação funcional requer mais estudos para investigar a extensão total dos efeitos. Poppendieck et al. (2013) e Pournot et al. (2011) relataram efeitos positivos em grupos atléticos de elite com resfriamento pós-exercício, sugerindo que a CCI acelera a recuperação quando administrada imediatamente pós-exercício, mas a evidência geral é limitada (Kępińska et al., 2013; Lombardi et al., 2017). Embora benefícios mínimos na recuperação funcional sejam relatados (Hornery et al., 2005; Zalewski et al., 2014), a recuperação subjetiva parece ser sustentada (Bleakley et al., 2014). Novos estudos devem investigar protocolos de recuperação funcional semelhantes aos de Kruger et al. (2015), que relataram a recuperação pós-exercício em atletas tratados com CCI e notaram melhorias na oxigenação do músculo de trabalho juntamente com reduções de esforço cardiovascular.

Crioterapia de corpo inteiro e lesão

Os escores de dor relacionados com a percepção da dor autorrelatada após exercícios extenuantes ou treinamento são reduzidos após a CCI (Pournot et al., 2011; Russell et al., 2017; Ziemann et al., 2014). Muitos outros estudos investigaram o efeito da CCI no DMIE (Banfi et al., 2009; Ferreira-Junior et al., 2014) em comparação ao seu efeito nas lesões esportivas pós-traumáticas. Portanto, só é possível fazer suposições teóricas quanto aos efeitos anti-inflamatórios relatados da CCI em lesões agudas.

Crioterapia de corpo inteiro e psicologia

O impacto relatado das exposições à CCI em fatores psicológicos é, geralmente, positivo. Menor fadiga, melhora do humor junto com a redução das síndromes de depressão clínica e melhor sono e qualidade do sono são descritos após repetidos tratamentos com CCI (Rymaszewska et al., 2007; Sieroń et al., 2007).

Pournot et al. (2011) encontraram percepções psicológicas reduzidas de dor e cansaço muscular após a exposição à CCI. Isso foi apoiado por Schaal et al. (2015), que encontraram melhorias na tolerância à carga de treinamento devido a um sono melhor após tratamentos diários com CCI por 3 minutos a –110°C. Esse estudo randomizado controlado propôs que os efeitos vantajosos da CCI na duração e na latência do sono se deviam à reativação parassimpática pós-exercício. Contrastando com os estudos citados, Russell et al. (2017) não relataram nenhum efeito na recuperação ou na percepção de dor após uma única exposição à CCI a –135°C por 2 minutos. Mais uma vez, é difícil comparar os resultados de Russell et al. (2017) aos de Schaal et al. (2015) devido às disparidades tanto no sexo dos participantes quanto na quantidade de exposições à CCI.

Discrepâncias nos resultados da pesquisa parecem estar relacionadas com a variação na exposição à CCI, variando de múltiplas exposições em curtos períodos de tempo, por exemplo, períodos semelhantes aos de campos de treinamento (Ziemann

Parte | 1 | Conceitos Básicos Importantes em Esportes

et al., 2014) a exposições repetidas durante as sessões de treinamento fora de temporada (Russell et al., 2017; Schaal et al., 2015). É importante notar, no entanto, que foi demonstrado que a CCI melhora significativamente o bem-estar e o humor do paciente; Szczepanska-Gieracha et al. (2014) relataram melhorias nos aspectos psicológicos e somáticos resultando em melhora da qualidade de vida.

Crioterapia de corpo inteiro e patologias sistêmicas

O uso da crioterapia no tratamento de uma série de doenças inflamatórias é amplamente aceito e bem documentado. Foram relatadas reações fisiológicas como efeitos analgésicos, anti-inflamatórios, vasoconstritores, antiedematosos e antioxidantes (Demoulin e Vanderthommen, 2012; Guillot et al., 2014; Oosterveld e Rasker, 1994). Embora a crioterapia possa ser usada em doenças reumatológicas, como artrite reumatoide (AR), espondiloartrite e gota (Oosterveld e Rasker, 1994), ela também é recomendada para artropatias dolorosas, como osteoartrite, capsulite e fibromialgia (Bettoni et al., 2013; Chatap et al., 2007; Demoulin e Vanderthommen, 2012). Além disso, descobriu-se que a CCI afeta biomarcadores ósseos (Galliera et al., 2012) e é útil em distúrbios neurológicos, incluindo esclerose múltipla (EM), devido ao seu efeito sobre os antioxidantes. O estresse oxidativo é uma marca registrada de muitas doenças crônicas, incluindo distúrbios neurodegenerativos e cardiovasculares (Miller et al., 2010a; 2012), e tem uma influência nos distúrbios depressivos e de ansiedade (Rymaszewska et al., 2008). A CCI tem sido utilizada como um complemento para melhorar os protocolos farmacológicos e de reabilitação em muitas doenças do sistema musculoesquelético. Os mecanismos precisos desses tratamentos, especialmente a CCI e a influência de temperaturas extremamente baixas no corpo humano e nas reações fisiológicas, ainda não são totalmente compreendidos (Lange et al. 2008; Lubkowska et al., 2010; Miller et al. 2010a; 2010b; 2010c; Stanek et al., 2010).

Estudos clínicos e em modelos animais sugerem que a hipotermia leve tem um efeito anti-inflamatório (Lubkowska et al., 2011) que pode inibir formação de infiltrado de leucócitos, transcrição de gene de citocina pró-inflamatória e vias enzimáticas (Guillot et al., 2014). Níveis elevados de marcadores inflamatórios, como proteína C reativa sérica (PCR), mucoproteínas, concentração de fibrinogênio plasmático, bem como velocidade de hemossedimentação (VHS) presentes na espondilite anquilosante (EA), foram reduzidos a um grau estatisticamente significativo após a exposição a um ciclo de 10 sessões diárias de CCI a –120°C por 2 minutos; resultados semelhantes também foram encontrados em indivíduos saudáveis (Stanek et al., 2010). Guillot et al. (2014) comprovaram esses achados positivos em sua revisão sistemática, na qual também observaram que os leucócitos tendem a diminuir os níveis séricos de IL-6 e histamina em pacientes com AR.

Esses achados sugerem um efeito terapêutico potencial para doenças reumáticas inflamatórias, como a AR, nas quais essas vias moleculares estão relacionadas com dor, escores reduzidos de atividade da doença, como o *Disease Activity Score* usando 28 contagens de articulações (DAS28), marcadores inflamatórios biológicos e alterações articulares visíveis em exames de imagem. Foi demonstrado que a CCI reduz significativamente os relatos de dor e o escore DAS28 em pacientes com AR (Guillot et al., 2014).

Miller et al. (2010a; 2010b; 2010c) relataram que uma série de 10 sessões de CCI teve um efeito significativo e positivo em pacientes com esclerose múltipla com déficits neurológicos em relação ao aumento de força muscular e níveis de *status* antioxidante, com redução da espasticidade e da incapacidade. Conforme descrito anteriormente, a hipotermia tem efeitos anti-inflamatórios e é um neuroprotetor, reduzindo a acidose intracelular e a isquemia. A hipotermia também inibe a geração de radicais livres de oxigênio envolvidos em danos secundários de reperfusão, ligados à inibição de espécies reativas de oxigênio (EROS) (Gilgun-Sherki et al., 2004; Miller et al., 2010a). EROS são uma causa de danos às estruturas celulares, como proteínas, ácidos nucleicos (p. ex., DNA) e lipídios; está implicada em danos neuronais, resultando em necrose celular e subsequente patogênese da EM (Gilgun-Sherki et al., 2004; Miller et al., 2010a).

Perigos, contraindicações e relatos de eventos adversos para crioterapia

Embora de baixo risco, as reações adversas à aplicação de crioterapia local são relatadas (Cipollaro, 1992; Cuthill e Cuthill, 2006; O'Toole e Rayatt, 1999; Selfe et al., 2007), incluindo reduções na função muscular, danos aos nervos e cicatrizes na pele. As contraindicações devido às mudanças fisiológicas causadas por resfriamento mais extenso, como a CCI como tratamento de saúde, são observadas e os profissionais da saúde devem seguir as diretrizes atuais (Boxe 7.3). Os médicos devem estar cientes das contraindicações antes da aplicação da crioterapia e monitorar cuidadosamente os pacientes quanto a quaisquer reações adversas durante a aplicação da crioterapia.

Até o momento, apenas um estudo relatou reações adversas durante a exposição à CCI (Selfe et al., 2014). Selfe et al. (2014) investigaram os efeitos da CCI em um grupo de jogadores de elite da liga de *rugby* e relataram uma leve queimadura superficial em um jogador de Samoa com intolerância ao frio. Esse jogador não divulgou essa informação antes da exposição à CCI, apesar de uma triagem cuidadosa. A queimadura superficial resultou em pequenas bolhas e eritema bilateralmente na parte anterior da coxa do jogador. Embora seja capaz de treinar e jogar competitivamente após essa reação adversa, é necessário enfatizar a importância de uma triagem cuidadosa de atletas ou pacientes antes de aplicar qualquer forma de crioterapia.

Boxe 7.3 Contraindicações para crioterapia

- Distúrbios cardiovasculares agudos
- Distúrbios respiratórios agudos
- Quaisquer transtornos mentais que possam afetar a cooperação do protocolo de exposição
- Caquexia
- Claustrofobia
- Intolerância ao frio
- Crioglobulinemia
- Hipotermia
- Hipotireoidismo
- Distúrbios do fluxo sanguíneo local
- Lesões cutâneas purulentas ou gangrenadas
- Síndrome de Raynaud
- Neuropatias simpáticas.

Adaptado de Lombardi, G., Ziemann, E., Banfi, G., 2017. Whole-body cryotherapy in athletes: from therapy to stimulation. An updated review of the literature. Frontiers in Physiology 8 (258), 1-16.

Referências bibliográficas

Abaïdia, A.E., Lambin, J., Delecroix, B., Leduc, C., McCall, A., Nédélec, M., et al., 2017. Recovery from exercise-induced muscle damage: cold-water immersion versus whole-body cryotherapy. International Journal of Sports Physiology and Performance 12 (3), 402-409.

Alexander, J., Selfe, J., Oliver, B., Mee, D., Carter, A., Scott, M., et al., 2016. An exploratory study into the effects of a 20 minute crushed ice application on knee joint position sense during a small knee bend. Physical Therapy Sport 18, 21-26.

Alexander, J., Richards, J., Attah, O., Cheema, S., Snook, J., Wisdell, C., et al., 2018. Delayed effects of a 20-min crushed ice application on knee joint position sense assessed by a functional task during a re-warming period. Gait & Posture 62, 173-178.

Alexander, J., Selfe, J., Oliver, B., Mee, D., Carter, A., Scott, M., et al., 2016. The effects of a 20 minute crushed ice application on knee joint position sense during a small knee bend. Physical Therapy Sport 18, 21-26.

Algafly, A., George, K., 2007. The effect of cryotherapy on nerve conduction velocity, pain threshold and pain tolerance. British Journal of Sports Medicine 41 (6), 365-369.

Allan, R., Mawhinney, C., 2017. Is the ice bath finally melting? Cold water immersion is no greater than active recovery upon local and systemic inflammatory cellular stress in humans. The Journal of Physiology 595 (6), 1857-1858.

Ammer, K., 2012. Temperature of the human knee – a review. Thermology International 22 (4), 137-151.

Anderson, M., Hall, S., 1995. Sports Injury Management. Lippincott Williams and Wilkins, Baltimore, MD.

Banfi, G., Lombardi, G., Columbini, A., Melegati, G., 2010. Whole-body cryotherapy in athletes. Sports Medicine 40 (6), 509-517.

Banfi, G., Melegati, G., Barassi, A., Dogliotti, G., d'Egril, G., Dugue, B., Corsi Romanelli, M., 2009. Effects of whole-body cryotherapy on serum mediators of inflammation and serum muscle enzymes in athletes. Journal of Thermal Biology 34 (2), 55-59.

Baranov, A., Malyseva, T., 2006. Thermophysical processes of cryotherapy. In: Podbielska, H., Strek, W., Bialy, D. (Eds.), Whole-Body Cryotherapy. Acta of Biomedical Engineering. Kriotechnika Medyczna Sp., Warsaw, pp. 27-33.

Bettoni, L., Bonomi, F., Zani, V., Manisco, L., Indelicato, A., Lanteri, P., et al., 2013. Effects of 15 consecutive cryotherapy sessions on the clinical output of fibromyalgia patients. Clinical Rheumatology 32 (9), 1337-1345.

Bleakley, C., Costello, J.T., Glasgow, P.D., 2012a. Should athletes return to sport after applying ice. A systematic review of the effect of local cooling on functional performance. Sports Medicine 42 (1), 69-87.

Bleakley, C., McDonough, S., MacAuley, D., 2006. Cryotherapy for acute ankle sprains: a randomised controlled study of two different icing protocols. British Journal of Sports Medicine 40, 700-705.

Bleakley, C., McDonough, S., Gardner, E., Baxter, G.D., Hopkins, J.T., Davison, G.W., 2012b. Cold-water immersion (cryotherapy) for preventing and treating muscle soreness after exercise. Cochrane Database of Systematic Reviews (2), CD008262.

Bleakley, C., McDonough, S., MacAuley, D., 2004. The use of ice in the treatment of acute soft-tissue injury: a systematic review of randomized controlled trials. American Journal of Sports Medicine 32 (1), 251-261.

Bleakley, C.M., Costello, J.T., 2013. Do thermal agents affect range of movement and mechanical properties in soft tissues? A systematic review. Archives of Physical Medicine and Rehabilitation 94 (1), 149-163.

Bleakley, C.M., Glasgow, P.D., Philips, N., Hanna, L., Callaghan, M.J., Davison, G.W., et al., 2011. Management of Acute Soft Tissue Injury Using Protection Rest Ice Compression and Elevation: Recommendations from the Association of Chartered Physiotherapists in Sports Medicine (ACPSM). ACPSM, London.

Bleakley, C.M., Hopkins, J.T., 2010. Is it possible to achieve optimal levels of tissue cooling in cryotherapy? Physical Therapy Reviews 15 (4), 344-351.

Bleakley, C.M., O'Connor, S., Tully, M.A., Rocke, L.G., Macauley, D.C., McDonough, S.M., 2007. The PRICE study (Protection Rest Ice Compression Elevation): design of a randomised controlled trial comparing standard versus cryokinetic ice applications in the management of acute ankle sprain [ISRCTN13903946]. BMC Musculoskeletal Disorders 8, 125.

Bleakley, C., Bieuzen, F., Davison, G.W., Costello, J.T., 2014. Whole-body cryotherapy: empirical evidence and theoretical perspectives. Journal of Sports Medicine 5, 25-36.

Bleakley, C.M., Glasgow, P., MacAuley, D.C., 2012c. PRICE needs updating should we call the POLICE? British Journal of Sports Medicine 46 (4), 220-221.

Bugaj, R., 1975. The cooling, analgesic, and rewarming effects of ice massage on localized skin. Physical Therapy 55 (1), 11-1.

Burgh, U., Ekblom, B., 1979. Influence of muscle temperature on maximal muscle strength and power output in human skeletal muscles. Acta Physiologica Scandinavica 107 (1), 33-37.

Cameron, M., 1999. Physical Agents in Rehabilitation. From Research to Practice. W.B. Saunders Company, Philadelphia, PA.

Chatap, G., De Sousa, A., Giraud, K., Vincent, J.P., 2007. Pain in the elderly: prospective study of hyperbaric CO2 cryotherapy (neurocryostimulation). Joint Bone Spine 74 (6), 617-621.

Cipollaro, V.A., 1992. Cryogenic injury due to local application of a reusable cold compress. Cutis 50 (2), 111-112.

Costello, J.T., Algar, L.A., Donnelly, A.E., 2012a. Effects of whole-body cryotherapy (–110°C) on proprioception and indices of muscle damage. Scandinavian Journal of Medicine & Science in Sports 22 (2), 190-198.

Costello, J.T., Culligan, K., Selfe, J., Donnelly, A.E., 2012b. Muscle, skin and core temperature after –110°C cold air and 8°C water treatment. PLoS One 7 (11):e48190.

Costello, J.T., Donnelly, A.E., Karki, A., Selfe, J., 2014. Effects of whole body cryotherapy and cold water immersion on knee skin temperature. International Journal of Sports Medicine 35 (1), 35-40.

Costello, J., Donnelly, A.E., 2011. Effects of cold water immersion on knee joint position sense in healthy volunteers. Journal of Sports Science 29 (5), 449-456.

Costello, J.T., Donnelly, A.E., 2010. Cryotherapy and joint position sense in healthy participants: a systematic review. Journal of Athletic Training 45 (3), 306-316.

Costello, J.T., Baker, P.R.A., Minett, G.M., Bieuzen, F., Stewart, I.B., Bleakley, C., 2015. Whole-Body cryotherapy (extreme cold air exposure) for preventing and treating muscle soreness after exercise in adults (Review). Cochrane Database of Systematic Reviews (9), CD010789.

Costello, J.T., McInerney, C., Bleakley, C., Selfe, J., Donnelly, A.E., 2012c. The use of thermal imaging in assessing skin temperature following cryotherapy: a review. Journal of Thermal Biology 37 (2), 103-110.

Crystal, N.J., Townson, D.H., Cook, S.B., LaRoche, D.P., 2013. Effect of cryotherapy on muscle recovery and inflammation following a bout of damaging exercise. European Journal of Applied Physiology 113 (10), 2577-2586.

Cuthill, J.A., Cuthill, G.S., 2006. Partial-thickness burn to the leg following application of a cold pack: case report and results of a questionnaire survey of Scottish physiotherapists in private practice. Physiotherapy 92 (1), 61-65.

Cuttell, S., Hammond, L., Langdon, D., Costello, J., 2017. Individualising the exposure of –110°C whole body cryotherapy: the effects of sex and body composition. Journal of Thermal Biology 65, 41-47.

De Nardi, M., Pizzigalli, L., Benis, R., Caffaro, F., Cremasco, M., Micheletti, M., 2017. Acute effects of partial-body cryotherapy on isometric strength: maximum handgrip strength evaluation. Journal of Strength and Conditioning Research 31 (12), 3497-3502.

Demoulin, C., Vanderthommen, M., 2012. Cryotherapy in rheumatic diseases. Joint Bone Spine 79 (2), 117-118.

Dewhurst, S., Macaluso, A., Gizzi, L., Felici, F., Forina, D., De Vito, G., 2010. Effects of altered muscle temperature on neuromuscular properties in young and older women. European Journal of Applied Physiology 108 (3), 451-458.

Dover, G., Powers, M.E., 2004. Cryotherapy does not impair shoulder joint position sense. Archives of Physical Medicine and Rehabiliation 85, 1241-1246.

Dykstra, J.H., Hill, H.M., Miller, M.G., Cheatham, C.C., Michael, T.J., Baker, R.J., 2009. Comparisons of cubed ice, crushed ice, and wetted ice on intramuscular and surface temperature changes. Journal of Athletic Training 44 (2), 136-141.

Erande, R., Dey, M., Richards, J., Selfe, J., 2016. An investigation of the relationship between thermal imaging and digital thermometer testing at the knee. Physiotherapy Practice and Research 37 (1), 41-47.

FDA, 2016. Whole Body Cryotherapy (WBC): a 'Cool' trend that lacks evidence, poses risks. Available at: https://www.fda.gov/ForConsumers/ConsumerUpdates/ucm508739.htm.

FDA, 2017. https://www.accessdata.fda.gov/scripts/cdrh/cfdocs/cfRL/rl.cfm.

Ferreira-Junior, J.B., Bottaro, M., Loenneke, J.P., Vieira, A., Vieira, C., Bemben, M.G., 2014. Could whole-body cryotherapy (below −100°C) improve muscle recovery from muscle damage? Frontiers in Physiology 5, 247.

Ferretti, G., 1992. Cold and muscle performance. International Journal of Sports Medicine 13 (Suppl. 1), S185-S187.

Fonda, B., Sarabon, N., 2013. Effects of whole-body cryotherapy on recovery after hamstring damaging exercise: a crossover study. Scandinavian Journal of Medicine and Science in Sports 23 (5), 270-278.

Fu, M., Weng, W., Chen, W., Luo, N., 2016. Review on modelling heat transfer and thermoregulatory responses in the human body. Journal of Thermal Biology 62, 189-200.

Fullam, K., Caulfield, B., Coughlan, G.F., McGroarty, M., Delahunt, E., 2015. Dynamic postural-stability deficits after cryotherapy to the ankle joint. Journal of Athletic Training 50 (9), 893-904.

Furmanek, M.P., Slomka, K., Juras, G., 2014. The effects of cryotherapy on proprioception system. Biomed Research International 2014, 696397.

Galliera, E., Dogliotti, D., Melegati, G., Corsi Romanelli, M.M., Cabitza, P., Banfi, G., 2012. Bone remodelling biomarkers after whole-body cryotherapy (WBC) in elite rugby players. Injury 44 (8), 1117-1121.

Gilgun-Sherki, Y., Melamed, E., Offen, D., 2004. The role of oxidative stress in the pathogenesis of multiple sclerosis. The need for the effective antioxidant therapy. Journal of Neurology 251 (3), 261-268.

Gonzalez, C., 2015. What's the difference between conduction, convection, and radiation? machine design. Available at: http://machinedesign.com/whats-difference-between/what-s-difference-between-conduction-convection-and-radiation.

Grasso, D., Lanteri, P., Di Bernardo, C., Mauri, C., Porcelli, S., Colombini, A., et al., 2014. Salivary steroid hormones response to whole-body cryotherapy in elite rugby players. Journal of Biological Regulators and Homeostatic Agents 28 (2), 291-300.

Green, J.H., 1981. An Introduction to Human Physiology, Forth ed, Oxford University Press, Oxford.

Grob, K.R., Kuster, M.S., Higgins, S.A., Lloyd, D.G., Yata, H., 2002. Lack of correlation between different measurements of proprioception in the knee. The Journal of Bone and Joint Surgery British 84 (4), 614-618.

Guillot, X., Tordi, N., Mourot, L., Demougeot, C., Dugue, B., Prati, C., et al., 2014. Cryotherapy in inflammatory rheumatic diseases: a systematic review. Expert Review of Clinical Immunology 10 (2), 281-294.

Hammond, L.E., Cuttell, S., Nunley, P., Meyler, J., 2014. Anthropometric characteristics and sex influence magnitude of skin cooling following exposure to whole body cryotherapy. Biomed Research International 2014, 628724.

Hardaker, N., Moss, A., Richards, J., Jarvis, S., McEwan, I., Selfe, J., 2007. The relationship between skin surface temperatures measured via non-contact thermal imaging and intra-muscular temperature of the rectus femoris muscle. Thermology International 17 (1), 45-50.

Hardy, M., Woodall, W., 1998. Therapeutic effects of heat, cold and stretch and connective tissue. Journal of Hand Therapy 11 (2), 148-156.

Hawkins, J.R., 2016. Is the clinical use of ice still relevant? Experimental Physiology 101, 789-789.

Hawkins, S.W., Hawkins, J.R., 2016. Clinical applications of cryotherapy among sports physical therapists. International Journal of Sports Physical Therapy 11 (1), 141-148.

Herrera, E., Sandoval, M.C., Camargo, D.M., Salvini, T.F., 2010. Motor and sensory nerve conduction are affected differently via ice pack, ice massage and cold water immersion. Physical Therapy 90 (4), 581-591.

Hildebrandt, C., Raschner, C., Ammer, K., 2010. An overview of recent application of medical infrared thermography in sports medicine in Austria. Sensors 10 (5), 4700-4715.

Hohenauer, E., Taeymans, J., Baeyens, J.P., Clarys, P., Clijsen, R., 2015. The effect of post-exercise cryotherapy on recovery characteristics: a systematic review and meta-analysis. PLoS One 10 (9):e0139028.

Holmes, M., Willoughby, D.S., 2016. The effectiveness of whole body cryotherapy compared to cold water immersion: implications for sports and exercise recovery. International Journal of Kinesiology and Sports Science 4 (4), 32-39.

Hopper, D., Whittington, D., Davies, J., 1997. Does ice immersion influence ankle joint position sense? Physiotherapy Research International 2 (4), 223-236.

Hornery, D.J., Papalia, S., Mujika, I., Hann, A., 2005. Physiological and performance of half-time cooling. Journal of Science and Medicine in Sport 8 (1), 15-25.

Jutte, L.S., Merrick, M.A., Ingersoll, C.D., Edwards, J.E., 2001. The relationship between intramuscular temperature, skin temperature, and adipose thickness during cryotherapy and rewarming. Archives of Physical Medicine and Rehabilitation 82 (6), 845-850.

Jutte, L.S., Merrick, M.A., Ingersoll, C.D., Edwards, J.E., 2001. The relationship between intramuscular temperature, skin temperature, and adipose thickness during cryotherapy and rewarming. Archives of Physical Medicine and Rehabilitation 82 (6), 845-850.

Kaynak, H., Altun, M., Tok, S., 2019. Effect of force sense to active joint position sense and relationships between active joint position sense, force sense, jumping and muscle strength. Journal of Motor Behavior 1-10.

Kelman, G.R., 1980. Physiology: a Clinical Approach, third ed, Churchill Livingstone, Edinburgh.

Kennet, J., Hardaker, N., Hobbs, S., Selfe, J., 2007. A comparison of four cryotherapeutic modalities on skin temperature reduction in the healthy ankle. Journal of Athletic Training 42 (3), 343-348.

Kępińska, M., Bednarek, J., Szygua, Z., Teleglow, A., Dabrowski, Z., 2013. A comparison of the efficacy of three different cryotherapy treatments used in the athletic recovery of sports people – literature review. Medicina Sportiva 17 (3), 142-146.

Knight, K.L., 1995. Cryotherapy in Sport Injury Management. Human Kinetics, Champaign, IL.

Knight, K.L., Brucker, J.B., Stoneman, P.D., Rubley, M.D., 2000. Muscle injury management with cryotherapy. Athletic Therapy Today 5 (4), 26-30.

Kruger, M., de Marees, M., Dittmar, K., Sperlich, B., Mester, J., 2015. Whole-body cryotherapy's enhancement of acute recovery of running performance in well-trained athletes. International Journal of Sports Physiology and Performance 10 (5), 605-612.

Lange, U., Uhlemann, C., Muller-Ladner, U., 2008. [Serial whole-body cryotherapy in the criostream for inflammatory rheumatic diseases. A pilot study]. Med Klin 103 (6), 383-388.

LaRiviere, J., Osternig, L.R., 1994. The effect of ice immersion on joint position sense. Journal of Sport Rehabilitation 3 (1), 58-67.

LaVelle, B.E., Snyder, M., 1985. Differential conduction of cold though barriers. Journal of Advanced Nursing 10 (1), 55-61.

Lephart, S.M., Pincivero, D.M., Giraldo, J.L., Fu, F.H., 1997. The role of proprioception in the management and rehabilitation of athletic injuries. The American Journal of Sports Medicine 25, 130-137.

Lombardi, G., Ziemann, E., Banfi, G., 2017. Whole-body cryotherapy in athletes: from therapy to stimulation. an updated review of the literature. Frontiers in Physiology 8 (258), 1-16.

Louis, J., Schaal, K., Bieuzen, F., Le Meur, Y., Filliard, J.R., Volondat, M., et al., 2015. Head exposure to cold during whole body cryostimulation: Influence on thermal response and autonomic modulation. PLoS One 10 (4), 1-18.

Lubkowska, A., Banfi, G., Doidgowska, B., Melzi d'Eril, V.G., Guczak, J., Barassi, A., 2010. Changes in lipid profile in response to three different protocols of whole-body cryostimulation treatments. Cryobiology 61 (1), 22-26.

Lubkowska, A., Szygula, Z., Chlubek, D., Banfi, G., 2011. The effect of prolonged whole body cryostimulation treatment with different amounts of sessions on chosen pro- and anti-inflammatory cytokines levels in healthy men. Scandinavian Journal of Clinical and Laboratory Investigation 71 (5), 419-425.

Lubkowska, A., Szygula, Z., Klimek, A.J., Torii, M., 2010. Do sessions of cryostimulation have influence on white blood cell count, level of IL6 and total oxidative and antioxidative status in healthy men? European Journal of Applied Physiology 109 (1), 67-72.

MacAuley, D.C., 2001. lce therapy: how good is the evidence? International Journal of Sports Medicine 22 (5), 379-384.

Markovic, G., Fonda, B., Nejc, Š., 2014. Does whole-body cryotherapy affect the recovery process after hamstring damaging exercise: A crossover study. British Journal of Sports Medicine 48 (7), 633.

McMaster, W.C., Liddle, S., 1980. Cryotherapy influence on posttraumatic limb edema. Clinical Orthopaedics and Related Research 150, 283-287.

Meeusen, R., Lievens, P., 1986. The use of cryotherapy in sports injuries. Journal of Sports Medicine 3 (6), 398-414.

Merrick, M., 2007. Physiological basis of physical agents. In: Magee, D.J., Zachazewski, J.E., Quillen, W.S. (Eds.), Scientific Foundations and Principles of Practice in Musculoskeletal Rehabilitation. Saunders, St Louis, MO.

Merrick, M., Jutte, L., Smith, M., 2003. Cold modalities with different thermodynamic properties produce different surface and intramuscular temperatures. Journal of Athletic Training 38 (1), 28-33.

Merrick, M., Knight, K., Ingersoll, C., Potteiger, J., 1993. The effects of ice and compression wraps on intramuscular temperatures at various depths. Journal of Athletic Training 28 (3), 236-245.

Merrick, M.A., 2002. Secondary injury after musculoskeletal trauma: a review and update. Journal of Athletic Training 37 (2), 209-217.

Miller, E., Mrowicka, M., Malinowska, K., Mrowicki, J., Saluk-Juszczak, J., Kędziora, J., 2010a. Effects of whole-body cryotherapy on a total antioxidative status and activities of antioxidative enzymes in blood of depressive multiple sclerosis patients. World Journal of Biological Psychiatry 12 (3), 223-227.

Miller, E., Mrowicka, M., Malinowska, K., Saluk-Juszczak, J., Kędziora, J., 2010c. Effects of whole body cryotherapy on oxidative stress in multiple sclerosis patients. Journal of Thermal Biology 35 (8), 406-410.

Miller, E., Mrowicka, M., Malinowska, K., Zołyński, K., Kędziora, J., 2010b. Effects of the whole-body cryotherapy on a total antioxidative status and activities of some antioxidative enzymes in blood of patients with multiple sclerosis. Journal of Medical Investigation 57 (1-2), 168-173.

Miller, E., Markiewicz, L., Saluk, J., Majsterek, I., 2012. Effect of short-term cryostimulation on antioxidative status and its clinical application in humans. European Journal of Applied Physiology 112 (5), 1645-1652.

Moreira, D.G., Costello, J.T., Brito, C.J., Adamczyk, J.G., Ammer, K., Bach, A.J.E., et al., 2017. Thermographic imaging in sports and exercise medicine: A Delphi study and consensus statement on the measurement of human skin temperature. Journal of Thermal Biology 69, 155-162.

Myrer, J.W., Myrer, K.A., Meason, G.J., Fellingham, G.W., Evers, S.L., 2001. Muscle temperature is affected by overlying adipose when cryotherapy is administered. Journal of Athletic Training 36 (1), 32-36.

O'Toole, G., Rayatt, S., 1999. Frostbite at the gym: a case report of an ice pack burn. British Journal of Sports Medicine 33 (4), 278-279.

Oksa, J., Rintamaki, H., Rissanen, S., Rytky, S., Tolonen, U., Kami, P., 2000. Stretch and H-Reflexes of the lower leg during whole body cooling and local warming. Aviation Space and Environmental Medicine 71 (2), 156-161.

Oosterveld, F.G., Rasker, J.J., 1994. Treating arthritis with locally applied heat or cold. Seminars in Arthritis and Rheumatism 24 (2), 82-90.

Otte, J.W., Merrick, M.A., Ingersoll, C.D., Cordova, M.L., 2002. Subcutaneous adipose tissue thickness alters cooling time during cryotherapy. Archives of Physical Medicine and Rehabilitation 83 (11), 1501-1505.

Palmieri-Smith, R., Leanard-Frye, J., Garrison, C., Welman, A., Ingersoll, C., 2007. Peripheral joint cooling increases spinal reflex excitability and serum norepinephrine. International Journal of Neuroscience 117 (2), 229-242.

Pathak, H.,M., 2014. Effect of cryotherapy on the intrinsic muscle strength of the hand. Indian Journal of Physiotherapy and Occupational Therapy 8 (4), 202-206.

Peake, J.M., Roberts, L.A., Figueiredo, V.C., Egner, I., Krog, S., Aas, S.N., et al., 2017. The effects of cold water immersion and active recovery on inflammation and cell stress responses in human skeletal muscle after resistance exercise. Journal of Physiotherapy 595 (3), 695-711.

Point, M., Gulhem, G., Hug, F., Nordez, A., Frey, A., Lacourpaille, L., 2017. Cryotherapy induces an increase in muscle stiffness. Scandinavian Journal of Medicine and Science in Sports 28 (1), 260-266.

Pointon, M., Duffield, R., Cannon, J., Marino, F.E., 2012. Cold water immersion recovery following intermittent-sprint exercise in the heat. European Journal of Applied Physiology 112, 2483-2494.

Poppendieck, W., Faude, O., Wegmann, M., Meyer, T., 2013. Cooling and performance recovery of trained athletes: a meta-analytical review. International Journal of Sports Physiology and Performance 8 (3), 227-242.

Pournot, H., Bieuzen, F., Louis, J., Fillard, J.R., Barbiche, E., Hausswirth, C., 2011. Time-course of changes in inflammatory response after whole-body cryotherapy multi exposures following severe exercise. PLoS One 6 (7), 227-248.

Rabelo, P., Botelho, K., Oliveria, F., 2016. Grip strength after forearm cooling in healthy subjects. Fisiotherapia em Movimento 29 (4), 685-692.

Ranatunga, K.W., Sharpe, B., Turnbull, B., 1987. Contractions of human skeletal muscle at different temperatures. Jounal of Physiology (London) 390, 383-395.

Ring, Ammer, K., 2000. The technique of infrared imaging in medicine. Thermology International 10 (1), 7-14.

Roberts, L.A., Noska, K., Coombes, J.S., Peake, J.M., 2014. Cold water immersion enhances recovery of submaximal muscle function after resistance exercise. American Journal of Physiology. Regulatory, Integrative and Comparative Physiology 307 (8), R998-R1008.

Russell, M., Birch, J., Love, T., Cook, C.J., Bracken, R.M., Taylor, T., et al., 2017. The effects of a single whole-body cryotherapy exposure on physiological, performance, and perceptual responses of professional academy soccer players after repeated sprint exercise. Journal of Strength and Conditioning Research 31 (2), 415-421.

Rutkove, S.B., 2001. Effects of temperature on neuromuscular electrophysiology. Muscle Nerve 24, 867-882.

Rymaszewska, J., Ramse, D., Chladzinska-Kiejna, S., 2007. Whole-body cryotherapy as an adjunct treatment of depressive and anxiety disorders. Archive Immunologia et Therapiae Experimentalis 56 (1), 63-68.

Sanya, A., Bello, A., 1999. Effects of cold application on isometric strength and endurance of quadriceps femoris muscle. African Journal of Medicine and Medical Sciences 28, 195-198.

Sawka, M., Wegner, C., 1988. Physiological responses to acute-exercise heat stress. In: Pandolf, K.B., Gonzalez, R.R., Sawka, M.N. (Eds.), Human Performance Physiology and Environmental Medicine at Terrestrial Extremes. Benchmark Press, Indianapolis, IN.

Schaal, K., Le Meur, Y., Louis, J., Filliard, J.R., Hellanrd, P., Casazza, G., Hausswirth, C., 2015. Whole-body cryostimulation limits overreaching in elite synchronised swimmers. Medicine and Science in Sports and Exercise 47 (7), 1416-1425.

Selfe, J., Hardaker, N., Whittaker, J., Hayes, C., 2007. Thermal imaging of an ice burn over the patella following clinically relevant cryotherapy application during a clinical research study. Physical Therapy in Sport 8 (3), 153-158.

Selfe, J., Hardaker, N., Thewlis, D., Karki, A., 2006. An accurate and reliable method of thermal data analysis in thermal imaging of the anterior knee for use in cryotherapy research. Archives of Physical Medicine and Rehabilitation 87 (12), 1630-1635.

Selfe, J., Alexander, J., Costello, J., May, K., Garratt, N., Atkins, S., et al., 2014. The effect of three different (–135°C) whole body cryotherapy exposure durations on elite rugby league players. PLoS One (9), 1-8 1.

Selfe, J., Hardaker, N., Whittaker, J., Hayes, C., 2009. An investigation into the effect on skin surface temperature of three cryotherapy modalities. Thermology International 19 (4), 121-126.

Sieroń, A., Stanek, A., Cieślar, G., Pasek, J., 2007. Cryorehabilitation – Role of cryotherapy in the contemporary rehabilitation. Fizjoterapia 15 (2), 3-8.

Smith, M., 2005. A review of the initial management of soft tissue sports injuries. Journal of Orthopaedic Nursing 9 (2), 103-107.

Song, M., Sun, X., Tian, X., Zhang, X., Shi, T., Sun, R., et al., 2016. Compressive cryotherapy versus cryotherapy alone in patients undergoing knee surgery: a meta-analysis. Springerplus 5 (1), 1074.

Stanek, A., Cieslar, G., Strzelczyk, J., Kasperczyk, S., Sieron-Stoltny, K., Wiczkowski, A., et al., 2010. Influence of cryogenic temperatures on inflammatory markers in patients with ankylosing spondylitis. Polish Journal of Environmental Studies 19 (1), 167-175.

Stephens, J.M., Halson, S., Miller, J., Slater, G.J., Askew, C.D., 2017. Cold-water immersion for athletic recovery: one size does not fit all. International Journal of Sports Physiology and Performance 12 (1), 2-9.

Sürenkök, Ö., Aytar, A., Tüzün, E.H., Akman, M.N., 2008. Cryotherapy impairs knee joint position sense and balance. Isokinetics and Exercise Science 16 (1), 69-73.

Sutkowy, P., Augustunska, B., Wozniak, A., Rakowski, A., 2014. Physical exercise combined with whole-body cryotherapy in evaluating the level of lipid peroxidation products and other oxidant stress indicators in kayakers. Oxidative Medicine and Cellular Longevity 2014, 402631.

Szczepańska-Gierachaa, J., Borsuka, P., Pawika, M., Rymaszewskaa, J., 2014. Mental state and quality of life after 10 session whole-body cryotherapy. Psychology, Health & Medicine 19 (1), 40-46.

Thain, P., Bleakley, C., Mitchell, A.C., 2015. Muscle reaction time during a simulated lateral ankle sprain after wet-ice application or cold-water immersion. Journal of Athletic Training 50 (7), 697-703.

Thornley, L., Ledford, E., Jacks, D., 2003. Local tissue temperature effects on peak torque and muscular endurance during isometric knee extension. European Journal of Applied Physiology 90 (5-6), 588-594.

Tomchuk, D., Rubley, M.D., Holcomb, W.R., Guadagnoli, M., Tarno, J.M., 2010. The magnitude of tissue cooling during cryotherapy with varied types of compression. Journal of Athletic Training 45 (3), 230-237.

Topp, C., Hesselholt, P., Trier, MR., Nielsen, PV., 2003. Influence of geometry of thermal manikins on room airflow. Proceedings of the 7th International Conference on Healthy Buildings 2003, vol. 2. Singapore, pp. 339-344.

Torres, R., Silva, F., Pedrosa, V., Ferreira, J., Lopes, A., 2017. The acute effect of cryotherapy on muscle strength and shoulder proprioception. Journal of Sports Rehabilitation 26 (6), 497-506.

Twist, C., Waldron, M., Highton, J., Burt, D., Daniels, M., 2012. Neuromuscular, biochemical and perceptual post-match fatigue in professional rugby league forwards and backs. Journal of Sports Science 30 (4), 359-367.

Uchio, Y., Ochi, M., Fujihara, A., Adachi, N., Iwasa, J., Sakai, Y., 2003. Cryotherapy influences joint laxity and position sense of the healthy knee joint. Archives of Physical Medicine and Rehabilitation 84 (1), 131-135.

Vincent, M., Tipton, M., 1988. The effect of cold immersion and hand protection on grip strength. Aviation, Space and Environmental Medicine 59 (8), 738-741.

Wassinger, C.A., Myers, J.B., Gatti, J.M., Conley, K.M., Lephart, S.M., 2007. Proprioception and throwing accuracy in the dominant shoulder after cryotherapy. Journal of Athletic Training 42 (1), 84-89.

Watsford, M.L., Murphey, A.J., McLachlan, K.A., 2010. A prospective study of the relationship between lower body stiffness and hamstring injury in professional Australian rules footballers. American Journal of Sports Medicine 38 (10), 2058-2064.

Watson, P., Watson, I., Batt, R., 1980. Total body water volumes for adult males and females estimated from simple anthropometric measurements. The American Journal of Clinical Nutrition 33 (1), 27-39.

White, G.E., Wells, G.D., 2013. Cold-water immersion and other forms of cryotherapy: physiological changes potentially affecting recovery from high-intensity exercise. Extreme Physiology and Medicine 2 (1), 26.

Wozniak, A., Mila-Kierzenkowska, C., Szpinda, M., Chwalbinska-Moneta, J., Augustynska, B., Jurecka, A., 2013. Whole-body cryostimulation and oxidative stress in rowers: the preliminary results. Archives of Medicine & Science 9 (2), 303-308.

Wozniak, A., Wozniak, B., Drewa, G., Mila-Kierzenkowska, C., Rokowski, A., 2007. The effect of whole-body cryostimulation on lysosomal enzyme activity in kayakers during training. European Journal of Applied Physiology 100 (2), 137-142.

Yamauchi, T., Kim, S., Nogami, S., Kwano, A.D., 1981a. Extreme cold treatment (−150°C) on the whole body in rheumatoid arthritis. Reviews in Rheumatology 48 (Suppl.), 1054.

Yamauchi, T., Nogami, S., Miura, K., 1981b. Various applications of the extreme cryotherapy and strenuous exercise program. Physiotherapy Rehabilitation 5, 35-39.

Young, A., 1988. Human adaptation to cold. In: Pandolf, K.B., Gonzalez, R.R., Sawka, M.N. (Eds.), Human Performance Physiology and Environmental Medicine at Terrestrial Extremes. Benchmark Press, Indianapolis, IN.

Zalewski, P., Bitner, A., Slomko, J., Szrajda, J., Klawe, J.J., Tafil-Klawe, M., et al., 2014. Whole-body cryostimulation increases parasympathetic outflow and decreases core body temperature. Journal of Thermal Biology 45, 75-80.

Ziemann, E., Olek, R.A., Grzywacz, T., Kaczor, J.J., Antosiewicz, J., Skrobot, W., et al., 2014. Whole-body cryostimulation as an effective way of reducing exercise-induced inflammation and blood cholesterol in young men. European Cytokine Network 25 (1), 14-23.

Ziemann, E., Olek, R.A., Kujach, S., Grzywacz, T., Antosiewicz, J., Garrsztka, T., et al., 2012. Five-day whole-body cryostimulation, blood inflammatory markers, and performance in high-ranking professional tennis players. Journal of Athletic Training 47 (6), 664-672.

Capítulo | 8 |

Fisiologia da Recuperação Esportiva e Atlética

Tony Tompos

Introdução

Atualmente, os campos mais pesquisados do desempenho atlético estão focados nas melhorias disponíveis por meio de vários modos de treinamento físico, enquanto a fisiologia da recuperação foi pouco pesquisada, apesar da possibilidade de muitos atletas profissionais gastarem o mesmo tempo em recuperação, se não mais, do que em treinamento ativo (Hausswirth e Mujika, 2013). O objetivo deste capítulo é fornecer ao leitor abordagens baseadas em evidências para o período de recuperação e como elas podem ser utilizadas de forma prática em seu campo de trabalho.

Nos campos dos esportes profissionais, muitos métodos de recuperação foram propostos e são, atualmente, usados na prática diária, incluindo, mas não se limitando a, imersão em água fria, banho de contraste, massagem e fisioterapia, treinamento cruzado, eletroestimulação, estratégias de nutrição e hidratação, modificação do treinamento, periodização do treinamento, alongamento, vestimentas de compressão, crioterapia de corpo inteiro, *laser*, sauna e outras aplicações térmicas (Howatson et al., 2016). As evidências e as aplicações de algumas dessas modalidades serão discutidas com o objetivo de fornecer ao leitor mensagens claras e concisas para serem aplicadas ao seu ambiente esportivo específico.

Todos os membros da equipe multiprofissional (EMP) de ciências do esporte têm a responsabilidade de garantir que cada atleta sob seus cuidados não atinja um estado de excesso de treinamento, o que pode levar a perdas significativas no tempo de treinamento e competição. É provável que as EMP que planejam oportunidades realistas de recuperação entre as programações de treinamento ativo sejam recompensadas com atletas de capacidades superiores e com menor risco de lesões (Hausswirth e Mujika, 2013).

A discussão e a avaliação da periodização do treinamento como assuntos não estão no escopo deste capítulo; em vez disso, ele enfocará e consolidará as evidências atuais sobre adjuntos de recuperação e fornecerá recomendações para a prática com base na literatura atual.

Alimentos funcionais

A utilização de alimentos funcionais, com suposta capacidade antioxidante, tem recebido muita atenção recentemente, uma vez que suplementos, como o concentrado de cereja ácida *Montmorency*,

foram encontrados para auxiliar na recuperação em ciclismo (Bell et al., 2014), corrida (Howatson et al., 2010), treinamento de força (Bowtell et al., 2011) e exercício prolongado e intermitente (Bell et al., 2016). Também foi sugerido que os efeitos benéficos do concentrado de cereja ácida *Montmorency* se devem aos seus altos níveis de compostos polifenólicos, incluindo flavonoides e antocianinas, possuindo propriedades antioxidantes e anti-inflamatórias (Bowtell et al., 2011).

Outras pesquisas descobriram que cerejas e framboesas têm efeito anti-inflamatório semelhante ao do ibuprofeno e do naproxeno, devido aos altos níveis de atividade dos inibidores de ciclo-oxigenase (COX) (Seeram et al., 2001).

Hyldahl et al. (2014) postularam que o dano muscular após atividade de *sprint* repetida pode ser devido ao dano na membrana muscular, à desorganização do sarcômero e à inflamação. Também foi sugerido que, após exercícios intensos, ocorrem rápidas perturbações nos sistemas nervoso, endócrino, imunológico e musculoesquelético, com um aumento da formação de espécies reativas de oxigênio (EROS) (Bogdanis et al., 2013). A geração de EROS após exercícios intensos é uma consequência provável de processos de reparo mediados por inflamação, que podem exacerbar o dano muscular existente. É possível que o sistema antioxidante endógeno seja incapaz de lidar com as demandas excessivas colocadas sobre ele durante o exercício intenso. Isso leva à possibilidade de que suplementos que controlam o estresse oxidativo, como alimentos funcionais antioxidantes, podem ajudar a acelerar a recuperação muscular após exercícios intensos (Clifford et al., 2016). Estratégias legais e não invasivas que podem ter impacto sobre o estresse oxidativo e sobre a inflamação induzidos por exercício podem, portanto, ser benéficas para o atleta profissional (Cockburn e Bell, 2017), devendo sempre ter atenção à legislação do *dopping*.

Bell et al. (2016), em estudo recente, mostraram que os participantes que ingeriram concentrado de cereja ácida *Montmorency* pré e pós-exercício, durante um período de 7 dias, tiveram melhorias significativas nos marcadores de recuperação em comparação àqueles no grupo placebo. Os indivíduos que ingeriram o concentrado de cereja ácida tiveram decréscimos significativamente menores no desempenho durante o salto de contramovimento (SCM) (6%), o *sprint* de 20 metros (4%), a força isométrica do quadríceps (17%) e a agilidade (3%) 72 horas após o teste.

Pesquisas adicionais apoiaram o uso de suplementos de concentrado de cereja ácida *Montmorency* para melhorar o tempo total de sono e a eficiência do sono em um ensaio clínico randomizado (ECR). Os indivíduos que ingeriram suco de cereja ácida por um período de 7 dias melhoraram significativamente o sono em termos de eficiência e duração. Os autores postularam que isso foi devido aos níveis mais elevados de melatonina exógena encontrados durante o teste (Howatson et al., 2012).

A ingestão a curto prazo de cerejas ácidas *Montmorency* em pó também beneficia os indivíduos ao completarem exercícios pesados de resistência. Em um ECR mais recente, verificou-se que, ao suplementar 480 mg/dia durante 10 dias, as cerejas ácidas *Montmorency* pareceram atenuar a dor muscular, a diminuição da força durante a recuperação e também os marcadores de catabolismo muscular (cortisol sérico) (Levers et al., 2015). Um estudo anterior também descobriu que, ao suplementar corredores de longa distância com suco de cereja 2 vezes/dia, durante 7 dias, antes de uma corrida de revezamento de longa distância, os participantes relataram um aumento significativamente menor na dor pós-prova em comparação àqueles que ingeriram uma bebida placebo (Kuehl et al., 2010).

O suco de beterraba também tem sido objeto de atenção recente, em parte devido aos seus supostos efeitos antioxidantes e ao conteúdo de nitrato. O suco de beterraba também é uma fonte benéfica de polifenóis e fornece betaína que dá ao vegetal sua cor vermelha/violeta. Betalaínas são fitoquímicos solúveis em água; elas têm propriedades anti-inflamatórias e antioxidantes e podem atenuar a lesão mediada por EROS (Clifford et al., 2016). Foi demonstrado que os compostos fitonutrientes contidos no suco de beterraba eliminam as EROS, o que pode limitar a lesão celular (El Gamal, 2014). Além disso, Jadert et al. (2012) propõem que pode haver um efeito antioxidante indireto devido ao alto teor de nitrato nas beterrabas suprimindo os principais produtores de EROS, os leucócitos.

Os estudos científicos sobre o uso de suco de beterraba como um auxiliar de recuperação existem em menor quantidade do que aqueles com concentrado de cereja ácida. No entanto, um estudo recente sugere que a suplementação aguda de beterraba pode atenuar a dor muscular e os decréscimos no desempenho do SCM após uma sessão de exercícios pliométricos, quando o suco é ingerido imediatamente, 24 horas e 48 horas após o exercício. Embora o desempenho tenha sido recuperado mais rapidamente em SCM (em relação à linha de base) e o limiar de dor à pressão foi reduzido em comparação ao grupo placebo, não houve diferença entre os grupos para medições dos marcadores inflamatórios creatinoquinase (CK), interleucina-6 (IL-6), interleucina-8 (IL-8) e fator de necrose tumoral-α (Clifford et al., 2015).

O mesmo grupo de pesquisa também realizou um estudo sobre a função muscular após exercícios de *sprint* repetidos, em que os indivíduos consumiram suco de beterraba por 3 dias após esses exercícios e foram comparados a um grupo correspondente que ingeriu uma bebida placebo. Em comparação ao grupo placebo, aqueles que ingeriram o suco de beterraba apresentaram melhorias no SCM (7,6% menos decréscimo) e no índice de força reativa (13,8% menos decréscimo) (Clifford et al., 2016).

Em resumo, há resultados promissores de pesquisas sobre os benefícios do suco de beterraba e do concentrado de cereja ácida *Montmorency* após a suplementação pré e pós-exercício em diferentes aspectos da recuperação atlética. Estes incluem diminuição da dor muscular de início tardio (DMIT); atenuação de perdas de potência, velocidade e agilidade; padrões de sono melhorados; e diminuição da dor após corrida de longa distância. Seria interessante ver se outros alimentos ricos em polifenóis com alto teor de antioxidantes, como romã, uva, amora ou mirtilo, tem efeitos semelhantes nos marcadores de recuperação após a ingestão pré e pós-exercício.

Roupas de compressão

O dano muscular induzido pelo exercício (DMIE) é uma consequência frequente do treinamento e da competição, com a quantidade de dano dependendo do tipo, da duração e da intensidade do exercício (Tee et al., 2007). Estratégias que permitem a redução de DMIE são, portanto, de importância para atletas de elite com o objetivo de se recuperar de forma otimizada entre as sessões.

Foi proposto que o uso de vestimentas de compressão pós-exercício pode ter um benefício fisiológico devido à criação de um gradiente de pressão externa e ao aumento do fluxo sanguíneo; isso pode reduzir qualquer inchaço e também aumentar a remoção de produtos residuais, como CK, um marcador indireto de lesão muscular (Baird et al., 2012), lactato e IL-6 (Davies et al., 2009).

Por causa disso, as roupas de compressão receberam recentemente muita atenção, com os pesquisadores se concentrando no impacto que essas roupas podem ter sobre a DMIT, os níveis de CK, a recuperação da força máxima, o lactato sanguíneo, os danos musculares e as outras respostas inflamatórias. Alguns resultados mostraram benefícios positivos. Um estudo recente sugeriu que a DMIT e a recuperação da força isométrica máxima foram significativamente melhoradas em indivíduos que usavam mangas de compressão que forneciam compressão de 5 a 10 mmHg sobre o bíceps imediatamente após uma sessão de exercícios excêntricos de bíceps (Kim et al., 2017). Embora tenha havido uma melhora em DMIT e força isométrica máxima, não houve melhora significativa na atividade de CK ou no fator de necrose tumoral-α (TNF-α), sugerindo que a resposta inflamatória não está associada à redução de DMIT (Kim et al., 2017). É importante notar que esse estudo foi realizado em uma pequena quantidade (n = 16) de alunos não treinados que não eram cegos para o grupo em que faziam parte; portanto, pode ter havido um efeito psicológico com sua recuperação percebida.

Resultados semelhantes foram encontrados em um estudo comparativo de diferentes vestimentas de compressão de corpo inteiro, em que jogadores de críquete realizaram uma série de exercícios de *sprint* e de arremesso com os membros superiores (Duffield e Portus, 2007). Os resultados mostraram que a maioria dos marcadores fisiológicos, incluindo lactato sanguíneo, pH, massa corporal, saturação de O_2 e pressão parcial de O_2, não diferiu com o uso ou não de cinta de compressão. Curiosamente, no entanto, esse estudo encontrou uma redução nos valores absolutos de CK ao usar roupas de compressão em comparação ao controle e também uma redução na classificação de dor muscular percebida e autorrelatada para membros superiores e inferiores (Duffield e Portus, 2007).

Essa diminuição nos níveis de CK foi observada em outros estudos (Gill et al., 2006; Kraemer et al., 2001) com ambos os grupos de autores sugerindo que isso pode ser devido à compressão fornecida para reduzir o inchaço e, portanto, limitar a resposta inflamatória aos danos musculares causados pelo exercício.

Em um estudo recente, Goto et al. (2017) avaliaram a eficácia dos benefícios potenciais das roupas de compressão na recuperação do desempenho atlético em um período de 24 horas, já que muitos atletas são obrigados a realizar exercícios extenuantes 2 vezes/dia com menos de 12 horas de descanso entre as sessões de exercício. Após duas sessões de exercício (com foco em força, potência e *sprints* repetidos), verificou-se que marcadores fisiológicos de danos musculares de mioglobina sérica, CK, leptina e plasma não eram diferentes entre os dois grupos (roupa de compressão de corpo inteiro vs. roupa normal sem compressão). Também não houve diferença na força muscular observada entre os grupos. No entanto, uma diferença significativa foi observada

Fisiologia da Recuperação Esportiva e Atlética **Capítulo** | 8 |

para a dor muscular subjetiva, com melhora no grupo de vestimenta de compressão em comparação ao grupo controle. Dado que o dano muscular e os marcadores inflamatórios alcançam o pico 24 a 48 horas após o exercício (Fatouros et al., 2010), mas as medições de sangue foram feitas antes desse período; a falta de cegamento (característica importante para o estudo) e de medição do nível de pressão aplicada aos participantes resultados desse estudo devem ser interpretados com cautela, por serem vieses metodológicos.

Marqués-Jiménez et al. (2017) compararam o uso de três tipos diferentes de vestimentas de compressão em jogadores de futebol semiprofissionais: meias de compressão, *shorts* e *collants* de perna inteira. As medições de DMIT, biomarcadores de DMIE e inchaço foram coletadas antes da partida e 24, 48 e 72 horas após a partida. Com semelhanças com outros estudos mencionados, todas as três roupas de compressão atenuaram os biomarcadores de DMIE de uma maneira positiva, mas não significativa, quando comparadas a não usar uma roupa de compressão, embora as meias de compressão de perna inteira tenham mostrado a maior melhora. Os autores sugerem que isso possivelmente se deva a um maior retorno venoso, melhorando, assim, a remoção de proteínas miofibrilares e outros produtos residuais. O inchaço e a DMIT também foram atenuados após a partida ao usar roupas de compressão. Isso sugere que durante períodos de altas cargas e volumes de treinamento, como a pré-temporada, as roupas de compressão podem oferecer um benefício positivo, se não significativo, para jogadores de futebol após a partida.

Imersão em água fria

A imersão em água fria (IAF) surgiu como uma das intervenções de recuperação mais populares para atletas e equipes de medicina esportiva em um esforço para melhorar a taxa de recuperação atlética (Bleakley e Davison, 2010). Foi sugerido que os mecanismos que sustentam os benefícios da IAF estão relacionados com a temperatura, as alterações induzidas por pressão no fluxo sanguíneo e a temperatura muscular reduzida, levando a uma diminuição na inflamação pós-exercício e subsequente DMIT (Leeder et al., 2012). Também foi proposto que a IAF melhora a DMIT por meio de resfriamento localizado, pressões hidrostáticas e redirecionamento do fluxo sanguíneo (Ihsan et al., 2016). Por exemplo, o edema dentro do músculo pós-exercício impede o fornecimento de oxigênio aos músculos, pois a compressão dos capilares locais aumenta, resultando em um aumento da distância entre os capilares e as fibras musculares para a troca de oxigênio. A vasoconstrição induzida pelo frio e as alterações hidrostáticas aumentam o volume sanguíneo central, elevando a pressão venosa central e facilitando, assim, o movimento de fluidos dos espaços intracelular e intersticial para os compartimentos intravasculares.

Esse movimento fluido, portanto, incentiva e facilita a eliminação de detritos celulares por meio de um gradiente osmótico intracelular-extracelular (Ihsan et al., 2016). A IAF pode, assim, melhorar a DMIT reduzindo o edema por meio da vasoconstrição induzida pelo frio, o que facilita a depuração de fluido periférico e atenua a inflamação da DMIT e os decréscimos na função muscular (Ihsan et al., 2016).

A IAF foi observada fornecendo melhorias na DMIT (Ingram et al., 2009; Jakeman et al., 2009; Vaile et al., 2008), diminuindo os níveis de CK (Goodall, 2008; Vaile, 2008) e melhorando a taxa de recuperação para potência muscular (Eston 1999; Vaile, 2008). Apesar do crescente corpo de evidências para apoiar a IAF como uma ferramenta de recuperação, permanece uma certa resistência ao seu uso devido à falta de diretrizes claras sobre o tempo, a profundidade e a temperatura de imersão, o que pode colocar o atleta em risco de suportar temperaturas extremas por mais do que o necessário (Bleakley e Davison, 2010). Uma revisão sistemática da literatura relacionada com a IAF descobriu que os estudos usaram temperaturas de água de 5 a 15°C para séries contínuas ou intermitentes de 5 a 24 minutos (Bleakley et al., 2012).

Buscando esclarecer quais temperaturas e tempos de imersão podem ser mais benéficos para os atletas, um estudo avaliou a eficácia de cinco protocolos de IAF diferentes em 50 alunos (1 min 38°C/1 min 10°C × 3; 1 min IAF em 10°C, seguido de nenhuma imersão por 1 min × 3; 10 min IAF em 10°C; 10 min IAF em 6°C; ou controle [repouso sentado]). Todos os quatro protocolos da IAF tiveram um efeito benéfico sobre a DMIT em comparação ao grupo controle. No entanto, não houve diferença estatística significativa entre esses quatro grupos. Em contrapartida, houve uma tendência positiva para 10 minutos de imersão em água a 6°C, demonstrando os maiores resultados para DMIT em 96 horas pós-exercício (Glasgow et al., 2014). Uma revisão sistemática encontrou resultados semelhantes em que a IAF pós-exercício em uma gama de 14 estudos demonstrou resultados favoráveis para DMIT em 24, 48, 72 e 96 horas pós-exercício (Bleakley et al., 2012).

Outra revisão sistemática descobriu que, em uma série de estudos que relataram um resultado significativo favorecendo a IAF em vez de intervenções passivas, a temperatura média para aliviar os sintomas subjetivos de DMIT foi de 10°C e o tempo médio de imersão sugerido foi de 13 minutos (Hohenauer et al., 2015). Uma revisão semelhante também encontrou resultados comparáveis ao investigar a IAF *versus* as terapias passivas. Os resultados indicaram que a IAF com uma temperatura da água de 11 a 15°C e com um tempo de imersão de 11 a 15 minutos forneceu os melhores resultados para DMIT (Machado et al., 2016).

Um estudo anterior de Leeder et al. (2012) também descobriu que a IAF aliviou os sintomas de DMIT em 24, 48, 72 e 96 horas pós-exercício, diminuiu significativamente os níveis de CK e também mostrou recuperação melhorada da potência muscular em 24, 48 e 72 horas pós-exercício, mas não da força muscular. Os resultados desse estudo mostraram que a IAF reduziu a percepção de DMIT em uma média de 16% e que parece ser mais eficaz como analgésico após exercícios de alta intensidade do que exercícios de viés excêntrico.

Dadas essas metanálises e revisões sistemáticas, torna-se razoável sugerir que a IAF pode ser benéfica para atletas que buscam diminuir a DMIT e reduzir a perda de potência entre o treinamento e a competição. No entanto, compreender os mecanismos pelos quais a IAF beneficia os atletas é de importância crítica ao profissional do esporte para garantir que a periodização da recuperação esteja entrelaçada com os objetivos a longo prazo para a adaptação induzida pelo treinamento (Ihsan et al., 2016).

Banho de contraste

A terapia com banho de contraste (TBC) é outra estratégia de recuperação que se tornou uma modalidade comum disponível para atletas de esportes de alto desempenho. Tem o suposto benefício de diminuir a DMIT por meio de uma "ação de bombeamento" criada por vasoconstrição e vasodilatação após imersões em água fria e quente, respectivamente (Vaile et al., 2007). Além disso, foi sugerido que a TBC pode auxiliar na recuperação, reduzindo o espasmo muscular, a inflamação e melhorando a amplitude de movimento (Biuzen et al., 2013). Os métodos comumente praticados incluem proporções de banhos quentes

Parte | 1 | Conceitos Básicos Importantes em Esportes

para frios de 3:1 ou 4:1, respectivamente, terminando com tratamento frio para estimular vasoconstrição suficiente (Cochrane, 2004). No entanto, essas estratégias foram desafiadas com a sugestão de que 1 minuto de exposição ao frio não é suficiente para diminuir a temperatura muscular após a imersão em água quente, anulando assim quaisquer efeitos fisiológicos (Higgins e Kaminski, 1998).

Atualmente, há uma acentuada falta de pesquisas na área de TBC em comparação às outras abordagens de recuperação. Em uma tentativa de estabelecer os efeitos da TBC na recuperação após o exercício, um estudo comparou a recuperação passiva (15 minutos sentado) a um protocolo de banho de contraste de 60 segundos de imersão em água fria (8 a 10°C), seguidos de 120 segundos de imersão em água quente (40 a 42°C). Em comparação ao grupo de recuperação passiva, o grupo de TBC demonstrou uma perda significativamente menor da capacidade de geração de força isométrica e dinâmica (avaliada por meio de agachamento isométrico e agachamento com salto), um aumento significativamente menor no volume da coxa (inchaço) e uma tendência a níveis mais baixos de dor (dor percebida) e de concentração de CK em 48 e 72 horas (Vaile et al., 2007).

Em uma revisão sistemática e metanálise comparando a TBC às outras técnicas de recuperação após o exercício, a dor muscular foi significativamente menor nos grupos de TBC em comparação aos de recuperação passiva em todos os 13 estudos analisados na revisão e em todos os tempos de acompanhamento (< 6, 24, 48, 72, > 96 horas). A força muscular (seis estudos) e a potência muscular (nove estudos) também foram significativamente melhoradas na TBC em comparação aos grupos de recuperação passiva quando comparados aos escores basais. Os autores sugerem que, devido à maioria dos estudos encerrando seu protocolo de TBC com imersão em água fria, isso pode ter tido um efeito analgésico ao diminuir a velocidade de condução nervosa e a excitabilidade, além de reduzir a transmissão neural (nociceptiva). Outra teoria postulada é que, após a imersão em água fria, há ativação de nociceptores térmicos que causam mudança na atividade nervosa simpática; isso reduz o fluxo sanguíneo arterial, causando diminuição no fluxo sanguíneo microvascular ao redor do local danificado e reduzindo edema e eventos inflamatórios. No entanto, o principal achado dessa revisão sistemática e metanálise é que, quando comparado aos outros métodos de recuperação, incluindo IAF, compressão e recuperação ativa, houve pouca diferença entre os grupos, com todos dando resultados superiores na recuperação em comparação à recuperação passiva (Bieuzen et al., 2013).

Crioterapia de corpo inteiro

A crioterapia de corpo inteiro (CCI) também se tornou um método de tratamento popular e tem sido cada vez mais usada como uma ferramenta de recuperação para atletas. Em uma sala com ambiente controlado, os atletas entram em uma câmara vestíbula a –60°C por aproximadamente 30 segundos para adaptação corporal antes de entrar na câmara criostática, na qual são expostos ao ar extremamente frio e seco (geralmente entre –100 e –140°C) por 2 a 5 minutos, usando roupas mínimas e uma máscara de ar para se proteger de lesões relacionadas com o frio (Bleakley et al., 2014).

Inicialmente, a CCI foi planejada para uso em ambiente clínico com o intuito de ajudar pacientes com doenças como esclerose múltipla e artrite reumatoide. No entanto, mais recentemente, os atletas começaram a usar a CCI na tentativa de ganhar uma vantagem competitiva por meio de recuperação aprimorada (Costello et al., 2015). A CCI é usada com frequência imediatamente após ou logo após (dentro de 24 horas) exercícios intensivos, com o tratamento sendo muitas vezes repetido no mesmo dia ou por vários dias (Costello et al., 2012).

Verificou-se que a CCI como uma ferramenta de recuperação após exercícios intensos diminui os níveis de CK (Banfi et al., 2009), melhora a recuperação psicológica, incluindo a percepção de cansaço e dor em corredores (Hausswirth et al., 2011), diminui os marcadores inflamatórios e melhora a recuperação muscular (Pournot et al., 2011). Foi sugerido que as temperaturas significativamente frias provocadas durante a CCI em comparação às da IAF podem levar os atletas a acreditar que a recuperação é aprimorada, contribuindo para alguns ou todos os efeitos observados. Os benefícios fisiológicos da CCI foram presumidos como relacionados com a vasoconstrição, limitando, assim, o edema e a inflamação e causando um efeito analgésico devido ao ar frio, o qual pode limitar a dor muscular após o exercício (Cockburn e Bell, 2017).

Em uma recente revisão da literatura (Lombardi et al., 2017), os autores observaram uma recuperação psicológica significativamente melhorada em corredores, após uma corrida em trilha simulada, relacionada com as percepções de dor e cansaço depois da primeira sessão de CCI (Hausswirth et al., 2011). Na revisão, também foi observado que os níveis de CK foram reduzidos em até 40% nos jogadores de rúgbi após cinco sessões em dias alternados de CCI quando comparados aos níveis em condição sem CCI (Banfi et al., 2009). Resultados semelhantes foram observados em canoístas, com uma diminuição de 34% nos níveis de CK após 3 sessões diárias de CCI, durante um ciclo de treinamento de 10 dias (Wozniak et al., 2007). Os níveis de CK, de IL-6 (60%) e de fator de necrose tumoral (63%) também diminuíram em jogadores de tênis profissionais após 5 dias de sessões de CCI, 2 vezes/dia, em uma câmara criogênica durante um cronograma de treinamento de intensidade moderada em comparação ao de treinamento sem CCI (Ziemann et al., 2012); a eficácia do lançamento e a recuperação do desempenho também melhoraram no grupo com CCI.

Quando os atletas foram aleatoriamente designados para recuperação com CCI ou sem CCI, após sessões de treinamento, verificou-se também que a CCI tem um impacto benéfico na duração do sono dos atletas e na limitação da latência do sono em praticantes de nado sincronizado (Schaal et al., 2015). Os autores desta revisão sistemática sugeriram que a CCI melhora a recuperação aguda por meio de efeitos benéficos na inflamação, no aumento da oxigenação e na redução da tensão cardiovascular causada pela vasoconstrição periférica (Lombardi et al., 2017).

Em uma revisão das evidências atuais sobre a CCI, os pesquisadores descobriram que havia evidências para apoiar a noção de que a CCI poderia melhorar as medidas subjetivas de resultados de recuperação percebida e de dor muscular, ao mesmo tempo tendo um efeito analgésico se o resfriamento da pele fosse suficiente (< 13°C) (Bleakley et al., 2014). Um objetivo fundamental para a revisão de Bleakley et al. (2014) foi determinar a magnitude das reduções de temperatura do tecido associadas à CCI em comparação aos outros métodos tradicionais de resfriamento. Pode-se sugerir que, devido às temperaturas significativamente mais baixas associadas à CCI, esse método pode ser superior à aplicação de gelo picado ou IAF. No entanto, devido à baixa condutividade térmica do ar e da água, a aplicação de gelo é mais eficiente na extração de energia térmica do corpo (Bleakley et al., 2014). Apesar disso, uma vantagem potencial pode ser que a CCI é capaz de resfriar áreas maiores da superfície do corpo simultaneamente.

Em 2015, uma revisão sistemática estudou os efeitos de CCI na dor muscular após o exercício. Os autores encontraram uma redução da dor muscular entre 7 e 20% nos estudos analisados, ao passo que quatro estudos encontraram redução significativa da dor em 1, 24, 48 e 72 horas após o exercício, isso quando com repouso ou sem CCI são comparados (Costello et al., 2015). Devido à falta de ensaios clínicos randomizados de alta qualidade nessa área, ao alto risco de viés nos estudos incluídos, à falta de evidências sobre eventos adversos e de estudos em mulheres ou atletas de elite, os autores sugerem que há pouca ou nenhuma evidência que informe sobre os efeitos relevantes da CCI *versus* outras intervenções, como a IAF (Costello et al., 2015). Até que mais pesquisas estejam disponíveis, os atletas devem estar cientes de que modos menos caros de crioterapia, como IAF ou aplicação de bolsa de gelo, parecem oferecer benefícios fisiológicos e clínicos comparáveis aos da CCI (Bleakley et al., 2014).

Sono

O sono é um componente essencial da saúde e do bem-estar e há evidências acumuladas que sugerem que a melhoria da qualidade e a duração do sono em atletas está correlacionada com o melhor desempenho, o sucesso competitivo e um risco reduzido de lesões e doenças (Watson, 2017). O sono é, portanto, considerado o principal método de recuperação para os atletas. O sono ruim persistente em atletas está associado a uma série de resultados adversos à saúde (Biggins et al., 2018). O manejo do sono de um atleta é especialmente importante durante os períodos de treinamento e competição intensos, com os atletas frequentemente relatando o sono como sua estratégia de recuperação mais importante (Halson, 2008). Infelizmente, no entanto, foi relatado que atletas de elite costumam ter sono inadequado em comparação aos não atletas (Simpson et al., 2017). Isso é ainda apoiado sobre um estudo com atletas dos Jogos Olímpicos 3 meses antes das Olimpíadas de 2016, que descobriu que até 49% dos atletas apresentavam sono de má qualidade, conforme medido pelo Índice de Qualidade do Sono de Pittsburgh (Drew et al., 2018).

Em uma tentativa de esclarecer a importância do sono para os atletas como uma ferramenta de recuperação pós-competição, um estudo foi realizado em jogadores amadores da liga de rúgbi, nele os participantes foram randomizados para um grupo de privação de sono (0 hora de sono) ou controle (8 horas de sono) após uma partida competitiva da liga de rúgbi. Os resultados indicaram que para o grupo privado de sono houve uma diminuição na recuperação neuromuscular (média e pico de distância do salto com contramovimento); recuperação bioquímica (aumento dos níveis de CK e proteína C reativa); e função cognitiva (recuperação retardada de respostas de tempo de reação para tarefas cognitivas de palavras de cores) (Skein et al., 2013).

Um estudo semelhante descobriu que a privação de sono tem um efeito significativamente prejudicial no processo de recuperação fisiológica, produzindo aumento do volume-minuto e do consumo de oxigênio durante o período de recuperação (McMurray e Brown, 1984). Outras pesquisas sugeriram que reduções significativas na quantidade e qualidade do sono estão associadas ao aumento da fadiga e à diminuição da capacidade de exercício em praticantes de nado sincronizado de elite (Schaal et al., 2015). A perda de sono também tem sido associada ao acúmulo de proteínas musculares prejudicadas, à diminuição do humor e do vigor, à síndrome do sobretreinamento e às maiores taxas de infecções do trato respiratório superior; além disso, também pode prejudicar o aprendizado de novas habilidades (Fullagar et al., 2015).

Uma redução na duração e na qualidade do sono tem sido relatada em atletas individuais e de equipe, especialmente em tempos de competição congestionada, durante viagens de curta e longa duração e durante o treinamento e jogo à noite (Fullagar et al., 2015). Um estudo recente avaliou a quantidade objetiva de sono e calculou a associação à carga de treinamento percebida em atletas de elite; embora os resultados indicassem durações de sono saudáveis, houve aumento da vigília após o início do sono (quantidade de tempo gasto acordado após adormecer inicialmente), sugerindo a necessidade de otimização do sono (Knufinke et al., 2017). Resultados semelhantes foram encontrados em jogadores de escolas de futebol durante períodos de treinamento intensivo, em que os jovens não atendiam às diretrizes nacionais de sono de 8 a 10 horas para adolescentes de 14 a 17 anos, sugerindo ainda a necessidade de educação e intervenções sobre o sono (Fowler et al., 2017). A diminuição do tempo total de sono também foi correlacionada com a diminuição do desempenho em ginastas de elite ao avaliar o sono como uma ferramenta de recuperação em 26 ginastas (Dumortier et al., 2018).

A educação do sono foi proposta como um método para melhorar o sono em pacientes com insônia (Stepanski et al., 2003). O'Donnell e Driller (2017) iniciaram um estudo utilizando a educação do sono como uma intervenção em jogadores de *netball* de elite. Nesse estudo, usaram um desenho experimental pré-pós de um único grupo em que os atletas receberam uma apresentação de educação sobre higiene do sono no meio de um período de teste de 2 semanas, em que os participantes foram educados sobre a manutenção da hora de dormir e de acordar regulares, garantindo um quarto silencioso e fresco, evitando estimulantes e a tecnologia de emissão de luz antes de dormir e usando estratégias de relaxamento antes de dormir. Os resultados indicaram que a apresentação da educação sobre higiene do sono resultou em uma melhora significativa no tempo total de sono e na variação da vigília. Os resultados também indicaram tendências positivas, embora não significativas, para as melhorias no tempo total na cama, na eficiência e na latência do sono.

A educação sobre higiene do sono também demonstrou ter um efeito benéfico e significativo na quantidade de sono em jogadores de tênis altamente treinados (Duffield et al., 2014).

Outro método proposto para melhorar a recuperação foi o cochilo restaurador quando o sono estava esgotado. Os indivíduos em um estado de depleção/ esgotamento do sono (< 4 horas de sono na noite anterior) cochilaram ou descansaram por 30 minutos após o almoço e foram comparados ao grupo controle que não o fez. O cochilo foi associado às melhorias significativas no estado de alerta, na sonolência e na memória a curto prazo, com melhorias positivas nos tempos de *sprint* de 20 metros em comparação ao grupo de controle sem cochilo (Waterhouse et al., 2007). Também foi sugerido que tirar uma soneca no meio da tarde, entre 13:00 e 15:00, pode ser o momento ideal devido a um pico no ritmo circadiano produzindo um aumento da fissura e uma necessidade de dormir se estiver em um estado de sono esgotado (Littlehales, 2016).

Períodos muito mais curtos de sono, de apenas 6 minutos, também foram sugeridos para melhorar o desempenho cognitivo (Lahl et al., 2008), enquanto cochilos de 10 minutos produziram os resultados mais imediatos para sonolência subjetiva, fadiga, vigor e desempenho cognitivo quando em comparação às outras durações de cochilo (Brooks e Lack, 2006).

Embora o sono seja frequentemente relatado como de importância crítica para a recuperação, atualmente, esse é um aspecto pouco pesquisado, com estudos limitados avaliando sua eficácia na recuperação atlética. A pesquisa limitada que existe sugere que os atletas frequentemente apresentam reduções na qualidade do sono e na duração após períodos de excesso de partidas, jogos e treinamentos noturnos e durante períodos de excesso de viagens. As intervenções que podem melhorar a recuperação dos atletas incluem educação sobre higiene do sono, com foco na melhoria da rotina de pré-sono dos atletas, e cochilos à tarde quando o atleta está privado de sono.

Referências bibliográficas

Baird, M., Graham, S., Baker, J., Bickerstaff, G., 2012. Creatine kinase- and exercise-related muscle damage implications for muscle performance and recovery. Journal of Nutrition and Metabolism 2012, 1-13.

Banfi, G., Melegati, G., Barassi, A., Dogliotti, G., Melzi d'Eril, G., Dugué, B., et al., 2009. Effects of whole-body cryotherapy on serum mediators of inflammation and serum muscle enzymes in athletes. Journal of Thermal Biology 34 (2), 55-59.

Bell, P., Stevenson, E., Davison, G., Howatson, G., 2016. The effects of montmorency tart cherry concentrate supplementation on recovery following prolonged, intermittent exercise. Nutrients 8 (8), 441.

Bell, P., Walshe, I., Davison, G., Stevenson, E., Howatson, G., 2014. Montmorency cherries reduce the oxidative stress and inflammatory responses to repeated days high-intensity stochastic cycling. Nutrients 6 (2), 829-843.

Bieuzen, F., Bleakley, C., Costello, J., 2013. Contrast water therapy and exercise induced muscle damage: a systematic review and meta-analysis. PLoS ONE 8 (4), e62356.

Biggins, M., Cahalan, R., Comyns, T., Purtill, H., O'Sullivan, K., 2018. Poor sleep is related to lower general health, increased stress and increased confusion in elite Gaelic athletes. The Physician and Sportsmedicine 46 (1), 14-20.

Bleakley, C., Davison, G., 2010. What is the biochemical and physiological rationale for using cold-water immersion in sports recovery? A systematic review. British Journal of Sports Medicine 44 (3), 179-187.

Bleakley, C., Bieuzen, F., Davison, G., Costello, J., 2014. Whole-body cryotherapy: empirical evidence and theoretical perspectives. Open Access Journal of Sports Medicine 5, 25-36.

Bleakley, C., McDonough, S., Gardner, E., Baxter, G., Hopkins, J., Davison, G., 2012. Cold-water immersion (cryotherapy) for preventing and treating muscle soreness after exercise. Cochrane Database of Systematic Reviews 2012 (2), CD008262.

Bogdanis, G.C., Stavrinou, P., Fatouros, I.G., Philippou, A., Chatzinikolaou, A., Draganidis, D., et al., 2013. Short-term high-intensity interval exercise training attenuates oxidative stress responses and improves antioxidant status in healthy humans. Food and Chemical Toxicology 61, 171-177.

Bowtell, J., Sumners, D., Dyer, A., Fox, P., Mileva, K., 2011. Montmorency cherry juice reduces muscle damage caused by intensive strength exercise. Medicine and Science in Sports and Exercise 43 (8), 1544-1551.

Brooks, A., Lack, L., 2006. A Brief afternoon nap following nocturnal sleep restriction: which nap duration is most recuperative? Sleep 29 (6), 831-840.

Clifford, T., Bell, O., West, D., Howatson, G., Stevenson, E., 2015. The effects of beetroot juice supplementation on indices of muscle damage following eccentric exercise. European Journal of Applied Physiology 116 (2), 353-362.

Clifford, T., Berntzen, B., Davison, G., West, D., Howatson, G., Stevenson, E., 2016. Effects of beetroot juice on recovery of muscle function and performance between bouts of repeated sprint exercise. Nutrients 8 (8), 506.

Cochrane, D., 2004. Alternating hot and cold-water immersion for athlete recovery: a review. Physical Therapy in Sport 5 (1), 26-32.

Cockburn, E., Bell, P., 2017. Strategies to enhance athlete recovery. In: Turner, A., Comfort, P. (Eds.), Advanced Strength and Conditioning – An Evidence Based Approach, first st ed. Routledge, Oxon, p. 168.

Costello, J.T., Baker, P.R.A., Minett, G.M., Bieuzen, F., Stewart, I.B., Bleakley, C., 2015. Whole-body cryotherapy (extreme cold air exposure) for preventing and treating muscle soreness after exercise in adults. Cochrane Database of Systematic Reviews. Issue 9. Art. No.: CD010789.

Costello, J., Culligan, K., Selfe, J., Donnelly, A., 2012. Muscle, skin and core temperature after −110°C cold air and 8°C water treatment. PLoS ONE 7 (11), e48190.

Davies, V., Thompson, K., Cooper, S., 2009. The effects of compression garments on recovery. Journal of Strength and Conditioning Research 23 (6), 1786-1794.

Drew, M., Vlahovich, N., Hughes, D., Appaneal, R., Burke, L., Lundy, B., et al., 2018. Prevalence of illness, poor mental health and sleep quality and low energy availability prior to the 2016 Summer Olympic Games. British Journal of Sports Medicine 52 (1), 47-53.

Duffield, R., Portus, M., 2007. Comparison of three types of full-body compression garments on throwing and repeat-sprint performance in cricket players. British Journal of Sports Medicine 41, 409-414.

Duffield, R., Murphy, A., Kellett, A., Reid, M., 2014. Recovery from repeated on-court tennis sessions: combining cold-water immersion, compression, and sleep interventions. International Journal of Sports Physiology and Performance 9 (2), 273-282.

Dumortier, J., Mariman, A. Boone, J., Delesie, L., Tobback, E., Vogelaers, D., Bourgois, J.G., 2018. Sleep, training load and performance in elite female gymnasts. European Journal of Sport Science.18(2),151-161.

El Gamal, A., AL Said, M., Raish, M., Al-Sohaibani, M., Al-Massarani, S., Ahmad, A., et al., 2014. Beetroot (Beta vulgaris L.) Extract ameliorates gentamicin-induced nephrotoxicity associated oxidative stress, inflammation, and apoptosis in rodent model. Mediators of Inflammation 2014, 983952.

Eston, R., Peters, D., 1999. Effects of cold water immersion on the symptoms of exercise induced muscle damage. Journal Sports Sciences 17 (3), 231-238.

Fatouros, I.G., Chatzinikolaou, A., Douroudos, I.I., Nikolaidis, M.G., Kyparos, A., Margonis, K., et al., 2010. Time-course of changes in oxidative stress and antioxidant status responses following a soccer game. The Journal of Strength and Conditioning Research 24 (12), 3278-3286.

Fowler, P., Paul, D., Tomazoli, G., Farooq, A., Akenhead, R., Taylor, L., 2017. Evidence of sub-optimal sleep in adolescent Middle Eastern academy soccer players which is exacerbated by sleep intermission proximal to dawn. European Journal of Sport Science 17 (9), 1110-1118.

Fullagar, H., Duffield, R., Skorski, S., Coutts, A., Julian, R., Meyer, T., 2015. Sleep and recovery in team sport: current sleep-related issues facing professional team-sport athletes. International Journal of Sports Physiology and Performance 10 (8), 950-957.

Gill, N., Beavan, C., Cook, c., 2006. Effectiveness of post-match recovery strategies in rugby players. British Journal of Sports Medicine 40 (3), 260-263.

Glasgow, P., Ferris, R., Bleakley, C., 2014. Cold water immersion in the management of delayed-onset muscle soreness: Is dose important? A randomised controlled trial. Physical Therapy in Sport 15 (4), 228-233.

Goodall, S., Howatson, G., 2008. The effects of multiple cold-water immersions on indices of muscle damage. Journal of Sports Science and Medicine 7, 235-241.

Goto, K., Mizuno, S., Mori, A., 2017. Efficacy of wearing compression garments during post-exercise period after two repeated bouts of strenuous exercise: a randomized crossover design in healthy, active males. Sports Medicine - Open 3 (1), 25.

Halson, S.L., 2008. Nutrition, sleep and recovery. European Journal Sports Science 8 (2), 119-126.

Hausswirth, C., Mujika, I., 2013. Recovery for Performance in Sport. The National Institute of Sport for Expertise and Performance (INSEP), Leeds, UK, Human Kinetics p. xi.

Hausswirth, C., Louis, J., Bieuzen, F., Pournot, H., Fournier, J., Filliard, J., et al., 2011. Effects of whole-body cryotherapy vs. far-infrared vs. passive modalities on recovery from exercise-induced muscle damage in highly trained runners. PLoS One 6 (12), e27749.

Higgins, D., Kaminski, T.W., 1998. Contrast therapy does not cause fluctuations in human gastrocnemius. Journal of Athletic Training 33 (4), 336-340.

Hohenauer, E., Taeymans, J., Baeyens, J., Clarys, P., Clijsen, R., 2015. The effect of post-exercise cryotherapy on recovery characteristics: a systematic review and meta-analysis. PLoS One 10 (9), e0139028.

Howatson, G., Bells, P.G., Tallent, J., Middleton, B., McHugh, M.P., Ellis, J., 2012. Effect of tart cherry juice (Prunus cerasus) on melatonin levels and enhanced sleep quality. European Journal of Nutrition. 51 (8), 909-916.

Howatson, G., Leeder, J., van Someren, K., 2016. The BASES Expert Statement on Athletic Recovery Strategies. British Association of Sport and Exercise Sciences (BASES), Leeds, UK. Available at: https://www.bases.org.uk/imgs/tses_expert_statement_spread_recovery_strategies947.pdf.

Howatson, G., McHugh, M.P., Hill, J.A., Brouner, J., Jewell, A.P., Van Someren, K.A., et al., 2010. Influence of tart cherry juice on indices of recovery following marathon running. Scandinavian Journal of Medicine and Science in Sports 20 (6), 843-852.

Hyldahl, R.D., Hubal, M.J., 2014. Lengthening our perspective: morphological, cellular, and molecular responses to eccentric exercise. Muscle and Nerve Journal 49 (2), 155-170.

Ihsan, M., Watson, G., Abiss, C.R., 2016. What are the physiological mechanisms for post exercise cold water immersion in the recovery from prolonged endurance and intermittent exercise? Sports Medicine 46 (8), 1095-1109.

Ingram, J., Dawson, B., Goodman, C., Wallman, K., Beilby, J., 2009. Effect of water immersion methods on post-exercise recovery from simulated team sport exercise. Journal of Science and Medicine in Sport 12 (3), 417-421.

Jadert, C., Petersson, J., Massena, S., Ahl, D., Grapensparr, L., Holm, L., et al., 2012. Decreased leukocyte recruitment by inorganic nitrate and nitrite in microvascular inflammation and NSAID-induced intestinal injury. Free Radical Biology and Medicine 52 (3), 683-692.

Jakeman, J.R., Macrae, R., Eston, R., 2009. A single 10-min bout of cold-water immersion therapy after strenuous plyometric exercise has no beneficial effect on recovery from the symptoms of exercise-induced muscle damage. Ergonomics 52 (4), 456-460.

Kim, J., Kim, J., Lee, J., 2017. Effect of compression garments on delayed-onset muscle soreness and blood inflammatory markers after eccentric exercise: a randomized controlled trial. Journal of Exercise Rehabilitation 13 (5), 541-545.

Knufinke, M., Nieuwenhuys, A., Geurts, S., Møst, E., Maase, K., Moen, M., et al., 2017. Train hard, sleep well? perceived training load, sleep quantity and sleep stage distribution in elite level athletes. Journal of Science and Medicine in Sport.

Kraemer, W.J., Bush, J.A., Wickham, R.B., Denegar, C.R., Gómez, A.L., Gotshalk, L.A., et al., 2001. Influence of compression therapy on symptoms following soft tissue injury from maximal eccentric exercise. Journal of Orthopaedic Sports Physical Therapy 31 (6), 282-290.

Kuehl, K., Perrier, E., 2010. Efficacy of tart cherry juice in reducing muscle pain during running. Journey of The International Society of Sports Nutrition 7, 17.

Lahl, O., Wispel, C., Willigens, B., Pietrowsky, R., 2008. An ultra-short episode of sleep is sufficient to promote declarative memory performance. Journal of Sleep Research 17 (1), 3-10.

Leeder, J., Gissane, C., van Someren, K., Gregson, W., Howatson, G., 2012. Cold water immersion and recovery from strenuous exercise: a meta-analysis. British Journal of Sports Medicine 46 (4), 233-240.

Levers, K., Dalton, R., Galvan, E., Goodenough, C., O'Connor, A., Simbo, S., Barringer, N., Mertens-Talcott, S.U., Rasmussen, C., Greenwood, M., Riechman, S., Crouse, S., Kreider, R.B., 2015. Effects of powdered Montmorency tart cherry supplementation on an acute bout of intense lower body strength exercise in resistance trained males. Journal of the International Society of Sports Nutrition. 12, 41.

Littlehales, N., 2016. Sleep, first ed. Penguin Random House, London, UK, p. 60.

Lombardi, G., Ziemann, E., Banfi, G., 2017. Whole-body cryotherapy in athletes: from therapy to stimulation. an updated review of the literature. Frontiers in Physiology 8, 258.

Machado, A.F., Ferreira, P.H., Micheletti, J.K., De Almeida, A.C., Lemes, I.R., Vanderlei, F.M., et al., 2016. Can water temperature and immersion time influence the effect of cold water immersion on muscle soreness? a systematic review and meta-analysis. Sports Medicine 46 (4), 503-514.

Marqués-Jiménez, D., Calleja-González, J., Arratibel-Imaz, I., Delextrat, A., Uriarte, F., Terrados, N., 2017. Influence of different types of compression garments on exercise-induced muscle damage markers after a soccer match. Research in Sports Medicine 26 (1), 27-42.

McMurray, R.G., Brown, C.F., 1984. The effect of sleep loss on high intensity exercise and recovery. Aviation, Space and Environmental Medicine 55 (11), 1031-1035.

O'Donnell, S., Driller, M.W., 2017. Sleep-hygiene education improves sleep indices in elite female athletes. International Journal of Exercise Science 10 (4), 522-530.

Pournot, H., Bieuzen, F., Louis, J., Mounier, R., Fillard, J.R., Barbiche, E., et al., 2011. Time-course of changes in inflammatory response after whole-body cryotherapy multi exposures following severe exercise. PLos One 6, e22748.

Schaal, K., Le Meur, Y., Louis, J., Filliard, J., Hellard, P., Casazza, G., et al., 2015. Whole-body cryostimulation limits overreaching in elite synchronized swimmers. Medicine and Science in Sports and Exercise 47 (7), 1416-1425.

Seeram, N.P., Momin, R.A., Nair, M.G., Bourquin, L.D., 2001. Cyclooxygenase inhibitory and antioxidant cyaniding glycosides in cherries and berries. Phytomedicine 8 (5), 362-369.

Simpson, N.S., Gibbs, E.L., Matheson, G.O., 2017. Optimizing sleep to maximize performance: implications and recommendations for elite athletes. Scandinavian Journal of Medicine and Science in Sports 27 (3), 266-274.

Skein, M., Duffield, R., Minett, G., Snape, A., Murphy, A., 2013. The effect of overnight sleep deprivation after competitive rugby league matches on post-match physiological and perceptual recovery. International Journal of Sports Physiology and Performance 8 (5), 556-564.

Stepanski, E., Wyatt, J., 2003. Use of sleep hygiene in the treatment of insomnia. Sleep Medicine Reviews 7 (3), 215-225.

Tee, J.C., Bosch, A.N., Lambert, M.I., 2007. Metabolic consequences of exercise-induced muscle thrombosis: a randomized cross-over trial. Journal of Thrombosis and Haemostasis 1, 494-499.

Vaile, J.M., Gill, N.D., Blazevich, A.J., 2007. The effect of contrast water therapy on symptoms of delayed onset muscle soreness. Journal of Strength and Conditioning Research 21 (3), 697-702.

Vaile, J., Halson, S., Gill, N., Dawson, B., 2008. Effect of hydrotherapy on recovery from fatigue. International Journal of Sports Medicine 29 (7), 539-544.

Waterhouse, J., Atkinson, G., Edwards, B., Reilly, T., 2007. The role of a short post-lunch nap in improving cognitive, motor, and sprint performance in participants with partial sleep deprivation. Journal of Sports Science 25 (14), 1557-1566.

Watson, A.M., 2017. Sleep and athletic performance. Current Sports Medicine Reports 16 (6), 413-418.

Wozniak, A., Wozniakn, B., Drewa, G., Mila-Kierzenkowska, C. Rakowski, A., 2007. The effect of whole-body cryostimulation on lysosomal enzyme activity in kayakers during training. European Journal of Applied Physiology. 100 (2), 137-142.

Ziemann, E., Olek, R.A., Kujach, S., Grzywacz, T., Antosiewicz, J., Garsztka, T., et al., 2012. Five-day whole-body cryostimulation, blood inflammatory markers, and performance in high-ranking professional tennis players. Journal of Athletic Training 47 (6), 664-672.

Capítulo | 9 |

Como Entender a Dor na Fisioterapia Esportiva: Aplicação do Modelo de Raciocínio para a Dor e o Movimento

Des O'Shaughnessy e Lester E. Jones

Introdução

O manejo clínico de lesões esportivas e reabilitação incorpora uma compreensão da ciência da dor (Hainline et al., 2017a; 2017b). A complexidade das experiências de dor em treinamento, competição e todos os estágios de recuperação é relevante para os médicos que trabalham na arena esportiva. Como em todos os campos dos cuidados musculoesqueléticos, é importante compreender o funcionamento dos mecanismos da dor para que os atletas de todos os níveis recebam cuidados personalizados e baseados em evidências, muitas vezes considerando o modelo biopsicossocial. Atualmente, é reconhecido que o sistema nervoso central (SNC) está sempre envolvido na maneira como a dor é percebida. Isso se reflete em estudos clínicos de atletas, os quais mostram que, embora o limiar dos atletas para reconhecer a dor seja semelhante ao da população em geral, sua capacidade de tolerá-la é diferente (Hainline et al., 2017b). Combinar os princípios de reabilitação relevantes ao indivíduo requer a compreensão de como apresentações aparentemente semelhantes podem surgir de diferentes mecanismos fisiológicos. Também exige um conhecimento de como os processos de avaliação podem discernir esses vários mecanismos, bem como um processo de raciocínio sólido que facilite o atendimento personalizado. Por exemplo, a recuperação retardada pode ser devido aos processos inflamatórios em andamento, à biomecânica alterada ou à falta de confiança do atleta no processo. Uma estratégia de raciocínio clínico que pode funcionar em mais de um domínio é considerada importante.

Reformulação da relação entre dor e dano ao tecido

Embora haja evidências suficientes para sugerir que a dor não é um bom indicador da saúde do tecido, para a maioria das pessoas a atribuição da dor a uma estrutura danificada é automática. Esse é especialmente o caso quando o dano ao tecido traz uma inflamação visível. Portanto, é fácil desenvolver a crença de que apenas a ruptura do tecido é responsável pela percepção da dor. É amplamente reconhecido que o objetivo principal da dor é estimular o comportamento de segurança do atleta lesionado ou em risco. No entanto, a relação entre a dor e o estado de saúde do tecido é indiscutivelmente incidental a isso. Nos últimos anos, tem existido uma aceitação crescente de que os sinais nervosos que vêm dos tecidos em resposta ao estresse ou à lesão do tecido não são sinais de dor. Em vez disso, eles devem ser considerados simplesmente como mensagens para os processadores do SNC de que há perigo potencial (Catley et al., 2019), podendo ser interpretado como parte da experiência dolorosa.

Praticantes de reabilitação experientes reconheceram que lesões aparentemente semelhantes podem impactar diferentes esportistas de maneiras distintas e podem até mesmo variar para a mesma pessoa, dependendo de como o indivíduo está se saindo ou da pressão que pode estar sentindo. Portanto, uma visão mais robusta da dor é que ela faz parte do sistema de proteção do corpo (Janig et al., 2006). A dor ocorre quando a avaliação do ambiente interno, junto com as memórias, os contexto, a atenção, o humor e a autoconfiança, traz a percepção consciente de que uma área do corpo é vulnerável (Baliki e Apkarian, 2015).

Isso significa que a dor é como outros estados internos de consciência, como sentir-se ansioso, com frio, fome ou sede, nos quais a informação é filtrada de acordo com o que é considerado importante reagir naquele momento (Legrain et al., 2011; Wallwork et al., 2016). Esses estados são percepções e são experimentados quando informações razoáveis sugerem que o corpo está em perigo. É importante ressaltar que a sensação de sede para aumentar a ingestão de água é baseada em mais do que apenas níveis de volume sanguíneo. A dor é semelhante no sentido de que não depende apenas de uma única fonte de entrada (i. e., nocicepção) para determinar o nível de intensidade, ou mesmo a qualidade, da dor sentida, além das relações entre a fonte de entrada e o sistema que irá interpretá-la. Isso reforça a necessidade de reformular a dor como parte de um conjunto de respostas protetoras.

Onde as cargas no tecido podem colocar o tecido em risco de lesão, faz sentido que um sistema de proteção do corpo produza dor a fim de alterar o comportamento e, dessa maneira, proteger o tecido sob estresse. Quando ocorre uma lesão, os processos inflamatórios de sensibilização subsequentes ao dano ao tecido aumentam essa percepção de vulnerabilidade e a dor novamente facilita a proteção do tecido. Esses mecanismos nociceptivos indicam uma ameaça à segurança e se coordenam com outros processos para que o atleta possa se proteger – por meio de padrões motores responsivos adequados, comportamentos, estratégias psicológicas e funções autonômicas, imunológicas e endócrinas (Baliki e Apkarian, 2015; Cortelli et al., 2013; Legrain et al., 2011; Melzack, 2005; Sullivan e Vowles, 2017).

Reformulação da relação entre dor e movimento

O processamento protetor da fisiologia do movimento é complexo, e os modelos teóricos contemporâneos explicam como o processamento da dor e das saídas motoras ocorre de maneira simultânea, em vez de sequencialmente, como em geral se pensa (Melzack, 2005; Wallwork et al., 2016). Há uma avaliação simultânea, contínua e inconsciente da atividade nociceptiva e dos comportamentos motores associados, trabalhando para minimizar quaisquer ameaças à saúde dos tecidos (Baliki e Apkarian, 2015; Hodges, 2011; Sullivan e Vowles, 2017). As respostas associadas à dor podem incluir alterações na atividade muscular, como acelerar o movimento para que uma parte do corpo seja removida de um perigo ambiental, trazendo contração para imobilizar internamente um segmento do corpo, inibindo a atividade para distanciar o corpo de um perigo, vocalizando um pedido de ajuda ou fazendo uma expressão facial para obter apoio para gerenciar a ameaça (Hodges e Smeets, 2015). Assim, de uma perspectiva neurológica, a dor é considerada uma experiência sensorimotora (Sullivan e Vowles, 2017).

A sensibilização pós-lesão ocorre na periferia e dentro do SNC, facilitando maior vigilância dos ambientes interno e externo (Arendt-Nielsen et al., 2018; Pelletier et al., 2015a). Esse processamento amplificado de estímulos potencialmente ameaçadores envolve, de maneira mais fácil, as saídas de proteção adequadas, incluindo mudanças na padronização motora e nocicepção aprimorada pela glia (Grace et al., 2014; Meulders et al., 2011; Nijs et al., 2014b; Schabrun et al., 2015a). As adaptações de movimento de uma pessoa são individualizadas de acordo com sua percepção da dor, seu corpo, suas estratégias motoras disponíveis e suas experiências, bem como a tarefa desejada (Falla e Hodges, 2017; Hodges, 2011). Quando esses ajustes duram mais que um período de ameaça do tecido, ocorrem mudanças subsequentes a longo prazo no processamento neurológico da informação sensorial, na coordenação motora e na atividade nos centros superiores relevantes envolvidos (Baliki et al., 2011; Moseley e Flor, 2012; Vrana et al., 2015; Zusman, 2008a). Esse processamento central de entradas periféricas permite a modulação em ambas as direções; ou mais sensibilidade ou, às vezes, mais inibição.

Processamento central para a produção da dor

A neurociência identificou que a dor existe quando as vias talâmicas e somatossensoriais são estimuladas, mas ela também depende da atividade em vários centros de processamento emocional e de pensamento, incluindo a ínsula, o córtex cingulado, o sistema límbico e o córtex pré-frontal, bem como áreas dedicadas a saídas motoras (Apkarian et al., 2011; Bushnell et al., 2013). Essa complexidade neurológica da dor é acompanhada pela atividade de modulação das células gliais dentro do SNC, que se ligam ao sistema imunológico do corpo e às substâncias endógenas, como endorfinas, ocitocina e os hormônios do estresse (Grace et al., 2014; Jones, 2017). Consequentemente, uma experiência de dor é um evento neuroimunoendócrino.

Com uma interação tão complexa de processos motores, de saliência, emocionais, cognitivos e imunológicos, não é surpreendente que as experiências de dor possam variar tanto (Apkarian et al., 2011; Baliki e Apkarian, 2015). Como resultado, o mesmo estímulo pode ser percebido de modo muito diferente, os atletas podem continuar a se mover apesar da ocorrência de impulso nociceptivo (p. ex., no campo esportivo) e a dor pode ser relatada na ausência de nocicepção (p. ex., dor de membro fantasma).

Modelo de raciocínio de dor e movimento

A avaliação apoiada por um raciocínio clínico abrangente é necessária para capturar essa fisiologia sofisticada. Uma abordagem baseada em mecanismo que considera todos os contribuintes para a experiência de dor permite que as principais influências sejam identificadas e abordadas no tratamento (Falla e Hodges, 2017; Hush et al., 2013; Nijs et al., 2014b; Smart et al., 2010; Stanos et al., 2016; Wijma et al., 2016). Isso requer experiência em avaliação e também uma estratégia que incorpore todas as informações relevantes coletadas na interação clínica. Os autores desenvolveram o *modelo de raciocínio para dor e movimento* com objetivo de facilitar o raciocínio clínico em que vários mecanismos podem estar implicados em estados de dor (Figura 9.1) (Jones e O'Shaughnessy, 2014). Acredita-se que haja três categorias potencialmente coexistentes de mecanismos de dor que requerem avaliação e assimilação em um plano de manejo. Isso inclui (1) o estado da matriz neuroimunológica central, (2) questões discretamente locais e (3) um agrupamento rotulado como "fatores regionais". Estando cientes do potencial de sobreposição dessas três categorias, os profissionais da saúde são orientados a combinar o seu tratamento com o que julgam ser o componente predominante na apresentação de uma pessoa. Para os que apoiam os esportistas que trabalham para otimizar o desempenho motor, é importante reconhecer que os mecanismos fisiológicos de movimento alterado podem ser captados de modo semelhante – influências centrais, regionais e locais.

Estimulação local

A nocicepção leva à transmissão de sinais que chegam ao SNC, os quais surgem de atividades relacionadas com a deformação biomecânica e com a estimulação química.

O disparo de nociceptores mecânicos de alto limiar pode ocorrer com compressão de tecidos, por meio de uma força externa,

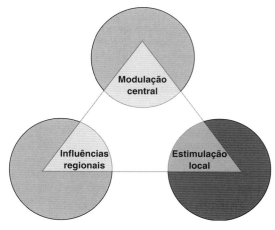

Figura 9.1 Categorias do modelo de raciocínio para a dor e o movimento. (*The Pain and Movement Reasoning Model*, de Des O'Shaughnessy e Lester Jones, sob uma licença *Creative Commons Attribution-NonCommercial-Share Alike 4.0 International [CC BY-NC-SA 4.0] License*.)

ou quando o movimento é restringido pelo movimento translacional em uma articulação ou com tração de tecidos, por exemplo, quando as estruturas são estendidas perto de faixas onde as cargas excederão a integridade do tecido (Smart et al., 2010). Isso, às vezes, pode ocorrer abaixo do limiar da percepção da dor (Baliki e Apkarian, 2015). Em nível significativo de agravamento, a dor provavelmente surgirá em decorrência de, por exemplo, uma luxação do ombro ou uma contusão do quadríceps.

Quando qualquer tecido é danificado, a inflamação é produzida enquanto o corpo trabalha para se curar. Felizmente, os mediadores químicos envolvidos nessa mistura inflamatória, como várias citocinas, também são pró-nociceptivos (Smart et al., 2012a). Isso apoia o comportamento protetor, como ficar em guarda ou reduzir as cargas teciduais, facilitando a cicatrização do tecido.

Há evidências de que os nociceptores químicos também são sensíveis ao excesso de trifosfato de adenosina (ATP) associado a espasmo muscular e desequilíbrios de pH decorrentes de isquemia (McGill et al., 2000; Mense, 2008; Rio et al., 2014). Essas mudanças bioquímicas locais adicionais podem ocorrer por meio da ativação dos músculos em posturas estáticas ou de proteção prolongadas ou como resultado de um espasmo muscular forte e persistente em resposta a uma lesão ou dor.

Além disso, a inflamação sensibiliza os nociceptores mecânicos, os quais, então, são capazes de enviar sinais de perigo com baixos níveis de pressão nos tecidos. Portanto, mesmo pequenos movimentos podem ser dolorosos, promovendo comportamentos de proteção com o mínimo de perturbação (Jones e O'Shaughnessy, 2014). À medida que a cicatrização do tecido avança pelos estágios, com a diminuição dos mediadores químicos pró-nociceptivos, a experiência da dor, geralmente, desaparece.

Nota clínica

As características que sugerem que os fatores de estimulação locais são predominantes incluem a presença de lesão no tecido e a demonstração de um padrão mecânico claro que corresponde ao raciocínio clínico da nocicepção em um tecido alvo (Figura 9.2) (Smart et al., 2012a). A melhora ocorre com processos de cura esperados ou observados e em resposta ao cuidado que enfatiza uma causa local, como proteção do movimento, terapia com foco mecânico, uso de anti-inflamatório não esteroide (AINE) ou cirurgia. Para que a dor seja considerada decorrente, principalmente, de mecanismos locais, as contribuições de outros fatores (i. e., influências regionais ou modulação central) são determinadas como menos significativas (Nijs et al., 2014b; Smart et al., 2012a). A presença de uma contribuição predominantemente nociceptiva para a dor não significa que apenas uma única estrutura seja afetada. Na maioria das apresentações de dor na lombar, não há causa anatomopatológica identificável (Müller-Schwefe et al., 2017). Para os casos em que a dor se deve, sobretudo, à estimulação local, acredita-se que a reabilitação mais adequada deva concentrar-se em aliviar qualquer inflamação presente e prescrever exercícios que abordem anomalias de carga ou reduzam a ativação muscular excessiva para normalizar o fluxo sanguíneo e restabelecer os níveis de oxigênio do tecido (Falla e Hodges, 2017; McGill et al., 2000).

Influências regionais

Esta categoria reconhece que a dor pode surgir remotamente à localização real da patologia ou disfunção. Três subcategorias de mecanismos são consideradas como "influências regionais": cadeia cinética, neuropatodinâmica e convergência do SNC. A relação entre

dor e movimento e a necessidade de considerar os mecanismos de dor e movimento em paralelo são indiscutivelmente mais bem exibidas nesta categoria.

Cadeia cinética

Os atletas se moverão de maneiras bastante individuais e a atividade escolhida exigirá uma variedade de posturas e variações de movimento em múltiplos segmentos corporais. No local em que a dor é atribuída ao movimento da cadeia cinética, a suposição é que as forças em uma região estão desencadeando padrões alterados de estresse e estimulação local de nociceptores no local dos sintomas. Um exemplo clínico pode ser um atleta experimentando padrões alterados de tensão nas articulações e dor nos joelhos; o profissional da saúde deve determinar se também há mudanças no comprimento da panturrilha, nas forças glúteas ou na capacidade proprioceptiva do tornozelo. A cadeia pode se estender ainda mais para incluir a coluna vertebral e a fáscia toracolombar, a qual, por sua vez, tem ligações com vários músculos, bem como tecido fascial visceral relacionado (Standring, 2015). Parece apropriado que o impacto das modificações da força mecânica causadas por equipamentos, órteses e outros dispositivos de suporte também seja considerado nesta subcategoria.

Neuropatodinâmica

Uma segunda subcategoria de influências regionais é a presença de alterações na sensibilidade do tecido neural periférico ou a mobilidade do tecido conjuntivo circundante ao longo de todo o nervo (Schmid et al., 2013; 2018). Neuropatia periférica, ou seja, doença ou dano ao tecido nervoso, caberia aqui. Mais comumente para praticantes musculoesqueléticos, isso envolve compressão ou encarceramento do nervo e as ramificações fisiopatológicas, também descritas como alterações *neuropatodinâmicas* (Jones e O'Shaughnessy, 2014). Muitas vezes, pode envolver mais do que um simples efeito biomecânico, como movimento ou restrição do nervo, e pode ocorrer quando parte do tecido conjuntivo adjacente ao leito do nervo perde sua mobilidade e as células de Schwann degeneram no ponto de tensão. Isso, por sua vez, leva a uma resposta inflamatória para promover a cura, novamente com a liberação de mediadores químicos pró-nociceptivos (Schmid et al., 2013; 2018; Smart et al., 2012b; Zusman, 2008b; 2009). Os potenciais de ação são criados bidirecionalmente no nervo. Ortodromicamente (i. e., distal para proximal), eles afetam neurônios de segunda ordem no corno dorsal que conduzem sinais para centros superiores. Antidromicamente (i. e., proximal para distal), a mudança no potencial atinge o local do receptor e causa uma liberação de mediadores químicos. Estes, por sua vez, são capazes de reestimular potenciais de ação, bem como de criar uma resposta inflamatória neurogênica, de modo que um elemento de edema possa ocorrer em um local distal à lesão original.

Esse é um bom exemplo de influências regionais, em que uma tensão ou lesão do tecido leva a uma atribuição de dor em um local remoto. Na verdade, a dor pode se tornar bastante disseminada, com respostas na medula espinal, processos corticais e gliais, depois de alguns dias dos processos periféricos iniciais (Arendt-Nielsen et al., 2018; Baliki e Apkarian, 2015; Grace et al., 2014; Nijs et al., 2017a; Schmid et al., 2013; 2018; Zusman, 2008b). A padronização motora também pode ser afetada, pois esses eventos podem alterar a capacidade contrátil do músculo adjacente (Hodges, 2011).

Essas apresentações são mais facilmente identificadas quando a dor segue estruturas ao longo de um leito nervoso e com a presença de testes neurodinâmicos positivos (Smart et al., 2012b). Outras pistas potenciais incluem local onde há um conjunto de

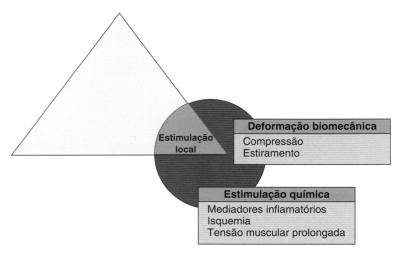

Figura 9.2 Subcategorias de estimulação local. (*The Pain and Movement Reasoning Model*, de Des O'Shaughnessy e Lester Jones, licenciado sob uma licença *Creative Commons Attribution-NonCommercial-Share Alike 4.0 International [CC BY-NC-SA 4.0] License*.)

alterações de dor, parestesia, alterações proprioceptiva e de energia; local onde a dor é descrita como tendo uma qualidade de queimação; ou quando há uma conexão, potencialmente apenas vaga, entre sintomas em diferentes partes do corpo (Smart et al., 2010). A triagem neurológica avalia as mudanças nos reflexos dos neurônios motores inferiores, na potência, na sensação ou no movimento dos leitos nervosos. Essencialmente, testa-se todo o sistema nervoso; portanto, se houver alterações no SNC, a capacidade de discernir disfunções no sistema nervoso periférico especificamente é reduzida. Também é difícil discriminar se uma limitação está no nível do nervo periférico e/ou do plexo e/ou da raiz nervosa (Nee e Butler, 2006; Schmid et al., 2013; 2018). Da mesma maneira, determinar o nível da raiz nervosa responsável é difícil devido ao grau de variação anatômica entre os indivíduos e ao alto nível de cruzamento entre os níveis, o qual se torna ampliado na presença de neuropatias de compressão (Anderberg et al., 2006; Schmid et al., 2013; 2018; Smart et al., 2012b). O exame neurodinâmico envolve alongar o tecido no local da dor percebida inicialmente e, em seguida, mover uma parte distante do corpo para ver se os sintomas estão alterados (Nee e Butler, 2006). Essa rotina de avaliação não é perfeita, pois casos de neuropatias por encarceramento ainda podem ser perdidos se procurarmos apenas sinais neurológicos como confirmação (Baselgia et al., 2017).

Os especialistas musculoesqueléticos verão regularmente casos como: apresentações semelhantes a um túnel do carpo quando o punho está sob carga, sendo resolvidas por meio de interfaces de endereçamento na coluna cervicotorácica e ao longo do leito do nervo mediano; sintomas de isquiotibiais que ocorrem devido à compressão do leito do nervo ciático surgindo na coluna lombar ou no piriforme; e manejo da articulação tibiofibular superior, melhorando o movimento dos nervos da perna e, como resultado, abordando a disfunção do pé e do tornozelo.

Convergência do sistema nervoso central

O cuidado musculoesquelético abrangente também considera o papel dos sinais nervosos periféricos distantes que convergem dentro do SNC (Graven-Nielsen e Arendt-Nielsen, 2010). Esse mecanismo de rede cruzada melhora a resiliência do corpo com o intuito de evitar a dependência de um caminho solitário para informações aferentes. Novamente, esse processo pode limitar a capacidade dos profissionais de identificar as estruturas exatas afetadas. Um exemplo comum é a dor lombar inespecífica com sintomas nas pernas, em que os padrões de referência podem ser semelhantes para os tecidos adjacentes, como articulações facetárias, músculos paravertebrais, periósteo ou estruturas sacroilíacas (LaPlante et al., 2012; Schwarzer et al., 1994). Localizar a fonte predominante de sintomas é ainda mais complicado quando as áreas de referência para estruturas aumentam na presença de disfunções, como distúrbios associados à síndrome do chicote ou às artropatias (Graven-Nielsen e Arendt-Nielsen, 2010).

Para aumentar a complexidade, os mecanismos de convergência nem sempre são somatossomáticos; o encaminhamento viscerossomático também pode ocorrer. Esse último é um mecanismo de dor que possibilita a identificação de patologias de vísceras (Giamberardino et al., 2010). As estruturas mesentéricas viscerais são relatadas como a fonte da dor referida, e a terapia manual que visa as vísceras pode melhorar os resultados da dor lombar, presumivelmente, por meio de processos de convergência ou conectividade estrutural (Gebhart e Bielefeldt, 2016; McSweeney et al., 2012; Tozzi et al., 2012).

Nota clínica

As características que sugerem que as influências regionais são predominantes em um caso incluem limitações de movimento associadas ao local da dor por cadeia cinética, sensibilidade ou mobilidade reduzida em estruturas neurais relevantes e evidência de patologia ou estresse em tecidos com inervação convergente (Figura 9.3). Estabelecer a extensão e a localização das limitações regionais em uma apresentação clínica requer uma avaliação abrangente das estruturas potencialmente implicadas. Por exemplo, um atleta que pula com sintomas laterais na coxa pode ser tratado levando-se em consideração as estruturas locais, como a tensão da banda iliotibial (BIT). No entanto, a investigação de influências mais amplas (*i. e.*, remotas ao local da dor) pode incluir desequilíbrio glúteo; mobilidade do nervo ciático com tendência para o nervo fibular comum; tensão do piriforme e encaminhamento da coluna lombar. Não seria uma apresentação incomum ter todos esses envolvidos. Um processo de raciocínio dedutivo pode ser mais apropriado quando uma medida objetiva válida e relevante é avaliada para alterações pré e pós-tratamento com várias técnicas. Abordar essas estruturas remotas sequencialmente com avaliação direcionada e observar a alteração dos sintomas determinam quais estruturas estão provavelmente associadas à disfunção relatada.

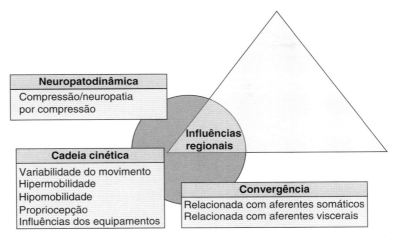

Figura 9.3 Subcategorias de modulação central. *(The Pain and Movement Reasoning Model*, de Des O'Shaughnessy e Lester Jones, licenciado sob uma licença *Creative Commons Attribution-NonCommercial-Share Alike 4.0 International [CC BY-NC-SA 4.0] License.)*

Modulação central

Esta categoria inclui mecanismos que podem sensibilizar ou inibir o sistema de proteção do corpo. Componentes centrais, envolvendo predominantemente o SNC, desempenham um papel crítico tanto no processamento da dor quanto na padronização motora.

Fatores de predisposição

Os níveis de dor e os padrões de movimento podem ser significativamente afetados pelo estado preexistente dos sistemas centrais antes de um evento de carga no sistema musculoesquelético. A modulação central pode ser influenciada pela plasticidade do sistema nervoso, bem como dos sistemas imunológico e endócrino. Os sistemas podem se tornar pró ou anti-inflamatórios e a responsividade nervosa pode ser estimulada ou atenuada, o que influencia o grau em que um indivíduo pode ser considerado vulnerável à dor (Flor et al., 2001; Generaal et al., 2016; Grace et al., 2014).

O termo "sensibilização central" é cada vez mais usado para descrever qualquer amplificação da nocicepção por mecanismos do SNC (medula espinal ou cortical) e é cada vez mais entendido como sendo influenciado por mecanismos imunológicos e endócrinos. Tem sido relatado como fator significativo em uma variedade de condições de dor, incluindo tendinopatias, lesão ligamentar, artropatias, dor lombar, disfunção de cotovelo, distúrbio de dor pélvica e fibromialgia (Arendt-Nielsen et al., 2018; Kapreli et al., 2009; Murphy et al., 2012; Needle et al., 2017; Pelletier et al., 2015a; Plinsinga et al., 2015; Rio et al., 2014; Sluka e Clauw, 2016; Wolfe et al., 2016). É importante ressaltar que os processos de sensibilização central podem ocorrer na fase aguda de uma lesão e, portanto, o termo não deve ser usado apenas para descrever apresentações de dor crônica ou persistente. O novo termo "nociplástico" foi recentemente introduzido para descrever esse tipo de influência na dor. No entanto, observe que a definição de *dor nociplástica* da International Association for the Study of Pain (IASP) é de exclusão (*i. e.*, nenhuma contribuição nociceptiva ou neuropática identificada) e, portanto, não reflete as apresentações clínicas em que a dor pode ser atribuída a múltiplos mecanismos (Aydede e Shriver, 2018).

As pessoas estarão predispostas a sentir dor em diferentes graus, dependendo de suas linhas de base de saúde física, psicológica e social anteriores. Conclui-se que a sensibilidade à dor é uma expressão da sensibilidade global aos vários sinais do corpo para manter o equilíbrio em resposta às ameaças internas e externas à fisiologia (Arendt-Nielsen et al., 2018; Yunus, 2015). A dor é apenas um sistema de alerta entre outros, como sinais para descansar e dormir, para renovar os níveis de energia, para evitar estímulos que possam danificar órgãos dos sentidos, como os olhos, para esvaziar o intestino de mediadores residuais, para manter o equilíbrio ereto, para reduzir o fluxo sanguíneo para a periferia a fim de manter a temperatura central ou para lidar com riscos socioambientais (Gracely e Schweinhardt, 2015). Em vez de ver a dor persistente como uma comorbidade frequente ao lado de outras síndromes de sensibilidade funcional (*i. e.*, síndrome de fadiga crônica, fotofobia, intestino irritável, vertigem posicional paroxística benigna, fenômeno de Raynaud ou transtorno de estresse pós-traumático), ela e essas síndromes são vistas como uma coleção de respostas amplificadas aos processos homeostáticos inconscientes, impulsionados por um SNC sensibilizado (Gracely e Schweinhardt, 2015; Maixner et al., 2016).

Escalas de medição para determinar a suscetibilidade de uma pessoa a respostas aumentadas aos estímulos incluem avaliar não apenas a sensibilidade a experiências dolorosas, mas também sensações de fadiga, experiências anteriores de dor, mudanças de humor, uma história de trauma, outros sintomas físicos e habilidades de concentração (Scerbo et al., 2018; Wolfe et al., 2016). As análises da prevalência dessas síndromes nas populações revelam que, em vez de estarem presentes ou não de modo binário, parece que todas as pessoas estão em um espectro e experimentam uma constelação de sintomas em vários graus (Wolfe et al., 2013). De algum modo, isso explica como as pessoas consideradas saudáveis demonstram uma amplitude dos níveis de dor relatados em experimentos. Parece que a extensão da sensibilização ou inibição central antes de uma experiência dolorosa afeta os níveis de dor subsequentes e os resultados funcionais após um evento de dor ou cirurgia (Clark et al., 2017; Coghill et al., 2003). Esse é o caso mesmo para aqueles que não têm nenhum diagnóstico de síndrome de sensibilização (Brummett et al., 2013; 2015).

A saúde de um indivíduo também afeta sua suscetibilidade à dor por meio de três expressões diferentes do sistema imunológico: (1) a presença de doenças autoimunes pode elevar a sensibilidade à dor; (2) há um aumento da sensibilidade na presença de atividade imunológica elevada, como o combate a uma infecção; e (3) parece haver uma relação entre os sintomas da síndrome de sensibilidade amplificada e um grande desafio imunológico recente, como a febre pós-glandular (Jones, 2017; Klein et al., 2012; Phillips e Clauw, 2013).

Parte | 1 | Conceitos Básicos Importantes em Esportes

Pesquisas recentes estão trazendo à luz a fisiologia complexa que está por trás dessa interação do sistema imunológico-nervoso, e um foco principal está na interface fornecida pelo sistema glial. As glias são consideradas células protetoras especializadas do SNC, as quais respondem não apenas às infecções em potencial, mas também aos outros estados de coação, como estresse atual e passado ou privação de sono (Grace et al., 2014; Loggia et al., 2015; Nijs et al., 2017b). Quando o SNC é confrontado por esses desafios, a glia torna-se ativada para lidar com esse estado de ameaça, liberando mediadores químicos que promovem a neuroinflamação e, ao fazer isso, aumentam a sensibilidade à dor (Grace et al., 2014; Nijs et al., 2017b). Esse processo também foi sugerido como um dos responsáveis pelo desenvolvimento da hiperalgesia induzida por opioides, em que o uso de medicamentos opiáceos leva a um aumento da sensibilidade do SNC (Grace et al., 2014). É importante ressaltar que essas células, após responderem a um risco percebido, não reduzem seus níveis de atividade aos níveis pré-tratamento, de modo que a sensibilidade à dor permanecerá ligeiramente elevada (Grace et al., 2014; Nicotra et al., 2012). Esse ciclo de declínio incompleto de estímulo pode ser repetido ao longo do tempo e, portanto, quando ameaças imunológicas-neurológicas são enfrentadas em várias ocasiões, o resultado final é um sistema de dor que se tornou mais responsivo ao movimento das estruturas musculoesqueléticas. Esse é um mecanismo provável para o impacto de traumas nos escores de sensibilidade central, fadiga muscular e dor (Burke et al., 2017; Generaal et al., 2016; Keller-Ross et al., 2014; Sueki et al., 2014; Tsur et al., 2017).

Também importante para a proteção do corpo é o sistema endócrino. Tanto os níveis elevados quanto os reduzidos do hormônio do estresse cortisol estão associados às condições de dor. Além disso, as substâncias tampão de estresse, como a ocitocina e as endorfinas, alteram a percepção da dor (Chapman et al., 2008; Hannibal e Bishop, 2014; Wippert et al., 2017). A disfunção do sistema respiratório altera a capacidade do diafragma de realizar as funções de controle da respiração e da coluna vertebral (Hodges et al., 2001), além de afetar os níveis de oxigenação dos tecidos em conjunto com o sistema cardiovascular. A saúde do sistema intestinal recentemente ganhou atenção na compreensão dos estados de dor por meio do que foi denominado eixo intestino-cérebro, predominantemente impulsionado pelo nervo vago (Farmer et al., 2014; Moloney et al., 2014).

Acredita-se que as características herdadas possuem um papel nas habilidades básicas de desempenho motor e na sensibilidade à dor de um indivíduo. A expressão de genes, influenciada por eventos externos e internos, está ganhando muita atenção na área de pesquisa conhecida como epigenética (Denk e McMahon, 2012; Huijnen et al., 2015). Os pesquisadores estão explorando os mecanismos que levam aos fenótipos individuais da dor, em particular como a interação entre a genética e o ambiente pode alterar características como a sensibilidade à dor, inclusive por meio dos mecanismos neuroimunes e neuroendócrinos descritos aqui.

Juntos, as experiências anteriores de uma pessoa, o estado imunológico, o meio ambiente, a genética e a saúde geral definem um nível de amplificação individual de sensibilidade mediada centralmente. Esses fatores predisponentes ditam como e em que grau os estímulos, incluindo aqueles relacionados com o movimento e com o sistema musculoesquelético, são interpretados (Phillips e Clauw, 2013; Yunus, 2015).

Plasticidade dependente de atividade

Outra grande influência sobre como o movimento e a dor são codificados no SNC é o papel dos padrões de atividade aprendidos.

Isso pode ser descrito como plasticidade dependente da atividade, pois o aprendizado depende da atividade nos neurônios e nas vias nervosas. Padrões persistentes de ativação reforçam a capacidade de resposta dos neurônios e as funções imunológicas e endócrinas associadas, levando a conexões neurais fortalecidas e transmissão aprimorada. A reabilitação esportiva é encorajada a utilizar esse conhecimento para a recuperação de lesões esportivas (Wallwork et al., 2016).

Há um reconhecimento de que mudanças na medula espinal e nos centros superiores (i. e., estruturais, químicos e conectividade) têm influência na percepção da dor que se relaciona com a duração de uma condição dolorosa (Apkarian et al., 2011; Arendt-Nielsen et al., 2018; Baliki et al., 2011; Coppieters et al., 2016; Kuner e Flor, 2017; Pelletier et al., 2015a; Pomares et al., 2017). Em particular, a transição de um estado de dor aguda para um persistente está relacionada com um maior envolvimento dos centros de processamento emocional e com menor envolvimento dos centros corticais somatossensoriais (Baliki e Apkarian, 2015; Hashmi et al., 2013; Vachon-Presseau et al., 2016). Mais importante ainda, essas mudanças são refletidas por alterações adicionais no córtex motor, mais uma vez reforçando a intimidade da relação entre a dor e o movimento (Hodges e Smeets, 2015; Moseley e Flor, 2012; Pelletier et al., 2015a; Vrana et al., 2015). Isso inclui aumento da atividade para aqueles com dor contínua ao antecipar a dor ou simplesmente ao imaginar movimentos, sem sinalização nociceptiva periférica (Tucker et al., 2012; Zusman, 2008a). Talvez sem surpresa, essas transformações em centros superiores envolvidos no processamento da dor e do desempenho motor foram encontradas para se correlacionar com os níveis de intensidade da dor em um amplo escopo de condições (Boudreau et al., 2010; Meeus et al., 2012; Pelletier et al., 2015a; Schabrun et al., 2015b; 2017; Stanton et al., 2012; Te et al., 2017; Tsao et al., 2011; Ung et al., 2012).

O processamento da dor aguda provoca tanto alterações do padrão motor, para encontrar a ativação muscular mais adequada, quanto mecanismos de sensibilização, que juntos minimizam o risco e promovem a cura (Boudreau et al., 2010; Hodges, 2011; Nijs et al., 2014a; Sullivan e Vowles, 2017; van Dieën et al., 2017). Quando essa ativação persiste, novos aprendizados biomecânicos ocorrem, que podem variar de uma redistribuição sutil de carga a novos padrões de movimento para completar uma ação, passando por comportamentos evitativos e posições antálgicas (Hodges e Smeets, 2015). Com a cura ou a resolução da condição de saúde disfuncional, geralmente há uma separação da necessidade de minimizar a dor dessas estratégias motoras aprendidas (Zusman, 2012). No entanto, se a sensação de vulnerabilidade permanecer alta, a repetição poderá levar a um aprendizado de que a biomecânica é ameaçadora e de quais são os comportamentos evitativos apropriados (den Hollander et al., 2010; Hodges e Smeets, 2015; Madden et al., 2015; Nijs et al., 2017a; van Dieën et al., 2017; Zusman, 2008a). Se não for contestado, isso pode eventualmente levar a alterações na quantidade e na variedade de padrões de movimento acessíveis à disposição de uma pessoa e a uma expansão dos comportamentos de evitação em um conjunto mais amplo de movimentos, podendo se elevar de acordo com a falta de reabilitação adequada (Meulders et al., 2011; Vlaeyen et al., 2016; Wallwork et al., 2016).

Modelos de evitação/proteção por medo evoluíram para ver essas aprendizagens não como patológicas, mas sim como uma resposta normal associada a uma sensação intensificada de dano e vigilância e a uma ênfase na remoção da dor como foco principal (Bunzli et al., 2015; Crombez et al., 2012; Wideman et al., 2013). Essas atitudes podem ter sido obtidas de várias fontes bem-intencionadas, como colegas de equipe, treinadores, familiares ou vários profissionais de saúde. Quando se acredita que a entrada mecânica sutil é uma representação da vulnerabilidade atual ou futura do tecido, isso encoraja alguém a se mover de maneira diferente e evitar as ações que ativam a dor e que são percebidas como causadoras de danos. À medida que o SNC se torna mais responsivo às informações aferentes e acentua o valor de ameaça de tais informações, a neuroplasticidade facilita que esse padrão sensibilizado seja inicialmente adquirido, depois incorporado, eventualmente, automatizado e, então, transferido para outros movimentos semelhantes ou estruturas vizinhas. Essa proteção excessivamente aplicada faz com que a dor seja sentida mais prontamente, percebida em estruturas antes não dolorosas e provocada por uma gama maior de movimentos e posturas.

Estado cognitivo-emocional-social

A aprendizagem de padrões neurais alterados, seja uma habilidade motora fina ou adaptação para minimizar os níveis de dor, dependerá do tempo, mas também do estado psicossocial de uma pessoa, levando em consideração mitos e crenças limitantes. A ativação dos centros cognitivos e emocionais está implicada na resistência da condição de apresentação do atleta ao tratamento (Bushnell et al., 2013; Malfliet et al., 2017; Nijs et al., 2014a). Isso atravessa uma variedade de domínios em que a dor e os níveis funcionais que a acompanham se relacionam não apenas com o medo, mas também com memórias de eventos semelhantes de dor ou cuidados anteriormente malsucedidos; tendência para catastrofização; resiliência; grau de percepção emocional; senso de injustiça; aceitação; culpa; estratégias de enfrentamento; ansiedade social; autoeficácia; suporte social; depressão; tensões atuais relacionadas com o desempenho ou seleção potencial; cinesiofobia; ou outros estresses ocupacionais, familiares ou pessoais (Bunzli et al., 2015; Gatchel et al., 2007; Hasenbring et al., 2012; Linton e Shaw, 2011; Lumley et al., 2011; Quartana et al., 2009; Serbic e Pincus, 2017; Sullivan et al., 2012; Wippert et al., 2017; Wurm et al., 2016). Esses fatores influenciam um espectro de cenários, incluindo situações experimentais envolvendo participantes sem dor, alguém em recuperação de um evento doloroso e onde a dor está em andamento.

Do mesmo modo, o desempenho motor também se baseou em fatores psicossociais e fornece a base para a psicologia do esporte ter um papel na maximização do desempenho motor (Benedetti, 2013; Pelletier et al., 2015b; Swinkels-Meewisse et al., 2006). Um sistema de "bandeiras amarelas" foi desenvolvido para ajudar a identificar fatores de risco psicológicos que têm o potencial de retardar a recuperação se deixados sem solução durante a reabilitação (Nicholas et al., 2011).[1]

Nota clínica

Foi destacado que, independentemente do estágio de cura que o atleta apresente, os fatores centrais estão sempre envolvidos em algum grau (Hainline et al., 2017a). A prática musculoesquelética que identifica as interações e influências complexas que levam à dor e ao movimento estará em melhor posição para abordar as mudanças neuroimunológicas centrais associadas às experiências passadas de um indivíduo, ao estado de saúde, às crenças e às emoções em todos os estágios de apresentação para a clínica (Figura 9.4) (Wallwork et al., 2016; Wijma et al., 2016). Isso ajudará os profissionais a reconhecer os vários fatores que podem fazer com que a dor seja experimentada e expressada em uma miríade de formas e sensibilidades. Adotar uma abordagem

biopsicossocial, incluindo a promoção de uma parceria terapêutica com o atleta, pode influenciar os resultados do SNC, imunológicos e endócrinos (Benedetti, 2013; Diener et al., 2016; Nijs et al., 2014a; O'Keeffe et al., 2016). Por exemplo, para pessoas que buscam cuidados para um episódio agudo de dor lombar, construir a confiança e fornecer informações tranquilizadoras sobre a resiliência da coluna e sobre os resultados normais para exames de imagem facilitam uma melhora nos resultados a longo prazo (Frederiksen et al., 2017; Hasenbring e Pincus, 2015).

A avaliação dos fatores contribuintes centrais é uma área emergente. Questionários que ajudam a identificar níveis de autoeficácia, medo, catastrofização, depressão, ansiedade e estresse podem ser usados como parte do julgamento clínico, mas é difícil traduzir e relacionar isso com a experiência de dor. Pode-se esperar que alguém com pontuação alta nessas escalas tenha maior sensibilização central, contribuindo para a dor, mas é improvável que haja uma relação nítida. A validade das estratégias de teste sensorial que avaliam a acuidade tátil, incluindo discriminação de dois pontos, e a hiperalgesia ao frio estão sendo exploradas (Harvie et al., 2017; Hübscher et al., 2014; Moss et al., 2016).

Uma maior consciência do impacto dos fatores moduladores centrais permite uma reinterpretação dos programas de exercícios. Em vez de atribuir resultados apenas às eficiências biomecânicas, à coordenação e à produção cardiovascular, torna-se importante maximizar os benefícios de direcionar as influências centrais. Além disso, permite que os prescritores de exercícios desenvolvam a autoconfiança de uma pessoa em sua capacidade de alcançar o padrão de movimento desejado ou realizar uma atividade sem desencadear respostas dolorosas (Wallwork et al., 2016). Embora a carga possa variar muito, caso a intenção seja melhorar a confiança em um movimento altamente qualificado ou ser mais capaz de realizar as atividades cotidianas, os princípios da progressão gradual são os mesmos (Moseley, 2003). Na presença de dor persistente, o incentivo ao exercício para facilitar a liberação de endorfina é, agora, visto como um objetivo inadequado, uma vez que a resposta hipoalgésica normal induzida por opioides é suprimida (Brellenthin et al., 2016). Da mesma maneira, o foco principal para ganhos de atividade funcional não é mais considerado como direcionamento ao descondicionamento, mas uma reversão da cautela sensorimotora e uma vigilância fisiológica relacionada com senso elevado de vulnerabilidade estrutural (Hodges e Smeets, 2015; Sullivan e Vowles, 2017; Vlaeyen et al., 2016; Wideman et al., 2013).

Esses cuidados não farmacológicos requerem que o profissional de saúde e o atleta trabalhem para adaptar habilmente os sistemas de proteção do corpo para serem menos reativos. Isso inclui reforçar que a dor é uma percepção e uma experiência personalizada e alterar as crenças sobre os níveis de segurança que são apropriados (Louw et al., 2016). A aprendizagem experiencial integra técnicas cognitivo-comportamentais com os princípios de exposição gradativa, em que a linha de base dos níveis de ameaça associados aos movimentos progride gradualmente (Blickenstaff e Pearson, 2016; Louw et al., 2016; Moseley, 2003; Nijs et al., 2017a; Pelletier et al., 2015a; Sullivan e Vowles, 2017).

A adaptação das expectativas é essencial com base no grau de pensamentos catastrofizantes e crenças de medo, bem como explorar como se mover sem os centros de ativação de resposta ao medo aprendidos da matriz de dor (Blickenstaff e Pearson, 2016; Huijnen et al., 2015; Moseley, 2003; Nijs et al., 2015; Wijma et al., 2016; Zusman, 2008a). Pode ser necessário iniciar os mecanismos neuroplásticos adequados de recuperação na ausência de movimento quando os processos de cura ou a sensibilidade ao movimento impedem a carga normal. Isso pode ser alcançado

---

[1] O sistema de bandeiras é muito utilizado para a classificação de subgrupos no tratamento de dorsalgias.

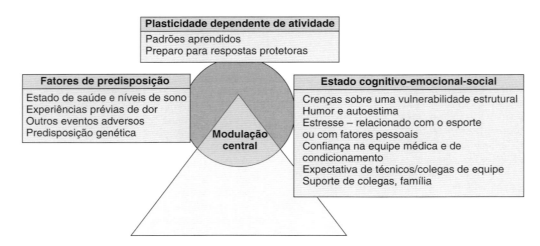

Figura 9.4 O espectro de fatores que influenciam a dor e o movimento e o efeito das mudanças neuroimunológicas centrais incluem experiências passadas de um indivíduo, seu estado de saúde, suas crenças e emoções. (*The Pain and Movement Reasoning Model*, de Des O'Shaughnessy e Lester Jones, licenciado sob uma licença *Creative Commons Attribution-NonCommercial-Share Alike 4.0 International [CC BY-NC-SA 4.0] License.*)

usando imagens motoras graduadas, antes de avançar para movimentos espelhados ou, então, maximizando o *feedback* visual (Daffada et al., 2015; Guillot e Collet, 2008; Moseley e Flor, 2012; Wallwork et al., 2016). As atividades podem progredir aumentando a repetição ou a duração do tempo gasto em uma tarefa, mesmo na presença de dor, embora a taxa de aumento, frequentemente, precise ser muito baixa. A progressão também pode ser alcançada desafiando o sistema a lidar com mudanças na carga musculoesquelética, no ambiente físico ou social, nas demandas cognitivo-emocionais e nos níveis de confiança, ou introduzindo movimento no local onde a dor é provocada (Moseley, 2003; Nijs et al., 2015; O'Sullivan et al., 2015; Pelletier et al., 2015b; Sullivan e Vowles, 2017).

Implicações para a reabilitação esportiva integrada

Um conhecimento aplicado da fisiologia da dor é importante para alcançar os melhores resultados para o atleta lesionado. O raciocínio clínico eficaz requer a consideração de todos os mecanismos potenciais que afetam o desempenho. A dor pode ser vista como um sinal de mudança e isso pode ocorrer em resposta aos problemas biomecânicos ou aos regimes de treinamento. Além disso, agora, é definida como uma percepção de ameaça e o julgamento de que algo precisa ser abordado pode ser sensibilizado por outros fatores musculoesqueléticos regionais ou modulado por uma miríade de estresses pessoais, relacionados com esporte ou com outras pressões, crenças, memórias e expectativas.

Abordagens de manejo baseadas em princípios centrais de sensibilização e focos psicossociais trouxeram melhorias funcionais nos resultados para as pessoas, com mudanças associadas nos centros superiores dentro da matriz de dor (Boudreau et al., 2010; Kregel et al., 2017; Nijs et al., 2017a; Pelletier et al., 2015b; Richmond et al., 2015; Seminowicz et al., 2013; Shpaner et al., 2014; Snodgrass et al., 2014; Veehof et al., 2016; Vowles et al., 2017; Wälti et al., 2015). Os processos de abordar esses mecanismos centrais e direcionar os medos individuais devem ocorrer em todos os estágios da reabilitação, incluindo os estágios iniciais (Boudreau et al., 2010; Pelletier et al., 2015b; Wallwork et al., 2016). É reconhecido que isso requer habilidades especializadas, experiência e tempo. Quando esses cuidados são necessários, pode ser apropriado encaminhar os esportistas para clínicas multidisciplinares de dor, mesmo em um estágio inicial da reabilitação. Na Austrália, o encaminhamento para fisioterapeutas de *dor* reconhecidos fornece outro caminho para aumentar a recuperação, no qual a dor é, de modo predominante, modulada centralmente. Estar ciente da modulação central da dor e das opções de encaminhamento disponíveis pode ser o primeiro passo importante para melhorar o controle da dor no esporte.

Buscar atividades de desenvolvimento profissional para aprimorar o conhecimento e as habilidades no tratamento da dor é incentivado, embora seja importante que o impacto na prática clínica seja mais do que apenas um acréscimo a um paradigma biomédico.

Resumo

Reconhecendo que múltiplas disfunções estão em jogo, o Modelo de Raciocínio para a Dor e o Movimento é projetado para auxiliar os profissionais da saúde a examinar todos os possíveis contribuintes e permite que as prioridades de intervenção sejam estabelecidas. Isso garante que o médico esportivo direcione o manejo para o fator mais significativo. É importante ressaltar que se alguém apresenta pontuações psicométricas altas, sugerindo fatores centrais em jogo, não se pode presumir que outros mecanismos estejam excluídos. Da mesma maneira, quando alguém apresenta dano franco ao tecido, o potencial para influências moduladoras centrais pode ser relevante, particularmente em relação à autoidentidade (Hainline et al., 2017a). A descrição da dor como aguda ou crônica aumenta o risco desse erro de raciocínio. Toda dor é complexa e, provavelmente, provocada pelos múltiplos mecanismos concorrentes que foram discutidos anteriormente.

Por meio da prestação de cuidados musculoesqueléticos, os quais levam em consideração os vários elementos envolvidos na experiência multifatorial de dor e movimento, tornam-se possíveis resultados mais sustentáveis para atletas e outros que acessam o atendimento.

Referências bibliográficas

Anderberg, L., Annertz, M., Rydholm, U., Brandt, L., Säveland, H., 2006. Selective diagnostic nerve root block for the evaluation of radicular pain in the multilevel degenerated cervical spine. European Spine Journal 15 (6), 794-801.

Apkarian, A.V., Hashmi, J.A., Baliki, M.N., 2011. Pain and the brain: specificity and plasticity of the brain in clinical chronic pain. Pain 152 (3, Suppl. 1), S49-S64.

Arendt–Nielsen, L., Morlion, B., Perrot, S., Dahan, A., Dickenson, A., Kress, H., et al., 2018. Assessment and manifestation of central sensitisation across different chronic pain conditions. European Journal of Pain 22 (2), 216-241.

Aydede, M., Shriver, A., 2018. Recently introduced definition of 'nociplastic pain' by the international association for the study of pain needs better formulation. Pain 159 (6), 1176-1177.

Baliki, M.N., Apkarian, A.V., 2015. Nociception, pain, negative moods, and behavior selection. Neuron 87 (3), 474-491.

Baliki, M.N., Schnitzer, T.J., Bauer, W.R., Apkarian, A.V., 2011. Brain morphological signatures for chronic pain. PloS ONE 6 (10), e26010.

Baselgia, L.T., Bennett, D.L., Silbiger, R.M., Schmid, A.B., 2017. Negative neurodynamic tests do not exclude neural dysfunction in patients with entrapment neuropathies. Archives of Physical Medicine and Rehabilitation 98 (3), 480-486.

Benedetti, F., 2013. Placebo and the new physiology of the doctor-patient relationship. Physiological Reviews 93 (3), 1207-1246.

Blickenstaff, C., Pearson, N., 2016. Reconciling movement and exercise with pain neuroscience education: a case for consistent education. Physiotherapy Theory and Practice 32 (5), 396-407.

Boudreau, S.A., Farina, D., Falla, D., 2010. The role of motor learning and neuroplasticity in designing rehabilitation approaches for musculoskeletal pain disorders. Manual Therapy 15 (5), 410-414.

Brellenthin, A.G., Crombie, K.M., Cook, D.B., Sehgal, N., Koltyn, K.F., 2016. Psychosocial influences on exercise-induced hypoalgesia. Pain Medicine 18 (3), 538-550.

Brummett, C.M., Janda, A.M., Schueller, C.M., Tsodikov, A., Morris, M., Williams, D.A., et al., 2013. Survey criteria for fibromyalgia independently predict increased postoperative opioid consumption after lower-extremity joint arthroplastya prospective, observational cohort study. The Journal of the American Society of Anesthesiologists 119 (6), 1434-1443.

Brummett, C.M., Urquhart, A.G., Hassett, A.L., Tsodikov, A., Hallstrom, B.R., Wood, N.I., et al., 2015. Characteristics of fibromyalgia independently predict poorer long–term analgesic outcomes following total knee and hip arthroplasty. Arthritis & Rheumatology 67 (5), 1386-1394.

Bunzli, S., Smith, A., Schütze, R., O'Sullivan, P., 2015. Beliefs underlying pain-related fear and how they evolve: a qualitative investigation in people with chronic back pain and high pain-related fear. BMJ Open 5 (10), e008847.

Burke, N.N., Finn, D.P., McGuire, B.E., Roche, M., 2017. Psychological stress in early life as a predisposing factor for the development of chronic pain: clinical and preclinical evidence and neurobiological mechanisms. Journal of Neuroscience Research 95 (6), 1257-1270.

Bushnell, M.C., Čeko, M., Low, L.A., 2013. Cognitive and emotional control of pain and its disruption in chronic pain. Nature Reviews Neuroscience 14 (7), 502-511.

Catley, M.J., Moseley, G.L., Jones, M.A., 2019. Understanding pain in order to treat patients in pain. In: Jones, M.A., Rivett, D.A. (Eds.), Clinical Reasoning in Musculoskeletal Practice, second ed. Elsevier Health Sciences, Oxford, p. 32.

Chapman, C.R., Tuckett, R.P., Song, C.W., 2008. Pain and stress in a systems perspective: reciprocal neural, endocrine, and immune interactions. The Journal of Pain 9 (2), 122-145.

Clark, J., Nijs, J., Yeowell, G., Goodwin, P., 2017. What are the predictors of altered central pain modulation in chronic musculoskeletal pain populations? A systematic review. Pain Physician 20 (6), 487-500.

Coghill, R.C., McHaffie, J.G., Yen, Y.-F., 2003. Neural correlates of interindividual differences in the subjective experience of pain. Proceedings of the National Academy of Sciences 100 (14), 8538-8542.

Coppieters, I., Meeus, M., Kregel, J., Caeyenberghs, K., De Pauw, R., Goubert, D., et al., 2016. Relations between brain alterations and clinical pain measures in chronic musculoskeletal pain: a systematic review. The Journal of Pain 17 (9), 949-962.

Cortelli, P., Giannini, G., Favoni, V., Cevoli, S., Pierangeli, G., 2013. Nociception and autonomic nervous system. Neurological Sciences 34 (1), 41-46.

Crombez, G., Eccleston, C., Van Damme, S., Vlaeyen, J.W., Karoly, P., 2012. Fear-avoidance model of chronic pain: the next generation. The Clinical Journal of Pain 28 (6), 475-483.

Daffada, P., Walsh, N., McCabe, C., Palmer, S., 2015. The impact of cortical remapping interventions on pain and disability in chronic low back pain: a systematic review. Physiotherapy 101 (1), 25-33.

den Hollander, M., De Jong, J.R., Volders, S., Goossens, M.E., Smeets, R.J., Vlaeyen, J.W., 2010. Fear reduction in patients with chronic pain: a learning theory perspective. Expert Review of Neurotherapeutics 10 (11), 1733-1745.

Denk, F., McMahon, S.B., 2012. Chronic pain: emerging evidence for the involvement of epigenetics. Neuron 73 (3), 435-444.

Diener, I., Kargela, M., Louw, A., 2016. Listening is therapy: patient interviewing from a pain science perspective. Physiotherapy Theory and Practice 32 (5), 356-367.

Falla, D., Hodges, P.W., 2017. Individualized exercise interventions for spinal pain. Exercise and Sport Sciences Reviews 45 (2), 105-115.

Farmer, A.D., Randall, H.A., Aziz, Q., 2014. It's a gut feeling: how the gut microbiota affects the state of mind. The Journal of Physiology 592 (14), 2981-2988.

Flor, H., Denke, C., Schaefer, M., Grusser, S., 2001. Effect of sensory discrimination training on cortical reorganisation and phantom limb pain. Lancet 357 (9270), 1763-1764.

Frederiksen, P., Indahl, A., Andersen, L.L., Burton, K., Hertzum-Larsen, R., Bendix, T., 2017. Can group-based reassuring information alter low back pain behavior? A cluster-randomized controlled trial. PloS One 12 (3), e0172003.

Gatchel, R.J., Peng, Y.B., Peters, M.L., Fuchs, P.N., Turk, D.C., 2007. The biopsychosocial approach to chronic pain: scientific advances and future directions. Psychological Bulletin 133 (4), 581.

Gebhart, G., Bielefeldt, K., 2016. Physiology of visceral pain. Comprehensive Physiology 6 (4), 1609-1633.

Generaal, E., Vogelzangs, N., Macfarlane, G.J., Geenen, R., Smit, J.H., de Geus, E.J., et al., 2016. Biological stress systems, adverse life events and the onset of chronic multisite musculoskeletal pain: a 6-year cohort study. Annals of the Rheumatic Diseases 75 (5), 847-854.

Giamberardino, M.A., Affaitati, G., Costantini, R., 2010. Visceral referred pain. Journal of Musculoskeletal Pain 18 (4), 403-410.

Grace, P.M., Hutchinson, M.R., Maier, S.F., Watkins, L.R., 2014. Pathological pain and the neuroimmune interface. Nature Reviews Immunology 14 (4), 217-231.

Gracely, R.H., Schweinhardt, P., 2015. Programmed symptoms: disparate effects united by purpose. Current Rheumatology Reviews 11 (2), 116-130.

Graven-Nielsen, T., Arendt-Nielsen, L., 2010. Assessment of mechanisms in localized and widespread musculoskeletal pain. Nature Reviews Rheumatology 6 (10), 599-606.

Guillot, A., Collet, C., 2008. Construction of the motor imagery integrative model in sport: a review and theoretical investigation of motor imagery use. International Review of Sport and Exercise Psychology 1 (1), 31-44.

Hainline, B., Derman, W., Vernec, A., Budgett, R., Deie, M., Dvořák, J., et al., 2017a. International olympic committee consensus statement on pain management in elite athletes. British Journal of Sports Medicine 51 (17), 1245-1258.

Hainline, B., Turner, J.A., Caneiro, J., Stewart, M., Moseley, G.L., 2017b. Pain in elite athletes –neurophysiological, biomechanical and psychosocial considerations: a narrative review. British Journal of Sports Medicine 51 (17), 1259-1264.

Hannibal, K.E., Bishop, M.D., 2014. Chronic stress, cortisol dysfunction, and pain: a psychoneuroendocrine rationale for stress management in pain rehabilitation. Physical Therapy 94 (12), 1816-1825.

Harvie, D.S., Kelly, J., Buckman, H., Chan, J., Sutherland, G., Catley, M., et al., 2017. Tactile acuity testing at the neck: a comparison of methods. Musculoskeletal Science and Practice 32, 23-30.

Hasenbring, M.I., Hallner, D., Klasen, B., Streitlein-Böhme, I., Willburger, R., Rusche, H., 2012. Pain-related avoidance versus endurance in primary care patients with subacute back pain: psychological characteristics and outcome at a 6-month follow-up. Pain 153 (1), 211-217.

Hasenbring, M.I., Pincus, T., 2015. Effective reassurance in primary care of low back pain: what messages from clinicians are most beneficial at early stages? The Clinical Journal of Pain 31 (2), 133-136.

Hashmi, J.A., Baliki, M.N., Huang, L., Baria, A.T., Torbey, S., Hermann, K.M., et al., 2013. Shape shifting pain: chronification of back pain shifts brain representation from nociceptive to emotional circuits. Brain 136 (9), 2751-2768.

Hodges, P.W., Heijnen, I., Gandevia, S.C., 2001. Postural activity of the diaphragm is reduced in humans when respiratory demand increases. The Journal of Physiology 537 (3), 999-1008.

Hodges, P.W., Smeets, R.J., 2015. Interaction between pain, movement, and physical activity: short-term benefits, long-term consequences, and targets for treatment. The Clinical Journal of Pain 31 (2), 97-107.

Hodges, P.W., 2011. Pain and motor control: from the laboratory to rehabilitation. Journal of Electromyography and Kinesiology 21 (2), 220-228.

Hübscher, M., Moloney, N., Rebbeck, T., Traeger, A., Refshauge, K.M., 2014. Contributions of mood, pain catastrophizing, and cold hyperalgesia in acute and chronic low back pain: a comparison with pain-free controls. The Clinical Journal of Pain 30 (10), 886-893.

Huijnen, I.P., Rusu, A.C., Scholich, S., Meloto, C.B., Diatchenko, L., 2015. Subgrouping of low back pain patients for targeting treatments: evidence from genetic, psychological, and activity-related behavioral approaches. The Clinical Journal of Pain 31 (2), 123-132.

Hush, J.M., Stanton, T.R., Siddall, P., Marcuzzi, A., Attal, N., 2013. Untangling nociceptive, neuropathic and neuroplastic mechanisms underlying the biological domain of back pain. Pain 3 (3), 223-236.

Janig, W., Chapman, C., Green, P., 2006. Pain and body protection: sensory, autonomic, neuroendocrine and behavioural mechanisms in control of inflammation and hyperalgesia. In: Flor, H., Kaslo, E., Dostrovsky, J.O. (Eds.), Proceedings of the 11th World Congress on Pain. IASP Press, Seattle.

Jones, L.E., 2017. Stress, pain and recovery: neuro-immune-endocrine interactions and clinical practice. In: Porter, S. (Ed.), Psychologically Informed Physiotherapy: Embedding Psychosocial Perspectives Within Clinical Management. Elsevier, Edinburgh, pp. 78-106.

bib55Jones, L.E., O'Shaughnessy, D.F., 2014. The Pain and Movement Reasoning Model: introduction to a simple tool for integrated pain assessment. Manual Therapy 19 (3), 270-276.

Kapreli, E., Athanasopoulos, S., Gliatis, J., Papathanasiou, M., Peeters, R., Strimpakos, N., et al., 2009. Anterior cruciate ligament deficiency causes brain plasticity: a functional MRI study. The American Journal of Sports Medicine 37 (12), 2419-2426.

Keller-Ross, M.L., Schlinder-Delap, B., Doyel, R., Larson, G., Hunter, S.K., 2014. Muscle fatigability and control of force in men with post-traumatic stress disorder. Medicine and Science in Sports and Exercise 46 (7), 1302-1313.

Klein, C.J., Lennon, V.A., Aston, P.A., McKeon, A., Pittock, S.J., 2012. Chronic pain as a manifestation of potassium channel-complex autoimmunity. Neurology 79 (11), 1136-1144.

Kregel, J., Coppieters, I., De Pauw, R., Malfliet, A., Danneels, L., Nijs, J., et al., 2017. Does conservative treatment change the brain in patients with chronic musculoskeletal pain? A systematic review. Pain Physician 20 (3), 139-154.

Kuner, R., Flor, H., 2017. Structural plasticity and reorganisation in chronic pain. Nature Reviews Neuroscience 18 (1), 20-30.

LaPlante, B.L., Ketchum, J.M., Saullo, T.R., DePalma, M.J., 2012. Multi-variable analysis of the relationship between pain referral patterns and the source of chronic low back pain. Pain Physician 15, 171-178.

Legrain, V., Iannetti, G.D., Plaghki, L., Mouraux, A., 2011. The pain matrix reloaded: a salience detection system for the body. Progress in Neurobiology 93 (1), 111-124.

Linton, S.J., Shaw, W.S., 2011. Impact of psychological factors in the experience of pain. Physical Therapy 91 (5), 700-711.

Loggia, M.L., Chonde, D.B., Akeju, O., Arabasz, G., Catana, C., Edwards, R.R., et al., 2015. Evidence for brain glial activation in chronic pain patients. Brain 138 (3), 604-615.

Louw, A., Zimney, K., Puentedura, E.J., Diener, I., 2016. The efficacy of pain neuroscience education on musculoskeletal pain: a systematic review of the literature. Physiotherapy Theory and Practice 32 (5), 332-355.

Lumley, M.A., Cohen, J.L., Borszcz, G.S., Cano, A., Radcliffe, A.M., Porter, L.S., et al., 2011. Pain and emotion: a biopsychosocial review of recent research. Journal of Clinical Psychology 67 (9), 942-968.

Madden, V.J., Harvie, D.S., Parker, R., Jensen, K.B., Vlaeyen, J.W., Moseley, G.L., et al., 2015. Can pain or hyperalgesia be a classically conditioned response in humans? A systematic review and meta-analysis. Pain Medicine 17 (6), 1094-1111.

Maixner, W., Fillingim, R.B., Williams, D.A., Smith, S.B., Slade, G.D., 2016. Overlapping chronic pain conditions: implications for diagnosis and classification. The Journal of Pain 17 (9), T93-T107.

Malfliet, A., Coppieters, I., Van Wilgen, P., Kregel, J., De Pauw, R., Dolphens, M., et al., 2017. Brain changes associated with cognitive and emotional factors in chronic pain: a systematic review. European Journal of Pain 21 (5), 769-786.

McGill, S.M., Hughson, R.L., Parks, K., 2000. Lumbar erector spinae oxygenation during prolonged contractions: implications for prolonged work. Ergonomics 43 (4), 486-493.

McSweeney, T.P., Thomson, O.P., Johnston, R., 2012. The immediate effects of sigmoid colon manipulation on pressure pain thresholds in the lumbar spine. Journal of Bodywork and Movement Therapies 16 (4), 416-423.

Meeus M., Vervisch S., De Clerck, L.S., Moorkens G., Hans G., Nijs J., editors., 2012. Central sensitization in patients with rheumatoid arthritis: a systematic literature review. Seminars in Arthritis and Rheumatism 41 (4), 556-567.

Melzack, R., 2005. Evolution of the neuromatrix theory of pain. The Prithvi Raj lecture: presented at the third world congress of world institute of pain, barcelona 2004. Pain Practice 5 (2), 85-94.

Mense, S., 2008. Muscle pain: mechanisms and clinical significance. Deutsches Ärzteblatt International 105 (12), 214.

Meulders, A., Vansteenwegen, D., Vlaeyen, J.W., 2011. The acquisition of fear of movement-related pain and associative learning: a novel pain-relevant human fear conditioning paradigm. Pain 152 (11), 2460-2469.

Moloney, R.D., Desbonnet, L., Clarke, G., Dinan, T.G., Cryan, J.F., 2014. The microbiome: stress, health and disease. Mammalian Genome 25 (1-2), 49-74.

Moseley, G., 2003. A pain neuromatrix approach to patients with chronic pain. Manual Therapy 8 (3), 130-140.

Moseley, G.L., Flor, H., 2012. Targeting cortical representations in the treatment of chronic pain: a review. Neurorehabilitation and Neural Repair 26 (6), 646-652.

Moss, P., Knight, E., Wright, A., 2016. Subjects with knee osteoarthritis exhibit widespread hyperalgesia to pressure and cold. PloS One 11 (1), e0147526.

Müller-Schwefe, G., Morlion, B., Ahlbeck, K., Alon, E., Coaccioli, S., Coluzzi, F., et al., 2017. Treatment for chronic low back pain: the focus should change to multimodal management that reflects the underlying pain mechanisms. Current Medical Research and Opinion 33 (7), 1199-1210.

Murphy, S.L., Phillips, K., Williams, D.A., Clauw, D.J., 2012. The role of the central nervous system in osteoarthritis pain and implications for rehabilitation. Current Rheumatology Reports 14 (6), 576-582.

Nee, R.J., Butler, D., 2006. Management of peripheral neuropathic pain: integrating neurobiology, neurodynamics, and clinical evidence. Physical Therapy in Sport 7 (1), 36-49.

Needle, A.R., Lepley, A.S., Grooms, D.R., 2017. Central nervous system adaptation after ligamentous injury: a summary of theories, evidence, and clinical interpretation. Sports Medicine 47 (7), 1271-1288.

Nicholas, M.K., Linton, S.J., Watson, P.J., Main, C.J., 'Decade of the flags' working group, 2011. Early identification and management of psychological risk factors ('yellow flags') in patients with low back pain: a reappraisal. Physical Therapy 91 (5), 737-753.

Nicotra, L., Loram, L.C., Watkins, L.R., Hutchinson, M.R., 2012. Toll-like receptors in chronic pain. Experimental Neurology 234 (2), 316-329.

Nijs, J., Clark, J., Malfliet, A., Ickmans, K., Voogt, L., Don, S., et al., 2017a. In the spine or in the brain? Recent advances in pain neuroscience applied in the intervention for low back pain. Clinical and Experimental Rheumatology 35 (5), 108-115.

Nijs, J., Girbés, E.L., Lundberg, M., Malfliet, A., Sterling, M., 2015. Exercise therapy for chronic musculoskeletal pain: innovation by altering pain memories. Manual Therapy 20 (1), 216-220.

Nijs, J., Loggia, M.L., Polli, A., Moens, M., Huysmans, E., Goudman, L., et al., 2017b. Sleep disturbances and severe stress as glial activators: key targets for treating central sensitization in chronic pain patients? Expert Opinion on Therapeutic Targets 21 (8), 817-826.

Nijs, J., Meeus, M., Cagnie, B., Roussel, N.A., Dolphens, M., Van Oosterwijck, J., et al., 2014a. A modern neuroscience approach to chronic spinal pain: combining pain neuroscience education with cognition-targeted motor control training. Physical Therapy 94 (5), 730-738.

Nijs, J., Torres-Cueco, R., van Wilgen, P., Lluch Girbés, E., Struyf, F., Roussel, N., et al., 2014b. Applying modern pain neuroscience in clinical practice: criteria for the classification of central sensitization pain. Pain Physician 17 (5), 447-457.

O'Keeffe, M., Cullinane, P., Hurley, J., Leahy, I., Bunzli, S., O'Sullivan, P.B., et al., 2016. What influences patient–therapist interactions in musculoskeletal physical therapy? Qualitative systematic review and meta-synthesis. Physical Therapy 96 (5), 609-622.

O'Sullivan, K., Dankaerts, W., O'Sullivan, L., O'Sullivan, P.B., 2015. Cognitive functional therapy for disabling nonspecific chronic low back pain: multiple case-cohort study. Physical Therapy 95 (11), 1478-1488.

Pelletier, R., Higgins, J., Bourbonnais, D., 2015a. Addressing neuroplastic changes in distributed areas of the nervous system associated with chronic musculoskeletal disorders. Physical Therapy 95 (11), 1582-1591.

Pelletier, R., Higgins, J., Bourbonnais, D., 2015b. Is neuroplasticity in the central nervous system the missing link to our understanding of chronic musculoskeletal disorders? BMC Musculoskeletal Disorders 16 (1), 25.

Phillips, K., Clauw, D.J., 2013. Central pain mechanisms in the rheumatic diseases: future directions. Arthritis & Rheumatology 65 (2), 291-302.

Plinsinga, M.L., Brink, M.S., Vicenzino, B., Van Wilgen, C.P., 2015. Evidence of nervous system sensitization in commonly presenting and persistent painful tendinopathies: a systematic review. Journal of Orthopaedic & Sports Physical Therapy 45 (11), 864-875.

Pomares, F.B., Funck, T., Feier, N.A., Roy, S., Daigle-Martel, A., Ceko, M., et al., 2017. Histological underpinnings of grey matter changes in fibromyalgia investigated using multimodal brain imaging. Journal of Neuroscience 37 (5), 1090-1101.

Quartana, P.J., Campbell, C.M., Edwards, R.R., 2009. Pain catastrophizing: a critical review. Expert Review of Neurotherapeutics 9 (5), 745-758.

Richmond, H., Hall, A.M., Copsey, B., Hansen, Z., Williamson, E., Hoxey-Thomas, N., et al., 2015. The effectiveness of cognitive behavioural treatment for non-specific low back pain: a systematic review and meta-analysis. PloS One 10 (8), e0134192.

Rio, E., Moseley, L., Purdam, C., Samiric, T., Kidgell, D., Pearce, A.J., et al., 2014. The pain of tendinopathy: physiological or pathophysiological? Sports Medicine 44 (1), 9-23.

Scerbo, T., Colasurdo, J., Dunn, S., Unger, J., Nijs, J., Cook, C., 2018. Measurement properties of the central sensitization inventory: a systematic review. Pain Practice 18 (4), 544-554.

Schabrun, S.M., Christensen, S.W., Mrachacz-Kersting, N., Graven-Nielsen, T., 2015a. Motor cortex reorganization and impaired function in the transition to sustained muscle pain. Cerebral Cortex 26 (5), 1878-1890.

Schabrun, S.M., Elgueta-Cancino, E.L., Hodges, P.W., 2017. Smudging of the motor cortex is related to the severity of low back pain. Spine 42 (15), 1172-1178.

Schabrun, S.M., Hodges, P.W., Vicenzino, B., Jones, E., Chipchase, L.S., 2015b. Novel adaptations in motor cortical maps: the relationship to persistent elbow pain. Medicine and Science in Sports and Exercise 47 (4), 681-690.

Schmid, A.B., Hailey, L., Tampin, B., 2018. Entrapment neuropathies: challenging common beliefs with novel evidence. Journal of Orthopaedic & Sports Physical Therapy 48 (2), 58-62.

Schmid, A.B., Nee, R.J., Coppieters, M.W., 2013. Reappraising entrapment neuropathies – mechanisms, diagnosis and management. Manual Therapy 18 (6), 449-457.

Schwarzer, A.C., Aprill, C.N., Derby, R., Fortin, J., Kine, G., Bogduk, N., 1994. The relative contributions of the disc and zygapophyseal joint in chronic low back pain. Spine 19 (7), 801-806.

Seminowicz, D.A., Shpaner, M., Keaser, M.L., Krauthamer, G.M., Mantegna, J., Dumas, J.A., et al., 2013. Cognitive-behavioral therapy increases prefrontal cortex gray matter in patients with chronic pain. The Journal of Pain 14 (12), 1573-1584.

Serbic D., Pincus T., 2017. The relationship between pain, disability, guilt and acceptance in low back pain: a mediation analysis. Journal of Behavioral Medicine 40 (4), 651-658. 119.

Sturgeon J.A., Zautra, A.J., 2013. Psychological resilience, pain catastrophizing, and positive emotions: perspectives on comprehensive modeling of individual pain adaptation. Current Pain and Headache Reports 17 (3), 317.

Shpaner, M., Kelly, C., Lieberman, G., Perelman, H., Davis, M., Keefe, F.J., et al., 2014. Unlearning chronic pain: a randomized controlled trial to investigate changes in intrinsic brain connectivity following cognitive behavioral therapy. NeuroImage: Clinical 5, 365-376.

Sluka, K.A., Clauw, D.J., 2016. Neurobiology of fibromyalgia and chronic widespread pain. Neuroscience 338, 114-129.

Smart, K.M., Blake, C., Staines, A., Doody, C., 2010. Clinical indicators of 'nociceptive', 'peripheral neuropathic' and 'central' mechanisms of musculoskeletal pain. A Delphi survey of expert clinicians. Manual Therapy 15 (1), 80-87.

Smart, K.M., Blake, C., Staines, A., Thacker, M., Doody, C., 2012a. Mechanisms-based classifications of musculoskeletal pain: part 3 of 3: symptoms and signs of nociceptive pain in patients with low back (±leg) pain. Manual Therapy 17 (4), 352-357.

Smart, K.M., Blake, C., Staines, A., Thacker, M., Doody, C., 2012b. Mechanisms-based classifications of musculoskeletal pain: part 2 of 3: symptoms and signs of peripheral neuropathic pain in patients with low back (±leg) pain. Manual Therapy 17 (4), 345-351.

Snodgrass, S.J., Heneghan, N.R., Tsao, H., Stanwell, P.T., Rivett, D.A., Van Vliet, P.M., 2014. Recognising neuroplasticity in musculoskeletal rehabilitation: a basis for greater collaboration between musculoskeletal and neurological physiotherapists Manual Therapy 19 (6), 614-617.

Standring, S., 2015. Gray's Anatomy: The Anatomical Basis of Clinical Practice, forty-first ed. Elsevier Health Sciences, Oxford.

Stanos, S., Brodsky, M., Argoff, C., Clauw, D.J., D'Arcy, Y., Donevan, S., et al., 2016. Rethinking chronic pain in a primary care setting. Postgraduate Medicine 128 (5), 502-515.

Stanton, T.R., Lin, C.-W.C., Smeets, R.J., Taylor, D., Law, R., Moseley, G.L., 2012. Spatially defined disruption of motor imagery performance in people with osteoarthritis. Rheumatology 51 (8), 1455-1464.

Sueki, D., Dunleavy, K., Puentedura, E., Spielholz, N., Cheng, M., 2014. The role of associative learning and fear in the development of chronic pain–a comparison of chronic pain and post-traumatic stress disorder. Physical Therapy Reviews 19 (5), 352-366.

Sullivan, M.D., Vowles, K.E., 2017. Patient action: as means and end for chronic pain care. Pain 158 (8), 1405-1407.

Sullivan, M.J., Scott, W., Trost, Z., 2012. Perceived injustice: a risk factor for problematic pain outcomes. The Clinical Journal of Pain 28 (6), 484-488.

Swinkels-Meewisse, I.E., Roelofs, J., Oostendorp, R.A., Verbeek, A.L., Vlaeyen, J.W., 2006. Acute low back pain: pain-related fear and pain catastrophizing influence physical performance and perceived disability. Pain 120 (1), 36-43.

Te, M., Baptista, A.F., Chipchase, L.S., Schabrun, S.M., 2017. Primary motor cortex organization is altered in persistent patellofemoral pain. Pain Medicine 18 (11), 2224-2234.

Tozzi, P., Bongiorno, D., Vitturini, C., 2012. Low back pain and kidney mobility: local osteopathic fascial manipulation decreases pain perception and improves renal mobility. Journal of Bodywork and Movement Therapies 16 (3), 381-391.

Tsao, H., Danneels, L.A., Hodges, P.W., 2011. ISSLS prize winner: smudging the motor brain in young adults with recurrent low back pain. Spine 36 (21), 1721-1727.

Tsur, N., Defrin, R., Ginzburg, K., 2017. Posttraumatic stress disorder, orientation to pain, and pain perception in ex-prisoners of war who underwent torture. Psychosomatic Medicine 79 (6), 655-663.

Tucker, K., Larsson, A.-K., Oknelid, S., Hodges, P., 2012. Similar alteration of motor unit recruitment strategies during the anticipation and experience of pain. Pain 153 (3), 636-643.

Ung, H., Brown, J.E., Johnson, K.A., Younger, J., Hush, J., Mackey, S., 2012. Multivariate classification of structural MRI data detects chronic low back pain. Cerebral Cortex 24 (4), 1037-1044.

Vachon-Presseau, E., Tétreault, P., Petre, B., Huang, L., Berger, S.E., Torbey, S., et al., 2016. Corticolimbic anatomical characteristics predetermine risk for chronic pain. Brain 139 (7), 1958-1970.

van Dieën, J.H., Flor, H., Hodges, P.W., 2017. Low-back pain patients learn to adapt motor behavior with adverse secondary consequences. Exercise and Sport Sciences Reviews 45 (4), 223-229.

Veehof, M., Trompetter, H., Bohlmeijer, E.T., Schreurs, K.M.G., 2016. Acceptance- and mindfulness-based interventions for the treatment of chronic pain: a meta-analytic review. Cognitive Behaviour Therapy 45 (1), 5-31.

Vlaeyen, J.W., Morley, S., Crombez, G., 2016. The experimental analysis of the interruptive, interfering, and identity-distorting effects of chronic pain. Behaviour Research and Therapy 86, 23-34.

Vowles, K.E., Witkiewitz, K., Levell, J., Sowden, G., Ashworth, J., 2017. Are reductions in pain intensity and pain-related distress necessary? An analysis of within-treatment change trajectories in relation to improved functioning following interdisciplinary acceptance and commitment therapy for adults with chronic pain. Journal of Consulting and Clinical Psychology 85 (2), 87.

Vrana, A., Hotz-Boendermaker, S., Stämpfli, P., Hänggi, J., Seifritz, E., Humphreys, B.K., et al., 2015. Differential neural processing during motor imagery of daily activities in chronic low back pain patients. PloS One 10 (11), e0142391.

Wallwork, S.B., Bellan, V., Catley, M.J., Moseley, G.L., 2016. Neural representations and the cortical body matrix: implications for sports medicine and future directions. British Journal of Sports Medicine 50, 990-996.

Wälti, P., Kool, J., Luomajoki, H., 2015. Short-term effect on pain and function of neurophysiological education and sensorimotor retraining compared to usual physiotherapy in patients with chronic or recurrent nonspecific low back pain, a pilot randomized controlled trial. BMC Musculoskeletal Disorders 16 (1), 83.

Wideman, T.H., Asmundson, G.G., Smeets, R.J.M., Zautra, A.J., Simmonds, M.J., Sullivan, M.J., et al., 2013. Re-thinking the fear avoidance model: toward a multi-dimensional framework of pain-related disability. Pain 154 (11), 2262-2265.

Wijma, A.J., van Wilgen, C.P., Meeus, M., Nijs, J., 2016. Clinical biopsychosocial physiotherapy assessment of patients with chronic pain: the first step in pain neuroscience education. Physiotherapy Theory and Practice 32 (5), 368-384.

Wippert, P.-M., Fliesser, M., Krause, M., 2017. Risk and protective factors in the clinical rehabilitation of chronic back pain. Journal of Pain Research 10, 1569-1579.

Wolfe, F., Brähler, E., Hinz, A., Häuser, W., 2013. Fibromyalgia prevalence, somatic symptom reporting, and the dimensionality of polysympto-matic distress: results from a survey of the general population. Arthritis Care & Research 65 (5), 777-785.

Wolfe, F., Clauw, D.J., Fitzcharles, M.-A., Goldenberg, D.L., Häuser, W., Katz, R.L., et al., 2016. Revisions to the 2010/2011 fibromyalgia diagnostic criteria. Seminars in Arthritis and Rheumatism 46 (3), 319-329.

Wurm, M., Edlund, S., Tillfors, M., Boersma, K., 2016. Characteristics and consequences of the co-occurrence between social anxiety and pain-related fear in chronic pain patients receiving multimodal pain rehabilitation treatment. Scandinavian Journal of Pain 12, 45-52.

Yunus, M.B., 2015. Editorial review (Thematic issue: an update on central sensitivity syndromes and the issues of nosology and psychobiology). Current Rheumatology Reviews 11 (2), 70-85.

Zusman, M., 2012. A review of the proposal that innocuous proprioceptive input may maintain movement-evoked joint pain. Physical Therapy Reviews 17 (5), 346-349.

Zusman, M., 2008a. Associative memory for movement-evoked chronic back pain and its extinction with musculoskeletal physiotherapy. Physical Therapy Reviews 13 (1), 57-68.

Zusman, M., 2008b. Mechanisms of peripheral neuropathic pain: implications for musculoskeletal physiotherapy. Physical Therapy Reviews 13 (5), 313-323.

Zusman, M., 2009. Pain science and mobilization of painful compressive neuropathies. Physical Therapy Reviews 14 (4), 285-289.

Capítulo | 10 |

Fisiologia da Terapia Manual

Christopher J. McCarthy, Elaine Lonnemann, Jackie Hindle, Ruth MacDonald e Ioannis Paneris

Introdução

A terapia manual (TM) é considerada um método de intervenção terapêutica que envolve a aplicação habilidosa do movimento ao corpo. Isso, geralmente, assume a forma de movimento que é aplicado ao receptor em vez de movimento gerado pelo receptor e, portanto, é denominado movimento passivo (Maitland, 1986; Vicenzino et al., 2007). No entanto, as formas de movimento ativo guiado e contrações musculares isométricas (Day e Nitz, 2012; Sharman et al., 2006; Smith e Fryer, 2008) também são consideradas como abrangendo o termo geral de terapia manual. A TM se destina a ter um ou todos os seguintes efeitos: melhorar a extensibilidade do tecido; aumentar a amplitude de movimento; mobilizar ou manipular tecidos moles e articulações; induzir relaxamento; alterar a função muscular; estabilizar o complexo articular; modular a dor; reduzir o inchaço dos tecidos moles, inflamação ou restrição de movimento (IFOMPT Standards, 2016). Existem numerosos textos que descrevem mobilizações articulares (Maitland, 1986; McCarthy, 2010; Vicenzino et al., 2007), técnicas musculares (Smith e Fryer, 2008) e técnicas nervosas (Shacklock, 2005). A aplicação de contato com o corpo na intenção de guiar ou evocar movimento irá influenciar pele, fáscia, tecido neural, vascular, linfático, miogênico e artrogênico e, portanto, esses rótulos são um pouco artificiais.

A TM também pode ser subcategorizada com base nos parâmetros do movimento produzido. Não localizado, leve pressão, grande amplitude, "massagem de tecidos moles" (Lindgren et al., 2010), enquanto movimento de pequena amplitude e alta velocidade seria considerado típico de técnicas de "impulso de manipulação" ou *Thrust*, difundido pela osteopatia ou quiropraxia (Evans, 2010; McCarthy et al., 2015). Embora existam diferenças nos métodos pelos quais alguém pode introduzir o movimento no corpo, parece haver algumas respostas comuns ao toque e ao movimento aplicados que podem oferecer benefícios terapêuticos para aqueles que sentem dor. Certamente, a consideração da TM (como um componente de um pacote multimodal de cuidados) é recomendada na maioria das diretrizes internacionais para o tratamento da dor lombar e ciática e seu uso é considerado de baixo custo (Chou et al. 2007; NICE, 2016).

Efeitos na dor

O estímulo mecânico do movimento aplicado gera uma série de respostas neurofisiológicas de vários sistemas, incluindo o sistema nervoso periférico, a medula espinal e as estruturas supraespinais (Bialosky et al., 2009; Lascurain-Aguirrebena et al., 2016; Pickar, 2002). Além dos efeitos neurofisiológicos, alguns efeitos biomecânicos foram observados. Estes incluem alterações de curto prazo a permanentes no comprimento e na rigidez do tecido conjuntivo (Bialosky et al., 2009; Martinez-Segura et al., 2006; 2012). O simples ato de aplicar o toque na pele pode ter efeitos benéficos na percepção da dor (Mancini et al., 2015). Breves aplicações de movimento leve, de pequena amplitude e de baixa pressão podem evocar estimulação aferente suficiente para reduzir a sensibilização e a amplificação do corno dorsal, resultando em uma redução no fenômeno de somação temporal, um índice observável em um "segmento" do corno dorsal (Mancini et al., 2015). Mediação inibitória semelhante do sistema nervoso central (SNC) também é observada após estimulação de alta velocidade e pequena amplitude (manipulação espinal) (Bishop et al., 2011). Além disso, o toque da pele de grande amplitude e leve pressão, estimulando os receptores C-táteis da pele, demonstrou reduzir a dor. Isso está ligado a respostas no córtex orbitofrontal associadas ao prazer, sugerindo uma inibição da dor em um nível supraespinal, sendo produzida no contexto de uma sensação de toque agradável (Leknes e Tracey, 2008; Liljencrantz e Olausson, 2014). A comunicação e o *feedback* de "efeitos práticos", a atenção pessoal e o exame são partes do processo de manejo clínico de um terapeuta manual. Esses fatores podem produzir um efeito placebo que deve ser considerado nos mecanismos plausíveis de melhora.

Há um corpo considerável de evidências que descreve a influência da estimulação aferente de vários tipos de TM na mediação de mecanismos de dor inibitórios orquestrados pelo SNC (Bialosky et al., 2009; Bishop et al., 2011; Coronado et al., 2012; Skyba et al., 2003; Vicenzino et al., 1999; Wright, 1999; Wright e Sluka, 2001; Yeo e Wright, 2011). O tipo preciso de estimulação aferente não parece ser crítico, com respostas semelhantes sendo relatadas com técnicas de mobilização (movimentos lentos, não localizados, de grande amplitude, baixa pressão) e técnicas de manipulação com manobra de alta velocidade e baixa amplitude (localizado, rápido, alta pressão, pequenos movimentos de amplitude) (Bishop et al., 2015; Moulson e Watson, 2006). Uma resposta simpática-excitatória de ação rápida e a curto prazo à TM foi bem documentada (Zusman, 2012), com esse mecanismo de "luta ou fuga" proporcionando reduções na percepção de informações aferentes nociceptivas locais para a região de aplicação e, em menor grau, sistemicamente (Hegedus et al., 2011; Voogt et al., 2015).

Há algumas evidências que sugerem que a aplicação de toque de pressão profunda e movimento suficiente para estimular mecanorreceptores de alto limiar e nociceptores locais pode evocar alterações corticais de controle inibitório nocivo difuso (DNIC, do inglês *diffuse noxious inhibitory control*) (Granot et al., 2008; Kunz et al., 2006; Peters et al., 1992; Ram et al., 2008; Staud et al., 2003). O desvio da atenção cortical da dor patológica para um estímulo nociceptivo não ameaçador e "menos significativo" (semelhante ao observado com a inserção de agulhas de acupuntura) pode reduzir os estados dolorosos (Staud et al., 2003). Além disso, evidências de ressonância magnética funcional mostraram que a percepção de desconforto não ameaçador pode ser interpretada na neuromatriz da dor (Moseley, 2003) como prazer, resultando em uma hipoalgesia sistêmica (Leknes e Tracey, 2008).

O alívio da dor após a aplicação da TM pode ser interpretado pelo cérebro como uma recompensa, principalmente se for inesperado ou maior do que o esperado (Bissonette e Roesch, 2016; Leknes et al., 2011; 2013; Morita et al., 2013; Navratilova e Porreca, 2014; Wise, 2005). Sensações de recompensa inesperadas resultam na liberação fásica do neurotransmissor dopamina que, além de contribuir para a hipoalgesia sistêmica, facilitará a motivação para buscar aquela sensação de recompensa novamente (Navratilova e Porreca, 2014). Assim, a motivação para repetir o movimento pode ser facilitada e um processo de exposição gradual ao movimento realizado (Jones et al., 2002). Uma atualização gradual do movimento levará a adaptações neurofisiológicas, facilitando a habituação ao estímulo nociceptivo e resultando em uma redução gradual da dor (Zusman, 2004).

A influência da TM no sistema neuroendócrino não é clara e é relativamente pouco pesquisada. O estímulo mecânico inicial afeta o sistema nervoso periférico e pode causar uma redução nos mediadores inflamatórios, como as citocinas (Kovanur Sampath et al., 2015; Teodorczyk-Injeyan et al., 2006; 2010). Alterações nos níveis de neuropeptídeos e no fator de crescimento do nervo também foram observadas (Bialosky et al., 2018). A resposta do sistema nervoso periférico ao estímulo mecânico não afeta apenas a medula espinal, mas também porções do cérebro que modulam a dor, como o córtex cingulado anterior, a substância cinzenta periaquedutal e a medula ventromedial rostral. Essas áreas afetam o sistema nervoso autônomo e causam alterações na temperatura e na condução da pele, nos níveis de cortisol e na frequência cardíaca (Coronado e Bialosky, 2017). Elas também estimulam uma resposta endócrina produzindo β-endorfinas e opioides endógenos. Além disso, as áreas do cérebro que modulam a dor criam efeitos placebo e mudanças psicológicas na catastrofização da dor, na cinesiofobia e no medo (Coronado e Bialosky, 2017).

Há alguma sugestão de que a manipulação espinal pode resultar em pequenos aumentos nos níveis de opioides endógenos (Vernon, 1989; Vernon et al., 1986) e em pequenas reduções nas citocinas inflamatórias (Kovanur Sampath et al., 2015; Teodorczyk-Injeyan et al., 2006; 2010). No entanto, são necessários mais estudos para estabelecer se esses achados terão qualquer relevância clínica para a dor na coluna lombar. Assim, as evidências sugerem que a introdução do toque e do movimento passivo/ativo pode influenciar a percepção da dor por meio de uma série de interações complexas do sistema nervoso periférico, sistema nervoso central e sistema neuroendócrino.

Efeitos mecânicos

Há um crescente corpo de evidências indicando que as interações mecânicas entre as células e a sua matriz extracelular (MEC) têm um efeito significativo no desenvolvimento e na função das células, tão importante quanto a sinalização bioquímica (Ingber, 2010; Swanson, 2013). Essa noção dá à TM, assim como às outras terapias mecânicas (como eletroterapia) e aos exercícios, outra base para influenciar a cura do tecido e melhorar a função. Tecidos e células traduzem cargas mecânicas em processos bioquímicos que ativam e desativam funções celulares, como inflamação, proliferação e migração celulares, diferenciação e maturação de células-tronco e remodelamento e reparo de tecidos; esse processo é denominado "mecanotransdução" (Chaitow, 2013; Dunn e Olmedo, 2016). Chalkias e Xanthos (2013) afirmam que "a mecanotransdução descreve os mecanismos moleculares pelos quais as células respondem a mudanças mecânicas em seu ambiente físico. Ela reflete o processo pelo qual as forças mecânicas são convertidas em sinais bioquímicos ou elétricos que são capazes de promover o remodelamento estrutural e funcional em células e tecidos".

O papel da carga mecânica e do exercício é há muito reconhecido no aumento das propriedades estruturais e na morfologia do osso, enquanto o exercício vigoroso pode reduzir a taxa de perda óssea associada à osteoporose. A estimulação mecânica também pode acelerar a consolidação óssea. A adição de compressão rítmica às fraturas imobilizadas acelerou a formação de calos e melhorou a qualidade do tecido ósseo recém-formado (Challis et al., 2006; Henstock et al., 2014), a potência muscular e a amplitude de movimento articular pós-imobilização (Challis et al., 2007). Na cartilagem articular, a estimulação mecânica na forma de compressão cíclica de baixo grau demonstrou suprimir a produção de reguladores pró-inflamatórios e antagonizar os processos inflamatórios e catabólicos da matriz *in vitro* (Leong et al., 2011). Além disso, estudos têm mostrado que os estresses compressivo e de tração produzem mudanças na forma celular que aumentam o acúmulo de proteoglicanos recentemente sintetizados, a produção de moléculas de matriz e colágeno tipo II, induzem a proliferação celular e aumentam a síntese da glicoproteína lubrificante lubricina (Jaumard et al., 2011).

A carga mecânica afeta o tecido conjuntivo de várias maneiras. A tensão induz o remodelamento citoesquelético e morfológico do fibroblasto, permitindo que o tecido conjuntivo relaxe e atinja níveis mais baixos de tensão de repouso em um curto período de tempo (Langevin et al., 2011). As células também respondem de maneira semelhante às cargas cíclicas que, se aplicadas por um período de tempo mais longo, podem levar à redução do estresse ainda mais em direção aos valores pré-carregados (Humphrey et al., 2014). O carregamento mecânico também tem efeitos positivos no *turnover* da MEC, pois aumenta a produção celular de constituintes estruturais da MEC e acelera a remoção de MEC antiga (Chiquet et al., 2003; Humphrey et al., 2014; Jaumard et al., 2011). No entanto, a conformidade com a MEC (Abbott et al., 2013) e o pré-esforço do citoesqueleto do fibroblasto (Chiquet et al., 2003) são pré-requisitos para as respostas acima dos fibroblastos. Nos tendões, o alongamento e o carregamento cíclico aumentaram a proliferação de fibroblastos do tendão e a expressão gênica do colágeno tipo I, enquanto o alongamento cíclico de baixo grau produziu um efeito anti-inflamatório no tendão e aumentou a proliferação de células-tronco do tendão (CTT), a produção de colágeno das CTT e a diferenciação das CTT em tenócitos (Wang et al., 2012).

A estimulação mecânica pode produzir efeitos adversos que parecem depender da magnitude da estimulação. Enquanto um alongamento cíclico de 4% parece ter um efeito anti-inflamatório no tendão, reduzindo a expressão gênica de citocinas pró-inflamatórias, aumentar o alongamento para 8% promove a expressão dessas citocinas (Wang et al., 2012). Além disso, um grande alongamento mecânico leva à diferenciação de CTT em não enócitos, como adipócitos, condrócitos e osteócitos (Wang et al., 2012). A taxa de aplicação da carga mecânica aos tecidos também parece ser importante. Aumentos agudos na tensão e no estresse podem levar à falha do mecanismo de homeostase da tensão celular e podem resultar em enrijecimento e fibrose contínuos da MEC (Humphrey et al., 2014).

Efeitos no controle motor

Além da redução da dor, os efeitos relatados da TM incluem melhorias na amplitude de movimento, reduções na resistência ao movimento passivo (rigidez da coluna) e alterações na atividade do músculo paraespinal (Edgecombe et al., 2015; Pickar, 2002). No entanto, esse corpo de evidências é surpreendentemente pequeno e, às vezes, contraditório. Curiosamente, há evidências que sugerem que o efeito da TM na rigidez pode não ser uniforme em toda a coluna, com diferenças regionais nas reduções da rigidez sendo observadas em modelos animais (Edgecombe et al., 2015). Há um debate sobre a mediação da atividade motora após a manipulação espinal, com evidências para apoiar tanto a facilitação a curto prazo quanto a atenuação das alças reflexas espinais e da atividade muscular paraespinal (DeVocht et al., 2005; Keller e Colloca, 2000).

Como a TM influencia o aprendizado do controle motor, essa é uma área importante a ser desenvolvida. Existem várias teorias de aprendizagem motora sugerindo que a TM tem um papel em influenciar a entrada, a interpretação e as integrações biopsicossociais necessárias para o movimento controlado. Uma dessas teorias é a teoria de aprendizagem motora, "otimização do desempenho por meio da motivação intrínseca e da atenção para o aprendizado" (OPTIMAL, do inglês *optimizing performance through intrinsic motivation and attention for learning*) (Figura 10.1).

Isso se baseia na premissa de que a aprendizagem motora não pode ser compreendida sem considerar as influências motivacionais (p. ex., sociocognitivas e afetivas) e a atenção no comportamento (Wulf e Lewthwaite, 2016) e oferece uma estrutura útil para a otimização do desempenho motor em relação com o uso da "terapia" do movimento. Isso é feito adaptando-se a aliança terapêutica de maneira que aborde o perfil sociocognitivo e afetivo (biopsicossocial) do paciente para permitir:

- Condições terapêuticas que aumentam as expectativas de efeito
- Escolha do paciente no movimento terapêutico, aumentando assim seu senso de autonomia
- Promoção de foco externo de atenção para o retreinamento do movimento, direcionando a concentração para um objetivo externo relevante e apropriado.

Ao fazer isso, a reaprendizagem motora e as reduções concomitantes na deficiência podem ser otimizadas (Figura 10.1).

Essas estratégias incorporam *feedback* comparativo positivo e social sobre o desempenho, a atenção seletiva (foco externo na terapia e não na dor) e a autonomia e a autoeficácia do aluno. No contexto da TM, isso inclui o estabelecimento de metas funcionais realistas em conjunto com o paciente, a reabilitação baseada em cotas graduadas e o reforço positivo de participação ativa e de comportamentos positivos de dor (Bunzli et al., 2011). Dentro do condicionamento clássico, associar a TM a uma experiência positiva pode ter um impacto marcante na resposta de um indivíduo e pode ser integrada a mais motivação intrínseca e a mais mudança comportamental (Fordyce et al., 1968).

Conclusão

Embora haja confiança de que a TM é uma modalidade eficaz no alívio da dor e na redução da incapacidade, suas influências e interações biomédicas, psicológicas e sociais específicas ainda precisam ser totalmente compreendidas. A TM é uma intervenção complexa e exigirá mais pesquisas de metodologia mista para avaliar plenamente seu papel no manejo biopsicossocial da dor e da incapacidade. A utilização eficaz da TM requer a síntese de fatores do paciente e do terapeuta, o que inclui características pessoais e específicas do paciente e também os preconceitos culturais, as crenças e as experiências do paciente e do terapeuta (Coronado e Bialosky, 2017). Além disso, é importante usar métodos para integrar intervenções auxiliares, como estratégias de aprendizagem motora psicossocial, educação em dor e exercícios que aumentam a eficácia da TM na redução da dor e da incapacidade (Coronado e Bialosky, 2017) (Figura 10.2). O raciocínio clínico para o uso da TM requer uma avaliação da influência do toque e do movimento no perfil psicológico, biomecânico e neurofisiológico do paciente. Uma compreensão da interação biopsicossocial pessoal desses mecanismos permite a integração eficaz e eficiente da TM com outras abordagens de reabilitação no tratamento da disfunção musculoesquelética.

| Parte | |1| Conceitos Básicos Importantes em Esportes

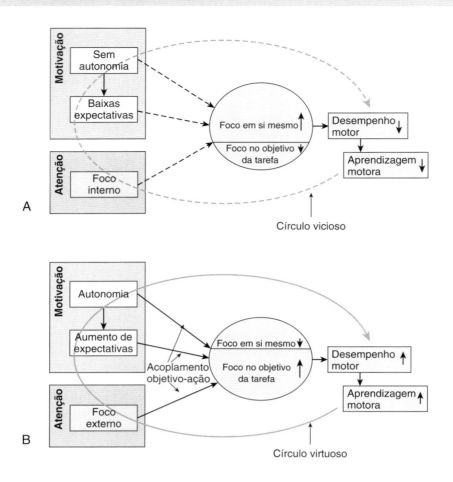

Figura 10.1 Otimização do desempenho por intermédio da teoria da aprendizagem motora com motivação intrínseca e atenção para a aprendizagem (OPTIMAL). A. Condições que falham em aumentar as expectativas do paciente, apoiar sua necessidade de autonomia e promover um foco interno de atenção resultam em um círculo vicioso de aprendizagem não ideal. **B.** Em contrapartida, as condições que aumentam as expectativas, fornecem suporte à autonomia e promovem um foco externo resultam em um círculo virtuoso de aprendizagem motora aprimorada.

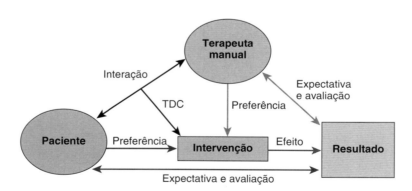

Figura 10.2 Abordagem abrangente para a eficácia da fisioterapia manual. Leva em consideração a interação entre paciente, terapeuta e fatores de intervenção. Exemplos desses fatores incluem preferências, expectativas, avaliação de resultados e tomada de decisão compartilhada (*TDC*). (De Coronado R.A., Bialosky, J.E., 2017. Manual physical therapy for chronic pain: the complex whole is greater than the sum of its parts. Journal of Manual & Manipulative Therapy 25, 115-117.)

Referências bibliográficas

Abbott, R.D., Koptiuch, C., Iatridis, J.C., Howe, A.K., Badger, G.J., Langevin, H.M., 2013. Stress and matrix-responsive cytoskeletal remodeling in fibroblasts. Journal of Cellular Physiology 228, 50-57.

Bialosky, J.E., Beneciuk, J.M., Bishop, M.D., Coronado, R.A., Penza, C.W., Simon, C.B., et al., 2018. Unraveling the mechanisms of manual therapy: modeling an approach. The Journal of Orthopaedic and Sports Physical Therapy 48, 8-18.

Bialosky, J.E., Bishop, M.D., Price, D.D., Robinson, M.E., George, S.Z., 2009. The mechanisms of manual therapy in the treatment of musculoskeletal pain: a comprehensive model. Manual Therapy 14, 531-538.

Bishop, M.D., Beneciuk, J.M., George, S.Z., 2011. Immediate reduction in temporal sensory summation after thoracic spinal manipulation. Spine Journal 11, 440-446.

Bishop, M.D., Torres-Cueco, R., Gay, C.W., Lluch-Girbes, E., Beneciuk, J.M., Bialosky, J.E., 2015. What effect can manual therapy have on a patient's pain experience? Pain Management 5, 455-464.

Bissonette, G.B., Roesch, M.R., 2016. Neurophysiology of reward-guided behavior: correlates related to predictions, value, motivation, errors, attention, and action. Current Topics in Behavioral Neurosciences 27, 199-230.

Bunzli, E., Gillham, D., Esterman, A., 2011. Physiothrapy-provided operant conditioning in the management of low back pain: a systematic review. Physiotherapy Research International 16 (1), 4-19.

Chaitow, L., 2013. Understanding mechanotransduction and biotensegrity from an adaptation perspective. Journal of Bodywork and Movement Therapies 17, 141-142.

Chalkias, A., Xanthos, T., 2013. Mechanotransduction and cardiac arrest during marathon running. American Journal of Medicine 126 (3), e23.

Challis, M.J., Gaston, P., Wilson, K., Jull, G.A., Crawford, R., 2006. Cyclic pneumatic soft-tissue compression accelerates the union of distal radial osteotomies in an ovine model. Journal of Bone and Joint Surgery British 88, 411-415.

Challis, M.J., Jull, G.J., Stanton, W.R., Welsh, M.K., 2007. Cyclic pneumatic soft-tissue compression enhances recovery following fracture of the distal radius: a randomised controlled trial. Australian Journal of Physiotherapy 53, 247-252.

Chiquet, M., Renedo, A.S., Huber, F., Flück, M., 2003. How do fibroblasts translate mechanical signals into changes in extracellular matrix production? Matrix Biology 22, 73-80.

Chou, R., Qaseem, A., Snow, V., et al. 2007. Diagnosis and treatment of low back pain: a joint clinical practice guideline from the American College of Physicians and the American Pain Society [published correction appears in Annals of Internal Medicine. 2008 Feb 5;148(3):247-8. Annals of Internal Medicine. 147 (7), 478-491.

Coronado, R.A., Bialosky, J.E., 2017. Manual physical therapy for chronic pain: the complex whole is greater than the sum of its parts. Journal of Manual & Manipulative Therapy 25, 115-117.

Coronado, R.A., Gay, C.W., Bialosky, J.E., Carnaby, G.D., Bishop, M.D., George, S.Z., 2012. Changes in pain sensitivity following spinal manipulation: a systematic review and meta-analysis. Journal of Electromyography & Kinesiology 22, 752-767.

Day, J.M., Nitz, A.J., 2012. The effect of muscle energy techniques on disability and pain scores in individuals with low back pain. Journal of Sport Rehabilitation 21, 194-198.

DeVocht, J.W., Pickar, J.G., Wilder, D.G., 2005. Spinal manipulation alters electromyographic activity of paraspinal muscles: a descriptive study. Journal of Manipulative and Physiological Therapeutics 28, 465-471.

Dunn, S.L., Olmedo, M.L., 2016. Mechanotransduction: relevance to physical therapist practice – understanding our ability to affect genetic expression through mechanical forces. Physical Therapy 96, 712-721.

Edgecombe, T.L., Kawchuk, G.N., Long, C.R., Pickar, J.G., 2015. The effect of application site of spinal manipulative therapy (SMT) on spinal stiffness. Spine Journal 15, 1332-1338.

Evans, D.W., 2010. Why do spinal manipulation techniques take the form they do? towards a general model of spinal manipulation. Manual Therapy 15, 212-219.

Fordyce, W.E., Fowler, R., Delateur, B., 1968. An application of behaviour modification technique to a problem of chronic pain. Behaviour Research and Therapy 6 (1), 105-107.

Granot, M., Weissman-Fogel, I., Crispel, Y., Pud, D., Granovsky, Y., Sprecher, E., et al., 2008. Determinants of endogenous analgesia magnitude in a diffuse noxious inhibitory control (DNIC) paradigm: do conditioning stimulus painfulness, gender and personality variables matter? Pain 136, 142-149.

Hegedus, E.J., Goode, A., Butler, R.J., Slaven, E., 2011. The neurophysiological effects of a single session of spinal joint mobilization: does the effect last? The Journal of Manual & Manipulative Therapy 19, 143-151.

Henstock, J.R., Rotherham, M., Rashidi, H., Shakesheff, K.M., El Haj, A.J., 2014. Remotely activated mechanotransduction via magnetic nanoparticles promotes mineralization synergistically with bone morphogenetic protein 2: applications for injectable cell therapy. Stem Cells Translational Medicine 3, 1363-1374.

Humphrey, J.D., Dufresne, E.R., Schwartz, M.A., 2014. Mechanotransduction and extracellular matrix homeostasis. Nature Reviews Molecular Cell Biology 15 (12), 802-812.

IFOMPT Standards, 2016. Educational Standards In Orthopaedic Manipulative Therapy. International Federation of Orthopaedic Manipulative Physical Therapists, Auckland, New Zealand. Available at: https://www.ifompt.org/site/ifompt/IFOMPT%20Standards%20Document%20definitive%202016.pdf.

Ingber, D.E., 2010. From cellular mechanotransduction to biologically inspired engineering: 2009 Pritzker Award Lecture, BMES annual meeting October 10, 2009. Journal of Biomechanical Engineering 38 (3), 1148-1161.

Jaumard, N.V., Welch, W.C., Winkelstein, B.A., 2011. Spinal facet joint biomechanics and mechanotransduction in normal, injury and degenerative conditions. Journal of Biomechanical Engineering 133 (7), 071010.

Jones, M., Edwards, I., Gifford, L., 2002. Conceptual models for implementing biopsychosocial theory in clinical practice. Manual Therapy 7 (1), 2-9.

Keller, T.S., Colloca, C.J., 2000. Mechanical force spinal manipulation increases trunk muscle strength assessed by electromyography: a comparative clinical trial. Journal of Manipulative and Physiological Therapeutics 23, 585-595.

Kovanur Sampath, K., Mani, R., Cotter, J.D., Tumilty, S., 2015. Measureable changes in the neuro-endocrinal mechanism following spinal manipulation. Medical Hypotheses 85, 819-824.

Kunz, M., Scholl, K.E., Schu, U., Lautenbacher, S., 2006. GABAergic modulation of diffuse noxious inhibitory controls (DNIC): a test by use of lorazepam. Experimental Brain Research 175, 363-371.

Langevin, H.M., Bouffard, N.A., Fox, J.R., Palmer, B.M., Wu, J., Iatridis, J.C., et al., 2011. Fibroblast cytoskeletal remodeling contributes to connective tissue tension. Journal of Cellular Physiology 226, 1166-1175.

Lascurain-Aguirrebena, I., Newham, D., Critchley, D.J., 2016. Mechanism of action of spinal mobilizations: a systematic review. Spine (Phila Pa 1976) 41, 159-172.

Leknes, S., Berna, C., Lee, M.C., Snyder, G.D., Biele, G., Tracey, I., 2013. The importance of context: when relative relief renders pain pleasant. Pain 154, 402-410.

Leknes, S., Lee, M., Berna, C., Andersson, J., Tracey, I., 2011. Relief as a reward: hedonic and neural responses to safety from pain. PLoS One 6, e17870.

Leknes, S., Tracey, I., 2008. A common neurobiology for pain and pleasure. Nature Reviews Neuroscience 9, 314-320.

Leong, D.J., Hardin, J.A., Cobelli, N.J., Sun, H.B., 2011. Mechanotransduction and cartilage integrity. Annals of the New York Academy of Sciences 1240, 32-37.

Liljencrantz, J., Olausson, H., 2014. Tactile C fibers and their contributions to pleasant sensations and to tactile allodynia. Frontiers in Behavioral Neuroscience 8, 37.

Lindgren, L., Rundgren, S., Winsö, O., Lehtipalo, S., Wiklund, U., Karlsson, M., et al., 2010. Physiological responses to touch massage in healthy volunteers. Autonomic Neuroscience 158, 105-110.

Maitland, G.D., 1986. Vertebral Manipulation, fifth ed. Butterworth-Heinemann, Oxford.

Mancini, F., Beaumont, A.L., Hu, L., Haggard, P., Iannetti, G.D., 2015. Touch inhibits subcortical and cortical nociceptive responses. Pain 156, 1936-1944.

Martinez-Segura, R., De-la-Llave-Rincon, A.I., Ortega-Santiago, R., Cleland, J.A., Fernandez-de-Las-Penas, C., 2012. Immediate changes in widespread pressure pain sensitivity, neck pain, and cervical range of motion after cervical or thoracic thrust manipulation in patients with bilateral chronic mechanical neck pain: a randomized clinical trial. Journal of Orthopaedic & Sports Physical Therapy 42, 806-814.

Martinez-Segura, R., Fernandez-de-las-Penas, C., Ruiz-Saez, M., Lopez-Jimenez, C., Rodriguez-Blanco, C., 2006. Immediate effects on neck pain and active range of motion after a single cervical high-velocity low-amplitude manipulation in subjects presenting with mechanical neck pain: a randomized controlled trial. Journal of Manipulative and Physiological Therapeutics 29, 511-517.

McCarthy, C.J., Bialoski, J., Rivett, D., 2015. Spinal manipulation. In: Jull, G., Moore, A., Falla, D., Lewis, J., McCarthy, C., Sterling, M. (Eds.), Grieve's Modern Musculoskeletal Physiotherapy, fourth ed. Elsevier, Oxford.

McCarthy, C.J., 2010. Combined Movement Theory: Rational Mobilization and Manipulation of the Vertebral Column. Elsevier Health Sciences, Oxford.

Morita, K., Morishima, M., Sakai, K., Kawaguchi, Y., 2013. Dopaminergic control of motivation and reinforcement learning: a closed-circuit account for reward-oriented behavior. Journal of Neuroscience 33, 8866-8890.

Moseley, G.L., 2003. A pain neuromatrix approach to patients with chronic pain. Manual Therapy 8, 130-140.

Moulson, A., Watson, T., 2006. A preliminary investigation into the relationship between cervical snags and sympathetic nervous system activity in the upper limbs of an asymptomatic population. Manual Therapy 11, 214-224.

Navratilova, E., Porreca, F., 2014. Reward and motivation in pain and pain relief. Nature Neuroscience 17, 1304-1312.

NICE, 2016. Low Back Pain and Sciatica in Over 16s: Assessment and Management. NICE Guideline, No. 59. National Institute for Health and Care Excellence, London.

Peters, M.L., Schmidt, A.J., Van den Hout, M.A., Koopmans, R., Sluijter, M.E., 1992. Chronic back pain, acute postoperative pain and the activation of diffuse noxious inhibitory controls (DNIC). Pain 50, 177-187.

Pickar, J.G., 2002. Neurophysiological effects of spinal manipulation. Spine Journal 2, 357-371.

Ram, K.C., Eisenberg, E., Haddad, M., Pud, D., 2008. Oral opioid use alters DNIC but not cold pain perception in patients with chronic pain – new perspective of opioid-induced hyperalgesia. Pain 139, 431-438.

Shacklock, M., 2005. Improving application of neurodynamic (neural tension) testing and treatments: a message to researchers and clinicians. Manual Therapy 10, 175-179.

Sharman, M.J., Cresswell, A.G., Riek, S., 2006. Proprioceptive neuromuscular facilitation stretching: mechanisms and clinical implications. Sports Medicine 36, 929-939.

Skyba, D.A., Radhakrishnan, R., Rohlwing, J.J., Wright, A., Sluka, K.A., 2003. Joint manipulation reduces hyperalgesia by activation of monoamine receptors but not opioid or GABA receptors in the spinal cord. Pain 106, 159-168.

Smith, M., Fryer, G., 2008. A comparison of two muscle energy techniques for increasing flexibility of the hamstring muscle group. Journal of Bodywork and Movement Therapies 12, 312-317.

Staud, R., Robinson, M.E., Vierck Jr., C.J., Price, D.D., 2003. Diffuse noxious inhibitory controls (DNIC) attenuate temporal summation of second pain in normal males but not in normal females or fibromyalgia patients. Pain 101, 167-174.

Swanson 2nd., R. L., 2013. Biotensegrity: a unifying theory of biological architecture with applications to osteopathic practice, education, and research – a review and analysis. Journal of the American Osteopathic Association 113 (1), 34-52.

Teodorczyk-Injeyan, J.A., Injeyan, H.S., Ruegg, R., 2006. Spinal manipulative therapy reduces inflammatory cytokines but not substance p production in normal subjects. Journal of Manipulative and Physiological Therapeutics 29, 14-21.

Teodorczyk-Injeyan, J.A., McGregor, M., Ruegg, R., Injeyan, H.S., 2010. Interleukin 2-regulated in vitro antibody production following a single spinal manipulative treatment in normal subjects. Chiropractic & Osteopathy 18, 26.

Vernon, H., 1989. Exploring the effect of a spinal manipulation on plasma beta-endorphin levels in normal men. Spine (Phila Pa 1976) 14, 1272-1273.

Vernon, H.T., Dhami, M.S., Howley, T.P., Annett, R., 1986. Spinal manipulation and beta-endorphin: a controlled study of the effect of a spinal manipulation on plasma beta-endorphin levels in normal males. Journal of Manipulative and Physiological Therapeutics 9, 115-123.

Vicenzino, B., Cartwright, T., Collins, D., Wright, A., 1999. An investigation of stress and pain perception during manual therapy in asymptomatic subjects. European Journal of Pain 3, 13-18.

Vicenzino, B., Paungmali, A., Teys, P., 2007. Mulligan's mobilization-with-movement, positional faults and pain relief: current concepts from a critical review of literature. Manual Therapy 12, 98-108.

Voogt, L., de Vries, J., Meeus, M., Struyf, F., Meuffels, D., Nijs, J., 2015. Analgesic effects of manual therapy in patients with musculoskeletal pain: a systematic review. Manual Therapy 20, 250-256.

Wang, J.H., Guo, Q., Li, B., 2012. Tendon biomechanics and mechanobiology – a minireview of basic concepts and recent advancements. Journal of Hand Therapy 25, 133-140; Quiz 141.

Wise, R.A., 2005. Forebrain substrates of reward and motivation. Journal of Comparative Neurology 493, 115-121.

Wright, A., Sluka, K.A., 2001. Nonpharmacological treatments for musculoskeletal pain. Clinical Journal of Pain 17, 33-46.

Wright, A., 1999. Recent concepts in the neurophysiology of pain. Manual Therapy 4, 196-202.

Wulf, G., Lewthwaite, R., 2016. Optimizing performance through intrinsic motivation and attention for learning: The OPTIMAL theory of motor learning. Psychonomic Bulletin & Review 23, 1382-1414.

Yeo, H.K., Wright, A., 2011. Hypoalgesic effect of a passive accessory mobilisation technique in patients with lateral ankle pain. Manual Therapy 16, 373-377.

Zusman, M., 2012. A note to the musculoskeletal physiotherapist. Journal of Back and Musculoskeletal Rehabilitation 25, 103-107.

Zusman, M., 2004. Mechanisms of musculoskeletal physiotherapy. Physical Therapy Reviews 9 (1), 39-49.

Capítulo | 11 |

Fisiologia da Analgesia por Acupuntura

Jonathan Hobbs

Introdução

As primeiras pesquisas sobre os mecanismos fisiológicos da analgesia por acupuntura (AA) começaram no final da década de 1960 (Zhao, 2008). Nas últimas décadas, a quantidade de pessoas que buscam a acupuntura como modalidade de tratamento tem crescido constantemente. A análise do National Health Interview Survey (NHIS) de 2002 e 2007 demonstrou que o uso da acupuntura aumentou de 0,4% da população em 1990 para 1,01% em 1998 nos EUA. Esse número aumentou de 1,1% em 2002 para 1,4% em 2007 (Barnes et al., 2004; 2009; Eisenberg et al., 1998). Esses resultados demonstram um aumento modesto, mas persistente, no uso geral e regular da acupuntura em 2007, que equivale a uma estimativa de mais de 14 milhões de indivíduos nos EUA (Burke et al., 2006). Dados da pesquisa de 2007 sugerem que a maioria dos indivíduos buscava a acupuntura para o tratamento da dor, que incluía dores musculoesqueléticas, dores de cabeça e fibromialgia (Barnes et al., 2009).

Embora haja um crescimento documentado na utilização da acupuntura, há um debate relevante quanto ao seu valor, à natureza dos seus mecanismos propostos e à importância para a prática clínica (Colquhoun e Novella, 2013). Há algumas evidências que sugerem que a expectativa e a crença afetam a experiência da dor e o seu manejo e que esses componentes existem na resposta placebo à analgesia (Richardson e Vincent, 1986; Wager et al., 2004). O trabalho inicial de Price et al. (1984) destacou esses aspectos e reconheceu que existem fatores psicológicos na analgesia da acupuntura, mas as propriedades analgésicas dessa técnica têm uma base neurofisiológica (Zhao, 2008). Uma recente revisão sistemática e metanálise de ensaios de acupuntura para dor lombar inespecífica concluiu que a acupuntura placebo é mais eficaz do que os cuidados de rotina ou estar na lista de espera para o tratamento (Xiang et al., 2017). A existência de um componente tátil, que pode criar uma resposta fisiológica semelhante à acupuntura com a técnica *verum*, pode causar problemas ao tentar avaliar e compreender os vários componentes do tratamento com acupuntura (Makary et al., 2018). Esses achados podem colocar em questão o uso da acupuntura *sham* ou placebo como intervenção em ensaios de pesquisa, nos quais são comparados com a acupuntura *verum*. A avaliação precoce do efeito do placebo e da acupuntura no tratamento da dor crônica sugeriu que essa terapia poderia ser eficaz em 50 a 80% dos pacientes. Essas são sugestões significativas quando comparadas à morfina, que ajudou 30% dos avaliados (Lewith e Machin, 1983; Richardson e Vincent, 1986).

Aplicação e mecanismos

Durante a acupuntura e o agulhamento seco (AS), uma agulha filiforme de calibre estreito, que normalmente varia entre 0,16 e 0,35 mm de diâmetro, é inserida no corpo para estimular os efeitos locais e sistêmicos propostos. Embora alguns busquem diferenciar os processos e técnicas de acupuntura e AS, sugerindo diferenças fundamentais de ideologia, ambas as abordagens podem ser consideradas para compartilhar componentes significativos, incluindo a própria agulha e o cruzamento entre pontos de acupuntura clássicos e locais de AS. Dorscher (2006) sugeriu uma correlação anatômica significativa de mais de 93% entre os pontos-gatilho miofasciais e os de acupuntura clássica. Abordagens como a acupuntura médica ocidental (AMO) podem usar a técnica da acupuntura chinesa tradicional (ACT) para sustentar a prática com explicação fisiológica e teoria mecanicista, deixando de lado conceitos esotéricos como *yin*, *yang* e *qi*.

Tanto a acupuntura tradicional quanto a AS utilizam o conceito de locais específicos para agulhamento e uma série de técnicas de inserção e manipulação da agulha para criar um estímulo e resposta subsequente do paciente. Foi demonstrado que a inserção de uma agulha filiforme no tecido do músculo esquelético estimula aferentes primários A delta (Aδ) ou aferentes primários mielinizados de pequeno diâmetro do grupo III na pele e no músculo (Pomeranz, 1987). Essas fibras são responsáveis pela sensação inicial de picada da agulha. Os primeiros estudos em primatas demonstraram que a estimulação das fibras Aδ tinha efeitos significativos na inibição da dor por meio do trato espinotalâmico (Chung et al., 1984). Após a inserção, as agulhas são manipuladas por rotação ou penetração repetida nas fibras musculares subjacentes, criando trauma localizado e forte estimulação mecânica. O nível de manipulação dita o nível de estímulo (Zhao, 2008). Acredita-se que a dormência, o peso e a distensão experimentados durante o estímulo mecânico de agulhamento de tecidos mais profundos sejam atribuídos à estimulação de uma combinação de fibras A beta (Aβ) e Aδ (Zhang et al., 2012). O trauma causado pela penetração e manipulação da agulha também desencadeia uma resposta inflamatória que estimula a liberação de uma variedade de mediadores pró-inflamatórios. Estes incluem serotonina, bradicinina, histamina, trifosfato de adenosina (ATP), prostaglandina E2 e peptídeo relacionado com o gene da calcitonina (*CGRP*, do inglês *calcitonin gene-related peptide*) que pode excitar nociceptores locais (Boucher et al., 2000; Meyer et al., 2006).

105

Durante o agulhamento de acupuntura, as fibras C responsáveis pela sensação dolorosa também são estimuladas (Pomeranz, 1987). As fibras amielínicas do tipo C têm uma condução mais lenta, são as responsáveis por uma dor surda, mais ardente e latejante que geralmente é sentida após o estímulo inicial agudo da inserção da agulha (Wilkinson, 2001). Acredita-se que as fibras C contribuam para o efeito analgésico geral gerado pela acupuntura e o fenômeno associado de *qi*, pois causam uma sensação de peso e dor (Wang et al., 1985; 1989). No entanto, Wang et al. (1990) concluíram que a ativação da fibra C não era necessária para AA, após a denervação química das fibras C não afetar negativamente a AA subsequentemente.

Desde o trabalho seminal de Pomeranz e Chiu (1976), vários estudos demonstraram que a analgesia da acupuntura em humanos e animais poderia ser revertida ou abolida pela naloxona, o antagonista do receptor opioide. Esse processo sugere que o mecanismo da acupuntura é opioidérgico. O grupo de opioides endógenos que influenciam a analgesia da acupuntura consiste em Leu-encefalina, Met-encefalina, β-endorfina e dinorfinas. Há um tempo considerável, existem evidências que comprovam o envolvimento de uma série de monoaminas, incluindo norepinefrina, serotonina (5 HT), dopamina e substância P (Han e Terenius, 1982). Também foi demonstrado que, quando um nervo é bloqueado pela anestesia local, a acupuntura é ineficaz na região inervada por esse nervo. A conclusão é de que o efeito da acupuntura está sendo transmitido por meio de vias neurais (Stux et al., 2003; Stux e Hammerschlag, 2001). O trabalho seminal de Chiang et al. (1973) demonstrou que o agulhamento do ventre do primeiro músculo interósseo dorsal (ponto meridiano: Intestino Grosso 4) aumentou o limiar de dor nos participantes do estudo. Após a administração de procaína nos ramos cutâneos do nervo radial, não houve alteração no limiar de resposta. No entanto, a administração da mesma aplicação de procaína aos ramos musculares mais profundos dos nervos ulnar e mediano, neutralizou o efeito da analgesia, sugerindo que, na verdade, era derivado da inervação aferente dos músculos.

Langevin et al. (2001a; 2002) demonstraram que a manipulação da agulha via rotação causa a sensação de preensão da agulha associada à acupuntura e um subsequente acoplamento mecânico da agulha e seu tecido conjuntivo circundante. Acredita-se que este fenômeno transmita sinais para as células do tecido conjuntivo adjacentes por meio de mecanotransdução e apoia os efeitos terapêuticos propostos pela acupuntura (Langevin et al., 2001b). As evidências sugerem que um estímulo significativamente maior da fibra C é elicitado em mecanorreceptores superficiais e profundos por meio da rotação do que é alcançado com empurrar, sacudir ou raspar a agulha (Zhang et al., 2012). Zhang et al. (2008) concluíram que os mastócitos tiveram um papel significativo no mecanismo analgésico da acupuntura, pois a analgesia foi diminuída após a destruição química dos mastócitos.

Analgesia por acupuntura

A manipulação mecânica da agulha dentro do tecido-alvo desencadeia uma resposta em fibras aferentes Aδ mielinizadas de pequeno diâmetro (Figura 11.1). Ao atingir a medula espinal, esses neurônios Aδ de primeira ordem fazem sinapses principalmente no corno dorsal superficial (lâminas I e V) da medula espinal com células do trato anterolateral (TAL). As fibras Aδ também enviam ramos curtos para células endorfinérgicas intermediárias da substância gelatinosa dentro do mesmo segmento espinal (Sugiura et al., 1986). O TAL prossegue em sentido cefálico para se comunicar com o mesencéfalo e o complexo hipotalâmico hipofisário (CHH). A sinapse das fibras Aδ dentro da medula espinal estimula a liberação das endorfinas encefalina e dinorfina. Embora também se considere que a β-endorfina desempenha um papel na analgesia da acupuntura, ela não está envolvida na resposta mediada pela medula espinal. A liberação de endorfinas da medula espinal gera um efeito inibitório pré-sináptico na região segmentar local, limitando a transmissão dos sinais de dor iniciados pelas fibras C para o trato espinotalâmico (TET) (Stux e Hammerschlag, 2001).

O TAL sobe, se comunica com o mesencéfalo e estimula as células da substância cinza periaquadutal (CPA). Muitos estudos destacam o papel do CPA no tratamento da dor, com Wang et al. (1990) demonstrando que as lesões do CPA abolem a AA no modelo de dor em ratos. Os estímulos que descem do núcleo arqueado do hipotálamo geram a liberação de β-endorfina. O sistema límbico, considerado influente na percepção da dor devido ao seu papel na emoção, também fornece estímulos ao CPA. A modulação da atividade nas estruturas límbica e subcortical foi demonstrada anteriormente em uma variedade de estudos que examinam os efeitos da especificidade do ponto por meio de varredura de ressonância magnética funcional (Li et al., 2000; Wu et al., 1999; Yan et al., 2005).

Também ocorre a excitação de células dentro do núcleo da rafe no bulbo. Esses impulsos disparam ao longo do trato dorsolateral (TDL), que iniciam a liberação das monoaminas serotonina e norepinefrina. A liberação de monoaminas na medula espinal apoia outros mecanismos analgésicos. Em um mecanismo descendente, a norepinefrina atua inibindo a membrana pós-sináptica da célula de transmissão dentro do TET, e limita a propagação da entrada nociceptiva das fibras C (Pomeranz, 1987; Stux e Hammerschlag, 2001; Zhao, 2008). Esse sistema atua difusamente em toda a medula espinal. Dentro do outro sistema inibitório descendente, a serotonina apoia ainda mais a inibição pré-sináptica, estimula as células intermediárias segmentares e reforça a liberação de Met-encefalina. Uma ou ambas as monoaminas liberadas podem suportar a supressão da transmissão nociceptiva (Stux e Hammerschlag, 2001). O estímulo ascendente adicional que é transportado por meio do TAL atinge as células dentro do CHH e dispara a liberação do hormônio adrenocorticotrófico (ACTH) e β-endorfina na circulação em igual medida. O ACTH influencia o córtex adrenal e modula a produção de cortisol, que é considerado uma influência para as respostas inflamatórias dentro do corpo (Stux e Hammerschlag, 2001).

Efeito de camadas

Quando a acupuntura é realizada em uma região próxima ao local da dor ou pontos sensíveis nos tecidos moles locais, tanto a resposta inflamatória local quanto os circuitos segmentares operando no mesmo segmento da medula espinal são utilizados como mecanismos analgésicos primários (Baeumler et al., 2015). Agulhamento local em pontos de dor miofascial ocorre tanto na prática da acupuntura quanto no AS, com um cruzamento significativo nas áreas-alvo para a inserção (Dorsher, 2006). Dentro do AS, os pontos-gatilho são pontos sensíveis localizados nos tecidos moles locais que são usados para aliviar os sintomas de dor miofascial (Cagnie et al., 2013). Uma revisão sistemática conduzida por Wong et al. (2014) concluiu que os pontos dolorosos locais são benéficos para o alívio da dor a curto prazo no tratamento da dor miofascial crônica.

A acupuntura, tanto ATC quanto AMO, também pode empregar agulhas colocadas em pontos distais a alguma distância da região dolorosa, seja dentro do mesmo dermátomo ou miótomo ou completamente heterossegmental em localização (White et al., 2018). O AS concentra-se no tecido miofascial alvo local

Fisiologia da Analgesia por Acupuntura — Capítulo | 11 |

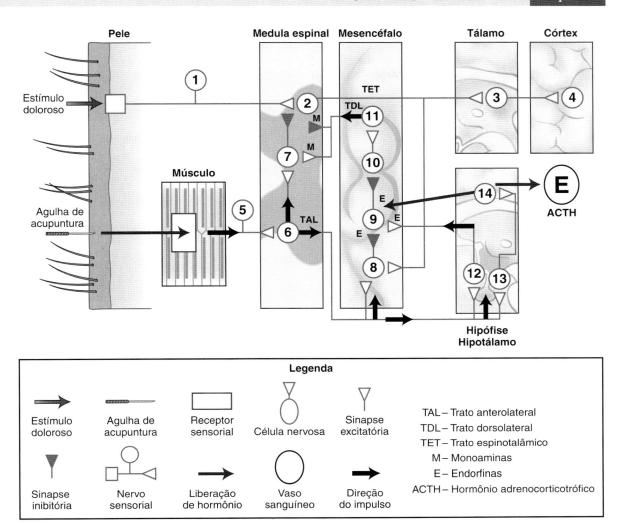

Figura 11.1 Mecanismo de analgesia por acupuntura. Dor: estímulo doloroso de pequenas fibras nervosas aferentes Aδ e C (1) fazem sinapse no corno dorsal da medula espinal (2) antes de subir do trato espinotalâmico (TET) para o tálamo (3) e terminar no córtex (4) onde a dor pode ser percebida em um nível consciente. Agulhamento: agulhamento do músculo estimula as fibras Aδ (5) que fazem sinapse na medula espinal (6) e estimulam a célula (7) onde a encefalina é liberada causando inibição pré-sináptica da célula (1). A célula (6) também faz sinapses com o trato anterolateral (TAL) para o mesencéfalo, estimulando células (8) e (9) na substância cinza periaquaductal (CPA) que liberam β-endorfina para excitar a célula (10) do núcleo da rafe e a célula (11), desencadeando impulsos ao longo do trato dorsolateral (TDL) para liberar monoaminas (M) nas células (2) e (7) da medula espinal. A célula (1) é inibida pré-sinapticamente por M (serotonina) por intermédio da célula (7), enquanto a célula (2) é inibida pós-sinapticamente por M (norepinefrina). O estímulo de TAL nas células (12) e (13) dentro do complexo hipotalâmico hipofisário libera hormônio adrenocorticotrófico (ACTH) e β-endorfina na circulação em medidas iguais. O ACTH modula a resposta anti-inflamatória. A estimulação da célula (8) pela célula (2) via TET também causa analgesia pelo mecanismo de controle inibitório nocivo difuso (CIND), onde um estímulo nocivo pode inibir outro. (*Esta figura se encontra reproduzida em cores no Encarte.*)

e geralmente não busca utilizar estímulos iniciados distalmente. A adição de agulhas distais pode contribuir para uma ativação mais profunda do estímulo para as regiões supraespinais do sistema nervoso central. Ao combinar os benefícios documentados dos efeitos segmentais e locais do agulhamento com os do agulhamento distal, propõe-se que o efeito geral da acupuntura pode ser aumentado (Bradnam, 2007a; 2007b). Esse conceito de efeito de camadas é considerado para criar o potencial para analgesia generalizada por todo o corpo (Stux e Hammerschlag, 2001). Portanto, o agulhamento segmentar local geralmente fornece analgesia mais intensiva do que o agulhamento não segmentar distal, porque usa todos os três centros. Os pontos distais são menos propensos a caírem no mesmo segmento, embora isso ocorra em alguns casos. Um estudo conduzido por Srbely et al. (2010) demonstrou que agulhando uma área de dor miofascial definida como um ponto-gatilho, houve uma resposta antinociceptiva a curto prazo em um músculo adjacente. Eles concluíram que havia um mecanismo segmentar de analgesia em vigor.

O trabalho de Baeumler et al. (2015) também apoia a conclusão de que as alterações do limiar de dor com eletroacupuntura (EA) são mediadas por inibição segmentar em nível segmentar na medula espinal. Outro estudo examinando agulhas para dor miofascial demonstrou que pontos de gatilho miofasciais distantes podem reduzir a irritabilidade de áreas dolorosas em músculos mais proximais dentro do mesmo miótomo por meio do mecanismo proposto de inibição segmentar da medula espinal (Hsieh et al., 2014).

Um estudo sobre a dor neuropática em um modelo murino de nervo espinal ligado demonstrou com o uso de naloxona que o sistema opioide estava envolvido na hipersensibilidade reduzida pela acupuntura. A acupuntura também apresentou eficácia semelhante à gabapentina no mesmo modelo e não houve aumento subsequente na tolerância com a continuação do tratamento, sugerindo seu papel potencial positivo no tratamento da dor neuropática (Cidral-Filho et al., 2011). O efeito heterossegmental do agulhamento é provocado por um mecanismo

Parte | 1 | Conceitos Básicos Importantes em Esportes

neuro-hormonal que envolve a liberação de β-endorfina e os dois mecanismos neuronais descendentes que são serotoninérgicos e adrenérgicos. Também é considerado que existe algum envolvimento do controle inibitório nocivo difuso (CIND) no efeito analgésico geral, onde uma dor pode inibir outra (Filshie e White, 1998).

Inflamação e cura

Em uma série de estudos em ratos, foi demonstrado que a acupuntura manual pode aumentar o fluxo sanguíneo muscular local por meio da liberação de óxido nítrico, CGRP, difosfato de adenosina (ADP) e ATP (Nagaoka et al., 2016; Shinbara et al., 2013; 2015; 2017). Shinbara et al. (2017) concluíram que a adenosina também pode ter influência no efeito analgésico da acupuntura, e auxilia na remoção de substâncias algésicas. Foi sugerido que, devido ao seu papel no aumento do fluxo sanguíneo muscular local, a acupuntura também pode ter um papel a desempenhar na cura do tecido (White et al., 2018). Em estudos que examinaram o papel da acupuntura na inflamação, foi demonstrado que a eletroacupuntura (EA) aumentou os níveis de hormônio liberador de corticotrofina e ACTH em ratos por meio da estimulação do eixo hipotálamo-hipófise-adrenal (Li et al., 2008). Um estudo anterior também mostrou que o bloqueio experimental

dos receptores de corticosterona resultou em uma perda mensurável dos efeitos anti-inflamatórios da EA (Li et al., 2007). Um estudo mais recente de Yang et al. (2017) demonstrou que a EA reduziu significativamente a hiperalgesia mecânica e térmica crônica no modelo de dor inflamatória crônica em camundongos quando comparada à simulação de EA. Isso fornece algum nível de evidência para apoiar a aplicação clínica da EA no tratamento da dor inflamatória crônica.

Resumo

Com avanços na pesquisa investigativa e compreensão mais profunda da neurofisiologia, há novas evidências destacando os mecanismos subjacentes da acupuntura e os benefícios potenciais de sua aplicação clínica. Alguns dos mecanismos mais estabelecidos de analgesia por acupuntura foram mencionados nesse capítulo, mas os efeitos fisiológicos da acupuntura são propostos como muito mais amplos. Fora do espectro da dor miofascial, existem evidências para o uso da acupuntura no tratamento de uma variedade de condições de saúde, incluindo náuseas, dores de cabeça, enxaquecas e bexiga hiperativa, para citar apenas alguns (Carlsson et al., 2000; Linde et al., 2016a; 2016b; Wang et al., 2012). Com mais pesquisas ainda, um conhecimento mais profundo dos mecanismos e aplicações certamente será possível.

Referências bibliográficas

Baeumler, P.I., Fleckensteina, J.B., Benedikta, F., Badera, J., Irnicha, D., 2015. Acupuncture-induced changes of pressure pain threshold are mediated by segmental inhibition – A randomized controlled trial. Pain 156 (11), 2245-2255.

Barnes, P.M., Bloom, B., Nahin, R.L., 2009. Complementary and alternative medicine use among adults and children: United States, 2007. National Health Statistics Reports (12), 1-23.

Barnes, P.M., Powell-Griner, E., McFann, K., Nahin, R.L., 2004. Complementary and alternative medicine use among adults: United States, 2002. Advance Data (343), 1-19.

Boucher, T.J., Okuse, K., Bennett, D.L., Munson, J.B., Wood, J.N., McMahon, S.B., 2000. Potent analgesic effects of GDNF in neuropathic pain states. Science 290, 124-127.

Bradnam, L., 2007a. A proposed clinical reasoning model for western acupuncture. Journal of the Acupuncture Association of Chartered Physiotherapists 21-30.

Bradnam, L., 2007b. A physiological underpinning for treatment progression of western acupuncture. Journal of the Acupuncture Association of Chartered Physiotherapists 25-33 Autumn.

Burke, D., Upchurch, M., Dye, C., Chyu, L., 2006. Acupuncture use in the United States: findings from the national health interview survey. Journal of Alternative and Complementary Medicine 12 (7), 639-648.

Cagnie, B., Dewitte, V., Barbe, T., Timmermans, F., Delrue, N., Meeus, M., 2013. Physiologic effects of dry needling. Current Pain and Headache Reports 17, 348.

Carlsson, C.P.O., Axemo, P., Bodin, A., Carstensen, H., Ehrenroth, B., Madegård-Lind, I., et al., 2000. Manual acupuncture reduces hyperemesis gravidarum: a placebo-controlled, randomized, single-blind, crossover study. Journal of Pain and Symptom Management 20 (4), 273-279.

Chiang, C.Y., Chang, C.T., Chu, H.C., Yang, L.F., 1973. Peripheral afferent pathway for acupuncture analgesia. Scientia Sinica - Series B 16, 210-217.

Chung, J.M., Willis, W.D., Lee, K.H., 1984. Factors influencing peripheral nerve stimulation produced inhibition of primate spinothalamic tract cells. Pain 19, 227-293.

Cidral-Filho, F.J., da Silva, M.D., Moré, A.O., Córdova, M.M., Werner, M.F., Santos, A.R., 2011. Manual acupuncture inhibits mechanical hypersensitivity induced by spinal nerve ligation in rats. Neuroscience 193, 370-376.

Colquhoun, D., Novella, S.P., 2013. Acupuncture is theatrical placebo. Anesthesia & Analgesia 116 (6), 1360-1363.

Dorsher, P.T., 2006. Trigger points and acupuncture points: anatomic and clinical correlations. Medical Acupuncture 17, 21-24.

Eisenberg, D.M., Davis, R.B., Ettner, S.L., 1998. Trends in alternative medicine use in the United States, 1990-1997: results of a follow-up national survey. Journal of the American Medical Association 280 (18), 1569-1575.

Filshie, J., White, 1998. Medical Acupuncture – a Western Scientific Approach. Churchill Livingstone, Edinburgh.

Han, J.S., Terenius, L., 1982. Neurochemical basis of acupuncture analgesia. Annual Review of Pharmacology and Toxicology 22, 193-220.

Hsieh, Y.L., Yang, C.C., Liu, S.Y., Chou, L.W., Hong, C.Z., 2014. Remote dose-dependent effects of dry needling at distant myofascial trigger spots of rabbit skeletal muscles on reduction of substance p levels of proximal muscle and spinal cords. Biomedical Research International 2014, 982121.

Langevin, H.M., Churchill, D.L., Cipolla, M.J., 2001a. Mechanical signalling through connective tissue: a mechanism for the therapeutic effect of acupuncture. FASEB Journal 15, 2275-2282.

Langevin, H.M., Churchill, D.L., Fox, J.R., Badger, G.J., Garra, B.S., Krag, M.H., 2001b. Biomechanical response to acupuncture needling in humans. Journal of Applied Physiology 91, 2471-2478.

Langevin, H.M., Churchill, D.L., Wu, J., Badger, G.J., Yandow, J.A., Fox, J.R., et al., 2002. Evidence of connective tissue involvement in acupuncture. FASEB Journal 16, 872-874.

Lewith, G.T., Machin, D., 1983. On the evaluation of the clinical effects of acupuncture. Pain 16, 111-127.

Li, A., Lao, L., Wang, Y., Xin, J., Ren, K., 2008. Electroacupuncture activates corticotrophin-releasing hormone-containing neurons in the paraventricular nucleus of the hypothalamus to alleviate edema in a rat model of inflammation. BMC Complementary and Alternative Medicine 8, 20.

Li, A., Zhang, R.X., Wang, Y., Zhang, H., Ren, K., 2007. Corticosterone mediates electroacupuncture-produced anti-edema in a rat model of inflammation. BMC Complementary and Alternative Medicine 7, 27.

Li, W.C., Hung, D.L., Kalnin, A., Holodny, A., Komisaruk, B., 2000. Brain activation of acupuncture induced analgesia. Neuroimage 11, S701.

Linde, K., Allais, G., Brinkhaus, B., Fei, Y., Mehring, M., Shin, B.C., et al., 2016a. Acupuncture for the prevention of tension-type headache. Cochrane Database of Systematic Reviews 4, CD007587.

Linde, K., Allais, G., Brinkhaus, B., Fei, Y., Mehring, M., Vertosick, E.A., et al., 2016b. Acupuncture for the prevention of episodic migraine. Cochrane Database of Systematic Reviews 2016 (6), CD001218 2016.

Makary, M.M., Lee, J., Lee, E., Eun, S., Kim, J., Jahng, G.H., et al., 2018. Phantom acupuncture induces placebo credibility and vicarious sensations: a parallel fMRI study of low back pain patients. Scientific Reports 8 (1), 930.

Meyer, R.A., Ringkamp, M., Campbell, J.N., Raja, S.N., 2006. Peripheral mechanisms of cutaneous nociception. In: McMahon, S.B., Koltzenburg, M. (Eds.), Wall and Melzack's Textbook of Pain, fifth ed. Elsevier/Churchill Livingstone, Edinburgh, pp. 3-34.

Nagaoka, S., Shinbara, H., Okubo, M., Kawita, T., Hino, K., Sumiya, E., 2016. Contributions of ADP and ATP to the increase in skeletal muscle blood flow after manual acupuncture stimulation in rats. Acupuncture in Medicine 2016 34 (3), 229-234.

Pomeranz, B., 1987. Scientific basis of acupuncture. In: Stux, G., Pomeranz, B. (Eds.), Acupuncture Textbook and Atlas. Springer-Verlag; 1987, Heidelberg, pp. 1-18.

Pomeranz, B., Chiu, D., 1976. Naloxone blocks acupuncture analgesia and causes hyperalgesia: endorphin is implicated. Life Sciences 19 (11), 1757-1762.

Price, D.D., Rafii, A., Watkins, L.R., Buckingham, B., 1984. A psychophysical analysis of acupuncture analgesia. Pain 19 (1), 27-42.

Richardson, H., Vincent, C.A., 1986. Acupuncture for the treatment of pain: a review of evaluative research. Pain 24, 15-40.

Shinbara, H., Nagaoka, S., Izutani, Y., Okubo, M., Kimura, K, Mizunuma, K., Sumiya, E., (2017) Contributions of adenosine to the increase in muscle blood flow caused by manual acupuncture in rats. Acupuncture in Medicine 35 (4), 284-288.

Shinbara, H., Okubo, M., Kimura, K., Mizunuma, K., Sumiya, E., 2013. Participation of calcitonin gene related peptide released via axon reflex in the local increase in muscle blood flow following manual acupuncture. Acupuncture in Medicine 31 (1), 81-87.

Shinbara, H., Okubo, M., Kimura, K, Mizunuma, K., Sumiya, E., 2015. Contributions of nitric oxide and prostaglandins to the local increase in muscle blood flow following manual acupuncture in rats. Acupuncture in Medicine 33 (1), 65-71.

Srbely, J.Z., Dickey, J.P., Lee, D., Lowerison, M., 2010. Dry needle stimulation of myofascial trigger points evokes segmental anti-nociceptive effects. Journal of Rehabilitation Medicine 42, 463-468.

Stux, G., Berman, B., Pomeranz, B., 2003. Basics of Acupuncture, fifth ed. Springer, Berlin.

Stux, G., Hammerschlag, R. (Eds.), 2001. Clinical Acupuncture: Scientific Basis. Springer, Berlin.

Sugiura, Y., Lee, C.L., Perl, E.R., 1986. Central projection of identified, unmyelinated (C) afferent fibers innervating mammalian skin. Science 234, 358-361.

Wager, T.D., Riling, J.K., Smith, E.E., Sokolik, A., Casey, K.L., Davidson, R.J., et al., 2004. Placebo-induced changes in FMRI in the anticipation and experience of pain. Science 303, 1162-1167.

Wang, H., Tanaka, Y., Kawauchi, A., Miki, T., Kayama, Y., Koyama, Y., 2012. Acupuncture of the sacral vertebrae suppresses bladder activity and bladder activity-related neurons in the brainstem micturition center. Neuroscience Research 72 (1), 43-49.

Wang, K.M., Liu, J., 1989. Needling sensation receptor of an acupoint supplied by the median nerve studies of their electro-physiological characteristics. The American Journal of Chinese Medicine 17 (3-4), 145-156.

Wang, K.M., Yao, S.M., Xian, Y.L., Hou, Z.L., 1985. A study on the receptive field of acupoints and the relationship between characteristics of needling sensation and groups of afferent fibres. Scientia Sinica Series B 28 (9), 963-971.

Wang, Q., Mao, L., Han, J.S., 1990. The arcuate nucleus of hypothalamus mediates low but not high frequency electroacupuncture in rats. Brain Research 513, 60-66.

White, A., Cummings, M., Filshie, J., 2018. An Introduction to Western Medical Acupuncture, second ed. Churchill Livingstone/Elsevier, Edinburgh.

Wilkinson, P.R., 2001. Neurophysiology of pain. Part 1: mechanisms of pain in the peripheral nervous system. CPD Anaesthesia 3 (3), 103-108.

Wong Lit Wan, D., Wang, Y., Xue, C.C., Wang, L.P., Liang, F.R., Zheng, Z., 2015. Local and distant acupuncture points stimulation for chronic musculoskeletal pain: A systematic review on the comparative effects. European Journal of Pain 19 (9), 1232-1247.

Wu, M.T., Hsieh, J.C., Xiong, J., Yang, C.F., Pan, H.B., Chen, Y.C., et al., 1999. Central nervous pathway for acupuncture stimulation: localization of processing with functional MR imaging of the brain—preliminary experience. Radiology 212, 133-141.

Xiang, Y., He, J.Y., Li, R., 2017. Appropriateness of sham or placebo acupuncture for randomised controlled trials of acupuncture for nonspecific low back pain: a systematic review and meta-analysis. Journal of Pain Research 11, 83-94.

Yan, B., Li, K., Xu, J.X., Wang, W., Li, K., Liu, H., et al., 2005. Acupoint specific fMRI patterns in human brain. Neuroscience Letters 383, 236-240.

Yang, J., Hsieh, C.L., Lin, Y.W., 2017. Role of transient receptor potential vanilloid 1 in electroacupuncture analgesia on chronic inflammatory pain in mice. BioMed Research International 2017, 5068347.

Zhang, D., Ding, G., Shen, X., Yao, W., Zhang, Z., Zhang, Y., et al., 2008. Role of mast cells in acupuncture effect: a pilot study. Explore 4 (3), 170-177.

Zhang, Z.J., Wang, X.M., McAlonan, G.M., 2012. Neural acupuncture unit: a new concept for interpreting effects and mechanisms of acupuncture. Evidence-Based Complementary and Alternative Medicine 2012, 429412.

Zhao, Z.Q., 2008. Neural mechanism underlying acupuncture analgesia. Progress in Neurobiology 85, 355-375.

Capítulo | 12 |

Determinantes Fisiológicos para o Desempenho de Resistência: Consumo Máximo de Oxigênio – Teste, Treinamento e Aplicação Prática

Paul Sindall

Introdução

A capacidade de perseverar é uma característica essencial que sustenta os resultados ideais em uma variedade de esportes organizados. Além disso, um requisito fundamental para a resistência cardiorrespiratória e muscular está por trás do desempenho e da função ótimos na vida cotidiana. Uma série de fatores fisiológicos determinam o desempenho de resistência, principalmente a disponibilidade de oxigênio (Weltman et al., 1978), altitude (Wehrlin e Hallén, 2006), economia [consumo de oxigênio (VO_2) em uma determinada taxa de trabalho] (Saunders et al., 2004), eficiência mecânica (Kyröläinen et al., 1995), tipo de fibra muscular (Taylor e Bachman, 1999), quantidade e tamanho das mitocôndrias (Meinild Lundby et al., 2018), limiares de transição de lactato sanguíneo (Yoshida et al., 1987), reservas de energia (Bjorntorp, 1991), hidratação (Goulet, 2012), táticas (Hanley, 2015) e resiliência mental (Crust e Clough, 2005). No entanto, o consumo máximo de oxigênio ($\dot{V}O_{2máx}$) é geralmente aceito como o determinante mais importante. Como $\dot{V}O_{2máx}$ é definido como o volume máximo de oxigênio que o corpo pode captar e utilizar ao nível do mar durante exercícios dinâmicos de alta intensidade, ele representa a capacidade máxima de um indivíduo para o metabolismo aeróbico (Kavcic et al., 2012; Tran, 2018). Embora "consumo máximo de oxigênio" seja a descrição preferida de $\dot{V}O_{2máx}$, vários termos são usados indistintamente para descrever o mesmo fenômeno, dependendo da configuração e do(s) grupo(s) populacional(is) envolvido(s):
- Capacidade aeróbica de pico/máxima
- Consumo de oxigênio de pico/máximo
- Potência aeróbica máxima
- Fitness aeróbico
- Capacidade funcional
- Resistência, capacidade e/ou aptidão cardiorrespiratória
- Resistência, capacidade e/ou aptidão cardiovascular.

Este capítulo descreve os métodos mais comuns pelos quais o $\dot{V}O_{2máx}$ pode ser medido e, posteriormente, utilizado para oferecer orientação sobre as intensidades do treinamento físico para a otimização dos resultados de saúde e desempenho em diferentes esportes/funções. Como um volume considerável de informações de alta qualidade está disponível na avaliação de $\dot{V}O_{2máx}$ e cinética de consumo de oxigênio durante o exercício, é apresentada uma visão geral das opções de teste comumente disponíveis, para que os profissionais possam aplicá-las com relativa facilidade, de modo que é apropriado para o contexto de teste e grupo(s) de população envolvida. Dados de exemplo também são apresentados na forma de um estudo de caso para delinear o processo de prescrição do treinamento de exercício para solicitar aumentos no $\dot{V}O_{2máx}$ e melhorar os marcadores fisiológicos associados.

Considerações centrais *versus* periféricas

A equação de Fick afirma que em qualquer estado fisiológico, seja em repouso ou sob esforço, o $\dot{V}O_{2máx}$ é o produto do débito cardíaco (Q) multiplicado pela diferença arteriovenosa de oxigênio (a – $\dot{V}O_{2dif}$). Como Q é um produto da frequência cardíaca (FC) multiplicado pelo volume sistólico do ventrículo esquerdo (= volume diastólico final – volume sistólico final), o $\dot{V}O_{2máx}$ é determinado, em parte, por fatores centrais, ou seja, o transporte de O_2 do ar ambiente para os pulmões, difusão para o suprimento de sangue arterial e subsequente translocação para a periferia por meio de mecanismos circulatórios sistêmicos. Em contraste, a –$\dot{V}O_{2dif}$ está relacionada com processos celulares e moleculares dentro do músculo esquelético, por meio dos quais o O_2 é difundido na mitocôndria a partir do sangue arterial para permitir a ressíntese de trifosfato de adenosina (ATP) e promover a produção de energia aeróbica. Portanto, o $\dot{V}O_{2máx}$ também é determinado por fatores periféricos. Então, se $\dot{V}O_{2máx}$ é um produto de Q × a – $\dot{V}O_{2dif}$, $\dot{V}O_{2máx}$ é simplesmente o produto coletivo de Q máximo (suprimento de oxigênio) e a – $\dot{V}O_{2dif}$ máxima (extração de oxigênio).

No entanto, a questão de quais fatores limitam o $\dot{V}O_{2máx}$ não é tão simples e permanece um tópico controverso e sem clareza (Noakes, 2008). A visão tradicional de que os fatores centrais predominam na realização do pico de esforço fisiológico (Bassett e Howley, 1997; 2000) tem sido questionada; alguns argumentam que as características do músculo e seu potencial oxidativo atuam como o determinante primário (Noakes, 1998; 2008; Sloth et al., 2013).

$\dot{V}O_{2máx}$ e sua associação com desempenho esportivo ideal

As partes interessadas no mundo do esporte de elite exigem informações sobre a capacidade máxima de resistência para identificação de talentos (Burgess e Naughton, 2010), para estabelecer a aptidão básica em pontos específicos dentro do calendário competitivo e para ajustar o desempenho para a competição (Ishak et al., 2016) com o objetivo de garantir uma "vantagem" fisiológica sobre os concorrentes. Um $\dot{V}O_{2máx}$ alto oferece uma vantagem distinta para a competição em esportes individuais, como corrida de longa distância (Sjödin e Svedenhag, 1985), tênis (Kovacs, 2006), e esportes coletivos, como basquete (Metaxas et al., 2009), futebol (Metaxas et al., 2009), hóquei sobre grama (Reilly e Borrie, 1992), hóquei no gelo (Cox et al., 1995; Ransdell et al., 2013), netball (Bell et al., 1994), rugby de 13 (Brewer e Davis, 1995; Gabbett et al., 2013) e rugby de quinze (Duthie et al., 2003; Vaz et al., 2016). Atletas de elite normalmente têm valores de $\dot{V}O_{2máx}$ 50 a 100% acima daqueles observados em pessoas ativas (Joyner e Coyle, 2008). Portanto, as populações atléticas podem essencialmente sustentar o dobro da taxa de trabalho de suas contrapartes menos treinadas. Em termos de desempenho, isso confere uma vantagem significativa, pois os participantes são capazes de sustentar a atividade aeróbica por um período mais longo e/ou uma proporção maior de um evento esportivo competitivo.

Embora seja prudente notar que $\dot{V}O_{2máx}$ não é o único fator fisiológico implicado na decisão dos resultados de desempenho (Coyle, 1995; Sjödin e Svedenhag, 1985), ele está intimamente relacionado com os tempos de desempenho em triatletas (Butts et al., 1991) e em corredores treinados em resistência, qualquer que seja o esporte (Freeman, 1990; Hagan et al., 1981; 1987). Outros indicadores de desempenho em esportes baseados em resistência foram propostos. Por exemplo, a velocidade de corrida em $\dot{V}O_{2máx}$ (Hill e Rowell, 1996) foi considerada útil devido à sua capacidade de combinar efetivamente $\dot{V}O_{2máx}$ e economia em um único fator (Billat e Koralsztein, 1996). O conceito de potência crítica tem sido discutido mais recentemente (Jones et al., 2010), referindo-se ao ponto em que as respostas fisiológicas não podem ser estabilizadas com o aumento da intensidade do exercício. Embora isso tenha sido contestado, principalmente devido à sua aplicação de terminologia potencialmente inadequada (Winter, 2011), ainda existe possibilidade para a aplicação de potência crítica para a otimização de programas de treinamento atlético (Poole et al., 2016).

Em um sentido mais holístico, o esporte deve ser considerado um veículo para a atividade física e é uma opção viável para aqueles que desejam e têm interesse em um ambiente de atividade física mais competitivo. Por exemplo, mudanças positivas no $\dot{V}O_{2máx}$ foram relatadas para futebol recreativo (Milanović et al., 2015a; 2015b), com potencial considerável para efeitos de melhoria da saúde (Bangsbo et al., 2015; Eime et al., 2015b). Os níveis de aptidão são normalmente mais baixos em pessoas de meia-idade (Lindgren et al., 2016) e meninas (Bohr et al., 2013) com baixo nível socioeconômico (NSE). Porém, há algumas evidências de que a participação em esportes coletivos é maior para pessoas com baixo NSE e para aqueles que vivem em áreas remotas (Eime et al., 2015a). Ainda assim, o fornecimento de instalações (Eime et al., 2017) e a acessibilidade (Karusisi et al., 2013) são barreiras consideráveis à participação.

$\dot{V}O_{2máx}$ e sua associação com a saúde ideal

Existe uma correlação negativa entre $\dot{V}O_{2máx}$ e idade devido a diminuições crônicas no débito cardíaco e um declínio na capacidade oxidativa do músculo esquelético, que ocasionam diminuições na utilização de oxigênio nos tecidos periféricos (Betik e Hepple, 2008). Esse declínio natural no $\dot{V}O_{2máx}$ é esperado com o aumento da idade em homens e mulheres (0,45 e 0,30 m$\ell \cdot$ kg $\cdot$ min^{-1} por ano, respectivamente) a partir dos 25 anos de idade (Stamford, 1988). No entanto, e além disso, a prevalência de comportamento sedentário e obesidade em adolescentes (Carnethon et al., 2005; Pate et al., 2006), adultos (Carnethon et al., 2005; Wang et al., 2010) e aqueles com deficiência intelectual (Oppewal et al., 2013) ou física (van den Berg-Emons et al., 2008), exacerbou e acelerou desnecessariamente o declínio do $\dot{V}O_{2máx}$ em nível populacional. O nível de atividade para homens e mulheres diminui com o aumento da idade (MacAuley et al., 1998). Isso colocou uma carga considerável sobre os sistemas de saúde em todo o mundo, visto que $\dot{V}O_{2máx}$ é aceito como o mais forte preditor da mortalidade por todas as causas e, especificamente, cardiovascular (Keteyian et al., 2008; Myers et al., 2002). Consequentemente, nunca houve um momento mais oportuno para o exame e crítica das metodologias de teste e treinamento para a respectiva identificação e aumento da capacidade aeróbica.

Tem sido dada uma atenção considerável na literatura científica para as associações feitas entre o $\dot{V}O_{2máx}$ e a saúde ideal. Um $\dot{V}O_{2máx}$ elevado oferece um efeito protetor à saúde, com incidência reduzida de mortalidade por todas as causas e doença coronariana naqueles com um $\dot{V}O_{2máx}$ alto (Kodama et al., 2009). Em contraste, um baixo $\dot{V}O_{2máx}$ foi fortemente associado à morte prematura (Lee et al., 2010). O estudo com ex-alunos da Universidade de Harvard focou a atenção nas características da atividade física para ganhos ótimos de saúde, com uma redução na mortalidade e nas taxas de acidente vascular cerebral associadas com atividade vigorosa crônica (Lee e Paffenbarger, 1998; 2000; Lee et al., 1995). Podem ser obtidos grandes ganhos em forma física e funcional por meio do compromisso com os exercícios, com um cruzamento considerável no estado de saúde individual e na qualidade de vida. Em termos de expectativa de vida, aumentos no $\dot{V}O_{2máx}$ são profundos, com um aumento tão pequeno quanto 3,5 m$\ell \cdot$ kg $\cdot$ min^{-1} (~1 MET) associado a grandes aumentos (10 a 25%) na taxa de sobrevivência (Kaminsky et al., 2013). Portanto, $\dot{V}O_{2máx}$ não deve ser considerado apenas uma preservação do mundo atlético. Além disso $\dot{V}O_{2máx}$ deve ser usado como uma ferramenta por profissionais que trabalham com populações em geral (*i. e.*, inaptos, descondicionados, sedentários aparentemente saudáveis) para informar a prescrição de exercícios relacionados com a saúde, orientação de estilo de vida e educação baseada na saúde.

Avaliação fisiológica de $\dot{V}O_{2máx}$

Abordagens baseadas em laboratório

A avaliação do $\dot{V}O_{2máx}$ é feita convencionalmente em condições laboratoriais com clima controlado, onde uma análise direta do ar expirado é realizada durante o exercício progressivo. Quando coletado, o $\dot{V}O_{2máx}$ é expresso em unidades absolutas (L $\cdot$ min^{-1}) ou relativas (m$\ell \cdot$ kg $\cdot$ min^{-1}), com a última permitindo a comparação entre indivíduos de diferentes massas corporais. Uma abordagem tradicional envolvendo a coleta manual de ar expirado usando bolsas de Douglas (Figura 12.1 A) seguida pela análise das concentrações de oxigênio e dióxido de carbono usando os respectivos analisadores paramagnéticos e infravermelhos ainda é adotada em alguns ambientes de teste. No entanto, os analisadores modernos permitem a medição da troca gasosa pulmonar respiração a respiração (Figura 12.1 B) e, portanto, são mais comumente usados para avaliar o custo fisiológico durante o teste incremental para pesquisa e consultoria fisiológica aplicada.

Os carrinhos metabólicos são facilmente calibrados (Macfarlane, 2001), permitem tempos de resposta rápidos, possibilitam relatórios e *feedback* de dados mais ágeis (Macfarlane, 2001) e oferecem dados válidos e confiáveis em comparação com métodos manuais (Lee et al., 2011; Nieman et al., 2007). Os valores de referência para $\dot{V}O_{2máx}$ são fornecidos com relativa facilidade e precisão (Macfarlane, 2001), o resultado do teste é utilizado para informar a prescrição de treinamento (Figura 12.1), e atua como uma linha de base para avaliar as respostas de treinamento

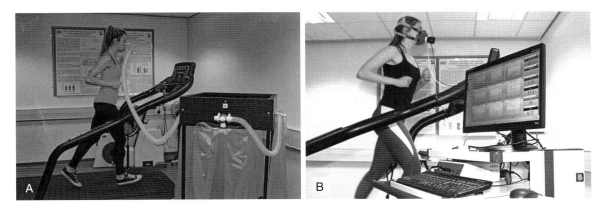

Figura 12.1 Coleta de amostras de ar expirado em ambiente de laboratório controlado utilizando bolsas de Douglas (A) e analisador *online* respiração a respiração (B).

crônico ou para detectar irregularidades e diagnosticar condições de saúde específicas. No entanto, esses testes requerem equipamentos caros, pessoal treinado para coleta de dados, assim como posterior interpretação e consomem tempo (Abut e Akay, 2015). Além disso, a identificação das variáveis fisiológicas de pico demanda um esforço máximo por parte do participante. Atingir o desempenho máximo é um processo complexo que requer a aplicação de critérios de término de teste fisiológico que é afetado pela idade (Huggett et al., 2005) e influenciado por fatores psicobiológicos (Midgley et al., 2017), principalmente motivação e compromisso com realizar um esforço máximo (Moffatt et al., 1994).

Considerações na seleção da modalidade de teste de exercício

Como a modalidade de exercício influencia a determinação de $\dot{V}O_{2máx}$ (Keren et al., 1980; Millet et al., 2009) e as prioridades de treinamento subsequentes (Sousa et al., 2015), deve-se considerar cuidadosamente esse aspecto antes do teste. O teste em esteira é a modalidade mais comumente usada, pois a locomoção ereta é um movimento familiar que envolve a ativação de todos os principais grupos musculares (McConnell, 1988; Weiglein et al., 2011). Esta modalidade está, portanto, associada aos maiores valores observados em estudos comparando os modos (Keren et al., 1980), com corredores (Caputo e Denadai, 2004; Millet et al., 2009), triatletas (Caputo e Denadai, 2004) e populações não treinadas (Caputo e Denadai, 2004) obtendo valores mais elevados por meio de uma esteira motorizada em comparação com a bicicleta ergométrica. Corredores altamente treinados devem, portanto, ser testados, sempre que possível, usando esta modalidade.

Enquanto o ciclismo de estrada é uma atividade motora complexa que envolve pedalar, frear e dirigir, a ação do ciclismo é uma tarefa de habilidade relativamente baixa e fácil de aprender, pois envolve um ritmo motor voluntário inato (Hansen, 2015). O uso de uma bicicleta ergométrica vertical estática, que não requer essas respostas a estímulos externos, representa uma opção de teste ideal para grupos de baixa habilidade ou ajuste. Os protocolos de ciclismo são uma opção popular para aqueles com limitações ou deficiências, pois esses grupos podem ser testados facilmente (Beltz et al., 2016), embora valores mais baixos para $\dot{V}O_{2máx}$ sejam provavelmente relatados devido ao recrutamento exclusivo da musculatura do membro inferior (Loftin et al., 2004; McKay e Bannister, 1976).

Os ciclistas treinados exigirão uma configuração de teste mais específica. O uso de um aparelho do tipo *turbo trainer* permite uma configuração personalizada, em que o ciclista é testado em sua própria bicicleta. Isso facilita uma coleta de dados mais específica e válida sem compensação em eficiência mecânica *versus* uma avaliação de ciclo baseada em esteira (Arkesteijn et al., 2013). No entanto, quando a repetição do teste é necessária (p. ex., intervenção pré e pós-treinamento), é preferível usar uma bicicleta ergométrica, pois o protocolo, a potência de saída e a configuração do piloto podem ser replicados com mais facilidade de um teste para o outro. Ciclistas treinados alcançam resultados de pico mais altos em uma bicicleta ergométrica estática do que em uma esteira (Caputo e Denadai, 2004; Ricci e Léger, 1983), mesmo sendo limitados por uma quantidade menor de massa muscular ativa, os eles podem atingir um $\dot{V}O_{2máx}$ semelhante ao de corredores que usam esta modalidade (Millet et al., 2009). Isso se deve às adaptações periféricas consideráveis provocadas por esforços repetidos na musculatura dos membros inferiores (Atkinson et al., 2003).

Atletas que treinam os braços (p. ex., remadores, nadadores, esquiadores de *cross-country*) podem atingir um $\dot{V}O_{2máx}$ da parte superior do corpo que supera seu desempenho equivalente em um teste da parte inferior do corpo (Secher e Volianitis, 2006) e, portanto, ergometria de braço do tipo manivela é a modalidade preferida para essas populações, junto com aqueles que são incapazes de pedalar (Orr et al., 2013). Diferenças sutis nas características do movimento também podem influenciar o desempenho do teste. Por exemplo, o $\dot{V}O_{2máx}$ de ciclistas de elite é 10% menor durante o teste em um ergômetro de manivela em padrão assíncrono quando comparado com seu padrão síncrono mais familiar no mesmo ergômetro (Goosey-Tolfrey e Sindall, 2007). Portanto, a determinação de $\dot{V}O_{2máx}$ é altamente modo-específica (Millet et al., 2009) e dependente da tarefa (Smirmaul et al., 2013); por isso, deve-se pensar cuidadosamente na seleção do modo com base na situação (i. e., recursos, instalações), considerações e restrições individuais (i. e., esporte, posição) antes do teste. A cadência do pedal também é um fator que influencia a economia (Hansen e Smith, 2009), assim como a carga fisiológica interna. A cadência preferida e "escolhida livremente" de um indivíduo tende a ser mais alta do que sua frequência de pedal mais econômica (Marsh e Martin, 1997; Vercruyssen e Brisswalter, 2010). Portanto, a falta de padronização da cadência potencialmente introduz viés em cenários de um teste para outro. Os não ciclistas, menos treinados, podem inconscientemente escolher taxas de pedal mais baixas para minimizar a demanda aeróbica (Marsh e Martin, 1997). Em contrapartida, a cadência escolhida livremente por ciclistas bem treinados está mais próxima das taxas de pedal energeticamente ideais (Brisswalter et al., 2000). Portanto, a decisão de corrigir ou permitir a cadência escolhida livremente deve ser feita antes da implementação do teste de exercício baseado em bicicleta e ser informada pelo *status* do treinamento.

Considerações na seleção e no desenho do protocolo de teste

Para garantir uma determinação precisa do $\dot{V}O_{2máx}$, e que recomendações apropriadas sejam feitas com relação ao treinamento, o protocolo do teste deve ser cuidadosamente considerado (Riboli et al., 2017). As durações dos testes entre aproximadamente 7 e 12 minutos são consideradas ótimas (Astorino et al., 2004; McConnell, 1988; Poole e Jones, 2012; Yoon et al., 2007). Embora isso represente um alvo geral apropriado, é útil observar que a inclinação mais íngreme da taxa $\Delta VO_2/\Delta trabalho$ em protocolos mais curtos pode ser um desafio para indivíduos de baixo ajuste, com fadiga prematura potencialmente confundindo os resultados (Beltz et al., 2016). Dessa maneira, a seleção deve sempre ser ditada pelo cenário de teste e pelo indivíduo a ser testado. Por exemplo, um atleta competitivo exigirá um estímulo comparativamente maior (p. ex., velocidade e gradiente em um teste de corrida em esteira) para alcançar um esforço máximo do que uma contraparte com baixa aptidão ou deficiência funcional. A Figura 12.2 apresenta uma comparação de protocolos de teste de esteira comumente usados, em que os incrementos são fixos. Estão incluídos dois exemplos de protocolos de teste utilizados dentro do laboratório do autor deste capítulo para avaliação de jogadores de futebol profissional de elite e boxeadores. Eles podem ser facilmente aplicados em um ambiente controlado e mostram como a velocidade e o gradiente podem ser manipulados para solicitar a progressão final para o esforço máximo. Em ambos os casos, o gradiente é fixado em 1% para melhor representar o custo energético da corrida ao ar livre (Jones e Doust, 1996).

Os protocolos atléticos, como os mostrados na Figura 12.2, podem parecer experimentais. Porém, sua aplicação pode fornecer um meio mais simples, rápido e eficaz para determinar os atributos fisiológicos de pico do que protocolos mais estabelecidos (Hamlin et al., 2012). Uma abordagem alternativa é que os indivíduos selecionem o ritmo, com a duração especificada e as escalas de esforço percebido (EEP) (Borg, 1982), empregadas como uma âncora para capacitar a autosseleção do ritmo/intensidade-alvo. Essa abordagem se compara favoravelmente aos protocolos tradicionais de rampa incremental para quantificação de $\dot{V}O_{2máx}$ (Chidnok et al., 2013; Straub et al., 2014) e oferece um meio simples e confiável de administrar o teste de exercício graduado (Beltz et al., 2016).

Identificação do pico de esforço fisiológico durante o teste de exercício em laboratório

$\dot{V}O_{2máx}$ aumenta linearmente com a taxa de trabalho. Portanto, a observação de um patamar de $\dot{V}O_{2máx}$ com aumento da taxa de trabalho é geralmente aceita como o método principal para definir a capacidade de pico (Howley et al., 1995). De fato, a ausência de um aumento no $\dot{V}O_{2máx}$ com incrementos adicionais na carga de trabalho durante o exercício foi o meio pelo qual o $\dot{V}O_{2máx}$ foi definido pela primeira vez nos trabalhos seminais de Hill e Lupton (1923). No entanto, um platô não é visto em todos os indivíduos. Em um estudo envolvendo 804 participantes com idades entre 20 e 85 anos, um platô foi observado em apenas 43% (Edvardsen et al., 2014). Nesses casos, o termo $\dot{V}O_{2pico}$ é defendido em preferência a $\dot{V}O_{2máx}$ e critérios secundários, como lactato sanguíneo (SLa^-), FC máxima, razão de troca respiratória (RTR) e EEP são usados para criar a identificação do pico de esforço fisiológico (Duncan et al., 1997; Howley et al., 1995).

Critérios secundários propostos para apoiar o término do teste e identificação de $\dot{V}O_{2máx}$:
- $SLa^- \geq 8$ mmol·ℓ^{-1}
- FC máxima $\geq$ (220 – idade)
- RTR $\geq 1,15$
- EEP ≥ 19.

Deve-se notar, no entanto, que esses parâmetros são frequentemente alcançados em intensidades abaixo de $\dot{V}O_{2máx}$ (Edvardsen et al., 2014; Schaun, 2017) e há uma variação considerável na maneira como esses critérios são aplicados, tanto na literatura quanto na prática (Howley et al., 1995). Por exemplo, a prática é aceitar dois critérios para representar o ponto de término do teste final, embora nem sempre seja esse o caso. Além disso, a exaustão voluntária é altamente variável e gerada intrinsecamente. Consequentemente, uma outra opção mais rigorosa é administrar um estágio de verificação pós-teste (Poole e Jones, 2017) em que uma sessão de exercício supramáximo adicional (~110% da carga de trabalho final) pós-teste para verificar o estágio final de $\dot{V}O_{2máx}$. Embora algumas evidências sugiram que valores semelhantes para $\dot{V}O_{2máx}$ são obtidos durante os testes convencionais e supramáximos (Hawkins et al., 2007), outros afirmam que esta abordagem aumenta a precisão das medições de $\dot{V}O_{2máx}$ em populações atléticas e aparentemente saudáveis (Midgley e Carroll, 2009; Mier et al., 2012). No entanto, a tolerância ao esforço supramáximo em grupos menos capazes (i. e., crianças, pessoas obesas e idosos) pode ser questionada (Midgley e Carroll, 2009). Portanto, onde a verificação é aplicada, ela deve ser específica para a população e um trabalho adicional deve ser concluído para refinar e padronizar os protocolos para esse fim (Schaun, 2017).

Abordagens baseadas em campo

As vantagens de testar o $\dot{V}O_{2máx}$ em um ambiente controlado de laboratório estão bem documentadas (Beltz et al., 2016). As condições podem ser facilmente replicadas de um teste para outro, oferecendo um meio ideal para monitorar a eficácia do programa de treinamento e para fins de pesquisa, onde a necessidade de limitar os fatores de confusão é a principal preocupação (McConnell, 1988; Skelly et al., 2012). Todavia, uma abordagem mecanicista para testes fisiológicos nem sempre é apropriada, nem viável.

Devido às características exclusivas e altamente especializadas de tarefas esportivas específicas, os testes de laboratório nem sempre são a opção mais atraente para treinadores que estão mais focados nas demandas de movimento específicas e nas características fisiológicas que sustentam o desempenho atlético em um determinado domínio esportivo. Juntamente com o fato de que o teste direto é muitas vezes impraticável (Lindberg et al., 2014) e invasivo (Nakagaichi et al., 2001), questões como o custo e a necessidade de pessoal treinado podem representar um desafio para acessar as instalações (Barbieri et al., 2017). Novos testes de campo envolvendo a avaliação em um ambiente esportivo "simulado" mais natural se tornaram cada vez mais populares nos últimos anos, com precisão aceitável e confiabilidade comprovada para uma variedade de esportes populares, incluindo, mas não se limitando a, ciclismo em pista coberta (González-Haro et al., 2007; Karsten et al., 2014), futebol (Castagna et al., 2014; Da Silva et al., 2011; Teixeira et al., 2014), futsal (Barbieri et al., 2017), caratê (Tabben et al., 2014), rugby de quinze (Moore e Murphy, 2003), tênis (Fernandez, 2005) e uma variedade de esportes em cadeira de rodas (Goosey-Tolfrey e Leicht, 2013), por exemplo, vôlei sentado (Marszalek et al., 2015).

Observações positivas semelhantes foram descritas para uma gama de testes aeróbicos de campo altamente específicos em um contexto de saúde, com boa reprodutibilidade e repetibilidade relatadas para o teste de caminhada de 6 minutos em pacientes com doença pulmonar obstrutiva crônica (DPOC) (Fotheringham et al., 2015; Jenkins e Čečins, 2011; Poulain et al., 2003), em um ambiente ocupacional para bombeiros (Lindberg et al., 2013; 2014; Michaelides et al., 2011) e militares (Hauschild et al., 2017; Weiglein et al., 2011). Essas abordagens de teste têm um valor considerável em termos de validade ecológica e, portanto, não devem ser negligenciadas (Goosey-Tolfrey e Leicht, 2013). De fato, em alguns casos, os testes de campo podem oferecer um meio

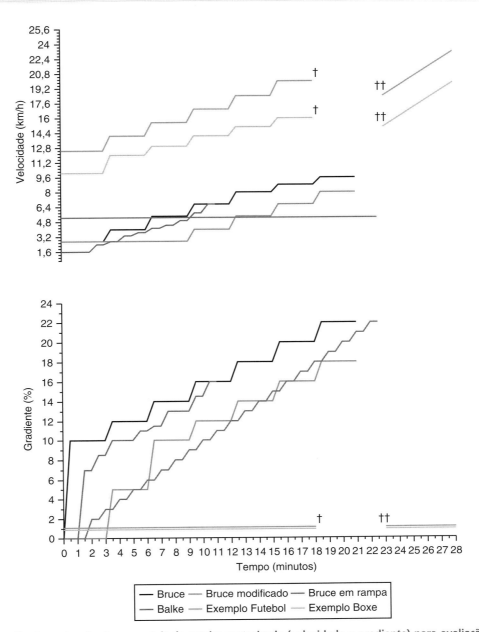

Figura 12.2 Comparação de protocolos incrementais de esteira motorizada (velocidade e gradiente) para avaliação do consumo de oxigênio durante o exercício. Protocolos comuns (Bruce, Bruce modificado, Bruce em rampa e Balke) são apresentados contra dois exemplos de protocolos usados com jogadores de futebol profissional e boxeadores. †, fim do teste graduado submáximo seguido por um período de recuperação de 5 minutos antes de ††, início do teste de pico até a exaustão. (*Esta figura se encontra reproduzida em cores no Encarte.*)

mais eficaz de avaliar o desempenho real (Rylands et al., 2015; Wells et al., 2012) e simular de maneira mais eficaz as demandas de qualquer esporte (Fernandez, 2005). Este argumento deve ser contrabalançado, pois os testes submáximos podem subestimar (Bennett et al., 2016a; Fitchett, 1985; Hartung et al., 1993; Jamnick et al., 2016) ou superestimar (Bennett et al., 2016b) o $\dot{V}O_{2máx}$ observado e dependem de monitoramento adequado durante o exercício (Caputo e Denadai, 2004). Além disso, os testes de campo não se mostraram eficazes para todos os subgrupos da população, com resultados questionáveis em algumas crianças e naquelas com deficiência intelectual (Wouters et al., 2017). Portanto, deve-se ter cuidado ao interpretar os resultados dos testes, particularmente aqueles relacionados à validade.

Doenças crônicas, deficiências físicas e estilos de vida sedentários estão todos associados com uma redução na função. Apesar disso, quando esses grupos embarcam em um regime de exercícios, a modalidade de teste deve ser adequada e de baixo risco. Em ambientes de lazer com base na saúde ou recreativos, é improvável que haja equipamento de teste especializado disponível. Além disso, o teste que envolve um esforço máximo pode ser contraindicado para indivíduos com intolerância ao esforço. Nesses casos, a previsão de $\dot{V}O_{2máx}$ usando teste submáximo oferece uma opção de baixo custo, baixo risco e baixa supervisão (Sartor et al., 2013). Em resumo, uma consideração cuidadosa deve ser dada ao contexto em que o teste é concluído, ou seja, esportes, clínicas, instalações de lazer, comunidade (Sartor et al., 2013); o objetivo do teste (West et al., 2015); movimento específico ou requisitos/restrições de atividade; equipamento disponível; a quantidade de participantes; e quaisquer restrições temporais. Para facilidade de referência, uma variedade de opções de teste populares e suas características estão resumidas na Tabela 12.1.

Tabela 12.1 Resumo dos testes baseados em campo ou laboratório comumente usados para quantificação de $\dot{V}O_{2máx}$.

	TESTE		DETALHES DO TESTE		
Tipo	**Nome(s)**	**Método**	**Modo**	**Esforço necessário**	**Equipamento**
Análise gasosa		Direto	Bicicleta, esteira, ergômetro (i. e., remador, manivela, cadeira de rodas)	100% (máximo)	a) Bolsas de Douglas, medidor de gás seco, bocal/máscara, monitor de FC, EEP b) Carrinho metabólico, bocal/máscara, monitor de FC, EEP
Corrida	Cooper	Indireto	Corrida no solo	100% (máximo)	Pista de atletismo[c], fita métrica
	Shuttle run com múltiplos estágios	Indireto	Corrida no solo	100% (máximo)	Pavilhão de esportes ou espaço equivalente (plano e antiderrapante[d]), cones, fita métrica de 20 m, folhas de relatório específicas, faixa de áudio com sistema para reprodução
	Teste Yo-yo	Indireto	Corrida no solo	100% (máximo)	Pavilhão de esportes ou espaço equivalente (plano e não deslizante[d]), cones, fita métrica de 20 m, folhas de relatório específicas, faixa de áudio com sistema para reprodução
	Resistência de 2,4 km	Indireto	Caminhada no solo, corrida leve ou corrida intensa	Livremente escolhido	Cronômetro, balanças de pesagem, pista de corrida[c], monitores de Fc[c], superfície plana
Teste de caminhada	Rockport; Fox	Indireto	Caminhada no solo	Baixo, mas variável (ritmo de caminhada)	Superfície lisa e nivelada[d], pista marcada[c], cronômetro, balanças, monitores de FC[c]
Passo	McArdle, Chester	Indireto	Step	< 85% FC máxima	Caixas de step, monitores de FC, EEP, planilha de pontuação/relatório dedicada
Teste de bicicleta ergométrica	Astrand-Rhyming, ACM, Ekblom-Bak	Indireto	Bicicleta estática	Baixo (submáximo)	Ciclo estático, monitores de FC[c], EEP, monitor de PA[c]
Predição		Não é exercício	Nenhum	Nenhum	Calculadora, balanças, escalas de pontuação de atividade física específica

Os tempos de teste são baseados na avaliação de um indivíduo e são aproximados. [a]Depende do protocolo. [b]Duração da análise variável (i. e., tempo mais curto se o investigador usar ferramentas de relatório integradas, tempo maior se os cálculos forem feitos e relatados manualmente). [c]Desejável (não essencial). [d]Essencial. PA, pressão arterial; FC, frequência cardíaca; EEP, escalas de esforço percebido.

Escopo	Ambiente	TEMPO			
		Calibração e configuração	Implementação de teste	Processamento de dados, análise, *feedback*	Total geral
Limitado a um indivíduo e acesso/ disponibilidade de equipamento/ pessoal especializado	Ambiente controlado de laboratório	~20 min	12 a 20 min[a]	10 a 90 min[b]	~40 a 130 min
Limitado apenas pelo espaço disponível	Externo	Insignificante	12 min	8 min	~20 min
Limitado pelo equipamento e espaço disponíveis	Interno/externo	~10 min	22 min (máximo)	5 min	~20 a 40 min
Limitado pelo equipamento e espaço disponíveis	Interno/externo	~10 min	Nível 1: 6 a 20 min	5 min	25 a 40 min
Limitado apenas pelo espaço disponível	Interno/externo	Insignificante	Nível 2: 2 a 10 min	5 min	< 40 min
Limitado apenas pelo espaço disponível	Interno/externo	Insignificante	< 20 min	5 min	< 30 min
Limitado pelo equipamento e espaço disponíveis	Interno/externo	Insignificante	< 20 min	10 min	< 35 min
Limitado apenas pelo espaço disponível	Interno	Insignificante	~30 min	10 min	~40 min
Ilimitado	Qualquer um	Nenhum	Nenhum	5 min	~5 min

Testes de caminhada

Caminhar é um modo de atividade familiar e facilmente acessível para uma grande parte da população e, portanto, é uma modalidade altamente aplicável para teste de esforço, abrangendo um amplo espectro de indivíduos. Os testes podem ser realizados em ambientes internos ou externos, com valores semelhantes obtidos (Brooks et al., 2003). Um teste de caminhada *Rockport* simples é ideal para aqueles com baixo condicionamento físico devido aos seus atributos de baixo risco (Kline et al., 1987). Os participantes caminham em um ritmo autosselecionado por 1,6 quilômetro, com peso, idade, sexo, tempo de caminhada e FC inseridos em uma equação de regressão para determinar o $\dot{V}O_{2máx}$. A validade foi confirmada com uma concordância aceitável com um protocolo de teste em esteira com base em laboratório (Weiglein et al., 2011) e a duração do teste e os tempos de processamento de dados se comparam favoravelmente com outros métodos mais intensivos em tempo e trabalho (ver Tabela 12.1). Alguns testes também podem ser personalizados de acordo com o participante. Por exemplo, o teste de caminhada *Fox* permite que o indivíduo autosselecione a distância do teste, com velocidade e gradiente inseridos na equação de regressão para determinação do $\dot{V}O_{2máx}$ (Nordgren et al., 2014). Como os resultados são confiáveis em uma base de teste a teste (Verberkt et al., 2012), os indivíduos podem efetivamente assumir o controle do processo de teste de aptidão, rastreando as mudanças no $\dot{V}O_{2máx}$ ao longo do tempo. Onde as restrições de tempo são um problema, testes muito curtos (cerca de 3 minutos) podem ser administrados com facilidade e com uma relação aceitável com as medidas de referência (Cao et al., 2013).

Testes de corrida

Devido à grande quantidade de massa muscular recrutada durante a corrida, este modo de exercício oferece indiscutivelmente a melhor indicação de potência aeróbica, especialmente em corredores treinados que replicam esse movimento em treinamento e desempenho (McConnell, 1988). O teste de aptidão multiestágio é uma opção viável e válida para adultos envolvidos com esportes baseados em corrida (Léger, 1982) e para crianças (variante de 20 m) (Artero et al., 2011; Batista et al., 2017; Castro-Piñero et al., 2010), com confiabilidade teste a teste aceitável contramedidas de referência (Léger, 1982; Metsios et al., 2008). A taxa de trabalho inicial é baixa (trote leve), progredindo para corrida e, por fim, esforço máximo. Como os incrementos de velocidade são fixos, indivíduos não qualificados ou descondicionados podem achar os testes desafiadores e desmotivadores se participarem com colegas mais capazes. Uma versão quadrada (*i. e.*, movimento linear com 4 voltas × 90° *versus* movimento linear padrão com 2 voltas × 180°) do mesmo teste pode ser aplicada onde a previsão de $\dot{V}O_{2máx}$ é importante (Flouris et al., 2009; Metsios et al., 2008) ou algoritmos revisados podem ser aplicados ao teste tradicional para aumentar a precisão (Flouris et al., 2005).

A maneira como os testes de corrida em campo são aplicados também é uma consideração importante. Oferecer *feedback* de desempenho durante os testes de 20 m lineares ou em *shuttle* reduz os limites de concordância e coeficiente de variação, produzindo resultados mais precisos (Metsios et al., 2006). Alternativamente, o teste de resistência de 2,4 km permite que os indivíduos selecionem o ritmo, optando por caminhar, correr devagar ou correr rapidamente. Esse tipo de teste é ideal para avaliação de grandes grupos com diferentes níveis de aptidão ou quando a avaliação laboratorial não é uma opção disponível (Mayorga-Vega et al., 2016). $\dot{V}O_{2máx}$ é predito com precisão (R = 0,86, SEE [erro padrão de estimativa, do inglês *standard error of estimation*] = 3,4 mℓ · kg · min^{-1}) usando a duração do teste, com melhorias marginais se a FC também for incluída no modelo (R = 0,90, SEE = 2,9 mℓ · kg · min^{-1}) (Larsen et al., 2002). O teste de yo-yo é uma escolha popular para esportes coletivos, principalmente futebol, onde sua aplicação permite a formação de um programa de treinamento eficaz, fornecendo dados úteis para monitorar o progresso do jogador na capacidade de exercício (Krustrup et al., 2003; Metaxas et al., 2005). Além disso, a variante de nível 2 é sensível à posição do jogador e ao nível de competição (*i. e.*, elite internacional *versus* elite moderada) (Krustrup et al., 2006), o que é útil dado que atletas de *resistência* de elite normalmente têm um $\dot{V}O_{2máx}$ mais alto do que atletas não de elite (Lorenz et al., 2013; Metaxas et al., 2009).

Teste de escada

Se executado de forma correta e adequada, o teste de escada pode fornecer dados confiáveis que não se desviam significativamente das medidas de referência para $\dot{V}O_{2máx}$ (Keren et al., 1980). A técnica deve ser padronizada e, o mais importante para praticantes inexperientes, um teste de familiarização prévio deve ser realizado para garantir resultados ideais. Nessas condições, os testes de escada fornecem resultados ecologicamente válidos e adequadamente robustos (Bennett et al., 2016). O teste de degrau de *Chester* (TDC) é um bom exemplo de um teste de campo de escada fácil de administrar. Um mínimo de duas FC submáximas é coletado, regredidas contra o $\dot{V}O_{2máx}$ e extrapoladas para a FC máxima prevista para a idade. Como a FC máxima coincide com o $\dot{V}O_{2máx}$ máximo, isso permite estimar o $\dot{V}O_{2máx}$. A validade de face foi confirmada (Sykes e Roberts, 2004). No entanto, devido à subestimação dos valores de referência baseados em laboratório e à falta de linearidade nas respostas de FC e $\dot{V}O_{2máx}$ durante o trabalho progressivo e incremental (Buckley et al., 2004), a precisão do TDC na identificação do verdadeiro $\dot{V}O_{2máx}$ é questionável. Contudo, como a confiabilidade teste a teste é aceitável (viés de interteste e limites de concordância de 95% (LC): −0,8 e 3,7 mℓ · kg · min^{-1}, respectivamente) (Buckley et al., 2004), o TDC tem considerável aplicabilidade para testar cenários onde o objetivo é monitorar as alterações temporais no desempenho ou na saúde induzidas pelo treinamento (Bennett et al., 2016). Além disso, como uma grande quantidade de pessoas pode ser acomodada em sessões de teste individuais, equipes/esquadrões completos podem ser avaliados simultaneamente. Testes mais curtos foram validados, onde a pressão do tempo é um problema, como o teste de escada contínuo de 5 minutos de estágio único, que relata excelente associação com medidas de referência (Keren et al., 1980). Tem aplicação para praticantes que definem programas de exercícios em ambientes de lazer recreativo, que não dispõem de instalações ou equipamentos de alta tecnologia e possuem um tempo limitado para a indução de novos clientes.

Testes de ciclismo submáximo

Os testes de ciclismo têm sido usados com bom efeito para predizer o desempenho de pico em indivíduos treinados (Lamberts et al., 2011) e para informar a prescrição de treinamento nesses grupos (Lamberts, 2014). O teste de *Astrand-Ryhming* (Astrand e Ryhming, 1954) foi considerado um teste submáximo apropriado para estimativa da capacidade de pico por muitos anos, com níveis de erro preferencialmente baixos e alta validade observada em comparação com outros métodos (Grant et al., 1999). Além disso, o teste de ciclismo da ACM é um método estabelecido há muito tempo e uma opção popular em ambientes recreativos e clínicos para testar populações em geral devido à sua relativa facilidade de aplicação e atributos de baixo risco (Garatachea et al., 2007). A pressão arterial, a FC e a EEP são monitoradas no final de uma série de estágios de exercício em estado estacionário

Determinantes Fisiológicos para o Desempenho de Resistência: Consumo Máximo de Oxigênio... | Capítulo | 12 |

de 3 minutos. Em contraste, o teste *Ekblom-Bak* (Björkman et al., 2016; Ekblom-Bak et al., 2012) inclui uma carga de trabalho submáxima fixa e uma escolhida individualmente. Este teste confere vantagens semelhantes a testes mais estabelecidos e compara-se favoravelmente com o $\dot{V}O_{2máx}$ observado (R = 0,91, SEE = 0,302 $\ell \cdot min^{-1}$). Na verdade, ele supera o teste de *Astrand-Ryhming* (Björkman et al., 2016; Ekblom-Bak et al., 2012). A disponibilidade de testes de ciclismo submáximo recentemente validados enfatiza a importância da crítica apropriada da literatura ao decidir sobre o tipo de teste, em oposição a uma posição padrão em que um teste é selecionado, pois tem sido usado por muitos anos. Entretanto, o consenso é que quaisquer que sejam os testes de ciclismo aplicados, eles devem ser minimamente invasivos e de curta duração (Capostagno et al., 2016).

Equações de predição sem exercício

A quantificação do $\dot{V}O_{2máx}$ sem exercício confere vantagens consideráveis quando os recursos e/ou equipamentos de teste são restritos ou as condições médicas impedem o esforço; uma vasta gama de equações é validada na literatura. Na maioria das vezes, as equações de regressão dependem de medidas quantitativas básicas, como porcentagem de gordura corporal (Robert McComb et al., 2006) e/ou estimativas autorrelatadas de função e/ou níveis de atividade física (Bradshaw et al., 2005; Malek et al., 2004; Schembre e Riebe, 2011). Como consequência, são particularmente fáceis de administrar e podem ser usados com

níveis aceitáveis de precisão. Porém, a ressalva é que para garantir a validade, a aplicação deve ser feita apenas para o(s) grupo(s) populacional(is) declarado(s) (Evans et al., 2015). Alguns exemplos de equações estão listados no Boxe 12.1 em ordem de força de associação entre a equação de regressão e os valores de referência para $\dot{V}O_{2máx}$ (R) (Boxe 12.1).

Prescrição de treinamento físico

$\dot{V}O_{2máx}$ é altamente responsivo ao treinamento físico em todas as idades, mesmo na vida adulta (Chodzko-Zajko et al., 2009; Stamford, 1988), com aumento do débito cardíaco, volume sanguíneo e densidade capilar e mitocondrial realizada por meio de atividade aeróbica regular (Costill et al., 1976). Portanto, os cientistas do esporte e do exercício que trabalham em todo o espectro de níveis de condicionamento físico (*i. e.*, descondicionados, aparentemente saudáveis, mas inativos, doenças crônicas, praticantes de atividades recreativas, populações atléticas) dedicam tempo e atenção consideráveis ao desenho, entrega e revisão de planos sob medida para promover alterações positivas no $\dot{V}O_{2máx}$.

A coleta de FC e EEP junto com a medição de $\dot{V}O_{2máx}$ durante os testes laboratoriais permite que uma prescrição de treinamento seja definida e traduzida na prática. Essas variáveis são facilmente monitoradas durante o treinamento e as condições de jogo, possibilita um entendimento da carga fisiológica interna e facilita um ambiente de treinamento propício para as adaptações

---

Boxe 12.1 Equações de predição sem exercício

Adultos saudáveis com idade entre 18 e 65 anos

$$\dot{V}O_{2máx} \sim 40 \pm 10\ m\ell\ kg\ min^{-1}$$
$$(R = 0,93,\ SEE = 3,5\ m\ell\ kg\ min^{-1}):$$

$$\dot{V}O_{2máx} = 48,0730 + (6,1779 \times S) -$$
$$(0,2463 \times I) - (0,6186 \times IMC) +$$
$$(0,7115 \times HFP) + (0,6709 \times PA\text{-}R)$$

em que S = sexo (feminino = 0, masculino = 1); I = idade (anos); IMC = índice de massa corporal (kg · m²); HFP = habilidade funcional percebida; PA-R = avaliação da atividade física (Bradshaw et al., 2005). Os procedimentos para a determinação de HFP (George, 1996) e PA-R (Jackson et al., 1990) foram previamente definidos e oferecem um meio rápido e fácil de quantificar os níveis de função e atividade.

Mulheres treinadas com idade de 38 ± 10 anos (intervalo indisponível)

$$\dot{V}O_{2máx} \sim 43 \pm 7\ m\ell\ kg\ min^{-1}$$
$$(R = 0,83,\ SEE = 259\ m\ell\ min^{-1}):$$

$$\dot{V}O_{2máx} = (18,528 \times P) + (11,993 \times H) -$$
$$(17,197 \times I) + (23,522 \times D) + (62,118 \times T)$$
$$+ (278,262 \times A) - 1375,878$$

em que P = peso (kg); H = altura (cm); I = idade (anos); D = duração do treinamento (h · semana⁻¹); T = intensidade de treinamento usando a escala de Borg 6 a 20; A = anos de treinamento (Malek et al., 2004).

Homens treinados com idade de 40 ± 12 anos (intervalo não disponível)

$$\dot{V}O_{2máx} \sim 53 \pm 9\ m\ell\ kg\ min^{-1}$$
$$(R = 0,82,\ SEE = 382\ m\ell\ min^{-1}):$$

$$\dot{V}O_{2máx} = (27,387 \times P) + (26,634 \times H) -$$
$$(27,572 \times I) + (26,161 \times D) + (114,094 \times T)$$
$$+ (506,752 \times A) - 4609,791$$

em que P = peso (kg); H = altura (cm); I = idade (anos); D = duração do treinamento (h · semana⁻¹); T = intensidade de treinamento usando a escala de Borg 6 a 20; A = anos de treinamento (Malek et al., 2005).

Adultos saudáveis com idade entre 46 ± 13 anos (intervalo não disponível)

$$\dot{V}O_{2máx} \sim 34 \pm 12\ m\ell\ kg\ min^{-1}$$
$$(R = 0,79,\ SEE = 7,2\ m\ell\ kg\ min^{-1}):$$

$$\dot{V}O_{2máx} = 79,9 - (0,39 \times I) -$$
$$(13,7 \times S) + (0,127 \times P)$$

em que I = idade (anos); S = sexo (feminino = 1, masculino = 0); P = peso (lb) (Myers et al., 2017).

Adultos saudáveis com idade entre 18 e 25 anos

$$\dot{V}O_{2máx} \sim 42 \pm 7\ m\ell\ kg\ min^{-1}$$
$$(R = 0,65,\ SEE = 5,5\ m\ell\ kg\ min^{-1}):$$

$$\dot{V}O_{2máx} = 47,749 - (6,493 \times S) + (0,140 \times AV)$$

onde S = sexo (feminino = 2, masculino = 1); AV = atividade vigorosa (Schembre e Riebe, 2011).

O cálculo da AV é direto, usando os resultados da aplicação do Questionário Internacional de Atividade Física – Short Form (IPAQ-SF) (Craig et al., 2003) (AV (MET min · semana⁻¹) = 8 MET × AV min por dia × AV dias por semana).

necessárias. Isso é de suma importância, visto que alguns pesquisadores identificaram insuficiências na carga fisiológica experimentada pelos jogadores durante o treinamento (Eniseler, 2005; Fulton et al., 2010). Embora a EEP tenha um valor prático considerável em um contexto de desempenho esportivo (Lambert e Borresen, 2010), ele não é comumente utilizado para prescrição de exercícios em atletas. No entanto, pode ser administrado com bons resultados com populações em geral que pretendem desenvolver aptidão cardiorrespiratória e muscular (Garnacho-Castaño et al., 2018) e pode atuar como uma medida auxiliar útil para aumentar a precisão das determinações indiretas de $\dot{V}O_{2máx}$ (Davies et al., 2008).

Observe que, em um contexto esportivo, a resistência cardiorrespiratória é apenas um aspecto do desempenho. Onde os programas são elaborados para o aprimoramento desse aspecto, outros atributos importantes definidos pelo esporte, ou seja, velocidade total, velocidade-resistência (Iaia e Bangsbo, 2010), força e potência musculares (Suchomel et al., 2016), agilidade (Sheppard e Young, 2006), habilidade motora (Annett, 1994), equilíbrio (Hrysomallis, 2011; Zemková, 2014), coordenação (Lech et al., 2011), também devem ser periodizados no plano do atleta. Embora esses atributos estejam fora do escopo deste capítulo, eles exigem a devida consideração por parte dos cientistas do esporte e do exercício.

Relações dose-resposta e $\dot{V}O_{2máx}$

A carga de treinamento pode ser simplificada e resumida por suas características em termos de estresse fisiológico (dose) e resultados obtidos (resposta) (Lambert e Borresen, 2010). Em termos gerais, um maior volume semanal de atividade física equivale a uma maior melhora na aptidão cardiorrespiratória (Oja, 2001). Consequentemente, diz-se que existe uma relação dose-resposta linear inversa entre o volume de atividade física e todas as causas de mortalidade (Lee e Skerrett, 2001). No entanto, a dose para a realização de alterações positivas no $\dot{V}O_{2máx}$ provavelmente não será consistente em todas as populações. Uma magnitude maior de benefício é experimentada ao longo do tempo para pessoas menos ativas quando comparadas a contrapartes altamente ativas (Haskell, 1994). Consequentemente, os praticantes de exercícios iniciantes e descondicionados experimentarão melhoras maiores em um período mais curto do que as populações mais bem condicionadas, que normalmente têm um $\dot{V}O_{2máx}$ mais alto (Rankovic et al., 2010). Em uma amostra mista de indivíduos aparentemente saudáveis de 20 a 60 anos de idade, os grupos de exercícios de caminhada de intensidade baixa e duração moderada ou alta (< 200 e > 200 min por semana, respectivamente) exibiram um $\dot{V}O_{2máx}$ maior do que aqueles que não faziam exercícios (Gim e Choi, 2016). Além disso, o treinamento aeróbico a 63 a 73% da reserva de FC por 40 a 50 min, 3 a 4 dias por semana é eficaz na otimização dos benefícios cardiorrespiratórios em idosos aparentemente saudáveis, mas sedentários (Huang et al., 2016). Portanto, podem ser vistas adaptações positivas com níveis relativamente baixos de atividade física em grupos de baixo preparo físico. Isso é encorajador, visto que esses indivíduos lutam para manter o compromisso com os programas de exercícios (Dishman, 2001), com uma porcentagem considerável (cerca de 50%) desistindo após 6 meses (Robinson e Rogers, 1994). No entanto, essas doses são provavelmente insuficientes para ganhos atléticos, ou até mesmo para um praticante de exercícios recreativos que está treinando para um evento como uma maratona ou triatlo.

Fatores que confundem e limitam as alterações crônicas no $\dot{V}O_{2máx}$

Embora existam evidências claras para apoiar a "treinabilidade" do $\dot{V}O_{2máx}$, os cientistas do esporte e do exercício não devem esperar automaticamente aumentos exponenciais na capacidade de exercício com o treinamento crônico. Com relação à programação de exercícios, existe uma variabilidade interindividual considerável nas respostas de treinamento (Williams et al., 2017). Além do programa de exercícios, muitos fatores influenciarão a predisposição de um indivíduo para uma elevação no $\dot{V}O_{2máx}$. Fatores como idade (Legaz Arrese et al., 2005), lesão, desuso e destreinamento (Neufer, 1989; Petibois e Déléris, 2003), posição do jogador (Duthie et al., 2003; Ransdell et al., 2013) e modalidade esportiva (Metaxas et al., 2009) irão influenciar a capacidade de pico. Além disso, atletas altamente treinados acabarão por atingir um "teto" genético para $\dot{V}O_{2máx}$ (Sjödin e Svedenhag, 1985). Ademais, os genes responsáveis pela codificação do subsistema muscular, equilíbrio eletrolítico, metabolismo lipídico, fosforilação oxidativa e entrega de oxigênio se combinam para construir um perfil individual único caracterizado pela variabilidade sistêmica inerente no desempenho motor (Bray et al., 2009; Williams et al., 2017). Esta assinatura individualmente única será um dos principais fatores que definem o potencial de desempenho e limitam os ganhos de desempenho. Este motivo, juntamente com o fato de que melhorias nas variáveis fisiológicas submáximas (p. ex., limiar ventilatório) podem ser vistas sem mudanças no $\dot{V}O_{2máx}$ (Millet et al., 2009) enfatizam a importância de evitar uma dependência exclusiva da capacidade máxima. Portanto, marcadores fisiológicos submáximos de desempenho, mais notavelmente limiares de transição SLa⁻ $\dot{V}O_{2máx}$ em cargas de trabalho submáximas e eficiência mecânica, também devem ser examinados para garantir que uma imagem completa e precisa do desempenho ou potencial funcional seja obtida.

Prescrição de exercícios para promover aumentos em $\dot{V}O_{2máx}$

As abordagens tradicionais de treinamento têm favorecido exercícios de resistência contínuo e de alto volume, envolvendo atividade rítmica de grandes grupos musculares para a elevação do $\dot{V}O_{2máx}$. No entanto, essas atividades consomem tempo e não se alinham naturalmente com as complexas demandas específicas do esporte, que muitas vezes requerem esforço intermitente, em vez de contínuo. Uma abordagem mais moderna é administrar o treinamento intervalado de alta intensidade (HIIT, do inglês *high intensity interval training*), em que sessões de trabalho de alta intensidade são intercaladas com períodos de recuperação ativa. Essa abordagem de treinamento se tornou popular devido à sua considerável eficiência de tempo (Burgomaster et al., 2008; Gibala et al., 2006; Gist et al., 2014) e ao impacto positivo na fisiologia do músculo estriado esquelético (Burgomaster et al., 2008; Cochran et al., 2014; Gibala et al., 2006; Little et al., 2010; Sjödin e Svedenhag, 1985). Especificamente, são observadas após o treinamento de alta intensidade aumentos na capacidade oxidativa do músculo (Burgomaster et al., 2008; Gibala et al., 2006), capacidade de tamponamento muscular (Gibala et al., 2006), conteúdo de glicogênio (Gibala et al., 2006; Little et al., 2010), a atividade da enzima glicogenolítica muscular (Kubukeli et al., 2002) e a capacidade de transporte sarcolemal de lactato (Kubukeli et al., 2002). Na verdade, as adaptações fisiológicas são consistentes com aquelas observadas durante um regime de resistência contínuo, mas o volume de treinamento é consideravelmente menor (cerca de 90%) (Gibala et al., 2006), com grandes aumentos em $\dot{V}O_{2máx}$ (cerca de 10%) esperados em curtos períodos de tempo usando esta abordagem (Munoz et al., 2015; Støren et al., 2012). Portanto, de uma perspectiva prática, as estratégias de treinamento de alta intensidade devem ser consideradas igualmente eficazes como o treinamento de resistência em estado estacionário e contínuo tradicional (Burgomaster et al., 2008; Gibala et al., 2006; Gist et al., 2014; Macpherson et al., 2011; Milanović et al., 2015c;

Determinantes Fisiológicos para o Desempenho de Resistência: Consumo Máximo de Oxigênio... **Capítulo** | 12 |

Sloth et al., 2013), com aplicabilidade clara para atletas de elite (Iaia e Bangsbo, 2010; Ní Chéilleachair et al., 2017), indivíduos ativos (não atléticos) (Weston et al., 2014) e indivíduos sedentários (Weston et al., 2014).

A manipulação de intensidade, duração e relação trabalho-repouso permite que o cientista do esporte e do exercício otimize estratégias de treinamento de alta intensidade para aumentar o $\dot{V}O_{2máx}$, com o treinamento de *sprint* sendo uma opção desejável. Durações entre 10 e 30 segundos são eficazes na elevação de $\dot{V}O_{2máx}$ (Hazell et al., 2010; McKie et al., 2018) e os efeitos podem ser percebidos em intervalos de tempo relativamente curtos (3 a 4 semanas) (Astorino et al., 2013; McKie et al., 2018; Rønnestad et al., 2014). De fato, *sprints* de curta duração (~5 s), concluídos em mais repetições podem representar uma estratégia ideal devido ao maior prazer percebido em estratégias de *sprints* mais longos (Islam et al., 2017; Townsend et al., 2017).

Resumo

Este capítulo explora o papel relativo e o propósito do $\dot{V}O_{2máx}$ como o principal determinante fisiológico da capacidade de resistência. Existem vários métodos para a quantificação deste parâmetro, com uma variedade de métodos baseados em campo e em laboratório disponíveis, cada um caracterizado por seus pontos fortes e fracos inerentes. O cientista do esporte e exercício deve considerar a população, o ambiente, a viabilidade da aplicação do teste e a disponibilidade de recursos onde os testes são aplicados. Posteriormente, os dados devem ser cuidadosamente analisados e interpretados para garantir que as metas e modos de treinamento apropriados possam ser determinados e otimizados para ganhos de saúde ou desempenho.

Estudo de caso

O exemplo a seguir ilustra como a coleta de medidas fisiológicas, especificamente $\dot{V}O_{2máx}$, pode ser usada para individualizar e melhorar a prescrição de treinamento.

Perfil do participante e protocolo de teste

Características	Homem de 56 anos aparentemente saudável Ciclista recreativo treinado Ciclismo rodoviário diário de longa distância e velocidade baixa (sessões de ≥ 60 min)
Peso	79 kg
Altura	176 cm
Protocolo de teste	Todos os testes concluídos usando bicicleta ergométrica (Lode BV, Holanda) configurada pelo participante para a posição desejada Teste de exercício graduado envolvendo oito estágios submáximos de 3 min (30 a 240 W, incrementos de 30 W); recuperação ativa de 10 min Teste de pico de exercício até a exaustão (0 a 345 W, incrementos de 15 W aplicados a cada 30 s)
Medidas	FC, $\dot{V}O_{2máx}$ e parâmetros respiratórios ($\dot{V}O_{2máx}$, V_E, RTR) monitorados continuamente usando um carrinho metabólico *online*. EEP no final de cada estágio submáximo e imediatamente após o teste de pico

Determinação de $\dot{V}O_{2máx}$

Os critérios primários foram atendidos para a determinação do pico de esforço fisiológico com um platô de $\dot{V}O_{2máx}$ observado. Portanto, não havia necessidade de um estágio de verificação nem consideração de critérios secundários. No entanto, neste caso, eles são listados para referência:

$\dot{V}O_{2máx}$ (absoluto)	3,84 $\ell \cdot min^{-1}$
$\dot{V}O_{2máx}$ (relativo)	49 $m\ell \cdot kg \cdot min^{-1}$
SLa^-_{pico}	7,49 $mmol \cdot \ell^{-1}$
FC_{pico}	169 $b \cdot min^{-1}$ (cerca de 103% do máximo previsto para a idade)
RTR_{pico}	1,25
EEP_{pico}	EEP geral de 20 (EEP 6 a 20: Borg, 1982)

Comparações com dados normativos

Uma vez identificado, o $\dot{V}O_{2máx}$ deve ser comparado aos dados normativos para facilitar o feedback para o atleta. Nesse caso, uma classificação funcional superior foi definida (> 45,3 $m\ell \cdot kg \cdot min^{-1}$) usando dados normativos aceitos para populações em geral (Heyward e Gibson, 2014). No entanto, como a maioria dos sistemas de classificação está relacionada com associações entre $\dot{V}O_{2máx}$ e o estado de saúde cardiovascular (Duncan et al., 2005; Heyward e Gibson, 2014; Sanders e Duncan, 2006), eles têm aplicação limitada para populações atléticas que apresentam um $\dot{V}O_{2máx}$ significativamente maior (Rankovic et al., 2010). Dados normativos úteis existem para uma série de esportes, incluindo jogadores de futebol masculino (Helgerud et al., 2011; Hoff, 2005; Tønnessen et al., 2013; Ziogas et al., 2011), jogadoras de futebol (Haugen et al., 2014), rúgbi de sete (Higham et al., 2013), rúgbi de 13 (Brewer e Davis, 1995) e corredores treinados (Barnes e Kilding, 2015). Além disso, dados fisiológicos estão disponíveis para alguns esportes para permitir a comparação com os padrões em fases específicas do ciclo competitivo (Miller et al., 2011). No entanto, os dados normativos não estão disponíveis para todas as disciplinas esportivas discretas ou para permitir perfis específicos de sexo em todos os casos. Quando dados coletados de atletas competindo dentro do mesmo esporte estão disponíveis, uma comparação mais específica pode, e deve, ser feita de acordo com a posição do jogador, liga e/ou disciplina.

Usando a relação FC e $\dot{V}O_{2máx}$ para informar a prescrição de treinamento

As medidas fisiológicas obtidas durante o teste podem ser usadas para identificar as intensidades-alvo de treinamento para otimizar os efeitos crônicos. Uma das abordagens mais comumente aplicadas para esse propósito é realizar a regressão linear básica de FC e $\dot{V}O_{2máx}$ (Figura 12.3). Em qualquer porcentagem dada de $\dot{V}O_{2máx}$, um alvo de FC ou em EEP pode ser fornecido, dependendo de qual variável é plotada no eixo y. Neste caso, como o cliente tinha acesso a um monitor de FC, foram disponibilizadas zonas de treino à sua medida.

Respostas de lactato sanguíneo e prescrição de treinamento

Devido às limitações de escopo, este capítulo não considerou a importância dos limiares de transição de lactato sanguíneo em detalhes, mas seu papel relativo na demarcação de fenômenos fisiológicos importantes não deve ser subestimado. A coleta de dados de SLa^- durante o teste de esforço graduado oferece uma alternativa válida e confiável aos limiares ventilatórios identificados

(continua)

(Continuação)

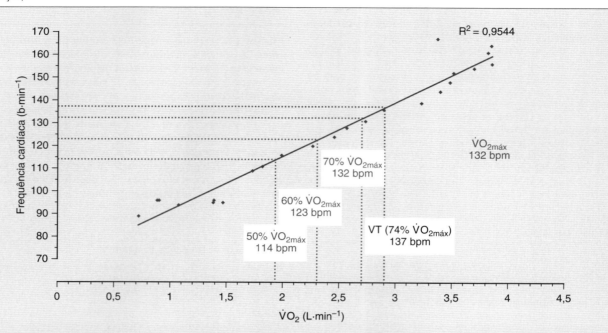

Figura 12.3 Regressão linear simples da frequência cardíaca (FC) e $\dot{V}O_{2máx}$ durante o teste de exercício graduado em laboratório. A *linha pontilhada vermelha* indica o processo de extrapolação da FC (y) a partir do $\dot{V}O_{2máx}$ (x) usando porcentagens fixas. A *linha pontilhada azul* indica o limiar ventilatório (LV), conforme definido pela análise separada das respostas respiratórias ao trabalho incremental até a exaustão. bpm, batimentos por minuto. (*Esta figura se encontra reproduzida em cores no Encarte.*)

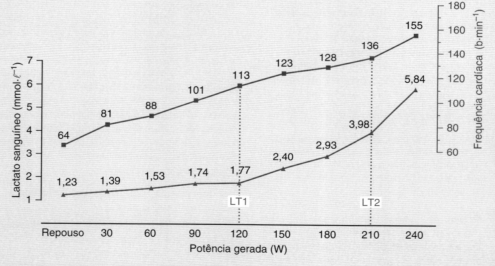

Figura 12.4 Resposta do lactato sanguíneo e da frequência cardíaca ao exercício incremental durante um teste de exercício graduado em uma bicicleta ergométrica. As linhas pontilhadas indicam o limiar de lactato (LT_1) e o ponto de virada (LT_2), respectivamente, conforme definido pela inspeção visual da curva de lactato.

por meio de medidas respiratórias (Pallarés et al., 2016). Portanto, o teste pode ser muito útil na definição da prescrição do treinamento de exercício. Um perfil de lactato de velocidade curvilínea (ou taxa de trabalho) (Figura 12.4) é gerado pela coleta de uma pequena amostra de sangue do lóbulo da orelha ou ponta do dedo, com medidas obtidas no final de cada estágio submáximo de estado estacionário (duração do estágio de 3 ou 4 min com um intervalo de repouso de 1 min é o ideal).

A inspeção visual desses dados permite a determinação do limiar de lactato (LT_1) onde uma elevação em SLa^- do repouso é observada pela primeira vez (< 1 mmol·ℓ^{-1}), e o ponto de inflexão de lactato (LT_2), onde a produção e depuração de lactato não estão mais em equilíbrio durante o exercício (ver Figura 12.4). Após a identificação de LT_1 e LT_2, três zonas de treinamento podem ser facilmente definidas (Faude et al., 2009) e foram aplicadas a este estudo de caso (Figura 12.5).

Determinantes Fisiológicos para o Desempenho de Resistência: Consumo Máximo de Oxigênio... | Capítulo | 12 |

(continuação)

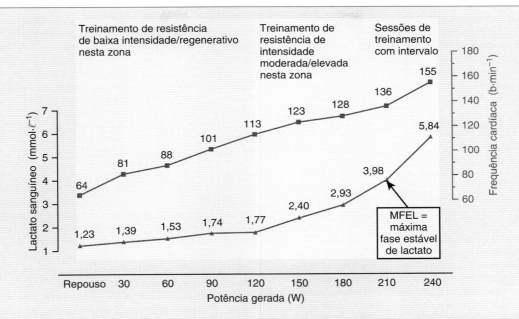

Figura 12.5 Zonas de treinamento de frequência cardíaca, conforme definido pelos limiares de transição de lactato sanguíneo identificados durante o trabalho incremental. (Adaptada de Faude, O., Kindermann, W., Meyer, T., 2009. Lactate threshold concepts: how valid are they? Sports Medicine, 39 (6), 469-490.)

Antes de atingir o LT_1, a produção de lactato é insignificante e, portanto, a carga fisiológica está em seu nível mais baixo. Para este exemplo de estudo de caso, isso equivale a uma FC de 113 b·min^{-1} (ver Figura 12.4) e uma intensidade de exercício relativa, taxa de trabalho e EEP de 50% $\dot{V}O_{2máx}$, 120 W e 10, respectivamente (Tabela 12.2). Portanto, exercícios com essa intensidade ou abaixo dela devem ser recomendados para sessões de aquecimento e sessões de recuperação ativa intercaladas entre intervalos de alta intensidade. Após o LT_1, mas abaixo do LT_2, o lactato começa a aumentar. No entanto, os aumentos estão alinhados às mudanças na intensidade do exercício e um equilíbrio fisiológico permanece (i. e., aumenta a taxa de trabalho = aumenta o lactato; a taxa de trabalho permanece constante = lactato permanece constante). Com relação ao exemplo de caso, FC de 114 a 137 b·min^{-1} W; EEP de 11 a 12) devem, portanto, ser aconselhados para treinamento lento de longa distância (ver Figura 12.5), com as prováveis adaptações crônicas sendo: aumento da densidade capilar e complacência arterial, diminuição da FC de repouso e submáxima,

Tabela 12.2 Resumo da prescrição de treinamento de exercício com base na porcentagem de $\dot{V}O_{2máx}$.

Tipo de treinamento	Observações	Intensidade de treino-alvo % $\dot{V}O_{2máx}$	Potência da saída Watts	FC b·min^{-1}	$\dot{V}O_{2máx}$ mℓ·kg·min^{-1}	EEP
Aquecimento/ relaxamento	Menor que LT_1	< 50%	< 120	≤ 113	24 a 29	10
Resistência – nível 1	Ciclismo com acúmulo de lactato – fácil	50 a 60%	125 a 160	114 a 123	24 a 29	11
Resistência – nível 2	Ciclismo com acúmulo de lactato – moderado	60 a 74%	161 a 210	124 a 137	29 a 34	12
Limiar anaeróbico (LT_2)	Transfira para o trabalho anaeróbico – treine até este nível	74%	210 a 225	137	34	13
Intervalos	Treinamento intervalado de alta intensidade (HIIT) – trabalhe neste nível intercalado com recuperação ativa (< 50%)	> 74%	225 a 345	137 a 169	34 a 49	≤ 13
Capacidade de pico	Esforço máximo	100%	345	169	49	20

EEP, escala de esforço percebido; *FC*, frequência cardíaca; *LT1*, limiar de lactato; *LT2*, ponto de inflexão do lactato.

(continua)

Parte | 1 | Conceitos Básicos Importantes em Esportes

(Continuação)

aumento do Q e da fração de ejeção do ventrículo esquerdo (Clausen, 1977).

Em condições de exercício em que o O_2 não está mais disponível em quantidades suficientes, grandes quantidades de lactato começam a se acumular por meio da dependência predominante dos sistemas anaeróbicos. Para este estudo de caso, isso pode ser visto nas taxas de trabalho além do LT_2, onde os níveis de SLa^{-1} aumentam desproporcionalmente ao longo do tempo, com a taxa de produção excedendo a sua depuração (ver Figura 12.4). Embora este ponto tenha sido descrito como o "limiar anaeróbico", e usado para demarcar a progressão do metabolismo aeróbico para o anaeróbico (Wasserman, 1986), o uso desta terminologia pode ser enganoso, pois os sistemas de energia e sua contribuição relativa ao resultado fisiológico líquido geral não são mutuamente exclusivos. No entanto, os eventos fisiológicos que ocorrem em torno deste ponto são geralmente aceitos como representativos da transição de carga fisiológica interna moderada para vigorosa; portanto, este ponto é altamente significativo. A capacidade de sustentar um alto componente faccional de $\dot{V}O_{2máx}$ por um período prolongado retarda a acidose metabólica (Ghosh, 2004) e, portanto, o limiar anaeróbico está altamente correlacionado ao desempenho em corridas de longa distância. Exceder esse limite é tipificado por concentrações excessivas de dióxido de carbono no plasma e íons de hidrogênio, produzidos como consequência do aumento da atividade metabólica dentro do músculo, causando uma redução no pH sanguíneo. Isso estimula um aumento imediato no volume-minuto (V_E), pois a eliminação do excesso de CO_2 produzido pelo tamponamento dos íons de hidrogênio torna-se uma prioridade para evitar a acidose metabólica. Portanto, a análise

dos gases respiratórios (*i. e.*, V_E VO_2, V_{CO2}) e, especificamente, as mudanças na linearidade nessas relações apoiam a identificação do limiar; portanto, o termo "limiar ventilatório" (LV) pode ser mais apropriado. Neste estudo de caso, determinou-se que o LV ocorria a 74% $\dot{V}O_{2máx}$ (137 b · min^{-1}). O cruzamento dos dados de SLa^- (ver Figura 12.4) revela que LT_2 ocorreu no mesmo ponto (136 b · min^{-1}) durante o teste graduado. Além disso, a concentração de SLa^- antes da quebra na linearidade observada durante e antes do estado estacionário máximo de lactato foi ~4 mmol·ℓ^{-1} (ver Figura 12.4), que é geralmente aceito para representar o início do acúmulo de lactato sanguíneo (OBLA, do inglês *onset of blood lactate accumulation*) entre indivíduos. Coletivamente, esses dados reforçam a premissa de que os processos anaeróbicos se tornam dominantes em 137 b · min^{-1} e que 210 W é representativo da potência crítica.

Como o LT_2 ocorre em uma porcentagem mais alta de $\dot{V}O_{2máx}$ em atletas de elite do que os equivalentes ativos não elite (Joyner e Coyle, 2008), é geralmente aceito que a elevação de LT_2/LV se traduz diretamente em melhor desempenho em esportes baseados em resistência. A elevação é alcançada por meio do treinamento de limiar, no ou ligeiramente acima do limiar anaeróbico (Ghosh, 2004). Essa intensidade tem o efeito adicional de aumentar o $\dot{V}O_{2máx}$, conforme declarado anteriormente. A natureza intermitente do treinamento intervalado, particularmente usando intensidades muito altas, mas baixo volume, é importante para maximizar as adaptações do músculo esquelético (Cochran et al., 2014), aumentando assim o $\dot{V}O_{2máx}$. Portanto, o cliente deve incorporar intervalos de alta intensidade em seu plano de treinamento, elevando a FC além de 137 b · min^{-1}, idealmente em direção ao limite superior da faixa (169 b · min^{-1}).

Referências bibliográficas

Abut, F., Akay, M.F., 2015. Machine learning and statistical methods for the prediction of maximal oxygen uptake: recent advances. Medical Devices (Auckland) 8, 369-379.

Annett, J., 1994. The learning of motor skills: sports science and ergonomics perspectives. Ergonomics 37 (1), 5-16.

Arkesteijn, M., Hopker, J., Jobson, S.A., Passfield, L., 2013. The effect of turbo trainer cycling on pedalling technique and cycling efficiency. International Journal of Sports Medicine 34 (6), 520-525.

Artero, E.G., España-Romero, V., Castro-Piñero, J., Ortega, F.B., Suni, J., Castillo-Garzon, M.J., et al., 2011. Reliability of field-based fitness tests in youth. International Journal of Sports Medicine 32 (3), 159-169.

Astorino, T., Rietschel, J.C., Tam, P.A., Taylor, K., Johnson, S.M., Freedman, T.P., et al., 2004. Reinvestigation of optimal duration of testing. Journal of Exercise Physiology 7 (6), 1-8.

Astorino, T.A., Schubert, M.M., Palumbo, E., Stirling, D., McMillan, D.W., Cooper, C., et al., 2013. Magnitude and time course of changes in maximal oxygen uptake in response to distinct regimens of chronic interval training in sedentary women. European Journal of Applied Physiology 113 (9), 2361-2369.

Astrand, P.O., Ryhming, I., 1954. A nomogram for calculation of aerobic capacity (physical fitness) from pulse rate during submaximal work. Journal of Applied Physiology 7, 218-221.

Atkinson, G., Davison, R., Jeukendrup, A., Passfield, L., 2003. Science and cycling: current knowledge and future directions for research. Journal of Sports Science 21 (9), 767-787.

Bangsbo, J., Hansen, P.R., Dvorak, J., Krustrup, P., 2015. Recreational football for disease prevention and treatment in untrained men: a narrative review examining cardiovascular health, lipid profile, body composition, muscle strength and functional capacity. British Journal of Sports Medicine 49 (9), 568-576.

Barbieri, R., Barbieri, F., Milioni, F., Dos-Santos, J., Soares, M., Zagatto, A., et al., 2017. Reliability and validity of a new specific field test of aerobic capacity with the ball for futsal players. International Journal of Sports Medicine 38 (3), 233-240.

Barnes, K.R., Kilding, A.E., 2015. Running economy: measurement, norms, and determining factors. Sports Medicine Open 1, 8.

Bassett, D.R., Howley, E.T., 1997. Maximal oxygen uptake: "classical" versus "contemporary" viewpoints. Medicine and Science in Sports and Exercise 29 (5), 591-603.

Bassett, D.R., Howley, E.T., 2000. Limiting factors for maximum oxygen uptake and determinants of endurance performance. Medicine and Science in Sports and Exercise 32 (1), 70-84.

Batista, M.B., Romanzini, C.L.P., Castro-Piñero, J., Vaz Ronque, E.R., 2017. Validity of field tests to estimate cardiorespiratory fitness in children and adolescents: a systematic review. Revista Paulista de Pediatria 35 (2), 222-233.

Bell, W., Cooper, S.M., Cobner, D., Longville, J., 1994. Physiological changes arising from a training programme in under-21 international netball players. Ergonomics 37 (1), 149-157.

Beltz, N.M., Gibson, A.L., Janot, J.M., Kravitz, L., Mermier, C.M., Dalleck, L.C., et al., 2016. Graded exercise testing protocols for the determination of: historical perspectives, progress, and future considerations. Journal of Sports Medicine. https://doi.org/10.1155/2016/3968393.

Bennett, H., Davison, K., Parfitt, G., Eston, R., 2016a. Validity of a perceptually-regulated step test protocol for assessing cardiorespiratory fitness in healthy adults. European Journal of Applied Physiology 116 (11-12), 2337-2344.

Bennett, H., Parfitt, G., Davison, K., Eston, R., 2016b. Validity of submaximal step tests to estimate maximal oxygen uptake in healthy adults. Sports Medicine 46 (5), 737-750.

Betik, A.C., Hepple, R.T., 2008. Determinants of decline with aging: an integrated perspective. Applied Physiology, Nutrition and Metabolism 33 (1), 130-140.

Billat, L.V., Koralsztein, J.P., 1996. Significance of the velocity at and time to exhaustion at this velocity. Sports Medicine 22 (2), 90-108.

Björkman, F., Ekblom-Bak, E., Ekblom, O., Ekblom, B., 2016. Validity of the revised Ekblom Bak cycle ergometer test in adults. European Journal of Applied Physiology 116, 1627-1638.

Bjorntorp, P., 1991. Importance of fat as a support nutrient for energy: metabolism of athletes. Journal of Sports Science 9 (7), 1-6.

Bohr, A.D., Brown, D.D., Laurson, K.R., Smith, P.J., Bass, R.W., 2013. Relationship between socioeconomic status and physical fitness in junior high school students. Journal of School Health 83 (8), 542-547.

Borg, G.A., 1982. Psychophysical bases of perceived exertion. Medicine and Science in Sports and Exercise 14, 377-381.

Bradshaw, D.I., George, J.D., Hyde, A., LaMonte, M.J., Vehrs, P.R., Hager, R.L., et al., 2005. An accurate nonexercise regression model for 18-65-year-old adults. Research Quarterly for Exercise and Sport 76 (4), 426-432.

Bray, M.S., Hagberg, J.M., Pérusse, L., Rankinen, T., Roth, S.M., Wolfarth, B., et al., 2009. The human gene map for performance and health-related fitness phenotypes: the 2006–2007 update. Medicine and Science in Sports and Exercise 41 (1), 35-73.

Brewer, J., Davis, J., 1995. Applied physiology of rugby league. Sports Medicine 20 (3), 129-135.

Brisswalter, J., Hausswirth, C., Smith, D., Vercruyssen, F., Vallier, J.M., 2000. Energetically optimal cadence vs. freely-chosen cadence during cycling: effect of exercise duration. International Journal of Sports Medicine 21 (1), 60-64.

Brooks, D., Solway, S., Weinacht, K., Wang, D., Thomas, S., 2003. Comparison between an indoor and an outdoor 6-minute walk test among individuals with chronic obstructive pulmonary disease. Archives of Physical Medicine and Rehabilitation 84 (6), 873-876.

Buckley, J.P., Sim, J., Eston, R.G., Hession, R., Fox, R., 2004. Reliability and validity of measures taken during the Chester step test to predict aerobic power and to prescribe aerobic exercise. British Journal of Sports Medicine 38, 197-205.

Burgess, D.J., Naughton, G.A., 2010. Talent development in adolescent team sports: a review. International Journal of Sports Physiology and Performance 5 (1), 103-116.

Burgomaster, K.A., Howarth, K.R., Phillips, S.M., Rakobowchuk, M., Macdonald, M.J., McGee, S.L., et al., 2008. Similar metabolic adaptations during exercise after low volume sprint interval and traditional endurance training in humans. Journal of Physiology 586 (1), 151-160.

Butts, N.K., Henry, B.A., Mclean, D., 1991. Correlations between and performance times of recreational triathletes. Journal of Sports Medicine and Physical Fitness 31 (3), 339-344.

Cao, Z.B., Miyatake, N., Aoyama, T., Higuchi, M., Tabata, I., 2013. Prediction of maximal oxygen uptake from a 3-minute walk based on gender, age, and body composition. Journal of Physical Activity and Health 10 (2), 280-287.

Capostagno, B., Lambert, M.I., Lamberts, R.P., 2016. Systematic review of submaximal cycle tests to predict, monitor and optimize cycling performance. International Journal of Sports Physiology and Performance 11 (6), 707-714.

Caputo, F., Denadai, B.S., 2004. Effects of aerobic endurance training status and specificity on oxygen uptake kinetics during maximal exercise. European Journal of Applied Physiology 93 (1-2), 87-95.

Carnethon, M.R., Gulati, M., Greenland, P., 2005. Prevalence and cardiovascular disease correlates of low cardiorespiratory fitness in adolescents and adults. The Journal of the American Medical Association 294 (23), 2981-2988.

Castagna, C., Iellamo, F., Impellizzeri, F.M., Manzi, V., 2014. Validity and reliability of the 45-15 test for aerobic fitness in young soccer players. International Journal of Sports Physiology and Performance 9 (3), 525-531.

Castro-Piñero, J., Artero, E.G., España-Romero, V., Ortega, F.B., Sjöström, M., Suni, J., et al., 2010. Criterion-related validity of field-based fitness tests in youth: a systematic review. British Journal of Sports Medicine 44 (13), 934-943.

Chidnok, W., Dimenna, F.J., Bailey, S.J., Burnley, M., Wilkerson, D.P., Vanhatalo, A., et al., 2013. is not altered by self-pacing during incremental exercise. European Journal of Applied Physiology 113 (2), 529-539.

Chodzko-Zajko, W.J., Proctor, D.N., Fiatarone Singh, M.A., Minson, C.T., Nigg, C.R., Salem, G.J., et al., 2009. American College of Sports Medicine position stand. Exercise and physical activity for older adults. Medicine and Science in Sports and Exercise 41 (7), 1510-1530.

Clausen, J.P., 1977. Effect of physical training on cardiovascular adjustments to exercise in man. Physiological Reviews 57 (4), 779-815.

Cochran, A.J., Percival, M.E., Tricarico, S., Little, J.P., Cermak, N., Gillen, J.B., et al., 2014. Intermittent and continuous high-intensity exercise training induce similar acute but different chronic muscle adaptations. Experimental Physiology 99 (5), 782-791.

Costill, D., Fink, W.J., Pollock, M.L., 1976. Muscle fiber composition and enzyme activities of elite distance runners. Medicine and Science in Sports and Exercise 8, 96-100.

Cox, M.H., Miles, D.S., Verde, T.J., Rhodes, E.C., 1995. Applied physiology of ice hockey. Sports Medicine 19 (3), 184-201.

Coyle, E.F., 1995. Integration of the physiological factors determining endurance performance ability. Exercise and Sports Science Reviews 23, 25-63.

Craig, C.L., Marshall, A.L., Sjostrom, M., Bauman, A., Booth, M.L., Ainsworth, B.E., et al., 2003. International Physical Activity Questionnaire: 12-country reliability and validity. Medicine and Science in Sports and Exercise 35, 1381-1395.

Crust, L., Clough, P.J., 2005. Relationship between mental toughness and physical endurance. Perception and Motor Skills 100 (1), 192-194.

Da Silva, J.F., Guglielmo, L.G., Carminatti, L.J., De Oliveira, F.R., Dittrich, N., Paton, C.D., et al., 2011. Validity and reliability of a new field test (Carminatti's test) for soccer players compared with laboratory-based measures. Journal of Sports Science 29 (15), 1621-1628.

Davies, R.C., Rowlands, A.V., Eston, R.G., 2008. The prediction of maximal oxygen uptake from submaximal ratings of perceived exertion elicited during the multistage fitness test. British Journal of Sports Medicine 42 (12), 1006-1010.

Dishman, R.K., 2001. The problem exercise adherence: fighting sloth in nations with market economics. Quest 53, 279-294.

Duncan, G.E., Howley, E.T., Johnson, B.N., 1997. Applicability of criteria: discontinuous versus continuous protocols. Medicine and Science in Sports and Exercise 29 (2), 273-278.

Duncan, G.E., Li, S.M., Zhou, X.H., 2005. Cardiovascular fitness among U.S. adults: NHANES 1999–2000 and 2001–2002. Medicine and Science in Sports and Exercise 37 (8), 1324-1328.

Duthie, G.1, Pyne, D., Hooper, S., 2003. Applied physiology and game analysis of rugby union. Journal of Sports Medicine 33 (13), 973-991.

Edvardsen, E., Hem, E., Anderssen, S.A., 2014. End criteria for reaching maximal oxygen uptake must be strict and adjusted to sex and age: a cross-sectional study. PLoS One 9 (1), e85276.

Eime, R.M., Charity, M.J., Harvey, J.T., Payne, W.R., 2015a. Participation in sport and physical activity: associations with socio-economic status and geographical remoteness. BMC Public Health 15, 434.

Eime, R.M., Harvey, J., Charity, M.J., Casey, M., Westerbeek, H., Payne, W.R., et al., 2017. The relationship of sport participation to provision of sports facilities and socioeconomic status: a geographical analysis. Australian and New Zealand Journal of Public Health 41 (3), 248-255.

Eime, R.M., Harvey, J.T., Charity, M.J., Casey, M.M., van Uffelen, J.G.Z., Payne, W.R., et al., 2015b. The contribution of sport participation to overall health enhancing physical activity levels in Australia: a population-based study. BMC Public Health 15, 806.

Ekblom-Bak, E., Björkman, F., Hellenius, M.L., Ekblom, B., 2012. A new submaximal cycle ergometer test for prediction of. Scandinavian Journal of Medicine and Science in Sports 24 (2), 319-326.

Eniseler, N., 2005. Heart rate and blood lactate concentrations as predictors of physiological load on elite soccer players during various soccer training activities. Journal of Strength and Conditioning Research 19 (4), 799-804.

Evans, H.J.L., Ferrar, K.E., Smith, A.E., Parfitta, G., Eston, R.G., 2015. A systematic review of methods to predict maximal oxygen uptake from submaximal, open circuit spirometry in healthy adults. Journal of Science and Medicine in Sport 18, 183-188.

Faude, O., Kindermann, W., Meyer, T., 2009. Lactate threshold concepts: how valid are they? Sports Medicine 39 (6), 469-490.

Fernandez, J., 2005. Specific field tests for tennis players. Medicine and Science in Tennis 10, 22-23.

Fitchett, M.A., 1985. Predictability of from submaximal cycle ergometer and bench stepping tests. British Journal of Sports Medicine 19, 85-88.

Flouris, A.D., Metsios, G.S., Koutedakis, Y., 2005. Enhancing the efficacy of the 20 m multistage shuttle run test. British Journal of Sports Medicine 39 (3), 166-170.

Flouris, A.D., Metsios, G.S., Famisis, K., Geladas, N., Koutedakis, Y., 2009. Prediction of from a new field test based on portable indirect calorimetry. Journal of Science and Medicine in Sport 13 (1), 70-73.

Fotheringham, I., Meakin, G., Punekar, Y.S., Riley, J.H., Cockle, S.M., Singh, S.J., et al., 2015. Comparison of laboratory- and field-based exercise tests for COPD: a systematic review. International Journal of Chronic Obstructive Pulmonary Disease 10, 625-643.

Freeman, W., Williams, C., Nute, M.G., 1990. Endurance running performance in athletes with asthma. Journal of Sports Science 8 (2), 103-117.

Fulton, S.K., Pyne, D.B., Hopkins, W.G., Burkett, B., 2010. Training characteristics of paralympic swimmers. Journal of Strength and Conditioning Research 24 (2), 471-478.

Gabbett, T.J., Stein, J.G., Kemp, J.G., Lorenzen, C., 2013. Relationship between tests of physical qualities and physical match performance in elite rugby league players. Journal of Strength and Conditioning Research 27 (6), 1539-1545.

Garatachea, N., Cavalcanti, E., García-López, D., González-Gallego, J., de Paz, J.A., 2007. Estimation of energy expenditure in healthy adults from the YMCA submaximal cycle ergometer test. Evaluation and the Health Professions 30 (2), 138-149.

Garnacho-Castaño, M.V., Domínguez, R., Muñoz González, A., Feliu-Ruano, R., Serra-Payá, N., Maté-Muñoz, J.L., et al., 2018. Exercise prescription using the Borg rating of perceived exertion to improve fitness. International Journal of Sports Medicine 39 (2), 115-123.

George, J.D., 1996. Alternative approach to maximal exercise testing and prediction in college students. Research Quarterly for Exercise and Sport 67 (4), 452-457.

Ghosh, A.K., 2004. Anaerobic threshold: its concept and role in endurance sport. Malaysian Journal of Medical Sciences 11 (1), 24-36.

Gibala, M.J., Little, J.P., van Essen, M., Wilkin, G.P., Burgomaster, K.A., Safdar, A., et al., 2006. Short-term sprint interval versus traditional endurance training: similar initial adaptations in human skeletal muscle and exercise performance. Journal of Physiology 575 (3), 901-911.

Gim, M.N., Choi, J.H., 2016. The effects of weekly exercise time on and resting metabolic rate in normal adults. Journal of Physical Therapy Science 28 (4), 1359-1363.

Gist, N.H., Fedewa, M.V., Dishman, R.K., Cureton, K.J., 2014. Sprint interval training effects on aerobic capacity: a systematic review and meta-analysis. Sport Medicine 44 (2), 269-279.

González-Haro, C., Galilea, P.A., Drobnic, F., Escanero, J.F., 2007. Validation of a field test to determine the maximal aerobic power in triathletes and endurance cyclists. British Journal of Sports Medicine 41 (3), 174-179.

Goosey-Tolfrey, V.L., Leicht, C.A., 2013. Field-based physiological testing of wheelchair athletes. Sports Medicine 43 (2), 77-91.

Goosey-Tolfrey, V.L., Sindall, P., 2007. The effects of arm crank strategy on physiological responses and mechanical efficiency during submaximal exercise. Journal of Sports Science 25 (4), 453-460.

Goulet, E.D., 2012. Dehydration and endurance performance in competitive athletes. Nutrition Reviews 70 (2), S132-S136.

Grant, J.A., Joseph, A.M., Campagna, P.D., 1999. The prediction of: a comparison of 7 indirect tests of aerobic power. Journal of Strength and Conditioning Research 13 (4), 346-352.

Hagan, R.D., Smith, M.G., Gettman, L.R., 1981. Marathon performance in relation to maximal aerobic power and training indices. Medicine and Science in Sports and Exercise 13 (3), 185-189.

Hagan, R.D., Upton, S.J., Duncan, J.J., Gettman, L.R., 1987. Marathon performance in relation to maximal aerobic power and training indices in female distance runners. British Journal of Sports Medicine 21 (1), 3-7.

Hamlin, M.J., Draper, N., Blackwell, G., Shearman, J.P., Kimber, N.E., 2012. Determination of maximal oxygen uptake using the Bruce or a novel athlete-led protocol in a mixed population. Journal of Human Kinetics 31, 97-104.

Hanley, B., 2015. Pacing profiles and pack running at the IAAF World Half Marathon Championships. Journal of Sports Science 33 (11), 1189-1195.

Hansen, E.A., 2015. On voluntary rhythmic leg movement behaviour and control during pedalling. Acta Physiologica 214 (702), 1-18.

Hansen, E.A., Smith, G., 2009. Factors affecting cadence choice during submaximal cycling and cadence influence on performance. International Journal of Sports Physiology and Performance 4 (1), 3-17.

Hartung, G.H., Krock, L.P., Crandall, C.G., Bisson, R.U., Myhre, L.G., 1993. Prediction of maximal oxygen uptake from submaximal exercise testing in aerobically fit and non-fit men. Aviation Space and Environmental Medicine 64 (8), 735-740.

Haskell, W.L., 1994. Health consequences of physical activity: understanding and challenges regarding dose-response. Medicine and Science in Sports and Exercise 26, 649-660.

Haugen, T.A., Tønnessen, E., Hem, E., Leirstein, S., Seiler, S., 2014. characteristics of elite female soccer players, 1989-2007. International Journal of Sports Physiology and Performance 9 (3), 515-521.

Hauschild, V.D., DeGroot, D.W., Hall, S.M., Grier, T.L., Deaver, K.D., Hauret, K.G., et al., 2017. Fitness tests and occupational tasks of military interest: a systematic review of correlations. Occupational and Environmental Medicine 74 (2), 144-153.

Hawkins, M.N., Raven, P.B., Snell, P.G., Stray-Gundersen, J., Levine, B.D., 2007. Maximal oxygen uptake as a parametric measure of cardiorespiratory capacity. Medicine and Science in Sports and Exercise 39 (1), 103-107.

Hazell, T.J., Macpherson, R.E., Gravelle, B.M., Lemon, P.W., 2010. 10 or 30-s sprint interval training bouts enhance both aerobic and anaerobic performance. European Journal of Applied Physiology 110 (1), 153-160.

Helgerud, J., Rodas, G., Kemi, O.J., Hoff, J., 2011. Strength and endurance in elite football players. International Journal of Sports Medicine 32 (9), 677-682.

Heyward, V.H., Gibson, A.L., 2014. Advanced Fitness Assessment and Exercise Prescription, seventh ed. Human Kinetics, Champaign, IL.

Higham, D.G., Pyne, D.B., Anson, J.M., Eddy, A., 2013. Physiological, anthropometric, and performance characteristics of rugby sevens players. International Journal of Sports Physiology and Performance 8 (1), 19-27.

Hill, A.V., Lupton, H., 1923. Muscular exercise, lactic acid, and the supply and utilization of oxygen. QJM. An International Journal of Medicine 16 (62), 135-171.

Hill, D.W., Rowell, A.L., 1996. Running velocity at. Medicine and Science in Sports and Exercise 28 (1), 114-119.

Hoff, J., 2005. Training and testing physical capacities for elite soccer players. Journal of Sports Science 23 (6), 573-582.

Howley, E.T., Bassett Jr., D.R., Welch, H.G., 1995. Criteria for maximal oxygen uptake: review and commentary. Medicine and Science in Sports and Exercise 27 (9), 1292-1301.

Hrysomallis, C., 2011. Balance ability and athletic performance. Journal of Sports Medicine 41 (3), 221-232.

Huang, G., Wang, R., Chen, P., Huang, S.C., Donnelly, J.E., Mehlferber, J.P., et al., 2016. Dose-response relationship of cardiorespiratory fitness adaptation to controlled endurance training in sedentary older adults. European Journal of Preventative Cardiology 23 (5), 518-529.

Huggett, D.L., Connelly, D.M., Overend, T.J., 2005. Maximal aerobic capacity testing of older adults: a critical review. Journal of Gerontology 60A (1), 57-66.

Iaia, F.M., Bangsbo, J., 2010. Speed endurance training is a powerful stimulus for physiological adaptations and performance improvements of athletes. Scandinavian Journal of Medicine and Science in Sports 20 (S2), 11-23.

Ishak, A., Hashim, H.A., Krasilshchikov, O., 2016. The effects of modified exponential tapering technique on perceived exertion, heart rate, time trial performance, and power output among highly trained junior cyclists. Journal of Sports Medicine and Physical Fitness 56 (9), 961-967.

Islam, H., Townsend, L.K., Hazell, T.J., 2017. Modified sprint interval training protocols. Part I: physiological responses. Applied Physiology, Nutrition and Metabolism 42 (4), 339-346.

Jackson, A.S., Blair, S.N., Maher, M.T., Wier, L.T., Ross, R.M., Stuteville, J.E., et al., 1990. Prediction of functional aerobic capacity without exercise testing. Medicine and Science in Sports and Exercise 22, 863-870.

Jamnick, N.A., By, S., Pettitt, C.D., Pettitt, R.W., 2016. Comparison of the YMCA and a custom submaximal exercise test for determining. Medicine and Science in Sports and Exercise 48 (2), 254-259.

Jenkins, S., Čečins, N., 2011. Six-minute walk test: observed adverse events and oxygen desaturation in a large cohort of patients with chronic lung disease. International Medicine Journal 41 (5), 416-422.

Jones, A.M., Doust, J.H., 1996. A 1% treadmill grade most accurately reflects the energetic cost of outdoor running. Journal of Sports Science 14 (4), 321-327.

Jones, A.M., Vanhatalo, A., Burnley, M., Morton, R.H., Poole, D.C., 2010. Critical power: implications for determination of and exercise tolerance. Medicine and Science in Sports and Exercise 42 (10), 1876-1890.

Joyner, M.J., Coyle, E.F., 2008. Endurance exercise performance: the physiology of champions. Journal of Physiology 586 (1), 35-44.

Kaminsky, L.A., Arena, R., Beckie, T.M., Brubaker, P.H., Church, T.S., Forman, D.E., et al., 2013. The importance of cardiorespiratory fitness in the United States: the need for a national registry: a policy statement from the American Heart Association. Circulation 127, 652-662.

Karsten, B., Jobson, S.A., Hopker, J., Jimenez, A., Beedie, C., 2014. High agreement between laboratory and field estimates of critical power in cycling. International Journal of Sports Medicine 35 (4), 298-303.

Karusisi, N., Thomas, F., Méline, J., Chaix, B., 2013. Spatial accessibility to specific sport facilities and corresponding sport practice: the RECORD Study. International Journal of Behavioural Nutrition and Physical Activity 20, 10-48.

Kavcic, I., Milic, R., Jourkesh, M., Ostojic, S.M., Ozkol, M.Z., 2012. Comparative study of measured and predicted during a multi-stage fitness test with junior soccer players. Kinesiology 44 (1), 18-23.

Keren, G., Magazanik, A., Epstein, Y., 1980. A comparison of various methods for the determination of. European Journal of Applied Physiology and Occupational Physiology 45 (2-3), 117-124.

Keteyian, S.J., Brawner, C.A., Savage, P.D., Ehrman, J.K., Schairer, J., Divine, G., et al., 2008. Peak aerobic capacity predicts prognosis in patients with coronary heart disease. American Heart Journal 156, 292-300.

Kline, G.M., Porcari, J.P., Hintermeister, R., Freedson, P.S., Ward, A., McCarron, R.F., et al., 1987. Estimation of from a one mile track walk, gender, age and body weight. Medicine and Science in Sports and Exercise 19, 253-259.

Kodama, S., Saito, K., Tanaka, S., Maki, M., Yachi, Y., Asumi, M., et al., 2009. Cardiorespiratory fitness as a quantitative predictor of all-cause mortality and cardiovascular events in healthy men and women. The Journal of the American Medical Association 301, 2024-2035.

Kovacs, M.S., 2006. Applied physiology of tennis performance. British Journal of Sports Medicine 40 (5), 381-386.

Krustrup, P., Mohr, M., Amstrup, T., Rysgaard, T., Johansen, J., Steensberg, A., et al., 2003. The Yo-Yo intermittent recovery test: physiological response, reliability, and validity. Medicine and Science in Sports and Exercise 35 (4), 697-705.

Krustrup, P., Mohr, M., Nybo, L., Jensen, J.M., Nielsen, J.J., Bangsbo, J., et al., 2006. The Yo-Yo IR2 test: physiological response, reliability, and application to elite soccer. 48. Medicine and Science in Sports and Exercise 38 (9), 1666-1673.

Kubukeli, Z.N., Noakes, T.D., Dennis, S.C., 2002. Training techniques to improve endurance exercise performances. Sports Medicine 32 (8), 489-509.

Kyröläinen, H., Komi, P.V., Belli, A., 1995. Mechanical efficiency in athletes during running. Scandinavian Journal of Medicine and Science in Sports 5 (4), 200-208.

Lambert, M.I., Borresen, J., 2010. Measuring training load in sports. International Journal of Sports Physiology and Performance 5 (3), 406-411.

Lamberts, R.P., 2014. Predicting cycling performance in trained to elite male and female cyclists. 223. International Journal of Sports Physiology and Performance 9 (4), 610-614.

Lamberts, R.P., Swart, J., Noakes, T.D., Lambert, M.I., 2011. A novel submaximal cycle test to monitor fatigue and predict cycling performance. British Journal of Sports Medicine 45 (10), 797-804.

Larsen, G.E., George, J.D., Alexander, J.L., Fellingham, G.W., Aldana, S.G., Parcell, A.C., et al., 2002. Prediction of maximum oxygen consumption from walking, jogging, or running. Research Quarterly for Exercise and Sport 73 (1), 66-72.

Lech, G., Jaworski, J., Lyakh, V., Krawczyk, R., 2011. Effect of the level of coordinated motor abilities on performance in junior judokas. Journal of Human Kinetics 30, 153-160.

Lee, D., Artero, E.G., Sui, X., Blair, S.N., 2010. Mortality trends in the general population: the importance of cardiorespiratory fitness. Psychopharmacology 24 (4), 27-35.

Lee, I.M., Paffenbarger Jr., R.S., 1998. Physical activity and stroke incidence: the Harvard Alumni Health Study. Stroke 29 (10), 2049-2054.

Lee, I.M., Paffenbarger Jr., R.S., 2000. Associations of light, moderate, and vigorous intensity physical activity with longevity. The Harvard Alumni Health Study. American Journal of Epidemiology 151 (3), 293-299.

Lee, I.M., Skerrett, P.J., 2001. Physical activity and all-cause mortality: what is the dose–response relation? Medicine and Science in Sports and Exercise 33 (S6), 459-471.

Lee, I.M., Hsieh, C.C., Paffenbarger Jr., R.S., 1995. Exercise intensity and longevity in men. The Harvard Alumni Health Study. The Journal of the American Medical Association 273 (15), 1179-1184.

Lee, J.M., Bassett Jr., D.R., Thompson, D.L., Fitzhugh, E.C., 2011. Validation of the Cosmed Fitmate for prediction of maximal oxygen consumption. Journal of Strength and Conditioning Research 25 (9), 2573-2579.

Legaz Arrese, A., Serrano Ostáriz, E., Casajús Mallén, J.A., Munguía Izquierdo, D., 2005. The changes in running performance and maximal oxygen uptake after long-term training in elite athletes. Journal of Sports Medicine and Physical Fitness 45 (4), 435-440.

Léger, L.A., 1982. A maximal multistage 20-m shuttle run test to predict. European Journal of Applied Physiology and Occupational Physiology 49 (1), 1-12.

Lindberg, A.S., Oksa, J., Malm, C., 2014. Laboratory or field tests for evaluating firefighters' work capacity? PLoS One 9 (3), e91215.

Lindberg, A.S., Oksa, J., Gavhed, D., Malm, C., 2013. Field tests for evaluating the aerobic work capacity of firefighters. PLoS One 8 (7), e68047.

Lindgren, M., Börjesson, M., Ekblom, Ö., Bergström, G., Lappas, G., Rosengrena, A., et al., 2016. Physical activity pattern, cardiorespiratory fitness, and socioeconomic status in the SCAPIS pilot trial: a cross-sectional study. Preventative Medicine Reports 4, 44-49.

Little, J.P., Safdar, A., Wilkin, G.P., Tarnopolsky, M.A., Gibala, M.J., 2010. A practical model of low-volume high-intensity interval training induces mitochondrial biogenesis in human skeletal muscle: potential mechanisms. Journal of Physiology 588 (6), 1011-1022.

Loftin, M., Sothern, M., Warren, B., Udall, J., 2004. Comparison of during treadmill and cycle ergometry in severely overweight youth. Journal of Sports Science and Medicine 3 (4), 554-560.

Lorenz, D.S., Reiman, M.P., Lehecka, B.J., Naylor, A., 2013. What performance characteristics determine elite versus nonelite athletes in the same sport? Sports Health 5 (6), 542-547.

MacAuley, D., McCrum, E.E., Stott, G., Evans, A.E., Gamble, R.P., McRoberts, B., et al., 1998. Levels of physical activity, physical fitness and their relationship in the Northern Ireland Health and Activity Survey. International Journal of Sports Medicine 19 (7), 503-511.

Macfarlane, D.J., 2001. Automated metabolic gas analysis systems: a review. Journal of Sports Medicine 31 (12), 841-861.

Macpherson, R.E., Hazell, T.J., Olver, T.D., Paterson, D.H., Lemon, P.W., 2011. Run sprint interval training improves aerobic performance but not maximal cardiac output. Medicine and Science in Sports and Exercise 43 (1), 115-122.

Malek, M.H., Housh, T.J., Berger, D.E., Coburn, J.W., Beck, T.W., 2005. A new non-exercise-based prediction equation for aerobically trained men. Journal of Strength and Conditioning Research 19 (3), 559-565.

Malek, M.H., Housh, T.J., Berger, D.E., Coburn, J.W., Beck, T.W., 2004. A new nonexercise-based equation for aerobically trained females. Medicine and Science in Sports and Exercise 36 (10), 1804-1810.

Marsh, A.P., Martin, P.E., 1997. Effect of cycling experience, aerobic power, and power output on preferred and most economical cycling cadences. Medicine and Science in Sports and Exercise 29 (9), 1225-1232.

Marszalek, J., Molik, B., Gomez, M.A., Skučas, K., Lencse-Mucha, J., Rekowski, W., et al., 2015. Relationships between anaerobic performance, field tests and game performance of sitting volleyball players. Journal of Human Kinetics 48, 25-32.

Mayorga-Vega, D., Bocanegra-Parrilla, R., Ornelas, M., Viciana, J., 2016. Criterion-related validity of the distance- and time-based walk/run field tests for estimating cardiorespiratory fitness: a systematic review and meta-analysis. PLoS One 11 (3), e0151671.

McConnell, T.R., 1988. Practical considerations in the testing of in runners. Journal of Sports Medicine 5 (1), 57-68.

McKay, G.A., Bannister, E.W., 1976. A comparison of maximum oxygen uptake determination by bicycle ergometry at various pedaling frequencies and by treadmill running at various speeds. European Journal of Applied Physiology 35, 191-200.

McKie, G.L., Islam, H., Townsend, L.K., Robertson-Wilson, J., Eys, M., Hazell, T.J., et al., 2018. Modified sprint interval training protocols: physiological and psychological responses to four weeks of training. Applied Physiology, Nutrition and Metabolism 43 (6), 595-601.

Meinild Lundby, A.K., Jacobs, R.A., Gehrig, S., de Leur, J., Hauser, M., Bonne, T.C., et al., 2018. Exercise training increases skeletal muscle mitochondrial volume density by enlargement of existing mitochondria and not de novo biogenesis. Acta Physiologica 222 (1), e12976.

Metaxas, T., Koutlianos, N., Sendelides, T., Mandrouka, A., 2009. Preseason physiological profile of soccer and basketball players in different divisions. 182. Journal of Strength and Conditioning Research 23 (6), 1704-1713.

Metaxas, T.I., Koutlianos, N.A., Kouidi, E.J., Deligiannis, A.P., 2005. Comparative study of field and laboratory tests for the evaluation of aerobic capacity in soccer players. Journal of Strength and Conditioning Research 19 (1), 79-84.

Metsios, G.S., Flouris, A.D., Koutedakis, Y., Nevill, A., 2008. Criterion-related validity and test-retest reliability of the 20-m square shuttle test. Journal of Science and Medicine in Sport 2008 11 (2), 214-217.

Metsios, G.S., Flouris, A.D., Koutedakis, Y., Theodorakis, Y., 2006. The effect of performance feedback on cardiorespiratory fitness field tests. Journal of Science and Medicine in Sport 9 (3), 263-266.

Michaelides, M.A., Parpa, K.M., Henry, L.J., Thompson, G.B., Brown, B.S., 2011. Assessment of physical fitness aspects and their relationship to firefighters' job abilities. Journal of Strength and Conditioning Research 25 (4), 956-965.

Midgley, A.W., Carroll, S., 2009. Emergence of the verification phase procedure for confirming 'true'. Scandinavian Journal of Medicine and Science in Sports 19 (3), 313-322.

Midgley, A.W., Earle, K., McNaughton, L.R., Siegler, J.C., Clough, P., Earle, F., et al., 2017. Exercise tolerance during testing is a multifactorial psychobiological phenomenon. Research in Sports Medicine 25 (4), 480-494.

Mier, C.M., Alexander, R.P., Mageean, A.L., 2012. Achievement of criteria during a continuous graded exercise test and a verification stage performed by college athletes. Journal of Strength and Conditioning Research 26 (10), 2648-2654.

Milanović, Z., Pantelić, S., Čović, N., Sporiš, G., Krustrup, P., 2015a. Is recreational soccer effective for improving? A systematic review and meta-analysis. Journal of Sports Medicine 45 (9), 1339-1353.

Milanović, Z., Pantelić, S., Sporiš, G., Mohr, M., Krustrup, P., 2015b. Health-related physical fitness in healthy untrained men: effects on, jump performance and flexibility of soccer and moderate-intensity continuous running. PLoS One 10 (8), e0135319.

Milanović, Z., Sporiš, G., Weston, M., 2015c. Effectiveness of high-intensity interval training (HIT) and continuous endurance training for improvements: a systematic review and meta-analysis of controlled trials. Journal of Sports Medicine 45 (10), 1469-1481.

Miller, D.K., Kieffer, H.S., Kemp, H.E., Torres, S.E., 2011. Off-season physiological profiles of elite National Collegiate Athletic Association Division III male soccer players. Journal of Strength and Conditioning Research 25 (6), 1508-1513.

Millet, G.P., Vleck, V.E., Bentley, D.J., 2009. Physiological differences between cycling and running: lessons from triathletes. Journal of Sports Medicine 39 (3), 179-206.

Moffatt, R.J., Chitwood, L.F., Biggerstaff, K.D., 1994. The influence of verbal encouragement during assessment of maximal oxygen uptake. Journal of Sports Medicine and Physical Fitness 34 (1), 45-49.

Moore, A., Murphy, A., 2003. Development of an anaerobic capacity test for field sport athletes. Journal of Science and Medicine in Sport 6 (3), 275-284.

Munoz, I., Seiler, S., Alcocer, A., Carr, N., Esteve-Lanao, J., 2015. Specific intensity for peaking: is race pace the best option? Asian Journal of Sports Medicine 6 (3), e24900.

Myers, J., Kaminsky, L.A., Lima, R., Christle, J.W., Ashley, E., Arena, R., et al., 2017. A reference equation for normal standards for: analysis from the Fitness Registry and the Importance of Exercise National Database (FRIEND Registry). Progress in Cardiovascular Diseases 60 (1), 21-29.

Myers, J., Prakash, M., Froelicher, V., Do, D., Partington, S., Atwood, J.E., et al., 2002. Exercise capacity and mortality among men referred for exercise testing. New England Journal of Medicine 346, 793-801.

Nakagaichi, M., Lee, M.S., Tanaka, K., 2001. Accuracy of two simple methods for the assessment of health-related physical fitness. Perception and Motor Skills 92 (1), 37-49.

Neufer, P.D., 1989. The effect of detraining and reduced training on the physiological adaptations to aerobic exercise training. Journal of Sports Medicine 8 (5), 302-320.

Ní Chéilleachair, N.J., Harrison, A.J., Warrington, G.D., 2017. HIIT enhances endurance performance and aerobic characteristics more than high-volume training in trained rowers. Journal of Sports Science 35 (11), 1052-1058.

Nieman, D.C., Lasasso, H., Austin, M.D., Pearce, S., McInnis, T., Unick, J., et al., 2007. Validation of Cosmed's FitMate in measuring exercise metabolism. Research in Sports Medicine 15 (1), 67-75.

Noakes, T.D., 1998. Maximal oxygen uptake: "classical" versus "contemporary" viewpoints: a rebuttal. Medicine and Science in Sports and Exercise 30 (9), 1381-1398.

Noakes, T.D., 2008. How did A V Hill understand the and the "plateau phenomenon"? Still no clarity? British Journal of Sports Medicine 42 (7), 574-580.

Nordgren, B., Fridén, C., Jansson, E., Österlund, T., Wilhelmus, J.G., Opava, C.H., et al., 2014. Criterion validation of two submaximal aerobic fitness tests, the self-monitoring Fox-walk test and the Åstrand cycle test in people with rheumatoid arthritis. BMC Musculoskeletal Disorders 15, 305.

Oja, P., 2001. Dose response between total volume of physical activity and health and fitness. Medicine and Science in Sports and Exercise 33 (S6), 428-437.

Oppewal, A., Hilgenkamp, T.I., van Wijck, R., Evenhuis, H.M., 2013. Cardiorespiratory fitness in individuals with intellectual disabilities: a review. Research in Developmental Disabilities 34 (10), 3301-3316.

Orr, J.L., Williamson, P., Anderson, W., Ross, R., McCafferty, S., Fettes, P., et al., 2013. Cardiopulmonary exercise testing: arm crank vs cycle ergometry. Anasthesia 68 (5), 497-501.

Pallarés, J.G., Morán-Navarro, R., Ortega, J.F., Fernández-Elías, V.E., Mora-Rodriguez, R., 2016. Validity and reliability of ventilatory and blood lactate thresholds in well-trained cyclists. PLoS One 11 (9), e0163389.

Pate, R.R., Wang, C.Y., Dowda, M., Farrell, S.W., O'Neill, J.R., 2006. Cardiorespiratory fitness levels among US youth 12 to 19 years of age: findings from the 1999–2002 National Health and Nutrition Examination Survey. Archives of Paediatric and Adolescent Medicine 160 (10), 1005-1012.

Petibois, C., Déléris, G., 2003. Effects of short- and long-term detraining on the metabolic response to endurance exercise. International Journal of Sports Medicine 24 (5), 320-325.

Poole, D.C., Jones, A.M., 2012. Oxygen uptake kinetics. Comprehensive Physiology 2, 933-996.

Poole, D.C., Jones, A.M., 2017. Measurement of the maximum oxygen uptake: is no longer acceptable. Journal of Applied Physiology 122 (4), 997-1002.

Poole, D.C., Burnley, M., Vanhatalo, A., Rossiter, H.B., Jones, A.M., 2016. Critical power: an important fatigue threshold in exercise physiology. Medicine and Science in Sports and Exercise 48 (11), 2320-2334.

Poulain, M., Durand, F., Palomba, B., Ceugniet, F., Desplan, J., Varray, A., et al., 2003. 6-Minute walk testing is more sensitive than maximal incremental cycle testing for detecting oxygen desaturation in patients with COPD. Chest 123 (5), 1401-1407.

Rankovic, G., Mutavdzic, V., Toskic, D., Preljevic, A., Kocic, M., Nedin Rankovic, G., et al., 2010. Aerobic capacity as an indicator in different kinds of sports. Bosnian Journal of Basic Medical Science 10 (1), 44-48.

Ransdell, L.B., Murray, T.M., Gao, Y., 2013. Off-ice fitness of elite female ice hockey players by team success, age, and player position. Journal of Strength and Conditioning Research 27 (4), 875-884.

Reilly, T., Borrie, A., 1992. Physiology applied to field hockey. Journal of Sports Medicine 14 (1), 10-26.

Riboli, A., Cè, E., Rampichini, S., Venturelli, M., Alberti, G., Limonta, E., et al., 2017. Comparison between continuous and discontinuous incremental treadmill test to assess velocity at. Journal of Sports Medicine and Physical Fitness 57 (9), 1119-1125.

Ricci, J., Léger, L.A., 1983. of cyclists from treadmill, bicycle ergometer and velodrome tests. European Journal of Applied Physiology and Occupational Physiology 50 (2), 283-289.

Robert McComb, J.J., Roh, D., Williams, J.S., 2006. Explanatory variance in maximal oxygen uptake. Journal of Sports Science and Medicine 5 (2), 296-303.

Robison, J.I., Rogers, M.A., 1994. Adherence to exercise programmes. Recommendations. Sports Medicine 17 (1), 39-52.

Rønnestad, B.R., Hansen, J., Ellefsen, S., 2014. Block periodization of high-intensity aerobic intervals provides superior training effects in trained cyclists. Scandinavian Journal of Medicine and Science in Sports 24 (1), 34-42.

Rylands, L.P., Roberts, S.J., Hurst, H.T., 2015. Variability in laboratory vs. field testing of peak power, torque, and time of peak power production among elite bicycle motocross cyclists. Journal of Strength and Conditioning Research 29 (9), 2635-2640.

Sanders, L.F., Duncan, G.E., 2006. Population-based reference standards for cardiovascular fitness among U.S. adults: NHANES 1999–2000 and 2001–2002. Medicine and Science in Sports and Exercise 38 (4), 701-707.

Sartor, F., Vernillo, G., de Morree, H.M., Bonomi, A.G., La Torre, A., Kubis, H.P., et al., 2013. Estimation of maximal oxygen uptake via submaximal exercise testing in sports, clinical, and home settings. Journal of Sports Medicine 43 (9), 865-873.

Saunders, P.U., Pyne, D.B., Telford, R.D., Hawley, J.A., 2004. Factors affecting running economy in trained distance runners. Journal of Sports Medicine 34 (7), 465-485.

Schaun, G.Z., 2017. The maximal oxygen uptake verification phase: a light at the end of the tunnel? Sports Medicine – Open 3 (1), 44.

Schembre, S.M., Riebe, D.A., 2011. Non-exercise estimation of using the International Physical Activity Questionnaire. Measurement in Physical Education and Exercise Science 15 (3), 168-181.

Secher, N.H., Volianitis, S., 2006. Are the arms and legs in competition for cardiac output? Medicine and Science in Sports and Exercise 38 (10), 1797-1803.

Sheppard, J.M., Young, W.B., 2006. Agility literature review: classifications, training and testing. Journal of Sports Science 24 (9), 919-932.

Sjödin, B., Svedenhag, J., 1985. Applied physiology of marathon running. Journal of Sports Medicine 2 (2), 83-99.

Skelly, A.C., Dettori, J.R., Brodt, E.D., 2012. Assessing bias: the importance of considering confounding. Evidence Based Spine Care Journal 3 (1), 9-12.

Sloth, M., Sloth, D., Overgaard, K., Dalgas, U., 2013. Effects of sprint interval training on and aerobic exercise performance: a systematic review and meta-analysis. Scandinavian Journal of Medicine and Science in Sports 23 (6), 341-352.

Smirmaul, B.P.C., Bertucci, D.R., Teixeira, I.P., 2013. Is the that we measure really maximal? Frontiers in Physiology 4, 203.

Sousa, A., Rodríguez, F.A., Machado, L., Vilas-Boas, J.P., Fernandes, R.J., 2015. Exercise modality effect on oxygen uptake off-transient kinetics at maximal oxygen uptake intensity. Experimental Physiology 100 (6), 719-729.

Stamford, B.A., 1988. Exercise and the elderly. Exercise and Sports Science Reviews 16, 341-379.

Støren, Ø., Bratland-Sanda, S., Haave, M., Helgerud, J., 2012. Improved and time trial performance with more high aerobic intensity interval training and reduced training volume: a case study on an elite national cyclist. Journal of Strength and Conditioning Research 26 (10), 2705-2711.

Straub, A.M., Midgley, A.W., Zavorsky, G.S., Hillman, A.R., 2014. Ramp-incremented and RPE-clamped test protocols elicit similar values in trained cyclists. European Journal of Applied Physiology 114 (8), 1581-1590.

Suchomel, T.J., Nimphius, S., Stone, M.H., 2016. The importance of muscular strength in athletic performance. Journal of Sports Medicine 46 (10), 1419-1449.

Sykes, K., Roberts, A., 2004. The Chester step test: a simple yet effective tool for the prediction of aerobic capacity. Physiotherapy 90, 183-188.

Tabben, M., Coquart, J., Chaabène, H., Franchini, E., Chamari, K., Tourny, C., et al., 2014. Validity and reliability of new karate-specific aerobic test for karatekas. International Journal of Sports Physiology and Performance 9 (6), 953-958.

Taylor, A.W., Bachman, L., 1999. The effects of endurance training on muscle fibre types and enzyme activities. Canadian Journal of Applied Physiology 24 (1), 41-53.

Teixeira, A.S., da Silva, J.F., Carminatti, L.J., Dittrich, N., Castagna, C., Guglielmo, L.G., et al., 2014. Reliability and validity of the Carminatti's test for aerobic fitness in youth soccer players. Journal of Strength and Conditioning Research 28 (11), 3264-3273.

Tønnessen, E., Hem, E., Leirstein, S., Haugen, T., Seiler, S., 2013. Maximal aerobic power characteristics of male professional soccer players, 1989–2012. International Journal of Sports Physiology and Performance 8 (3), 323-329.

Townsend, L.K., Islam, H., Dunn, E., Eys, M., Robertson-Wilson, J., Hazell, T.J., et al., 2017. Modified sprint interval training protocols. Part II: psychological responses. Applied Physiology, Nutrition and Metabolism 42 (4), 347-353.

Tran, D., 2018. Cardiopulmonary exercise testing. Methods in Molecular Biology 67 (1735), 285-295.

van den Berg-Emons, R.J., Bussmann, J.B., Haisma, J.A., Sluis, T.A., van der Woude, L.H., Bergen, M.P., et al., 2008. A prospective study on physical activity levels after spinal cord injury during inpatient rehabilitation and the year after discharge. Archives of Physical Medicine and Rehabilitation 89, 2094-2101.

Vaz, L., Vasilica, I., Carreras, D., Kraak, W., Nakamura, F.Y., 2016. Physical fitness profiles of elite under-19 rugby union players. Journal of Sports Medicine and Physical Fitness 56 (4), 415-421.

Verberkt, C.A., Fridén, C., Grooten, W.J., Opava, C.H., 2012. Reliability of the Fox-walk test in patients with rheumatoid arthritis. Disability and Rehabilitation 34 (23), 2001-2006.

Vercruyssen, F., Brisswalter, J., 2010. Which factors determine the freely chosen cadence during submaximal cycling? Journal of Science and Medicine in Sport 13 (2), 225-231.

Wang, C.Y., Haskell, W.L., Farrell, S.W., Lamonte, M.J., Blair, S.N., Curtin, L.R., et al., 2010. Cardiorespiratory fitness levels among US adults 20–49 years of age: findings from the 1999–2004 National Health and Nutrition Examination Survey. American Journal of Epidemiology 171 (4), 426-435.

Wasserman, K., 1986. The anaerobic threshold: definition, physiological significance and identification. Advances in Cardiology 35, 1-23.

Wehrlin, J.P., Hallén, J., 2006. Linear decrease in and performance with increasing altitude in endurance athletes. European Journal of Applied Physiology 96 (4), 404-412.

Weiglein, L., Herrick, J., Kirk, S., Kirk, E.P., 2011. The 1-mile walk test is a valid predictor of and is a reliable alternative fitness test to the 1.5-mile run in U.S. Air Force males. Military Medicine 176 (6), 669-673.

Wells, C.M., Edwards, A.M., Winter, E.M., Fysh, M.L., Drust, B., 2012. Sport-specific fitness testing differentiates professional from amateur soccer players where and kinetics do not. Journal of Sports Medicine and Physical Fitness 52 (3), 245-254.

Weltman, A., Katch, V., Sady, S., 1978. Effects of increasing oxygen availability on bicycle ergometer endurance performance. Ergonomics 21 (6), 427-437.

West, C.R., Leicht, C.A., Goosey-Tolfrey, V.L., Romer, L.M., 2015. Perspective: does laboratory-based maximal incremental exercise testing elicit maximum physiological responses in highly-trained athletes with cervical spinal cord injury? Frontiers in Physiology 6, 419.

Weston, M., Taylor, K.L., Batterham, A.M., Hopkins, W.G., 2014. Effects of low-volume high-intensity interval training (HIT) on fitness in adults: a meta-analysis of controlled and non-controlled trials. Journal of Sports Medicine 44 (7), 1005-1017.

Williams, C.J., Williams, M.G., Eynon, N., Ashton, K.J., Little, J.P., Wisloff, U., et al., 2017. Genes to predict trainability: a systematic review. BMC Genomics 18 (S8), 831.

Winter, E.M., 2011. "Critical power": time to abandon. Medicine and Science in Sports and Exercise 43 (3), 552.

Wouters, M., Evenhuis, H.M., Hilgenkamp, T.I., 2017. Systematic review of field-based physical fitness tests for children and adolescents with intellectual disabilities. Research in Developmental Disabilities 61, 77-94.

Yoon, B.K., Kravitz, L., Robergs, R., 2007., protocol duration, and the plateau. Medicine and Science in Sports and Exercise 39 (7), 1186-1192.

Yoshida, T., Chida, M., Ichioka, M., Suda, Y., 1987. Blood lactate parameters related to aerobic capacity and endurance performance. European Journal of Applied Physiology and Occupational Physiology 56 (1), 7-11.

Zemková, E., 2014. Sport-specific balance. Journal of Sports Medicine 44 (5), 579-590.

Ziogas, G.G., Patras, K.N., Stergiou, N.,Georgoulis, A.D., 2011. Velocity at lactate threshold and running economy must also be considered along with maximal oxygen uptake when testing elite soccer players during preseason. Journal of Strength and Conditioning Research 25 (2), 414-419.

Capítulo | 13 |

Imagem de Ultrassonografia em Lesões na Virilha

Amanda Parry

Neste capítulo, são apresentados os tipos de lesões na virilha prevalentes em atletas profissionais, alguns dos acertos e armadilhas no uso da ultrassonografia diagnóstica (USD), como ela pode ser utilizada para ajudar no diagnóstico e quando outras modalidades de imagem são mais apropriadas. A ultrassonografia é uma modalidade que requer experiência clínica. Os resultados podem ser facilmente mal interpretados por um olho não treinado, devido à má manipulação da máquina e seus artefatos e à natureza da física da ultrassonografia. Indivíduos que aplicam ultrassonografia devem ser qualificados ou estar estudando para fazê-lo. Muitos cursos já estão disponíveis e o incentivo para a realização de um curso credenciado pelo Consórcio para o Credenciamento de Educação Sonográfica (CASE, do inglês *Accreditation of Sonographic Education*) é altamente recomendado antes de incorporar a USD na prática.

Lesões na virilha são altamente prevalentes em atletas, particularmente em esportes que envolvem corrida em alta velocidade, mudanças rápidas de direção e chutes. Atletas de elite podem ser afastados por várias semanas ou mais se não forem clara e prontamente diagnosticados, tratados e gerenciados. A dificuldade pode estar em detectar a origem e extensão exatas da lesão na virilha, pois é uma área complexa de tecido mole e anatomia óssea. O exame clínico completo é essencial e sempre a primeira linha de análise em qualquer lesão, possibilitando ao profissional da saúde restringir a área suspeita e o mecanismo da lesão. No entanto, esta não é uma tarefa simples, pois a dor na virilha pode irradiar-se de várias regiões diferentes, como lombar, abdominal, inguinal ou do quadril. Para investigação posterior, pacientes com dor na virilha são frequentemente encaminhados para ressonância magnética (RM), que tem suas vantagens e continua a ser aceita como o padrão-ouro, mas tem algumas limitações. Com os avanços na tecnologia de USD e o aumento do conhecimento e experiência dos operadores, o uso de USD por praticantes de esportes de primeira linha está mais eficaz para um diagnóstico preciso. Também está gradualmente se tornando a modalidade de imagem *inicial* de escolha para dor na virilha do atleta.

Ferramenta de exclusão

Atualmente, há pesquisas limitadas disponíveis sobre USD para a avaliação da dor na virilha do atleta. No entanto, USD é uma área de imagem que tem muitas vantagens para avaliação da virilha e seu uso é encorajado como uma ferramenta de "exclusão" antes de solicitar uma investigação mais aprofundada. Essa modalidade de imagem é móvel, o que significa que as varreduras podem ser realizadas no local, e possibilita a conferência entre vários médicos e outras pessoas envolvidas no momento da varredura.

Tempo ideal para fazer o exame

O tempo ideal para escanear lesões esportivas é geralmente entre 48 e 72 horas após a lesão. Embora haja pressões crescentes para diagnosticar jogadores imediatamente após a lesão, tanto dos próprios jogadores quanto de outras partes interessadas envolvidas com o atleta, ainda é uma prática recomendada aguardar esse período de tempo para obtenção de imagens mais precisas. Na fase aguda pós-lesão estão presentes inchaço e edema. Isso fornece uma complicação adicional para a imagem em que os tecidos superficiais têm densidade aumentada e, portanto, o feixe de ultrassonografia é atenuado (*i. e.*, enfraquecido) por meio desses tecidos, o que resulta em uma visualização mais pobre das estruturas subjacentes. Deixar que a lesão acalme de 48 a 72 horas permite uma avaliação mais precisa e dinâmica.

Se a cirurgia for considerada, o diagnóstico precoce é vantajoso. O melhor prognóstico de recuperação é registrado se a cirurgia for realizada nos estágios iniciais. O raciocínio e a justificativa por trás disso serão discutidos de maneira detalhada no Capítulo 15.

Revisão dinâmica

A USD é relativamente barata e geralmente rápida de realizar quando comparada com a RM, além de atualmente existirem aparelhos portáteis. A sonopalpação, o uso da compressão do transdutor, pode ajudar a determinar áreas de dor com relação ao que é demonstrado em uma imagem e é uma ferramenta útil para avaliar se o que é visualizado é realmente sintomático. Também permite que o clínico perceba o que acontece com a estrutura anatômica enquanto a manipulação está em andamento. A revisão dinâmica pode auxiliar no diagnóstico pela abertura de rupturas de tecidos moles, simplesmente pelo próprio movimento ou pela distensão do líquido ao mover a região afetada, ou seja, a rotação interna ou externa do quadril pode introduzir líquido em uma ruptura do tendão adutor, tornando a lesão mais óbvia. A avaliação dinâmica também ajuda a diferenciar entre rupturas de espessura total e parcial.

Rupturas de espessura total *versus* parcial

Em caso de incerteza, se uma ruptura demonstrada for de espessura parcial ou total, deve-se flexionar/estender e girar o membro afetado. Se um tendão se mover com a manipulação da área de inserção, uma ruptura de espessura total poderá ser descartada; caso contrário, uma ruptura completa será indicada. As rupturas de espessura total do tendão adutor longo são geralmente óbvias devido ao fluido livre, um vazio na aparência de ultrassonografia do padrão fibrilar e retração das fibras. Ainda assim, caso mais esclarecimentos sejam necessários, deve-se examinar a perna em uma posição neutra e em uma posição de perna de rã abduzida (abdução com rotação externa e flexão de quadril) ou em forma de quatro (lembrando a posição do teste de Patrick Fabere). A ruptura deve ser mais óbvia quando abduzida, pois a inserção do tendão foi esticada e, portanto, separará as fibras rasgadas.

Planos de imageamento

A USD tem a capacidade de escanear em qualquer plano. As estruturas devem sempre ser visualizadas, avaliadas e fotografadas em dois planos a 90° entre si, a fim de distinguir a extensão total da lesão. Ser capaz de constatar uma ruptura em todo o seu comprimento é vantajoso, mas não essencial para o diagnóstico. Uma função de campo de visão estendido está disponível na maioria das máquinas.

Acompanhamento

As varreduras de acompanhamento são rápidas, simples e de baixo custo, sem riscos para o paciente. Elas são úteis, pois medições precisas podem ser obtidas a partir de marcos consistentes, tornando-as ideais para avaliar a progressão/regressão das estruturas lesionadas.

Imageamento

Radiografias simples: ainda são úteis?

Sim. Às vezes, o simples não deve ser esquecido. Se houver suspeita de dor na virilha relacionada com o quadril (DVRQ), a radiografia ainda deve ser uma investigação de primeira linha. Embora alterações ósseas discretas sejam bem visualizadas com ultrassonografia, não é possível enxergar toda a cabeça femoral dentro da articulação, o que é vantajoso para um diagnóstico preciso. A avaliação radiográfica é essencial para confirmar o diagnóstico e excluir lesões ou distúrbios ósseos ou da articulação coxofemoral (Pesquer et al., 2015).

Tomografia computadorizada

A tomografia computadorizada (TC) geralmente não é usada para avaliação do quadril e da virilha, devido à RM ser capaz de fornecer um quadro mais completo e também à dose de radiação envolvida, especificamente na região gonadal de jovens adolescentes e adultos envolvidos no esporte profissional.

Ressonância magnética

A RM continua sendo o padrão de referência para a imagem de muitas áreas e a virilha não é exceção, especialmente ao avaliar anormalidades sutis, lesões intra-articulares e alterações ósseas, como edema de medula óssea (EMO). Também é útil nos casos em que nenhuma causa para os sintomas foi identificada, usando outras modalidades de imagem, mas os sintomas persistem. A RM é superior na identificação de anormalidades sutis, especialmente para dor na virilha relacionada ao púbis, onde pode haver envolvimento de outras estruturas, como nervos. Ela é mais precisa para demonstrar neuropatias e, se houver suspeita, recomenda-se que o paciente seja encaminhado diretamente para a RM (Boxe 13.1).

Experiência do operador

O profissional da saúde que realiza a USD é o mesmo que a relata; portanto, os resultados e a interpretação dependem muito do operador. Isso pode ser uma vantagem ou desvantagem, dependendo do conjunto de habilidades do médico. É essencial que os profissionais de saúde sejam qualificados para realizar a varredura e interpretar os resultados. É provável que haja pequenas discrepâncias entre os usuários, mas isso não deve ser significativo. O desenvolvimento profissional contínuo e a revisão/auditoria por pares podem ajudar a garantir que este seja o caso. O conhecimento anatômico é a chave para obter resultados precisos de uma ultrassonografia musculoesquelética (ME). O Boxe 13.2 fornece orientação para obter resultados ideais ao realizar a USD.

O tipo e a data de fabricação da máquina de ultrassonografia também terão impacto nos resultados obtidos. Obviamente, é preferível usar uma máquina atualizada e de alta qualidade e trabalhar em conjunto com a equipe de aplicativos para criar configurações adequadas às necessidades do seu departamento. Geralmente, para ultrassonografia ME de frequência mais alta, o transdutor linear é a sonda de escolha, devido à natureza superficial da maioria das estruturas escaneadas. No entanto, a região da virilha e do quadril podem ser a exceção, dependendo da constituição corporal do paciente. Um transdutor linear de frequência mais baixa pode ser suficiente e, em alguns casos, um transdutor curvo será necessário – porém, isso é improvável em profissionais do esporte.

Boxe 13.1 Comparação entre ressonância magnética e ultrassonografia

- *Planos de imagem*: a RM pode visualizar a anatomia em planos padrão, enquanto a ultrassonografia pode visualizar a área em quase qualquer plano
- *Posições de imagem*: a RM é realizada principalmente em posições sem apoio de peso/não provocativas, geralmente em decúbito dorsal, em comparação com a ultrassonografia na qual o paciente pode ser fotografado em uma posição que replica seus sintomas ou coloca estresse na área afetada
- *Avaliação dinâmica*: a RM é limitada a uma visão estática, enquanto a ultrassonografia possibilita a avaliação dinâmica do complexo do quadril e virilha
- *Custo e disponibilidade*: a RM é cara em comparação com o exame de ultrassonografia. Ambos estão disponíveis para atletas de elite, mas a ultrassonografia tem a vantagem de poder ser realizada no local
- *Interpretação*: a RM depende de um radiologista externo, enquanto a ultrassonografia depende de um clínico que faz parte da equipe multiprofissional.

Imagem de Ultrassonografia em Lesões na Virilha | **Capítulo** | **13** |

> **Boxe 13.2 Pontos-chave para resultados ideais ao se realizar ultrassonografia diagnóstica**
>
> - Mantenha o feixe de ultrassonografia perpendicular às fibras do tendão/músculo e aos planos da fáscia, sempre que possível. Isso possibilita melhor visualização e evita a anisotropia (um vazio artificial que é criado quando o feixe de ultrassonografia deixa de ser perpendicular ao plano de imagem desejado, isto é, fibras de tendão, que podem imitar ruptura) (Sanders, 1998). Manipule a posição do transdutor, a pressão e o agite, inclinando-o no sentido de seu eixo longo (colocando suavemente mais pressão em uma das extremidades) do transdutor para conseguir isso
> - Use uma pressão suave para ultrassonografia musculoesquelética, de modo a não comprimir fluido/rupturas ou neovascularização. No entanto, muitas vezes é necessário haver uma pressão mais forte para a região da virilha/quadril devido ao aumento da profundidade das estruturas a serem avaliadas e, possivelmente, da constituição corporal
> - Use avaliação dinâmica para auxiliar no diagnóstico, isto é, use Valsalva ou esforço para avaliar herniação. Utilize a flexão, extensão e rotação interna/externa do quadril para auxiliar no diagnóstico, alongando e relaxando as fibras do tendão e, possivelmente, introduzindo fluido em uma interface rompida
> - Considere diminuir a frequência ou trocar os transdutores. A região da virilha/quadril em qualquer paciente é um desafio, particularmente em pacientes maiores, e a penetração pode ser limitada em um transdutor linear de alta frequência
> - As zonas focais auxiliam na visualização da região de interesse. Uma zona focal corresponde à largura mais estreita do feixe de ultrassonografia. Como as ondas sonoras estão mais próximas neste ponto, maior resolução é alcançada; portanto, sua zona focal deve ser igual ao ponto de interesse. Isso é automático nas máquinas de ultrassonografia mais recentes
> - Esteja ciente do artefato. Existem muitos tipos de artefatos de ultrassonografia que podem comprometer sua imagem e, portanto, seu diagnóstico. O artefato é um efeito indesejável em uma imagem e se deve a um dos três motivos:
>   - Instrumentação – ao equipamento não funcionar como deveria ou ao tipo de instrumento que está sendo utilizado
>   - Técnica – à falta de experiência e conhecimento do operador
>   - Interação com o tecido – à maneira como o som é afetado pelo tipo de tecido; esses artefatos são inevitáveis (Sanders, 1998)
> - Sempre examine toda a anatomia em dois planos para evitar muitas armadilhas de imagem, particularmente para imagens dinâmicas quando a região anatômica muda de aparência.

Ultrassonografia

Um exame completo da virilha e do quadril pode ser realizado em um período de tempo relativamente curto (em comparação com outras técnicas) e, se a lesão *suspeita* não for demonstrada, a ultrassonografia tem a vantagem de passar para a área adjacente para descartar qualquer lesão relacionada. Ela também tem a capacidade de comparar qualquer anormalidade suspeita com o lado não sintomático, rapidamente e sem riscos. Isso tem uma grande vantagem em descobrir o que é clinicamente significativo.

Suspeita de dor na virilha relacionada com o adutor

As lesões mais prevalentes em jogadores de futebol – e em praticantes de esportes de natureza semelhante – estão relacionadas com os adutores devido à rápida mudança de direção, chutes e movimentos repetitivos de um lado para o outro. Para descartar dor na virilha relacionada com o adutor (DVRA), deve ser realizado um exame completo da região do adutor, incluindo avaliação da aponeurose comum, quando possível.

O que se deve considerar:
- Existe ruptura? Em caso afirmativo, é de espessura parcial ou total? Há fluido livre presente? Uma ruptura aparece como um defeito hipoecoico focal onde as fibras do tendão foram rompidas
- Há evidência de tendinopatia? Isso se manifestará como espessamento do tendão com perda do padrão fibrilar normal e frequentemente de natureza hipoecoica. A vascularização (neovascularização) não é frequentemente identificada na região do quadril devido à profundidade das estruturas
- Existe alguma miosite ossificante, entesopatia ou calcificação presente? Existem focos ecogênicos dentro das fibras do tendão ou irregularidade óssea?
- Como o lado sintomático se compara ao lado não sintomático?

Protocolo de adutor

O paciente deve ser avaliado inicialmente na posição supina, idealmente com a perna abduzida e girada externamente em uma posição em formato de quatro. Aqui, a inserção dos tendões adutores pode ser mais facilmente identificada.

A porção anterior do tendão adutor longo é razoavelmente pequena e contínua com o reto abdominal com uma bainha comum, a aponeurose comum. A aponeurose do reto abdominal-adutor longo (RA-AL) se mistura com o disco fibrocartilaginoso subjacente e a cápsula da sínfise púbica. Esses achados anatômicos revelam porque a dor pode irradiar da estrutura afetada e se espalhar para a coxa ou para o abdome (Pesquer et al., 2015).

Em um plano longitudinal do tendão e dos músculos, faça a varredura das inserções dos adutores no ventre do músculo. Ruptura e lesão podem ocorrer em qualquer ponto da progressão do tendão através da junção musculotendínea e no ventre muscular. O tendão adutor longo é notado superficialmente no tubérculo púbico e forma um triângulo hipoecoico na inserção. Deve-se ter cuidado para não introduzir anisotropia, que pode ser confundida com ruptura. A mesma região deve então ser avaliada no plano transversal do tendão/músculo. A comparação com o outro lado ajudará a determinar o significado de qualquer irregularidade, seja nas estruturas dos tecidos moles ou nos ossos. É importante identificar a localização exata da lesão ao longo do tendão/músculo para o manejo contínuo, o que pode fazer diferença no tempo de retorno ao jogo. Se houver uma lesão adutora aguda, a avulsão do osso púbico também pode estar presente, que será claramente visível na investigação de ultrassonografia como uma pequena área ecogênica, possivelmente com alguma sombra acústica, que parece estar dentro do tendão, adjacente à inserção. Alguma reação circundante também pode ser identificada, geralmente hipoecogenicidade de tecidos, algum líquido livre e possivelmente aumento da vascularização com imagens de Doppler colorido ou *power* Doppler. A irregularidade cortical óssea também é frequentemente identificada, mas nem sempre é sintomática, daí a necessidade de comparação.

133

A aponeurose comum da virilha pode ser difícil de demonstrar, mas a ultrassonografia pode ser usada como ferramenta de exclusão para lesões graves na região. A avaliação pode ser feita na área de tecido mole ao redor da sínfise púbica, onde as inserções do tendão adutor se tornam contínuas com a bainha do reto abdominal. Se houver suspeita de anormalidade, ou seja, qualquer coisa diferente do comum, como qualquer uma das anormalidades listadas, a comparação com o lado contralateral deve ser feita. As lesões nos adutores, em primeiro lugar, podem ser escaneadas por ultrassonografia; se nenhuma causa para os sintomas for identificada ou os achados forem inconclusivos, será recomendada a RM para avaliar lesões discretas e anormalidades intra-articulares.

Suspeita de dor inguinal na virilha

Para lesões esportivas, a dor na virilha de origem inguinal (DVOI) não é tão comum quanto a do adutor, mas ainda precisa ser descartada como uma fonte do problema se nenhuma outra causa for encontrada ou se os sintomas persistirem apesar do tratamento. Isso é relativamente rápido e simples de fazer com a ultrassonografia e tem a vantagem adicional de poder ser realizado dinamicamente e permitir uma comparação fácil com o lado contralateral.

O exame ultrassonográfico normalmente começa com a interrogação dos canais femoral e inguinal e da parede abdominal inferior, para descartar hérnia ou qualquer outra anormalidade do canal inguinal.

O que se deve considerar:
- Foi identificada uma hérnia? Em caso afirmativo, é femoral, originando-se no canal femoral, ou inguinal, originando-se medialmente ou lateralmente ao anel inguinal profundo?
- Se houver hérnia inguinal, é direta, surgindo medialmente aos vasos epigástricos inferiores, ou indireta, surgindo lateralmente aos vasos epigástricos inferiores? Uma hérnia direta é geralmente chamada de formato de cogumelo, enquanto uma hérnia indireta segue a linha longitudinal do canal
- O que a hérnia contém: intestino e/ou omento (gordura abdominal)?
- É redutível? Quando a compressão é aplicada à área, se o conteúdo da hérnia puder ser comprimido completamente de volta através do defeito, então ele é considerado redutível. Essas hérnias são menos preocupantes para os médicos, pois há menos risco de intestino encarcerado ou, em casos extremos, estrangulado. Se toda ou parte da hérnia não voltar por meio do defeito, ela será considerada não redutível.

Região femoral

O exame começa com o paciente em decúbito dorsal. Um plano transversal é o melhor lugar para começar e definir a orientação. Localize os vasos femorais. O canal femoral encontra-se medial e superior à junção femoral superficial. Avalie o canal com Valsalva e em repouso. Com Valsalva, a veia femoral deve dilatar. Se houver uma hérnia femoral presente, a veia femoral se comprimirá e será observada uma protuberância. O transdutor pode então ser girado 90° em um plano longitudinal e a hérnia será vista empurrando ao longo do canal. As hérnias femorais são menos comuns do que as inguinais, mas podem ser uma emergência médica se ficarem encarceradas; portanto, o diagnóstico preciso é essencial (Figura 13.1).

Região inguinal

Do canal femoral, o transdutor é movido superiormente para onde os vasos epigástricos inferiores bifurcam dos vasos ilíacos externos e seguem medialmente. Os vasos epigástricos inferiores são um ponto de referência crítico para a avaliação ultrassonográfica da virilha. Eles se originam da artéria e veia ilíaca externa imediatamente acima do ligamento inguinal (Yoong et al., 2013). O canal inguinal está situado na metade medial do ligamento. O anel profundo do canal, portanto, fica lateral à artéria epigástrica inferior (AEI).

O transdutor deve estar em um plano ligeiramente oblíquo para visualizar o comprimento do canal inguinal. Localize o anel

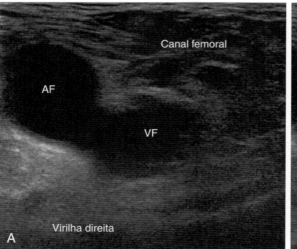 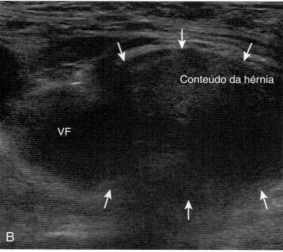

Figura 13.1 Imagem de ultrassonografia transversal demonstrando hérnia femoral direita típica emergindo medialmente a uma veia femoral comprimida com aumento da pressão intra-abdominal. Tomada em repouso (**A**) e durante Valsalva (**B**). *AF*, artéria femoral; *VF*, veia femoral. (Adaptada de De Yoong, P., Duffy, S., Marshall, T.J., 2013. The inguinal and femoral canals: a practical step by step approach to accurate sonographic assessment. Indian Journal of Radiology and Imaging 23 (4), 391-395.)

profundo, lateral à AEI e imediatamente superior ao ligamento inguinal. Novamente, avalie o canal em repouso e com Valsalva ou distensão. Se houver uma hérnia indireta, uma massa de omento/intestino ou ambos será vista movendo-se medialmente através do anel profundo e ao longo do canal (Figuras 13.2 e 13.3).

Uma hérnia direta é vista medialmente à AEI, pois é um defeito na parede posterior. Deslize o transdutor, no mesmo plano, ligeiramente medial e novamente peça ao paciente para realizar Valsalva ou distensão. Se houver uma hérnia direta, uma aparência do tipo cogumelo será observada de profunda a superficial através da parede posterior do canal. O plano transverso costuma ser comum na avaliação da hérnia.

As hérnias costumam ser visualizadas com mais clareza com o paciente em pé. Se nenhuma hérnia for identificada com o paciente em decúbito dorsal, um exame ereto deve ser realizado.

Suspeita de dor na virilha relacionada com o quadril

DVRQ em atletas é menos comumente vista, mas se não houver outra causa para os sintomas identificados, a ultrassonografia pode ajudar a descartar as estruturas do quadril como causa da dor.

O que se deve considerar:
- Há evidência de laceração ou inflamação dos tendões (tendinopatia)?
- Existe algum fluido livre? Existe derrame no quadril no recesso anterior?
- Há evidência de calcificação?
- Lembre-se de também avaliar dinamicamente as estruturas do quadril.

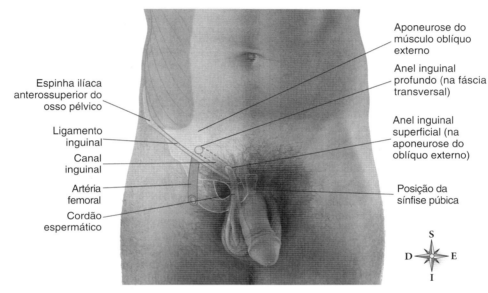

Figura 13.2 Anatomia da região inguinal. (*Esta figura se encontra reproduzida em cores no Encarte.*)

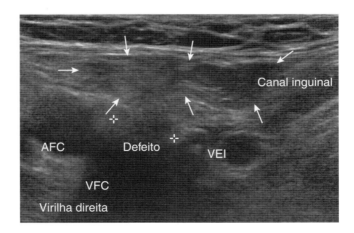

Figura 13.3 Ultrassonografia em eixo longo pelo canal inguinal direito. A hérnia inguinal indireta (*setas*) emerge lateral aos vasos epigástricos inferiores (*VEI*) através do anel profundo (*cruzes*), passando sobre os vasos e descendo pelo canal em direção ao anel superficial. *AFC*, artéria femoral comum; *VFC*, veia femoral comum. (Adaptada de De Yoong, P., Duffy, S., Marshall, T.J., 2013. The inguinal and femoral canals: a practical step by step approach to accurate sonographic assessment. Indian Journal of Radiology and Imaging 23 (4), 391-395.)

Região do quadril

Um exame de ultrassonografia de rotina do quadril começa com o paciente em posição supina, neutra e pernas estendidas.

Com o transdutor em um plano longitudinal do colo femoral, a articulação anterior é analisada. Em primeiro lugar, avalie o contorno do acetábulo e da cabeça e pescoço femorais para quaisquer irregularidades ósseas que instigariam uma investigação mais aprofundada dos tecidos moles circundantes. Irregularidades ósseas e entesopatia aumentam a probabilidade de problemas nos tendões.

A região do labrum anterior pode ser avaliada para cistos e líquido labiais, que são facilmente visualizados na ultrassonografia se houver penetração e profundidade adequadas. Os cistos aparecem como estruturas anecoicas (pretas) de paredes finas, de aparência arredondada ou oval. O fluido livre segue e preenche a linha da articulação. Seguindo o colo femoral no plano longitudinal, a cápsula articular pode ser identificada e avaliada para derrame articular do quadril no recesso do colo femoral. Explore a mesma área em um plano transversal também. Na ultrassonografia, a bursite do iliopsoas pode ser confundida com derrame articular do quadril e vice-versa. Se houver comunicação com a articulação do quadril – uma trilha definida de fluido para dentro da articulação – o derrame estará presente. Nenhuma conexão indica bursite em vez de efusão.

Deslize o transdutor para a espinha ilíaca anteroinferior (EIAI); a cabeça do reto femoral pode ser visualizada nos planos transverso e longitudinal. Muitas vezes, isso pode ser difícil de avaliar no plano longitudinal devido à anisotropia e é necessário ter cuidado para tentar garantir que o feixe de ultrassonografia seja perpendicular às fibras. Novamente, a comparação com o lado não sintomático é útil para determinar a significância de quaisquer achados. O Doppler colorido ou *power* Doppler pode ser introduzido para verificar se há qualquer neovascularização, mas isso também pode ser difícil de visualizar, dependendo da constituição física do paciente e da configuração da máquina. As configurações podem não ter sido instaladas adequadamente e podem precisar ser manipuladas. Mantenha a caixa colorida tão pequena quanto razoavelmente possível para manter a taxa de quadros compatível com o diagnóstico.

Em um plano transversal, siga o tendão reto femoral distalmente e continue a interrogar o músculo. Volte para a porção proximal para avaliar a porção indireta do tendão reto femoral, procurando qualquer espessamento ou laceração adjacente. Uma visão longitudinal da cabeça indireta do tendão reto femoral pode ser obtida, mas é difícil conseguir sem uma máquina de qualidade superior. Aduza a perna afetada, geralmente cruzando os tornozelos. Com o transdutor no plano transversal, comece no EIAI e rastreie inferiormente, deslize o transdutor lateralmente e incline para trás em direção à articulação do quadril para obter a visualização necessária. A porção indireta do tendão é notada como uma faixa hipoecoica. A pressão firme revelará seu padrão fibrilar. Lesões suspeitas na porção indireta requerem encaminhamento por RM; porém, se a ultrassonografia estiver disponível, novamente será uma boa ferramenta inicial de exclusão.

Na visão anterior do quadril, o músculo psoas e o tendão podem ser visualizados junto com o músculo ilíaco. Outras estruturas a serem consideradas em torno da articulação do quadril são as estruturas laterais: tendões e músculos glúteos, tensor da fáscia lata e bursas na região. Os achados mais comuns do quadril lateral são tendinopatia e bursite. A Sociedade Europeia de Radiologia Musculoesquelética (ESSR, do inglês European Society of Musculoskeletal Radiology) fornece diretrizes para a região de ultrassonografia do quadril (Beggs et al., 2010).

Aparências de achados comuns na ultrassonografia

Tendinopatia. Isso pode ser visto com frequência nas inserções do tendão do adutor longo e reto femoral. Na ultrassonografia, a aparência do tendão pode parecer desgastada, heterogênea (não uniforme) e hipoecoica. Alguma degeneração cística também pode ser observada. O tendão pode parecer espessado e a neovascularização pode ser identificada, mas nem sempre (Figura 13.4). Deve-se

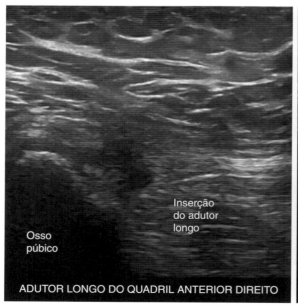 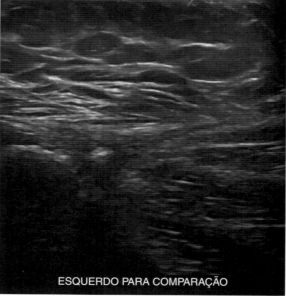

Figura 13.4 Tendinopatia adutora. A imagem (**A**) mostra a inserção sintomática do tendão adutor longo do lado direito, que está espessado e hipoecoico com perda do padrão fibrilar normal em comparação com o lado esquerdo não sintomático (**B**).

observar que não há consenso sobre a fisiopatologia da tendinopatia e que os achados de imagem anterior também podem estar presentes em pacientes não sintomáticos. Em resumo, é importante tratar o paciente e não basear seus achados apenas em exames de imagem.

Ruptura. Isso aparece como uma fenda ou vazio dentro da estrutura do músculo ou tendão. Na fase aguda, geralmente está cheio de líquido e, portanto, hipoecoico na ultrassonografia. Na fase crônica, um tendão torna-se fino. Em um músculo, o tecido cicatricial pode ser observado. Este se apresenta como uma área hiperecoica, com alguma irregularidade no padrão fibrilar do músculo (Figura 13.5).

Distensão. Existem vários graus de distensão muscular observados na ultrassonografia. Geralmente é descrita como uma área de hiperecogenicidade na região de interesse. Pode haver alteração mínima da estrutura fibrilar.

Derrame. Este é o fluido articular e tem uma aparência hipoecoica na ultrassonografia. Detritos dentro do fluido às vezes

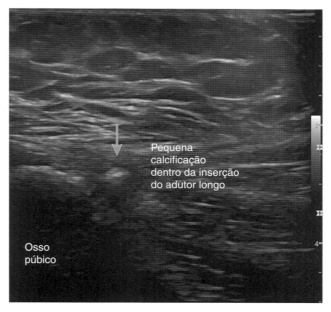

Figura 13.7 Calcificação. A imagem mostra um pequeno foco ecogênico no tendão adutor longo na inserção (seta), consistente com depósito calcificado.

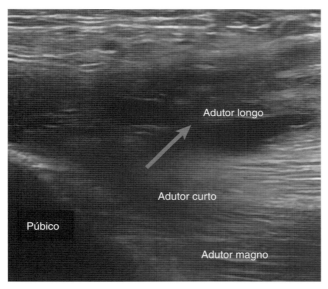

Figura 13.5 Ruptura do adutor. A ultrassonografia no plano longitudinal do osso púbico e dos músculos do grupo adutor demonstra ruptura e hematoma do adutor longo com o tendão retraído (seta). (Adaptada de De McNally, E.G., 2014. Practical Musculoskeletal Ultrasound, second ed. Churchill Livingstone, Edinburgh.)

também podem ser identificados. Com um derrame anterior do quadril, uma coleção de líquido seria observada na região anterior do colo do fêmur. Maior que 7 mm é considerado um derrame significativo (Figura 13.6).

Calcificação. O acúmulo de calcificação nos tendões pode ser o resultado de microtrauma repetido, chamado de tendinopatia calcárea. São observadas áreas ecogênicas dentro do tendão. O sombreamento é notado se for calcificação dura. A calcificação suave também é reconhecida. Ainda é ecogênica, mas não tão brilhante e mínima e, se houver, sombreamento é notado. Podem ser pequenas manchas ou quantidades substanciais. Isso geralmente é encontrado em conjunto com tendinopatia. É menos comum no adutor longo e mais frequentemente vista nas inserções dos isquiotibiais (Figura 13.7).

Avulsão. Descreve onde uma pequena área do osso foi arrancada do osso principal como resultado de uma ruptura do tendão ou ligamento. Uma pequena área ecogênica é vista como uma entidade separada e a reação circundante é provável. Isso mudará dependendo da idade da lesão, mas pode incluir fluido hipoecoico e retração das fibras, ou seja, um tendão flácido hipoecoico (Figura 13.8).

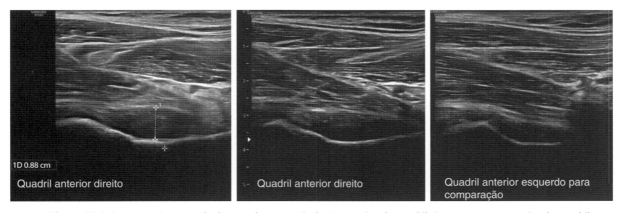

Figura 13.6 Derrame. Imagens de derrame leve na articulação anterior do quadril visto no recesso anterior do quadril.

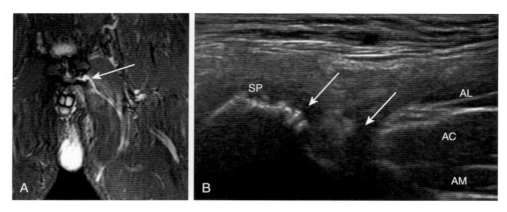

Figura 13.8 Avulsão. Imagens de ultrassonografia longitudinais do músculo adutor longo e do tendão (**B**) mostram defeito hipoecoico focal do tendão na inserção no osso púbico, consistente com ruptura do tendão (*setas*). A imagem de ressonância magnética de T2 com saturação de gordura axial (**A**) demonstra mais claramente a avulsão parcial do tendão longo do adutor direito (*seta*). *AC*, adutor curto; *AL*, adutor longo; *AM*, adutor magno; *SP*, sínfise púbica.

Miosite ossificante. Isso é definido como a "formação de tecido ósseo dentro do tecido muscular após uma lesão traumática na área" (www.marshfieldclinic.org). Aparece como estruturas ecogênicas irregulares que sombream o tecido muscular. Elas são comuns na região do adutor longo.

Conclusão

A lesão na virilha é complexa devido à composição anatômica da área. Várias técnicas de imagem podem ser usadas para ajudar o médico a administrar melhor esses tipos de lesões. Uma combinação de modalidades pode ser necessária para melhores resultados, mas a ultrassonografia está se tornando mais comumente utilizada como a modalidade de imagem inicial de escolha, devido à sua facilidade de disponibilidade, às informações práticas do médico e à capacidade de auxiliar técnicas terapêuticas no local. No entanto, é essencial que os médicos sejam treinados adequadamente ou que trabalhem em conjunto com uma equipe multiprofissional, incluindo profissionais de imagem, para obter resultados ideais. A RM continua sendo o padrão de referência, mas com mais instalações médicas esportivas fornecendo imagens de ultrassonografia, não há prejuízo para o paciente ao realizar primeiro um exame de ultrassonografia como método de exclusão.

Referências bibliográficas

Beggs, I., Bianchi, S., Bueno, A., Cohen, M., Court-Payen, M., Grainger, A., et al., 2010. Musculoskeletal ultrasound technical guideline IV. Hip. European Society of Musculoskeletal Radiology. Available at: https://www.essr.org/subcommittees/ultrasound/.

Pesquer, L., Reboul, A., Silvestre, A., Poussange, N., Meyer, P., Dallaudiere, B., 2015. Imaging of adductor-related groin pain. Diagnostic and Interventional Imaging 96 (9), 861-869.

Sanders, R.C., 1998. Clinical Sonography: A Practical Guide, third ed. Lippincott Williams and Wilkins, Philadelphia, PA.

Yoong, P., Duffy, S., Marshall, T.J., 2013. The inguinal and femoral canals: a practical step by step approach to accurate sonographic assessment. Indian Journal of Radiology and Imaging 23 (4), 391-395.

Leitura adicional

McNally, E.G., 2014. Practical Musculoskeletal Ultrasound, second ed. Churchill Livingstone, Edinburgh.

Miller, M.D., Hart, J.A., MacKnight, J.M. (Eds.), 2019. Essential Orthopaedics, second ed. Elsevier, Amsterdam.

www.asum.com.au.
www.sonographers.org.

Recursos online

www.ultrasoundtraining.co.uk.
www.theultrasoundsite.co.uk
www.jacobsonmskus.com.
www.essr.org.
www.aium.org.
www.bmus.org.

Parte | 2 | Aplicação Clínica

Seção | 1 | Problemas Regionais

Capítulo | 14 |

Manejo Conservador de Lesões Agudas e Crônicas na Virilha

James Moore e Michael Giakoumis

Este capítulo evidencia o tratamento conservador da dor aguda e crônica na virilha. São abrangidos o diagnóstico diferencial de dor na virilha; a incidência e a epidemiologia; os principais fatores de diagnóstico; além disso, é apresentada uma compreensão das áreas que influenciam o funcionamento da região, assim como o conhecimento e a estrutura que permitirão ao profissional da saúde receber o conteúdo necessário para reabilitar adequadamente o indivíduo que apresenta dor aguda ou crônica na virilha.

Introdução

A dor na virilha pode ser uma lesão debilitante na população esportiva. Em casos crônicos, os jogadores podem continuar a treinar e jogar com frequência, mas com desempenho reduzido. Por muitos anos, a lesão na virilha teve conotações mais negativas do que outros tipos de lesão esportiva e está associada ao termo comumente utilizado "osteíte púbica", que não abrange todo o espectro de patologias que podem ser responsáveis pela dor na virilha (Verrall et al., 2008).

O manejo conservador das lesões e dores na virilha requer compreensão adequada da área circundante, especialmente o papel do quadril, que não será abordado neste capítulo. O leitor deve reconhecer sua contribuição nas apresentações de dor na virilha e é direcionado ao Capítulo 16 para obter mais informações.

Incidência e epidemiologia

A dor na virilha é comum em atletas de uma variedade de modalidades de futebol, esqui, corridas de obstáculos e hóquei. Todos esses esportes envolvem torção do tronco em alta velocidade, corte lateral, chute, mudanças súbitas de direção, corrida e requerem o uso específico (ou uso excessivo) da musculatura proximal da coxa e dos músculos inferiores do abdome. Em uma

revisão sistemática, observou-se que, no futebol, a dor na virilha foi responsável por 4 a 19% de todas as lesões, sendo os homens duas vezes mais prováveis de serem afetados do que as mulheres (Walden et al., 2015). Na extremidade superior das estatísticas, uma lesão na virilha pode ocorrer 2,1 vezes a cada 1.000 horas de treinamento. É importante notar que a lesão na virilha pode não ser relatada; como mencionado anteriormente, muitos atletas que sofrem de dor crônica na virilha podem continuar a jogar e treinar.

No futebol, 4 em cada 10 casos de dores na virilha serão de natureza aguda (Hölmich et al., 2014). Para destacar a prevalência de lesões agudas na virilha no hóquei no gelo, Mölsä et al. (1997) demonstraram que 43% de todas as lesões musculares ocorreram na região dos adutores. Estudos mais recentes descobriram que a dor na virilha diagnosticada como lesão por estresse no osso púbico (LEOP) ou dor na virilha relacionada com o adutor raramente ocorre de forma isolada; em vez disso, está associada a patologias concomitantes, como quadril, psoas, abdominal etc. (Bradshaw et al., 2008; Hölmich, 2007).

Ao contrário das lesões do quadríceps, que costumam ser encontradas no início da pré-temporada (Orchard, 2001), não há tendência sazonal associada às lesões na virilha. No entanto, a taxa de recorrência é alta (Tyler et al., 2001; 2010), sendo de difícil manejo e com elevada chance de cronificação.

Etiologia

O mecanismo mais comum de lesão, especialmente em um cenário agudo, é chutar (40%), seguido por mudança de direção e alongamento excessivo (17% cada) e, finalmente, corrida (15%). Das lesões relacionadas ao adutor, 93% envolveram o adutor longo (AL), enquanto o adutor curto (AC) e o pectíneo estavam envolvidos em 19 e 17% dos casos, respectivamente (Serner et al., 2015). Quando apresentado com lesões envolvendo o AC ou o pectíneo, o clínico deve observar que isso pode ser

Parte | 2 | Aplicação Clínica

considerado um mecanismo incomum e, portanto, ele deve avaliar as articulações associadas para disfunção e revisar a cadeia cinética, tanto aberta quanto fechada.

A etiologia das apresentações crônicas ou "agudas sobre crônicas" está frequentemente associada a uma incapacidade do sistema de lidar com a carga apresentada – melhor resumida como "capacidade excedente". Frequentemente, está relacionada com muitos fatores, não apenas à resposta de um tecido sensível à dor ou patológico.

Diagnóstico

É extremamente importante que um diagnóstico apropriado seja estabelecido. A Reunião do acordo de Doha sobre terminologia e definições em dores na virilha em atletas (Weir et al., 2015) foi um grande avanço no estabelecimento de um vocabulário preciso e consistente; no entanto, é necessário mais trabalho para ganhar especificidade no processo de diagnóstico. Uma apresentação aguda, crônica ou aguda sobre crônica não pode ser tratada do mesmo modo, ainda que envolva a mesma entidade clínica. Não se reabilitaria a dor patela-femoral e a tendinopatia patelar da mesma maneira, apesar de ambas serem rotuladas como "dor anterior do joelho". Embora o resultado de retornar ao esporte em um nível de alto desempenho seja o intuito de ambos, os objetivos específicos e o raciocínio para eles dependem fortemente do diagnóstico correto.

A Tabela 14.1 fornece uma lista das apresentações musculoesqueléticas que podem se manifestar como dor na virilha, e a Tabela 14.2 apresenta vários diagnósticos diferenciais que podem ser mascarados como dor na virilha. É nessa área que a vasta experiência é valiosa e, muitas vezes, nesses casos, a imagem e a avaliação clínica apropriada podem ajudar no diagnóstico correto.

A natureza subjetiva da lesão é pertinente ao processo de exame e formula a maior parte do raciocínio clínico. Ouça atentamente o paciente e a escolha das palavras, pois isso geralmente pode dar uma indicação das estruturas envolvidas (articulação, músculo, nervo). Em geral, uma dor vaga, profunda e inespecífica (i. e., que cobre uma área) pode envolver a articulação (quadril ou articulação púbica). Uma dor pontual aguda provocada por um movimento específico pode ser indicativa de um problema muscular (ou específico do tecido). Basta perguntar "Você pode colocar um dedo onde está o problema?". Se puderem, isso é mais indicativo de um problema de tecido específico ou, por exemplo,

virilha, adutor ou tendinopatia do músculo reto abdominal (RA) de um esportista. No entanto, se eles usam a palma da mão ou não conseguem localizá-la, isso pode indicar um problema mais profundo da articulação ou entidades clínicas sobrepostas.

A idade do paciente pode ser um indicador significativo para o tipo de patologia. Diferentes condições ocorrem em diferentes grupos de idade, por exemplo, apofisite púbica < 23 anos de idade. Sempre pergunte se houve um incidente ou mecanismo específico de lesão. Frequentemente, a lesão ocorreu durante um movimento esportivo e, portanto, o mecanismo exato nem sempre pode ser lembrado, ou houve um início gradual ou piora dos sintomas que não impediu o envolvimento esportivo, mas resultou em desempenho reduzido. Como resultado, o paciente pode apresentar sintomas alguns meses (ou até anos) depois. Nesses cenários, é importante tentar diferenciar o máximo possível.

Bradshaw et al. (2008) conseguiram mostrar que diferentes tipos de atividade se correlacionam com diferentes patologias. Por exemplo, em pessoas envolvidas em um esporte de chute, há uma maior incidência de patologia púbica. No entanto, para atletas envolvidos em um esporte de torção (sem chutar) ou correndo em linha reta, a incidência de patologia do quadril é maior.

Ao tentar averiguar a irritabilidade, não pergunte apenas sobre os fatores agravantes e atenuantes; seja específico com suas questões funcionais (ver os exemplos a seguir). Procure saber quais os movimentos que o paciente evita, aqueles que sente fraqueza ou perda de força ao realizar, ou mesmo apenas falta de confiança e cinesiofobia. O paciente pode muito bem ter evitado certos movimentos por algum tempo para funcionar e ter esquecido no momento em que se apresenta para a consulta. Observe que as lesões por uso excessivo representam até 80% dos atletas que apresentam dor no quadril e na virilha (Lloyd-Smith et al., 1985).

Faça perguntas específicas sobre os seguintes cenários:
- Calçar meias e sapatos/calças – isso geralmente é feito no mesmo horário todos os dias, portanto, fornece um nível de resultado funcional e elucidará o impacto do quadril e da virilha
- Subir e descer escadas – oferece um resultado funcional de postura unipodal e carga no quadril e na hemipelve
- Entrar e sair do carro/cama – mostra um possível componente inflamatório se logo pela manhã, ou apenas o mecanismo de colisão do quadril e carga de tração da virilha
- Dirigir por longos períodos – indica carga compressiva sustentada no quadril ou hiperatividade dos flexores do quadril em relação à disfunção pélvica sutil

Tabela 14.1 **Patologias musculoesqueléticas que causam dor na virilha.**

Relacionada com a articulação do quadril	Relacionada com a articulação púbica e com o adutor	Relacionada com o abdome
Intra-articular – laceração labral ou lesão na borda	Resposta ao estresse púbico	Tendinopatia do reto abdominal
Acetábulo delaminado	Fratura por estresse púbico	Distensões e rupturas miofasciais retais e oblíquas
Lesão ou defeito osteo condral	Degeneração do disco púbico	Encarceramento do nervo abdominal/ neuropatia
Corpo livre osteo condral	Sinfisite púbica	"Neuralgia do ligamento inguinal"
Cistos	Instabilidade púbica	Hérnia verdadeira
Distensão ou ruptura do ligamento redondo	Entesopatia adutora ou tendinopatia	Defeito na virilha/parede abdominal posterior de Gilmore
Capsulite ou sinovite	Distensão da junção miofascial e miotendínea	Dor relacionada ao iliopsoas
Entorse ou ruptura do ligamento periarticular	Torção ou ruptura de ligamento	
Osteoartrite	Lesão secundária de fenda	
Síndrome do ressalto – "coxa saltans"	Lesão CPLA	
Bursite do iliopsoas e do trocânter maior	Neuropatia obturadora	
	Apofisite púbica	

CPLA, complexo piramidal-ligamento púbico anterior-adutor longo.

140

Manejo Conservador de Lesões Agudas e Crônicas na Virilha **Capítulo** | 14 |

- Dormir/rolar na cama – os problemas aqui são classicamente relacionados à articulação do quadril, mas podem ser de natureza púbica
- Trabalho abdominal, por exemplo, sentar-se/tossir – classicamente relacionado à virilha de um esportista, mas também pode estar associado a uma lesão na articulação púbica
- Movimentos acelerados/desprotegidos – estão associados a rompimento da virilha

Tabela 14.2 Patologias não musculoesqueléticas que causam dor na virilha.

Neoplasias benignas de osso ou tecido mole
Condrocalcinose
Endometriose
Neoplasias malignas de osso ou tecido mole
Doença metastática do osso
Osteomielite
Cisto no ovário
Doença de Paget
Doença vascular periférica
Sinovite vilonodular pigmentada
Hiperparatireoidismo primário
Abscesso do músculo psoas
Artrite psoriática
Síndrome de Reiter
Artrite reumatoide
Artrite séptica
Dor referida na coluna
Condromatose sinovial
Osteoporose transitória do quadril

- Pegar/ceder/"sinal de agarrar" – classicamente associado à patologia da articulação do quadril.

O exame objetivo deve ser usado para apoiar ou negar suas hipóteses formuladas durante seu exame subjetivo (Tabela 14.3). A confirmação da hipótese é construída agrupando-se uma série de testes para melhorar a probabilidade de que a hipótese nula seja verdadeira. Não se pode ser 100% positivo, mas sim melhorar a probabilidade de ser positivo. Seguir um bom processo e avaliação demonstrou melhorar a confiabilidade intra e interexaminador para diagnosticar com precisão diferentes entidades clínicas (Hölmich et al., 2004). Seja sistemático e lembre-se de que na maioria das vezes pode haver duas ou mais patologias presentes no exame (Bradshaw et al., 2008; Hölmich, 2007).

Apesar da discussão em torno da palpação e da falta de fatores diagnósticos em certas tendinopatias e patologias de membros inferiores, na região da virilha é necessária uma boa habilidade palpatória para diferenciar (Drew et al., 2016; Falvey et al., 2009). Falvey et al. (2009) usam o termo "localizar e recriar" e foram capazes de mostrar uma correlação com a localização da dor em referência ao triângulo da virilha e sua associação com a patologia subjacente. No PhD de Michael Drew, aqueles que apresentam patologia relacionada ao adutor demonstraram hiperalgesia mecânica (Drew et al., 2016). Para complicar as coisas, quando o AL foi mecanicamente sensibilizado por meio de uma injeção de solução salina, os indivíduos descreveram uma disseminação dos sintomas ao longo do triângulo da virilha superior lateral que viajou ao longo da borda inferior da linha inguinal e, em casos raros, a parte inferior do abdome (Drew et al., 2017). Portanto, o clínico deve ser específico com sua palpação para distinguir entre estruturas sensíveis à dor e áreas subjetivas de sintomas, uma vez que podem não ser sinônimos.

Tabela 14.3 **Exame objetivo de dor na virilha.**

Articulação púbica e adutores	Abdome
Palpação: de marcos ósseos, como ramos (tubérculos) púbicos superiores e inferiores, linha articular púbica, ligamentos púbicos superior e inferior	**Palpação:** de todas as intersecções abdominais – inserção do reto no osso púbico, ao longo do ligamento inguinal, a aponeurose oblíqua
Palpação: dos ventres musculares, junções miotendíneas e origens do tendão, especialmente origem do tendão adutor longo e consistência do adutor magno e área transversal	**Testes de provocação resistida:** plano sagital dominante Resista à flexão de joelhos e flexões de perna esticada Resista ao aumento da perna reta dupla
Teste de compressão: feito em três posições	**Teste de provocação resistida:** plano transversal dominante
0°: média masculina 200 a 220 mmHg	Em posição sentada com rotação de 20°
45 a 60°: média masculina 220 a 240 mmHg	Resista à rotação direita e esquerda no lado direito e repita no lado esquerdo
90°: média masculina 200 a 220 mmHg (para mulheres espere em média 20 mmHg menos para cada)	**Teste de "batidas de tesoura":** levante ambas as pernas do chão (aproximadamente 15 cm) e, em seguida, abduza e aduza repetidamente por 1 min, alternando a perna superior
Teste de compressão: realizado em uma elevação dupla da perna reta a 30°	**Teste de Thomas para a flexão do quadril:** semelhante a um aspecto do TESP, o paciente realiza um pequeno *sit up* e, em seguida, produz a flexão do quadril que pode carregar o reto abdominal, bem como o CPLA
Provocação de alta carga de IAP	
Teste do sistema (*sling*) oblíquo anterior – também um critério para o retorno à corrida	
Queda de joelho dobrado: para defesa	
Procure simetria e suavidade de movimento, bem como amplitude	
Capacidade de força: medir a produção de força em:	
Alcance externo de alavanca curta (FARE)	
Alcance externo de alavanca longa (abdução FDA)	
TESP: provocação em um teste modificado de Thomas ao realizar:	
Extensão passiva total do quadril	
Extensão passiva total do quadril e flexão resistida à abdução do quadril em extensão passiva total	
Adução resistida em extensão total e abdução	

CPLA, complexo piramidal-ligamento púbico anterior-adutor longo; *FARE*, flexão-abdução-rotação externa; *FDA*, fim da amplitude; *IAP*, instabilidade da articulação púbica; *TESP*, teste de estresse da sínfise púbica.

Parte | 2 | Aplicação Clínica

Evolução do complexo piramidal-ligamento púbico anterior-adutor longo

Recentemente, tem havido discussões e consciência crescentes sobre o que antes era chamado de placa aponeurótica adutora, mas aqui denominado como complexo piramidal-ligamento púbico anterior-adutor longo (CPLA). Anteriormente, pensava-se que os tendões do RA se mesclavam com o AL contralateral (Norton-Old et al., 2013). A lesão dessa estrutura foi previamente anotada como fenda secundária ou lesão de tração do adutor (Branci et al., 2013). No entanto, Schilders e colegas (2017) realizaram avaliações anatômicas em cadáveres e mostraram que este complexo pensado anteriormente não envolvia o tendão do RA.

O piramidal é o único músculo anterior ao osso púbico e tem anexos na linha alba. Apenas por sua anatomia, seu papel pode ser visto em fornecer tensão e estrutura para a ação do RA e do sistema abdominal, proporcionando rigidez para as inserções aponeuróticas de RA e oblíquos para trabalhar. Portanto, é o piramidal e o AL cujos tendões se comunicam para formar o ligamento púbico anterior. Na superfície profunda entre o AL e a crista púbica, uma estrutura fibrocartilaginosa é encontrada. Quando interrompida, é essa estrutura e a cavidade preenchida com fluido resultante que são vistas como uma região hiperecoica na varredura.

O ligamento púbico anterior fornece um ponto de ancoragem para os oblíquos e é uma estrutura integral para a estabilidade mecânica do anel púbico. Foi demonstrado que a maior parte do movimento ocorre no plano transverso da articulação púbica, portanto, o CPLA atua como um estabilizador (Birmingham et al., 2012). Combinando seu papel na estabilidade com seu papel na transmissão e resistência de forças de alta tensão, pode-se ver que é um complexo integral da região pélvica.

Exames de imagem

A obtenção de imagens nessa área pode ser complicada, pois os achados anatômicos nem sempre correspondem aos achados clínicos. Portanto, a imagem é de grande valor para descartar patologia alternativa ou não musculoesquelética. Quando capaz de fornecer um diagnóstico claro, a imagem tem um valor inestimável. No entanto, deve sempre ser usada em conjunto com a hipótese clínica do exame físico e do histórico. É importante entender que muitos falsos positivos são gerados na imagem da região pélvica, como no quadril (Branci et al., 2015).

A pesquisa até agora forneceu resultados variados sobre a prevalência de edema da medula óssea púbica em indivíduos assintomáticos, mas sua presença foi confirmada em 72% dos jovens jogadores de futebol de elite assintomáticos na coorte de um estudo (Lovell et al., 2006). Há uma variedade de opções disponíveis ao profissional da saúde, isso sempre deve ser discutido com a equipe de saúde e radiologistas para determinar a série mais apropriada de investigações necessárias.

Função muscular e miocinemática

Como este capítulo se concentra no tratamento conservador da dor na virilha, serão abordados apenas os músculos que cruzam o complexo articular púbico.

Função do músculo adutor

O foco principal do grupo de músculos adutores é por meio do AL, magno e grácil; no entanto, deve-se reconhecer que adução significativa pode ser produzida pelos adutores curtos, psoas e isquiotibiais mediais (Neumann, 2010).

Todos os adutores produzem um braço de momento de adução. No entanto, quando a coxa se move para a flexão do quadril (> 60°), todos eles têm um braço de momento de extensão, com o adutor magno (AM) se tornando o extensor mais forte na flexão do quadril além de 45° (Vigotsky, 2016). Quando a coxa se move em extensão, todos os adutores (exceto o magno) produzem um braço de momento de flexão, com o AL sendo um flexor-chave atrás do iliopsoas. O grupo adutor também tem a capacidade de produzir um braço de momento de rotação medial em torno do quadril.

De todos os adutores, o AM tem a maior área da seção transversal (AST) e é o terceiro maior músculo do membro inferior. Possui fibras de comprimento longo e, portanto, a capacidade de produzir altos níveis de força em uma grande amplitude de movimento. O AM pode ser dividido em dois ou quatro elementos distintos. Dois elementos são definidos por diferentes inervações: proximalmente pelo nervo obturador e distalmente pelo nervo ciático. Quatro elementos são definidos pelos diferentes ângulos de penação, os compartimentos do músculo e as ações subsequentes (Takizawa et al., 2014). Portanto, o AM tem um braço de alavanca para adução, extensão do quadril, flexão do joelho e tem um papel de estabilidade local no quadril e na articulação púbica com seu compartimento mais proximal.

O grácil possui o maior braço de momento adutor, bem como o segundo maior comprimento de fibra muscular no membro inferior, proporcionando sua capacidade de trabalhar em alta velocidade (Neumann, 2010; Ward et al., 2009).

O AL tem o maior braço de momento de flexão no grupo de músculos adutores, que aumenta quando colocado em extensão posterior do quadril, daí o seu papel na flexão do quadril na corrida. Ele funciona sinergicamente ao lado do iliopsoas para produzir a flexão do quadril após o início da flexão do quadril. O AL também atua isometricamente na fase intermediária da marcha, tanto na caminhada quanto na corrida, para estabilizar a pelve em sinergia com os glúteos. Finalmente, o AL demonstrou amortecer a ação dos abdutores após a propulsão; portanto, tem uma grande função excêntrica sobre o quadril para desacelerar a extensão do quadril (Mann e Hagy, 1980).

Como já discutido anteriormente, os adutores não contribuem apenas para a adução, que é o terceiro movimento mais forte em torno do quadril, mas contribuem extensivamente para os torques de alta flexão (o segundo mais forte) e extensão (o mais forte) que podem ser produzidos (Neumann, 2010).

Função do músculo abdominal

De maneira semelhante aos adutores, os abdominais, em particular o RA, desempenham um papel fundamental na resistência aos torques baseados em extensão. O RA, por sua natureza linear (fusiforme) e fibras musculares curtas, está mais bem equipado para controlar a extensão do tronco e, ao lado dos isquiotibiais, resistir à inclinação anterior da pelve durante a locomoção. O ângulo multipenado dos oblíquos (interno e externo), juntamente com sua grande área de seção transversal e braço de alavanca, permite que eles não apenas controlem, produzam e resistam à rotação, mas também têm uma influência significativa na flexão do tronco, controlando a rotação posterior de cada osso inominado ipsilateral e fornecem estabilidade à pelve por meio de fechamento forçado.

Função da virilha no esporte

A primeira coisa a notar é que a pelve é um anel fechado, fornecendo uma base estável para a coluna e os membros inferiores e é uma parte integrante do complexo da virilha. Foi estabelecido que o eixo de todo movimento da pelve ocorre na face superior da articulação púbica (Alderink, 1991). Por meio disso, pode-se observar que seu papel funcional primário é transferir força. Ela fornece suporte para o impulso para baixo e para frente do tronco, ao mesmo tempo em que absorve as forças propulsivas transmitidas dos membros inferiores em uma direção recíproca (Gracovetsky e Iacono, 1987). Portanto, qualquer instabilidade, disfunção ou dor na região lombopélvica pode sobrecarregar a área levando a lesões do CPLA, do osso ou dos tecidos moles.

Cinética e cinemática da tarefa esportiva

Corrida

Fora do chute em movimento, os adutores não precisam gerar altos níveis de força no plano coronal. Mann e Hagy (1980) mostraram que durante o *jogging* e a corrida, os adutores eram os únicos músculos a trabalhar durante e imediatamente antes do período de retirada do pé. No *sprint* eles foram acompanhados durante este período pelo RA. Portanto, sua função primária durante a corrida é controlar a extensão terminal do quadril e neutralizar o torque de extensão e rotação externa produzido durante a postura terminal pela musculatura glútea (Schache et al., 2011). Eles também têm o papel de ajudar a reacelerar a coxa no plano sagital e agir como sinergistas para os flexores primários do quadril, como fica evidente pelos altos níveis de força produzidos durante a fase inicial de balanço (Schache et al., 2011). Eles também trabalham sinergicamente com os abdutores para manter a estabilidade pélvica durante a fase de apoio (Torry et al., 2006).

Mudança de direção

A maneira como um indivíduo corta e gira influencia fortemente as demandas na região da virilha. Foi demonstrado em pesquisas recentes que diferentes indivíduos têm um padrão de movimento preferencial de mudança de direção (MDD) que causa resultados cinemáticos variados (Franklyn-Miller et al., 2017).

Durante o movimento de rotação, é mostrado que o iliopsoas e o AL têm funções importantes tanto na reorientação da perna oscilante quanto na orientação da pelve de sustentação por meio de ações opostas ao sentido de inserção à origem (Ventura et al., 2015).

Deve-se considerar toda a cadeia cinética, especialmente o complexo do pé e tornozelo, em quem apresenta dor na virilha em esportes que envolvem MDD. Foi demonstrado que o complexo da panturrilha e, em particular, sua capacidade de produzir potência (potência = força × velocidade) é o principal determinante físico no desempenho da MDD (Marshall et al., 2014).

Chute

A região pélvica torna-se o principal gerador de força, uma vez que se torna o ponto pivô para a energia a ser transferida da região proximal para a distal e é responsável por uma grande geração de torque. Durante o chute, a coxa se move a até 500° por segundo e, de toda a energia cinética gerada, apenas 15% é absorvida pela bola; o resto da energia é absorvida pelo corpo (Barfield, 1998).

Durante a fase de armar, grandes quantidades de tração e carga excêntrica ocorrem na virilha, coincidindo com o fato de que a ativação máxima ocorre no pico de extensão do quadril (Charnock et al., 2009). A carga de trabalho sobre os adutores durante o chute no futebol australiano é mostrada posteriormente por Baczkowski et al. (2006). Em média, o AL passou pelo segundo maior nível de trabalho metabólico no grupo de adutores atrás do grácil e a maior alteração metabólica registrada foi no AL em um de seus participantes.

A técnica empregada durante os chutes no futebol europeu (chutes coma porção interna ou externa do pé) dita os requisitos espaciais e temporais do AL. Foi determinado que durante o chute lateral, um maior nível de atividade é observado no AL antes do impacto; em contraste, o chute na etapa demonstra maior atividade de AL pós-impacto (Ikeda et al., 2011).

Outros músculos que contribuem para a função de chute incluem o iliopsoas, uma vez que o pico de torque do quadril gerado durante o chute coincide com o pico da atividade do iliopsoas; também contribui com o reto femoral em seu papel na desaceleração da extensão do quadril (Dörge et al., 1999). Dado que os músculos flexores do quadril produzem mais de 90% da força gerada durante o chute, ter a capacidade não apenas de gerar, mas também de tolerar esses altos níveis de força é essencial (Robertson e Mosher, 1985).

Intervenção médica/farmacoterapia

A terapia de injeção pode ser usada como um complemento para ajudar no controle da dor e provocar uma mudança no ambiente bioquímico para evocar uma melhor resposta do tecido na apresentação aguda ou crônica de lesão na virilha. Várias opções estão listadas abaixo; entretanto, está além do escopo deste capítulo discutir seu valor e méritos relativos. Esse problema deve ser discutido com sua equipe de saúde ou encaminhado por um profissional adequado. Exemplos de possíveis injeções incluem:

- Cortisona
  - Injeção na bainha do adutor
  - Injeção na fenda púbica
- *Traumeel*
- Sangue autólogo
- Plasma rico em plaquetas
- Bisfosfonatos.

Reabilitação

A reabilitação e o tratamento de lesões agudas e persistentes na virilha podem ser divididos em cinco estágios principais. Esses estágios se sobrepõem, semelhantes às cores mutáveis de um arco-íris que se mesclam coesivamente. À medida que os estágios progridem, a seleção de exercícios geralmente passa de ações isoladas para exercícios e movimentos mais globais, cobrindo vários planos de movimento. O protocolo para reabilitação de lesão muscular adutora é mostrado na Figura 14.1.

Os três primeiros estágios estão sempre presentes em uma lesão aguda. No entanto, eles nem sempre estão presentes na dor persistente na virilha, a menos que o problema seja um cenário agudo sobre crônico ou o profissional da saúde tenha deliberadamente iniciado um processo inflamatório "estressando" o tecido, por exemplo, se eles acreditam que houve uma falha no processo de cicatrização do tecido de uma lesão anterior que inibe o retorno total ao jogo. O profissional da saúde deve mover-se com fluidez pelos estágios, dependendo da necessidade e da resposta.

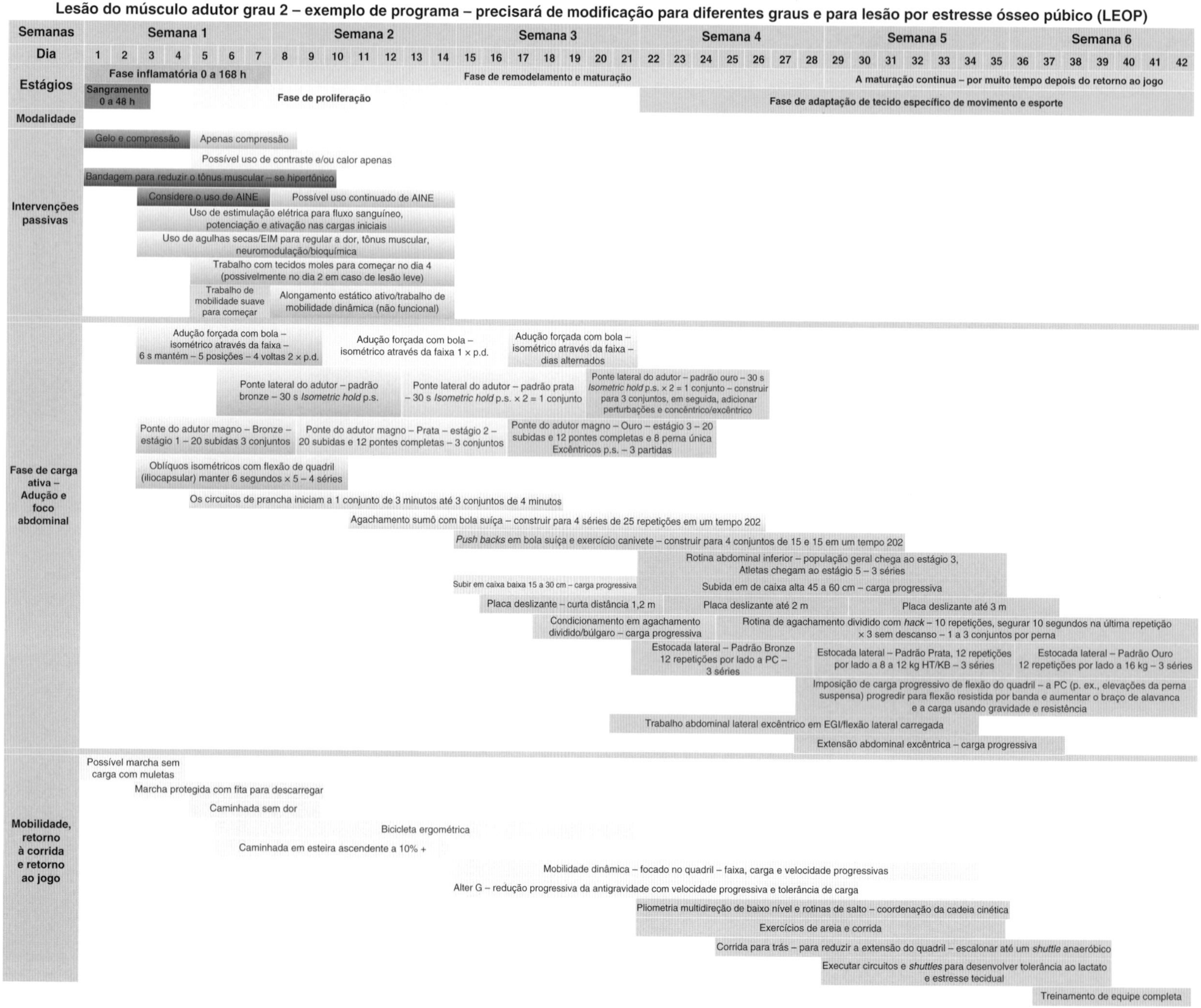

Figura 14.1 **Protocolo de lesão do músculo adutor.** *AINE*, anti-inflamatórios não esteroidais; *EGI*, elevação do glúteo-isquiotibiais; *EIM*, estimulação intramuscular; *HT*, halteres; *KB*, kettlebell; *PC*, peso corporal; *p.d.*, por dia; *p.s.*, por série. (*Esta figura se encontra reproduzida em cores no Encarte.*)

Estágios do manejo no contexto agudo

No contexto agudo, o uso de farmacoterapia pode ser extremamente útil não apenas na modulação da dor, mas também na regulação da resposta bioquímica à lesão e na estimulação das citocinas certas para o reparo.

É importante compreender as três fases primárias associadas a qualquer lesão tecidual.

Estágio 1: fase de sangramento (0 a 48 horas)

Esta etapa é uma das etapas às quais se aplica o ditado "menos é mais". O manejo adequado nesta fase envolve:
- Evitar o uso de anti-inflamatórios não esteroidais (AINE)
- Gelo e compressão
- Movimento precoce, mas evitando alongamento
- Evitar o trabalho direto com tecidos moles
- Evitar viagens excessivas.

A nível bioquímico, esta fase é caracterizada por um aumento na produção de neutrófilos para regular o dano tecidual. Há toda uma cascata química por trás disso, mas o foco deve ser direcionado para dois mediadores químicos ou citocinas vitais: fator de crescimento endotelial vascular (VEGF) e óxido nítrico (NO). O primeiro pode ajudar a regular os neurotransmissores da dor, como a substância P e o peptídeo relacionado com o gene da calcitonina (CRGP), enquanto o último pode ajudar na dor não contrátil do tecido e melhorar o reparo do tecido.

Permitir que a química se regule e encontre um equilíbrio homeostático é fundamental, portanto, as estratégias aqui são "descarregar" e permitir que o trauma do tecido "se estabilize".

Estágio 2: fase inflamatória (dias 0 a 5/6/7)

A resposta inflamatória aguda à lesão está agora se instalando e pode ser regulada com o uso de AINE ou outra farmacoterapia. É nesse estágio que é provável que haja edema residual do estágio 1, que causará inibição reflexa e dor tanto pela pressão do edema (hiperalgesia secundária) quanto pelas alterações químicas (hiperalgesia primária). Isso pode resultar em movimento e amplitude reduzidos, bem como atrofia muscular (um fator de risco chave em novas lesões) e inibição da unidade motora.

A chave nesta fase é manter a área em movimento e sob carga leve e restaurar a amplitude e a elasticidade do tecido e da articulação. Mais importante ainda, é necessário recuperar os limiares de recrutamento na unidade motora. Isso pode ser facilitado com a contração isométrica que pode permitir forças maiores (que recrutarão a unidade motora), mas sem movimento e, portanto, menos tensão do tecido. Outros acessórios úteis são os dispositivos de estimulação elétrica, como o Compex.

Estágio 3: fase de condicionamento/ remodelamento do tecido

Nesta fase, a ênfase é colocada em restaurar a capacidade adequada ao tecido para que ele possa tolerar as atividades normais da vida diária, seguido pelo retorno à corrida e aos movimentos específicos dos esportes. É importante variar a carga sobre o tecido para sua tarefa ao considerar esse espectro, bem como a demanda que será colocada sobre eles em seu esporte. Os princípios-chave são restaurar o movimento e a força por meio do alcance no plano sagital, seguido pelo coronal e pelo transversal. A função muscular é mais bem restaurada por meio de movimentos isométricos (por toda a amplitude) e concêntricos, corrigindo qualquer perda de unidade motora e atrofia, antes de tentar restaurar a função excêntrica. Sabe-se que os movimentos do estilo concêntrico podem ter mais influência na AST do próprio ventre do músculo, enquanto o excêntrico pode ter mais influência na unidade do tendão do músculo e sarcômeros em série.

Antes de abordar os dois estágios finais da reabilitação, é importante considerar os princípios apropriados de carga em pacientes com dor aguda e persistente na virilha. Pode ter ocorrido uma falha na resposta de cicatrização do tecido com dor persistente na virilha em particular. Portanto, o tecido precisa ser carregado além de seu nível fisiológico normal para causar algum micro e possível macrotrauma para reiniciar a cura apropriada que pode ser regulada e, assim, obter uma melhor adaptação do tecido à carga.

Diferenças crônicas/agudas na apresentação crônica

Em apresentações crônicas, a adaptação adequada do tecido geralmente leva mais tempo, por isso, pode ser necessário um período prolongado ou contínuo de condicionamento do tecido. Novamente, isso não para a progressão, pois uma vez que os marcos são alcançados, a progressão pode continuar. Em vez disso, a chave para o sucesso da gestão a longo prazo é entender os prazos prováveis para que as adaptações ocorram. Uma armadilha que pode ocorrer nesta fase é que, quando um atleta descondicionado progride muito rapidamente de volta ao nível de competição, é mais provável que haja nova lesão e cronicidade.

Princípios do treino com carga

Conforme descrito anteriormente, é fundamental respeitar o processo e o prazo de cicatrização do tecido e determinar o momento certo para iniciar o treino com carga e o seu nível apropriado. Ficou claro desde o artigo seminal de Hölmich et al. (1999) que o tratamento passivo não evoca a resposta necessária ou adaptação em pessoas que sofrem de dor persistente na virilha; é necessário o treino com carga progressiva ativo.

Com isso em mente, é essencial entender os princípios da carga e distinguir entre carga para dor ou carga para restauração e capacidade do tecido.

Apesar das variações nos princípios do treino com carga para diferentes tecidos, o processo subjacente é o da mecanotransdução por meio da mecanoterapia e sua noção de sobrecarga progressiva (Khan e Scott, 2009). A mecanotransdução descreve a resposta da matriz extracelular (MEC) a estímulos mecânicos e a transformação dessas pistas em alterações na permeabilidade da membrana celular e consequente aumento na proliferação de citocinas nessas células. Conforme mencionado, existem várias citocinas diferentes, mas dois exemplos principais são o VEGF e o NO. Estas citocinas são expressas de modo mais eficaz sob certas condições, a saber, um ambiente hipóxico para VEGF ou usando treinamento de restrição de fluxo sanguíneo (RFS) para NO.

Os princípios da imposição de carga no tecido precisam ser compreendidos. O primeiro aspecto que deve ser considerado é a curva comprimento-tensão (CCT). Essa curva descreve a relação entre o comprimento do músculo e a tensão/força. Ela ilustra que os músculos orientados para o movimento geram uma força ótima na faixa média; no entanto, eles exibem capacidade de força reduzida na faixa externa por serem mecanicamente ineficientes e na faixa interna por serem fisiologicamente ineficientes. A eficiência está relacionada à aproximação da actina e da miosina dentro de um acoplamento de ação-contração. Portanto, o profissional da saúde é mais aconselhado a restaurar a

Parte | 2 | Aplicação Clínica

amplitude, então construir a força ótima na amplitude média e progredir para a força por meio da amplitude para equilibrar a curva e permitir movimentos esportivos, que frequentemente ocorrem nos extremos da amplitude.

Saindo da CCT, considera-se agora a curva tensão-deformação, em que a tensão representa a carga ou a força em Newton-metro (Nm) e a deformação é a porcentagem de alongamento do tecido sob carga. O gradiente da curva representa o módulo de Young, que é a medida da elasticidade. À medida em que a velocidade do movimento aumenta, o componente elástico do movimento também aumenta e, como tal, a eficiência do movimento, visto que a energia elástica é mais eficiente do que a mecânica (ver Capítulo 16). O profissional da saúde deve inicialmente progredir a carga dentro da faixa fisiológica disponível, depois começar a aumentar a carga e, em seguida, progredir a carga para a faixa externa, conforme descrito acima. Isso aumentará a capacidade da curva e, portanto, o módulo de Young.

A lei de Hooke e a lei de Wolff/Davis fornecem orientação adicional em termos de princípios de treino com carga: a deformação em um sólido é proporcional à tensão aplicada dentro do limite elástico desse sólido (lei de Hooke); a qualidade do sistema biológico e a orientação do tecido conjuntivo se adaptam ao estresse mecânico para melhor resistir às forças externas de "flexão dinâmica" (lei de Wolff/Davis). Essas leis dizem que, enquanto o clínico estressar progressivamente o tecido dentro de seus limites fisiológicos, ele continuará a se adaptar e a ficar mais forte.

Finalmente, o clínico deve entender a relação força-velocidade, que pode ser vista como uma extrapolação de uma variedade de CCT. Em resumo, quanto mais rápido um movimento, menos força pode ser gerada. Como a maioria dos esportes é conduzida em altas velocidades (chutando a até 500° por segundo ou correndo a mais de 7 m/s), os profissionais da saúde que trabalham com atletas de elite precisam treinar novamente a tolerância à velocidade antes de progredir para movimentos específicos do esporte. Os exemplos incluem correr para trás para aumentar a velocidade da coxa, pois reduz o momento de extensão do braço, ou balançar as pernas sem chutar para a tolerância do tecido.

Estratégias de treino com carga específicas podem ser vistas adiante.

Treino com carga do adutor

A funcionalidade dos adutores é bastante variada e, logo, a carga necessária para certos músculos também irá variar. Foi demonstrado que o AL não altera o recrutamento, haja sustentação de peso ou não, pois aumentar a carga em uma tarefa de cadeia cinética fechada de plano sagital de 10 para 50% do peso corporal apenas aumentou a produção de eletromiografia (EMG) do AL de 15 a 30%. No entanto, ao avaliar o AM, o mesmo aumento na carga resultou em um salto de 80% no registro EMG de 60 a 140% da contração voluntária máxima EMG (Hides et al., 2016). Isso significa que, para carregar AM, deve-se realizar exercícios de sustentação de peso em flexão idealmente além de 45° (como agachamento, split squat e afundo lateral), enquanto o treino com carga de adutor pode ser realizado em uma natureza sem sustentação de peso por meio de pontes laterais adutoras e apertos de bola.

Foi demonstrado que o aperto da bola adutora produz os maiores registros EMG do AL bilateralmente em comparação com uma série de outros exercícios, especialmente o exercício de adução de Copenhagen. Este último exercício tem maiores níveis de ativação em toda a funda lateral, com maiores aumentos de carga colocados nos oblíquos e glúteos (Serner et al., 2014).

Tanto a prancha com adução (ponte lateral) quanto a placa de deslizamento (patinação lateral) têm sido usadas na reabilitação progressiva de jovens jogadores de futebol europeu de elite durante seu retorno de lesões por estresse nos ossos púbicos. Em dados não publicados do Instituto de Esportes Australiano (AIS, do inglês Australian Institute of Sport), foi demonstrado que a prancha com adução tem características espaciais semelhantes ao chute, enquanto a prancha deslizante tem características temporais semelhantes. Esses exercícios têm relevância para a ação semelhante de aceleração e patinação e ajudam a entregar carga adutora excêntrica, que tem se mostrado um fator de diferenciação em pessoas com e sem dor na virilha (Thorborg et al., 2014).

O leitor é aconselhado a lembrar que músculos adicionais desempenham papéis importantes no trabalho com os adutores. Desse modo, a carga dos flexores do quadril em faixas de flexão do quadril de > 60° (Yoshio et al., 2002), bem como a carga dos isquiotibiais é recomendada.

Ao considerar outros marcos, a avaliação da relação adução-abdução tem se mostrado um importante fator de risco e deve fazer parte da fase de condicionamento do tecido e atuar como um marco para o plano coronal. Tyler et al. (2001) demonstraram que, em jogadores de hóquei no gelo, aqueles que passaram a ter lesões subsequentes relacionadas aos adutores tinham uma proporção de < 0,8 adutores-abdutores, com aqueles que não tiveram lesões subsequentes apresentando uma proporção próxima a 1. Conforme a demanda aumenta no quadril e na virilha, ou seja, chute ou corrida, há evidências que sugerem que a proporção precisa ser ponderada em direção à adução, por exemplo, mais força de adução pode ser necessária para chutar e correr rápido.

Com dor persistente na virilha de origem adutora (ou articulação púbica), o profissional da saúde é aconselhado a pensar em estratégias alternativas para promover uma adaptação eficaz do tecido. As intervenções sugeridas podem incluir: bandagem de descarga de adutor, shorts de compressão e cintos sacroilíacos (Mens et al., 2006) para reduzir o tônus muscular inadequado e melhorar a função muscular sinérgica; e terapia de tecidos moles, incluindo o uso de mobilização de tecidos moles e agulhas secas. Na patologia adutora recalcitrante, pode-se induzir um processo inflamatório por meio do uso de agulhas, principalmente na entesopatia, para promover aumento do fluxo sanguíneo. Foi demonstrado que o suprimento de sangue na entese e no meio do tendão é pobre e pode ser um fator para a cronicidade (Davis et al., 2012).

Treinamento com carga em musculatura abdominal

Para carregar os músculos abdominais de maneira ideal, o leitor deve consultar sua função, fisiologia e arquitetura. Devido à orientação variada das fibras dos oblíquos ao longo de seu curso proximal-distal, eles precisam ser treinados em vários planos de movimento. Por serem constituídos principalmente por fibras musculares do tipo 1 (Haggmark e Thorstensson, 1979), eles têm uma alta capacidade oxidativa e grande capacidade de recuperação após sessões de exercício. Em indivíduos que apresentam patologia relacionada à região inguinal, o ditado "engrossar ou falhar" se aplica; portanto, a hipertrofia e a taxa de deformação são fundamentais. A literatura de força e condicionamento demonstrou que a carga de volume é fundamental para a hipertrofia e mesmo com cargas de baixa magnitude, a hipertrofia pode ser alcançada (Mitchell et al., 2012). Devido à capacidade fisiológica esta área pode ser treinada diariamente e ainda assim se recuperar e se adaptar ao estímulo de carga.

Entretanto, o RA requer um momento de extensão para gerar resistência a fim de obter a adaptação adequada. Nesse momento, os exercícios podem evoluir de abaixamento lento durante

Manejo Conservador de Lesões Agudas e Crônicas na Virilha | Capítulo | 14 |

abdominais para atividades de ponta, como rolar ou abaixar as pernas, para os quais o braço de alavanca pode ser alterado para aumentar a dificuldade.

Estresse ósseo e tecido não contrátil

Está além do escopo desse capítulo cobrir os princípios da carga óssea e do tecido não contrátil em detalhes, mas como a patologia da virilha pode envolver edema da medula óssea púbica e tecidos não contráteis (p. ex., tendão; ligamento e fáscia), um breve resumo do que é considerado ótimo é fornecido na Tabela 14.4.

Estágio 4: esporte-específico com retorno à fase de corrida

Ao longo desse estágio, o clínico deve começar a abordar o movimento multiplanar. A chave é recuperar os extremos do movimento do plano sagital, tanto em termos de força, quanto em controle e velocidade. A próxima prioridade é a recuperação do plano coronal. Uma vez que esses dois planos estejam fixos, a restauração do controle rotacional será muito mais fácil. Isso permitirá que a complexidade dos movimentos específicos do esporte seja alcançada e dominada. Nesse ponto, o profissional da saúde deve incorporar a velocidade, frequência, magnitude e direção da carga.

Estágio 5: integração de volta ao treinamento completo

Durante esta fase, o clínico deve considerar o retorno progressivo e calculado ao treinamento completo e as habilidades e movimentos necessários a serem realizados. É nesse ponto que o condicionamento de tecidos realizado nos estágios anteriores fornece ao atleta a capacidade e o nível de resiliência necessários para progredir pelos critérios de retorno ao jogo. Esses critérios incluirão volume e intensidade da distância, velocidade, mudança de direção e chutes/habilidades específicas relacionadas ao esporte. Evite aumentar vários aspectos ao mesmo tempo, pois aumentar a velocidade e aumentar a intensidade ou volume do chute na mesma sessão duplica a demanda sobre a região da virilha. Para visualizar e compreender a progressão da carga, o clínico pode achar útil usar a média móvel aguda sobre crônica exponencialmente ponderada, cujo uso está bem estabelecido nos departamentos de ciência do esporte e medicina (Murray et al., 2017).

Processos de monitoramento adicionais para os tecidos locais podem incorporar os testes objetivos mencionados anteriormente, sem exacerbação dos sintomas e uma queda < 10% nos escores de compressão da virilha após o treinamento. Os escores de compressão da virilha são um produto da habilidade e disposição do sistema musculoesquelético ao redor da virilha para transferir força e não são testes de capacidade de força adutora. Embora um resultado não doloroso possa ser produzido, ele pode atuar como uma medida sensível para saber se a região da virilha está lidando com a carga.

Ao longo do processo de reabilitação, o clínico deve garantir que um nível consistente e alto de condicionamento físico seja mantido. É imperativo que o sistema total tenha capacidade aeróbica suficiente não apenas para suportar os rigores do retorno ao treinamento, de modo que o início da fadiga seja atrasado o suficiente e, portanto, os padrões de movimento não sejam alterados, mas também para garantir que haja uma maior capacidade de recuperação entre as sessões de exercício.

Tabela 14.4 Parâmetros de cargas e estresse tecidual.

Osso[a]	Tendão/tecido conectivo[b]
4 a 6 ciclos por dia	Força isométrica máxima e submáxima
Período de descanso de 3 a 4 h	Força isométrica ao longo da amplitude
Ciclos curtos com períodos de descanso mais longos	Tempo sob tensão
Alta magnitude e taxa para ativação de osteoclastos ideal	Fator chave de carga de volume
Cargas não lineares e não repetitivas	Pode ser carregado 2 vezes/dia
	Após a carga de alta dose requer resposta de 72 h para atingir a homeostase novamente

[a]Robling, A.G., Turner, C.H., 2009. Mechanical signaling for bone modeling and remodeling. Critical Reviews in Eukaryotic Gene Expression 19 (4), 319-338.
[b]Magnusson, S.P., Langberg, H., Kjaer, M., 2010. The pathogenesis of tendinopathy: balancing the response to loading. Nature Reviews Rheumatology 6 (5), 262-268.

O condicionamento deve abranger não apenas a aptidão cardiovascular, mas também deve abordar a capacidade do sistema anaeróbico e do sistema trifosfato de adenosina – fosfocreatina (ATP-FC) de acordo com as demandas do esporte. Além disso, o treinamento cruzado pode ser manipulado para fornecer um ambiente hormonal ideal para apoiar outros objetivos de adaptação do tecido, como níveis de hormônio do crescimento, fator de crescimento semelhante à insulina 1 (IGF-1) etc., que podem influenciar positivamente as adaptações no remodelamento do tecido conjuntivo (Wang, 2006).

É importante para a visão não reducionista do atleta entender que os músculos podem atuar como geradores de força, bem como dissipadores de força. Outros possíveis fatores contribuintes identificados durante a reabilitação devem ser tratados ao longo dos estágios, desde que isso não carregue excessivamente o tecido comprometido. Por exemplo, pode tornar-se aparente em um indivíduo que sofre de estresse nos ossos púbicos que melhorar a capacidade da panturrilha e do complexo quádruplo pode ser vantajoso. Sabe-se que o tornozelo e depois o joelho são os amortecedores de primeira e segunda fases que ajudam a absorver as forças (em todos os movimentos de sustentação de peso e dinâmicos) que são transferidas até as estruturas articulares e ósseas da pelve (Zhang et al., 2000).

Resumo

O tratamento agudo ou crônico da dor na virilha pode ser difícil, mas é mais simples com um processo sistemático de avaliação. O mais importante é obter um diagnóstico correto e estar atento, sabendo que pode haver múltiplas patologias presentes. É fundamental determinar qual é o principal e qual pode ser o secundário ou o terciário no processo de prioridade; não seguir a progressão terapêutica pode limitar a progressão. Com uma melhor compreensão da função da região da virilha, a seleção dos exercícios fica mais fácil. Finalmente, conhecer o perfil do atleta e o do evento ou esporte é fundamental para entender quais critérios devem ser atendidos.

O leitor deve considerar o uso de estratégias para otimizar o manejo. Assim como acontece com outras intervenções e tratamentos, garantir que o atleta compreenda o propósito dos métodos de reabilitação e tenha um certo nível de autonomia é um fator chave para o sucesso do engajamento.

Referências bibliográficas

Alderink, G.J., 1991. The sacroiliac joint: review of anatomy, mechanics, and function. The Journal of Orthopaedic and Sports Physical Therapy 13 (2), 71-84.

Baczkowski, K., Marks, P., Silberstein, M., Schneider-Kolsky, M.E., 2006. A new look into kicking a football: an investigation of muscle activity using MRI. Australasian Radiology 50 (4), 324-329.

Barfield, W.R., 1998. The biomechanics of kicking in soccer. Clinics in Sports Medicine 17 (4), 711-728, vi.

Birmingham, P.M., Kelly, B.T., Jacobs, R., McGrady, L., Wang, M., 2012. The effect of dynamic femoroacetabular impingement on pubic symphysis motion: a cadaveric study. The American Journal of Sports Medicine 40 (5), 1113-1118.

Bradshaw, C.J., Bundy, M., Falvey, E., 2008. The diagnosis of longstanding groin pain: a prospective clinical cohort study. British Journal of Sports Medicine 42 (10), 851-854.

Branci, S., Thorborg, K., Bech, B.H., Boesen, M., Nielsen, M.B., Hölmich, P., 2015. MRI findings in soccer players with long-standing adductor-related groin pain and asymptomatic controls. British Journal of Sports Medicine 49 (10), 681-691.

Branci, S., Thorborg, K., Nielsen, M.B., Hölmich, P., 2013. Radiological findings in symphyseal and adductor-related groin pain in athletes: a critical review of the literature. British Journal of Sports Medicine 47 (10), 611-619.

Charnock, B.L., Lewis, C.L., Garrett Jr., W.E., Queen, R.M., 2009. Adductor longus mechanics during the maximal effort soccer kick. Sports Biomechanics 8 (3), 223-234.

Davis, J.A., Stringer, M.D., Woodley, S.J., 2012. New insights into the proximal tendons of adductor longus, adductor brevis and gracilis. British Journal of Sports Medicine 46 (12), 871-876.

Dörge, H.C., Andersen, T.B., Sørensen, H., Simonsen, E.B., Aagaard, H., Dyhre-Poulsen, P., et al., 1999. EMG activity of the iliopsoas muscle and leg kinetics during the soccer place kick. Scandinavian Journal of Medicine & Science in Sports 9 (4), 195-200.

Drew, M.K., Lovell, G., Palsson, T.S., Chiarelli, P.E., Osmotherly, P.G., 2016. Do Australian football players have sensitive groins? Players with current groin pain exhibit mechanical hyperalgesia of the adductor tendon. Journal of Science and Medicine in Sport 19 (10), 784-788.

Drew, M.K., Palsson, T.S., Hirata, R.P., Izumi, M., Lovell, G., Welvaert, M., et al., 2017. Experimental pain in the groin may refer into the lower abdomen: Implications to clinical assessments. Journal of Science and Medicine in Sport 20 (10), 904-909.

Falvey, E.C., Franklyn-Miller, A., McCrory, P.R., 2009. The groin triangle: a patho-anatomical approach to the diagnosis of chronic groin pain in athletes. British Journal of Sports Medicine 43 (3), 213-220.

Franklyn-Miller, A., Richter, C., King, E., Gore, S., Moran, K., Strike, S., et al., 2017. Athletic groin pain (part 2): a prospective cohort study on the biomechanical evaluation of change of direction identifies three clusters of movement patterns. British Journal of Sports Medicine 51 (5), 460-468.

Gracovetsky, S.A., Iacono, S., 1987. Energy transfers in the spinal engine. Journal of Biomedical Engineering 9 (2), 99-114.

Haggmark, T., Thorstensson, A., 1979. Fibre types in human abdominal muscles. Acta Physiologica Scandinavica 107 (4), 319-325.

Hides, J.A., Beall, P., Franettovich Smith, M.M., Stanton, W., Miokovic, T., Richardson, C., 2016. Activation of the hip adductor muscles varies during a simulated weight-bearing task. Physical Therapy in Sport 17, 19-23.

Hölmich, P., Thorborg, K., Dehlendorff, C., Krogsgaard, K., Gluud, C., 2014. Incidence and clinical presentation of groin injuries in sub-elite male soccer. British Journal of Sports Medicine 48 (16), 1245-1250.

Hölmich, P., Uhrskou, P., Ulnits, L., Kanstrup, I.L., Nielsen, M.B., Bjerg, A.M., et al., 1999. Effectiveness of active physical training as treatment for long-standing adductor-related groin pain in athletes: randomised trial. Lancet 353 (9151), 439-443.

Hölmich, P., Hölmich, L.R., Bjerg, A.M., 2004. Clinical examination of athletes with groin pain: an intraobserver and interobserver reliability study. British Journal of Sports Medicine 38 (4), 446-451.

Hölmich, P., 2007. Long-standing groin pain in sportspeople falls into three primary patterns, a "clinical entity" approach: a prospective study of 207 patients. British Journal of Sports Medicine 41 (4), 247-252; discussion 252.

Ikeda, Y.Y., M, Sugawara, K., Katayose, M., 2011. The difference of hip adductor longus activity between side-foot kicks and instep kicks. British Journal of Sports Medicine 45 (4), 353.

Khan, K.M., Scott, A., 2009. Mechanotherapy: how physical therapists' prescription of exercise promotes tissue repair. British Journal of Sports Medicine 43 (4), 247-252.

Lloyd-Smith, R., Clement, D.B., McKenzie, D.C., Taunton, J.E., 1985. A survey of overuse and traumatic hip and pelvic injuries in athletes. The Physician and Sportsmedicine 13 (10), 131-141.

Lovell, G., Galloway, H., Hopkins, W., Harvey, A., 2006. Osteitis pubis and assessment of bone marrow edema at the pubic symphysis with MRI in an elite junior male soccer squad. Clinical Journal of Sport Medicine 16 (2), 117-122.

Mann, R.A., Hagy, J., 1980. Biomechanics of walking, running, and sprinting. The American Journal of Sports Medicine 8 (5), 345-350.

Marshall, B.M., Franklyn-Miller, A.D., King, E.A., Moran, K.A., Strike, S.C., Falvey, É.C., et al., 2014. Biomechanical factors associated with time to complete a change of direction cutting maneuver. Journal of Strength and Conditioning Research 28 (10), 2845-2851.

Mens, J.M., Damen, L., Snijders, C.J., Stam, H.J., 2006. The mechanical effect of a pelvic belt in patients with pregnancy-related pelvic pain. Clinical Biomechanics (Bristol, Avon) 21 (2), 122-127.

Mitchell, C.J., Churchward-Venne, T.A., West, D.W., Burd, N.A., Breen, L., Baker, S.K., et al., 2012. Resistance exercise load does not determine training-mediated hypertrophic gains in young men. Journal of Applied Physiology (1985) 113 (1), 71-77.

Mölsä, J., Airaksinen, O., Näsman, O., Torstila, I., 1997. Ice hockey injuries in Finland. A prospective epidemiologic study. The American Journal of Sports Medicine 25 (4), 495-499.

Murray, N.B., Gabbett, T.J., Townshend, A.D., Blanch, P., 2017. Calculating acute:chronic workload ratios using exponentially weighted moving averages provides a more sensitive indicator of injury likelihood than rolling averages. British Journal of Sports Medicine 51 (9), 749-754.

Neumann, D.A., 2010. Kinesiology of the hip: a focus on muscular actions. The Journal of Orthopaedic and Sports Physical Therapy 40 (2), 82-94.

Norton-Old, K.J., Schache, A.G., Barker, P.J., Clark, R.A., Harrison, S.M., Briggs, C.A., et al., 2013. Anatomical and mechanical relationship between the proximal attachment of adductor longus and the distal rectus sheath. Clinical Anatomy 26 (4), 522-530.

Orchard, J.W., 2001. Intrinsic and extrinsic risk factors for muscle strains in Australian football. The American Journal of Sports Medicine 29 (3), 300-303.

Robertson, D.G.E., Mosher, R.E., 1985. Work and power of the leg muscles in soccer kicking. In: Winter, D.A., Norman, R.W., Wells, R.P., Hayes, K.C., Patla, A.E. (Eds.), Biomechanics IX-B. Human Kinetics Publishers Inc., Champaign, IL, pp. 533-538.

Schache, A.G., Blanch, P.D., Dorn, T.W., Brown, N.A., Rosemond, D., Pandy, M.G., et al., 2011. Effect of running speed on lower limb joint kinetics. Medicine and Science in Sports and Exercise 43 (7), 1260-1271.

Schilders, E., Bharam, S., Golan, E., Dimitrakopoulou, A., Mitchell, A., Spaepen, M., et al., 2017. The pyramidalis–anterior pubic ligament–adductor longus complex (PLAC) and its role with adductor injuries: a new anatomical concept. Knee Surgery, Sports Traumatology, Arthroscopy 25 (12), 3969-3977.

Serner, A., Jakobsen, M.D., Andersen, L.L., Hölmich, P., Sundstrup, E., Thorborg, K., et al., 2014. EMG evaluation of hip adduction exercises for soccer players: implications for exercise selection in prevention and treatment of groin injuries. British Journal of Sports Medicine 48 (14), 1108-1114.

Serner, A., Tol, J.L., Jomaah, N., Weir, A., Whiteley, R., Thorborg, K., et al., 2015. Diagnosis of acute groin injuries: a prospective study of 110 athletes. The American Journal of Sports Medicine 43 (8), 1857-1864.

Takizawa, M., Suzuki, D., Ito, H., Fujimiya, M., Uchiyama, E., 2014. Why adductor magnus muscle is large: the function based on muscle morphology in cadavers. Scandinavian Journal of Medicine & Science in Sports 24 (1), 197-203.

Thorborg, K., Branci, S., Nielsen, M.P., Tang, L., Nielsen, M.B., Hölmich, P., et al., 2014. Eccentric and isometric hip adduction strength in male soccer players with and without adductor-related groin pain: an assessor-blinded comparison. Orthopaedic Journal of Sports Medicine 2 (2), 2325967114521778.

Torry, M.R., Schenker, M.L., Martin, H.D., Hogoboom, D., Philippon, M.J., 2006. Neuromuscular hip biomechanics and pathology in the athlete. Clinics in Sports Medicine 25 (2), 179-197, vii.

Tyler, T.F., Nicholas, S.J., Campbell, R.J., McHugh, M.P., 2001. The association of hip strength and flexibility with the incidence of adductor muscle strains in professional ice hockey players. The American Journal of Sports Medicine 29 (2), 124-128.

Tyler, T.F., Silvers, H.J., Gerhardt, M.B., Nicholas, S.J., 2010. Groin injuries in sports medicine. Sports Health 2 (3), 231-236.

Ventura, J.D., Klute, G.K., Neptune, R.R., 2015. Individual muscle contributions to circular turning mechanics. Journal of Biomechanics 48 (6), 1067-1074.

Verrall, G.M., Henry, L., Fazzalari, N.L., Slavotinek, J.P., Oakeshott, R.D., 2008. Bone biopsy of the parasymphyseal pubic bone region in athletes with chronic groin injury demonstrates new woven bone formation consistent with a diagnosis of pubic bone stress injury. The American Journal of Sports Medicine 36 (12), 2425-2431.

Vigotsky, A.D., Bryanton, M.A., 2016. Relative muscle contributions to net joint moments in the barbell back squat. 40 Annual Meeting of the American Society of Biomechanics, Raleigh, NC, USA, August 2-5, 2016.

Walden, M., Hagglund, M., Ekstrand, J., 2015. The epidemiology of groin injury in senior football: a systematic review of prospective studies. British Journal of Sports Medicine 49 (12), 792-797.

Wang, J.H., 2006. Mechanobiology of tendon. Journal of Biomechanics 39 (9), 1563-1582.

Ward, S.R., Eng, C.M., Smallwood, L.H., Lieber, R.L., 2009. Are current measurements of lower extremity muscle architecture accurate? Clinical Orthopaedics and Related Research 467 (4), 1074-1082.

Weir, A., Brukner, P., Delahunt, E., Ekstrand, J., Griffin, D., Khan, K.M., et al., 2015. Doha agreement meeting on terminology and definitions in groin pain in athletes. British Journal of Sports Medicine 49 (12), 768-774.

Yoshio, M., Murakami, G., Sato, T., Sato, S., Noriyasu, S., 2002. The function of the psoas major muscle: passive kinetics and morphological studies using donated cadavers. Journal of Orthopaedic Science 7 (2), 199-207.

Zhang, S.N., Bates, B.T., Dufek, J.S., 2000. Contributions of lower extremity joints to energy dissipation during landings. Medicine and Science in Sports and Exercise 32 (4), 812-819.

Capítulo | **15** |

Tratamento Cirúrgico de Lesões Esportivas na Virilha

Simon Marsh

Introdução

A síndrome de perturbação da virilha (virilha de Gilmore, hérnia de esportista, virilha de hóquei) foi reconhecida pela primeira vez pelo cirurgião londrino Jerry Gilmore em 1980 após o tratamento bem-sucedido de três jogadores profissionais de futebol, todos os quais estavam impossibilitados de jogar por meses por causa de dores na virilha não diagnosticadas (Dimitrakopoulou e Schilders, 2015; Paksoy e Sekmen, 2016).

O caso inicial foi de um jogador do Tottenham Hotspur que não pôde jogar durante 17 semanas devido a dores na virilha. Nesse caso, houve um episódio específico de lesão eversiva como causa da dor. O jogador descreveu um padrão característico de dor ao tentar correr, girar, tossir e espirrar. Ele havia recebido três pareceres ortopédicos, submetido a radiografias, tomografia computadorizada (TC) e ultrassonografia sem nenhuma causa óbvia encontrada. Os tratamentos anteriores incluíam repouso, manipulação e injeções de esteroides, sem sucesso. Quando foi examinado por Gilmore (sua quarta opinião), não havia nenhuma anormalidade visível na virilha e nada encontrado à palpação. Em particular, não houve hérnia. O achado crucial foi um anel inguinal superficial dilatado com um impulso de tosse e sensibilidade no canal inguinal quando comparado com o outro lado. Um padrão semelhante foi observado com o segundo caso: este indivíduo também sofreu uma lesão de eversão excessiva e ficou impossibilitado de jogar por 16 semanas. Esse paciente não conseguia fazer nada além de andar e sentia dor ao correr, chutar, fazer movimentos bruscos e também tossir e espirrar. Os achados clínicos foram semelhantes, com anel inguinal superficial dilatado e sensibilidade do canal inguinal com impulso de tosse quando comparados com o outro lado. O terceiro paciente sofreu dores na virilha por 72 semanas e ficou completamente impossibilitado de jogar durante 12 semanas. Nesse caso, não houve lesão específica, mas os sintomas e sinais foram semelhantes aos dos outros dois casos.

Todos os três foram submetidos a cirurgia para explorar a virilha e os achados característicos de ruptura da virilha (virilha de Gilmore) foram encontrados e reparados. Em todos os três casos, os achados na operação consistiram em rupturas no músculo oblíquo externo, resultando em um anel inguinal superficial dilatado, um tendão conjunto rompido e o músculo oblíquo interno sendo puxado para fora do ligamento inguinal (deiscência). A ruptura foi reparada com suturas. Em cada caso, o treinamento completo foi retomado após a terceira semana e o futebol de alto nível foi possível após 6 semanas, com um paciente retornando ao futebol internacional 7 semanas após a cirurgia. Não houve recorrências na coorte original.

Incidência

Dor na virilha é um sintoma comum em pessoas com lesões esportivas (Gilmore, 1996; 1998; Renstrome, 1992). Embora muitos desses casos sejam resolvidos com medidas conservadoras, há uma quantidade significativa que exigirá cirurgia. A virilha de Gilmore é mais comum em jogadores de futebol, mas pode ocorrer em muitos outros esportes, incluindo rúgbi (de 13 e de 15), jogos de raquete, atletismo, críquete e hóquei. Aqueles que simplesmente realizam um treinamento geral de condicionamento físico também podem sucumbir (Tabela 15.1). Os desportistas amadores estão mais conscientes dos potenciais tratamentos para lesões que antes significavam desistir dos seus passatempos.

Tabela 15.1 Diferentes esportes em que os profissionais têm sido tratados na Gilmore Groin and Hernia Clinic desde 1980.

Esporte	Percentual de pacientes
Futebol	56
Rúgbi de 13 e de 15	9
Atletismo	5
Esportes com raquete	4
Críquete	2
Hóquei sobre grama	2
Outros: Futebol americano Futebol australiano Futebol gaélico Handebol Esqui Artes marciais, incluindo MMA Basquetebol Esgrima Lacrosse Hóquei no gelo Ginástica Polo aquático Atletismo de força Boxe Levantamento de peso	12
Nenhum esporte	10

O sexo feminino representa 3% dos encaminhados e 1% dos que necessitam de cirurgia, refletindo as diferentes embriologia e anatomia da região inguinal (Schache et al., 2017).

Etiologia

A etiologia parece envolver um desequilíbrio entre os músculos abdominais e os da coxa. Os fortes flexores do quadril (o quadríceps) puxam a pelve para baixo e a pelve inclinada alonga os músculos abdominais. O músculo abdominal alongado (os oblíquos) torna-se fraco e não consegue mais estabilizar a pelve, resultando em lesões por uso excessivo e lacerações recorrentes, levando à descompensação da virilha. É importante notar que a incidência de rompimento na virilha está caindo em jogadores de futebol profissionais com o advento de um treinamento de estabilidade do core mais rigoroso (Walden et al., 2015). No entanto, está aumentando em desportistas amadores e em pessoas mais velhas, à medida que se mantêm em forma e tentam manter-se ativos e praticar esportes por mais tempo. A incidência em mulheres também está crescendo à medida que a popularidade do futebol feminino aumenta.

Apresentação e diagnóstico

Fazer um diagnóstico preciso é fundamental para o sucesso do tratamento (Bisciotti et al., 2016; Sheen et al., 2014). Como em todas as condições de saúde, o diagnóstico consiste em avaliar os sintomas físicos, examinar os sinais clínicos e realizar investigações especializadas. Fundamentalmente, é uma lesão esportiva e o paciente típico é um homem jovem e ativo que participa regularmente de atividades esportivas. O principal sintoma é a dor. Apenas em casos raros de hérnia coexistente haverá um nódulo (Ekberg, 1981; Lovell et al., 1990; Smedberg et al., 1985). Muito ocasionalmente, pode haver hematomas na parte inferior do abdome (Figura 15.1). Anteriormente, a condição era rara acima dos 45 anos, mas está se tornando mais comum em pessoas mais velhas que continuam a praticar esportes por mais tempo. O paciente mais velho operado com sucesso foi um ex-tenista internacional de 78 anos que voltou a jogar 3 semanas após a cirurgia. Em um terço dos pacientes, ocorre um evento definido que causa a dor, como alongamento excessivo, chute incorreto ou abdução ou lesões por eversão. Em dois terços, não há um evento definido e parece ser uma lesão de "uso excessivo", onde sucessivas lesões relativamente menores eventualmente resultam na "gota d'água que transborda o copo", de modo que a musculatura da virilha não pode mais realizar suas funções normais e resulta em dor.

Sintomas

Os sintomas geralmente se encaixam em dois grupos: aqueles durante o exercício e aqueles depois (Boxes 15.1 e 15.2). Durante o exercício, a dor na virilha aumenta com corridas lentas ou rápidas, passadas, torções e viradas, passos de lado e com movimentos bruscos. Pular, chutar uma bola parada e chutar tiro de meta também causam dor. Normalmente, o paciente fica rígido e dolorido por um período variável após o exercício. Além disso, a dor pode ocorrer com tosse, espirros, levantar-se de uma posição baixa (normalmente ao sair da cama ou do carro), bem como virar-se na cama ou com movimentos bruscos.

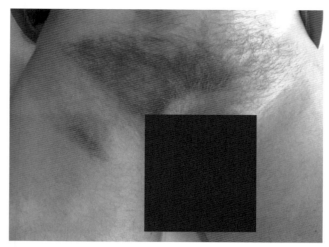

Figura 15.1 Padrão de hematoma que ocorre em uma lesão grave na virilha. Nesse paciente, jogador de futebol profissional, o hematoma delineia os limites anatômicos da região inguinal, acima da do sulco inguinal, além de demonstrar ruptura adutora concomitante com hematoma na parte superior da coxa. Em casos como este, não é apropriado operar na presença de hematomas significativos, pois os planos do tecido terão sido obliterados. Na verdade, esse paciente se recuperou completamente em um período de 8 semanas e não precisou de cirurgia. (*Esta figura se encontra reproduzida em cores no Encarte.*)

Boxe 15.1 Sintomas de lesão na virilha que ocorrem com o exercício

A dor na virilha aumenta com:
- Corrida
- Caminhada
- *Sprint*
- Movimento repentino
- Torção e giro
- Desvio lateral
- Salto
- Chute de bola parada
- Chute de tiro de meta.

Boxe 15.2 Sintomas de lesão na virilha que ocorrem após o exercício

A dor na virilha aumenta com:
- Virar na cama
- Sair da cama
- Sair de um carro
- Abdominais
- Tosse
- Espirros
- Movimentos repentinos.

Embora os sintomas sejam relativamente constantes, diferentes tipos de esportes suscitam padrões característicos. A apresentação clássica para um jogador de futebol é alguém que inicialmente joga em um sábado e depois fica rígido e dolorido por alguns dias, mas pode treinar no meio da semana antes de jogar novamente. Então, a rigidez e a dor após o jogo persistem, de modo que nenhum treinamento é possível durante esse período, mas a dor passa no fim de semana. Posteriormente, a dor surge antes do final do jogo, necessitando de substituição. Nenhum treinamento no meio da semana é possível e no próximo jogo a substituição ocorre mais cedo e, eventualmente, jogar e treinar tornam-se tarefas impossíveis, pois ocorre dor com qualquer tipo de exercício. Os jogadores do rúgbi de 15 têm um padrão semelhante de sintomas, com os jogadores das linhas atrasadas normalmente sentindo dor ao correr, torcer, girar, acelerar, dar passos largos, andar de lado e chutar bola parada, enquanto os atacantes também sentem dor ao pular ou se levantar após um *tackle* (placagem). No críquete, os jogadores de arremesso perdem o ritmo e desenvolvem dores na virilha ao pousar. Isso geralmente é pior na perna de arrastamento em comparação com a perna de aterrissagem. Os batedores sentem dor ao correr entre os postigos e ao girar e os defensores sentem dor na virilha com qualquer movimento repentino, empurrando, dando passos largos e mergulhando. O advento da forma T20 do jogo levou a um aumento na incidência de lesões na virilha entre os jogadores de críquete. Os atletas notam uma perda de ritmo e os corredores de longa distância notam especialmente a dor durante o *sprint* final. Também há perda de resistência e recuperação mais lenta. No hóquei sobre grama, os arremessos em grama sintética podem ter aumentado a incidência de lesões na virilha e isso ocorre particularmente em especialistas em canto, enquanto no hóquei no gelo os goleiros são mais propensos a lesões na virilha. Em contrapartida, a incidência de perturbações na virilha caiu em jogadores de futebol da *Premier League* (em até dois terços), possivelmente como consequência da adoção de exercícios regulares de estabilidade de core e eliminação de métodos de treinamento inadequados (Whittaker et al., 2015).

Sinais

No exame físico, geralmente não há nada para ver na inspeção, embora, com rupturas graves e agudas, hematomas possam ser aparentes e frequentemente demarquem as regiões anatômicas da virilha e do adutor naqueles que também têm rupturas de adutor (ver Figura 15.1). O local da dor é importante, pois em uma ruptura da virilha, o paciente apontará para a área do anel inguinal superficial. Outras áreas comuns onde a dor é sentida incluem a origem do adutor na parte interna da coxa, indicando uma possível ruptura do adutor ou prega na virilha (às vezes com radiação na nádega), sugerindo um problema no quadril (geralmente choque femoroacetabular). Flexão e rotação interna do quadril podem produzir rigidez que, novamente, pode vir do quadril. Apertar as pernas uma contra a outra cria uma resistência que pode causar dor na origem do adutor em casos de ruptura. Em casos de ruptura da virilha, a perna esticada levantando-se contra a resistência (com o médico apoiado nas coxas) normalmente causa dor sobre o anel inguinal superficial afetado, mas nem sempre. O achado característico é de um anel inguinal superficial dilatado, identificado pela invaginação do dedo mínimo na parte posterior do escroto e seguindo o cordão espermático até o anel inguinal superficial. Não apenas o anel está dilatado, indicativo de uma ruptura no músculo oblíquo externo, mas muitas vezes há sensibilidade intensa no próprio canal inguinal com um impulso de tosse acentuado, demonstrando uma falta de continuidade na parede posterior do canal inguinal (Gilmore, 1992). Frequentemente, o exame causa a dor sentida após o exercício, que então diminui com o repouso. Todos esses achados devem ser comparados com o lado normal, onde estarão ausentes (exceto no caso de rupturas bilaterais).

Lesões de adutor

Até 40% dos pacientes com ruptura da virilha terão ruptura adutora concomitante, embora também possa se apresentar como lesão isolada (Pesquera et al., 2015). Apesar de eles ainda experimentarem dor ao correr, girar e dar passos largos, ela é sentida na origem do adutor na parte interna da coxa, abaixo do ligamento inguinal. Há sensibilidade na inserção do adutor no lado afetado, com fraqueza e dor na adução resistida (teste de compressão). Ainda que muitos desses casos agora possam ser tratados de maneira conservadora usando técnicas de injeção guiada por imagem, cerca de um quarto exigirá cirurgia para liberar o tendão adutor, resultando em diminuição da tensão na origem do adutor. Isso é necessário em rupturas graves ou crônicas que não respondem ao tratamento conservador. Também pode ser realizada ao mesmo tempo que uma operação de reconstrução da virilha.

Investigações

Historicamente, muitos tipos diferentes de diagnóstico por imagem foram realizados para tentar torná-lo mais objetivo.

Radiografia simples

Embora as radiografias simples não mostrem diretamente os músculos da virilha, elas podem detectar patologias do quadril. Elas mostrarão alterações de osteoartrite ou a anatomia anormal do impacto femoroacetabular. Pode até haver uma fratura não deslocada do colo femoral ou fraturas do ramo púbico. As imagens adquiridas na "posição de cegonha", onde as radiografias pélvicas são obtidas em uma perna e depois na outra, podem desmascarar o caso raro de instabilidade da sínfise púbica com movimento excessivo visto na sínfise púbica. Fraturas por estresse dos ramos púbicos ou do colo femoral também podem ser observadas.

Cintilografia óssea com radionuclídeo

As varreduras ósseas com radionuclídeos anormais podem detectar lesão por estresse do osso púbico (osteíte púbica) ou fraturas por estresse, bem como alterações artríticas. Raramente o câncer metastático pode ser diagnosticado.

Ultrassonografia

A ultrassonografia nas mãos de um radiologista musculoesquelético experiente às vezes pode mostrar atenuação dos ligamentos inguinais. A protuberância da parede posterior na ultrassonografia é um achado quase universal e não acrescenta nada ao diagnóstico. Da mesma maneira, muitos exames de ultrassom pretendem mostrar uma hérnia quando ela está simplesmente mostrando gordura normal no canal inguinal (Morley et al., 2016).

Ressonância magnética

A investigação padrão ouro é uma ressonância magnética (RM) 3T olhando para os quadris, virilhas e adutores (Cross et al., 2013; Omar et al., 2008). Em casos de rompimento da virilha, isso quase sempre mostrará uma ruptura na aponeurose do adutor longo-reto abdominal com fendas secundárias ao redor do tubérculo púbico (Murphy et al., 2013). É vital que os exames de RM (ou qualquer imagem) sejam relatados por um radiologista

Parte | 2 | Aplicação Clínica

musculoesquelético especialista com experiência em rompimento da virilha, ou os resultados positivos podem ser perdidos. Da mesma maneira, um centro especializado é necessário para garantir que as sequências de imagem corretas sejam obtidas. Apesar de uma tomografia computadorizada poder fornecer informações semelhantes às de uma RM, a dose de raios X necessária é muito alta para justificar seu uso rotineiro.

Diagnóstico diferencial

A virilha é uma junção musculoesquelética complexa entre a perna e a musculatura abdominal. Embora a perturbação da virilha se apresente com os sintomas, sinais e achados de RM típicos, existem várias outras patologias que podem produzir sintomas semelhantes (Corrigan e Stenstone, 1985; Ekberg et al., 1988; Hackney, 1993; Zimmerman, 1988).

O impacto femoroacetabular (IFA) é cada vez mais reconhecido como uma causa potencial de dor na virilha (Munegato, 2015). Normalmente, isso se apresentará com dor na dobra da virilha, às vezes com radiação para as nádegas, e haverá dor à compressão e rotação interna do quadril. Alterações anatômicas do tipo formação de massa óssea adicional na cabeça do fêmur e pinça relacionadas com o IFA são frequentemente vistas em exames de RM, mas em muitos casos são simplesmente coincidentes e nenhum tratamento é necessário. A osteoartrite do quadril também pode se manifestar com dor na virilha e há uma correlação entre o IFA e a osteoartrite na vida adulta. As rupturas labrais no acetábulo também podem produzir sintomas semelhantes e um artrograma de quadril pode ser útil para fazer o diagnóstico nesses casos. Não é incomum ver pessoas cujos sintomas lembram os sintomas do quadril e da virilha. Nesses casos, uma injeção diagnóstica no quadril pode ser uma investigação útil para tentar determinar de onde vem a maior parte da dor. Uma injeção de anestésico local no quadril (realizada sob orientação de imagem) que alivia a dor seria o diagnóstico de patologia primária do quadril. Nos casos em que o diagnóstico ainda é ambíguo, é apropriado tratar primeiro a virilha, pois esse é o procedimento mais simples e com tempo de recuperação mais rápido. Esses pacientes precisam ser avisados de que a cirurgia pode não levar à resolução completa da dor e que investigações adicionais podem ser necessárias. Em pacientes mais jovens, a doença de Perthe e o deslizamento da epífise femoral também devem ser considerados como possíveis diagnósticos. Fraturas pélvicas, principalmente ao redor dos ramos púbicos (e especialmente fraturas por estresse), mas também do acetábulo, e mesmo fraturas não deslocadas do colo do fêmur, também podem apresentar sintomas semelhantes. Também podem ocorrer fraturas com a avulsão, geralmente relacionadas ao músculo adutor longo ou reto femoral.

Na sínfise púbica, a degeneração do disco e a protrusão posterior podem causar sintomas semelhantes às rupturas dos adutores, além de dor no períneo, e a osteíte púbica há muito é reconhecida como uma causa potencial de dor em atletas (Harris e Murray, 1974). Embora a osteíte púbica indubitavelmente possa ocorrer como uma condição primária, em alguns casos pode ser secundária ao estresse causado por uma ruptura na virilha. Além disso, apesar de ser denominado uma "ite" (inflamação), os estudos não mostram persistentemente marcadores inflamatórios elevados. Portando, é preferível utilizar o termo "lesão por estresse do osso púbico". A instabilidade púbica é uma causa rara de dor suprapúbica mais central e pode ser diagnosticada por meio de radiografias em "posição de cegonha". O movimento na sínfise de mais de 2 mm sugere instabilidade. Dor de sínfise púbica também pode ocorrer após trauma, incluindo cirurgia, e foi sugerido que pode haver uma causa infecciosa em alguns casos.

Outras causas possíveis incluem síndromes de compressão nervosa dos nervos ilioinguinal, genitofemoral, ílio-hipogástrico e obturador e bursite, particularmente do iliopsoas, mas também trocantérica. Além disso, precisam ser consideradas tensões musculares agudas do reto abdominal, adutores, reto femoral e iliopsoas. Uma hérnia inguinal ou femoral e linfadenopatia inguinal (secundária a infecção, infecções sexualmente transmissíveis e raramente linfoma) podem se apresentar como dor na virilha e também é importante lembrar que a dor pode ser referida à virilha pela coluna vertebral ou patologia urológica, testicular ou ginecológica.

Cirurgia

A cirurgia para reparar uma ruptura da virilha é chamada de reconstrução da virilha e é um reparo anatômico dos músculos da virilha rompidos. Uma abordagem anterior aberta é necessária, uma vez que o rompimento dessa região afeta os músculos da parede abdominal anterior. O objetivo é restaurar a anatomia e a função normais, por isso nenhuma tela é usada. Há uma sugestão de que o implante de uma tela pode enrijecer a musculatura abdominal e restringir a flexão do quadril. Além disso, a simples colocação de um remendo de tela sobre os músculos rompidos não repara a patologia primária e pode resultar em dor persistente, exigindo nova cirurgia para remoção da tela e reconstrução da virilha.

Indicações para a cirurgia

Para os profissionais do esporte, a cirurgia é indicada se o treino e o jogo forem inibidos, resultando em perda de velocidade e condicionamento físico. Muitos já terão feito as investigações apropriadas e o clube (ou geralmente o agente) solicitará a cirurgia.

Já para os amadores, a cirurgia é indicada se os sintomas afetarem o seu dia a dia ou sua qualidade de vida pela incapacidade de praticar esportes. Pacientes com uma perturbação moderada muitas vezes podem continuar a jogar usando uma combinação de analgésicos e medicamentos anti-inflamatórios não esteroidais até que sofram um episódio agudo ou um problema adicional de uma ruptura adutora. Em todos os casos, a cirurgia é indicada se os métodos de tratamento conservador falharem.

Técnica cirúrgica

O objetivo da cirurgia é explorar a virilha e reparar cada elemento da ruptura, restaurando a anatomia e a função normais. A operação é mais bem realizada sob anestesia geral. Geralmente, em grupo de pacientes jovens e em boa forma, o anestésico local não tem vantagens e com a anestesia geral pode-se induzir um grau de relaxamento muscular para facilitar o reparo, o que é impossível com o anestésico local. Depois de administrada a anestesia geral, um bloqueio do nervo ilioinguinal pode ser realizado sob orientação de ultrassom. Ele é colocado lateralmente para não obscurecer os planos cirúrgicos e ajudar no alívio da dor pós-operatória. Um bom bloqueio pode durar até 12 horas. Para os profissionais, é importante que recebam uma carta do anestesista com a relação de todos os medicamentos que foram usados durante a cirurgia para que possam ser relatados, se necessário, no caso de um teste antidoping aleatório. A técnica de reparo utilizada é baseada na técnica original e bem-sucedida de Gilmore com modificações (a modificação de Marsh da técnica de Gilmore).

Reconstrução da virilha (modificação de Marsh da técnica de Gilmore)

Uma incisão de 5 cm é usada, colocada na prega da virilha abaixo da "linha da cintura" apenas dentro da área onde os pelos púbicos podem escondê-la. A marcação deve ser feita no pré-operatório, com dois pontos nas extremidades da incisão proposta com o paciente em pé, para que ele veja onde ficará a incisão e para garantir um bom resultado cosmético. Uma vez na sala de cirurgia, toda a área é raspada. A incisão é então realizada, de acordo com as marcas feitas no pré-operatório, e a gordura subcutânea incisada até a aponeurose oblíqua externa. Ocorre então uma incisão ao longo do comprimento de suas fibras, por um comprimento de aproximadamente 4 cm, até o anel inguinal superficial, e as folhas superior e inferior refletidas para revelar o cordão espermático (ou ligamento redondo do útero nas mulheres). O cordão é então mobilizado para revelar a parede posterior do canal inguinal e a deiscência do músculo oblíquo interno e do ligamento inguinal que estará presente, juntamente com rupturas no tendão conjunto. Nas mulheres, o ligamento redondo do útero pode ser ligado e excisado.

A primeira etapa do reparo é realizar uma tenólise do ligamento inguinal no tubérculo púbico para aliviar a tensão do ligamento inguinal. Isso também permite que o "ponto âncora" primário seja colocado mais lateralmente, e não no próprio tubérculo púbico. Isso diminui a incidência de dor no tubérculo púbico no pós-operatório. A próxima etapa é plicar a fáscia transversal solta, exposta pela deiscência do músculo oblíquo interno do ligamento inguinal e, em seguida, o tendão conjunto e o oblíquo interno podem ser recolocados no próprio ligamento inguinal. Essas duas camadas são realizadas com suturas de Vicryl® que se dissolvem em cerca de 14 dias. A próxima etapa do reparo é realizada com uma sutura mais duradoura. Um ponto frouxo é colocado na parede posterior para reforçá-lo e manter a integridade do reparo conforme as suturas de Vicryl® se dissolvem, antes que a cura fisiológica completa tenha ocorrido. Sem essa sutura, existe o perigo de que a queda na resistência da ferida, que ocorre naturalmente em cerca de 2 semanas, possa levar à falha do reparo. A aponeurose oblíqua externa é então reparada com Vicryl®, reconstituindo e apertando o anel inguinal superficial antes que a camada subcutânea (fáscia de Scarpa) seja fechada e um ponto subcuticular dissolvível usado para suturar a pele (Figura 15.2). A ferida é curada com *Steri-Strips™*, um curativo não alergênico, e um curativo compressivo é aplicado por 24 horas. Para muitos pacientes, a operação pode ser realizada em regime diurno, com internação hospitalar inferior a 24 horas.

As quatro principais áreas de ruptura são deiscência (D), ligamento inguinal (I), tendão conjunto (C) e aponeurose oblíqua externa (E). Podem ser pontuadas como levemente (1), moderadamente (2) ou severamente (3) rotos, dando uma pontuação total de interrupção (DICE) de 12. Isso permite que o grau de ruptura seja registrado objetivamente, auxiliando na auditoria subsequente.

Tenotomia do adutor

A tenotomia do adutor pode ser realizada por meio de uma pequena incisão (2 cm) na prega da virilha localizada sobre o próprio tendão do adutor. Isso é marcado no pré-operatório com o paciente deitado, o quadril e o joelho flexionados e a perna em rotação externa. A incisão é aprofundada e a bainha do tendão (peritendão) é aberta longitudinalmente para expor os tendões

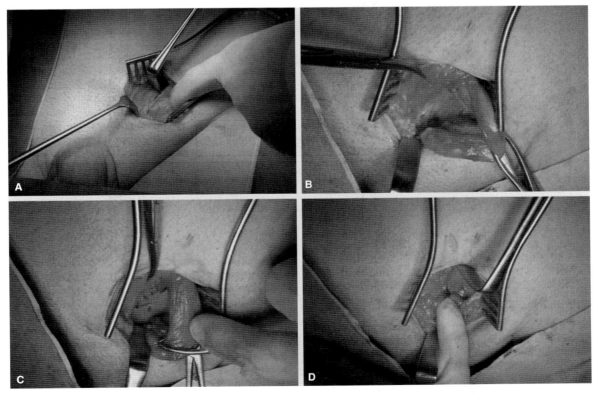

Figura 15.2 Fotografias operatórias durante a cirurgia de reconstrução da virilha esquerda. Em todas as fotos, a orientação é a mesma: a cabeça está voltada para o topo da foto com a perna esquerda voltada para o canto inferior direito. **A.** Aponeurose externa atenuada. **B.** Cordão espermático sendo retraído lateral e inferiormente, mostrando a ruptura muscular da parede posterior, visto como a área branca à esquerda do cordão. **C.** A mesma área após a parede posterior ter sido reparada – o músculo oblíquo interno foi recolocado no ligamento inguinal para que o defeito fosse fechado. **D.** Reparo completo com o anel inguinal superficial reconstituído. (*Esta figura se encontra reproduzida em cores no Encarte.*)

do adutor longo, adutor curto e grácil. O tendão é seccionado transversalmente para liberar a tensão no tubérculo púbico por baixo, antes que o peritendão seja reparado e a pele fechada com uma sutura subcuticular dissolvível.

Fisiologia da cicatrização de feridas

Existe muita discussão sobre a rapidez com que um paciente pode retornar ao esporte após a cirurgia. Fundamentalmente, isso está relacionado à rapidez com que as feridas cirúrgicas cicatrizam e quanto tempo demora para os tecidos se repararem após uma operação. Depois de uma operação em que a ferida é suturada, diz-se que a cura ocorre por "intenção primária". A fase inicial é caracterizada por *inflamação* e dura até 10 dias. Assim que a hemostasia ocorre, os vasos sanguíneos dilatam-se para permitir que os leucócitos, anticorpos e citocinas (proteínas que estimulam a cura) entrem na região. Durante essa fase, a ferida é caracteristicamente quente, vermelha e dolorida. Durante o segundo estágio, de *proliferação*, o colágeno reconstrói a ferida e novos vasos sanguíneos crescem na região para aumentar o suprimento de oxigênio e o tecido de granulação é formado. Essa fase dura até 1 mês. O estágio final é a *maturação*, onde a estrutura e a função normais dos tecidos são estabelecidas. O tipo de colágeno muda do tipo III para o tipo I e a quantidade de vasos sanguíneos diminui. Esta fase começa após 3 dias e, embora possa continuar por 3 meses, é amplamente concluída em 4 semanas (Ledingham e MacKay, 1988). A única parte de uma ferida que está totalmente curada em 2 semanas é a pele. Essa compreensão da cicatrização de feridas elucida por que um período de 4 a 6 semanas é recomendado para a recuperação total e o retorno ao esporte.

Resultado e recorrência

Em pacientes devidamente selecionados, 94% dos profissionais podem retomar suas atividades esportivas normais (Choi et al., 2016; Gilmore, 1992; Hackney, 1993; Horsky et al., 1984; Polglase et al., 1991). Em um período de 5 anos, 3% terão sintomas recorrentes no lado operado e em um período de 10 anos, 10% apresentarão dor no lado oposto. Nestes casos, os pacientes reconhecem os sintomas como idênticos ao problema do lado anterior e apresentam-se solicitando uma operação sabendo que curará seus sintomas. Nenhuma operação tem uma taxa de sucesso de 100%.

Reabilitação

O tratamento da ruptura da virilha não termina com a cirurgia. Um programa de reabilitação rigoroso é requisito fundamental para a recuperação plena, no qual o fisioterapeuta desempenha um papel integral. Tradicionalmente, os pacientes seguem um programa de 4 semanas elaborado para atender profissionais com acesso a um fisioterapeuta em tempo integral, muitos dos quais estão familiarizados com a condição e seu tratamento. Observar a operação também é incentivado, pois isso pode ajudar a compreender a reabilitação necessária. Os desportistas profissionais tendem a estar mais em forma do que a maioria no momento da cirurgia e isso reduz o tempo de recuperação. Classicamente, a primeira semana é passada caminhando, com exercícios de corrida e adutor sendo adicionados na semana 2. A semana 3 inclui ciclismo e corrida, com a semana 4 (para jogadores de futebol) adicionando torções, viradas e chutes, antes de voltar a jogar após a quarta semana. A eficácia desse programa é bem demonstrada pelo fato de que um capitão do futebol inglês conseguiu voltar a jogar 20 dias após a cirurgia de reconstrução bilateral da virilha.

O programa padrão de 4 semanas foi modificado para atender àqueles sem acesso à fisioterapia em tempo integral e aos amadores, para refletir o fato de que os indivíduos se recuperam em taxas diferentes e cada paciente recebe um guia de reabilitação completo por escrito. Em vez de usar um tempo específico (uma semana), a reabilitação pode ser considerada em estágios, com cada paciente passando para o próximo estágio em seu próprio tempo, conforme a recuperação permitir. Em termos gerais, os quatro estágios são: mobilidade, flexibilidade, força, seguidos de treinamento específico para o esporte antes de voltar a jogar. No primeiro estágio, as atividades em linha reta são incentivadas e o esforço abdominal é evitado. Dependendo do paciente, as atividades apropriadas incluem caminhada, nado *crawl*, ciclismo estático e treinamento cruzado. No estágio 2, movimentos de peso corporal como afundo, afundo lateral e agachamentos parciais podem ser adicionados junto com exercícios de flexão e extensão de quadril. No estágio 3, a intensidade do trabalho de estabilidade do core pode ser aumentada e a mudança de direção na velocidade pode começar incluindo séries com caixas, de habilidade com mudança de direção e rotinas de formar um "oito" com o quadril. Quando cada estágio é concluído, o treinamento específico do esporte constitui o estágio final antes de retornar ao jogo. Para os profissionais, o retorno ao esporte em 3 a 4 semanas pode ser possível; entretanto, para a maioria das pessoas, 6 a 8 semanas é mais realista. A adição de uma liberação de adutor adiciona cerca de 2 semanas ao período de recuperação.

Equipe multiprofissional

A associação de grupos de profissionais de saúde especializados em diferentes aspectos da medicina esportiva tem melhorado o diagnóstico e o tratamento de pessoas com problemas na virilha (Cross et al., 2013; Elattar et al., 2016). Além de cirurgiões gerais com experiência em cirurgia de virilha, a equipe deve ter acesso a praticantes de esportes e exercícios físicos especializados em técnicas não operatórias, cirurgiões ortopédicos especializados em problemas de quadril, fisioterapeutas e anestesistas familiarizados com relaxamento muscular, bem como especialistas em dor. Um consultor experiente em radiologia musculoesquelética é fundamental, pois não há mais lugar para o cirurgião fazer e relatar seus próprios exames de imagem. Os pacientes precisam de acesso a informações e conselhos em todas as fases, enfermeiros especializados também são uma parte importante da equipe. Todos aqueles que investigam e tratam pacientes com problemas na virilha devem agora fazer parte de uma equipe extensa.

Controvérsias

Uma série de outras técnicas foram descritas na tentativa de simplificar a cirurgia, particularmente à medida em que mais cirurgiões tentam realizar a reconstrução da virilha. Alguns dependem do reforço da parede posterior fraca, enquanto outros se concentram principalmente na aponeurose oblíqua externa. Todos eles carecem da robustez do reparo completo. Em alguns casos, a compressão do nervo ilioinguinal na aponeurose oblíqua externa pode contribuir para a dor (Ziprin et al., 1999). Um procedimento de neurólise (ou mesmo divisão do nervo) pode ser apropriado nesses casos. O papel dos nervos na etiologia da dor é controverso. Existem três nervos envolvidos em torno da área de reconstrução da virilha. O nervo ilioinguinal corre com o cordão espermático e é facilmente controlado com o próprio

Tratamento Cirúrgico de Lesões Esportivas na Virilha — Capítulo 15

cordão. O nervo ílio-hipogástrico tende a correr no músculo oblíquo interno sob a parte superior da aponeurose oblíqua externa e pode ser controlado levantando-o acima da borda superior. O ramo genital do nervo genitofemoral tende a correr na superfície do cordão espermático, enquanto o ramo femoral corre sob o ligamento inguinal mais profundamente e lateralmente. Alguns cirurgiões acham que a causa da dor é sempre devido ao estiramento do nervo e, portanto, os nervos devem sempre ser divididos. Embora isso possa permitir um retorno rápido ao esporte sem dor, há o risco de o esportista desmaiar se um distúrbio musculotendíneo subjacente não tiver sido reparado. Além disso, a dormência causada pela divisão dos nervos pode ser angustiante e a divisão do nervo pode resultar na formação de neuromas, o que pode realmente aumentar a dor pós-operatória (Minnich et al., 2011). O reparo laparoscópico reforçará a parede posterior fraca, mas não reparará a ruptura muscular anterior, e essa técnica foi amplamente abandonada na Austrália. A tenólise do ligamento inguinal pode ser realizada por laparoscopia e isso reduz o estresse do osso púbico. Postula-se que a tenólise do ligamento inguinal pode aumentar a incidência de hérnia femoral, mas não parece ser o caso.

Resumo

Dor na virilha em desportistas continua a ser um problema clínico difícil devido à quantidade e à variedade de condições que podem ser responsáveis (Bisciotti et al., 2016; Morales-Conde et al., 2010; Sheen et al., 2014; Weir et al., 2015). Atualmente, a abordagem mais científica do condicionamento físico e do treinamento com foco no equilíbrio e na estabilidade do core resultou em uma incidência reduzida de lesões na virilha. Embora muitas lesões na virilha possam ser tratadas de modo conservador com sucesso, uma proporção significativa não responderá e precisará de intervenção cirúrgica (Garvey et al., 2010). A chave para o sucesso do tratamento é um exame clínico completo, imagens e indicação do paciente adequadas. Se for aceito que a ruptura da virilha é uma lesão musculotendínea complexa, então um reparo anatômico, funcional e fisiológico é a abordagem lógica para o tratamento, seguido por um programa de reabilitação estruturado visando um retorno rápido, mas realista, ao esporte. A presença de uma equipe multiprofissional é fundamental (Cross et al., 2013; Elattar et al., 2016).

Referências bibliográficas

Bisciotti, G.N., Volpi, P., Zini, R., Auci, A., Aprato, A., Belli, A., et al., 2016. Groin Pain Syndrome Italian Consensus Conference on terminology, clinical evaluation and imaging assessment in groin pain in athlete. BMJ Open Sport & Exercise Medicine 2 (1), e000142.

Choi, H.R., Elatta, O., Dills, V.D., Busconi, B., 2016. Return to play after sports hernia surgery. Clinics in Sports Medicine 35 (4), 621.

Corrigan, B., Stenstone, B., 1985. Hip and groin problems in runners. Patients' Management 9, 33-42.

Cross, S.G., Rastogi, A., Ahmad, M., Carapeti, E., Marsh, S., Jalan, R., 2013. Sportsman's Groin: Importance of a Multidisciplinary Approach. ESSR 2013 Poster / P-0139. European Society for Musculoskeletal Radiology. Available at: https://doi.org/10.1594/essr2013/P-0139.

Dimitrakopoulou, A., Schilders, E., 2015. Sportsman's hernia? An ambiguous term. Journal of Hip Preservation Surgery 3 (1), 16-22. https://doi.org/10.1093/jhps/hnv083.

Ekberg, O., 1981. Inguinal herniography in adults: technique, normal anatomy and diagnostic criteria for hernias. Radiology 138 (1), 31-36.

Ekberg, O., Persson, N.H., Abrahamsson, P., Westlin, N.E., Lilja, B., 1988. Long standing groin pain in athletes. A multidisciplinary approach. Sports Med. 6, 56-61.

Elattar, O., Choi, H.R., Dills, V.D., Busconi, B., 2016. Groin injuries (athletic pubalgia) and return to play. Sports Health 8 (4), 313-323.

Garvey, J.F.W., Read, J.W., Turner, A., 2010. Sportsman hernia: What can we do? Hernia 14, 17-25.

Gilmore, J., 1996. A pain in the groin? Sports Med. 2, 1-3.

Gilmore, J., 1998. Groin pain in the soccer athlete: Fact, fiction, and treatment. Clinics in Sports Medicine 17, 787-793.

Gilmore, O.J.A., 1992. Gilmores' groin. Sports Medicine and Soft Tissue Trauma 3, 12-14.

Hackney, R.G., 1993. The sports hernia: a cause of chronic groin pain. British Journal of Sports Medicine 27, 58-62.

Harris, N.M., Murray, R.O., 1974. Lesions of the symphysis in athletes. British Medical Journal iv, 211-214.

Horsky, I., Huraj, E., 1984. Surgical treatment of the painful groin. Acta Chirugiae Orthopaedicae et Taumatologiae Cechoslovaca 52, 350-353.

Ledingham, IMcA., MacKay, C., 1988. Jamieson and Kay's Textbook of Surgical Physiology, fourth ed. Churchill Livingstone, Edinburgh.

Lovell, G., Malycha, P., Pieterse, S., 1990. Biopsy of the conjoint tendon in athletes with chronic groin pain. Australian Journal of Science and Medicine in Sport 22, 102-103.

Minnich, J.M., Hanks, J.B., Muschaweck, U., Brunt, L.M., Diduch, D., 2011. Sports hernia: Diagnosis and treatment highlighting a minimal repair surgical technique. American Journal of Sports Medicine 39, 1341-1349.

Morales-Conde, S., Socas, M., Barranco, A., 2010. Sportsmen hernia: what do we know? Hernia 14 (1), 5.

Morley, N., Grant, T., Blount, K., Omar, I., 2016. Sonographic evaluation of athletic pubalgia. Skeletal Radiology 45 (5), 689.

Munegato, D., 2015. Sports hernia and femoroacetabular impingement in athletes: a systematic review. World Journal of Clinical Cases 3 (9), 823.

Murphy, G., Foran, P., Murphy, D., Tobin, O., Moynagh, M., Eustace, S., 2013. "Superior cleft sign" as a marker of rectus abdominus/adductor longus tear in patients with suspected sportsman's hernia. Skeletal Radiology 42 (6), 819.

Omar, I.M., Zoga, A.C., Kavanagh, E.C., Koulouris, G., Bergin, D., Gopez, A.G., et al., 2008. Athletic pubalgia and "sports hernia": Optimal MR imaging technique and findings. Radiographics 28 (5), 1415.

Paksoy, M., Sekmen, U., 2016. Sportsman hernia; the review of current diagnosis and treatment modalities. Ulus Cerrahi Derg 32, 122-129.

Pesquera, L., Reboulb, G., Silvestre, A., Poussange, N., Meyer, P., Dallaudière, B., 2015. Imaging of adductor-related groin pain. Diagnostic and Interventional Imaging 96, 861-869.

Polglase, A.L., Frydman, G.M., Farmer, K.C., 1991. Inguinal surgery for debilitating chronic groin pain in athletes. Medical Journal of Australia 155, 674-677.

Renstrome, P.A., 1992. Tendon and muscle injuries in the groin area. Clinics in Sports Medicine 11, 815-831.

Schache, A.G., Woodley, S.J., Schilders, E., Orchard, J.W., Crossley, K.M., 2017. Anatomical and morphological characteristics may explain why groin pain is more common in male than female athletes. British Journal of Sports Medicine 51, 554-556.

Sheen, A.J., Stephenson, B.M., Lloyd, D.M., Robinson, P., Fevre, D., Paajanen, H., et al., 2014. 'Treatment of the sportsman's groin': British hernia society's 2014 position statement based on the manchester consensus conference. British Journal of Sports Medicine 48, 1079-1087. https://doi.org/10.1136/bjsports-2013-092872.

Smedberg, S.G., Broome, A.E.A., Elmer, O., Gullmo, A., Roos, H., 1985. Herniography in athletes with groin pain. The American Journal of Surgery 149, 378-382.

Walden, M., Hagglund, M., Ekstrand, J., 2015. The epidemiology of groin injury in senior football: a systematic review of prospective studies. British Journal of Sports Medicine 49, 792-797.

Weir, A., Brukner, P., Delahunt, A., Ekstrand, J., Griffin, D., Khan, K.M., et al., 2015. Doha agreement meeting on terminology and definitions in groin pain in athletes. British Journal of Sports Medicine 49 768-744.

Whittaker, J.L., Small, C., Maffrey, L., Emery, C.A., 2015. Risk factors for groin injury in sport: an updated systematic review. British Journal of Sports Medicine 49, 803-809.

Zimmerman, G., 1988. Groin pain in athletes. Australian Family Physician 17, 1046-1052.

Ziprin, P., Williams, P., Foster, M.E., 1999. External aponeurosis nerve entrapment as a cause of groin pain in the athelete. British Journal of Surgery 86 (4), 566-568.

Capítulo | **16** |

Quadril Esportivo

James Moore

Introdução

Este capítulo evidencia o papel da articulação do quadril no esporte, como ela é a chave para todos os movimentos esportivos e como a disfunção e a patologia podem causar dor e sobrecarga de uma série de outras estruturas.

Para isso, nos concentraremos na estrutura, função e mecânica do movimento da articulação do quadril para fornecer indicadores de onde o profissional pode intervir e melhorar a função geral à medida que exploramos cada aspecto. Finalmente, falaremos sobre patologia e suas incidências (que é bem abordada em vários textos diferentes) e quais testes podem ser realizados para determinar a causa raiz do problema. Discutiremos apenas o manejo por meio da prescrição correta de exercícios, pois isso foi abordado com mais detalhes no Capítulo 14.

Antes de começar, é importante definir que o quadril esportivo está focado principalmente em uma população jovem e atlética com uma faixa etária de ~18 a 40/45 anos. Antes disso, o quadril é considerado em uma faixa adolescente/em desenvolvimento e, depois, em uma faixa degenerativa.

> ### Ponto de aprendizagem
> Para entender o quadril, o clínico precisa considerar o equilíbrio da contribuição relativa de três pilares principais: estrutura, função e movimento.

Estrutura

Forma da articulação

O quadril é o melhor exemplo de uma articulação de esfera e soquete no corpo. É capaz de suportar forças muito grandes, sendo o impacto de 8 × o peso corporal (PC) descrito na corrida normal (Mann e Hagy, 1980). É geralmente considerada uma das articulações mais estáveis do corpo, em virtude da configuração óssea, a profundidade do acetábulo e do lábio e o forte complexo capsular-ligamentar que o cerca.

A estabilidade primária na articulação do quadril é decorrente do formato da articulação e como ela cobre a cabeça do fêmur. De um modo geral, um acetábulo orientado fica voltado lateralmente, inferior e anteriormente, e é côncavo com cobertura significativa superior e posteriormente, o que permite um bom suporte para a cabeça femoral na sustentação de peso, sobretudo durante a fase de contato inicial do calcanhar no chão até a fase de apoio médio durante a marcha. No entanto, o acetábulo tem cobertura reduzida anterior e inferiormente devido à incisura acetabular, o que é perfeito para permitir uma boa amplitude de movimento em flexão e a capacidade de agachar, avançar e engatinhar. Isso significa que na extensão, ou seja, correr e chutar, há cobertura e suporte ósseo reduzidos para a cabeça do fêmur (que é orientada medialmente, superiormente, mas também anteriormente) e, portanto, há um maior potencial para a translação anterior da cabeça dentro do soquete envolvendo as estruturas anteriores do lábio, cápsula e tecido miofascial.

Conforme descrito anteriormente, as superfícies articulares não se adaptam bem na posição vertical, com até 30% da cabeça do fêmur sendo exposta. Isso levou alguns anatomistas a afirmarem que a articulação do quadril não evoluiu e está mais bem posicionada para receber carga em uma marcha quadrúpede (flexão, abdução e rotação externa do fêmur no acetábulo), ou seja, a posição aberta da articulação do quadril.

A cabeça do fêmur é bem sustentada pelo acetábulo em flexão, abdução, adução e rotação interna. Artrocinematicamente, pode-se observar que a principal restrição à adução e rotação interna na flexão (impacto femoroacetabular) é o engajamento do colo femoral na face anterior e superior do acetábulo. Em extensão e rotação externa, a cabeça do fêmur fica exposta e envolve o lábio, estruturas periarticulares e estruturas miofasciais como contrastes para controlar o movimento.

A mecânica descrita anteriormente pode mudar significativamente com as mudanças na orientação da cabeça do fêmur e do acetábulo (ver seção *Radiologia*, mais adiante).

> ### Ponto de aprendizagem
> O formato da articulação pode influenciar significativamente o movimento e a função muscular e deve ser considerado ao elaborar todos os programas de exercícios e reabilitação.

Lábio

O lábio acetabular é uma estrutura fibrocartilaginosa, que aprofunda o soquete e ajuda a cobrir um terço extra da cabeça do fêmur. Ele é ricamente inervado com terminações nervosas livres não encapsuladas; isso significa que eles podem se tornar sensíveis a estímulos dolorosos e provavelmente apresentar um padrão de esclerodermia. O lábio cria uma vedação para o líquido sinovial, que combinada com a pressão atmosférica na articulação atua como um efeito de sucção na cabeça femoral, aumentando a estabilidade.

Mecânica periarticular e microinstabilidade

O sistema capsular-ligamentar pode ser considerado uma estrutura mista contínua ao redor da articulação do quadril. Os quatro ligamentos primários que devem ser considerados são: ligamento iliofemoral (ligamento de Bigelow); ligamento isquiofemoral; ligamento pubofemoral; e ligamento redondo. Argumenta-se que o ligamento iliofemoral é o mais forte do corpo, em forma de "Y" na face anterior da articulação do quadril, e está mais bem posicionado para apoiar a cabeça do fêmur no acetábulo em pé, corroborando assim a mecânica descrita anteriormente. O ligamento resiste à extensão e rotação externa do fêmur no acetábulo. A banda superior também resistirá à adução e rotação interna na posição neutra da articulação do quadril. Os aspectos anteroinferiores do ligamento fornecerão resistência à rotação externa em uma posição flexionada e abduzida.

O ligamento isquiofemoral oferece resistência à rotação interna tanto em adução com flexão, quanto em abdução em extensão, e também pouca ou nenhuma resistência à rotação externa. O ligamento pubofemoral fornece uma pequena quantidade de resistência à rotação externa em extensão com abdução; há um pouco mais de resistência à rotação interna em flexão com abdução. O ligamento redondo é estressado em abdução e rotação externa, mas é intracapsular e possui membrana sinovial. Ele foi comparado anatômica e biomecanicamente ao ligamento cruzado anterior no joelho.

A cápsula da articulação do quadril também é única: não é uma estrutura uniforme, com um aumento (de milímetros) significativo na espessura (Philippon et al., 2014; Walters et al., 2014) em 1 a 3 horas anteriormente (se considerado o acetábulo como um mostrador de relógio), mas ainda demonstrando aspectos mais grossos inferiormente das 4 às 7 horas, bem como às 12 horas. Isso pode ser visto como correspondendo à falta de cobertura da superfície acetabular. Há argumentos de que a espessura da cápsula fornece maior estabilidade à articulação do quadril e há algumas evidências radiográficas (ressonância magnética) (Magerkurth et al., 2013) contra frouxidão e estresse da articulação do quadril. Uma cápsula mais espessa não apenas proporciona suporte, mas também ajuda a controlar o movimento da cabeça do fêmur no acetábulo.

Uma cápsula intacta pode fornecer até 200 a 400 N de força para evitar distração da cabeça do fêmur no acetábulo (Khair et al., 2017). No entanto, após a capsulotomia (de até 8 cm), a força para deslocar a cabeça do fêmur pode cair para 119 N; se reparado, a força volta a 280 a 355 N. Isso implica que são necessários entre 20 e 40 kg de força para deslocar a cabeça do fêmur no acetábulo em uma cápsula intacta, mas apenas 12 kg de força em uma cápsula rompida.

A redução da integridade capsular pode levar a uma série de problemas (Wuerz et al., 2016): aumento da amplitude de movimento (ADM) de até 20%; aumento da área de histerese de até 29%; e aumento na zona neutra de até 147%. Além disso, foi demonstrado que qualquer derrame articular do quadril reduz a ADM de rotação em 0° e 90° de flexão ao tensionar a cápsula, com a perda mais significativa ocorrendo na rotação externa (RE) a 0°. Cada detalhe individual destacado anteriormente é

interessante por si só e fornece ao clínico os principais aspectos da função e do movimento. No entanto, essas estruturas devem sempre ser consideradas como uma unidade integrada e, desse modo, a atenção do leitor é direcionada para a noção de tensegridade. Descrita pela primeira vez pelo arquiteto Buckminster Fuller, em termos biológicos, refere-se a forças de tensão (contrátil e não contrátil) puxando estruturas (articulares) que ajudam a manter o corpo estável e eficiente em massa e movimento.

Esse conceito é demonstrado pelo fato de que, quando a cápsula e o lábio estão intactos, precisa-se até ~225 N de força para causar um deslocamento de 3 mm da cabeça do fêmur. No entanto, se a cápsula for removida e o lábio estiver intacto, a força cai para ~125 N e, com ambas as estruturas removidas, há menos de 5 N antes do deslocamento. Além disso, pode-se observar que o deslocamento inicial de até 3 mm é resistido pelo lábio; porém, em valores além de 3,5 mm, a cápsula começa a afrouxar e fornece a principal resistência ao deslocamento. Isso implicaria que a microinstabilidade do quadril (Harris, 2016) durante movimentos simples é suportada pelo lábio principalmente, mas conforme a ADM amplia, o sistema capsuloligamentar aumenta sua contribuição para as restrições de deslocamento (Nepple e Smith, 2015).

Finalmente, há evidências significativas de que os ligamentos capsulares se engajam para evitar o impacto e que as restrições rotacionais capsulares guiam a ADM disponível para essas posições livres de impacto (van Arkel et al., 2015).

O sistema miofascial é fundamental na estrutura da articulação do quadril; no entanto, a discussão desse aspecto é incorporada na cobertura de função e movimento, adiante, para torná-lo mais clinicamente aplicável.

> ### Ponto de aprendizagem
> - O sistema capsuloligamentar controla a amplitude de movimento
> - A cápsula e o lábio se combinam para fornecer tensegridade
> - A perda de qualquer uma das restrições resulta em aumento do jogo articular e microinstabilidade
> - Recuperar e melhorar a integridade do sistema capsuloligamentar ajuda a reduzir o impacto.

Função

A articulação do quadril é a articulação chave do membro inferior à coluna por meio da pelve. Por sua vez, a pelve é um anel fechado que fornece uma base estável para a coluna e os membros inferiores e atua para transferir força. Ela proporciona suporte para o impulso para baixo e para frente do tronco, ao mesmo tempo que absorve as forças propulsivas transmitidas dos membros inferiores em uma direção recíproca (Gracovetsky e Iacono, 1987). Portanto, qualquer instabilidade ou dor em um ponto pode ter um efeito direto em outro.

Desse modo, a articulação do quadril fornece a interface chave entre o membro inferior e o tronco, o que significa que os profissionais devem sempre ter uma visão global da área, avaliando a função de cima para baixo e de baixo para cima. A região deve ser considerada um complexo lombopélvico-quadril; qualquer disfunção dentro desse complexo pode ter um efeito cumulativo da mecânica e do movimento do quadril.

Como mencionado anteriormente, na marcha bípede, a articulação do quadril não está mais bem posicionada para suportar a carga. Isso é destacado por alguns trabalhos de laboratório de marcha, onde os pesquisadores mostraram que nos últimos 20% da postura (salto do calcanhar para a ponta do pé), a cabeça do fêmur envolve a borda acetabular anterossuperior e, portanto, o lábio, colocando uma força do tipo tração sobre o lábio (Bergmann et al. 2001). O quadril pode ficar em extensão por mais tempo durante a deambulação do que durante a corrida; consequentemente, a dor na extensão terminal do quadril devido ao esforço de tração labial pode ser mais significativa na deambulação normal e menos na corrida.

Trazendo o sistema capsuloligamentar em jogo, podemos ver como o ligamento iliofemoral resiste à extensão e rotação externa na fase de apoio terminal (últimos 20%); quando combinado com o ligamento redondo (que resiste à abdução e rotação externa), pode-se ver como ambos os ligamentos ajudam a "centralizar" a cabeça do fêmur no acetábulo e, assim, apoiar o lábio e as estruturas anteriores do quadril descritas anteriormente.

Durante a deambulação (Lewis et al., 2007), as forças anteriores e laterais na articulação do quadril atingem até 1 × PC em aproximadamente meia postura. As forças superiores podem atingir até 4 × PC. Isso é formado pela força de reação vertical do solo (FRVS) de 0,8 a 1,2 × PC e as forças musculares que atingem até 3 × PC. Se o indivíduo quisesse limitar a extensão do quadril encurtando o comprimento da passada, as forças anteriores do quadril seriam reduzidas. No entanto, se a extensão do quadril for maximizada, as forças anteriores aumentam significativamente. Com base na mecânica descrita anteriormente, aumenta a tensão relativa no lábio, sistema capsuloligamentar anterior (iliofemoral e ligamento redondo), além de colocar mais demanda no sistema miofascial.

As forças laterais do quadril no meio da postura alcançam até 1 × PC. O centro de massa (CM) passa medialmente à articulação do quadril, com um caminho sinusoidal lateral causando sua inclinação; há um grande braço de momento adutor em torno da articulação do quadril. Isso é suportado e moderado pelas estruturas laterais, à medida que controlam excentricamente esse movimento da pelve no quadril. O ângulo do colo do fêmur no corpo do fêmur (coxa vara ou coxa valga) pode influenciar a eficiência mecânica das estruturas laterais do quadril. Geralmente, um ângulo anormal é visto em crianças como uma deformidade congênita; vale observar se está presente em adultos, já que pode influenciar a eficiência dessas estruturas laterais.

As forças primárias no golpe do calcanhar até a postura intermediária são absorvidas no quadril e no joelho. No entanto, quando uma pessoa se move da elevação do calcanhar para a ponta do pé, vemos uma demanda proporcional no tornozelo e quadril, o que proporciona uma força igual e oposta na extensão antes do início da fase de balanço. O quadril sofre uma variedade de forças diferentes nas várias atividades da vida diária (Tabela 16.1). Foi demonstrado que com um aumento na propulsão (*pushoff*) da marcha em comparação com uma natural, há atividade mais precoce e aumentada tanto no gastrocnêmico medial quanto no sóleo, com uma redução relativa na demanda de iliopsoas (Lewis e Garibay, 2015). A partir desses dados, é razoável extrapolar que a cadeia cinética pode influenciar a carga e função anterior do quadril e, assim, sugestionar os sintomas, reduzindo a tensão nas estruturas anteriores do quadril. Após a cirurgia para a articulação do quadril, a cinemática pode mudar com uma redução na amplitude de movimento do plano frontal e sagital; menores momentos de abdução do quadril e rotação interna; e diminuição do pico de potência do quadril (Brisson et al., 2013). Portanto, é vital que o clínico compreenda as forças

Tabela **16.1** **Cargas nas articulações do quadril nas atividades da vida diária.**

Movimento	Percentual de carga do peso corporal
Ciclismo	25 a 50
Caminhada	80 a 120
Caminhada rápida	220 a 270
Subir escadas	300
Descer escadas	350
Corrida	500
Tropeçar	900

normais de deambulação e as restaure assim que a sintomatologia diminuir ou após a intervenção.

O foco na mecânica funcional tem sido a articulação do quadril com a pelve. Seria negligente não mencionar a influência que a pelve e o tronco têm sobre o quadril do ponto de vista cinético, e isso é mais bem descrito nos três planos de movimento.

No plano sagital, toda a pelve pode apresentar inclinação anterior, um inominado pode girar anteriormente ou a coluna lombar pode sofrer hiperlordose.

O impacto resultante na articulação do quadril será semelhante independentemente da causa e do início do movimento. A borda acetabular anterior aumentará sua cobertura da cabeça do fêmur e, assim, fornecerá mais suporte/estabilidade articular; esta poderia ser uma estratégia ativa para reduzir as cargas e a tensão de tração nas estruturas anteriores. A desvantagem disso é que pode haver uma tendência aumentada de choque das estruturas de tecidos moles ao redor dos aspectos anteriores da hemipelve (espinha ilíaca anterossuperior/espinha ilíaca ânteroinferior EIAS/EIAI), e aumento da carga na coluna lombar em extensão.

No plano coronal, o movimento primário que provavelmente ocorrerá é um aumento na inclinação para o lado contralateral na marcha, aumentando assim a excursão do trajeto sinusoidal. Esse movimento fará com que o quadril ipsilateral permaneça em rotação interna por mais tempo e seja visto como uma leve rotação para trás do complexo lombopélvico-quadril na postura terminal. Novamente, isso pode reduzir a tensão de tração e a instabilidade nas estruturas anteriores. A consequência desse movimento pode aumentar a força bruta e a tensão adutora na articulação púbica do quadril contralateral e no complexo muscular adutor, bem como a tensão na junção lombossacral. Finalmente, a mudança de peso precoce pode elevar a carga excêntrica relativa nas estruturas laterais do quadril contralateral, possivelmente predispondo ao estresse trocantérico e síndromes de dor.

O movimento do plano transversal sempre ocorre em conjunto com o movimento do plano coronal e, portanto, é improvável que haja rotação isolada. Se isso ocorrer na articulação do quadril, é provável que seja impulsionado do solo para cima, com um aumento no braço do momento pronatório, ou valgo e rotação interna do fêmur. Isso reduzirá novamente a carga nas estruturas articulares anteriores do quadril, mas aumentará uma carga correspondente nas estruturas anterior e medial do joelho e nas estruturas plantar e medial do pé.

Parte | 2 | Aplicação Clínica

> ### Ponto de aprendizagem
> - O quadril recebe grandes forças na marcha (superior 4 × PC, anterior 1 × PC)
> - Isso pode ser influenciado pelo formato da articulação e posição pélvica
> - Alterar o comprimento da passada pode influenciar a carga anterior no quadril
> - A função muscular e o tempo podem reduzir a carga anterior no quadril (propulsão melhorada, por meio de uma boa função da panturrilha).

Movimento no esporte

Para entender o quadril nos movimentos esportivos, precisamos entender quatro atividades principais: corrida (*i. e.*, corrida em velocidade lenta < 5 m/s, 18 km/h); corrida rápida (*i. e.*, corrida em alta velocidade > 7 m/s, ~24 km/h); mudança de direção; e chute.

À medida que fazemos a transição da marcha de caminhada para a corrida, passamos de uma fase de apoio duplo para uma fase de apoio único. Andar é descrito como um modelo de pêndulo invertido, onde o centro de massa atinge seu ponto alto na fase intermediária, e por períodos de forças de frenagem que armazenam energia cinética potencial e de liberação de propulsão (*pushoff*). Em contrapartida, a corrida é vista como um modelo de massa com mola, onde o centro de massa está em um ponto baixo no meio. Desta vez, a frenagem é detalhada por compressão, que armazena energia elástica, e propulsão, liberando o recuo da energia armazenada. Afirma-se que correr é 20% mais eficiente do que caminhar, pois é utilizada mais energia elástica do que mecânica.

Cineticamente, isso se parece com um tempo de contato do pé mais curto, com forças verticais muito mais altas, o que tem mais probabilidade de resultar no movimento da pelve no quadril na fase de apoio. Assim, o FRVS produzirá um braço de momento maior em torno do membro que suporta o peso, aumentando a carga nas estruturas laterais. Se houver energia de corrida positiva (o centro de massa está na frente da base de suporte), então há um braço de momento aumentado para a pelve estar em rotação anterior e a coluna lombar sofrer lordose, colocando uma maior demanda nos abdominais, isquiotibiais e extensores do quadril (glúteos e adutores) para controlar o complexo lombopélvico-quadril. Finalmente, o aumento da propulsão do braço fará com que a pelve gire em direção ao quadril que suporta o peso, colocando uma demanda muito maior nos músculos torcionais, como os oblíquos, glúteos e adutores.

Agora consideraremos o movimento pélvico do quadril durante diferentes velocidades de corrida. As demandas sobre a amplitude de movimento na articulação do quadril aumentam à medida que passam por diferentes velocidades. Além disso, há maior demanda nas restrições passivas ao redor do quadril, do lábio e, em maior medida, do complexo capsuloligamentar. Observe também que o formato da articulação do quadril influenciará a amplitude e a função muscular utilizada durante todas as velocidades de corrida.

Para o propósito deste capítulo, nos concentraremos nos músculos que cruzam a articulação do quadril. O leitor também deve consultar o Capítulo 14 para obter informações sobre as influências de outros músculos ao redor do complexo lombopélvico-quadril.

Durante a caminhada lenta, observamos que a demanda primária é no sóleo, com gastrocnêmico e glúteo médio seguindo de perto. À medida que o indivíduo se move em diferentes velocidades de caminhada, de lento para rápido, há um aumento proporcional na demanda no glúteo máximo, médio e gastrocnêmico. Conforme o indivíduo passa dessas velocidades de caminhada para a corrida lenta e para sua velocidade preferida de corrida, há um aumento acentuado na demanda no vasto em particular e sóleo dominando o pico de força muscular com até 7 × e 5 × PC, respectivamente (Pandy e Andriacchi, 2010).

Curiosamente, as demandas no quadril durante a corrida (3,4 a 5,3 m/s, 12 a 19 km/h), certamente no plano sagital, são muito baixas com até apenas 2 × PC sendo utilizado por ambos os psoas e o complexo de isquiotibiais (Dorn et al., 2012). No entanto, assim que o indivíduo atinge mais de 7 m/s (25 km/h), o quadril começa a assumir o controle, com isquiotibiais, psoas e o vasto contribuindo entre 5 e 6 × PC, enquanto o sóleo ainda é dominante em quase 9 × PC. Uma vez que o indivíduo está em velocidades muito altas (9 m/s, 32,4 km/h), o quadril é dominante, com sóleo e vasto caindo para 7 × e 5 × PC, respectivamente, enquanto os psoas e isquiotibiais estão na região de 9 × PC (Pandy e Andriacchi, 2010).

Com a mudança de direção, a força primária vem do complexo tornozelo-pé (ver Capítulo 14). Porém, o quadril tem um papel fundamental a desempenhar, principalmente com relação aos glúteos máximo e médio, pois controlam a criação de um momento de abdução no joelho e permitem que o CM se afaste da base de apoio.

No chute, o quadril tem a maior rede de força com impacto balístico, com forças relatadas em torno de 450 N e aceleração anterior ao contato de 25,5 m/s (91 km/h); a coxa atinge uma velocidade angular de até 500°/s. No entanto, apesar desses números muito elevados, é relatado que apenas 15% da energia cinética é transferida para a bola (Barfield, 1998). A força restante é perdida no contato do pé pela deformação da bola, perdida na forma de calor ou dissipada pelo corpo, aumentando a tração e a carga excêntrica no complexo lombopélvico-quadril. O que se observa é que a demanda máxima na articulação do quadril ocorre no pico de extensão do quadril, com ativação máxima e pico de carga excêntrica ocorrendo no complexo miofascial, especialmente no adutor longo. Com base na mecânica descrita anteriormente, conclui-se que se houver alguma disfunção ou frouxidão na articulação do quadril, principalmente no que diz respeito às estruturas anteriores, a demanda aumentará nas demais estruturas miofasciais, em particular no adutor longo.

> ### Ponto de aprendizagem
> - Diferentes velocidades de movimento requerem diferentes padrões de disparo muscular
> - Eles podem influenciar e serem influenciados pela cadeia cinética
> - O quadril está intimamente ligado à função tornozelo-pé
> - A mudança de direção requer funções diferentes no quadril em comparação com a corrida em linha reta
> - O chute requer maior controle da extensão, com maior demanda na musculatura anterior
> - Os programas de treinamento e reabilitação requerem uma compreensão das cargas necessárias para caminhar e correr, e construir capacidade para tolerar essas cargas
> - Considere uma sessão simples de chutes de rúgbi envolvendo 40 a 50 *drop kicks*; será claro observar como a demanda no complexo lombopélvico-quadril aumentará significativamente.

Retorno à atividade/esporte

Há uma série de aspectos diferentes específicos do esporte que precisam ser considerados. No entanto, os fundamentos para o retorno à atividade e ao esporte não mudam. Para ser capaz de funcionar no dia a dia, um indivíduo precisa primeiro tolerar as cargas colocadas no quadril na marcha normal e, como isso, aumentar cumulativamente durante o dia.

Vamos usar como exemplo um homem de 80 kg. As atividades normais da vida diária teriam alguém realizando entre 5.000 e 10.000 passos por dia. Se estimarmos que cada membro inferior representa 20% do peso corporal (16 kg), então na fase de balanço há uma demanda entre 40.000 e 80.000 kg de carga. Se estimarmos que a força de reação do solo é 0,8 a 1,2 × PC por contato do pé, então a força vertical será 1,6 a 4,8 mkg de carga. Observe que esses números são extremamente exagerados e consideram apenas a energia mecânica na fase de balanço e de apoio, respectivamente, e retira todas as outras variáveis. Esta carga será bastante reduzida quando se considera a eficiência do movimento, transferência de energia elástica, comprimento da passada, calçados, superfícies etc.

Vamos agora considerar a corrida em velocidade lenta, e de novo usando como exemplo um homem de 80 kg com um comprimento de passada moderado de 1,5 m. Isso significaria que em 400 m haveria 266,66 passadas (133,33 por lado). Podemos estimar que o FRVS será de 2 a 3 × PC por contato do pé. Assim, o seguinte pode ser estimado por membro:

$$400 \text{ m} = 26.600 \text{ kg}$$

$$1 \text{ milha} = 106.400 \text{ kg}$$

$$5 \text{ K sessão de treinamento} = 666.666 \text{ kg}$$

(uma sessão simples de treinamento de rúgbi)

Esses números não levam em consideração o *jogging* rápido ou a corrida em alta velocidade, são puramente de carga mecânica e seguem os mesmos princípios de eliminação de variáveis descritos anteriormente.

Se essas são as demandas fundamentais do corpo humano para caminhar por 1 dia ou para completar uma única sessão de treinamento, então existem algumas demandas básicas de força e *endurance* que precisam ser atendidas a fim de retornar à atividade. Logo, precisamos considerar as atividades de alta demanda na vida diária, como subir e descer escadas, sentar-se para ficar de pé ou vice-versa, as demandas esportivas de mudança de direção, corrida em alta velocidade ou chutes. Se um indivíduo não atendeu aos requisitos básicos, não é de se estranhar que, ao retornar à vida diária/ao esporte, ele pode se descontrolar à medida que as demandas de atividades aumentam.

Patologia

Diferenciar a fonte da dor quando um paciente se apresenta pode se tornar um desafio diagnóstico (Boxe 16.1).

Ao avaliar o quadril esportivo, é importante verificar a área usando uma abordagem estruturada e sistemática. O médico deve tentar criar um casamento entre o histórico obtido, as investigações solicitadas ou recebidas e o exame físico. Um histórico detalhado e completo é vital para ajudar a diagnosticar diferencialmente a origem da dor. O exame físico deve ser usado para confirmar ou negar a hipótese subjacente para a dor e a disfunção que já foi formulada por meio do histórico e das investigações.

> **Boxe 16.1 Dor no quadril relacionada à articulação do quadril**
>
> - Intra-articular – laceração labral ou lesão na borda
> - Acetábulo delaminado
> - Lesão ou defeito osteocondral
> - Corpo solto osteocondral
> - Cistos
> - Ruptura ou distensão do ligamento redondo
> - Capsulite ou sinovite
> - Entorse ou ruptura do ligamento periarticular
> - Osteoartrite
> - Coxa saltans
> - Bursite do iliopsoas e do trocânter maior.

Vários estudos mostram que o quadril pode ter patologia contínua (silenciosa) que pode ser responsável por parte da dor na maioria dos pacientes atendidos (até 44%) (Bradshaw et al., 2008). A chave é verificar se o quadril é um problema primário ou secundário, ou às vezes até mesmo uma pista falsa.

Geralmente, a patologia do quadril se apresenta como uma dor intensa profunda, vaga e inespecífica, sinônimo de dor somática/esclerodermal, ao contrário da patologia adutora/inguinal, que pode ser mais superficial e específica/localizada.

Foi demonstrado que todos os pacientes com patologia articular primária do quadril apresentam dor profunda na virilha que não conseguem identificar. Muitas vezes, é mostrado pelo paciente agarrando em torno dos aspectos laterais e anteriores da articulação do quadril, conhecido como um "sinal C" devido ao formato da mão do paciente ao realizar o movimento. Também é importante notar que a articulação do quadril pode referir dor longe da própria articulação/virilha, com até 6,4 locais de dor em média (Mitchell et al., 2003).

Como parte da obtenção do histórico, o esporte específico que o indivíduo pratica pode ser uma informação útil para o profissional da saúde. Embora a patologia do quadril seja comum em esportes de chute, há uma incidência muito maior de patologia pubiana/adutora nessa situação, então o clínico faria bem em diferenciar isso. Se o atleta está praticando um esporte de torção (*squash*, tênis, *badminton*, hóquei no gelo) ou correndo em linha reta (atletismo/triatlo), há uma maior incidência de patologia da articulação do quadril.

O trabalho foi realizado observando a incidência da articulação do quadril em comparação com outras patologias na população esportiva. Nos homens, verificou-se que 45% tinham patologia de quadril, contra 77% nas mulheres. Além disso, a patologia da articulação do quadril ocorreu com mais frequência como uma entidade isolada, quando comparada à dor relacionada com a articulação adutora ou púbica, que provavelmente ocorre com outra patologia. Os pesquisadores também conseguiram mostrar que a maior incidência de patologia nesta região ocorre na faixa etária de 19 a 40 anos e que esportes de chute (futebol e futebol gaélico) têm a maior incidência de patologia na virilha (Rankin et al., 2015). Esses dados ilustram que a idade e o esporte praticado são determinantes-chave na obtenção do histórico.

Ao realizar o exame físico para auxiliar no processo de reabilitação, o clínico é aconselhado a dividir o objetivo do exame físico em três partes:

1. Identificar a patologia estrutural anatômica que tem o potencial de ser uma fonte de dor.
2. Indicar o provável processo fisiopatológico (inflamação *versus* degeneração) que está causando a dor.

Parte | 2 | Aplicação Clínica

3. Determinar a sobrecarga funcional e disfunções de movimento contribuintes que podem evocar tensão e tensão contínua do tecido, perpetuando assim as duas anteriores.

A patologia labral é a alteração mais provável que um profissional da saúde encontrará em um jovem atleta com dor no quadril. O lábio é responsável por até 63% da patologia observada na artroscopia (Shetty e Villar, 2007).

Ao lidar com patologia labral, o clínico descobrirá que raramente há um histórico de trauma; normalmente é precipitado por estresse repetitivo, seja por flexão e rotação (impacto) ou por extensão (tração no lábio). O paciente pode reclamar de uma sensação de estalo ou pegada – isso precisa ser diferenciado de coxa saltans (síndrome do quadril com ressalto) – ou mesmo um sinal de "agarrar", caracterizado pela sensação de "perder um passo". Mais comumente, a dor é caracterizada por uma dor vaga e profunda, geralmente na prega da virilha, que o paciente não consegue atingir. Será em uma área não específica; em vez de ser capaz de apontar para o local com um dedo, o paciente segurará a articulação do quadril entre o dedo indicador e o polegar (o "sinal C") e comentará "Está bem lá dentro". Isso é apoiado por uma série de estudos que demonstraram que a localização da dor é a chave, descrevendo um "triângulo na virilha" (Falvey et al., 2009; Lovell, 1995).

Para uma visão geral dos princípios de teste, consulte a Tabela 16.2 (os valores normais são fornecidos); o processo do teste descrito não é exaustivo, mas fornece uma sugestão das avaliações principais.

Ao diagnosticar uma patologia do quadril, o histórico (sintomas) e o exame físico (sinais clínicos) são críticos. Há boas evidências que sugerem que, quando essas duas fontes de dados são combinadas com achados radiológicos, há uma forte indicação da fonte de dor (Peters et al., 2017). No primeiro caso, as radiografias simples são as mais úteis para elucidar a morfologia de came ou pinça (Griffin et al., 2016).

Mudanças morfológicas como came ou pinça (ver adiante) que envolvem/aproximam a superfície acetabular com o colo do fêmur dinamicamente em movimento foram descritas como impacto femoroacetabular (IFA). No entanto, isso pode acontecer em indivíduos assintomáticos e, portanto, o fenômeno do impacto mecânico não deve ser visto como patologia isoladamente.

Estudos demonstram que mais de 55% dos atletas terão uma deformidade em came (em comparação com a população em geral em 25%) e que ~50% dos atletas têm uma deformidade em pinça (na população em geral, mais perto de 80%). Mais importante ainda, mais de 60% de ambas as populações apresentam laceração labial. Em todos os casos nas populações amostradas, esses indivíduos eram assintomáticos (Frank et al., 2015). Portanto, o clínico deve estar ciente de que, embora possa haver sinais de patologia no quadril, mais informações serão necessárias antes que possa ser atribuída com segurança a verdadeira causa dos sintomas manifestos.

O leitor é guiado ao acordo de Warwick (Griffin et al., 2016), que descreve a tríade de sintomas, sinais e características radiológicas para fornecer um diagnóstico de síndrome IFA (SIFA). Pode ser adicionado mais peso para o processo de diagnóstico ao melhorar as investigações para incluir imagem em corte transversal (ressonância magnética [RM]; tomografia computadorizada [TC]). Houve algum trabalho adicional para examinar o movimento funcional e sua associação/correlação com a SIFA. Os resultados provisórios indicam que há algum mérito em fazer testes, como um agachamento máximo em pacientes sintomáticos; no entanto, mais estudos precisam ser realizados.

> **Ponto de aprendizagem**
> - O diagnóstico diferencial da patologia do quadril é complexo; uma abordagem sistemática é necessária
> - Equilibre os componentes da estrutura, fisiopatologia e função
> - A síndrome do impacto femoroacetabular (SIFA) é diagnosticada por sintomas, sinais e radiologia
> - A função deve ser esclarecida no processo de diagnóstico.

Radiologia

Ao examinar um paciente, é importante consultar todos os aspectos da imagem que foi realizada. Está além do escopo deste capítulo entrar em detalhes sobre a geração de imagens; o leitor é encaminhado para outros textos.

Para entender melhor a estrutura (formato) da articulação do quadril e como isso pode influenciar a patologia e os sintomas, é importante fazer uma combinação de radiografias com e sem suporte de peso, com ou sem uma TC 3D. Logo, o clínico está em posição de relacionar isso com a função do quadril por meio do exame físico realizado, de modo que o impacto do formato da articulação possa ser avaliado com relação à estabilidade e mobilidade avaliadas.

Os principais ângulos a serem observados são: coxa profunda (profundidade do acetábulo); sinal de cruzamento (acetábulo retro/antevertido); ângulo de Tönnis (teto do acetábulo); ângulo central lateral (cobertura da cabeça do fêmur); ângulo alfa (esfericidade da cabeça do fêmur; desenvolvimento de came). O formato da articulação é de vital importância, pois é considerada a causa de até 73% de todas as lesões labiais (Konrath et al., 1999).

Uma ressonância magnética e uma artrografia por ressonância magnética podem evidenciar muito sobre a articulação e as estruturas que estão danificadas. Quaisquer achados precisam ser correlacionados com o exame físico e a sintomatologia. Como mencionado anteriormente, é comum observar patologias nas imagens que não se relacionam com os sintomas.

Para ajudar no diagnóstico diferencial, especialmente em um padrão misto onde há patologia concomitante, o exame sob anestesia local (ESAL) pode ser extremamente útil. O clínico pode estar relativamente certo de que a articulação do quadril contribui consideravelmente para a apresentação, se a dor diminuir durante a intervenção (Frank et al., 2015).

> **Ponto de aprendizagem**
> - A varredura de radiografia e a tomografia computadorizada 3D são melhores para determinar o formato da articulação
> - A ressonância magnética e a artrografia por ressonância magnética ajudam a avaliar os danos aos tecidos
> - O exame sob anestesia local pode ajudar no processo de diagnóstico.

Reabilitação

O formato da articulação é crítico e afeta os padrões de recrutamento muscular e o movimento da articulação. O clínico deve sempre usar a radiologia disponível, mesmo em pacientes assintomáticos, para ajudar a orientar a seleção do exercício.

Quadril Esportivo **Capítulo** | **16** |

Tabela 16.2 **Procedimento de teste.**

Observação		
Estrutura do membro inferior Pode afetar a carga geral do quadril e da virilha	**Postura geral da coluna** Pode indicar como os músculos estão funcionando	**Visualização direta e inspeção da área** Pequenas áreas de inchaço e mudança de cor podem direcionar o exame
Avaliação do movimento		
Agachamento Procure simetria nos quadris e na capacidade funcional para controlar o movimento	**Afundo lateral ou agachamento unilateral** Procure simetria nos quadris e na capacidade funcional para controlar o movimento	**Corrida/girar a perna em exercício de cadeia aberta** O primeiro pode dizer muito sobre a função muscular e sinergia
Testes de supino – articulação do quadril		
Palpação de todas as proeminências ósseas e tecidos moles que se inserem na e ao redor da articulação do quadril		
ADM – flexão total – 130° Manter o movimento do plano sagital sem desvio		
ADM – rotação completa A proporção normal é 2:1 RE:RI Eixo de rotação – 90° = normal < 70° = restrito; > 100° = móvel		
ADM – abdução – 45 a 60° Porém, avalie também para proteção nos adutores		
Teste para Instabilidade Rotatória Póstero-Lateral (*Dial test*) – qualidade e ADM de rotação em neutro/leve flexão do quadril – procure por sinais de instabilidade/frouxidão		
Teste *log roll* – semelhante ao anterior, mas realizado com a perna apoiada no pedestal e avalia a "elasticidade para trás" do membro inferior		
Tração anterior – na posição aberta da articulação (*loose pack*), aplique um deslizamento posterior-anterior no CF		
Tração lateral – na posição aberta da articulação (*loose pack*), aplique um deslizamento lateral no CF		
Testes de impacto femoroacetabular		
FARIF – flexão, adução e RI e depois flexionar – teste suave em busca de provocação		
FARI – flexão, abdução e RI – em busca de provocação – tem um viés para o acetábulo superior		
Testes de pronação – articulação do quadril		
ADM – RI – ambos os joelhos dobrados buscando por RI passiva total Normal = 30 a 35°		
ADM – RE Em ligeira abdução, realizar RE do quadril Normal = 60° Na FDA, aplique um deslizamento posterior-anterior ao quadril para provocar estruturas anteriores		
ADM – extensão Avaliar alcance – 15 a 60° Avalie a sensação final da cápsula		
Provocação – EARE Na FDA aplique um deslizamento posterior-anterior ao quadril (trocânter maior) para provocar estruturas anteriores		
Restrição passiva – EARE e sensação final O mesmo que o anterior, mas avalie a sensação final da articulação/ligamento iliofemoral		

CF, colo do fêmur; *RE*, rotação externa; *FDA*, final da amplitude; *RI*, rotação interna; *ADM*, amplitude de movimento; *EARE*, extensão, abdução, rotação externa.

O formato do acetábulo é digno de nota (raso, profundo, antevertido ou retrovertido) e o formato do fêmur, em particular, o colo (deformidade em *came* ou um colo antevertido). Essas variações podem influenciar (aumentar ou inibir) a função muscular normal, bem como a função muscular em um estado patológico. A reabilitação não deve se concentrar apenas em restaurar o movimento funcional e a atividade muscular sinérgica, mas também retreinar os músculos para compensar o formato da articulação, esta última exigindo mais experiência clínica.

Se o acetábulo for raso, o recrutamento eficaz dos rotadores profundos e adutores do quadril pode ajudar a estabilizá-lo. Se o quadril é antevertido, então a musculatura posterior do quadril

165

e em particular os glúteos precisam ter melhor capacidade na amplitude externa e controle excêntrico do quadril para desacelerar o eixo de rotação interna natural, que é uma consequência do viés de movimento de ter um quadril antevertido.

Deve ser um pré-requisito de qualquer patologia de quadril e virilha restaurar a amplitude de movimento rotacional normal (a um nível equivalente ao do quadril contralateral). Em particular, é importante maximizar a amplitude de movimento rotacional interna e externa disponível no quadril, tanto em flexão quanto em extensão, não apenas de uma capacidade passiva, mas certificando-se de que haja amplitude de movimento rotacional efetiva em uma posição carregada. O médico também deve observar se o quadril é geralmente restrito (eixo de rotação total de 70° ou menos), normal (eixo de rotação de ~90°) ou móvel (eixo de rotação > 100°), pois isso afetará a prescrição de exercícios.

Finalmente, o clínico deve se concentrar em restabelecer a complacência miofascial normal das estruturas contráteis e não contráteis ao redor do quadril. Isto não se refere especificamente à flexibilidade e à capacidade de alongamento, mas à extensibilidade, ou seja, a capacidade do tecido de se alongar ativamente sem alterar o movimento em uma articulação ou região acima ou abaixo do tecido em questão. Uma vez que isso tenha sido restaurado em um estado ativo sem carga, o médico deve focar na restauração dessa capacidade muscular em um estado ativo com carga, o que é referido a seguir como capacidade de tração.

Ao projetar um programa de reabilitação do quadril, é comum pensar em termos de um paradigma típico de reabilitação com uma progressão linear; entretanto, esta nem sempre é a melhor maneira de restaurar a função. É importante identificar as áreas-chave que precisam ser abordadas e aplicar diferentes estratégias simultaneamente para evocar a resposta e a adaptação em torno da articulação. Em suma, o clínico deve se perguntar quais adaptações ou mudanças no quadril terão maior impacto na dor e na função. Uma vez verificadas, essas áreas devem ser priorizadas no processo de tomada de decisão e exercícios apropriados ou estratégias de tratamento devem ser atribuídos.

Por exemplo, é prática comum para um profissional da saúde restaurar a amplitude de movimento primeiro, em particular com o foco na restauração da rotação (levando em consideração o formato da articulação). Ao recompor o eixo de rotação de movimento, também é aconselhável recuperar a extensão adequada. A extensão é um componente vital do esporte para produzir um torque de extensão durante a corrida e para criar um braço de alavanca para uma força de flexão para chutar. É importante notar que a força anterior do quadril é maior quando ele está em extensão (Lewis e Garibay, 2015).

Como mencionado anteriormente, restaurar o intervalo mais cedo é uma prática comum; no entanto, o clínico deve observar que às vezes o que parece uma restrição de intervalo pode ser devido a uma perda de extensibilidade do tecido sob carga e recrutamento apropriado e função sinérgica sobre uma articulação. Portanto, a estratégia para restaurar a amplitude passivamente pode variar de capacidade de movimento articular à extensibilidade dos tecidos (complacência neurológica) *versus* recrutamento apropriado e função coordenada em torno de uma articulação permitindo que o eixo de movimento seja mantido.

Com esse paradigma em mente, o clínico deve pensar sobre o controle da translação sobre uma articulação, pois o aumento das forças de cisalhamento dentro da articulação pode ser responsável pelo aumento da carga do tecido e, portanto, pela dor. Uma estratégia importante em torno disso é colocar a articulação em uma posição ideal, ou seja, articulação solta; flexionar, abduzir e girar externamente a articulação pode fazer isso. Essa posição reduz o contato articular e aumenta a cobertura da cabeça do fêmur dentro do acetábulo e permite que os músculos ao redor da articulação otimizem o sentido da posição e a cocontração e coativação necessárias para fornecer estabilidade ideal.

Enquanto no esporte esta não é uma posição mantida regularmente, adotá-la para exercícios nos permite otimizar a adaptação do tecido, ou seja, a atividade muscular contínua vai estimular os mecanorreceptores na cápsula e ligamentos e, assim, modular a dor. Com o tempo, o tecido periarticular se adaptará e aumentará em integridade, proporcionando maior estabilidade passiva à articulação.

A maioria dos programas de reabilitação concentra-se em exercícios de levantamento de peso para a função do quadril. No entanto, conforme mencionado, a cabeça do fêmur pode ser exposta em até um terço quando em posição vertical. O clínico é aconselhado a construir exercícios que adotem uma variedade de posições, especialmente nos estágios iniciais, como ajoelhar em quatro apoios com "pernas de sapo" e posições estilo agachamento sumô, ou posições que se concentram na atividade de cadeia fechada na postura unipodal e leve flexão do tronco. Essas posições reduzem a atenuação da carga na linha e estruturas articulares anteriores e, assim, ajudam a restaurar o padrão motor e a sinergia ao redor do quadril.

O profissional da saúde pode trabalhar no equilíbrio da força ao redor do quadril ao mesmo tempo que trabalha na amplitude de movimento e otimiza o padrão motor. Esse equilíbrio de força, especialmente no plano coronal, é vital para o esporte, como foi demonstrado em vários artigos. A literatura do hóquei no gelo examinou extensivamente essa área e mostra claramente que se a força de adução fosse ≤ 78% da força de abdução, então o jogador tinha 17 vezes mais probabilidade de sustentar uma tensão muscular adutora (Tyler et al., 2001). Esses resultados foram apoiados por pesquisas semelhantes realizadas em jogadores de futebol de elite, que mostram que a força isométrica do quadril em adução é maior do que a de abdução para ambos os lados dominante e não dominante e que não há diferença de proporção entre os lados, mas a proporção é significativamente menor em jogadores com dor na virilha (Thorborg et al., 2014).

Embora a relação adução-abdução e o equilíbrio na perna dominante e não dominante sejam a pedra angular do processo de reabilitação, isso não significa apenas os músculos adutores *versus* os músculos abdutores. Trata-se de força de adução total *versus* força de abdução. Portanto, dentro desse modelo conceitual de vetores de força ao longo do quadril no plano coronal, é importante observar que outros músculos desempenham um papel importante em ajudar a produzir esses vetores de força, como os flexores do quadril. O'Connor (2004), ao estudar a dor na virilha, fez referência ao fato de que a força total do quadril envolveu os flexores do quadril, enquanto Lewis et al. (2009) afirmaram que uma diminuição na contribuição da força do iliopsoas durante a flexão resultou em um aumento nas forças anteriores da articulação do quadril.

Uma vez que o clínico tenha restaurado o equilíbrio ao longo do quadril, é hora de considerar a ADM, especialmente a rotação, a força ao longo da amplitude – em particular o plano coronal e a extensão, bem como a função muscular sinérgica ao longo do eixo da articulação. Para retornar a atividade esportiva plena, o clínico precisa transferir esses métodos para atividades e demandas específicas do esporte, seja na velocidade, nos extremos da extensão do quadril ou nas demandas específicas de resistência do quadril; precisa ser apropriado para o atleta e o esporte.

Os parâmetros de carregamento ao redor do quadril e da virilha são tratados no Capítulo 14. No entanto, o leitor deve considerar quatro aspectos principais a esse respeito, o papel do manguito rotador do quadril, o iliopsoas, os glúteos e o adutor magno.

Os rotadores profundos do quadril podem ser classificados de várias maneiras, mas provavelmente constituem uma combinação de glúteos mínimos; o tendão conjunto do obturador interno com os gêmeos superior e inferior; piriforme; quadrado femoral; obturador externo; reto femoral (cabeça curta); e iliocapsular. Está além do escopo deste capítulo cobrir sua função em detalhes. No entanto, é importante chamar a atenção do leitor para alguns aspectos importantes. O glúteo mínimo se comunica com a cápsula superiormente, enquanto o obturador externo e o tendão conjunto no obturador interno e o gêmeo (que flanqueia o obturador interno) se comunicam com a cápsula posteriormente. Glúteo mínimo, cabeça curta do reto femoral e iliocapsular, todos se comunicam anteriormente com a cápsula. Portanto, recuperar a eficiência do recrutamento, o controle e a tensão apropriada podem tensionar e controlar a cápsula, que pode guiar a cabeça do fêmur para posições livres de impacto. A tensão prolongada aplicada por meio da cápsula pode estimular a produção de colágeno e aumentar a resistência à tração e, portanto, a taxa de deformação, melhorando a estabilidade e os padrões de movimento na articulação.

Estratégias de reabilitação para ajudar a estimular o manguito rotador e a cápsula podem ser utilizadas fazendo trabalho isométrico submáximo sustentado nas principais posições de tração e, em seguida, mantendo essas posições por períodos de tempo para desenvolver a tensão de tração. Os exemplos incluem a posição em quatro apoios com "pernas de sapo" ou postura de "gorila de dorso prateado" e agachamento sumô trabalhado em intervalos mais profundos, mobilizando-se de um lado para o outro. É feita referência particular ao obturador externo (que curiosamente também tem um momento de adução); foi demonstrado que estabiliza a cabeça do fêmur no soquete e tem momento de rotação externa seletivo a 0° e 90°. A isometria é a chave novamente, pois o músculo não possui o comprimento da fibra muscular para produzir excursão.

O iliopsoas tem múltiplas funções, incluindo compressão axial (vertical) dos segmentos da coluna lombar; controle excêntrico da flexão lateral do tronco; controle do inominado, especialmente na rotação posterior; braço do momento de adução no quadril (em particular o psoas maior); e, a seguir, um grande momento flexor do quadril em extensão, sobretudo por usar a eminência iliopectínea como fulcro para aumentar o braço de alavanca e a eficiência mecânica na extensão. No entanto, como mencionado anteriormente, há um músculo adjuvante com iliopsoas no iliocapsular, que fica diretamente sobre a face medial anterior da cápsula. Este músculo demonstrou ter ativação seletiva na flexão de quadril em 90°, onde tensiona a cápsula para evitar o impacto.

O iliopsoas e seus auxiliares podem ser mais bem carregados e ativados com exercícios isométricos de flexão do quadril; trabalho de limiar de recrutamento a partir da estabilidade da coluna vertebral e "puxando o quadril para dentro do soquete" para estabilidade local do quadril; carga de adução estática no quadril (ponte lateral do adutor); carregamento lateral do tronco (pranchas laterais); e carregamento de flexão do quadril.

Os glúteos têm uma grande variedade de funções no quadril. O glúteo máximo é o maior produtor de força de extensão, abdução e rotação externa, com um grande braço de alavanca que permite influenciar a excursão. Embora o glúteo médio tenha um braço de momento para abduzir, seu eixo é próximo ao da articulação do quadril e, assim, não possui o braço de alavanca para produzir a abdução com eficiência. Além disso, o comprimento da fibra muscular é muito curto, o que implica que ele não pode produzir a excursão necessária. Em vez disso, o glúteo médio é mais bem projetado para produzir força na abdução ou por desaceleração/controle excêntrico da adução. Portanto, o glúteo máximo é mais bem treinado com uma variedade de movimentos que envolvem tanto a sustentação quanto a não sustentação de peso, em todos os três planos de movimento. No entanto, o glúteo médio pode ser mais bem treinado por meio de isometria pesada e momentos de resistência em adução, como um mergulho com uma perna, ou estocagem onde o centro de massa produz um braço de momento de adução no quadril.

O adutor magno foi bem descrito no Capítulo 14. Porém, a mensagem principal no quadril é que seu compartimento mais proximal tem um braço de momento para aproximar a cabeça do fêmur no acetábulo e, assim, fornecer estabilidade, puxando a cabeça para baixo, reduzindo as forças articulares superior e anterior descritas previamente. Além disso, devido à sua função multipenada e multicompartimental, ele tem um grande braço de momento na extensão do quadril e se torna um componente-chave em exercícios de aceleração, agachamento, *split squats*, afundo e *step-ups*.

O retorno ao esporte e ao treinamento/competição total está além do escopo desse capítulo. No entanto, ao projetar esse programa, é útil resumir e incorporar componentes-chave do esporte. Considere o seguinte:

- Estruturar e projetar um programa apropriado que permita que a mecânica seja compensada
- Compreender as cargas funcionais no quadril e os diferentes suportes musculares que podem ser fornecidos por meio das estruturas profundas e superficiais, especialmente a cápsula
- Compreender as cargas extremas de correr e chutar e dar tempo suficiente para adaptação nos tecidos para tolerar essas forças
- Construir um equilíbrio adequado ao longo do quadril, principalmente no plano sagital e coronal, de modo que haja pelo menos uma proporção de 1:1; o foco primário deve estar sempre no plano sagital e coronal, pois o movimento rotacional é terciário e um movimento combinado com o plano coronal. Assim, a restauração do equilíbrio do vetor de força do plano coronal irá restaurar a rotação. Se for necessária atenção especial para os rotadores profundos, isso pode ser resolvido, mas não às custas dos primeiros.

Referências bibliográficas

Barfield, W.R., 1998. The biomechanics of kicking in soccer. Clinics in Sports Medicine. 17 (4) 711-28.

Bergmann, G., Deuretzbacher, G., Heller, M., Graichen, F., Rohlmann, A.; Strauss, J., Duda, G.N.; 2001. Hip contact forces and gait patterns from routine activities. Journal of Biomechanics 34 (7), 859-871.

Bradshaw, C.J., Bundy, M., Falvey, E., 2008. The diagnosis of longstanding groin pain: a prospective clinical cohort study. British Journal of Sports Medicine 42 (10), 851-854.

Brisson, N., Lamontagne, M., Kennedy, M.J., Beaulé, P.E., 2013. The effects of cam femoroacetabular impingement corrective surgery on lower-extremity gait biomechanics. Gait Posture 37 (2), 258-263.

Dorn, T.W., Schache, A.G., Pandy, M.G., 2012. Muscular strategy shift in human running: dependence of running speed on hip and ankle muscle performance. The Journal of Experimental Biology 215 (Pt 11), 1944-1956.

Falvey, E.C., Franklyn-Miller, A., McCrory, P.R., 2009. The groin triangle: a patho-anatomical approach to the diagnosis of chronic groin pain in athletes. British Journal of Sports Medicine 43 (3), 213-220.

Frank, R.M., Lee, S., Bush-Joseph, C.A., Kelly, B.T., Salata, M.J., Nho, S.J., 2015. Improved outcomes after hip arthroscopic surgery in patients undergoing T-capsulotomy with complete repair versus partial repair for FAI; a comparative matched-pair analysis. The American Journal of Sports Medicine 42 (11), p2634-2642.

Gracovetsky, S.A., Iacono, S., 1987. Energy transfers in the spinal engine. Journal of Biomedical Enginering 9 (2), 99-114.

Griffin, D.R., Dickenson, E.J., O'Donnell, J., Agricola, R., Awan, T., Beck, M., et al., 2016. The Warwick agreement on femoroacetabular impingement syndrome (FAI syndrome): an international consensus statement. British Journal of Sports Medicine 50 (19), p1169-1176.

Harris, J.D., Gerrie, B.J., Lintner, D.M., Varner, K.E., McCulloch, P.C., 2016. Microinstability of the hip and the splits Radiograph. Orthopedics 39 (1), e169-e175.

Khair, M.M., Grzybowski, J.S., Kuhns, B.D., Wuerz, T.H., Shewman, E., Nho, S.J., 2017. The effect of capsulotomy and capsular repair on hip distraction a cadaveric investigation. Arthroscopy: The Journal of Arthroscopic and Related Surgery 33 (3), 559-565.

Konrath, G.A., Hamel, A.J., Olson, S.A., Bay, B., Sharkey, N.A., 1999. The role of the acetabular labrum and the transverse acetabular ligament in load transmission in the hip. The Journal of Bone and Joint Surgery 80 (12), 1781-1788.

Lewis, C.L., Garibay, E.J., 2015. Effect of increased pushoff during gait on hip joint forces. Journal of Biomechanics 48 (1), 181-185.

Lewis, C.L., Sahrmann, S.A., Moran, D.W., 2007. Anterior hip joint force increases with hip extension, decreased gluteal force, or decreased iliopsoas force. Journal of Biomechanics 40 (16), 3725-3731.

Lewis, C.L., Sahrmann, S.A., Moran, D.W., 2009. Effect of position and alteration in synergist muscle function contribution on hip forces when performing hip strengthening exercises. Clinical Biomechanics 24, 35-42.

Lovell, G., 1995. The diagnosis of chronic groin pain in athletes: a review of 189 cases. Australian Journal of Science and Medicine in Sport 27 (3), 76-79.

Magerkurth, O., Jacobson, J.A., Morag, Y., Caoili, E., Fessell, D., Sekiya, J.K., 2013. Capsular laxity of the Hip: findings at magnetic resonance arthrography. Arthroscopy: The Journal of Arthroscopic and Related Surgery 29 (10), 1615-1622.

Mann, R.A., Hagy, J., 1980. Biomechanics of walking, running, and sprinting. The American Journal of Sports Medicine 8 (5), 345-350.

Mitchell, B., McCrory, P., Brukner, P., O'Donnell, J., Colson, E., Howells, R., 2003. Hip joint pathology: clinical presentation and correlation between magnetic resonance arthrography, ultrasound, and arthroscopic findings in 25 consecutive cases. Clinical Journal of Sports Medicine 13,152-156.

Nepple, J.J., Smith, M.V., 2015. Biomechanics of the hip capsule and capsule management strategies in hip arthroscopy. Sports Medicine and Arthroscopy Review 23 (4), 164-168.

O'Connor, D., 2004. Groin injuries in professional rugby league players: a prospective study. Journal of Sports Science 22 (7), 629-636.

Pandy, M.G., Andriacchi, T.P., 2010. Muscle and joint function in human locomotion. Annual Review of Biomedical Engineering 12, 401-433.

Peters, S., Laing, A., Emerson, C., et al., 2017. Surgical criteria for femoroacetabular impingement syndrome: a scoping review. British Journal of Sports Medicine 51 (22), 1605-1610.

Philippon, M.J., Michalski, M.P., Campbell, K.J., Goldsmith, M.T., Devitt, B.M., Wijdicks, C.A., et al., 2014. Surgically relevant bony and soft tissue anatomy of the proximal femur. The Orthopedic Journal of Sports Medicine 2 (6), 1-9 DOI2325967114535188.

Rankin, A.T., Bleakley, C.M., Cullen, M., 2015. Hip Joint Pathology as a leading cause of groin pain in the sporting population; a 6 year review of 894 cases. The American Journal of Sports Medicine 43 (7), 1698-1703.

Shetty, V.D., Villar, R.N., 2007. Hip arthroscopy: current concepts and review of the literature. British Journal of Sports Medicine 41 (2), 64-68.

Thorborg, K., Branci, S., Nielsen, M.P., Tang, L., Nielsen, M.B., Hölmich, P., 2014. Eccentric and isometric hip adduction strength in male soccer players with and without adductor-related groin pain: an assessor-blinded comparison. Orthopaedic Journal of Sports Medicine 2 (2) 2325967114521778.

Tyler, T.F., Nicholas, S.J., Campbell, R.J., McHugh, M.P., 2001. The association of hip strength and flexibility with the incidence of adductor muscle strains in professional ice hockey players. American Journal of Sports Medicine 29 (2), 124-128.

van Arkel, R.J., Amis, A.A., Jeffers, J.R., 2015. The envelope of passive motion allowed by the capsular ligaments of the hip. Journal of Biomechanics. 48 (14), 3803-3809.

Walters, B.L., Cooper, J.H., Rodriguez, J.A., 2014. New findings in hip capsular anatomy: dimensions of capsular thickness and pericapsular contributions. Arthroscopy: The Journal of Arthroscopic and Related Surgery 30 (10), 1235-1245.

Wuerz, T.H., Song, S.H., Grzybowski, J.S., et al., 2016. Capsulotomy size affects hip joint kinematic stability. Arthroscopy: The Journal of Arthroscopic and Related Surgery 32 (8), 1571-1580.

Capítulo | 17 |

Disfunção Lombopélvica na População Esportiva: O "o Que", o "Porquê" e o "Como"

Neil Sullivan

Introdução

As práticas de tratamento, os métodos e as filosofias irão inevitavelmente evoluir ao longo de uma carreira. Isso dependerá de influências como cursos, pesquisas, colegas, opiniões de especialistas, experiências de resultados positivos e, definitivamente, experiências de resultados negativos. Minha própria prática clínica foi moldada muito cedo, passando um tempo com um fisioterapeuta que me ensinou a questionar tudo o que eu fazia e tudo o que eu pensava, que é, em essência, o ponto crucial do raciocínio clínico. Assistir às avaliações e aos tratamentos e falar sobre o raciocínio clínico nesta prática proporcionou uma grande visão e aprofundou o meu desejo de aprender mais sobre a disfunção lombopélvica.

Um capítulo sozinho não é suficiente para fornecer uma cobertura abrangente da função e da patologia da região lombopélvica, incluindo a anatomia detalhada e como isso fornece movimento e estabilidade. Em vez disso, neste capítulo, forneço orientação sobre como identificar a disfunção lombopélvica no atleta. São discutidos testes objetivos e técnicas de avaliação, possibilitando determinar a manifestação dos sintomas, a origem e, finalmente, por que o problema pode ter ocorrido em primeiro lugar – essencialmente, o "o que", o "porquê" e o "como".

A pelve é o ponto médio da máquina humana, é uma base para tudo o que está acima e uma plataforma significativa para tudo o que está abaixo. As estruturas que se conectam à pelve são vastas, variadas e essenciais para a locomoção, postura e função humanas. A pelve é frequentemente negligenciada como contribuinte para a dor, disfunção e lesões. Frequentemente, é mais fácil diagnosticar e tratar outras estruturas do que corrigir a causa raiz da lesão.

A região lombopélvica é complexa, pois transfere a carga da parte superior do corpo e fornece estabilidade e controle dinâmico. Consiste na coluna lombar, dois ossos inominados (ílio fundido, ísquio e púbis) e o sacro (Figura 17.1). O sacro e dois ossos inominados formam o anel pélvico, com duas articulações sacroilíacas posteriormente e a sínfise púbica anteriormente. A integridade do anel pélvico é proporcionada pelo fechamento forçado (sistema ativo usando músculo e fáscia) e pelo fechamento da forma (sistema passivo constituído de articulações e

ligamentos). A espinha ilíaca anterossuperior (EIAS), a espinha ilíaca posterossuperior (EIPS), as cristas ilíacas, o ligamento inguinal, a tuberosidade isquiática e o ramo púbico superior são os pontos de referência anatômicos que ajudam os profissionais da saúde a avaliarem e tratarem isso.

A chave para tratar com sucesso o paciente com problemas lombopélvicos é ampliar o ponto de vista de "Qual é a área lesionada em questão?" para "Por que esse problema ocorreu?". Precisamos olhar para as estruturas que podem contribuir para esse problema e restaurá-las para que funcionem sem dor. O componente final do processo é "Como isso aconteceu na primeira instância?", pois ser capaz de encontrar um contribuidor para o problema (o "como") nos possibilita, como clínicos, apreciar totalmente os motivadores por trás do problema e orientar os atletas adequadamente. Esses motivadores podem estar relacionados com o treinamento ativo ou com a competição, ou podem ser decorrentes de modificações passivas, de comportamentos habituais e/ou de posicionamento postural. Entender o *como* pode garantir que sejamos mais eficazes no tratamento do atleta. Isso nos permitirá aconselhar os atletas e, então, tratá-los de maneira eficaz, com a confiança de obter um resultado positivo.

No futebol e no rúgbi profissionais, e na prática privada, a disfunção lombopélvica pode contribuir para muitas apresentações musculoesqueléticas. Nem todas as avaliações desta área serão devido a sintomas locais. Os clínicos experientes que trabalham no esporte incluem o exame desta área como parte do processo de avaliação geral com várias apresentações diferentes, especialmente se forem insidiosas ou mesmo crônicas por natureza. Patologias e condições específicas, como dor lombar, distensões nos isquiotibiais e dor na virilha, também exigem o exame da região lombopélvica como um contribuinte para um quadro mais amplo. Pode ser o principal fator ou apenas um contribuinte para a disfunção ou dor do atleta, mas de qualquer maneira, ao incluir isso como parte de sua avaliação geral, como clínico, mune-se de mais informações para resolver o problema.

Por exemplo, a dor na virilha relacionada com o adutor é uma apresentação comum no futebol. A origem do adutor é encontrada no ramo púbico inferior, portanto, qualquer alinhamento pélvico alterado pode resultar em uma posição modificada do púbis e, portanto, ajudar o aumento da tensão e da carga do adutor. Por sua vez, a rotação posterior de um ílio também pode contribuir

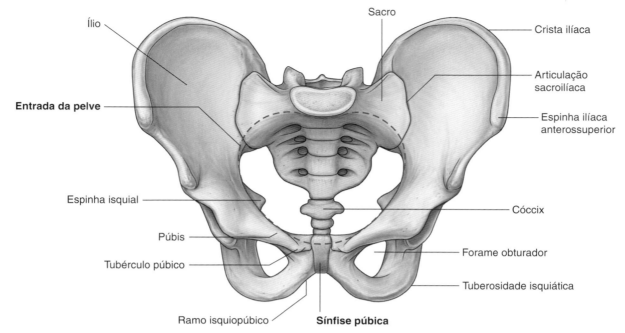

Figura 17.1 Pelve óssea.

para a virilha anterior ou dor púbica no lado ipsilateral, devido a um aumento potencial na tensão do ligamento inguinal.

Transversalmente, uma rotação anterior do ílio altera a posição da tuberosidade isquiática e, portanto, pode facilitar o aumento da tensão dos isquiotibiais. Mudanças sutis de posição da pelve ou aumentos na tensão das estruturas que se fixam e saem da pelve podem ter um efeito na função (Figura 17.2). Os treinamentos fasciais proximais e distais à pelve podem contribuir para a função ou posicionamento alterados ou serem afetados pela posição modificada da região lombopélvica.

Avaliação – identificação do "o que"

A avaliação deve ser metódica e estratégica. Se for feita dessa maneira, deve descobrir pistas que permitirão um diagnóstico preciso e, em última análise, um plano de tratamento eficaz. O processo deve começar com um histórico detalhado, antes de passar para um exame visual. O próximo estágio é colocar o paciente em alguns testes cinéticos ou de movimento, que são projetados para destacar quaisquer deficiências ou disfunções de movimento. Finalmente, há uma avaliação física, onde palpação e habilidades visuais são utilizadas para confirmar uma hipótese diagnóstica desenvolvida. O exame e a avaliação que se seguem foram desenvolvidos ao longo dos anos para se adequarem à minha prática clínica e são um híbrido de cursos e experiências pessoais.

Histórico do paciente

Como acontece com todas as boas avaliações, obter um histórico detalhado do atleta ou paciente é essencial. No ambiente esportivo, muitas vezes nos familiarizamos com as apresentações individuais dos atletas. Talvez eles sejam dominantes de um lado, tenham uma condição subjacente conhecida ou um histórico de lesões que os predispõe determinado padrão ou restrição de movimento. Todas essas informações são relevantes. A coisa mais importante a ser lembrada é que se está tentando montar o quebra-cabeça. O paciente pode relatar ao profissional da saúde uma lesão no tendão da coxa; este, por sua vez, precisará descobrir como é provável que ela tenha ocorrido e se a região lombopélvica contribuiu. Nesse momento, é possível fazer uma série de perguntas estruturadas para estabelecer um quadro:
- Qual foi o mecanismo?
- Qual foi a atividade no momento da lesão?
- Há quanto tempo o paciente está ciente do problema?
- O que o paciente estava fazendo nos dias anteriores àquele ponto que pode ter contribuído (exercícios e descanso)?

Avaliação visual e observação

A observação inicial pode revelar uma das anormalidades clássicas mostradas na Figura 17.3.

Com o paciente em pé, muitas vezes existem várias pistas que podem ser utilizadas para orientar o resto da avaliação. O Boxe 17.1 ilustra alguns marcadores de avaliação visual e fornece detalhes que devem ser examinados.

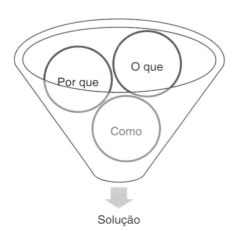

Figura 17.2 Componentes de uma intervenção bem-sucedida.

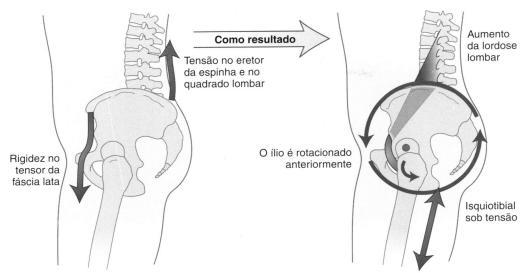

Figura 17.3 Efeitos da musculatura tensa no alinhamento da pelve. (*Esta figura se encontra reproduzida em cores no Encarte.*)

Nem todas as observações são relevantes para a disfunção lombopélvica, mas cada uma pode fornecer uma peça do quebra-cabeça que revela o quadro geral. Ao ligar as peças, não apenas será possível entender a apresentação do paciente, como também descobrir as razões pelas quais sua disfunção lombopélvica se manifestou em primeira instância.

A próxima etapa é passar para os testes cinéticos. Ao contrário dos testes de provocação de dor comumente usados para confirmar a dor na articulação sacroilíaca (ASI), esses testes são aplicados para considerar a qualidade do movimento da região lombopélvica e são elementos-chave da avaliação. Assim, ao avaliar a qualidade do movimento, podemos determinar se há uma disfunção contribuindo para o problema do nosso paciente ou que pode levar a um problema futuro. No entanto, neste ponto, vale a pena lembrar que há evidências limitadas para apoiar a confiabilidade ou validade desses testes isoladamente ao tentar identificar uma disfunção na ASI. Laslett (2008) sugere que um padrão de referência para testes de disfunção na ASI não foi estabelecido, portanto, a validade deles para este transtorno é desconhecida. No entanto, quando realizados em grupos, alguns estudos descobriram que a confiabilidade é aumentada (Laslett, 2008).

Ao realizar os seguintes testes regular e coletivamente, podemos começar a associar os resultados com a nossa avaliação visual. A partir daqui é possível criar uma imagem de quais estruturas estão envolvidas e/ou estão contribuindo para a apresentação. Por exemplo, um teste positivo (que mostra movimento alterado) direcionará o processo de tratamento que se segue: o lado positivo nem sempre é o que provoca dor e, muitas vezes, não está na área de onde o paciente percebe que estão vindo os sintomas, portanto, tenha isso em mente. No passado avaliei muitos pacientes com sintomas de isquiotibiais, por exemplo. Às vezes, é fácil concentrar-se na área sintomática em questão para a qual

---

Boxe 17.1 Postura – marcadores de avaliação visual

Postura do pé

O paciente fica em pé com postura de pé igual? A pronação do pé pode sugerir uma estratégia de compensação para um comprimento maior do membro ou uma rotação anterior do ílio (Figura 17.4 A). A supinação pode sugerir uma estratégia de compensação para um comprimento menor do membro ou uma rotação posterior do ílio (Figura 17.4 B).

Posição do joelho

Um paciente em pé com o joelho fletido de um lado pode indicar uma discrepância no comprimento da perna ou uma rotação anterior do ílio (Figura 17.4 C).

Alinhamento da crista ilíaca

Se houver uma diferença visível na altura, isso pode ser causado pelo aumento do tônus no paravertebral lombar ou no quadrado lombar. Também pode demonstrar uma discrepância no comprimento da perna – funcional ou estrutural (Figura 17.4 D).

Alinhamento do ombro

Aqui deve-se procurar por diferenças na altura dos ombros. Um lado fica mais alto? Em caso afirmativo, isso se deve à tensão localizada ou ao aumento do volume muscular? Também pode sugerir uma discrepância no comprimento da perna ou disfunção lombopélvica (Figura 17.4 E).

Massa muscular

Existem assimetrias óbvias no volume? Alguns atletas, pela natureza de seu esporte, apresentam assimetrias no volume, portanto, tome cuidado para não presumir que o volume alterado é uma anormalidade.

Alinhamento espinal

O atleta está com aumento da lordose ou cifose? Essas mudanças posturais podem ser duradouras se forem simétricas e podem ser algo a ser considerado para a restauração ao longo do tempo se afetarem a função e o desempenho. Mais importante ainda, há algum sinal de escoliose? Qualquer ligeira alteração ou desvio lateral da coluna vertebral pode ser uma discrepância estrutural ou funcional no comprimento da perna que precisará ser tratada para obter o melhor resultado possível (Figura 17.4 F).

Posição da cabeça e do pescoço

Procure algum tônus aumentado na musculatura do pescoço, especialmente unilateral. Isso pode indicar mudanças posturais e o aumento do tônus na linha posterior superficial pode alterar a dinâmica mais abaixo na cadeia.

(continua)

> **Boxe 17.1 Postura – marcadores de avaliação visual** (*Continuação*)

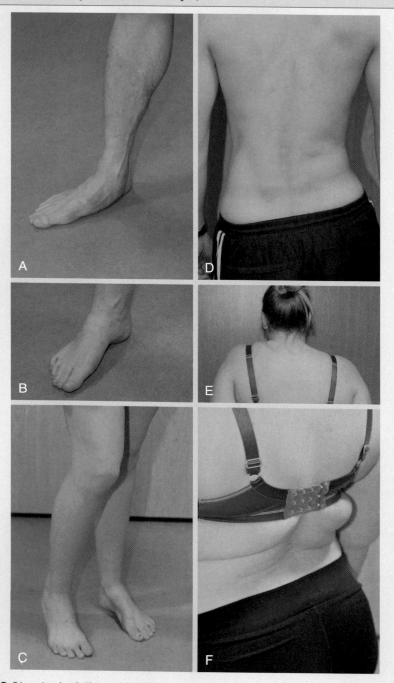

Figura 17.4 A. Pé pronado. **B.** Pé supinado. **C.** Flexão do joelho para acomodar o comprimento da perna. **D.** Lado direito da crista ilíaca elevada. **E.** Cintura omoplata elevada do lado esquerdo. **F.** Aumento da lordose lombar.

o paciente aponta. Ao examinar adicionalmente a região lombopélvica, é fácil ver como uma disfunção nessa área pode contribuir ou ser um fator causal nesta apresentação. Ao observar, compreender e corrigir essas disfunções, podemos facilitar um resultado bem-sucedido, acelerando a recuperação, auxiliando na reabilitação e até mesmo prevenindo lesões futuras.

Antes de pedir ao paciente que realize qualquer um desses testes de movimento, certifique-se de que ele é fisicamente capaz de realizá-los. Use suas habilidades de raciocínio clínico para determinar se exacerbará algum sintoma. Pode ser o caso de realizar apenas um ou dois dos testes, em vez de todos eles. Isso ainda pode ser suficiente para fornecer a você, como profissional de saúde, informações de diagnóstico suficientes.

Testes em pé ou testes cinéticos

Avaliação da flexão do tronco

Durante a realização deste teste, procuramos quaisquer assimetrias na amplitude e qualidade do movimento, pois estamos

Disfunção Lombopélvica na População Esportiva: O "o Que", o "Porquê" e o "Como"

avaliando o quão bem as articulações sacroilíacas se movem. Outros fatores a serem observados são a qualidade da flexão da coluna lombar e a tensão ou assimetria torácica. Mais informações sobre esse teste, sua sensibilidade e especificidade são fornecidas por Tong et al. (2006).

Método. Peça ao paciente que fique de costas com os pés afastados na largura do quadril. Neste ponto, será necessário palpar a EIPS. Prenda os polegares sob essas estruturas, isso ajudará a eliminar muitos erros ao monitorar o movimento e oferece um grau muito maior de *feedback*. Peça ao paciente que flexione para frente o máximo que puder confortavelmente. Procure um movimento suave e uniforme de ambas as EIPS à medida que o paciente se flexiona para a frente. A amplitude e a qualidade dos movimentos são fundamentais e devem ser simétricas. Se a EIPS de um lado se move mais longe do que o outro, isso pode sugerir que a ASI está hipomóvel desse lado. Essa avaliação fornece uma grande quantidade de informações ao clínico, mas também pode apresentar algumas pistas falsas, portanto, não tire conclusões precipitadas.

Avaliação da extensão do tronco

Para obter informações mais detalhadas sobre este teste, sua sensibilidade e especificidade, consulte Gibbons (2017).

Método. Peça ao paciente que fique de costas e se estenda para trás enquanto mantém a posição das mãos em sua EIPS. Procure um movimento ligeiramente inferior da EIPS. O movimento de extensão pode, às vezes, provocar dor e reproduzir sintomas em algumas etiologias, especialmente condições da coluna lombar, como dor discogênica ou dor nas articulações facetárias. Este também é o momento de realizar o teste de Michelis (extensão do tronco com flexão lateral, em postura unipodal no lado ipsilateral) para avaliar a integridade da *pars interarticularis*. A resposta ao estresse na *pars* é uma das causas mais comuns de dor lombar em atletas adolescentes. É uma condição crônica de uso excessivo que geralmente começa como uma leve dor nas costas unilateral e progride com a atividade. A progressão dessa condição pode levar a uma fratura por estresse na *pars*; a identificação precoce dessa apresentação é fundamental para o tratamento, pois um atraso pode causar um defeito permanente ou espondilólise.

Flexão lateral do tronco

Mais informações sobre este teste, sua sensibilidade e especificidade, são fornecidas em Gibbons (2017).

Método. O teste mostrará como o sacro se move em relação ao ílio. Coloque seus polegares na EIPS e, em seguida, mova um polegar para o centro do sacro no mesmo nível da EIPS. Peça ao paciente que flexione o lado para o lado em que seu polegar está palpando a EIPS. Deve ser observado um deslizamento superior sutil, mas suave, do sacro à medida que o lado do paciente se flexiona. A falta de movimento superior ao comparar um lado ao outro pode, novamente, sugerir uma ASI hipomóvel.

Teste de Gillet ou teste de cegonha

Esse teste comumente usado fornece muitas informações ao examinador ao avaliar a ASI. Não apenas fornece *feedback* sobre como a ASI se move, mas também como a perna de apoio atua para manter o alinhamento pélvico. Arab et al. (2009) fornecem mais detalhes sobre este teste, sua sensibilidade e especificidade.

Método. Para realizar o teste, fique atrás do paciente e apalpe a EIPS colocando um polegar no sacro no mesmo nível da EIPS.

Instrua o paciente a ficar em uma perna enquanto levanta a outra perna em 90° de flexão de joelho e quadril. Nesse caso, se ele estiver flexionando o quadril esquerdo, o examinador colocará o polegar esquerdo na EIPS esquerda enquanto o polegar direito palpa o sacro. Repita o teste do outro lado e compare a amplitude e a qualidade do movimento. Um movimento normal mostraria a EIPS deslizando inferiormente sobre o sacro. Qualquer restrição nesse movimento em comparação com o outro lado sugere que a ASI está hipomóvel nesse lado.

Teste de extensão do quadril

Gibbons (2017) fornece mais detalhes sobre este teste, sua sensibilidade e especificidade.

Método. Coloque um polegar na EIPS e o outro no centro do sacro, no mesmo nível da EIPS, da mesma maneira que no teste de Gillet ou cegonha. Peça ao paciente que fique em pé e, em seguida, em uma perna enquanto estende o quadril levando o calcanhar para trás em sua direção. Um movimento normal mostrará a EIPS deslizando em uma direção superior. Compare esquerda e direita.

Como em todos esses testes, um resultado positivo é determinado se um movimento for de menor amplitude, de pior qualidade ou provocar dor. Não importa se nesta fase o paciente não apresenta nenhum teste cinético positivo (K + ve). Continue com o processo de avaliação e construa um quadro completo da apresentação do paciente e qualquer disfunção pélvica antes de considerar o tratamento da coluna lombar.

Palpação

As habilidades de palpação são muito importantes no processo de avaliação. É fundamental entender o alinhamento dos pontos ósseos, a tensão na musculatura e as restrições dos tecidos para os corretos diagnóstico e tratamento do paciente.

Supino

Nesta posição, procure identificar se existem assimetrias de alinhamento: cristas ilíacas, EIAS, ramo púbico superior, trocânter maior e maléolo medial. Ao incluir o maléolo medial, é possível considerar se há alguma discrepância no comprimento da perna. Essa diferença pode ser estrutural ou funcional e precisará de mais investigações para confirmar posteriormente.

Prono

Com o paciente ou atleta deitado de frente, avalie o alinhamento das cristas ilíacas, EIPS, sulco sacral, ligamento sacrotuberal, tuberosidade isquiática e calcâneo. Nessa fase, também é recomendado fazer uma comparação da rotação interna dos quadris.

Nutação sacral, contranutação sacral ou inclinação sacral

Como sabemos, a pelve é composta por três ossos, dois inominados e o sacro. Até agora discutimos testes usados para identificar alterações na posição dos inominados, mas alterações na posição sacral também são apresentações comuns.

Existem várias maneiras de descrever esta próxima apresentação. Ocasionalmente, um paciente pode apresentar uma disfunção durante os testes cinéticos em pé, mas quando eles estão

Parte | 2 | Aplicação Clínica

no pedestal, há muito pouco que sugira qualquer variação de alinhamento. É quando a posição sacral precisa ser avaliada pela palpação do sulco sacral. A maneira mais simples de descrever isso, sem entrar em detalhes sobre a anatomia da pelve e das ASI, é uma inclinação do sacro para um lado ou para o outro. Agora, estamos avaliando como a posição sacral pode afetar a ASI K + ve. O sacro pode parecer mais alto ou raso (contranutado) no lado K + ve, em comparação com o lado funcional. Alternativamente, o sacro pode parecer mais baixo ou profundo (nutado) no lado K + ve em comparação com o lado funcional.

Posicionamento do paciente

A técnica usada para avaliar esta apresentação é com o paciente deitado em decúbito ventral, para colocar os polegares em cima de ambas as EIPS. Um de cada vez, role o polegar sobre a EIPS medialmente e sobre o sacro. Deve-se comparar a profundidade da queda da EIPS para o sacro e observar se há uma diferença da esquerda para a direita. Isso exigirá excelentes habilidades palpatórias. A diferença geralmente será sutil, mas deve-se tentar sentir a diferença com as mãos, em vez de visualizá-la com os olhos. Isso também pode ser avaliado na extensão lombar. Peça ao paciente que se estenda nos quadris, apoiando-se nos cotovelos. Além disso, na flexão lombar, solicite ao paciente que se sente sobre os calcanhares. Essas três posições de teste fornecerão uma imagem mais clara desta apresentação.

Testes em decúbito dorsal deitado

Elevação ativa da perna reta

Peça ao paciente que levante um pé da cama em 10 cm, depois abaixe-o novamente antes de levantar a perna oposta. Agora pergunte ao paciente se uma perna está mais pesada do que a outra ou se causa alguma dor. Se o paciente relatar qualquer um desses sintomas, isso pode destacar uma deficiência na força de fechamento da ASI. Existem dois sistemas que fornecem integridade estrutural ao anel pélvico, o fechamento forçado e o fechamento da forma. O fechamento da forma é um sistema passivo que utiliza articulações e ligamentos. Neste caso, estamos interessados no fechamento por força, que é o sistema ativo composto de músculo e fáscia, e como isso funciona para estabilizar a ASI. Mais informações sobre este teste, sua sensibilidade e especificidade, são fornecidas por Mens, Vleeming, Snijders et al. (1999).

O teste é então repetido com o avaliador aplicando uma pressão bilateral igual em ambos os lados do aspecto anterior, lateral ou posterior da pelve sistematicamente. Adicionar essa pressão igual enquanto o paciente realiza a elevação ativa da perna reta, dará ao avaliador algum *feedback* importante sobre se as estruturas anteriores (lateral ou posterior) estão falhando em ajudar no fechamento forçado da pelve.

Elevação passiva da perna reta

Ao levantar a perna para o paciente, estamos teoricamente enviesando as estruturas neurais em vez das contráteis, mas em vez de avaliar a amplitude do movimento perguntando ao paciente onde ele sente a tensão, sinta a tensão por meio do *feedback* de suas mãos para obter um quadro e avaliar se há uma restrição proximal ou distal.

Resultados da avaliação – estabelecimento do "porquê"

A parte mais difícil é criar um quadro claro do que exatamente foi descoberto durante a avaliação. Várias apresentações podem ser descobertas, e agora tentaremos juntá-las para ajudar nas opções de tratamento. Será necessário associar quaisquer achados dos testes cinéticos em pé com os achados palpatórios no pedestal. Este é o momento de descartar quaisquer discrepâncias estruturais no comprimento da perna. Para acomodar uma diferença no comprimento das pernas, a forma humana vai compensar de uma maneira ou de outra, e isso pode obscurecer o quadro. Algumas dessas apresentações podem ser vistas durante o exame, como pronação do pé, flexão do joelho em pé, crista ilíaca em uma posição superior e rotação anterior do ílio no lado contralateral. A Tabela 17.1 mostra a apresentação do lado da disfunção.

Prevenção – determinação do "como"

Então, o que causa uma disfunção lombopélvica? Existem diversos fatores que contribuem para uma disfunção lombopélvica e, portanto, várias razões pelas quais uma disfunção lombopélvica contribui para outras apresentações de lesão. Atividades e esportes de natureza unilateral causarão um viés

Tabela 17.1 Apresentação do lado da disfunção.

Disfunção	Crista ilíaca	EIAS	EIPS	Ramo púbico superior	Tuberosidade isquiática	Maléolo medial
Rotação anterior	Nivelada	Inferior	Superior	Nivelado	Superior	Inferior
Pós-rotação	Nivelada	Superior	Inferior	Nivelado	Inferior	Superior
Superioridade do ilíaco (*up-slip*)	Superior	Superior	Superior	Superior	Superior	Superior
Downslip	Inferior	Inferior	Inferior	Inferior	Inferior	Inferior
Rotação anterior com deslizamento para cima	Superior	Nivelada	Superior	Superior	Superior	Nivelado
Pós-rotação com *upslip*	Superior	Superior	Nivelada	Superior	Nivelada	Superior

EIAS, espinha ilíaca anterossuperior; *EIPS*, espinha ilíaca posterossuperior. (Adaptada de Gibbons, J., 2017. Functional Anatomy of the Pelvis and the Sacroiliac Joint. Lotus Publishing, Chichester, UK.)

Disfunção Lombopélvica na População Esportiva: O "o Que", o "Porquê" e o "Como"

físico no lado dominante, mas os atletas geralmente são desenvolvidos para funcionar de acordo com o esporte ou atividade que realizam. Desequilíbrios estruturais, como discrepâncias no comprimento das pernas, são comuns e devem ser identificados no processo de exame antes de serem resolvidos. Frequentemente, é o posicionamento postural habitual (que pode levar ao encurtamento da musculatura), causado pela maneira como os atletas usam seus corpos longe do ambiente esportivo, que muitas vezes são os precursores significativos de disfunções. Esses fatores contribuintes fora da arena esportiva podem explicar "como" os problemas se manifestam em primeira instância. Os atletas geralmente têm muito tempo livre para relaxar entre o treinamento e a competição e como um indivíduo passa seu tempo longe do esporte pode ser relevante para a apresentação. Isso pode parecer óbvio, mas para o atleta que pode ser descrito como um infrator reincidente, podemos precisar olhar para fora do ginásio ou do campo de jogo e focar em outras influências. Se nós, como profissionais da saúde, estivermos pensando dessa maneira, podemos destacar para o atleta qualquer alerta potencial relacionado à mudança postural. A posição de direção, a postura do sofá ou poltrona, o posicionamento da TV em relação à posição sentada, o uso do telefone celular, a disposição do quarto, jogos e viagens excessivas têm um papel a desempenhar como fatores contribuintes.

Papel do exame de imagem

Por experiência, sugere-se que o exame de imagem tem o papel de descartar qualquer condição ameaçadora na coluna lombar, ou se o paciente não consegue progredir no tratamento. Os pacientes com apresentações óbvias da coluna lombar precisam que a extensão da lesão seja confirmada. Populações atléticas, especialmente em esportes de elite, muitas vezes precisam de um diagnóstico rápido para permitir uma resolução rápida, selecionando o tratamento correto ou via de encaminhamento.

Radiografia, ressonância magnética e tomografia computadorizada fornecem uma grande quantidade de informações ao profissional de saúde que o encaminhou. Porém, essas informações precisam ser relevantes para a apresentação em questão e é extremamente importante a capacidade de casar a apresentação clínica com os achados em uma imagem.

Conclusão

A disfunção lombopélvica contribui para muitas apresentações em tecidos moles. Há vários testes que fornecem altos níveis de confiabilidade no diagnóstico de dor na ASI. No entanto, estamos tentando diagnosticar disfunção do movimento que contribuirá para a dor e/ou lesão. Com o manejo regular do alinhamento pélvico e lombar, independentemente das apresentações sintomáticas, existe a oportunidade de diminuir o número de lesões que podem ser atribuídas a essa região e limitar os casos de perda de tempo crônica que se propagam para os casos cirúrgicos. O problema é que muitas vezes o atleta não percebe nenhuma alteração precoce no alinhamento, por isso não busca a intervenção do tratamento. Aqueles atletas que entendem a ligação entre o alinhamento postural habitual e seus sinais e sintomas são os que buscam manutenção e intervenções regulares. A chave para tratar o paciente com sucesso é ampliar o ponto de vista. Nós, como profissionais da saúde, precisamos nos concentrar em "quais" são os sintomas da lesão, e também nos perguntar "por que" esse problema ocorreu em primeira instância. Precisamos olhar para as estruturas que contribuem para esse problema e restaurá-las para funcionar antes de podermos superar a lesão com eficácia. Entretando, isso não é o fim do processo. Compreender "como" a disfunção ocorreu em primeira instância nos permitirá tomar decisões que mudarão o resultado daqui para frente. Somente quando pudermos responder a essas três perguntas, poderemos tratar o paciente com sucesso, com a confiança de uma solução a longo prazo.

Referências bibliográficas

Arab, A.M., Abdollahi, I., Joghataei, M.T., Golafshani, Z., Kazemnejad, A., 2009. Inter- and intra-examiner reliability of single and composites of selected motion palpation and pain provocation tests for sacroiliac joint. Manual Therapy 14, 213-221.

Gibbons, J., 2017. Functional Anatomy of the Pelvis and the Sacroiliac Joint. Lotus Publishing, Chichester, UK.

Laslett, M., 2008. Evidence-based diagnosis and treatment of the painful sacroiliac joint. The Journal of Manual and Manipulative Therapy 16 (3).

Mens, J., Vleeming, A., Snijders, C., Stam, J.H., Ginai, A.Z., 1999. The active straight leg raising test and mobility of the pelvic joints. European Spine Journal 8, 469-473.

Tong, H.C., Heyman, O.G., Lado, D.A., Isser, M.M., 2006. Interexaminer reliability of three methods of combining test results to determine side of sacral restriction, sacral base position, and innominate bone position. Journal of the American Osteopathic Association 106 (8), 464-468.

Capítulo | 18 |

Reabilitação do Desempenho para Lesões dos Isquiotibiais – Abordagem de Sistemas Multimodais

Johnny Wilson, Paulina Czubacka e Neil Greig

Introdução

As lesões dos isquiotibiais (LITs) no futebol de elite continuam a ser um enigma desafiador e complexo. O aumento progressivo da incidência de LIT ao longo do tempo, sua tendência de recorrência após o retorno ao jogo (RAJ) e a evidente falta de consenso em ambos os critérios de avaliação, reabilitação e RAJ podem levar a um manejo inadequado.

As LITs continuam sendo as lesões mais prevalentes no futebol profissional, contribuindo com aproximadamente 12% de todas as lesões registradas (Ekstrand et al., 2013). Essa tendência de aumento (4% ao ano) representa um grande fardo para os clubes de futebol profissional, em torno de 18 dias de treinamento e três jogos perdidos por jogador e temporada (Woods et al., 2004). De maneira alarmante, 33% dessas lesões são recorrentes, e mais de 50% das novas lesões ocorrem dentro de 30 dias do RAJ inicial do jogador (Ekstrand et al., 2013). Ao observar que as taxas de recorrência não melhoraram nas últimas três décadas, sugere-se que os resultados ruins podem estar relacionados, em parte, à reabilitação inadequada, RAJ prematuro e falta de consenso sobre as melhores práticas (Orchard et al., 2013).

Esses fatores, aliados com as supostas demandas físicas crescentes do esporte no nível de elite, demonstram a necessidade de uma abordagem de equipe multiprofissional baseada em evidências e devidamente estruturada ao reabilitar LIT. No entanto, apesar das complexidades mencionadas anteriormente, a gestão de jogadores de futebol que sofrem de LIT, e seu subsequente RAJ, é influenciada por um grupo muito mais amplo de interessados do que simplesmente aqueles com formação médica – muitos dos quais podem ter interesses concorrentes em um determinado jogador retornando ao campo antes do previsto. Embora o clínico esportivo e o próprio jogador estejam em melhor posição para medir e monitorar o cumprimento dos critérios de RAJ, a influência dos treinadores, o estágio da temporada, os agentes e os termos contratuais etc., sugerem que um consenso mais amplo deve ser buscado a respeito das decisões finais do RAJ (Van Der Horst et al., 2017). Em última análise, um modelo centrado no atleta, que incorpore as opiniões daqueles que influenciam diretamente o manejo de risco médico pode servir para melhorar os resultados.

Do ponto de vista clínico, obter consenso sobre os critérios objetivos mais valiosos com os quais o progresso pode ser medido de modo mais eficaz, tem se mostrado um desafio que ainda não foi totalmente superado. Termos genéricos comumente utilizados, como "ausência de dor", "insignificância dos sinais clínicos", "força e flexibilidade semelhantes" e "boa função neuromuscular" não possuem qualquer grau de especificidade em que o clínico avaliador possa confiar. Alcançar "força semelhante" isoladamente, por exemplo, pode atrapalhar a tomada de decisão, em particular quando se considera que cerca de 70% das LITs reabilitadas com sucesso ainda demonstram déficits de força isocinética superiores a 10% após o RAJ (Tol et al., 2014). Da mesma maneira, a imagem isolada é uma ferramenta de diagnóstico valiosa, porém não demonstra grande valor ao prever o RAJ (De Vos et al., 2014; Reurink et al., 2015). Esses caprichos levaram à ausência de consenso e a grandes variações na avaliação e no manejo entre os casos e podem contribuir para as altas taxas de recorrência. Em termos práticos, nenhum critério clínico ou físico isolado é provavelmente específico ou sensível o suficiente para prever um RAJ seguro. O entendimento de que uma bateria de marcadores clínicos objetivos e de campo claramente definidos, específicos para o caso individual, junto com o *feedback* subjetivo do jogador, é mais confiável e pode oferecer uma visão significativa em um plano de reabilitação para o RAJ bem construído. Esses marcadores objetivos serão discutidos em detalhes neste capítulo.

Exigências anatômicas esportivas

Como um grupo de músculos biarticulares complexo, a função primária dos isquiotibiais é flexionar o joelho e/ou estender o quadril (Petersen e Hölmich, 2005). No esporte de rendimento, esse grupo de três (ou quatro quando se considera a assistência do adutor magno) músculos são colocados sob a maior demanda física durante a corrida, em comparação com a caminhada e a corrida leve (Schache et al., 2009). O pico de força excêntrica e alongamento ocorrem nos isquiotibiais durante a fase final de balanço do ciclo da marcha, pois eles trabalham excentricamente para controlar a extensão do joelho e se opor à atividade do quadríceps (Schache et al., 2012). No contato com o solo e durante a fase de apoio, os isquiotibiais mudam de função, contraindo-se concentricamente para estender o quadril e impulsionar o corpo para frente, antes de gerar grandes forças excêntricas durante a desaceleração para resistir ao movimento do tronco para frente (Chumanov et al., 2012; Schache et al., 2012).

Classificação de lesões de isquiotibiais

Dadas as demandas abordadas, é razoável esperar que haja grandes variações entre os tipos, localização e gravidade das lesões, sem falar na reabilitação subsequente. Pelo menos dois tipos distintos de LIT são discutidos na literatura (Brukner, 2012). O tipo I mais comum ocorre de modo predominante na corrida de alta velocidade (CAV), enquanto o tipo II, observado com menos frequência, tende a ocorrer durante o alongamento dos músculos com carga, como visto com chutes altos e carrinhos no futebol, e pode acontecer em velocidades mais lentas (Askling e Thorstensson, 2008; Woods et al., 2004). Em geral, lesões do tipo I envolvem a cabeça longa do bíceps femoral localizada lateralmente na junção músculo-tendínea proximal (JMT) e se recuperam bem. Em contrapartida, as lesões do tipo II normalmente envolvem o tendão livre proximal do músculo semimembranoso e resultam em uma recuperação prolongada (Brukner, 2012). Com isso em mente, o clínico esportivo criterioso com a tarefa de gerenciar atletas que sofrem de LIT deve considerar como seu plano de manejo apoia a recuperação dos atletas, dadas as grandes variações no tipo de lesão, localização, tecidos envolvidos e as diferentes demandas de seu esporte específico e/ou posição de jogo.

Importância da reabilitação adequada

A reabilitação inadequada é uma razão frequentemente citada para as altas taxas de recorrência associadas à LIT (De Visser et al., 2012; Wangensteen et al., 2016). Portanto, o objetivo desse capítulo é oferecer uma visão geral baseada em evidências, mas aplicada, dos principais aspectos da reabilitação de desempenho para LIT. A natureza multivariada das LITs deve direcionar o clínico para longe dos programas de reabilitação que falham ao considerar todas as nuances da lesão, para uma abordagem igualmente multivariada. As demandas físicas do futebol profissional, os fatores de risco associados às LITs, as abordagens de força e condicionamento para a seleção de exercícios e as demandas baseadas no campo de reabilitação de desempenho serão todos discutidos. Considerando essa visão geral, os autores pretendem estimular o leitor a repensar e evoluir sua prática atual, a fim de devolver seus atletas ao campo com capacidade de desempenho em nível de elite.

Criação de um ambiente para a melhora de desempenho

Não existe uma reabilitação perfeita. Um clínico sábio pode esperar chegar a um acordo ao concordar com os prazos de RAJ, adaptar-se às demandas irrealistas de jogadores, dirigentes e partes interessadas, lidar com as pressões de trabalhar em um ambiente esportivo de elite e estar preparado para cenários como contratempos durante o período de reabilitação e recorrência precoce de lesão no RAJ. Nós, como grupo de autores, entendemos que os profissionais da saúde devem despertar interesses por essas situações adversas e usá-las como uma oportunidade para melhorar a sua prática clínica. Este capítulo debate pesquisas atuais e opiniões de especialistas e discute os aspectos que consideramos imperativos para preparar os atletas para tolerar física e psicologicamente as demandas de desgaste do futebol profissional. Fundamental para a reabilitação de desempenho é a noção de que as sessões de reabilitação são intencionalmente projetadas para atender aos mais exigentes cenários de dias de jogo. Ao adotar essa metodologia, os atletas são capazes de se adaptarem aos estressores inesperados durante uma competição, são íntegros o suficiente para lidar com 60 jogos em um período de 10 meses e desenvolvem uma resiliência por meio de ultrapreparação durante a jornada de reabilitação.

Filosofia de reabilitação para a melhora de desempenho

A seguir estão listados os principais princípios que sustentam esta filosofia de reabilitação.

Melhora da habilidade atlética

O tempo gasto durante a recuperação de uma lesão é aquele que pode ser usado de maneira eficaz para tratar os déficits que não podem ser resolvidos ou que são difíceis de resolver durante a temporada. Todo atleta tem áreas a melhorar – o desempenho humano ainda não atingiu seu teto genético.

Redução do risco de lesões futuras

A recorrência de lesões é comum no esporte profissional; portanto, um aspecto importante da reabilitação de desempenho é mitigar o risco de nova lesão no RAJ. Dadas as altas cargas associadas ao desempenho no futebol, a reabilitação eficaz incorpora uma abordagem global, visando as áreas mais comumente lesionadas relacionadas com perdas de tempo significativas por temporada, ou seja, isquiotibiais, virilha, joelho e tornozelo.

Otimização do envolvimento do atleta

O envolvimento do atleta é crucial ao fornecer uma reabilitação eficaz. Isso pode ser facilitado pela melhora da compreensão do jogador de como a reabilitação se traduz em uma situação de jogo – na verdade, capacitando os atletas por meio da educação. As estratégias de reabilitação devem ser motivacionalmente sensíveis e a adesão à jornada de reabilitação pode ser melhorada tornando o processo novo, divertido e competitivo. O clínico deve possuir um alto nível de inteligência emocional para cultivar uma relação de trabalho eficaz em que o atleta e o terapeuta sejam criadores, gerentes, programadores e aprendizes reflexivos (Mulvany e Wilson, 2018). Finalmente, a incorporação de medidas de resultados que sejam relevantes e significativas para o atleta pode melhorar o envolvimento do atleta.

Reabilitação de desempenho: força

Desenvolvimento de uma variedade de qualidades de força de isquiotibiais

Conforme destacado na introdução, as LITs geralmente ocorrem devido a forças excêntricas de pico excessivas colocadas sobre eles durante atividades esportivas balísticas de alta intensidade, como corrida, desaceleração, chutes e alongamento. Portanto, se um músculo tem as características de força para suportar esses fatores, a probabilidade de se lesionar é reduzida. Como consequência, um programa de treinamento de força bem planejado e prescrito individualmente, projetado em torno da especificidade e da sobrecarga progressiva, é fundamental para nossa filosofia de reabilitação, pois produz as adaptações fisiológicas necessárias dentro do músculo para reduzir o risco de lesões. A força sustenta a potência e a potência sustenta a velocidade, e a velocidade é "rainha" no futebol profissional.

Princípios que sustentam a filosofia de reabilitação de força de isquiotibiais

Especificidade

O primeiro conceito fundamental que aderimos ao projetar um programa de força para nossos atletas é incorporar a especificidade às suas necessidades individuais e ao esporte que praticam. A especificidade foi cunhada pela primeira vez por DeLorme (1945). Em essência, refere-se a um método pelo qual reabilitamos o atleta de uma maneira específica para produzir a adaptação específica desejada, discutida posteriormente por Todd et al. (2012), por exemplo, implementar o exercício nórdico como um estímulo para melhorar a força excêntrica ou prescrever CAV para melhorar a velocidade de contração do atleta durante o pico de forças excêntricas. Jogar o jogo em si é, de fato, um modo de treinamento de força e fornece a maior oportunidade de melhorar a força específica do esporte e deve desempenhar um papel importante ao projetar o programa de força.

Sobrecarga progressiva

No ambiente com tempo escasso para a reabilitação de isquiotibiais, para esportes profissionais, aumentar a intensidade e/ou velocidade de um exercício, em vez do volume ou frequência (número de sessões por semana) é geralmente a maneira mais eficiente de aplicar o princípio de "sobrecarga progressiva" para alcançar melhorias nas qualidades de força (Bruton, 2002). Isso significa que precisamos expor continuamente o atleta a um estímulo maior do que o habitual (p. ex., aumento de peso, corrida em uma velocidade mais alta, dificuldade crescente da tarefa) durante a fase de reabilitação e durante seu RAJ. Ao aplicar este princípio corretamente, pode-se evitar o excesso de treinamento e maximizar o efeito do estímulo de força durante o seu RAJ (Bompa e Haff, 2009).

Para alcançar melhorias de força a longo prazo necessárias para tolerar as demandas de competir em quase 60 jogos durante uma temporada, é benéfica a integração de dois princípios científicos básicos: a lei de Hooke e a lei de Wolff. Elas afirmam que, ao se aplicar uma carga externa (exercício de força) a um objeto sólido (osso, tendão, ligamento ou músculo), ela irá adaptar-se especificamente às demandas impostas (adaptação específica às demandas impostas – princípio SAID, do inglês *specific adaptation to imposed demands*). Portanto, se quisermos progredir continuamente no estímulo externo (exercício), o objeto (isquiotibiais) continuará a se adaptar. No entanto, ao deixar de progredir no estímulo, não apenas os ganhos de força se estabilizarão, como também, eventualmente, começarão a declinar (Bruton, 2002). Portanto, dado que o período desde o início da lesão até o RAJ é tão breve, é imperativo que os atletas continuem a progredir na intensidade de seu programa de força por pelo menos 4 a 6 semanas após o RAJ. Após esse período, eles começam uma nova fase: um programa de força de sustentabilidade para mitigar o risco de lesões futuras.

Argumentou-se que todos nós temos um limite genético para a capacidade de força. No entanto, poucos atletas estão realmente próximos de seu limite genético, especialmente em esportes coletivos como o futebol, daí a necessidade de carregar jogadores de forma contínua e progressiva.

Seleção de exercícios

Os exercícios são prescritos individualmente para refletir as necessidades particulares de um jogador e dependem de muitos fatores, alguns exemplos sendo o *status* do treinamento, período da temporada, histórico de lesões, análise de risco do exercício, resultados de testes de força, perfil excêntrico. A variedade de exercícios e qualidades de movimento são essenciais no desenvolvimento da força para reduzir o risco de novas lesões (Mendiguchia et al., 2017). Exercícios como levantamento terra isométrico (Figura 18.1), variações de levantamento terra romeno unipodal (Figuras 18.2 e 18.3), controles deslizantes de isquiotibiais usando prancha deslizante (Figura 18.4), impulsos de quadril (Figura 18.5) e nórdicos (Figura 18.6) são alguns exemplos que podem ser utilizados.

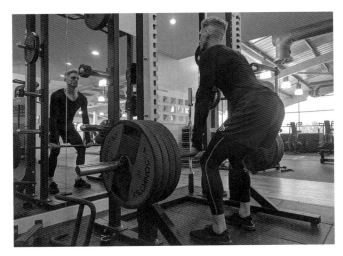

Figura 18.1 Levantamento terra isométrico.

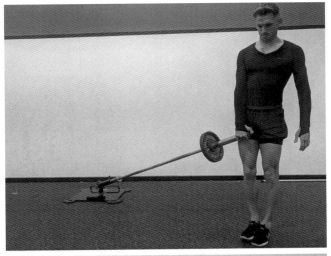

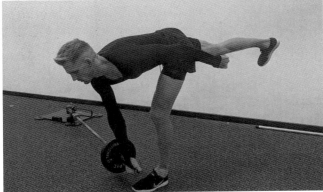

Figura 18.2 Levantamento terra romeno de uma perna com barra.

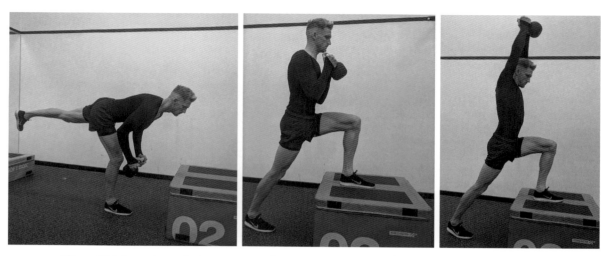

Figura 18.3 Levantamento terra romeno de uma perna com propulsão do joelho e supino frontal.

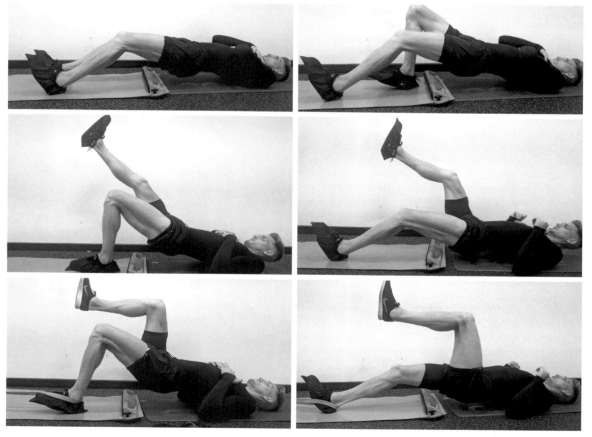

Figura 18.4 Variações do controle deslizante de isquiotibiais em uma prancha deslizante.

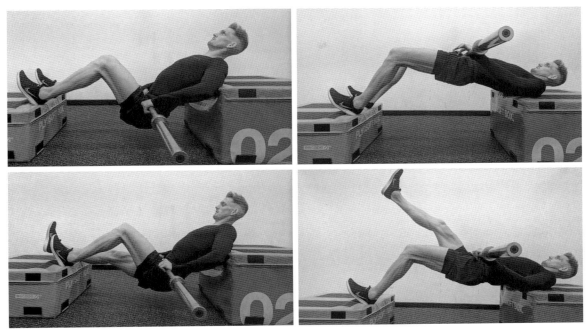

Figura 18.5 Impulso de quadril bipodal e unipodal.

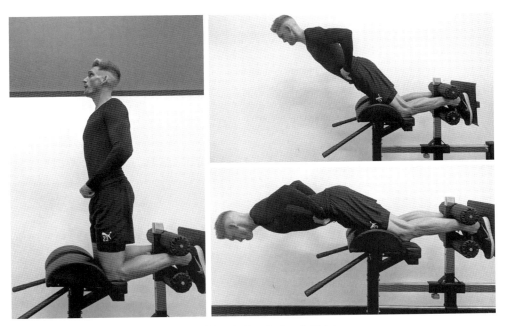

Figura 18.6 Exercício nórdico de isquiotibiais.

Parte | 2 | Aplicação Clínica

É essencial fornecer variação para desafiar o complexo dos isquiotibiais de várias maneiras: perturbação, unipodal, bipodal, dominante no joelho, dominante no quadril e proprioceptivamente. Uma variedade de estímulos inunda essa área altamente densa e rica em estruturas de recepção de informações. No entanto, a pesquisa é altamente focada na importância da força excêntrica. Estudos recentes mostram que o aumento do comprimento do fascículo pode ser fundamental para o sucesso da reabilitação dos isquiotibiais, embora haja algumas evidências conflitantes em relação a esse tópico (Bourne et al., 2017; Fukutani e Kurihara, 2015).

O alongamento excêntrico dos isquiotibiais aumenta o comprimento do fascículo, a área transversal e o pico de produção muscular e é considerado essencial para a reabilitação eficaz de LIT (Timmins et al., 2016). Esta intervenção demonstrou reduzir a incidência de lesão durante a temporada de isquiotibiais em muitos esportes baseados em corrida (Evans e Williams, 2017; Van Der Horst et al., 2015), bem como aumentar os marcadores de desempenho (Clark et al., 2005).

Os exercícios nórdicos são excêntricos simples, podem ser executados sem equipamentos caros e requerem proficiência mínima. O atleta pode trabalhar grandes variações de movimentos no joelho em um ritmo constante, de modo que o tempo muscular sob tensão aumenta. Embora usados como parte de nossa estratégia de reabilitação, os nórdicos nunca são utilizados isoladamente, pois a recuperação dos isquiotibiais precisa da exposição a diversos estímulos para desenvolver imunidade para as demandas de jogos de futebol em ritmo acelerado.

Nosso programa de força é mostrado na Tabela 18.1.

Tabela 18.1 Exemplos para seleção de exercícios de força.

Exercício	Variações	Faixa de séries	Faixa de repetições	Faixa de carga
Foco: isométrico – elevar o pico de estresse isométrico da fibra, aumentando o número de pontes cruzadas de actina-miosina por fibra e força por ponte cruzada. Como consequência, isso levará a um aumento na contração voluntária máxima e na taxa de desenvolvimento de torque				
Manter uma ponte	PC, bilateral, unilateral, alcance interno, alcance externo, elevado, resistido, perturbação			
Levantamento terra isométrico (ver Figura 18.1)	Bilateral, unilateral, médio alcance, resistido	1 a 3	6 × segurar 6 s	Contração máxima
Sustentação em máquina para glúteos/isquiotibiais ou exercícios nórdicos	Assistido, PC, resistido, alcance interno, alcance externo			
Foco: força geral – aumentar a área da secção transversal do músculo (sarcômeros em paralelo) e a força. Sincronização aprimorada do padrão de recrutamento e disparo das unidades motoras. Todos os exercícios devem ser concluídos ao longo do intervalo				
Variações de ponte	PC, bilateral, unilateral, alcance interno, alcance externo, elevado, com tornozelo, resistido			
Afundo reverso	PC, resistida, *jammer press*, para um nível acima	1 a 3	6 a 8	60 a 85% 6 RM
Variações de agachamento dividido	PC, resistido, agachamento dividido búlgaro, perturbação			
Foco: carregamento excêntrico – aumentar o número de sarcômeros em série, o comprimento do fascículo e o ângulo de penetração. Ação excêntrica para ser lenta e controlada				
LTR	PC, resistido, bilateral, unilateral (ver Figura 18.2)	1 a 3	4 a 6	60 a 85% 6 RM
Variações nórdicas	Assistido, não assistido (ver Figura 18.3), resistido	1 a 3	6 a 10	PC
Excêntricos em placa de deslizamento (*slide board*) (Figura 18.4)	Bilateral, alternado, unilateral, resistência	1 a 3	8 a 12	PC a 30% 6 RM
Foco: potência – elevar a taxa de desenvolvimento de força influenciando a ativação/recrutamento da unidade motora para aumentar a produção de força muscular				
Impulso do quadril (ver Figura 18.5)	PC, resistido, bilateral, unilateral			
LTR unipodal (ver Figura 18.6)	PC, resistido, bilateral, unilateral, com pressão acima da cabeça ou impulso de rotação do joelho, *step up*	1 a 3	4 a 6	≤ 30% 6 RM
Balanço de Kettlebell	Carregado	1 a 3	12 a 20	≤ 30% 6 RM

PC, peso corporal; *LTR*, levantamento terra romeno; *RM*, repetição máxima.

Reabilitação do Desempenho para Lesões dos Isquiotibiais – Abordagem de Sistemas Multimodais **Capítulo** | **18** |

Força explosiva: pliometria

Como mencionado anteriormente, as LITs ocorrem de um modo geral durante movimentos explosivos, de alta potência, quando o músculo é exposto a cargas de alta velocidade. Portanto, expor esse grupo de músculos às ações explosivas do treinamento pliométrico ajudará a habituar os isquiotibiais a tolerar atividades perigosas, melhorando sua capacidade de desacelerar efetivamente o membro durante ações de alta velocidade. Além de reduzir o risco de lesões futuras, há um forte corpo de evidências que sugere que o treinamento pliométrico também é muito eficaz em aumentar as características de velocidade, como aceleração, velocidade máxima e agilidade (Manouras et al., 2016; Sáez de Villarreal et al., 2015). Para correr em velocidade, saltar explosivamente e mudar de direção, os jogadores precisam combinar forças horizontais, verticais e laterais para gerar esses movimentos poderosos. Portanto, as pliometrias horizontal, vertical e lateral formam componentes importantes de nossa filosofia de reabilitação.

Pliometria de baixo limiar

Iniciamos nossos atletas apresentando-lhes a pliometria de baixo limiar na piscina, o que nos permite introduzir atividades de salto logo no 3º dia após a lesão, respeitando as restrições do tecido em cicatrização. A flutuabilidade da água permite uma redução da gravidade agindo sobre o corpo e reduz o suporte de peso e as forças de cisalhamento através do músculo afetado. Progredimos essas atividades para aterrissar muito rapidamente (geralmente no dia seguinte), onde exercícios submáximos como o salto agachado, salto em largura (salto para frente), saltos (salto lateral de um pé para o outro) e saltos unipodais (salto e aterrissagem na mesma perna), são introduzidos se tolerados pelo atleta.

Pliometria de alto limiar

A próxima etapa da reabilitação é apresentar ao jogador a pliometria de limiares elevados com o objetivo de desenvolver força, potência máxima e taxa de desenvolvimento de força para aprimorar habilidades atléticas explosivas. A pesquisa mostrou que os exercícios pliométricos horizontais têm uma maior transferência para melhorar a qualidade de aceleração, enquanto os pliométricos verticais têm mais efeito no desempenho da velocidade máxima acima de 30 a 40 m (Loturco et al., 2015). Portanto, expomos nossos atletas a um estímulo combinado de pliometria horizontal e vertical durante sua reabilitação. Ideias para progressões pliométricas para reabilitação de isquiotibiais podem ser vistas na Tabela 18.2.

Reabilitação de desempenho: importância da força lombopélvica-quadril

Complexo lombopélvico-quadril

A força do *core* e o controle neuromuscular (CNM) estão associados à diminuição do risco de desenvolver uma lesão nos membros inferiores (Willson et al., 2005). A ação coordenada de estabilizar e mobilizar grupos musculares sobre as regiões lombar, pélvica e do quadril permite a transferência de energia eficaz por

Tabela 18.2 **Exemplos para seleção de exercícios pliométricos.**

Exercício	Variações	Faixa de séries	Faixa de repetições	Faixa de carga
Foco: mecânica de pouso/pliometria de baixo limiar – melhorar as estratégias de ativação muscular e a excitabilidade do reflexo de alongamento por meio de adaptações neuromusculares aos sistemas de controle sensorial e motor				
Salto vertical	Hidro, PC, com uma volta de vários graus, perturbação	1 a 3	4 a 6	PC a 30% 6 RM
Salto horizontal	Hidro, PC, perturbação			
Salto unilateral UP	Hidro, PC, com uma volta de vários graus, perturbação			
Salto unilateral triplo	Hidro, PC			
Drop jump	PC, bilateral, unilateral			
Foco: pliometria de alto limiar – utilizar o ciclo de alongamento-encurtamento e melhorar a coordenação intermuscular para aumentar a taxa de desenvolvimento de força				
Salto vertical e horizontal	PC, resistido, excentricamente carregado, combinado	1 a 3	4 a 6	PC a 30% 6 RM
Salto com obstáculos	Unilateral, multidirecional			
Salto unilateral com barreira	PC, bilateral, unilateral, combinado, lateral, multidirecional			
Agachamento com salto	*Switches*, agachamento dividido búlgaro, carga excêntrica, salto de caixa após de agachamento dividido			
LTR unipodal para salto de caixa com uma única perna	PC, excentricamente carregado, resistido			

PC, peso corporal; *LTR*, levantamento terra romeno; *RM*, repetição máxima; *UP*, unipodal.

183

Parte | 2 | Aplicação Clínica

todo o corpo e possibilita o movimento ideal durante atividades como correr, pular, mudar de direção e chutar (De Blaiser et al., 2018). Também foi sugerido que a fraqueza sobre esta região anatômica pode ter um efeito negativo no alinhamento dos membros inferiores por meio da incapacidade de controlar a rotação interna do quadril, resultando em colapso do joelho valgo, o que pode predispor o jogador a um maior risco de lesões (Wilkerson e Colston, 2015). Em contrapartida, o CNM melhorado dessa região permite um maior controle da posição do corpo durante as ações de corte, corrida e salto (Zazulak et al., 2007).

A investigação científica mostra que os músculos glúteos, em particular o glúteo máximo (GM) (responsável pela extensão do quadril) e os músculos superficiais do tronco – especificamente os eretores da espinha (EE), podem reduzir o risco de lesão dos isquiotibiais (Schuermans et al., 2017). O GM e os EE também atuam como estabilizadores importantes do quadril, especialmente na postura unipodal (Lieberman et al., 2006), e fornecem uma base estável para os isquiotibiais gerarem uma força significativa durante a extensão do quadril. Isso é essencial para movimentos explosivos vitais para o sucesso no futebol. Assim como os isquiotibiais, o GM e os EE são projetados para absorver e gerar uma quantidade significativa de força para a extensão do quadril, de modo que a carga total dessa ação vital durante a corrida não seja suportada apenas pelos próprios isquiotibiais (Lieberman et al., 2006). Com efeito, eles ajudam a proteger os isquiotibiais contra as altas forças associadas à corrida em alta velocidade, aceleração rápida, mudança de direção (MDD) com força, salto máximo e chutes com força, atividades que podem danificar os isquiotibiais. A estabilidade lombopélvica-quadril, força e o CNM desempenham um papel vital na reabilitação dos isquiotibiais (Chumanov et al., 2007; Huxel Bliven e Anderson, 2013).

Controle neuromuscular e neurodinâmica

Para o sucesso do RAJ, os atletas de elite precisam ser capazes de realizar tarefas motoras complexas que reproduzam as demandas do esporte. O treinamento do CNM resulta em padrões de disparo muscular mais eficientes, melhora a estabilidade dinâmica das articulações e é fundamental para aprender ou reaprender padrões de movimento e habilidades essenciais para o futebol.

Propomos dois exercícios de CNM: moinho de vento (Figura 18.7) e mergulhador (Figura 18.8) como componentes-chave da reabilitação dos isquiotibiais. Incorporamos esses exercícios devido à sua natureza multiarticular e multiplanar; eles requerem uma série de grupos de músculos trabalhando em uníssono para ligar várias partes do corpo. Ambos os exercícios são altamente específicos para o futebol e enfocam o equilíbrio dinâmico na postura unipodal com o objetivo de melhorar o controle na transição da tripla flexão para a tripla extensão do quadril, joelho e tornozelo. Esses exercícios de CNM desafiam o atleta no plano transversal, que é o plano em que ocorre a maioria das LITs. O atleta é obrigado a controlar a rotação externa em um plano transversal ao executar os exercícios de CNM.

Após uma lesão no tendão da coxa, ramos do nervo ciático podem ficar sensibilizados e, como resultado, ocorrer um aumento da tensão neural nos músculos da cadeia posterior (Turl e George, 1998). Os exercícios neurodinâmicos, como uso de deslizadores neurais sobre a bola de estabilidade (Figura 18.9), facilitam o deslizamento distal e proximal alternado da cadeia de tecido neural, com o objetivo de manter ou melhorar a mobilidade neural ao se mover por meio das estruturas miofasciais.

Reabilitação de desempenho: exposição à corrida

Normalmente, os jogadores de futebol profissional da Liga Inglesa de Futebol cobrem, em média, 300 a 1000 m correndo a uma velocidade acima de $6,3$ ms^{-1} em arrancadas intermitentes durante um jogo. Isso tem o potencial de lesionar os músculos isquiotibiais (Bradley et al., 2013). Dada a natureza perigosa de correr rápido, é importante expor os jogadores a este tipo de estímulo o mais cedo possível como uma "vacinação" contra lesões nos isquiotibiais, conforme discutido por Malone et al. (2017). Os jogadores são apresentados à corrida na piscina já no 3º dia após a lesão, progredindo para a terra no 4º dia (corrida em estado estacionário). A intensidade e o volume do exercício progridem para CAV, corrida resistida e corrida tão logo o jogador seja capaz de tolerar as forças envolvidas em atividades explosivas. Idealmente, antes do retorno ao treinamento, os jogadores são expostos a cargas de corrida que excedem as demandas da partida para garantir que sejam capazes de tolerar as demandas de treinamento e jogo. Porém, no ambiente de alta pressão do futebol profissional, isso nem sempre ocorre e os jogadores voltam aos treinos prematuramente. Picos agudos de intensidade e volume para corrida em alta velocidade devem ser evitados e, em vez disso, um aumento gradual da carga de corrida é necessário para fazer a transição eficaz do jogador durante a reabilitação. A fim de fornecer o melhor preparo contra novas lesões, o objetivo é aplicar uma dose ideal de atividades baseadas em corrida. Algumas dessas atividades incluem:
- Corrida em piscina
- Corrida resistida
- Corrida assistida
- Operação de MDD explosiva
- Corrida e CAV.

Observe a Figura 18.10 como exemplo de nossa prescrição de corrida.

Corrida em piscina: a batalha contra o tempo começa

A maioria dos jogadores com lesões nos isquiotibiais no futebol profissional geralmente terá RAJ 18 a 24 dias após a lesão inicial (Dinnery e Wilson, 2018). Imediatamente após seu RAJ, eles deverão correr em alta velocidade, correr repetidamente, mudar de direção no ritmo, acelerar, desacelerar, pular ao máximo e golpear a bola com força centenas de vezes, não apenas em jogos, como também em sessões de treinamento consecutivas. Portanto, seu "cronômetro de RAJ" começa quando eles agarram a parte de trás da coxa em agonia. Os profissionais da saúde têm a tarefa nada invejável de tirar o máximo proveito de cada segundo para ajudar a planejar uma transição bem-sucedida de volta à arena volátil, acelerada e cheia de ação do futebol profissional em um curto período.

A hidroterapia foi conjecturada para reduzir os prazos de RAJ por meio de uma série de processos. Ela permite a restauração precoce da função, pois a flutuabilidade natural da água reduz a quantidade de força de sustentação de peso pelos isquiotibiais, permitindo a mobilização precoce e o carregamento do tecido para ajudar a alinhar o colágeno recém-formado com o tecido muscular existente (Kim e Choi, 2014; Nualon et al., 2013). A reeducação da marcha pode começar na piscina 48 horas após o incidente e, sistemicamente, pode ser utilizada durante todo o período de reabilitação para manter os níveis de $\dot{V}O_{2máx}$ e melhorar o limiar de lactato por meio da natação (braços apenas nos estágios iniciais).

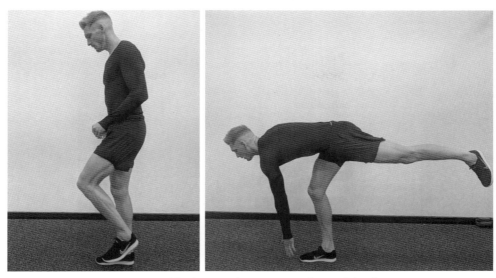

Figura 18.7 Exercício de controle neuromuscular: moinho de vento.

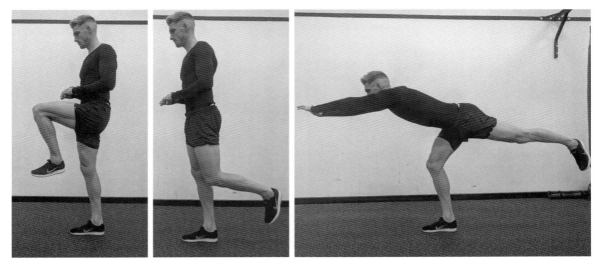

Figura 18.8 Exercício de controle neuromuscular: mergulhador.

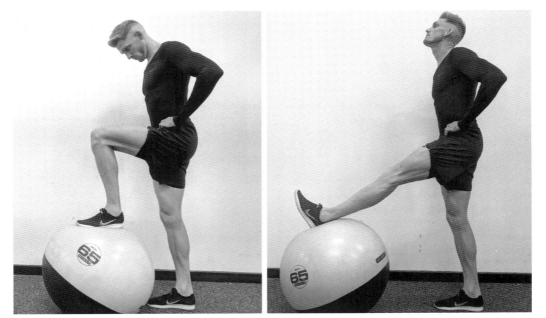

Figura 18.9 Neurodinâmica: controles deslizantes neurais de bola de estabilidade.

Exemplo de plano para a progressão de corrida

Tipo de estímulo	Frequência	Critérios de progressão				
		Fase 1	Fase 2	Fase 3	Fase 4	RAT baseado em corrida
Hidroterapia	2 a 3 sessões	Aumento gradual de até 8 minutos de corrida contínua	Estágios posteriores – utilizados como modalidade de recuperação			
Corrida leve 7,2 a 14,3 km/h	3-4× semana	Correr/caminhar 30 segundos começar/parar 2×8	Correr/caminhar 1 min 1:1 Razão T:R ×8 / 4 min ×3 a 4 / 1 min de descanso			
Corrida 14,4 a 19,7 km/h	3-4× semana		20 s 1:1 Razão T:R 8×2 / 3 min de descanso	30 s 1:1 Razão T:R 8×2 / 4 min de descanso		
CAV 19,8 a 25,1 km/h	3× semana			< 22 s. Comprimento do campo 8×2 / Razão T:R 1:1	< 20 s. Comprimento do campo 10×2 / Razão T:R 1:1	< 18 s. Comprimento do campo 10×2 / Razão T:R 1:1
Corrida de velocidade > 25,1 km/h	2× semana				Sprints 10 m × 4, 20 m / Recuperação total	Sprint 30 m 2×4; GPS velocidade máxima de 95% / Razão T:R 1:1
Corridas resistidas: trenó	1 a 2× semana			Corrida de trenó 10% PC 15 m 2×4 / Corrida de trenó 20% PC 5 m 2×4 / Recuperação total	Corrida de trenó 10% PC 15 m 2×6 / Corrida de trenó 20% PC 5 m 2×6 / Recuperação 60 s	Corrida de trenó 15% PC 15 m ×4 / Corrida de trenó 25% PC 5 m ×4 / Recuperação de 45 s	Corrida de trenó 15% PC 15 m 2×4 / Corrida de trenó 25% PC 15 m 2×4 / Recuperação de 45 s
Corridas assistidas: corrida em declive	1 a 2× semana			1×3×15 m	1×3×20m	1×3×25 m a uma desaceleração de 10 m	1×3×25 m a uma desaceleração de 5 m
Mudança de direção	3× semana	Por exemplo, corrida em ziguezague, viragem em uma curva, deslocamento lateral 1×4×10 m	Por exemplo, corte, giro de 90° 1×4×10 m; curva de 180° (meio campo/campo completo; cones de progressão a cada 20 a 10 m)	Por exemplo, exercícios de aceleração/desaceleração + viragem em vários planos, vários ângulos; ("Y", "L", "T" e "ziguezague", variações de teste "505 modificado" (2 a 3 exercícios por sessão) 1 a 2×4 razão T:R 1:1	Exercícios de agilidade reativa – introdução de componentes cognitivos e trabalho com bola, por exemplo, exercício de marcação shadow drill, exercícios com cones (2 a 3 exercícios por sessão) 1 a 2×4 razão T:R 1:1	Exercícios de agilidade – incorporação de sprint (2 a 3 exercícios por sessão) 1 a 2×4 (recuperação < 60 segundos)	Exercícios de agilidade específicos para esporte/posição, por exemplo, 1 contra 1, virar/receber sob pressão 1 a 2×4 (recuperação < 60 s)
Sprints repetidos	2× semana					5×6 s sprint máximo; GPS ≥ velocidade máxima de 95%

Aquecimento: aquecimento + mecânica de corrida, variações de marcha e salto específicos do esporte

	Fase 1	Fase 2	Fase 3	Fase 4	RAT baseado em corrida
	Subjetivamente: assintomático OU capaz de concluir com sintomas mínimos que não afetam a tarefa				
Diretrizes para progressões	Andar com marcha normal / Capaz de tolerar ritmo lento Introdução às atividades MDD	Capaz de tolerar curvas em vários ângulos	Capaz de tolerar tarefas multidirecionais em ritmo acelerado	Pontuação do teste MDD dentro de 10% da linha de base	Durante a sessão de reabilitação, cubra a distância correspondente às distâncias percorridas durante o jogo para: distância total, CAV e corrida (dados de GPS)
	Capaz de completar a matriz de jogo: perna dupla e única, amplitude interna	Capaz de completar a matriz de jogo: amplitude externa de perna dupla e única	Ponte elevada UP > 30 repetições e dentro de 20% ISM	Ponte elevada UP > 30 repetições e dentro de 10% ISM	Capaz de tolerar exercícios específicos para o esporte ou posição que replicam as demandas do jogo
	EAJ dentro de 10% ISM		Teste de força isométrica UP IT – manguito de pressão arterial; pontuação dentro de 10% ISM	Pontuação de potência da UP dentro de 10% ISM	Atingir > 90% da velocidade máxima a partir dos dados da linha de base

A transição por meio dos estágios de reabilitação é sempre conduzida pelo atleta e as decisões sobre seguir em frente ou permanecer na fase atual se resumem à prontidão mental do atleta. O atleta deve receber informações suficientes sobre as diretrizes de progressão para permitir que ele tome decisões informadas sobre seu processo de reabilitação. Medidas de resultados físicos por si só são insignificantes se o atleta não estiver psicologicamente pronto para avançar em sua jornada de reabilitação.

Figura 18.10 Exemplo de plano para a progressão de corrida. *EAJ*, extensão ativa de joelho; *PC*, peso corporal; *MDD*, mudança de direção; *GPS*, sistema de posicionamento global, do inglês *global positioning system*; *IT*, isquiotibiais; *CAV*, corrida em alta velocidade; *ISM*, índice de simetria de membros; *RAJ*, retorno ao jogo; *RAT*, retorno ao treinamento; *UP*, unipodal; *T:R*, trabalho/repouso.

Reabilitação do Desempenho para Lesões dos Isquiotibiais – Abordagem de Sistemas Multimodais

A dor é comumente usada como um guia para a progressão na reabilitação e, desse modo, pode atuar como uma barreira significativa para a progressão na reabilitação. Portanto, usamos a piscina 24 horas após a lesão para ajudar a reduzir os níveis de dor por meio do efeito da temperatura e da pressão da água nos termorreceptores e mecanorreceptores, respectivamente (Konlian, 1999). Este ambiente com otimização de carga ajuda a facilitar a transição para corridas e saltos em terra, tanto física quanto psicologicamente.

Corridas resistidas: quanta resistência é suficiente?

Talvez o parâmetro mais importante na corrida resistida seja o nível de carga aplicado ao atleta. Cargas altas podem potencialmente alterar a técnica de corrida e foi proposto que têm um efeito negativo no desempenho de *sprint*. Petrakos et al. (2016) defenderam o uso de cargas pesadas (20% da massa corporal) no trenó para melhorar a aceleração inicial onde a velocidade é lenta e as forças resistivas são altas, e uma carga mais leve (> 10% da massa corporal) para melhorar a velocidade máxima. Existem vários métodos de aplicação de resistência e a consideração para métodos de corrida resistida são discutidos mais detalhadamente na Tabela 18.3.

Corridas assistidas

A corrida assistida pode fornecer um estímulo de treinamento para melhorar a velocidade máxima, utilizando força externa para impulsionar o atleta para frente, onde a assistência pode ser fornecida por cordão elástico, faixa de resistência ou adaptação ambiental, como correr em declive. A corrida assistida provou ser eficaz no aumento da velocidade e aceleração máximas de corrida. A literatura saliente recomenda uma inclinação de 3,4 a 5,8° como ótima para desenvolver esta qualidade (Ebben et al., 2008). A assistência ao utilizar qualquer um dos métodos permite que o atleta atinja uma aceleração mais rápida até o pico de velocidade por meio da força gravitacional ou aplicada externamente. O aumento na aceleração e na velocidade de corrida pode ser uma consequência do aumento do comprimento e da frequência da passada durante a execução de corrida assistida e pela exposição do atleta à corrida supramáxima.

Mudança de direção e agilidade

Durante um jogo de futebol, os jogadores são expostos a cenários cognitivamente desafiadores que requerem movimentos rápidos e MDD em resposta a vários estímulos com e sem a posse de bola. A capacidade de acelerar, desacelerar e mudar de direção em velocidade por meio de uma série de movimentos em múltiplos planos e em resposta a um estímulo é definida como agilidade (Sheppard e Young, 2006). Esses momentos explosivos podem decidir o resultado do jogo, por exemplo, derrotar um adversário com a bola em uma oportunidade de gol. Na maioria das vezes, essas atividades explosivas também são a etiologia de muitas LITs. Portanto, a agilidade é um componente altamente importante do desempenho no futebol e um

Tabela 18.3 Considerações sobre métodos de corrida resistidos.

Método	Carga (% PC)	Desvantagens	Objetivo
Fundamentação: criar sobrecarga e aumentar a força dos membros inferiores, bem como maximizar as forças de propulsão durante as fases iniciais do *sprint*; promover inclinação para a frente e maior grau de flexão do quadril, joelho e tornozelo; desenvolvendo potência de força e resistência; melhorando qualidades anaeróbicas			
Faixa de resistência/ banda elástica	A resistência aplicada deve permitir que o atleta impulsione para a frente com uma inclinação frontal e uma corrida de velocidade moderada completa sem afetar negativamente a mecânica de corrida	Difícil de quantificar objetivamente a carga aplicada. Contando com a banda e com a resistência aplicada pela pessoa segurando a banda de resistência	Para melhorar a aceleração e a velocidade máxima
Vestimenta com peso	8 a 20% PC	Pode afetar negativamente a mecânica de funcionamento; extensão de quadril reduzida. A inclinação para a frente pode ser evitada pelo atleta (centro de massa transladado anteriormente durante a inclinação para a frente com colete pode desequilibrar o atleta)	
Paraquedas	Tamanho dependendo do peso corporal do atleta e das condições ambientais, por exemplo, vento ao completar corridas ao ar livre	Carga aplicada de difícil controle, tamanho do paraquedas *versus* peso corporal do atleta *versus* ambiente. Distância maior é executada apenas para permitir que o paraquedas abra totalmente	
Corridas de trenó	> 20% PC	Pode afetar negativamente a mecânica de funcionamento se a carga usada for muito alta	Para melhorar a aceleração inicial
	10 a 20% PC		Para melhorar a velocidade máxima

PC, peso corporal.

fator de risco significativo para LIT. Melhorar o desempenho de agilidade de um atleta é parte integrante de nossa filosofia de reabilitação de LIT.

Desaceleração e giro

Para uma MDD eficaz, os atletas precisam possuir a habilidade de desacelerar e frear rapidamente. Atletas que conseguem desacelerar com rapidez também serão capazes de mudar de direção do mesmo modo, já que a desaceleração influencia diretamente o tempo necessário para redirecionar a força para um novo plano de movimento. Isso permite que o atleta esteja um passo à frente e domine seu oponente. Movimentos de MDD de alta velocidade são gerados pelo GM enquanto os rotadores externos curtos trabalham para estabilizar a articulação do quadril. Com um pé plantado e o quadril em uma posição estável, a ação dos rotadores externos contralaterais do quadril (predominantemente GM) permite uma combinação eficiente de movimento de extensão e rotação criando uma ação de corte e propulsão; uma MDD durante a corrida (Neumann, 2010). A força excêntrica dos isquiotibiais parece ser um preditor de desempenho chave para desacelerar de forma eficaz (Naylor e Greig, 2015). Para atividades de MDD, os músculos isquiotibiais laterais (bíceps femoral) desempenham um papel importante em impulsionar o atleta para frente por sua capacidade de produzir altas forças de reação horizontal do solo (Morin et al., 2015).

Durante os movimentos de desaceleração, adotamos uma postura mais ereta e posterior inclinada, o que movimenta o centro de massa posteriormente em relação à base de apoio, permitindo a geração de maiores forças de ruptura horizontais (Dintiman e Ward, 2003). A flexão do quadril e do joelho e a dorsiflexão do tornozelo durante a desaceleração ajudam a dissipar a força de impacto excêntrica. O pé atinge o solo com o calcanhar para prolongar o tempo de contato com o solo, resistindo ao impulso do corpo para a frente. Durante esta ação de frenagem de estágio final, todos os músculos do membro inferior estão trabalhando excentricamente para absorver e dispersar a carga por meio do membro inferior (Hewit et al., 2011). Durante os jogos de futebol, os jogadores completam essas atividades repetidamente por 90 minutos ou mais; eles precisam possuir grandes habilidades de "frenagem" para resistir a altas forças externas e manter a estabilidade das articulações por meio de uma série de ações explosivas.

Aceleração

Os jogadores de futebol precisam de uma grande capacidade de aceleração; pesquisas sugerem que os músculos isquiotibiais desempenham um papel significativo na fase de aceleração do *sprint*, uma vez que a força de reação horizontal do solo durante as acelerações está associada com uma maior ativação do bíceps femoral antes do contato com o solo e pico de torque excêntrico dos flexores do joelho necessário para impulsionar o atleta para frente (Morin et al., 2015). Isso fornece a justificativa para sua inclusão durante a reabilitação. A posição do corpo durante a fase de aceleração da corrida é ajustada para permitir a produção de maiores forças horizontais e maximizar a propulsão (Morin et al., 2015). Essas adaptações incluem inclinação para a frente, preferência pelo contato do antepé com o solo (minimizando a frenagem), movimentos poderosos do braço (equilíbrio do momento angular das pernas) e tempo mínimo de voo (já que mais tempo no ar levará a uma diminuição da velocidade), conforme discutido por Hewit et al. (2011), Dintiman e Ward (2003) e Kreighbaum e Barthels (1996). Mais especificamente

para os isquiotibiais e sua contribuição para a fase de aceleração do *sprint*, a pesquisa mostrou que os indivíduos que são capazes de gerar forças de reação do solo horizontais de alto nível possuem alta capacidade de produção de torque para extensão do quadril e maior atividade eletromiográfica dos isquiotibiais durante o final da fase de balanço da aceleração do *sprint* (Morin et al., 2015). O grupo de músculos isquiotibiais também contribui para uma transferência líquida de força das articulações proximal para distal durante a extensão explosiva da perna (Jacobs et al., 1993) influenciando diretamente a transferência de energia por meio da cadeia cinética.

Implementar exercícios de aceleração na reabilitação desafiará os isquiotibiais a produzirem essa ação de alta intensidade. Um aumento gradual na intensidade e no volume é necessário para preparar o atleta para os *sprints* de aceleração repetidos aos quais ele será exposto no RAJ. As acelerações no futebol não são iniciadas apenas de uma posição estacionária, portanto, o atleta precisa ter a capacidade de completar uma aceleração inicial em "movimento", onde eles mudam o plano de movimento por meio de uma série de ações multiplanares em várias velocidades.

Agilidade

O treinamento de agilidade é parte integrante da reabilitação de desempenho. O foco desta intervenção é desenvolver a conexão entre os sistemas físicos e psicológicos necessários para realizar tarefas multidirecionais complexas em resposta a um estímulo com o objetivo de melhorar a conexão mente-corpo ao processar sinais e dicas do ambiente (Sheppard e Young, 2006). Desafiar a velocidade de processamento mental de um atleta durante tarefas específicas de esportes reforça o aprendizado de reação e permite que eles iniciem o movimento mais rápido e/ou com o tempo mais apropriado para alcançarem o melhor resultado (Pojskic et al., 2018). Para influenciar os componentes perceptivos e de tomada de decisão de agilidade, exercícios reativos, jogos pequenos ou 1 contra 1 podem ajudar a reduzir o tempo de resposta total, sugerindo o tempo necessário para reagir a um estímulo (processamento da entrada sensorial) e a duração do tempo necessária para realizar o movimento (resposta de controle motor) (Serpell et al., 2011; Young et al., 2015; Young e Rogers, 2014). Para uma discussão mais aprofundada sobre como treinar agilidade, consulte o Capítulo 33.

Corrida de alta velocidade e *sprint*

CAV e *sprint* são responsáveis por 8 a 12% da distância total de corrida coberta no futebol, com 90% de todos os *sprints* não excedendo 5 s de duração. Jogadores avançados com exposição significativamente maior a CAV e *sprint* durante todo o jogo (Andrzejewski et al., 2013; Bradley et al., 2013). A cada 3 a 5 segundos durante uma partida de futebol, os jogadores são expostos a ~1.200 mudanças imprevisíveis na atividade, que incluem vários *sprints*, *tackles* e saltos (Mohr et al., 2003), curvas (Bloomfield et al., 2007) e várias outras ações explosivas, como chutes e dribles. A reabilitação dos músculos isquiotibiais precisa de um aumento gradual da exposição à intensidade da corrida para progredir para a CAV e *sprint*, onde ocorre a maioria das lesões nos isquiotibiais (Askling et al., 2007).

A exposição a CAV, especialmente sob fadiga, é um componente importante da reabilitação de isquiotibiais em estágio final, uma vez que a pesquisa indica que a fadiga pode reduzir os ângulos de flexão do quadril e extensão do joelho, bem como aumentar a inclinação pélvica anterior durante a fase final de balanço, o que por sua vez pode aumentar a tensão nos isquiotibiais durante a corrida (Small et al., 2009).

Retorno ao jogo

O processo de reabilitação não termina quando o atleta é declarado apto e retorna ao treinamento e à competição. O monitoramento da exposição a CAV semanalmente, garantindo que o jogador conclua os exercícios de CAV (> 95% da velocidade máxima) ajudará a reduzir a ocorrência de lesões futuras nos isquiotibiais (Malone et al., 2017). Devido à variabilidade das demandas de jogo e treinamento, os jogadores podem nem sempre alcançar exposição suficiente à CAV durante essas atividades; portanto, é importante introduzir exercícios que permitam aos atletas atingir sua velocidade máxima regularmente para manter as adaptações alcançadas por meio da reabilitação. Também recomendamos esta abordagem como uma estratégia de mitigação de risco de lesão para todos os jogadores, com ou sem histórico de lesão no tendão da coxa. Os atletas precisam de exposição regular à CAV, que reproduz as demandas que eles encontrarão em campo; tolerar a corrida em um estado de fadiga fornece uma tradução eficaz da reabilitação para a competição.

Métricas de resultado

Métricas de resultado podem ajudar a determinar a prontidão de um jogador para retornar à competição. O teste de RAJ pode variar de clínico para clínico com base nos recursos disponíveis e restrições de tempo (Zambaldi et al., 2017). Os atletas devem receber informações suficientes sobre as diretrizes de progressão e critérios objetivos para permitir que tomem decisões informadas. Métricas de resultados físicos por si só não são significativas se o atleta não estiver psicologicamente pronto para retornar à competição. Várias métricas de resultados devem ser consideradas ao voltar a jogar após a lesão no tendão da coxa para minimizar as chances de nova lesão. Veja a Figura 18.10 e a Tabela 18.4 para saber como usamos marcadores objetivos como parte de nossa progressão de corrida e para métricas de resultado para RAJ.

Conclusão

A reabilitação de desempenho tem como objetivo preparar os atletas tanto física quanto psicologicamente, criando um ambiente de reabilitação flexível que atende às necessidades individuais dos atletas. Até o momento, ainda não há consenso para os critérios de avaliação, reabilitação e RAJ para LIT. A complexidade arquitetônica dos isquiotibiais e as crescentes demandas que os atletas colocam nesse grupo de músculos criam um desafio para os profissionais de saúde que tentam fazer com que seus atletas voltem a jogar com segurança.

Tabela 18.4 Considerações para métricas de resultado de lesão nos isquiotibiais no retorno ao jogo.

Testes clínicos			
Sem sensibilidade à palpação	Assintomático na queda	Teste de Elevação da Perna Estendida (*Straight leg raise*) Assintomático D = E	Extensão ativa do joelho D = E
Teste baseado em força			
Matriz de ponte: Faixa interna PD e UP Faixa externa PD e UP	Força isométrica do isquiotibial: (manguito de pressão arterial) dentro de 10% ISM Força geral: Estocada reversa 3 × 6 (75% 1RM) Ponte elevada UP 3 × 6 (75% 1RM) ou repetições máximas de ponte elevada UP > 30 dentro de 10% ISM	Força excêntrica: Nórdico 3 × 6 com peso de 10 kg Controle deslizante de isquiotibiais ponderado 3 × 8 (75% 1RM)	Força explosiva: Impulso de quadril UP 3 × 6 (30% 1RM) Salto de contramovimento PD e UP ou teste de salto vertical dentro de 10% ISM Salto triplo para distância dentro de 10% ISM
Teste baseado em campo			
Tempo de *sprint* em comparação com a linha de base: 10 m 30 m Tolerar 2 semanas de treinamento de equipe completa antes do RAJ	Tempo de teste MDD em comparação com a linha de base: Teste 5-0-5 modificado Teste T	Habilidade de *sprint* repetida: 6 × 6 *sprints* máximos com 24 s de recuperação entre cada *sprint* e alcance índice de fadiga de 85%+	Velocidade aeróbica máxima: Distância coberta em comparação com a linha de base correspondem aos dados Teste VAM de 1600 m GPS atinge 130% da CAV em 3 sessões de reabilitação antes do RAJ
Estabilidade lombopélvica-quadril e controle neuromuscular			
Exercício *dead bug* 20 reps com peso de 20 kg	Manter a estabilidade durante: moinho de vento, mergulhador, SEBT usando ferramenta de avaliação qualitativa de carregamento unipodal (QASLS).		

A maioria dos testes será comparada com dados de linha de base (se disponíveis) ou resultados de teste de membros não envolvidos. *MDD*, mudança de direção; *PD*, perna dupla; *GPS*, sistema de posicionamento global, do inglês *global positioning system*; *CAV*, corrida em alta velocidade; *ISM*, índice de simetria de membros; *VAM*, velocidade aeróbica máxima; *QASLS*, análise qualitativa do agachamento unipodal, do inglês *qualitative analysis of single leg squat*; *RM*, repetição máxima; *RAJ*, retorno ao jogo; *SEBT, star excursion balance test*; *UP*, unipodal. Ferramentas úteis para medições objetivas de força: Norbord®, dinamômetro portátil, teste isocinético.

Aplicação Clínica

A reabilitação eficaz dos isquiotibiais precisa ser de natureza multimodal para replicar as demandas do jogo, com o "cronômetro de RAJ" sendo ativado quando ocorre a lesão. Programas multimodais bem planejados, prescritos individualmente, projetados em torno da especificidade e da sobrecarga progressiva são fundamentais para a nossa filosofia de reabilitação. Um amplo espectro de exercícios deve ser considerado para atender às necessidades individuais dos atletas e não há uma receita que sirva para todos. O perfil de força excêntrica, bem como a exposição à corrida em alta velocidade são dois componentes significativos no tratamento de LIT. No entanto, muitos outros subcomponentes precisam ser direcionados para um RAJ bem-sucedido e seguro após a LIT e, como clínicos, precisamos ser capazes de nos adaptar e lidar com contratempos, recorrências e casos incomuns.

O objetivo da reabilitação de desempenho é construir a resiliência física e mental dos atletas, melhorar a capacidade atlética, reduzir o risco de lesões futuras e otimizar o envolvimento. Nenhuma intervenção única ou medida de resultado clínico ou físico provavelmente será específica ou sensível o suficiente para prever um RAJ seguro – dada a natureza perigosa do futebol – e uma bateria de marcadores objetivos clínicos, de ginástica e de campo específicos para o indivíduo, junto com *feedback* subjetivo do jogador, podem oferecer informações mais significativas ao tomar decisões para o RAJ.

Agradecimentos

Os autores deste capítulo gostariam de agradecer as contribuições de Andy Mitchell do Blackburn Rovers FC, Mike Edwards do Notts County FC, Simon Mulvany, Dave Orton do Leicester Tigers RFC e Lee Taylor do Peterborough United FC na redação deste conteúdo.

Referências bibliográficas

Andrzejewski, M., Chmura, J., Pluta, B., Strzelczyk, R., Kasprzak, A., 2013. Analysis of sprinting activities of professional soccer players. Journal of Strength and Conditioning Research 27, 2134-2140.

Askling, C.M., Tengvar, M., Saartok, T., Thorstensson, A., 2007. Acute first-time hamstring strains during high-speed running: a longitudinal study including clinical and magnetic resonance imaging findings. American Journal of Sports Medicine 35 (2), 197-206.

Askling, C., Thorstensson, A., 2008. Hamstring muscle strain in sprinters. N. Stud. Athl. 23, 67-79.

Bloomfield, J., Polman, R., O'Donoghue, P., 2007. Physical demands of different positions in FA premier League soccer. Journal of Sports Science and Medicine 6 (1), 63-70.

Bompa, T.O., Haff, G.G., 2009. Periodization: Theory and Methodology of Training, fifth ed. Human Kinetics, Champaign, Il, pp. 259-286.

Bourne, M.N., Duhig, S.J., Timmins, R.G., Williams, M.D., Opar, D.A., Al Najjar, A., et al., 2017. Impact of the Nordic hamstring and hip extension exercises on hamstring architecture and morphology: implications for injury prevention. British Journal of Sports Medicine 51 (5), 469-477.

Bradley, P.S., Carling, C., Diaz, A.G., Hood, P., Barnes, C., Ade, J., et al., 2013. Match performance and physical capacity of players in the top three competitive standards of English professional soccer. Human Movement Science 32, 808-821.

Brukner, P., 2012. Brukner & Khan's Clinical Sports Medicine. McGraw-Hill, North Ryde, Australia.

Bruton, A., 2002. Muscle plasticity: response to training and detraining. Physiotherapy 88 (7), 398-408.

Chumanov, E.S., Schache, A.G., Heiderscheit, B.C., Thelen, D.G., 2012. Hamstrings are most susceptible to injury during the late swing phase of sprinting. British Journal of Sports Medicine 46 (2), 90.

Chumanov, E.S., Heiderscheit, B.C., Thelen, D.G., 2007. The effect of speed and influence of individual muscles on hamstring mechanics during the swing phase of sprinting. Journal of Biomechanics 40 (16), 3555-3562.

Clark, R., Bryant, A., Culgan, J.-P., Hartley, B., 2005. The effects of eccentric hamstring strength training on dynamic jumping performance and isokinetic strength parameters: a pilot study on the implications for the prevention of hamstring injuries. Physical Therapy in Sport 6, 67-73.

De Blaiser, C., Roosen, P., Willems, T., Danneels, L., Bossche, L.V., De Ridder, R., 2018. Is core stability a risk factor for lower extremity injuries in an athletic population? A systematic review. Physical Therapy in Sport 30, 48-56.

De Visser, H., Reijman, M., Heijboer, M., Bos, P., 2012. Risk factors of recurrent hamstring injuries: a systematic review. British Journal of Sports Medicine 46, 124-130.

De Vos, R.J., Reurink, G., Goudswaard, G.J., Moen, M.H., Weir, A., Tol, J.L., 2014. Clinical findings just after return to play predict hamstring re-injury, but baseline MRI findings do not. British Journal of Sports Medicine 48 (18), 1377-1384.

Delorme, T.L., 1945. Restoration of muscle power by heavy-resistance exercises. Journal of Bone and Joint Surgery 27, 645-667.

Dinnery, B., Wilson, J., 2018. Return to Play Timeframes Following Hamstring Injury in the Premier League. www.premierinjuries.com/betting.php?.

Dintiman, G., Ward, B., 2003. Starting and stopping. In: Sports Speed, third ed. Human Kinetics, Champaign, IL, pp. 212-217.

Ebben, W.P., Davies, J.A., Clewien, R.W., 2008. Effect of the degree of hill slope on acute downhill running velocity and acceleration. Journal of Strength and Conditioning Research 22, 898-902.

Ekstrand, J., Hägglund, M., Kristenson, K., Magnusson, H., Waldén, M., 2013. Fewer ligament injuries but no preventive effect on muscle injuries and severe injuries: an 11-year follow-up of the UEFA Champions League injury study. British Journal of Sports Medicine 47, 732-737.

Evans, K., Williams, M., 2017. The effect of Nordic hamstring exercise on hamstring injury in professional rugby union. British Journal of Sports Medicine 51, 316-317.

Fukutani, A., Kurihara, T., 2015. Comparison of the muscle fascicle length between resistance-trained and untrained individuals: cross-sectional observation. SpringerPlus 4, 341.

Hewit, J., Cronin, J., Button, C., Hume, P., 2011. Understanding deceleration in sport. Strength and Conditioning Journal 33 (1), 47-52.

Huxel Bliven, K.C., Anderson, B.E., 2013. Core stability training for injury prevention. Sports Health 5 (6), 514-522.

Jacobs, R., Bobbert, M.F., van Ingen Schenau, G.J., 1993. Function of mono- and biarticular muscles in running. Medicine & Science in Sports & Exercise 25 (10), 1163-1173.

Kim, E., Choi, H., 2014. Aquatic physical therapy in the rehabilitation of athletic injuries: a systematic review of the literatures. Journal of Yoga and Physical Therapy 5.

Konlian, C., 1999. Aquatic therapy: making a wave in the treatment of low back injuries. Journal of Orthopaedic Nursing 3, 181.

Kreighbaum, E., Barthels, K.M., 1996. Biomechanics: A Qualitative Approach for Studying Human Movement. Allyn and Bacon, Boston, MA.

Lieberman, D.E., Raichlen, D.A., Pontzer, H., Bramble, D.M., Cutright-Smith, E., 2006. The human gluteus maximus and its role in running. Journal of Experimental Biology 209 (Pt 11), 2143-2155.

Loturco, I., Pereira, L.A., Kobal, R., Zanetti, V., Kitamura, K., Abad, C.C.C., et al., 2015. Transference effect of vertical and horizontal plyometrics on sprint performance of high-level U-20 soccer players. Journal of Sports Sciences 33, 2182-2191.

Malone, S., Roe, M., Doran, D.A., Gabbett, T.J., Collins, K., 2017. High chronic training loads and exposure to bouts of maximal velocity running reduce injury risk in elite Gaelic football. Journal of Science and Medicine in Sport 20, 250-254.

Manouras, N., Papanikolaou, Z., Karatrantou, K., Kouvarakis, P., Gerodimos, V., 2016. The efficacy of vertical vs. horizontal plyometric training on speed, jumping performance and agility in soccer players. International Journal of Sports Science & Coaching 11, 702-709.

Mendiguchia, J., Martinez-Ruiz, E., Edouard, P., Morin, J.-B., Martinez-Martinez, F., Idoate, F., et al., 2017. A multifactorial, criteria-based progressive algorithm for hamstring injury treatment. Medicine & Science in Sports & Exercise 49, 1482-1492.

Mohr, M., Krustrup, P., Bangsbo, J., 2003. Match performance of high-standard soccer players with special reference to development of fatigue. Journal of Sports Sciences 21, 519-528.

Morin, J.-B., Gimenez, P., Edouard, P., Arnal, P., Jiménez-Reyes, P., Samozino, P., et al., 2015. Sprint acceleration mechanics: the major role of hamstrings in horizontal force production. Frontiers in Physiology 6, 404.

Mulvany, S.T., Wilson, J., 2018. Complex-Adaptive Modeling in Sports Science & Sports Medicine. https://wilsonmulvany.wordpress.com/2018/10/18/model-number-1-neuromuscular-systems-conditioning-nsc-advantaged-stacked-over-preparedness-for-sport-specific-demand/

Naylor, J., Greig, M., 2015. A hierarchical model of factors influencing a battery of agility tests. Journal of Sports Medicine and Physical Fitness 55, 1329-1335.

Neumann, D.A., 2010. Kinesiology of the hip: a focus on muscular actions. Journal of Orthopaedic & Sports Physical Therapy 40, 82-94.

Nualon, P., Piriyaprasarth, P., Yuktanandana, P., 2013. The role of 6-week hydrotherapy and land-based therapy plus ankle taping in a preseason rehabilitation program for athletes with chronic ankle instability. Asian Biomedicine 7, 553-559.

Orchard, J.W., Seward, H., Orchard, J.J., 2013. Results of 2 decades of injury surveillance and public release of data in the Australian Football League. American Journal of Sports Medicine 41, 734-741.

Petersen, J., Hölmich, P., 2005. Evidence based prevention of hamstring injuries in sport. British Journal of Sports Medicine 39, 319-323.

Petrakos, G., Morin, J.-B., Egan, B., 2016. Resisted sled sprint training to improve sprint performance: a systematic review. Sports Medicine 46, 381-400.

Pojskic, H., Åslin, E., Krolo, A., Jukic, I., Uljevic, O., Spasic, M., et al., 2018. Importance of reactive agility and change of direction speed in differentiating performance levels in junior soccer players: reliability and validity of newly developed soccer-specific tests. Frontiers in Physiology 9, 506.

Reurink, G., Whiteley, R., Tol, J.L., 2015. Hamstring injuries and predicting return to play: 'bye-bye MRI?' British Journal of Sports Medicine 49 (18), 1162-1163.

Sáez De Villarreal, E., Suarez-Arrones, L., Requena, B., Haff, G.G., Ferrete, C., 2015. Effects of plyometric and sprint training on physical and technical skill performance in adolescent soccer players. Journal of Strength and Conditioning Research 29, 1894-1903.

Schache, A.G., Dorn, T.W., Blanch, P.D., Brown, N.A., Pandy, M.G., 2012. Mechanics of the human hamstring muscles during sprinting. Medicine & Science in Sports & Exercise 44, 647-658.

Schache, A.G., Wrigley, T.V., Baker, R., Pandy, M.G., 2009. Biomechanical response to hamstring muscle strain injury. Gait Posture 29, 332-338.

Schuermans, J., Van Tiggelen, D., Witvrouw, E., 2017. Prone hip extension muscle recruitment is associated with hamstring injury risk in amateur soccer. International Journal of Sports Medicine 38, 696-706.

Serpell, B.G., Young, W.B., Ford, M., 2011. Are the perceptual and decision-making components of agility trainable? A preliminary investigation. Journal of Strength and Conditioning Research 25 (5), 1240-1248.

Sheppard, J.M., Young, W.B., 2006. Agility literature review: classifications, training and testing. Journal of Sports Sciences 24, 919-932.

Small, K., Mcnaughton, L., Greig, M., Lohkamp, M., Lovell, R., 2009. Soccer fatigue, sprinting and hamstring injury risk. International Journal of Sports Medicine 30, 573.

Timmins, R.G., Bourne, M.N., Shield, A.J., Williams, M.D., Lorenzen, C., Opar, D.A., 2016. Short biceps femoris fascicles and eccentric knee flexor weakness increase the risk of hamstring injury in elite football (soccer): a prospective cohort study. British Journal of Sports Medicine 50 (24), 1524-1535.

Todd, J.S., Shurley, J.P., Todd, T.C., 2012. Thomas L. DeLorme and the science of progressive resistance exercise. Journal of Strength and Conditioning Research 26, 2913-2923.

Tol, J.L., Hamilton, B., Eirale, C., Muxart, P., Jacobsen, P., Whiteley, R., 2014. At return to play following hamstring injury the majority of professional football players have residual isokinetic deficits. British Journal of Sports Medicine 48 (18), 1364-1369.

Turl, S.E., George, K.P., 1998. Adverse neural tension: a factor in repetitive hamstring strain? Journal of Orthopaedic & Sports Physical Therapy 27, 16-21.

Van Der Horst, N., Backx, F., Goedhart, E.A., Huisstede, B.M., 2017. Return to play after hamstring injuries in football (soccer): a worldwide Delphi procedure regarding definition, medical criteria and decision-making. British Journal of Sports Medicine 51 (22), 1583-1591.

Van Der Horst, N., Smits, D.-W., Petersen, J., Goedhart, E.A., Backx, F. J.G., 2015. The preventive effect of the Nordic hamstring exercise on hamstring injuries in amateur soccer players: a randomized controlled trial. American Journal of Sports Medicine 43, 1316-1323.

Wangensteen, A., Tol, J.L., Witvrouw, E., Van Linschoten, R., Almusa, E., Hamilton, B., et al., 2016. Hamstring reinjuries occur at the same location and early after return to sport: a descriptive study of MRI-confirmed reinjuries. American Journal of Sports Medicine 44, 2112-2121.

Wilkerson, G.B., Colston, M.A., 2015. A refined prediction model for core and lower extremity sprains and strains among collegiate football players. Journal of Athletic Training 50, 643-650.

Willson, J.D., Dougherty, C.P., Ireland, M.L., Davis, I.M., 2005. Core stability and its relationship to lower extremity function and injury. JAAOS – Journal of the American Academy of Orthopaedic Surgeons 13, 316-325.

Woods, C., Hawkins, R., Maltby, S., Hulse, M., Thomas, A., Hodson, A., 2004. The Football Association Medical Research Programme: an audit of injuries in professional football—analysis of hamstring injuries. British Journal of Sports Medicine 38, 36-41.

Young, W., Rogers, N., 2014. Effects of small-sided game and change-of-direction training on reactive agility and change-of-direction speed. Journal of Sports Sciences 32 (4), 307-314.

Young, W.B., Dawson, B., Henry, G.J., 2015. Agility and change-of-direction speed are independent skills: implications for training for agility in invasion sports. International Journal of Sports Science and Coaching 10 (1), 159-169.

Zambaldi, M., Beasley, I., Rushton, A., 2017. Return to play criteria after hamstring muscle injury in professional football: a Delphi consensus study. British Journal of Sports Medicine 51 (16), 1221-1226.

Zazulak, B.T., Hewett, T.E., Reeves, N.P., Goldberg, B., Cholewicki, J., 2007. Deficits in neuromuscular control of the trunk predict knee injury risk:prospective biomechanical-epidemiologic study. American Journal of Sports Medicine 35, 1123-1130.

Capítulo | 19 |

Manejo de Ruptura dos Músculos Gastrocnêmico e Sóleo em Jogadores de Futebol Profissional

Paul Godfrey, Mike Beere e James Rowland

Introdução

Está além do escopo deste capítulo discutir todas as causas da dor na panturrilha no jogador de futebol profissional. Em vez disso, serão abordadas lesões comuns na panturrilha observadas nessa população: distensão ou ruptura dos músculos sóleo e gastrocnêmico. Há uma escassez de pesquisas relacionadas com esses tipos de lesões no ambiente do esporte de elite e menos ainda no futebol profissional. Das pesquisas que podem ser encontradas sobre o assunto (Dixon, 2009; Pedret et al., 2015), não há nenhuma que possa ser considerada de alta qualidade, ou seja, ensaios clínicos randomizados duplo-cegos e, portanto, muito do que foi escrito talvez precise ser visto com cautela considerável.

Os autores, que trabalham na "linha de frente" no futebol profissional e em outros esportes de elite, trataram muitas lesões nos músculos da panturrilha ao longo dos anos e conseguiram reduzi-las ao longo de temporada(s) de futebol profissional. Portanto, este capítulo representa muitos anos de experiência combinada, durante os quais os autores testaram várias abordagens para o tratamento de rupturas nos músculos da panturrilha. Os autores demonstram o que funciona a partir dessas várias abordagens e delineiam uma estratégia de manejo abrangente. Os estudos de caso fornecidos posteriormente no texto mostram exemplos de como os elementos dessa estratégia funcionam quando aplicados às circunstâncias de um indivíduo.

Este capítulo também abrange quando esperar essas lesões durante uma temporada, e suas possíveis causas – incluindo os "mitos" comumente considerados e a reabilitação inadequada resultante disso. É apresentada uma abordagem para a avaliação e a reabilitação dessas rupturas musculares usando métodos experimentados e testados conforme utilizados pelos autores. Além disso, este capítulo esclarece o significado de termos como "carga", "sobrecarga" e "manejo de carga", com o objetivo de fornecer ao leitor melhor compreensão do que cada um deles significa no contexto de rupturas na panturrilha. Ademais, o texto analisa o que esses termos de engenharia realmente significam e por que não devem ser confundidos com o conceito agora comum dentro da profissão de ciência do esporte de carga aguda *versus* carga crônica.

Dessa maneira, este capítulo examina quais são as diferenças relatadas na anatomia, fibras musculares e função de cada músculo e, se essas diferenças existem, como a reabilitação deve ser diferente para cada músculo e os diferentes métodos de treinamento aplicados.

Finalmente, os autores também discutem como o ambiente do futebol profissional e as pressões exercidas sobre os jogadores e equipe que trabalham em campo costumam influenciar o uso de imagens radiológicas, o processo de reabilitação e, em última instância, a eficácia dessa reabilitação. Na realidade, uma "abordagem ideal" para a reabilitação de rupturas no sóleo e no gastrocnêmico, como discutido nesse capítulo, nem sempre é possível, em detrimento de todos os envolvidos.

Conceito de estresse/tensão

Qualquer clínico que estudou fisiologia muscular estará familiarizado com o conceito de engenharia de estresse/tensão e a curva que descreve como o tecido humano responde a qualquer força ou carga, ou seja, como o tecido se alonga ou se comprime para tolerar um peso colocado sobre ele (Figura 19.1).

Cada tecido (p. ex., ligamento, tendão, músculo, osso) tem propriedades comuns a todos os tecidos do corpo – de elasticidade e plasticidade. A elasticidade está relacionada com a capacidade de um tecido de esticar (ou comprimir) sob carga e retornar ao seu estado original quando ela é removida (extrapola pela linha preta A–B na Figura 19.1). Já a plasticidade é um ponto em que a força/carga aplicada é tão grande que o tecido não consegue mais acomodá-la e perde sua capacidade de retornar ao estado original, permanecendo em seu estado deformado (alongado ou comprimido). Isso indica onde ocorreu o microtrauma no tecido; as propriedades de recuo foram excedidas (linha preta B–C na Figura 19.1). Os sintomas nesse ponto incluem inflamação leve e algum grau de desconforto – uma tensão de grau muito baixo pode ser diagnosticada.

A falha completa de um tecido ocorre quando a quantidade de força/carga ou sobrecarga excede as propriedades elásticas e plásticas do tecido, fazendo com que o tecido se danifique significativamente, ou seja, variando de uma ruptura considerável para uma completa (ponto além de C na Figura 19.1). Os sintomas seriam altos níveis de dor, inflamação considerável e uma perda significativa da função do tecido afetado.

Cabe aos departamentos de ciências da saúde e esportivas de um clube de futebol auxiliar a gestão no conceito de manejo de carga, ou seja, fornecer informações sobre a quantidade de trabalho atribuída a cada jogador durante o treinamento e qual é

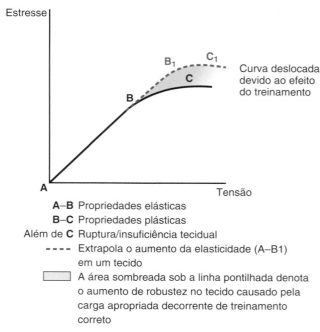

Figura 19.1 Curva de tensão/deformação simplificada em relação ao tecido humano e um efeito de treinamento.

o trabalho ou carga acumulativa conforme a semana de treinamento se desenvolve. A ideia é tentar determinar a quantidade ideal de trabalho/carga ou estímulo para produzir um efeito de treinamento para melhorar a aptidão cardiovascular, força, potência, capacidade de recuperação e repetição. Além disso, esses departamentos também devem aconselhar quanto descanso é necessário para permitir que os tecidos dos jogadores se recuperem e respondam ao estímulo, sem atingir o ponto crítico de falha de qualquer tecido ou supertreinamento como um todo. O objetivo final em termos da curva de tensão/deformação é mover a curva para cima e para a direita (extrapolada pela linha tracejada vermelha na Figura 19.1 e os novos pontos B_1 e C_1). Isso sugere que uma boa resposta de treinamento por meio de estímulo/carregamento repetido apropriado faz com que o tecido humano responda por aumentos em sua robustez (denotada pela área sombreada na Figura 19.1) para suportar forças/carga maiores antes que o tecido seja lesionado, alcançado pelo manejo da carga ideal.

Incidência de rupturas e o calendário do futebol

Em uma temporada de futebol, existem períodos com potencial para maior incidência de lesões de tecidos moles, sobretudo rupturas musculares – especificamente nos músculos da cadeia posterior (os grupos de músculos isquiotibiais e panturrilhas; Woods et al., 2002). Ainda não é bem compreendido por que esses grupos estão em maior risco; entretanto, na opinião dos autores, isso pode ser devido ao papel que esses músculos desempenham na atenuação e na propulsão do choque durante o ciclo da marcha. Além disso, eles têm que lidar com grandes forças ou carga, enquanto em posições alongadas, ao cruzarem o quadril e o joelho ou o joelho e o tornozelo.

Os dois períodos distintos em questão são a pré-temporada (julho e início de agosto no hemisfério Norte) e no final da temporada (março, abril e maio no hemisfério Norte). O primeiro é definido pela introdução de um aumento da demanda ou carga de trabalho no período que antecede o início da temporada. A pré-temporada sempre segue um período de verão (maio e junho no hemisfério Norte) de carga de trabalho muito reduzida, onde os jogadores estiveram de férias e tiveram um período de relativo descanso, permitindo que os músculos fiquem descondicionados devido à redução dos exercícios realizados. Julho tem um aumento repentino na demanda sendo colocado nos músculos das pernas enquanto eles tentam recuperar a forma física e o condicionamento perdidos em um curto período de tempo, ou seja, geralmente 6 semanas. Esse aumento da carga de trabalho, se muito intenso e aplicado muito cedo, sobrecarrega maciçamente os músculos, fazendo com que falhem (rompam), pois não conseguem lidar com a demanda que se espera deles. No entanto, o jogador de futebol profissional moderno está ciente das consequências de não se exercitar o suficiente durante as férias de verão e está (principalmente) feliz em seguir o programa de encerramento da temporada definido para eles pelos departamentos de ciências da saúde e esportivas do clube em uma tentativa de manter um nível de condicionamento que diminui a probabilidade de lesão durante a pré-temporada.

Apesar de esse período ser conhecido como um potencial de grande frequência de lesões, ainda existem alguns jogadores que preferem correr o risco de lesões na pré-temporada, tendo um descanso mais longo do que o recomendado do exercício no verão e muitas vezes pagam o preço durante a pré-temporada.

O outro período para maior risco de lesões, especialmente para rupturas musculares, são os meses finais de temporada. Estes são caracterizados por jogadores com um nível mais alto de fadiga acumulada e esta fadiga resulta de treinamentos inadequados ou volumes de supertreinamento definidos pela equipe técnica e/ou estratégias de recuperação inadequadas que não permitem que os jogadores descansem o suficiente e que os músculos se preparem para a próxima sessão de exercício. Isso significa que os jogadores vão para os últimos meses da temporada (quando a pressão para o desempenho e as apostas gerais são mais altas) em um estado inferior ao ideal para jogar, o que significa que os músculos correm um risco maior de não serem capazes de suportar a carga de trabalho exigida deles, então falham e se rompem.

No entanto, também deve ser observado que se os jogadores não forem treinados adequadamente quando entram no período de pré-temporada (*i. e.*, trabalharem duro o suficiente), e se essa falta de estímulo continuar na temporada, os jogadores estão tentando jogar partidas competitivas em um estado descondicionado. Isso significa que as lesões dos tecidos moles podem e invariavelmente ocorrerão a qualquer momento durante a temporada e não apenas durante os dois períodos destacados.

Avaliação e uso de imagens radiológicas

Existem muitos testes declarados em vários textos (Brukner e Kahn, 2012) sobre como as lesões musculares devem ser avaliadas para diagnosticar uma ruptura muscular e talvez até mesmo estabelecer a extensão da ruptura. No entanto, na realidade, as rupturas do sóleo e do gastrocnêmio precisam apenas de algumas perguntas ao realizar alguns testes simples para auxiliar no processo de diagnóstico (Boxe 19.1).

> **Boxe 19.1 Perguntas a serem feitas ao se realizar testes**
>
> - A dor/rigidez sentida na parte inferior da perna começou repentina ou gradualmente?
> - Sente dor/desconforto ao caminhar?
> - Há dor com a dorsiflexão ativa do tornozelo sem sustentação de peso (SSP)? Com o joelho reto e/ou flexionado?
> - Há dor com dorsiflexão passiva do tornozelo SSP? Com o joelho reto e/ou flexionado?
> - O jogador pode fazer uma elevação de calcanhar? Com o joelho reto e/ou flexionado?
> - O jogador consegue pular?
> - Que sintomas são desencadeados com a palpação e onde?

Para que uma ruptura muscular seja diagnosticada, a maioria dos testes mencionados anteriormente precisa ser positivo para produzir dor. Os sintomas produzidos com um joelho predominantemente flexionado, mas não quando o joelho está reto, sugerem mais um envolvimento do sóleo; o inverso é verdadeiro para o músculo gastrocnêmico. A capacidade de realizar um salto e/ou elevação do calcanhar sugere menos comprometimento muscular do que um jogador que é incapaz de elevar o calcanhar ou pular devido à dor e isso indica uma ruptura considerável em um dos dois principais músculos da panturrilha.

Na experiência dos autores, quanto mais testes são positivos e mais súbito é o início, maior é a probabilidade de ser uma ruptura grave. No entanto, no futebol profissional, devido às pressões para que os jogadores voltem a jogar no menor tempo possível, os departamentos médicos devem confirmar esse tipo de lesão por meio de imagens radiológicas, seja uma ultrassonografia, seja uma ressonância magnética (RM). Nesse ponto, a varredura tende a ser de rotina para apaziguar o jogador e a equipe, que esperam imagens como parte integrante do processo de diagnóstico. Pouquíssimos médicos experientes precisam de um exame para confirmar o que sua avaliação clínica disse a eles; a imagem apenas corrobora o diagnóstico da avaliação clínica.

Em geral, o imageamento de uma lesão não influencia o modo como é tratada; afinal, devem ser sempre os sintomas que ditam o tratamento. No entanto, um jogador lesionado e/ou a direção de um clube tende a ficar mais tranquilo se um exame for realizado e parece que os médicos que trabalham no futebol profissional simplesmente devem aceitar isso.

Causas comumente consideradas

Flexibilidade

A falta de flexibilidade (talvez mais fora do esporte de elite) é frequentemente considerada uma possível causa subjacente para a ocorrência de uma ruptura muscular. Existe a noção de que se os músculos sóleo e/ou gastrocnêmico não tiverem amplitude de movimento suficiente, eles não terão a capacidade necessária para se alongar e velocidade suficiente para impedir que o músculo se rasgue quando for aplicada força/carga sobre ele e, como resultado, as musculaturas se rompem.

A amplitude anatômica do tornozelo é considerada ~0 a 50° de flexão plantar e 0 a 20° de dorsiflexão (Standring, 2015). São esses 20° de dorsiflexão que dão origem a um teste do joelho à parede (JAP) com uma amplitude de 8 cm ou mais sendo o objetivo (Figura 19.2). A menos que um jogador de futebol profissional tenha sofrido uma lesão anterior no tornozelo que possa

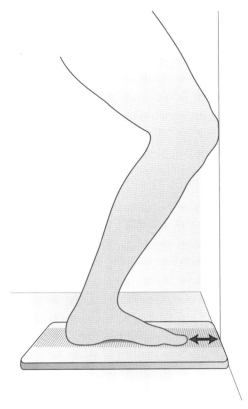

Figura 19.2 Posição de teste do joelho à parede (JAP). A *seta* extrapola a distância medida do dedão do pé à parede, com o joelho tocando a parede e o calcanhar permanecendo em contato com o chão.

limitar sua dorsiflexão, a maioria dos jogadores atinge facilmente uma pontuação de teste JAP ≥ 8 cm e, mesmo aqueles que não o fazem, raramente continuam e sofrem uma ruptura do músculo sóleo ou do gastrocnêmico.

A flexibilidade e sua possível relação com a lesão muscular foram estudadas com mais detalhes do que muitos outros fatores que podem contribuir para a lesão muscular (Cornwall et al., 2002; Ettema et al., 1996; Kubo et al., 2002; van Mechelen et al., 1993; Wilson et al., 1992; Witvrouw et al., 2003; 2004). No entanto, a pesquisa não parece apoiar a noção amplamente difundida de que a falta de flexibilidade predispõe o indivíduo a rupturas musculares. Isso é ecoado pelas próprias experiências dos autores até o momento. A clara maioria dos jogadores de futebol profissionais que sofrem rupturas do sóleo ou do gastrocnêmico o fazem sem perda adversa da flexibilidade desse músculo e isso sugere que há outros fatores etiológicos.

Inadequações de força

Juntamente com a falta de flexibilidade percebida, a falta de força ou fraqueza no complexo gastrocnêmico/sóleo é outra razão comumente considerada para o rompimento desses músculos. Ao contrário da flexibilidade como causa, é a experiência dos autores que se um jogador é incapaz de gerar força e potência suficientes para realizar todas as ações exigidas no futebol profissional, por exemplo, correr, acelerar, pular, pousar, as forças colocadas sobre esses músculos, quando essas atividades são realizadas, podem fazer com que um ou ambos os músculos falhem e se rompam. (Ver seção *Reabilitação*, com ginástica para o retorno ao jogo (RAJ) adiante para uma discussão sobre como corrigir esta deficiência.)

Mecânica do pé e uso de órteses

Se o pé não estiver funcionando como deveria e não estiver transferindo força do solo no impacto durante a marcha até o tornozelo e a parte inferior da perna, então outras estruturas na região podem ser sobrecarregadas e falhar.

As estruturas do pé devem manter sua forma, mas têm elasticidade suficiente para lidar com as forças de reação do solo colocadas sobre eles durante o ciclo da marcha – o pé atuando como um atenuador de choque durante a fase de apoio da marcha e garantindo que essas forças sejam empurradas para cima na parte inferior da perna. Da mesma maneira, as estruturas do pé também devem ser sólidas o suficiente para transferir as forças de propulsão dos músculos sóleo e gastrocnêmio para o solo, auxiliando no movimento efetivo até a fase de impulso da marcha para que a transferência de força máxima seja alcançada.

No entanto, muitos jogadores de futebol profissionais não têm uma mecânica de pé "ideal" por vários motivos, que vão desde a predisposição genética até uma lesão anterior e/ou cirurgia. Os autores acreditam que essa falta de função adequada do pé causa um aumento da carga do sóleo e do gastrocnêmio e que, se permitida a ocorrência repetidamente sem correção, pode levar à sobrecarga desses músculos a ponto de falhar; a ruptura desses músculos é um resultado possível.

Uma solução para a mecânica deficiente do pé é a prescrição de aparelhos ortopédicos feitos sob medida para o jogador individual e são consideravelmente mais do que apenas uma "palmilha". A órtese oferece suporte proprioceptivo e estrutural para as estruturas do pé em falha na tentativa de otimizar o seu funcionamento. Pode incluir uma elevação do calcanhar, cunha do pé traseiro ou corte do primeiro metatarso falangeano (MTF), todos com o objetivo de melhorar o papel que o pé desempenha durante a marcha e efetivamente alivia a força excessiva aplicada por meio dos músculos da panturrilha que pode levar à falha muscular.

Uma vez prescritas, as órteses são colocadas nos calçados dos jogadores para garantir uniformidade na função do pé em todos os momentos – não apenas durante o treinamento ou partidas. O desafio é encontrar um podólogo que possa fazer diferentes tipos de órteses para os calçados de treino e, especialmente, as chuteiras de um jogador. Quase sempre os jogadores usam suas chuteiras muito justas (possivelmente até meio número menor), não deixando espaço para a inserção de um dispositivo corretivo; portanto, esses jogadores simplesmente não usarão esses dispositivos em suas chuteiras e não se beneficiarão de sua correção durante os momentos-chave. Alguns jogadores têm a oportunidade de trabalhar com o fabricante da chuteira e ter um dispositivo ortótico incorporado ao design da chuteira, eliminando os problemas descritos anteriormente (Boxe 19.2).

> **Boxe 19.2 Estudo de caso 1**
>
> Um jogador de futebol profissional de 34 anos tinha um histórico de rupturas recorrentes na panturrilha, tanto no sóleo quanto no gastrocnêmico, durante um período de 12 meses e uma incapacidade de correr qualquer distância sem uma dor do tipo cãibra nas panturrilhas. Este jogador tinha boa mobilidade da panturrilha e tornozelo e foi tratado com várias técnicas de tecidos moles, uma máquina Compex para estimular a contração muscular e fluxo sanguíneo e um programa de força na academia para aumentar a força muscular isométrica, concêntrica e excêntrica. Apesar de tudo isso, ele ainda apresentava rupturas nos músculos da panturrilha. Este jogador foi enviado para avaliação de um podólogo que examinou sua função do pé e sentiu que um dispositivo ortótico era necessário, incluindo uma elevação do calcanhar para reduzir o alongamento por meio do complexo da panturrilha durante o ciclo da marcha. Após 1 semana de uso da órtese, os sintomas da panturrilha do jogador diminuíram completamente, permitindo que ele corresse sem restrições. Até o momento, ele não sofreu mais rupturas nos músculos da panturrilha.

Muitos médicos consideram que, se um jogador nasce com um tipo de pé que pode ser considerado "defeituoso" e sempre andou e correu com ele, então a sugestão de que essa seja a causa de qualquer laceração no sóleo ou no gastrocnêmico é sem fundamento, já que o jogador teve uma vida inteira para condicionar os membros inferiores ao desempenho de seus pés. Embora seja importante considerar, "se não está quebrado, não conserte", uma vez que ocorre uma laceração no sóleo ou no gastrocnêmico causada por forças internas, ou seja, não um golpe direto de outro jogador, mas por sobrecarga repetida, então a mecânica do pé é uma área que vale a pena avaliar como parte do processo de reabilitação.

Causas menos consideradas

Hidratação e seus efeitos na elasticidade muscular

Existem muitas pesquisas (Baker et al., 2014; Nuccio et al., 2017) sobre os efeitos da desidratação no desempenho esportivo – especificamente, os efeitos da hidratação inadequada antes, durante e após o exercício. É claro que o desempenho esportivo é drasticamente prejudicado tanto cognitiva quanto fisiologicamente por um atleta estar desidratado durante uma competição. Um estudo de Cleary et al. (2005) examinou a questão da dor muscular de início tardio (DMIT) e hidratação. Os pesquisadores descobriram que os atletas que foram desidratados durante o exercício sofreram um aumento na DMIT pós-exercício quando comparados ao grupo controle hidratado.

Embora a DMIT não seja considerada uma ruptura no(s) músculo(s), é um tipo de lesão muscular. Se, como foi demonstrado, a hidratação desempenha um papel muito importante na prevenção de DMIT durante o exercício, postula-se que a falta de elasticidade em um tecido causada pela desidratação pode aumentar a probabilidade de que o tecido possa falhar completamente, ou seja, sofra uma lesão ou ruptura. No entanto, atualmente existem poucas pesquisas que examinam a relação da desidratação e o seu papel nas rupturas musculares, como as dos músculos sóleo e gastrocnêmio.

É a opinião considerada dos autores a partir de suas próprias experiências clínicas que a desidratação e as rupturas musculares estão intimamente relacionadas em alguns jogadores de futebol profissionais. Embora todos os clubes de futebol profissional entendam a necessidade de um protocolo de hidratação para seus jogadores durante o treinamento e o jogo, ele é invariavelmente implementado por seu efeito no desempenho geral e não especificamente para a prevenção de lesões. Esses protocolos de hidratação muitas vezes serão do tipo "um protocolo serve para todos", e espera-se que todos os jogadores sigam isso com resultados iguais. Isso contrasta com uma maior individualização de outras áreas dos regimes de treinamento dos jogadores. Não se espera que os jogadores sigam o mesmo programa de treinamento de força na academia, pois é bem conhecido que cada um precisa de um programa que reflita as próprias necessidades. Os autores questionam por que essa mesma abordagem não está sendo adotada com a questão da hidratação.

Um dos clubes atuais dos autores instituiu recentemente uma política de criação de perfis de suor, em que cada jogador é submetido a um teste de suor para avaliar não apenas a quantidade total de fluido perdido durante o exercício, mas também o equilíbrio eletrolítico de sua transpiração. O que fica aparente ao testar uma equipe de 25 jogadores de futebol profissional da equipe principal é que pelo menos 5 dessa equipe são considerados "transpiradores elevados", o que significa que para cada mililitro de suor perdido, esses jogadores também estão perdendo uma quantidade maior do que o normal de eletrólitos como parte dessa perda de suor.

Se esse déficit de eletrólitos não for reposto corretamente, esses jogadores correm o risco de sentir os efeitos prejudiciais do desequilíbrio eletrolítico, apesar de repor o volume total de fluido perdido. Na opinião dos autores, o desequilíbrio eletrolítico, mais do que qualquer perda total de fluido, torna os músculos mais propensos a danos, aumentando o risco de rupturas musculares devido à elasticidade muscular reduzida e ao aumento da fadiga. Eletrólitos como sódio e cálcio são essenciais para a contração muscular. Portanto, qualquer déficit ou desequilíbrio significa que a função muscular está abaixo do ideal e o tecido pode não suportar os rigores do exercício (Boxe 19.3).

Manejo deficiente da carga de treinamento

Manejo de carga (ver *Conceito de estresse/tensão*, anteriormente), ou seja, monitoramento da quantidade de trabalho atribuída a um jogador e equipe em uma base diária e semanal para otimizar o treinamento e garantir que os jogadores estejam na melhor forma física possível no dia da partida, tornou-se o "Santo Graal" da ciência do esporte nos últimos anos.

Isso tem muito a ver com o trabalho do Dr. Tim Gabbett e sua pesquisa relacionada com a carga aguda/crônica (Gabbett, 2016). Gabbett postulou que se os atletas são expostos a picos agudos em excesso de carga durante o treinamento ou uma partida, então eles estão em maior risco de lesão (p. ex., rupturas musculares) do que aqueles que mantêm um alto volume de carga consistente, já que o último grupo é muito mais preparado para as demandas de uma sessão de exercícios intensos, por exemplo, durante uma partida.

No entanto, o conceito de carga de Gabbett se relaciona com todo o esforço colocado no corpo de um atleta durante o treinamento e as partidas e o esforço percebido que cada atleta sente que foi exposto. No entanto, para o propósito deste capítulo, os autores utilizam o conceito de manejo de carga especificamente como a quantidade de força (carga) aplicada aos músculos sóleo e gastrocnêmico durante o treinamento de resistência e sua capacidade de produzir as forças isométrica, concêntrica, excêntrica desejadas e aumentos de potência necessários para um desempenho no mais alto nível do futebol profissional de forma repetida e sem falhas, ou seja, sem lesões.

Reabilitação

Sala de tratamento para academia

A triagem da linha de base torna-se importante ao avaliar como um jogador está melhorando após qualquer tipo de lesão. Alguns exemplos de medidas de resultados comumente usados na prática clínica durante o monitoramento de lesões na panturrilha são fornecidos a seguir.

Teste do joelho à parede/teste de afundo com suporte de peso

O JAP é utilizado para avaliar os déficits da amplitude de movimento da dorsiflexão do tornozelo (ver Figura 19.2). Alcançar 8 cm parece ótimo entre os jogadores de futebol, com qualquer restrição significativa associada a alterações na cinemática do joelho e do tornozelo. Isso pode levar a padrões de movimento de alto risco comumente associados a lesões sem contato.

> **Boxe 19.3 Estudo de caso 2**
>
> Um jogador de futebol profissional de 27 anos que joga em nível internacional tinha histórico de rupturas intermitentes do músculo sóleo e episódios regulares de cãibras bilaterais nas panturrilhas nos últimos 30 minutos do jogo. Ele foi examinado por um podólogo para avaliação da função do pé e usava órteses. Ele se submeteu a um programa de força na academia para aumentar a força da panturrilha até ser capaz de levantar múltiplos do peso corporal durante a elevação do calcanhar e tinha boa mobilidade da articulação do tornozelo e dos músculos da panturrilha. Ele também era muito cuidadoso em seguir os protocolos de reidratação do clube pós-treino e para jogos. Mesmo assim, ele sofria de rupturas de sóleo.
>
> Esse jogador foi submetido a um teste de suor no início da temporada (ver seção *Hidratação e os seus efeitos na elasticidade muscular*) e está entre os cinco jogadores considerados "transpiradores elevados", tanto em termos de volume de suor perdido quanto de conteúdo de eletrólitos. Ele começou com uma bebida de reidratação específica que fornecia a reposição correta de eletrólitos; dentro de 1 semana, ele relatou ter percebido que as cãibras na panturrilha haviam desaparecido durante o treinamento e no final dos jogos. Ele relatou sentir-se muito mais revigorado no dia seguinte após o jogo, com dor muscular mínima de início tardio. Até o momento, ele não sofreu outra ruptura do sóleo.

Powden et al. (2015) descreveu o JAP como o teste de afundo com suporte de peso (TASP). Eles demonstraram confiabilidade intra e intertestes consistentes na medição da dorsiflexão do tornozelo, embora geralmente utilizando uma população saudável. No entanto, esses resultados são facilmente traduzíveis para a população esportiva. Aplicativos do iPhone® para medir a dorsiflexão do tornozelo estão surgindo e um deles foi estudado por Balsalobre-Fernandez et al. (2018). Embora esses pesquisadores concluam que o aplicativo avalia a dorsiflexão do tornozelo de modo fácil, preciso e confiável, amostras pequenas tornam suas descobertas pouco confiáveis.

Embora não haja literatura ligando JAP/TASP insatisfatório e lesões na panturrilha, medidas imediatas após a lesão e ao longo do processo de reabilitação podem indicar progresso. Para começar a corrida ao ar livre, esperaríamos que o atleta tivesse retornado à sua medição basal e tivesse uma assimetria < 2 cm, além de considerar outros marcadores discutidos posteriormente neste capítulo.

Teste de capacidade de trabalho muscular/resistência da panturrilha

Um teste de capacidade de trabalho muscular (CTP)/resistência da panturrilha pode ser usado para avaliar a capacidade funcional da musculatura tríceps sural. Usar uma fase concêntrica e excêntrica de 2 segundos parece obter os resultados mais precisos, com base na experiência pessoal dos autores. No ambiente aplicado, esse teste requer um exame cuidadoso para garantir que nenhuma compensação ocorra para obter pontuações falsas. A incapacidade de completar totalmente a fase concêntrica/excêntrica e/ou inversão/eversão excessiva indicaria a interrupção do teste.

Para participar de sessões de corrida ao ar livre, o atleta deve ser capaz de completar > 25 repetições com pontuação superior a 90% no índice de simetria do membro. Esse tipo de teste é vantajoso por ser realizado na posição de sustentação de peso, o que o torna, indiscutivelmente, uma medida de desfecho mais relevante do que a dinamometria isocinética. É frequentemente usado para triagem inicial, concluída na pré-temporada, para

Parte | 2 | Aplicação Clínica

garantir que o atleta esteja trabalhando em suas capacidades físicas ideais e possa retornar ao jogo/competição com segurança. Pode destacar os atletas que estão em maior risco, exibindo assimetrias ou pontuações baixas que podem aumentar o risco de sofrer uma lesão na panturrilha. Embora déficits de resistência da panturrilha tenham sido observados após o reparo do tendão de Aquiles (Bostick et al., 2010), mais pesquisas são necessárias para identificar melhor os atletas na população esportiva com maior risco de desenvolver uma lesão na panturrilha.

Dinamometria portátil

A dinamometria portátil (DMP) pode ser útil na medição da contração isométrica voluntária máxima (CIVM). No entanto, a base de evidências atual indica que existem alguns problemas de confiabilidade. Clarke et al. (2011) demonstraram confiabilidade intra-avaliador de moderada a excelente em contraste com confiabilidade entre avaliadores relativamente baixa a moderada usando o dispositivo MicroFET3®. Na experiência pessoal dos autores, essas medidas podem ser usadas periodicamente ao longo do processo de reabilitação para indicar progresso e assimetrias da direita para a esquerda. Ao alterar o ângulo do joelho, os profissionais da saúde são capazes de argumentar que podem isolar o sóleo em comparação com um posicionamento do joelho reto enviesando o gastrocnêmico. Isso claramente requer mais estudos longitudinais em atletas profissionais para padronizar os procedimentos de teste. Apesar disso, o MicroFET3® tem sido útil na identificação de déficits de força e assimetrias na reabilitação de lesões de longa duração.

Junto com os testes de capacidade, a DMP pode começar a criar um perfil de atleta, identificando sua força e necessidades de condicionamento. Ao coletar esses dados, a relação peso corporal:força também pode ser desenvolvida, e assimetrias entre os membros, calculadas. Não é razoável esperar que um atleta de 70 kg produza a mesma CIVM que um atleta de 90 kg. Isso pode ser proporcional usando categorias de peso. Ainda não foi estabelecido se as pontuações de DMP se correlacionam com as pontuações de MWC.

Protocolo AlterG

A esteira AlterG é um novo equipamento utilizado na maioria dos ambientes esportivos de alto desempenho. Ela usa tecnologia de pressão de ar diferencial para permitir que os atletas carreguem até 30% de seu peso corporal (PC), permitindo um retorno mais rápido à função normal, o que pode reduzir os tempos de recuperação.

Quando um atleta consegue tolerar as sustentações isométricas com um joelho reto e dobrado a 30% do seu PC na academia, começamos o protocolo AlterG de retorno ao protocolo de corrida ao ar livre. Para uma lesão na panturrilha de grau 1, 4 sessões podem ser adequadas. Em comparação, uma lesão de grau 2 pode exigir de 6 a 8 sessões progressivas. Quando um jogador pode tolerar 85 a 90% do PC por 4 × 4 minutos a 16 km/h, é considerado apropriado começar sessões em campo conduzidas por fisioterapia. Recentemente, foi demonstrado que a velocidade de corrida afeta amplamente as forças plantares criadas no AlterG (Thomson et al., 2017). Isso permite uma progressão objetiva do carregamento plantar durante a reabilitação. Por exemplo, correr a 16 km/h a 80% do PC produz 2,11 múltiplos de peso corporal. Isso permite que os treinadores de força e condicionamento planejem seu programa de força de acordo e nos ajuda a entender quanta carga o atleta pode tolerar com segurança.

O AlterG tem como objetivo aumentar a carga de trabalho crônica para preparar o atleta para o condicionamento em campo. Além de correr, o treinamento pliométrico pode ser iniciado usando uma variação de salto "pogo", contramovimento e pouso.

Um atleta muitas vezes descreverá um efeito de "pneu furado" ao correr pela primeira vez ao ar livre. O AlterG nos permite condicionar o complexo tríceps-sural e melhorar a rigidez do tornozelo. Por experiência, os atletas muitas vezes se queixam de rigidez na panturrilha durante os estágios iniciais da reabilitação ao ar livre. Ao aumentar as capacidades de trabalho muscular do gastrocnêmio e do sóleo para tolerar essas cargas, podemos erradicar esses problemas e criar um processo de reabilitação mais fluente.

O que e quem estamos reabilitando?

Existem diferentes tipos de fibras musculares no gastrocnêmio e no sóleo, afetando suas funções na locomoção. Estudos em humanos indicam que o sóleo consiste em uma porcentagem maior de fibras oxidativas de contração lenta (tipo I) em comparação com as fibras de contração rápida (tipo II) (70:30%). Os achados também revelam que o número de fibras do tipo II é muito maior no gastrocnêmio em comparação ao sóleo, sem diferença entre a cabeça medial ou lateral. Como isso afeta o modo como reabilitamos?

As lesões do sóleo requerem maior treinamento de resistência e são predominantemente responsáveis pela locomoção até cerca de 18 km/h ou 5 m/s. O gastrocnêmio é mais explosivo, exigindo treinamento de potência/força para ser capaz de sustentar esforços repetidos de *sprint* a > 18 km/h e poderosa extensão tripla da cadeia posterior.

O músculo sóleo gera maior força isométrica e dinâmica durante a corrida (Blazkiewicz et al., 2017) em comparação com o gastrocnêmio. Ele funciona excentricamente durante a postura intermediária para controlar o centro de gravidade do corpo; argumenta-se que, ao melhorar a eficiência de absorção de força do sóleo, a economia de funcionamento pode ser melhorada. O sóleo normalmente absorve 6 a 8 × o PC durante a corrida e produz o pico de força mais alto em comparação com outros músculos dos membros inferiores. O treinamento de força pesada deve começar assim que puder ser tolerado.

A reabilitação é um processo complexo no qual muitas variáveis, intrínsecas e extrínsecas, precisam ser consideradas. Tomemos, por exemplo, um zagueiro central comparado a um jogador atacante lateral. Como seus jogos diferem?

Um zagueiro central de 1,98 m que vence predominantemente os cabeceios opera em linhas retas em comparação com um ala habilidoso que precisa ser capaz de mudar de direção em alta velocidade e fazer jogadas explosivas repetidamente. Mas como sabemos o que é "normal"?

Os sistemas de posicionamento global (GPS, do inglês *global positioning systems*) são usados regularmente e estão disponíveis no esporte de elite. Eles permitem que a equipe de saúde esportiva veja a distância total percorrida, metros de alta intensidade > 19 km/h e número de *sprints* > 25 km/h. Essas informações podem ser usadas de várias maneiras, por exemplo, ao considerar a necessidade de treinamento extra, para diminuir gradualmente a carga e para identificar atletas em risco de supertreinamento ou *overreaching*.

A transição de um atleta da academia para a reabilitação em campo deve levar em consideração uma série de fatores:

- O atleta obteve amplitude de movimento completa?
- O atleta tem pontuações de pico de potência > 90%, sem assimetrias?

Manejo de Ruptura dos Músculos Gastrocnêmico e Sóleo em Jogadores de Futebol Profissional

- Ele é capaz de realizar uma elevação e salto unilateral do calcanhar, continuamente e sem dor, em posições retas/flexionadas dos joelhos?
- O atleta pode absorver carga, produzir força e completar os desafios pliométricos?

Se a resposta for "sim" a todas as perguntas anteriores, podemos raciocinar clinicamente que esse atleta está pronto para aumentar suas demandas físicas.

As sessões conduzidas por fisioterapia precisam cobrir todos os ângulos para garantir uma transferência segura para a equipe de ciências do esporte/reabilitação. Neste ponto, o atleta deve ser capaz de completar corrida de alta velocidade até 80% da velocidade máxima, mudança de direção no ritmo, esforços pliométricos específicos da posição e exercícios técnicos/com bola baseados em sua posição. Uma lesão de baixo grau/grau 1 pode exigir 2 a 3 sessões, enquanto uma lesão de grau 2 ou superior pode precisar de cuidado extra e 4 a 6 sessões.

O condicionamento intensivo e extensivo é o foco dos preparadores físicos de reabilitação nesta fase. O sóleo é responsável por ~80% da carga em níveis de velocidade mais baixos; portanto, o foco é menos na explosão, mas mais na robustez do sóleo e sua capacidade de tolerar cargas de trabalho crônicas. Em contraste, testes de velocidade repetidos e reativos precisam ser cobertos após uma lesão do gastrocnêmico. Um exemplo disso poderia ser *sprints* de 6 × 50 m trabalhando na proporção trabalho:descanso de 1:1. Isso pode progredir para um cenário reativo específico de posição, incluindo uma situação 1 contra 1 com a bola. Isso remove o elemento de previsibilidade e exige que o atleta responda a padrões de movimento aleatórios.

Existem outros fatores que precisamos considerar? Lesão recorrente? Mecanismo de lesão? O aspecto psicológico da reabilitação sempre merece consideração. Ocorreram adaptações inadequadas no tríceps sural, resultando em inibição neuromuscular? Podemos recriar o mecanismo para inspirar confiança, para prevenir quaisquer estratégias de evitar o medo no estilo de corrida ou padrão de movimento?

Por ser uma equipe multiprofissional, é importante discutir esses fatores e envolver o atleta no processo de tomada de decisão. Isso pode melhorar a conformidade e permite que o atleta aceite seu processo de pensamento e planejamento. Isso deve levar a uma rotina pré e pós-treinamento e ajudar a reduzir o risco de recorrência. Como na maioria dos ambientes de elite, o tempo gasto fora do centro de treinamento supera o tempo gasto dentro, destacando a importância da educação sobre preparação física, regeneração e recuperação.

Reabilitação em ginásio para o retorno ao jogo

Não existe um único fator que determina o RAJ após uma lesão muscular (Benito et al., 2014; Ekstrand et al., 2012). No entanto, o aumento da força muscular local e global e das capacidades de potência são fatores determinantes para um RAJ bem-sucedido. Particularmente em relação à panturrilha (gastrocnêmico e sóleo), muitos programas de retorno ao treinamento (RAT) ou RAJ frequentemente negligenciam as funções-chave determinantes do músculo individual e falham em fornecer estímulo suficiente para adaptação.

Durante a corrida, o complexo da panturrilha e do tornozelo absorvem e produzem forças de 5 a 13 × PC (Burdett, 2012). Sem carga progressiva suficiente, o atleta que retorna corre o risco de sofrer nova lesão não apenas na panturrilha, mas também potencialmente no tendão de Aquiles.

Muitos programas de reabilitação ignoram o fato de que a musculatura da panturrilha responde a cargas pesadas, e eles geralmente prescrevem exercícios ou alongamento somente com o PC. O perigo dessa abordagem de PC e baixa carga é que ela não prepara o atleta de modo suficiente e eficaz para as demandas dos próximos exercícios pliométricos baseados na academia e, mais importante, para o protocolo de retorno à corrida em campo.

Apesar do equívoco comum de que o gastrocnêmico é o principal produtor de força durante a corrida, pesquisas mostram que ele é, de fato, o sóleo, que produz até 50% da força vertical total (Albracht et al., 2008). O sóleo tem a maior capacidade de produção de força devido à sua grande área transversal fisiológica. O sóleo pode produzir forças reais em torno de 8 × PC em comparação ao gastrocnêmico, produzindo 3 × PC (Albracht et al., 2008). O fato de que o sóleo é um grande contribuidor de força leva à noção de que um treinamento pesado de resistência é necessário para treinar adequadamente a musculatura da panturrilha.

Juntamente com o treinamento de resistência pesada, os programas de RAJ também devem ter como objetivo incorporar exercícios pliométricos. Estes devem seguir um programa pliométrico progressivo e controlado prestando atenção aos exercícios de absorção de força (p. ex., aterrissagens de queda), exercícios de produção de força (p. ex., saltos) e saltos reativos contínuos (p. ex., pogos, pular corda ou saltos com rebote). Os exercícios pliométricos, especialmente os saltos reativos contínuos, só devem ser realizados quando o atleta que está retornando tiver completado o programa de força desejado e reduzido quaisquer inadequações e desequilíbrios de força.

Na opinião dos autores, durante a reabilitação e uma vez que o atleta comece a recuperar a amplitude total de movimento, um RAJ progressivo lógico deve seguir três etapas, embora haja sobreposição e continuidade entre esses estágios: (1) restaurar a força muscular concêntrica, (2) restaurar a força muscular excêntrica e (3) restaurar as capacidades de alta velocidade e potência. Cada estágio requer uma progressão de apenas PC para cargas externas mais altas, carga bilateral para unilateral, aumento no volume total e aumento na velocidade.

Como um atleta progride através desses estágios dependerá de uma série de fatores, como gravidade da lesão, força pré-lesão, lesão anterior, idade/exposição do treinamento anterior e tolerância sem dor.

Como carregar

Como mencionado anteriormente, para reabilitar adequadamente um músculo lesionado, é necessária uma carga progressiva. As diretrizes tradicionais para o treinamento de força sugerem usar uma carga de > 85% 1 repetição máxima (1RM), 4 a 6 repetições, 4 a 6 séries, com períodos de recuperação de 3 a 5 min (Fleck e Kraemer, 2003). Na opinião e experiência dos autores, isso é apenas parte do caminho para ajudar a aumentar a força muscular e o RAJ bem-sucedido. Devido ao envolvimento da panturrilha em quase todos os movimentos no campo de futebol (corrida, salto etc.), a panturrilha não só precisa de força máxima, como também de força, *endurance* e treinamento de taxa de desenvolvimento de força (TDF) para ajudar a prevenir o risco de lesões. Portanto, o treinamento de maior repetição, por exemplo, 10 a 15 repetições, ou volume aumentado, 8 a 12 séries, pode também ser necessário para ganhos de força adequados, bem como movimentos mais rápidos e poderosos para a TDF.

Considerando o aumento na pesquisa sobre a prevenção de lesões e os benefícios de desempenho de exercícios excêntricos e isométricos, especialmente nos isquiotibiais, seria negligência de qualquer treinador de força e condicionamento físico ou fisioterapeuta ignorar esses tipos de exercícios ao fortalecer ou reabilitar uma lesão relacionada à panturrilha.

Os exercícios excêntricos visam fortalecer o músculo quando ele está no seu comprimento mais fraco e longo. Nessas posições finais, os músculos geralmente correm o maior risco de rompimento. Estratégias excêntricas para enfatizar a geração de força e o controle do movimento podem ser importantes na normalização da função e força musculares, bem como no comportamento do movimento relacionado com lesões. O fortalecimento do músculo nesses movimentos excêntricos também ajuda a preparar o atleta para os próximos exercícios pliométricos e especialmente para os exercícios de aterrissagem. A pesquisa mostra que os exercícios excêntricos são superiores a outras formas de reabilitação ao lidar com lesões do tendão de Aquiles e, por associação, ajuda com o RAJ após lesões na panturrilha (Allison, 2009).

O treinamento isométrico é um método de treinamento que existe há muito tempo, mas ainda não é praticado por muitos. Assim como o treinamento excêntrico, a pesquisa sobre o treinamento isométrico geralmente se concentra no treinamento dos isquiotibiais (Van Hooren e Bosch, 2018). No entanto, a pesquisa mostrou grandes benefícios para a carga isométrica na tendinopatia de Aquiles (Cook, 2009) e evidências pessoais apoiam seu uso no treinamento da musculatura da panturrilha para melhorar o desempenho de *sprint*. O treinamento isométrico é essencialmente manter a tensão muscular em uma posição específica por um período de tempo desejado, com a contração máxima do músculo sendo treinado de modo ideal.

O sucesso da isometria é baseado na noção de tempo sob tensão (TST) e serve para melhorar a eficiência neural, ativação muscular, interação agonista e antagonista, bem como disparos musculares de alta frequência e, portanto, a TDF. Os dois tipos principais de treinamento isométrico são frequentemente chamados de sustentações isométricas e *push/pull* isométrico. As contenções isométricas referem-se a suportar ou sustentar a massa corporal e uma carga externa em uma posição estática por um determinado período de tempo (6 a 40 segundos).

Push/pull isométrico refere-se à aplicação de forças de empurrar/puxar muito altas contra um objeto imóvel, por exemplo, frequentemente visto em um teste de "levantamento" de peso em um aparelho isométrico a partir do meio da coxa. A intenção é aplicar força rapidamente até o máximo individual por um curto período de tempo (4 a 6 segundos) antes de descansar.

Embora um atleta deva ser excentricamente forte para obter o máximo do treinamento isométrico, a carga isométrica pode ser de grande benefício para atletas lesionados devido à amplitude limitada de movimento necessária e à falta de dor muscular residual (ou DMIT) gerada, que potencialmente agravaria o tecido já lesionado. Na opinião dos autores, portanto, o carregamento precoce sensível por meio de isometria pode servir bem ao atleta lesionado.

Uma vez que a força, a resistência muscular e a taxa de disparo atingem o nível desejado, a reabilitação da panturrilha deve se concentrar no retorno aos exercícios de alta velocidade, potência e TDF, ou seja, exercícios pliométricos. A iniciação de exercícios pliométricos deve seguir um programa controlado e progressivo, prestando atenção aos exercícios de absorção de força (p. ex., aterrissagens), exercícios de produção de força (p. ex., saltos) e saltos reativos contínuos (p. ex., pogos, pular corda ou salto com rebote).

Os exercícios de absorção de força são uma progressão funcional lógica dos exercícios excêntricos, pois fornecem uma sobrecarga de força excêntrica devido à ação da gravidade sobre o corpo. Antes que um atleta possa produzir força em velocidade (potência), é essencial que ele seja capaz de absorver com segurança sua força máxima de frenagem. Patamares lineares e laterais de alturas de caixa progressivas são um ponto de partida fundamental.

Está além do escopo desse capítulo fornecer uma revisão detalhada do ciclo de alongamento-encurtamento (CAE; ver Capítulos 1 e 4), mas a sua importância para o fortalecimento, a prevenção e a reabilitação de uma lesão na panturrilha é muito grande. A panturrilha e o tornozelo encontram forças enormes, as quais são reaplicadas com velocidade durante a corrida. Assegurar que um atleta possa realizar o salto duplo e único com uma perna do chão para uma caixa de altura pequena a média (15 a 45 cm) em um movimento de salto de agachamento e contramovimento é um teste essencial para um atleta que retorna de uma ruptura muscular da panturrilha.

O estágio final de um programa pliométrico bem-sucedido são os saltos reativos/contínuos, como pular corda ou pogo e, finalmente, *drop jumps* reativos. Esses exercícios combinam as funções de todos os anteriores, utilizando a força excêntrica e a produção de força concêntrica sob grande carga e velocidade. De acordo com os autores, são esses exercícios que ajudam o atleta que retorna a perder a sensação de "pneu furado", frequentemente associada a lesões na panturrilha e no tornozelo.

Elevação da panturrilha, exercícios isométricos e excêntricos são comumente realizados em duas posições de joelho em vários ângulos de flexão do joelho, em uma tentativa de isolar e direcionar ambos os músculos da panturrilha. Isso muitas vezes se origina do regime de treinamento original de Alfredson (Alfredson et al., 1998). Embora vários pesquisadores tenham relatado a inibição do gastrocnêmico com o aumento dos ângulos de flexão do joelho, há relatos limitados de alterações na atividade do sóleo pela polarização de certos ângulos do joelho (Reid et al., 2012). Essencialmente, o sóleo funciona igualmente (medido como uma porcentagem de sua contração voluntária máxima) na flexão ou na extensão do joelho. Reid et al. (2012) concluíram que parecia não haver benefício em usar a reabilitação excêntrica do joelho flexionado, já que o sóleo trabalhou igualmente durante a reabilitação estendida do joelho. No entanto, Price et al. (2003) relataram que o músculo gastrocnêmico medial parecia consideravelmente mais ativo durante o teste de posição de joelho totalmente estendido, enquanto a atividade do músculo sóleo foi significativamente menor. No entanto, a atividade do músculo sóleo pareceu maior durante a condição de joelho flexionado (90°) em comparação com o gastrocnêmio.

Embora não esteja claro se a atividade do sóleo aumenta com uma grande flexão do joelho, há uma sugestão de que a dominância do gastrocnêmico diminui com esses ângulos maiores de flexão do joelho, sugerindo uma justificativa para a utilização de uma variedade de ângulos de flexão do joelho para tratar lesões específicas da panturrilha.

Em última análise, é uma combinação desses fatores de treinamento de força, trabalhando todo o espectro de faixas de força, a curva de força-velocidade, o ângulo de flexão do joelho e uma manipulação da programação de RAJ que fornecerá a maior chance de um RAJ bem-sucedido (Figuras 19.3 a 19.8).

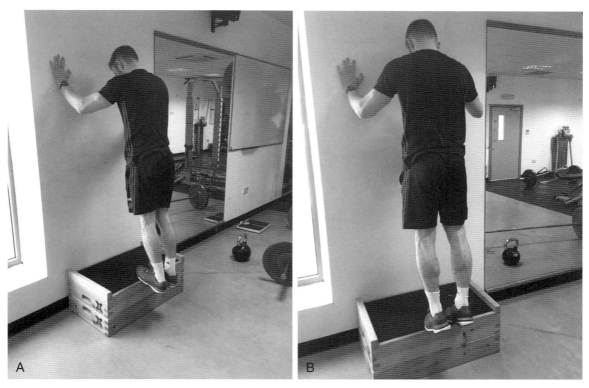

Figura 19.3 Levantamento da panturrilha de perna dupla com peso corporal (foco no gastrocnêmico). Carregue com halteres, barra ou máquina *Smith*. **A.** Início do movimento. **B.** Fim do movimento.

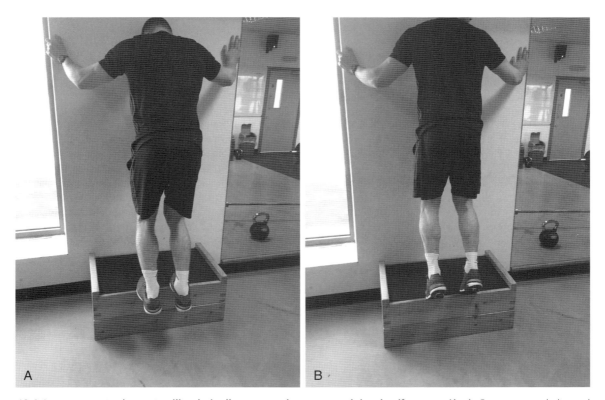

Figura 19.4 Levantamento da panturrilha do joelho com as duas pernas dobradas (foco no sóleo). Carregue com halteres, barra ou máquina *Smith*. **A.** Início do movimento. **B.** Fim do movimento.

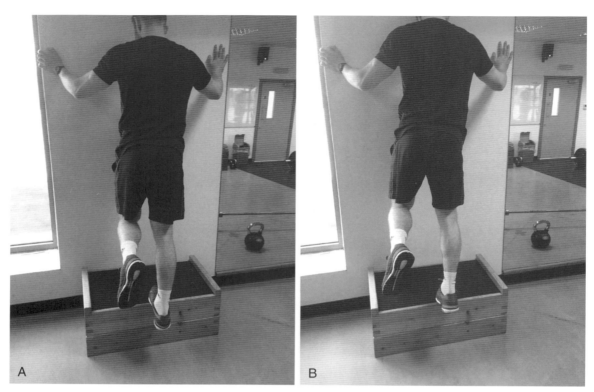

Figura 19.5 **Levantamento da panturrilha com peso corporal em uma perna (foco no gastrocnêmico).** Carregue com halteres, barra ou máquina *Smith*. **A.** Início do movimento. **B.** Fim do movimento.

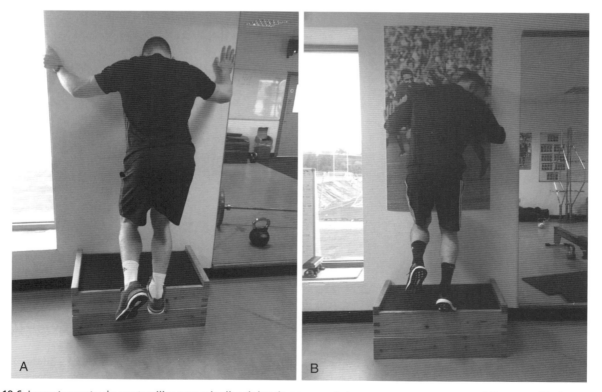

Figura 19.6 **Levantamento da panturrilha com o joelho dobrado em uma única perna com peso corporal (foco no sóleo).** Carregue com halteres, barra ou máquina *Smith*. **A.** Início do movimento. **B.** Fim do movimento.

Manejo de Ruptura dos Músculos Gastrocnêmico e Sóleo em Jogadores de Futebol Profissional | Capítulo | 19 |

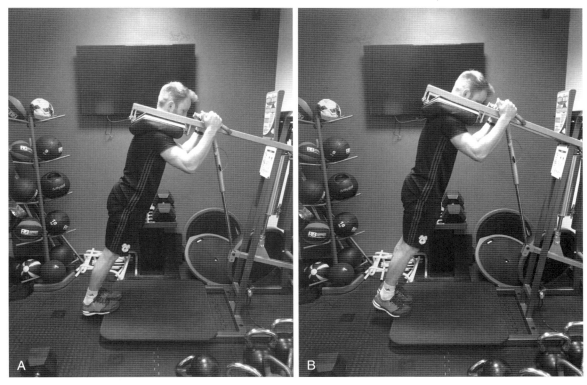

Figura 19.7 Apoios isométricos de perna dupla (usando a máquina Keizer, mas a barra ou a máquina *Smith* também são opções). **A.** Início do movimento. **B.** Fim do movimento.

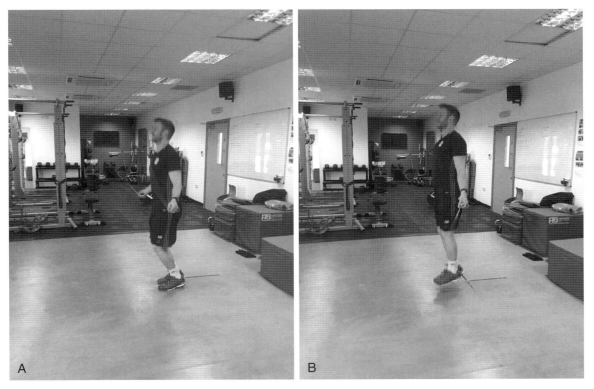

Figura 19.8 Salto (taxa de desenvolvimento de força, pliométrica). **A.** Início do movimento. **B.** Fim do movimento.

Sinais de alerta

Ao considerar as condições dos membros inferiores, é importante descartar patologias graves que, embora raras, podem existir na população esportiva. Portanto, é necessário garantir que os sinais de alerta sejam descartados com base no histórico subjetivo e no exame objetivo.

Trombose venosa profunda

A trombose venosa profunda (TVP) é um coágulo sanguíneo que se desenvolve em uma veia profunda na parte inferior da perna e pode se manifestar como dor, inchaço e sensibilidade na panturrilha. Isso pode levar a complicações graves, como embolia pulmonar. Dor, calor e vermelhidão são outros sintomas que podem se apresentar neste cenário. As TVP podem ser vistas no pós-operatório de um atleta, durante os períodos de inatividade ou após trauma em um vaso sanguíneo. Em atletas do sexo feminino, alguns medicamentos anticoncepcionais podem fazer com que o sangue coagule com mais facilidade. As TVP geralmente são diagnosticadas por meio de uma ultrassonografia por um radiologista experiente; o tratamento consiste em medicamentos anticoagulantes como a varfarina. Embora uma TVP geralmente seja resultado de cirurgia, seja inatividade, é importante descartar essa patologia em pacientes que apresentam sintomas vagos de dor na panturrilha e nenhum mecanismo de lesão.

Tumor

Massas de tecidos moles, como um tumor (maligno ou benigno), podem ocorrer em atletas de elite. Frequentemente, têm início insidioso e podem estar associadas a nódulo palpável e edema. É importante ressaltar que os tumores podem imitar condições como um cisto de Baker ou sarcoma sinovial, destacando a importância da RM ou outros testes para confirmar o diagnóstico. É importante considerar o histórico familiar, bem como sintomas como mal-estar geral, perda de peso inexplicada e causas desconhecidas ao considerar tumores malignos.

Fraturas por estresse

As fraturas por estresse do membro inferior tendem a ocorrer dentro da tíbia. Os sintomas geralmente incluem dor no terço inferior da tíbia com inchaço localizado ocasional e sensibilidade no local da fratura. Os atletas podem estar predispostos à fratura por estresse após um período de inatividade ou correndo longas distâncias extraordinárias em comparação com suas cargas normais. A sensibilidade geralmente estará presente diretamente na palpação da tíbia e é importante na diferenciação entre a síndrome de estresse tibial medial. As radiografias iniciais podem não detectar uma fratura por estresse, sendo a RM o padrão-ouro. Edema da medula óssea evidente em uma RM pode indicar uma fratura por estresse. A tomografia computadorizada (TC) também pode ser utilizada, se necessário, e a cintilografia óssea é um exame complementar que pode auxiliar no diagnóstico.

Síndrome do encarceramento da artéria poplítea

A síndrome do encarceramento da artéria poplítea (SEAP) é uma patologia incomum em atletas. É uma doença vascular rara que pode afetar particularmente jovens atletas. Pode ser causada por um defeito de desenvolvimento na panturrilha ou no músculo poplíteo, ou ocorrer ao longo do tempo como resultado da hipertrofia do músculo tríceps sural comprimindo a artéria poplítea. Frequentemente, esses casos são bilaterais, com sintomas que incluem dor nos músculos da panturrilha, cãibras e dormência nos pés. As investigações incluem varredura de RM e teste de pressão do compartimento pós-exercício. É importante ressaltar que um exame por um especialista vascular experiente é necessário se houver suspeita de SEAP.

Resumo

O manejo de lesões e patologia na panturrilha têm sido negligenciados na literatura até o momento. No entanto, existem evidências empíricas emergentes indicando a importância do músculo sóleo e seu papel na locomoção.

Usando uma bateria de testes, podemos construir perfis de atletas que identificam se existem diferenças/déficits sutis na força do gastrocnêmio em relação à força do sóleo, bem como assimetrias de membros. Podemos utilizar essas informações para implementar programas de força e condicionamento para aumentar a robustez da musculatura do tríceps sural. É fundamental adaptar cada programa de reabilitação ao indivíduo, garantindo que eles atendam ou excedam seus marcadores de linha de base e continuem após a lesão. O desenvolvimento de resiliência isométrica, produção de força de extensão tripla concêntrica, controle excêntrico e rigidez ideal do tornozelo podem contribuir para as demandas gerais necessárias para competir em um esporte de contato multidirecional de ritmo acelerado como o futebol.

Resumindo, a abordagem dos autores para as rupturas dos músculos gastrocnêmio e sóleo é a seguinte:

- Uma avaliação simples, mas completa é necessária para diagnosticar uma ruptura do músculo da panturrilha, embora no futebol profissional muitas vezes se espere que alguma forma de imagem seja "necessária" para confirmar a hipótese diagnóstica
- A flexibilidade não é causa de rupturas musculares
- A falta de força e potência torna os músculos mais suscetíveis a falhas, mas melhorar esses elementos requer um bom *design* de programa e mais sobrecarga do que a maioria faria em uma academia
- A desidratação reduz as propriedades elásticas do músculo, tornando-o mais sujeito a falhas. Faça o perfil de seus jogadores individualmente para que planos de reposição individuais possam ser implementados
- As órteses ajudam na otimização da mecânica do pé e, portanto, promovem uma boa transferência de força para cima e para baixo na perna
- O manejo ideal da carga de treinamento é fundamental para reduzir o risco de lesão muscular, tornando o tecido mais robusto e aumentando suas propriedades elásticas. Muito pouco carregamento deixa o jogador com treino insuficiente e muito treino deixa o jogador fatigado; ambos os cenários aumentam a suscetibilidade de um jogador a rompimento muscular
- Sempre descarte possíveis "sinais de alerta" como parte do diagnóstico diferencial para rupturas do músculo da panturrilha.

Referências bibliográficas

Albracht, K., Arampatzis, A., Baltzopoulos, V., 2008. Assessment of muscle volume and physiological cross-sectional area of the human triceps surae muscle in vivo. Journal of Biomechanics 41 (10), 2211-2218.

Alfredson, H., Pietila, T., Jonsson, P., Lorentzon, R., 1998. Heavy-load eccentric calf muscle training for the treatment of chronic Achilles tendinosis. American Journal of Sports Medicine 26 (3), 360-366.

Allison, G.T., Purdam, C., 2009. Eccentric loading for Achilles tendinopathy strengthening or stretching? British Journal of Sports Medicine 43 (4), 276.

Baker, LB., Jeukendrup, AE., 2014. Optimal composition of fluid-replacement beverages. Comprehensive Physiology 4 (2), 575-620.

Balsalobre-Fernandez, C., Romero-Franco, N., Jimenez-Reyes, P., 2018. Concurrent validity and reliability of an iPhone app for the measurement of ankle dorsiflexion and inter-limb asymmetries. Journal of Sports Sciences 37 (3), 1-5.

Benito, L., Ayan, C., Revuelta, G., Maestro, A., Fernandez, T., Sanchez, M., 2014. Influence of the soccer players' professional status on the frequency and severity of injuries: a comparative pilot study [in Spanish]. Apunts Medicine Esport 49 (181), 20-24.

Blazkiewicz, M., Wiszomirska, I., Kaczmarczyk, K., Naemi, R., Wit, A., 2017. Inter-individual similarities and variations in muscle forces acting on the ankle joint during gait. Gait & Posture 58, 166-170.

Bostick, G.P., Jomha, N.M., Suchak, A.A., Beaupre, L.A., 2010. Factors associated with calf muscle endurance recovery 1 year after Achilles tendon rupture repair. Journal of Orthopaedic & Sports Physical Therapy 40, 345-351.

Brukner, P., Kahn, K., 2012. Brukner & Khan's Clinical Sports Medicine, fourth ed. McGraw Hill Australia, Sydney, pp. 761-775. Chapter 36.

Burdett, R., 1981. Forces predicted at the ankle during running. Medicine & Science in Sports & Exercise 14, 308-316.

Clarke, M., Nimhuircheartaigh, D., Walsh, G., Walsh, J., Meldrum, D., 2011. Intra-tester and inter-tester reliability of the MicroFET 3 hand-held dynamometer. Physiotherapy Practice and Research 32, 13-18.

Cleary, M.A., Sweeney, L.A., Kendrick, Z.V., Sitler, M.R., 2005. Dehydration and symptoms of delayed onset muscle soreness in hyperthermic males. Journal of Athletic Training 40 (4), 288-297.

Cook, J.L., Purdam, C.R., 2009. Is tendon pathology a continuum? A pathology model to explain the clinical presentation of load-induced tendinopathy. British Journal of Sports Medicine 43 (6), 409-416.

Cornwell, A., Nelson, A.G., Sidaway, B., 2002. Acute effects of stretching on the neuromechanical properties of the triceps surae muscle complex. European Journal of Applied Physiology 86, 428-434.

Dixon, J.B., 2009. Gastrocnemius vs. soleus strain: how to differentiate and deal with calf muscle injuries. Current Reviews in Musculoskeletal Medicine 2, 74-77.

Ekstrand, J., Healy, J.C., Walden, M., Lee, J.C., English, B., Hagglund, M., 2012. Hamstring muscle injuries in professional football: the correlation of MRI findings with return to play. British Journal of Sports Medicine 46, 112-117.

Ettema, G.J.C., 1996. Mechanical efficiency and efficiency of storage and release of series elastic energy in skeletal muscle during stretch-shortening cycles. The Journal of Experimental Biology 199, 1983–1997.

Fleck, S.J., Kraemer, W.J., 2003. Designing Resistance Training Programs, third ed. Human Kinetics, Champaign, Il.

Gabbett, T.J., 2016. The training–injury prevention paradox: should athletes be training smarter and harder? British Journal of Sports Medicine (50), 5.

Kubo, K., Kanehisa, H., Fukunaga, T., 2002. Effects of resistance and stretching training programmes on the viscoelastic properties of human tendon structures in vivo. The Journal of Physiology 538, 219-226.

Nuccio, R.P., Barnes, K.A., Carter, J.M., Baker, L.B., 2017. Fluid balance in team sport athletes and the effect of hydration on cognitive, technical and physical performance. Sports Medicine 47, 1951-1982.

Pedret, C., Rodas, G., Balius, R., 2015. Return to play after soleus muscle injuries. Orthopaedic Journal of Sports Medicine 3 (7), 2325967115595802.

Powden, C.J., Hoch, J.M., Hoch, M.C., 2015. Reliability and minimal detectable change of the weight-bearing lunge test: a systematic review. Manual Therapy 20, 524-532.

Price, T.B., Kamen, G., Damon, B.M., Knight, C.A., Applegate, B., Gore, J.C., et al., 2003. Comparison of MRI with EMG to study muscle activity associated with dynamic plantar flexion. Magnetic Resonance Imaging 21 (8), 853-861.

Reid, D., McNair, P.J., Johnson, S., Potts, G., Witvrouw, E., Mahieu, N., 2012. Electromyographic analysis of an eccentric calf muscle exercise in persons with and without Achilles tendinopathy. Physical Therapy in Sport 13 (3), 150-155.

Standring, S., 2015. In: Gray's Anatomy 41st Edition, The Anatomical Basis of Clinical Practice. Elsevier.

Thomson, A., Einarsson, E., Witvrouw, E., Whiteley, R., 2017. Running speed increases plantar load more than per cent body weight on an AlterG® treadmill. Journal of Sports Sciences 35, 277-282.

Van Hooren, B., Bosch, F., 2018. Preventing hamstring injuries – Part 2: There is possibly an isometric action of the hamstrings in high-speed running and it does matter. Sport Performance & Science Reports.

van Mechelen, W., Hlobil, H., Kemper, H.C., Voorn, W.J., De Jongh, H.R., 1993. Prevention of running injuries by warm-up, cool-down, and stretching exercises. American Journal of Sports Medicine 21 (5), 711-719.

Wilson, G.J., Elliott, B.C., Wood, G.A., 1992. Stretch-shortening cycle performance enhancement through flexibility training. Medicine and Science in Sports and Exercise 24, 116-123.

Witvrouw, E., Danneels, L., Asselman, P., D'Have, T., Cambier, D., 2003. Muscle flexibility as a risk factor of developing muscle injuries in professional male soccer players. American Journal of Sports Medicine 31 (1), 41-46.

Witvrouw, E., Mahieu, N., Danneels, L., McNair, P., 2004. Stretching and injury prevention – an obscure relationship. Sports Medicine 34 (7), 443-449.

Woods, C., Hawkins, R., Hulse, M., Hodson, A., 2002. The Football Association Medical Research Programme: an audit of injuries in professional football – analysis of preseason injuries. British Journal of Sports Medicine 36 (6), 436-441.

Capítulo | 20 |

Lesões no Joelho no Futebol Profissional

Jon Fearn, Paco Biosca, Dimitris Kalogiannidis e Jason Palmer

Introdução

Neste capítulo, daremos ao leitor uma visão sobre a nossa experiência no futebol profissional e sobre os tipos de lesão no joelho a que estamos expostos em um ambiente de futebol de elite, ou seja, a realidade dos profissionais da saúde no futebol. Apresentaremos também a filosofia de abordagem do Departamento de Saúde do Chelsea Football Club, discutiremos alguns aspectos específicos de nossa progressão de reabilitação funcional e, finalmente, forneceremos com mais detalhes os tipos específicos de lesões no joelho. Reconhecemos que existem muitas maneiras de implementar programas de reabilitação de lesões com sucesso.

Lesões no joelho são uma ocorrência comum em um esporte multidirecional como o futebol (Majewski et al., 2006), em que os movimentos e as cargas exclusivas colocadas no complexo do joelho podem desafiar a integridade da articulação. Lesões no joelho são sofridas por contato direto, como ao derrubar outro jogador ou ao ser derrubado, ou durante incidentes sem contato, como quando um jogador salta e cai desajeitadamente, durante movimentos de giro, também chamados de pivô, e mudança de direção.

Epidemiologia

A chave para uma abordagem eficaz de reabilitação de lesões é registrar os resultados e desfechos. É importante documentar claramente os tipos de lesões sofridas e como são tratadas. As informações a seguir representam os dados de lesões no joelho da auditoria de lesões do time principal do Chelsea FC entre as temporadas de 2011/12 e 2016/17. É importante notar que, de acordo com nossos critérios de auditoria, uma "lesão no joelho" se refere à patologia do joelho em que um jogador não está disponível para jogar ou treinar por mais de 48 horas.

A revisão dos dados de auditoria durante as seis temporadas descritas anteriormente mostrou que o joelho foi a área mais comum (n = 66) de ferimentos, representando 23% de todas as lesões sofridas nessas seis temporadas. O segundo tipo mais comum foi nos músculos da coxa (n = 65), incluindo isquiotibiais e quadríceps.

Em geral, acredita-se que as lesões no tornozelo são uma das lesões musculoesqueléticas comuns no futebol, mas elas representam apenas 11% das lesões no Chelsea FC e 13% nos clubes da Liga dos Campeões da União das Federações Europeias de Futebol (UEFA). As lesões da estrutura articular do joelho constituem a maioria das sofridas no joelho (84%), sendo as lesões ligamentares (36%) e meniscais (1%) as mais prevalentes (Tabela 20.1).

A carga da lesão é uma medida combinada da frequência (taxa de lesões) e da gravidade (dias de ausência) das lesões, dando a carga da lesão para o jogador e as consequências para a equipe. Ela é geralmente expressa como o número de dias de ausência/1.000 horas de exposição. Exemplo: A equipe A com 10 lesões em 5.000 horas, cada uma resultando em uma ausência de 10 dias em média, tem uma carga de lesões de 20 dias/1.000 horas. A equipe B com 20 lesões em 5.000 horas, cada uma resultando em uma ausência de 5 dias em média, também tem uma carga de lesões de 20 dias/1.000 horas.

A carga de lesões no joelho muda consideravelmente com o tipo e grau de lesão, e varia entre apenas alguns dias de perda de tempo com problemas menores, a vários meses nos casos mais graves. Por exemplo, das 17 lesões do ligamento colateral medial (LCM) sofridas, o período em que houve absenteísmo no treinamento como consequência variou de 2 a 16 dias. Em contraste, com lesões mais graves no joelho, como lesões do ligamento cruzado anterior (LCA) (n = 4), a perda de tempo foi entre 146 e 193 dias.

Filosofia do departamento médico do Chelsea FC

Em nossa experiência, a chave para um serviço de qualidade no manejo de todas as lesões é ter uma abordagem lógica, progressiva e multidisciplinar na qual todos da equipe entendam e sigam. Isso, combinado com uma equipe multiprofissional e polivalente experiente e excelentes instalações, nos permite oferecer nosso serviço de reabilitação.

Um tema predominante em nossa filosofia da saúde é manter as coisas o mais simples possível. Quanto mais complexo for o processo, há mais chances de que as coisas deem errado, então tentamos não complicar as coisas. Outros aspectos que sustentam a filosofia do nosso departamento são:

- Trabalhar em equipe multiprofissional
- Ter uma equipe de profissionais da saúde experientes, com uma mistura de habilidades
- Alcançar um diagnóstico preciso; isso é essencial para garantir que o plano de manejo correto seja implementado
- Realizar a avaliação e decidir sobre o diagnóstico com vários profissionais, incluindo pelo menos um médico e um fisioterapeuta

Parte | 2 | Aplicação Clínica

Tabela 20.1 Lesões no joelho sofridas na equipe principal do Chelsea FC entre junho de 2011 e maio de 2017.

Temporada	LCM[a]	LCL	LCA[a]	LCP	CPL[a]	Menisco[a]	Tendão patelar	Articulação patelofemoral	Sinóvia/ efusão[a]	Outras
2011-12	4[b]	–	1	–	–	2	–	1	1	2
2012-13	2	–	1	1	1	2	–	–	–	–
2013-14	8	1	1	–	–	–	–	2	1	2
2014-15	–	–	–	–	1	2	1	–	1	2
2015-16	2	–	1	–	1	2	–	–	1	1
2016-17	1	2	–	–	1	–	1	–	1	1
Total	17	3	4	1	4	8	2	3	5	N/A

A principal estrutura envolvida é conhecida como o tecido de diagnóstico, embora outras estruturas também possam estar envolvidas. [a]Lesões mais comuns sofridas no joelho. [b]Indica um novo ferimento. *LCA*, ligamento cruzado anterior; *LCL*, ligamento colateral lateral; *LCM*, ligamento colateral medial; *LCP*, ligamento cruzado posterior; *CPL*, canto posterolateral.

- Entregar um diagnóstico consensual: após a avaliação do grupo, o jogador é convidado a deixar a sala enquanto os membros da equipe discutem as descobertas e chegam a um único diagnóstico e plano de tratamento. O jogador é então convidado a voltar para a sala e recebe um único diagnóstico da "equipe" e um plano sobre o qual ele também pode fazer perguntas e contribuir como desejar
- Outras investigações (ressonância magnética [RM] etc.) são realizadas conforme necessário, mas nem sempre são essenciais
- Um fisioterapeuta lidera a implementação do plano de tratamento de lesões
- *Feedback* e comunicação regulares com a equipe médica em relação ao progresso, desafios e manejo são discutidos diariamente, com revisões do grupo sendo realizadas conforme necessário.

Filosofia do Chelsea FC
"Movimento sem dor é terapêutico."

Uma vez que o diagnóstico tenha sido acordado, o objetivo de qualquer programa de reabilitação é retornar o indivíduo ao seu nível anterior de função assim que for possível com segurança, com risco mínimo de nova lesão. De acordo com nossa filosofia, a reabilitação é funcionalmente específica e, portanto, os padrões de movimentos específicos do futebol são introduzidos assim que for seguro fazê-los.

Começando com padrões de movimentos simples e sem dor, nossa abordagem orientada para a reabilitação funcional progride por meio de padrões mais complexos conforme a dor e a patologia permitem, culminando em desafios totalmente específicos para lesões, futebol e posições específicas. Novamente, o mais importante é que todas as progressões devem ser realizadas sem dor, mas uma vez que, por exemplo, o "estágio 7" pode ser realizado sem dor, começamos com o "estágio 8". Esta abordagem é usada pela equipe de saúde para todos os jogadores, ou seja, em todas as equipes, em todas as idades (equipe profissional, sistema de academia de U9 a U23, equipes femininas) e simplesmente adaptada aos indivíduos em conformidade.

Estrutura de tratamento

Em nossa abordagem, o tratamento específico do joelho é complementado com movimento funcional global em diferentes modalidades e ambientes. Os jogadores são supervisionados de perto e progredidos nesses ambientes de maneira lógica, o que permite a progressão gradual e controlada da carga e, portanto, desafia o tecido em cicatrização.

Os métodos de adaptação de carregamento incluem:
- Terapia aquática, na qual a profundidade variável de submersão e esteiras subaquáticas podem adaptar o carregamento
- Esteiras antigravidade, que permitem o controle do *status* relativo de sustentação de peso
- Reabilitação em campo, em que a atenção à estrutura do exercício pode possibilitar a progressão controlada.

A maioria dos jogadores começa sua progressão de movimento funcional na água, onde suas qualidades criam uma maneira segura e produtiva de evolução. Uma dessas qualidades da água é a de flutuabilidade, que atua para reduzir o *status* de carga relativa de um indivíduo de acordo com a profundidade submersa. Este efeito tem uma relação linear, em que quanto maior a profundidade de submersão, maior o grau de descarga relativa com suporte de peso. Portanto, muitas vezes os jogadores começam a andar na água na profundidade dos ombros, o que equivale a aproximadamente 20 a 25% de sustentação de peso. À medida que o conforto e a qualidade do padrão funcional melhoram em um nível de água, a profundidade da água é reduzida, aumentando, assim, a sustentação de peso relativo e progredindo o indivíduo em direção ao movimento funcional de sustentação de peso total. Assim que o jogador puder andar efetivamente e ficar livre de sintomas na água com 40 a 50% de sustentação de peso, ele será encaminhado para exercícios de corrida, que podem começar com águas mais profundas novamente, para reduzir a sustentação de peso relativo para o início dessa progressão. Esse efeito ocorre devido à propriedade física da água chamada de empuxo. Durante esse processo, a apresentação clínica do joelho é monitorada de perto pela equipe médica. A mobilização precoce na água não só permite que o joelho se mova funcionalmente em um ambiente seguro e estável, mas também possibilita que ocorra a estimulação proprioceptiva precoce, o que pode acelerar a capacidade do jogador de progredir com confiança.

Métodos de progressão funcional

Existem diferentes maneiras de progredir o movimento funcional. Alguns exemplos estão listados a seguir:
- Progresso de sustentação de peso parcial no ambiente aquático para sustentação de peso total

Lesões no Joelho no Futebol Profissional **Capítulo** | 20 |

- Progressão do padrão de movimento: uma progressão pode começar com movimentos lineares (linha reta) para proteger as estruturas do joelho afetadas antes de progredir para movimentos laterais, rotacionais ou multidirecionais que requerem mais controle do joelho
- Sessão de progresso e tempo de exercício, velocidade de movimento e intensidade de movimento: começando com um formato menos desafiador e progredindo conforme a tolerância do jogador ao movimento permitir.

Novamente, é importante monitorar regularmente a resposta da área ferida à intervenção. Esse monitoramento pode envolver observar qualquer dor durante ou após os exercícios, mudanças no inchaço/derrame, monitorar a mobilidade do joelho e/ou adaptar de acordo com a necessidade o conteúdo da sessão no futuro.

Esta abordagem de "reabilitação funcional" é combinada diariamente com terapia manual, técnicas de eletroterapia, exercícios de controle neuromuscular proprioceptivo e, em ocasiões específicas, podemos usar a terapia de injeção de plasma rico em plaquetas (PRP). Isso dependerá do local da lesão, do tipo de tecido envolvido e do grau de dano sofrido (ver seção *Lesões do ligamento colateral medial* para obter mais informações sobre a injeção de PRP).

Um dia típico para um jogador lesionado pode envolver 4 a 5 horas de trabalho e normalmente inclui atenção individual de um membro da equipe médica. Cada dia pode incluir:
- Revisão de avaliação de equipe multiprofissional
- Terapia manual
- Reabilitação com base funcional (p. ex., na piscina, no campo com a bola, no ginásio)
- Exercícios proprioceptivos
  - Eletroterapia.

> **Filosofia do Chelsea FC**
> "A melhor prevenção contra lesões no futebol é jogar futebol."

Nossa filosofia é baseada no princípio de que quanto mais cedo o jogador realizar o movimento funcional específico do futebol, melhor. Esse conceito se encaixa bem com as teorias de que as melhores estratégias de prevenção são muito específicas para a atividade pretendida. Nada é mais específico para jogar futebol do que jogar futebol.

O jogador estará mais bem preparado para o retorno competitivo ao jogo seguindo um abrangente processo de reabilitação orientado para a "função futebolística" para lesões no joelho, em que uma demanda gradualmente crescente é colocada nele para que execute movimentos funcionais. Acreditamos que essa abordagem é eficaz para minimizar o risco de novas lesões e casos de instabilidade, além de reduzir a necessidade de intervenção cirúrgica. Durante o período de seis temporadas discutido, tivemos apenas uma pequena lesão reincidente (lesão no ligamento), o que também nos garante que nossa abordagem não é excessivamente agressiva.

Intervenções direcionadas "específicas para o joelho"

Após um exame completo e um diagnóstico consensual, as principais áreas a serem levadas em consideração no desenvolvimento de um plano de tratamento são:
- Nível e extensão da lesão anatômica sofrida, para planejar a direção do tratamento, por exemplo, conservador ou cirúrgico

- Biotipo do jogador (p. ex., ectomorfo, mesomorfo, endomorfo) e patomecânica consequente (p. ex., pé cavo, joelho varo) que pode ter predisposto o indivíduo à lesão no joelho
- Mobilização do complexo articular do joelho em conjunto com outras estruturas circundantes envolvidas para obter amplitude de movimento ideal
- Fortalecimento dos músculos que podem afetar a função do joelho, incluindo aqueles ao redor de outras articulações que estarão envolvidas na cadeia cinética do membro inferior
- Controle neuromuscular e propriocepção do joelho, pelve e membro inferior.

A melhoria do controle neuromuscular pode começar com exercícios em ambientes controlados, como a piscina. Tornar os movimentos funcionais mais dinâmicos, como caminhar para a corrida e mudar os padrões de movimento de linear para multidirecional, pode aumentar a demanda proprioceptiva para o joelho e para o membro inferior.

As intervenções do tratamento precisam variar de acordo com o estágio e o estado do tecido em cicatrização. Por exemplo, diferentes intervenções são necessárias em diferentes estágios de cura e variam em sua eficácia, mas pequenos avanços podem ajudar coletivamente na progressão geral. Alguns exemplos incluem:
- Terapia manual para melhorar a mobilidade das articulações e dos tecidos moles
- Terapia de repouso/passiva para permitir que o tecido se cure, mas aumenta a mobilidade das articulações, por exemplo, máquinas de movimento passivo contínuo (MPC)
- Eletroterapia para otimizar a cicatrização e controlar a resposta inflamatória, por exemplo:
  - Diatermia por ondas curtas e terapia magnética nos estágios agudos (Peres et al., 2002)
  - Ultrassom terapêutico durante a fase proliferativa e de remodelamento, principalmente nas estruturas colágenas superficiais, como o LCM e o ligamento colateral lateral
  - Estimulação elétrica nervosa transcutânea (TENS, do inglês *transcutaneous electrical nerve stimulation*) para controle da dor (Atamaz et al., 2012)
- Terapia de exercícios para melhorar a propriocepção, o controle neuromuscular, a força do joelho e do membro inferior (Aman et al., 2018)
- Estimulação elétrica muscular local para músculos com risco de atrofia, como quadríceps. Isso pode ser combinado com exercícios dinâmicos, como ciclismo, elevações de perna esticada, agachamento ou *leg press* (Feil et al., 2011; Taradaj et al., 2013)
- Dispositivo de compressão pneumática intermitente para reduzir o inchaço excessivo e melhorar a drenagem linfática (Goats, 1989)
- Terapia térmica para amortecer a resposta inflamatória nos estágios iniciais (p. ex., frio/gelo) ou para facilitar ainda mais a resposta de cura de acordo, dependendo do estágio de cura
- Uso de medicamentos para o controle da dor, incluindo anti-inflamatórios não esteroidais (AINE), particularmente para facilitar a função efetiva, reduzindo a dor nos estágios iniciais (Ong et al., 2007)
- Terapia de injeção – especificamente terapia de PRP, para facilitar a resposta de cura (Miranda-Grajales, 2017). Por exemplo, todos os jogadores com lesões do LCM sofridas no Chelsea FC voltaram ao treinamento em 16 dias e, desses indivíduos, vários receberam injeções de PRP incluídas em seu plano de reabilitação. Consideramos o uso de injeções de PRP como um complemento do processo de reabilitação muito eficaz.

209

Lesões comuns no joelho

Após a análise das lesões sofridas no joelho dentro do time principal nas últimas seis temporadas, as quatro lesões mais comuns são a do ligamento medial, a do LCA, a do menisco e a do canto posterolateral (CPL).

Outras estruturas que podem ser lesionadas em torno do complexo do joelho incluem o ligamento colateral lateral (LCL), o ligamento cruzado posterior (LCP), o tendão patelar, a articulação patelofemoral e a sinóvia, bem como lesões por contusão. Essas são ocorrências relativamente raras, com apenas um ou dois incidentes por temporada no time. Além disso, muitas apenas impedem o jogador de participar dos jogos por alguns dias. Portanto, vamos nos concentrar nas lesões mais comuns nos joelhos.

Deve-se destacar que pode haver múltiplas estruturas envolvidas na maioria das lesões do joelho, mas nos concentraremos no problema principal e no diagnóstico consensual.

Lesões do ligamento colateral medial

Esse é o tipo mais comum de lesão sofrida no joelho no time principal nas últimas seis temporadas. A maioria dos movimentos de chute e bloqueios que um jogador executa é com o peito do pé, o que coloca mais pressão nos compartimentos mediais do membro inferior. A lesão do LCM geralmente ocorre por causa de uma disputa com um oponente ou um movimento de chute desconhecido estressando excessivamente o aspecto medial do joelho.

Nos estágios iniciais de uma lesão do LCM, os fundamentos de reabilitação usuais são seguidos (conforme descrito anteriormente), ou seja, restaurando a mobilidade total do joelho, potencializando sua força e propriocepção e maximizando o nível de função do jogador enquanto o tecido lesionado está se curando. Além desse processo, com quase todas as lesões do LCM, realizamos uma série de injeções semanais de PRP (Boxe 20.1 e Tabela 20.2). Acreditamos que isso seja muito eficaz para facilitar uma recuperação imediata após uma lesão.

Boxe 20.1 O que é plasma rico em plaquetas?

O PRP é isolado do sangue por meio de uma centrífuga. O mecanismo de ação proposto para o PRP é que ele auxilie no processo de cicatrização de um tendão lesado. O tecido conjuntivo do tendão tem um suprimento sanguíneo pobre e, portanto, propriedades curativas diminuídas. As plaquetas contêm fatores de crescimento endógenos. Esses fatores de crescimento são: fator de crescimento transformante-β1 (TGF-β1), fatores de crescimento semelhantes à insulina (IGF) 1 e 2, fator de crescimento endotelial vascular (VEGF), fator de crescimento de fibroblastos básico (BFGF) e fator de crescimento de hepatócitos (HGF).

Adaptado de Miranda-Grajales, H., 2017. Platelet-rich plasma. In: Pope, J., Deer, T. (Eds.), Treatment of Chronic Pain Conditions. Springer, New York, NY.

No caso de recuperação de uma lesão no LCM, mesmo após um período relativamente breve, o jogador é capaz de realizar movimentos lineares sem dor (para frente e para trás) com facilidade, pois o LCM não é excessivamente estressado por esses movimentos. Estes podem ser realizados inicialmente na piscina, mas podem progredir rapidamente para o campo, embora com algumas restrições de espaço, velocidade e movimentos na direção lateral ou rotacional. Com o tempo, isso pode progredir ainda mais, uma vez que o tecido lesionado pode sustentar cargas maiores e mais variadas. O jogador ainda estará realizando exercícios específicos na piscina ou academia visando o estresse do LCM sem dor, junto com movimentos funcionais no campo (como discutido mais adiante). É essencial diferenciar entre instabilidade, que provavelmente requer intervenção cirúrgica, e frouxidão.

À medida que o LCM se recupera, os dois movimentos mais provocativos que requerem atenção específica são chutar a bola e correr em uma curva onde o aspecto medial do joelho é excessivamente tenso e aberto. Ironicamente, as manobras de curta distância e às vezes rápidas no campo podem ser fáceis de executar relativamente no início de sua recuperação, mas as corridas mais longas em formato de S ou em círculo podem ser problemáticas. Começar os exercícios de chute com uma bola de voleibol leve ou menor, o uso de bola tamanho 3 pode ser uma nova maneira de estimular o complexo medial durante a ação de chutar sem dor e com o tempo isso pode ser construído até a bola tamanho 5 completo. Isso é feito inicialmente com pequenos exercícios de *"punch pass"* do rúgbi e progredindo para exercícios de passe, cruzamento e chute mais longos quando o jogador conseguir.

Lesões do ligamento cruzado anterior

Em muitos times de futebol profissional, pelo menos um jogador sofrerá uma lesão no LCA em qualquer temporada. Elas geralmente ocorrem como uma lesão sem contato, em que o jogador se move ou aterrissa desajeitadamente, girando excessivamente e estressando o complexo do LCA.

No time principal do Chelsea, sofremos quatro lesões no LCA em seis temporadas. Todas elas precisaram de reconstrução cirúrgica, mas curiosamente, um jogador que voltou à plena forma e ao jogo de nível de equipe principal o fez com um joelho com deficiência de LCA, ou seja, em algum ponto da cirurgia à investigação, que cobriu um período de 18 meses, o enxerto no LCA falhou. Apesar de o LCA estar rompido, ele foi capaz de jogar e competir em um futebol de alto nível, sem sintomas nos joelhos. Esses tipos de pacientes são frequentemente referidos como "sustentadores", *versus* "não sustentadores", ou "ligamento dependentes" e "ligamentos independentes", em que o joelho com deficiência de LCA não é capaz de lidar com a carga funcional e resulta em episódios de instabilidade.

Tabela 20.2 **Tempo de recuperação para lesões do ligamento colateral medial (LCM) recebendo injeções de plasma rico em plaquetas no Chelsea FC.**

Temporada	Nº de lesões do LCM	Dias de afastamento	Média de dias de afastamento
2011-12	4	3:7:16:13	10
2012-13	2	5:4	4
2013-14	8	15:5:15:4:13:15:7:2	9
2014-15	0	–	–
2015-16	2	13:16	14
2016-17	1	5	5

Devido às demandas multidirecionais do futebol e ao estresse excessivo colocado na articulação do joelho, a maioria dos jogadores faz cirurgias com o objetivo de restaurar a anatomia funcional do ligamento do LCA e estabilizar o complexo do joelho. Em muitos esportes, especialmente aqueles que não colocam tanto estresse rotacional no joelho, os atletas podem lidar com isso sem ter o LCA reconstruído e não têm episódios de instabilidade ou fraqueza durante a realização de seus esportes.

Em quase todos os casos de lesão do LCA, não apenas o LCA é rompido, mas outras estruturas costumam estar envolvidas. Danos ao menisco ou à cartilagem articular, bem como a outros ligamentos, como o LCP, o LCM e o complexo ligamentar posterolateral também podem ter ocorrido. É importante planejar o manejo de todos os aspectos da lesão e decidir quais intervenções são apropriadas. Isso pode ter um reflexo na hora de voltar aos treinos. Em uma lesão do LCA relativamente simples, com nenhum ou menor envolvimento meniscal, esperaríamos que um jogador retornasse ao treinamento por volta de 5 meses; no entanto, com lesões mais complexas, pode demorar muito mais devido aos danos estruturais no joelho.

A reabilitação de uma lesão do LCA leva tempo, pois o joelho está fortemente comprometido. Cada jogador reage à cirurgia de maneira diferente e, portanto, a reabilitação de um jogador com uma lesão no LCA é diferente em cada caso. Compilamos um protocolo de reabilitação do LCA (Apêndice 1) para orientar os médicos quanto à nossa abordagem no manejo desse tipo de lesão. Este guia é usado para todos os times do clube.

Lesões de menisco

É importante notar que não é incomum identificar problemas meniscais no exame clínico do joelho; costumam ser vistos em investigações como o exame de RM (Figura 20.1). Muitos desses achados são alterações meniscais crônicas antigas que estão presentes há algum tempo sem quaisquer sintomas e não requerem intervenção. Elas definitivamente não requerem cirurgia. A RM é prática aceita agora quando se lida com ruptura meniscal (*i. e.*, a presença de lesões ou degeneração) para evitar a realização de cirurgia, a menos que seja clinicamente indicado, por exemplo, em um joelho travado devido à ruptura meniscal. Uma cirurgia desnecessária pode tornar o jogador vulnerável a danos prematuros na cartilagem articular e, no caso de um jogador jovem, pode representar uma ameaça à carreira poucos anos após a cirurgia.

Uma vez que uma lesão meniscal é diagnosticada por exame clínico, que pode ou não ser apoiado por achados de RM, a equipe médica decide sobre a abordagem de tratamento indicada. Nas últimas seis temporadas, sofremos oito lesões meniscais, cinco das quais resultaram em cirurgia artroscópica (ressecção ou reparo) e esses jogadores faltaram entre 21 e 78 dias. Das três lesões meniscais restantes tratadas de maneira conservadora, todas receberam injeções de PRP, o que acreditamos que acelera a resposta de cura e o retorno dos jogadores ao jogo. Os jogadores tratados de modo conservador voltaram a jogar em 3 a 8 dias. A decisão sobre a necessidade de intervenção conservadora ou cirúrgica foi baseada no exame clínico e na extensão do dano meniscal.

A abordagem de reabilitação é fundamentalmente a mesma de todas as outras lesões do joelho, ou seja, reduzir o inchaço/derrame, restaurar a mobilidade total do joelho, normalizar a força e a propriocepção ao redor do complexo do joelho e progredir as capacidades funcionais do joelho específicas para as demandas do futebol e da posição do jogador. Durante a reabilitação de lesões meniscais, é dada atenção especial à presença ou à extensão de um derrame no joelho ou qualquer perda de mobilidade do joelho. Isso pode dar uma indicação clara se o joelho está lidando bem com o nível e o progresso do processo de reabilitação.

Lesões de canto posterolateral

O CPL tem uma estrutura anatômica complexa com músculos como o poplíteo, tendões incluindo o bíceps femoral e ligamentos como o ligamento arqueado e o ligamento poplíteofibular, todos contribuindo para sua capacidade de controlar a extensão do joelho, rotação lateral e estresse em varo.

As lesões geralmente ocorrem como resultado da restrição do complexo do CPL sendo estressado durante atividades forçadas de cadeia aberta ou fechada, como agarrar ou pousar desajeitadamente (Figura 20.2).

A reabilitação de lesões do CPL segue essencialmente um processo de manejo lógico e conservador, conforme descrito anteriormente, com cuidado para não mobilizar de modo excessivo as estruturas danificadas. Essa mobilização demasiada pode levar à frouxidão do complexo do CPL e problemas durante as atividades funcionais. Em nossa experiência, muitas dessas lesões se recuperam em poucas semanas. Um caso demorou 46 dias para retornar ao treinamento, mas isso foi complicado devido a uma ruptura parcial do tendão do bíceps.

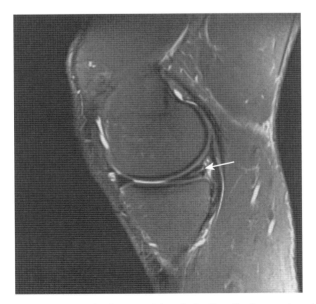

Figura 20.1 Ressonância magnética do joelho direito mostrando ruptura meniscal (*seta*).

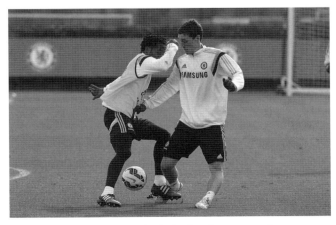

Figura 20.2 A hiperextensão do joelho é um mecanismo comum de lesões do canto posterolateral.

Parte | 2 | Aplicação Clínica

Reabilitação em campo

Se o jogador estiver incapaz de treinar ou realizar suas atividades esportivas normais, é importante otimizar o processo de recuperação de "reabilitação funcional" em um ambiente mais controlado. Isso pode assumir a forma de reabilitação em campo.

Assim que o jogador for capaz de completar padrões de movimento de qualidade em um ambiente de sustentação de peso reduzido, como a água, o clínico e o jogador terão confiança para fazer a transição para a função de sustentação de peso total. Se isso não for possível, será necessário apresentar a atividade em sua forma mais básica e aumentar a complexidade à medida que eles tolerem cada etapa.

Embora a abordagem do movimento funcional seja focada na função e não na patologia, a natureza e o tipo de movimento que se deve incluir em suas primeiras sessões na grama serão influenciados, em parte, pela patologia com a qual se está lidando.

Novamente, de acordo com a filosofia do movimento funcional, deve-se fazer algo assim que possível. Se, por exemplo, são realizados movimentos multidirecionais leves na água e o jogador os tolera bem, então pode-se introduzir versões de baixa intensidade desses movimentos no início, mesmo na primeira sessão em solo.

As sessões são então progredidas de acordo com o aumento da intensidade ou velocidade dos exercícios, a quantidade de tempo gasto no campo e o aumento da complexidade e estresse nas estruturas dos joelhos.

Como mencionado anteriormente, comece com exercícios lineares em linha reta em um ritmo lento, o que garante a proteção do complexo do joelho e a progressão do controle neuromuscular. A Figura 20.3 é um exemplo de um exercício linear inicial que um jogador pode executar no campo.

O jogador então progride para o corte lateral ou movimentos rotacionais com velocidade crescente. Além disso, a introdução de sinais e obstáculos externos, como a bola, fornece maneiras sutis de aumentar a complexidade e a demanda do exercício.

A Figura 20.4 é um exemplo de exercício de campo controlado mais avançado para um jogador de futebol atacante. Com a execução de exercícios sem problemas como este, o jogador estará perto de retornar ao treinamento modificado.

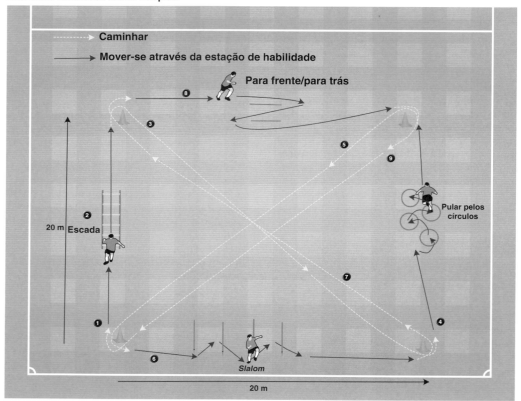

Figura 20.3 Diagrama de um exercício linear inicial. (*Esta figura se encontra reproduzida em cores no Encarte.*)

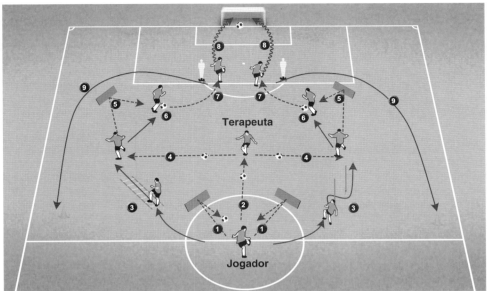

Figura 20.4 Diagrama de um exercício de campo controlado mais avançado para um jogador de futebol de ataque. (*Esta figura se encontra reproduzida em cores no Encarte.*)

Unidade de prevenção de lesões do Chelsea FC

No momento, estamos compilando uma "Unidade de Prevenção" para garantir que nossa filosofia de prevenção de lesões seja refletida em todo o Chelsea FC. Isso envolve todos os times de todas as idades, incluindo profissionais, academia e mulheres, bem como os times de base e de desenvolvimento.

A Unidade será multiprofissional, envolvendo médicos, fisioterapeutas, treinadores, preparadores físicos e cientistas do esporte que representam todas as equipes envolvidas.

Como um clube, há uma mensagem comum para todos os jogadores serem educados na importância dos princípios básicos de saúde, como nutrição, sono, estilo de vida e bem-estar físico e mental. É função da Unidade de Prevenção procurar maneiras de melhorar o controle locomotor e o desempenho de um jogador.

Por ter uma Unidade de Prevenção transmitindo a mesma mensagem, esperamos garantir que nossa filosofia seja seguida desde o time principal até o grupo de idade mais jovem (8 anos) em todo o clube e garantir que nossos jogadores possam jogar e desfrutar do futebol tanto quanto possível.

É importante notar que dentro do elenco principal, devido aos compromissos de jogo dos jogadores tanto para o clube quanto para as seleções, com períodos regulares em que há apenas 2 a 3 dias entre os jogos oficiais, ter tempo para implementar estratégias de prevenção de lesões pode ser um desafio.

Conclusão

Existem numerosos artigos, pesquisas e livros dedicados à epidemiologia e ao tratamento de lesões no joelho. Esses estudos tendem a ser oriundos de instituições acadêmicas ou hospitais, muito distantes da realidade de nossas experiências no futebol profissional. Nossa experiência evidencia que a metodologia científica de manejo de lesões geralmente não é um reflexo verdadeiro do que acontece dentro de um clube de futebol profissional.

Acreditamos que uma abordagem lógica, progressiva e funcional é o tratamento mais eficaz para lesões nos joelhos no futebol. Isso basicamente começa com um diagnóstico preciso envolvendo todos os membros da equipe médica após um exame completo e abrangente. A lesão do jogador é então manejada com intervenções direcionadas locais ou específicas do joelho, juntamente com estratégias de carga funcional precoce em ambientes seguros e controlados. O objetivo final é completar as tarefas relacionadas ao futebol relevantes para a posição individual do jogador com uma velocidade, intensidade e duração suficientes para permitir que eles retornem ao ambiente de treinamento. Em muitas ocasiões, ao retornar ao ambiente de treinamento do time, pode haver um período de modificação em que o envolvimento do jogador é adaptado de acordo com seus requisitos. Obviamente, isso requer uma discussão estreita com a equipe de manejo e a comissão técnica e pode ou não ser sempre necessário. Dito isto, não há alternativa ao se preparar para voltar a jogar futebol profissional do que jogar futebol profissional: os movimentos e decisões aleatórias e inesperadas que ocorrem no ambiente de treinamento e jogo não podem ser reproduzidos de outra maneira.

Agradecimentos

O conteúdo desse capítulo é um reflexo da abordagem de equipe que temos no departamento médico do Chelsea FC. Temos uma equipe médica muito experiente que representa diferentes origens, opiniões e habilidades, mas nosso objetivo é oferecer uma abordagem aceita pelo coletivo. Nós, autores, agradecemos a contribuição de toda a equipe de saúde neste capítulo.

Referências bibliográficas

Åman, M., Larsén, K., Forssblad, M., Näsmark, A., Waldén, M., Hägglund, M., 2018. A nationwide follow-up survey on the effectiveness of an implemented neuromuscular training program to reduce acute knee injuries in soccer players. Orthopaedic Journal of Sports Medicine 6 (12), 2325967118813841.

Atamaz, F.C., Durmaz, B., Baydar, M., et al., 2012. Comparison of the efficacy of transcutaneous electrical nerve stimulation, interferential currents, and shortwave diathermy in knee osteoarthritis: a double-blind, randomized, controlled, multicenter study. Archives of Physical Medicine and Rehabilitation 93 (5), 748-756.

Feil, S., Newell, J., Minogue, C., Paessler, H.H., 2011. The effectiveness of supplementing a standard rehabilitation program with superimposed neuromuscular electrical stimulation after anterior cruciate ligament reconstruction: a prospective, randomized, single-blind study. The American Journal of Sports Medicine 39 (6), 1238-1247.

Goats, G.C., 1989. Pulsed electromagnetic (short-wave) energy therapy. British Journal of Sports Medicine 23 (4), 213-216.

Majewski, M., Habelt, S., Steinbrück, K., 2006. Epidemiology of athletic knee injuries: a 10-year study. The Knee Journal 13 (3), 184-188.

Miranda-Grajales, H., 2017. Platelet-rich plasma. In: Pope, J., Deer, T. (Eds.), Treatment of Chronic Pain Conditions. Springer, New York, NY.

Ong, C.K.S., Lirk, P., Seymour, R.A., 2007. An evidence-based update on nonsteroidal anti-inflammatory drugs. Clinical Medicine & Research 5 (1), 19-34.

Peres, S.D., Knight, K., 2002. Pulsed shortwave diathermy and prolonged long-duration stretching increase dorsiflexion range of motion more than identical stretching without diathermy. Journal of Athletic Training 37(1), 43–50.

Taradaj, J., Halski, T., Kucharzewski, M., Walewicz, K., Smykla, A., Ozon, M., et al., 2013. The effect of neuromuscular electrical stimulation on quadriceps strength and knee function in professional soccer players: return to sport after ACL reconstruction. BioMed Research International 2013, 802534.

UEFA Champions League Injury Audit Data 2011–2017. Chelsea FC unpublished data.

Capítulo | 21 |

Tornozelo Esportivo: Entorse Lateral do Tornozelo – a Lesão Musculoesquelética de Membro Inferior mais Comum

Eamonn Delahunt

Introdução

Lesões na articulação do tornozelo são comumente sofridas por atletas que participam de esportes de campo e de quadra. A lesão articular do tornozelo mais frequentemente sustentada por atletas que participam desses esportes é uma entorse lateral do tornozelo. Tanto pela alta prevalência quanto pela elevada taxa de incidência de lesão e carga de lesão de entorse de tornozelo lateral, é essencial que os profissionais da saúde que trabalham com atletas de esportes de campo e de quadra sejam "especialistas" em avaliação, diagnóstico e reabilitação de lesões na articulação do tornozelo. Este capítulo detalha um estudo de caso de um jogador de futebol semiprofissional que sofreu uma lesão aguda na articulação do tornozelo. O estudo de caso detalha a avaliação clínica e os processos de raciocínio clínico associados a um diagnóstico de lesão e ao desenvolvimento de uma estrutura de reabilitação baseada na deficiência.

Descrição do caso

Um jogador de futebol da associação semiprofissional, do sexo masculino e de 22 anos (Jogador A) sofreu uma lesão de contato traumática na articulação do tornozelo. No momento da lesão, ele estava com a posse da bola e corria em alta velocidade em direção à grande área do time adversário. Em um esforço para impedi-lo de penetrar na grande área, um jogador defensor executou um carrinho, mas errou a bola de futebol e, em vez disso, fez contato com o jogador A na parte interna da canela, logo acima do maléolo medial. Este contato físico resultou em uma inversão substancial e rotação interna do complexo tornozelo/pé do Jogador A. Como resultado dessa lesão, o Jogador A foi substituído; no entanto, ele foi capaz de deambular fora do campo com a assistência mínima do fisioterapeuta em campo da equipe.

Epidemiologia das lesões

As lesões na articulação do tornozelo são responsáveis por 13% de todas as que são sofridas por jogadores de futebol de elite da Europa (Walden et al., 2013). Sua taxa de incidência é de 1/1.000 horas; isso significa que um time de futebol profissional com 25 jogadores incorre em sete lesões nas articulações do tornozelo por temporada. Lesões por entorse de tornozelo representam 68% de todas as que ocorrem nessa parte do corpo, com uma taxa de incidência de 0,7/1.000 horas, ou seja, um time de futebol profissional com 25 jogadores incorre em cinco lesões por entorse de tornozelo por temporada. Até 75% envolvem lesão do complexo ligamentar lateral, com apenas 5% classificadas como "entorses altas de tornozelo". A perda média de tempo devido à lesão da articulação do tornozelo é de 16 dias; no entanto, "entorses de tornozelo" têm uma perda de tempo médio substancialmente superior a 43 dias. Foi relatado que o "jogo sujo" (p. ex., jogadas de risco desnecessárias com alta agressividade) contribui para 40% das entorses de tornozelo relacionadas com o jogo. Assim, está claro que as lesões da articulação do tornozelo são preocupação substancial no futebol.

Mecanismo da lesão

Estabelecer o mecanismo da lesão é um componente fundamental de todas as avaliações clínicas. Isso dá aos profissionais da saúde uma indicação quanto às estruturas anatômicas que provavelmente sofreram lesão e, portanto, quais tecidos devem ser priorizados durante o componente físico da avaliação clínica.

Para desenvolver uma compreensão abrangente dos mecanismos de lesões na articulação do tornozelo e, em particular, entorses de tornozelo no futebol, Andersen et al. (2004) avaliaram gravações de vídeo de 26 entorses de tornozelo no futebol de elite norueguês e islandês nas temporadas de 1999 e 2000. Eles relataram que um dos mecanismos de lesão mais comuns incluía o contato jogador a jogador, com impacto de um oponente no aspecto medial da perna um pouco antes ou durante o encostar do pé no chão, resultando em uma força dirigida lateralmente causando uma inversão e rotação interna do complexo tornozelo/pé. Portanto, com base em um artigo publicado na literatura revisada por pares, o mecanismo de lesão descrito anteriormente é comum no futebol.

Os médicos devem suspeitar de lesão nos ligamentos laterais da articulação do tornozelo se um paciente relatar que o mecanismo

Parte | 2 | Aplicação Clínica

da lesão incluiu uma inversão rápida súbita baseada em contato ou sem contato e carga de rotação interna do complexo tornozelo/pé. Os mecanismos de lesão associados a "entorses altas de tornozelo" são menos claros, mas geralmente incluem rotação externa do pé e hiperdorsiflexão da articulação do tornozelo.

Avaliação clínica: o essencial

Fratura

Conforme demonstrado na descrição do caso, o Jogador A foi capaz de deambular fora do campo com a assistência mínima do fisioterapeuta da equipe. Isso indica que era improvável que uma fratura da articulação do tornozelo fosse sustentada. Um critério específico das regras de tornozelo de Ottawa refere-se ao estado de capacidade de sustentação de peso do paciente imediatamente após a lesão e na avaliação clínica (Stiell et al., 1993). Se, em vez disso, o Jogador A não tivesse conseguido suportar o peso imediatamente após a lesão ou no momento da avaliação clínica, a probabilidade de fratura da articulação do tornozelo teria aumentado. No entanto, devido à natureza do contato traumático do mecanismo de lesão, seria prudente realizar a avaliação clínica das regras de tornozelo de Ottawa (Stiell et al., 1993). Nesse caso, o objetivo principal é avaliar a sensibilidade óssea localizada ao longo dos 6 cm posteriores distais do maléolo medial ou lateral, que especificamente replica ou recria a "dor conhecida" do Jogador A. No momento da avaliação clínica, nenhuma sensibilidade óssea replicando a "dor conhecida" do Jogador A foi observada, negando assim a necessidade de radiografia da articulação do tornozelo. Esse achado de ausência de sensibilidade óssea específica replicando sua "dor conhecida" juntamente com sua capacidade de deambular imediatamente após a lesão (embora com ajuda) significa que a radiografia não era indicada, já que a probabilidade de fratura da articulação do tornozelo neste caso era menor do que 1%.

Ligamentos

O mecanismo de lesão delineado na descrição do caso indica alta probabilidade para a lesão dos ligamentos da articulação lateral do tornozelo. Dessa maneira, o ligamento talofibular anterior e o ligamento calcaneofibular devem ser priorizados durante o componente físico da avaliação clínica. Lesões por entorse de tornozelo são responsáveis por 68% de todas as lesões articulares do tornozelo no futebol, com 75% delas envolvendo danos nos tecidos dos ligamentos laterais da articulação do tornozelo (Waldén et al., 2013).

O ligamento talofibular anterior deve ser palpado e alongado (flexão plantar passiva da articulação do tornozelo combinada com inversão passiva e rotação interna do pé). A replicação ou recriação da "dor conhecida" do Jogador A à palpação ou ao alongamento do ligamento talofibular anterior é indicativa de dano ao tecido desse ligamento. Nesse caso, tanto a palpação quanto o alongamento do ligamento talofibular anterior recriaram a "dor conhecida" do Jogador A, indicando dano no tecido desse ligamento. Além da palpação e do alongamento do ligamento talofibular anterior, o teste da gaveta anterior de avaliação clínica pode ser realizado para determinar se o ligamento talofibular anterior está completamente rompido. A sensibilidade e a especificidade do teste são otimizadas se a avaliação clínica for realizada 4 a 6 dias após a lesão (van Dijk et al., 1996). Nessa situação, nenhum sinal de sulco foi observado na avaliação clínica durante a realização do teste da gaveta anterior, indicando

que o Jogador A não havia sofrido uma ruptura completa de seu ligamento talofibular anterior.

O ligamento calcaneofibular deve ser palpado e alongado (inversão passiva do retropé com a articulação do tornozelo em dorsiflexão). A replicação ou recriação da "dor conhecida" do Jogador A na palpação ou alongamento do ligamento calcaneofibular é indicativa de dano ao tecido deste ligamento. Neste caso, a palpação e o alongamento do ligamento calcaneofibular não recriaram a "dor conhecida" do Jogador A, indicando, portanto, que não há dano ao tecido deste ligamento.

Embora o mecanismo de lesão demonstrado no caso descritivo não seja compatível com o de uma "entorse alta de tornozelo", devido à natureza de contato traumático da lesão, é prudente realizar uma avaliação clínica dos ligamentos da sindesmose da articulação do tornozelo. Os dois testes de avaliação clínica mais importantes incluem a palpação do ligamento tibiofibular anterior inferior (mais sensível) e o teste de compressão (mais específico). As descobertas combinadas dessas avaliações clínicas podem guiar um clínico na determinação da probabilidade de um paciente ter dano tecidual sustentado aos ligamentos da sindesmose da articulação do tornozelo. Em caso de suspeita dessa lesão, a imagem diagnóstica (geralmente a ressonância magnética) pode ser utilizada para confirmar ou refutar a suspeita. No caso do Jogador A, a palpação do ligamento tibiofibular inferior anterior não recriou sua "dor conhecida", nem o teste de compressão. Esses resultados combinados de avaliação clínica negativa indicam que o dano ao tecido nos ligamentos da sindesmose da articulação do tornozelo era improvável.

Componente físico da avaliação clínica: resumo

Integrando as informações sobre o mecanismo de lesão e os achados primários da avaliação clínica detalhada anteriormente, concluiu-se que o Jogador A sofreu uma lesão isolada de seu ligamento talofibular anterior. Não foram utilizados exames de imagem médica para diagnóstico, pois não havia indicações da avaliação clínica de que isso fosse necessário.

Reabilitação do tornozelo do jogador de futebol

O objetivo principal é retornar o Jogador A ao seu nível de desempenho anterior à lesão sem colocar ele ou outros em risco indevido de lesão, ao mesmo tempo mitigando seu risco de lesão futura. Para atingir esse objetivo, é essencial que os profissionais da saúde considerem o paradigma das insuficiências sensorimotoras induzidas por lesão.

Insuficiências sensorimotoras: teoria

Sensorimotor é o sistema biológico que controla as contribuições das restrições dinâmicas (i. e., músculos) para a manutenção da estabilidade funcional da articulação. Compreende todos os componentes aferentes, eferentes, centrais de integração e processamento envolvidos na preservação da estabilidade funcional da articulação. Um fluxo constante de impulsos aferentes (i. e., entrada somatossensorial) de mecanorreceptores articulares, cutâneos e musculotendíneos entra na medula espinal por meio da raiz dorsal e são projetados para centros de processamento de ordem superior, incluindo o tronco cerebral, cerebelo e córtex somatossensorial. Uma resposta motora coordenada apropriada (*i. e.*, resposta eferente) com o objetivo de manter a estabilidade funcional da articulação é desenvolvida em resposta aos impulsos aferentes desses mecanorreceptores mencionados anteriormente. Assim, após uma perturbação articular (p. ex., supinação súbita inesperada do pé devido à colocação do pé em um tufo em um campo de futebol durante a corrida), mecanorreceptores articulares, cutâneos e musculotendíneos são estimulados. Em resposta, há transmissão neural de sinais aferentes para o sistema nervoso central, com o processamento desses sinais ocorrendo em centros de ordem superior. Os sinais eferentes resultantes iniciam a ativação muscular e a produção de força para manter a estabilidade funcional da articulação do tornozelo e prevenir lesões. A lesão da articulação do tornozelo pode causar lesões nos tecidos articulares, cutâneos e musculotendíneos. Portanto, é lógico concluir que a entrada somatossensorial para o sistema sensorimotor é interrompida após a lesão da articulação do tornozelo.

O desempenho seguro e eficiente das tarefas motoras depende da interação síncrona de mecanismos de *feedback* sensorimotor eferente e aferente pré-programados. A perturbação desta sincronia, como pode ocorrer após a interrupção das aferências somatossensoriais, pode ter a capacidade de distorcer a coordenação específica da tarefa motora pré-programada e as estratégias de movimento "armazenadas" pelo sistema sensorimotor. Por exemplo, foi proposto que as restrições orgânicas (p. ex., dor, inchaço, lesão de tecido) induzidas por uma lesão de entorse de tornozelo interrompem o fluxo de impulsos dos mecanorreceptores nos tecidos lesionados para o sistema nervoso central. Isso, por sua vez, pode desencadear padrões adaptativos de reorganização sensorimotora, "redefinindo" estratégias de coordenação e movimento previamente estabelecidas na adoção de novos padrões de coordenação e movimento. Então, essas alterações podem manifestar-se em um espectro de sintomas residuais que comprometem a estabilidade articular funcional e que aumentam o risco de lesões futuras. É importante notar que essas alterações não se resolvem rapidamente e continuam a se manifestar nas semanas e meses após a lesão, a menos que uma intervenção sensorimotora específica, direcionada e apropriada seja implementada.

Avaliação clínica de insuficiências sensorimotoras

As seções a seguir descrevem a justificativa e alguns mecanismos baseados em evidências propostos para realizar uma avaliação clínica abrangente, com o objetivo de estabelecer a presença de deficiências sensorimotoras.

Dor

A dor na articulação do tornozelo autorrelatada pelo Jogador A pode ser quantificada usando uma medida de resultado adequada orientada para o paciente. Existem várias opções para avaliar a dor nas articulações do tornozelo em ambientes clínicos. Uma escala numérica de avaliação da dor, que pode ser administrada verbalmente e por escrito, pode ser facilmente utilizada para quantificar a dor durante a realização de várias tarefas motoras. A quantificação da dor nas articulações do tornozelo autorrelatada pelo Jogador A pode ser usada como uma medida de resultado clinicamente orientada para a progressão de uma intervenção de reabilitação baseada em exercícios. Por exemplo, ao realizar um exercício de salto anterior, a distância do salto necessário não deve ser progredida até que o paciente possa executar a distância necessária do salto com o mínimo de dor. Se, por exemplo, o Jogador A notou um aumento na dor nas articulações do tornozelo em resposta a uma progressão de exercício específica envolvendo um aumento na distância de salto, então seria lógico concluir que esta progressão de exercício está sobrecarregando os tecidos lesionados e pode não ser apropriadamente alinhada com a fase de cicatrização do tecido. Nesses casos, um "sistema de semáforo" pode ser integrado à escala de classificação numérica para dor, permitindo uma orientação inequívoca da progressão do exercício (Figura 21.1). A quantificação da dor nas articulações do tornozelo autorrelatada do Jogador A serve a outro propósito. Também pode ser utilizada para avaliar a eficácia de qualquer tratamento implementado, ajudando assim a nortear a escolha adequada de intervenções terapêuticas.

Inchaço

O edema da articulação do tornozelo pode alterar o fluxo de impulsos aferentes para o sistema nervoso central, cuja manifestação primária é o desenvolvimento de inibição muscular artrogênica. Isso, por sua vez, pode comprometer a estabilidade funcional da articulação por meio de uma alteração na ativação muscular e consequente produção de força.

A magnitude do inchaço da articulação do tornozelo lesionado do Jogador A pode ser avaliada clinicamente por meio do mecanismo em forma de oito e, em seguida, utilizada como medida de resultado clinicamente orientada para a progressão de uma intervenção de reabilitação baseada em exercícios. Por exemplo, durante a reabilitação da técnica de salto, um aumento no inchaço da articulação do tornozelo (maior do que a mudança mínima detectável que foi estabelecida para a figura de oito: 9,6 mm) (Rohner-Spengler et al., 2007) seguido da progressão de aterrissagens com perna dupla para aterrissagem com uma única perna no tornozelo lesionado indicaria que essa progressão é prematura. Portanto, neste caso, pode ser mais apropriado adicionar uma "restrição ambiental" (p. ex., ter o Jogador A controlando uma bola de futebol em seu peito e passá-la de volta para o médico imediatamente após a aterrissagem ou ter o Jogador A realizando uma tarefa de cabeceio com um pouso com perna dupla), em vez de alterar a "restrição da tarefa" (*i. e.*, realizar uma aterrissagem com uma perna sobre o tornozelo lesionado).

Quantificar a magnitude do inchaço do tornozelo lesionado do Jogador A serve a outro propósito. Semelhantemente ao descrito no parágrafo anterior para dor, quantificar a magnitude do edema também pode ser usado para avaliar a eficácia de qualquer tratamento implementado, ajudando a orientar a escolha adequada de intervenções terapêuticas.

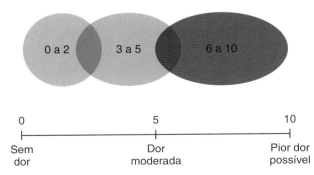

Figura 21.1 Escala numérica de classificação de dor "semáforo". *Verde*, provavelmente seguro para continuar o exercício; *laranja*, é necessário cuidado, pois o exercício pode exceder a tolerância dos tecidos carregados; *vermelho*, provavelmente inseguro para continuar o exercício, pois a tolerância dos tecidos carregados provavelmente foi excedida. (*Esta figura se encontra reproduzida em cores no Encarte.*)

Parte | 2 | Aplicação Clínica

Amplitude de movimento: osteocinemática e artrocinemática

A amplitude de movimento da articulação do tornozelo depende da interação da osteocinemática e da artrocinemática. Osteocinemática se refere aos movimentos que ocorrem em torno de um centro de rotação, ou seja, o eixo articular. Com relação à articulação do tornozelo, os movimentos osteocinemáticos primários incluem flexão plantar/dorsiflexão. Uma vez que o eixo de rotação da articulação do tornozelo não está situado em um plano cardinal, os movimentos que ocorrem na articulação do tornozelo são tipicamente descritos como triplanares; a flexão plantar está associada à inversão e rotação interna, enquanto a dorsiflexão está associada à eversão e abdução. Em contraste, artrocinemática se refere ao movimento das superfícies articulares, com o movimento normal da superfície articular sendo parte integrante da integridade articular a longo prazo. As superfícies das juntas movem-se em relação umas às outras, rolando, deslizando e girando simultaneamente. Com relação à articulação do tornozelo, o deslizamento posterior do tálus ocorre durante a dorsiflexão com o deslizamento oposto (i. e., deslizamento anterior) no decorrer da flexão plantar.

Um achado comum após lesão da articulação do tornozelo e, em particular, lesão por entorse lateral do tornozelo, é uma restrição temporária ou a longo prazo na amplitude de movimento de dorsiflexão. Isso é particularmente relevante e merece atenção considerável, uma vez que a amplitude de movimento de dorsiflexão explica até 28% da variância no desempenho do equilíbrio postural dinâmico, conforme avaliado pela direção de alcance anterior do SEBT (do inglês *star excursion balance test*) (Hoch et al., 2011). A amplitude de movimento de dorsiflexão da articulação do tornozelo do jogador A pode ser avaliada usando o teste de afundo com sustentação de peso, que é válido e confiável (Langarika-Rocafort et al., 2017). Para determinar se um déficit de dorsiflexão associado é principalmente osteocinemático ou artrocinemático, o clínico pode realizar uma série de mobilizações anteroposteriores aplicadas ao tálus. Nesse caso, se o déficit de dorsiflexão for principalmente artrocinemático, essa série de mobilizações resultará em melhora imediata na amplitude de movimento de dorsiflexão.

A pontuação do teste de afundo com sustentação de peso do Jogador A para a articulação do tornozelo machucada foi de 13 cm. Imediatamente após a aplicação de duas séries de 2 minutos de mobilizações da articulação talocrural com direção anterior-posterior de Maitland grau III com 1 minuto de descanso entre as séries, sua pontuação no teste de afundo com sustentação de peso melhorou 2 cm. Isso indicou que sua restrição na amplitude de movimento da dorsiflexão era principalmente de natureza artrocinemática.

Força muscular

Os músculos da articulação do tornozelo constituem as restrições dinâmicas para a manutenção da estabilidade funcional da articulação. Durante o processo contrátil, as unidades musculotendíneas geram rigidez, que contribuem para a proteção dinâmica da articulação sobre a qual atuam. Um déficit na força da articulação do tornozelo pode comprometer a integridade da articulação do tornozelo para suportar movimentos prejudiciais repentinos. Portanto, é importante que a avaliação clínica da força da articulação do tornozelo seja feita após a lesão. Um dinamômetro portátil pode ser utilizado em ambientes clínicos para quantificar de maneira confiável e objetiva a força da articulação do tornozelo (Kelln et al., 2008).

Os valores de força isométrica da articulação do tornozelo do Jogador A, conforme avaliados usando um dinamômetro portátil, são detalhados na Tabela 21.1.

Equilíbrio postural estático e dinâmico

O equilíbrio postural refere-se à capacidade de um indivíduo de controlar a posição do seu centro de massa em relação à sua base de apoio para evitar quedas. A diminuição do equilíbrio postural é comumente relatada como um fator de risco primário para lesões musculoesqueléticas de membros inferiores sem contato. Portanto, após uma lesão musculoesquelética, se o objetivo principal é mitigar o risco de lesão recorrente, então é lógico concluir que a avaliação do equilíbrio postural estático e dinâmico deve ser rotineiramente incorporada em qualquer avaliação clínica.

O desempenho do equilíbrio postural estático do Jogador A pode ser avaliado fazendo-o realizar cada um dos seis testes constituintes do sistema BESS (do inglês *Balance Error Scoring System*) (Figura 21.2). Avaliar o desempenho do Jogador A em cada um desses seis testes pode fornecer informações úteis para o desenvolvimento do componente de exercício de equilíbrio postural estático de seu programa de reabilitação.

O desempenho do equilíbrio postural estático do Jogador A pode ser avaliado fazendo-o executar as direções de alcance especificadas do SEBT (Figura 21.3). As três direções de alcance mais comumente utilizadas são as direções de alcance anterior, posterior-lateral e posterior-medial. Em cada caso, a distância de alcance é normalizada em relação ao comprimento da perna do paciente (conforme medido da espinha ilíaca anterossuperior até a ponta distal do maléolo medial) e multiplicada por 100, produzindo uma pontuação que representa a porcentagem do comprimento da perna (Equação 1). Além disso, uma pontuação composta também pode ser calculada (Equação 2).

Distância de alcance normalizada (% comprimento da perna) =

$$\frac{\text{Distância de alcance atingida (cm)}}{\text{Comprimento da perna (cm)}} \times 100 \qquad \text{Equação 1}$$

Distância de alcance normalizada composta (% comprimento da perna) =

$$\frac{[\text{Anterior (cm)} + \text{posterior} - \text{lateral (cm)} + \text{posterior} - \text{medial (cm)}]}{\text{Comprimento da perna (cm)} \times 3} \times 100 \qquad \text{Equação 2}$$

Tabela 21.1 Pontuações isométricas de força da articulação do tornozelo para articulações do tornozelo não lesionadas e lesionadas do Jogador A, conforme avaliado por meio de dinamometria portátil.

	Articulação do tornozelo não lesionada	Articulação do tornozelo lesionada	Diferença média
Inversão isométrica (N)	95	80	15
Eversão isométrica (N)	92	79	13
Dorsiflexão isométrica (N)	159	140	19

Os valores são medidos em Newtons (N).

218

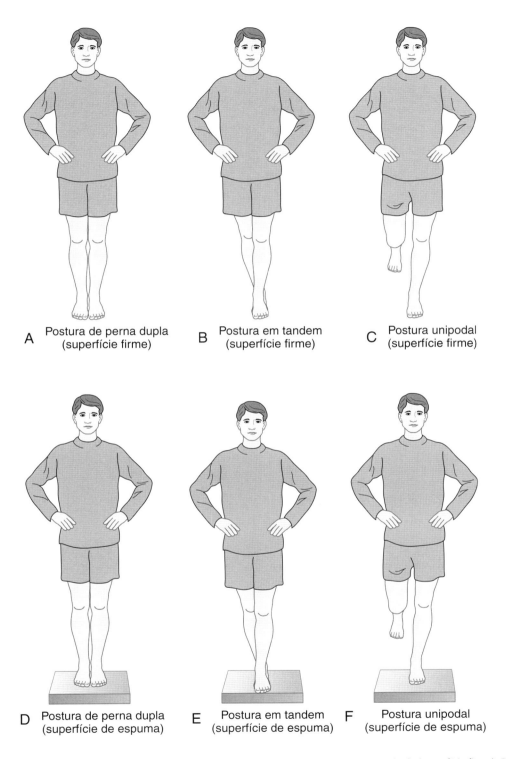

Figura 21.2 Os seis testes que constituem o *Balance Error Scoring System*. A. Postura de perna dupla (superfície firme). **B.** Postura em tandem (superfície firme). **C.** Postura unipodal (superfície firme). **D.** Postura de perna dupla (superfície de espuma). **E.** Postura em tandem (superfície de espuma). **F.** Postura unipodal (superfície de espuma). Todos os testes são iniciados e duram 20 segundos quando o paciente fecha os olhos.

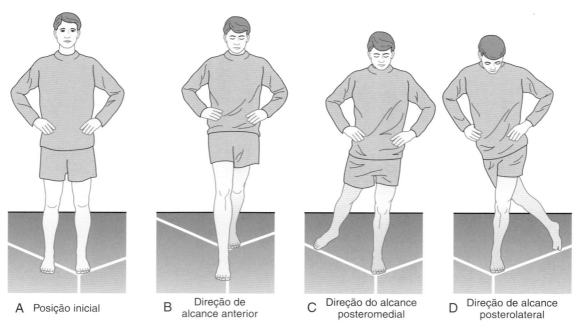

Figura 21.3 *Star excursion balance test* (também chamado de Y-teste, para essa variação). **A.** Posição inicial. **B.** Direção de alcance anterior. **C.** Direção do alcance posteromedial. **D.** Direção de alcance posterolateral.

O desempenho do Jogador A nessas direções de alcance poderia então ser utilizado como uma medida de resultado orientada clinicamente para avaliar a eficácia de qualquer tratamento implementado e para monitorar a recuperação de seu desempenho de equilíbrio postural dinâmico.

A Tabela 21.2 resume a quantidade de "erros" cometidos pelo Jogador A ao realizar cada um dos testes constituintes do BESS. A Tabela 21.3 resume as pontuações de distância de alcance normalizadas (i. e., percentual de comprimento da perna) obtidas pelo Jogador A ao realizar as direções de alcance anterior, posterior-medial e posterior-lateral do SEBT ou Y-teste.

Intervenções terapêuticas e reabilitação de insuficiências sensorimotoras identificadas

O objetivo de qualquer intervenção terapêutica pós-lesão e programa de reabilitação deve ser retornar o atleta lesionado para a prática ou competição sem colocar ele/ela ou outros em risco indevido de lesão, embora concomitantemente mitigando o risco de nova lesão. Na descrição do caso apresentada, diversas insuficiências sensorimotoras foram identificadas na avaliação clínica por meio de metodologias objetivas, válidas e confiáveis. Essas insuficiências sensorimotoras devem ser utilizadas para orientar quaisquer intervenções terapêuticas planejadas e reabilitação baseada em exercícios.

Amplitude de movimento: osteocinemática e artrocinemática

Usando uma abordagem de raciocínio clínico, foi determinado que a restrição do Jogador A na amplitude de movimento da dorsiflexão era principalmente artrocinemática. Dessa maneira, a utilização de mobilizações articulares com o objetivo específico de melhorar o deslizamento posterior do tálus deve ser implementada como intervenção terapêutica. Há uma série de técnicas de terapia manual que são apoiadas pela literatura revisada por

Tabela 21.2 Erros de equilíbrio cometidos pelo Jogador A avaliados por meio do desempenho no BESS.

	Postura de perna dupla (superfície firme)	Postura tandem (superfície firme)	Postura unipodal (superfície firme)	Postura de perna dupla (superfície de espuma)	Postura tandem (superfície de espuma)	Postura de perna única (superfície de espuma)
Erros	0	2	5	2	5	10

BESS, Balance Error Scoring System.

Tabela 21.3 Pontuações de distância de alcance normalizadas obtidas pelo Jogador A em três das direções de alcance do SEBT (Y-teste).

	Direção de alcance anterior	Direção de alcance posterior-medial	Direção de alcance posterior-lateral
Distância de alcance normalizada (% comprimento da perna)	58	94	83

SEBT, star excursion balance test.

pares, incluindo mobilizações da articulação talocrural anterior-posterior de Maitland (Hoch et al., 2012; Hoch e McKeon, 2011), bem como mobilizações de dorsiflexão com movimento (Collins et al., 2004; Vicenzino et al., 2006). O teste de afundo com sustentação de peso deve ser usado para avaliar clinicamente a resposta do Jogador A à aplicação de qualquer técnica de terapia manual. Nesse caso, o objetivo é minimizar qualquer assimetria entre os membros na amplitude de movimento da dorsiflexão. Observe que a dorsiflexão com sustentação de peso deve continuar a ser avaliada durante os estágios posteriores da reabilitação, visto que, anedoticamente, déficits artrocinemáticos na amplitude de movimento da dorsiflexão podem ressurgir quando a carga na articulação do tornozelo aumenta durante o desempenho de tarefas motoras específicas de esportes.

Força muscular

Conforme detalhado na Tabela 21.1, foi determinado usando dinamometria portátil que o Jogador A tinha deficiências na força isométrica de sua articulação do tornozelo lesionada. Foi relatado que o treinamento de força influencia o recrutamento de unidades motoras, a ativação seletiva dos músculos agonistas e suas unidades motoras e a coativação antagonista (Komi e Sale, 1992). Além disso, ao considerar o desempenho de exercícios dinâmicos e específicos do esporte, um nível fundamental de rigidez musculotendínea é necessário para a utilização ideal do processo do ciclo de alongamento-encurtamento. Como tal, exercícios multiplanares de fortalecimento da articulação do tornozelo devem ser incorporados como parte integrante de um programa de reabilitação baseado em exercícios. Numerosos programas de reabilitação baseados em exercícios foram detalhados na literatura publicada, incluindo exercícios de fortalecimento da articulação do tornozelo (Docherty et al., 1998; Hall et al., 2015).

Equilíbrio postural estático e dinâmico

Os resultados obtidos da avaliação clínica do desempenho do equilíbrio postural estático (ver Tabela 21.2) e dinâmico (ver Tabela 21.3) do Jogador A podem ser utilizados para desenvolver a base inicial para o componente de equilíbrio postural baseado em exercícios de seu programa de reabilitação. Com relação à interpretação dos escores de desempenho do equilíbrio postural estático descritos na Tabela 21.2, o seguinte seria uma abordagem de raciocínio clínico apropriado. Nenhum erro foi cometido pelo Jogador A ao completar a tarefa de postura de perna dupla (superfície firme). Portanto, esta tarefa não desafiará o sistema sensorimotor e sua incorporação em um programa de reabilitação seria redundante. O jogador A cometeu dois erros ao completar a tarefa de postura em tandem (superfície firme) e a tarefa de postura de perna dupla (superfície de espuma). Essa baixa quantidade de erros sugere que essas tarefas devem constituir apenas um componente minoritário (i. e., uma pequena porcentagem) do tempo total dedicado aos exercícios de equilíbrio postural. O jogador A cometeu cinco erros ao completar a tarefa de postura unilateral (superfície firme) e a tarefa de postura tandem (superfície de espuma). Este é uma quantidade substancial de erros para cada uma dessas tarefas e sugere que elas estão desafiando adequadamente o sistema sensorimotor, ou seja, não são tão fáceis que ele possa completá-las com erros mínimos, mas não são tão difíceis que ele não possa completá-las totalmente. Portanto, seria prudente incluir essas tarefas como exercícios-chave do componente de equilíbrio postural de seu programa de reabilitação. O Jogador A cometeu 10 erros (i. e., a quantidade máxima de erros) ao completar a tarefa de apoio de perna única (superfície de espuma). Isso sugere que essa tarefa é muito desafiadora (neste momento) para o sistema sensorimotor e não deve

ser incluída como um exercício inicial do componente de equilíbrio postural de seu programa de reabilitação.

Com relação à interpretação dos escores de desempenho do equilíbrio postural dinâmico descritos na Tabela 21.3, o seguinte seria uma abordagem de raciocínio clínico apropriado. Todas as pontuações de distância de alcance normalizadas são menores do que o que seria esperado de um jogador de futebol semiprofissional não lesionado (Butler et al., 2012; Stiffler et al., 2015), portanto, o Jogador A apresenta prejuízos substanciais no desempenho do equilíbrio postural dinâmico. O SEBT não deve ser considerado apenas como uma metodologia de avaliação clínica, mas também como um exercício de reabilitação do equilíbrio postural dinâmico. O desempenho das diferentes direções de alcance do SEBT desafia vários componentes do sistema sensorimotor (Gabriner et al., 2015).

Perfil do atleta

Ao avaliar a prontidão do Jogador A para retornar ao esporte, é necessário garantir que ele esteja adequadamente preparado para as demandas fisiológicas, táticas e psicológicas de seu esporte. Conforme declarado anteriormente, o objetivo principal de qualquer intervenção terapêutica e programa de reabilitação seria retornar o Jogador A ao seu nível de desempenho anterior à lesão sem colocar ele ou outros em risco indevido de lesão, ao mesmo tempo mitigando seu risco de lesão futura. Para isso, é vital que os médicos tenham uma compreensão abrangente das demandas fisiológicas, táticas e psicológicas do esporte. Esse entendimento reduzirá o risco do Jogador A ser exposto de maneira inadequada a demandas para as quais ele está mal preparado.

Outras lesões da articulação do tornozelo: breve comentário

Embora a entorse lateral do tornozelo seja a lesão do tornozelo mais frequente em atletas de campo e de quadra, os médicos devem estar cientes das características de outras lesões da articulação do tornozelo. O reconhecimento das características dessas lesões pode ajudá-los a direcionar de modo adequado a sua avaliação clínica para os tecidos/estruturas com maior probabilidade de sofrer lesões. Uma breve visão geral de algumas dessas outras lesões da articulação do tornozelo, juntamente com suas características, estão descritas na Tabela 21.4.

Conclusão e resumo

A entorse lateral do tornozelo é uma das lesões mais prevalentes em atletas que praticam esportes de campo e de quadra. Assim é vital que os profissionais da saúde que trabalham com os atletas que participam desses esportes sejam "especialistas" na avaliação, diagnóstico e reabilitação de lesões da articulação do tornozelo e, em particular, lesões por entorse lateral do tornozelo. Uma preocupação particular após essa lesão é a propensão de desenvolver uma variedade de deficiências sensorimotoras, que podem resultar na persistência de sintomas relacionados à lesão a longo prazo. O primeiro passo imperativo para o desenvolvimento de uma via de tratamento apropriada é avaliação clínica estruturada após lesão por entorse lateral aguda de tornozelo que considere deficiências sensorimotoras. Essa avaliação permitirá que os médicos concentrem o desenho e a progressão dos programas de tratamento e reabilitação em torno de deficiências identificadas de modo objetivo.

Parte | 2 | Aplicação Clínica

Tabela 21.4 Características de outras lesões da articulação do tornozelo experimentadas por atletas de esportes de campo e de quadra.

Lesão	Sintomas característicos de lesão relatados pelo paciente	Achados típicos da avaliação clínica
Impacto posterior do tornozelo	Dor sentida na flexão plantar de alcance final	Dor reproduzida na flexão plantar forçada
Tendinopatia de Aquiles da porção média	Rigidez matinal localizada na porção média do tendão de Aquiles	Dor localizada na porção média do tendão de Aquiles com atividades que carregam o tendão, como pular
Tendinopatia de Aquiles de inserção	Rigidez matinal localizada na região de inserção do tendão de Aquiles	Dor localizada na região de inserção do tendão de Aquiles com atividades que carregam o tendão
Ruptura do tendão de Aquiles	Sensação súbita de incapacitação no tendão de Aquiles. Um som audível ou sensação de ser chutado na parte de trás da perna é frequentemente descrito	Teste de compressão da panturrilha positivo
Instabilidade crônica do tornozelo	Múltiplas entorses laterais de tornozelo autorreferidas. Relatos de que a articulação do tornozelo está instável. Episódios autorrelatados de "ceder" na articulação do tornozelo	Uma combinação de insuficiências mecânicas (frouxidão patológica, hiper/hipomobilidade) e funcionais (deficiências no equilíbrio postural, força, propriocepção e controle neuromuscular)
Síndrome do seio do tarso	Dor sentida na face lateral da articulação do tornozelo anterior e inferior ao maléolo lateral	Sensibilidade e inchaço no seio do tarso. Dor com inversão do retropé
Impacto anterior do tornozelo	Dor sentida na dorsiflexão final	Dor reproduzida na dorsiflexão forçada
Dor plantar no calcanhar	Dor sentida sob o calcanhar com o "primeiro passo" pela manhã	Sensibilidade na tuberosidade medial do calcâneo

Referências bibliográficas

Andersen, T.E., Floerenes, T.W., Arnason, A., Bahr, R., 2004. Video analysis of the mechanisms for ankle injuries in football. The American Journal of Sports Medicine 32 (1 Suppl. l), 69S-79S.

Butler, R.J., Southers, C., Gorman, P.P., Kiesel, K.B., Plisky, P.J., 2012. Differences in soccer players' dynamic balance across levels of competition. Journal of Athletic Training 47 (6), 616-620.

Collins, N., Teys, P., Vicenzino, B., 2004. The initial effects of a Mulligan's mobilization with movement technique on dorsiflexion and pain in subacute ankle sprains. Manual Therapy 9 (2), 77-82.

Docherty, C.L., Moore, J.H., Arnold, B.L., 1998. Effects of strength training on strength development and joint position sense in functionally unstable ankles. Journal of Athletic Training 33 (4), 310-314.

Gabriner, M.L., Houston, M.N., Kirby, J.L., Hoch, M.C., 2015. Contributing factors to star excursion balance test performance in individuals with chronic ankle instability. Gait & Posture 41 (4), 912-916.

Hall, E.A., Docherty, C.L., Simon, J., Kingma, J.J., Klossner, J.C., 2015. Strength-training protocols to improve deficits in participants with chronic ankle instability: a randomized controlled trial. Journal of Athletic Training 50 (1), 36-44.

Hoch, M.C., Andreatta, R.D., Mullineaux, D.R., English, R.A., Medina McKeon, J.M., Mattacola, C.G., et al., 2012. Two-week joint mobilization intervention improves self-reported function, range of motion, and dynamic balance in those with chronic ankle instability. Journal of Orthopaedic Research 30 (11), 1798-1804.

Hoch, M.C., McKeon, P.O., 2011. Joint mobilization improves spatiotemporal postural control and range of motion in those with chronic ankle instability. Journal of Orthopaedic Research 29 (3), 326–332.

Hoch, M.C., Staton, G.S., McKeon, P.O., 2011. Dorsiflexion range of motion significantly influences dynamic balance. Journal of Science and Medicine in Sport 14 (1), 90-92.

Kelln, B.M., McKeon, P.O., Gontkof, L.M., Hertel, J., 2008. Hand-held dynamometry: reliability of lower extremity muscle testing in healthy, physically active, young adults. Journal of Sport Rehabilitation 17 (2), 160-170.

Komi, P.V., Sale, D.G., 1992. Neural adaptation to strength training. In: Strength and Power in Sport. Blackwell Scientific Publications, Oxford, pp. 249-265.

Langarika-Rocafort, A., Emparanza, J.I., Aramendi, J.F., Castellano, J., Calleja-González, J., 2017. Intra-rater reliability and agreement of various methods of measurement to assess dorsiflexion in the Weight Bearing Dorsiflexion Lunge Test (WBLT) among female athletes. Physical Therapy in Sport 23, 37-44.

Rohner-Spengler, M., Mannion, A.F., Babst, R., 2007. Reliability and minimal detectable change for the figure-of-eight-20 method of measurement of ankle edema. Journal of Orthopaedic & Sports Physical Therapy 37 (4), 199-205.

Stiell, I.G., Greenberg, G.H., McKnight, R.D., Nair, R.C., McDowell, I., Reardon, M., et al., 1993. Decision rules for the use of radiography in acute ankle injuries. Refinement and prospective validation. Journal of the American Medical Association 269 (9), 1127-1132.

Stiffler, M.R., Sanfilippo, J.L., Brooks, M.A., Heiderscheit, B.C., 2015. Star excursion balance test performance varies by sport in healthy division I collegiate athletes. Journal of Orthopaedic & Sports Physical Therapy 45 (10), 772-780.

van Dijk, C.N., Lim, L.S., Bossuyt, P.M., Marti, R.K., 1996. Physical examination is sufficient for the diagnosis of sprained ankles. The Journal of Bone and Joint Surgery. British Volume 78 (6), 958-962.

Vicenzino, B., Branjerdporn, M., Teys, P., Jordan, K., 2006. Initial changes in posterior talar glide and dorsiflexion of the ankle after mobilization with movement in individuals with recurrent ankle sprain. Journal of Orthopaedic & Sports Physical Therapy 36 (7), 464-471.

Waldén, M., Hägglund, M., Ekstrand, J., 2013. Time-trends and circumstances surrounding ankle injuries in men's professional football: an 11-year follow-up of the UEFA Champions League injury study. British Journal of Sports Medicine 47 (12), 748-753.

Capítulo | 22 |

Reabilitação do Ombro no Rúgbi: Proposta de Abordagem para o Manejo

Keith Thornhill e Marc Beggs

Introdução

O objetivo deste capítulo é apresentar um modelo de reabilitação progressiva e flexível que pode ser adaptado e utilizado com uma variedade de atletas em diferentes estágios de seu retorno ao jogo (RAJ) após uma lesão. Um desafio significativo no esporte profissional é devolver os atletas lesionados para jogar o mais rápido e seguramente possível e, ao mesmo tempo, promover a saúde dos ombros para ajudar na redução do risco de lesões em atletas ilesos. Isso impulsionou a evolução de nossa abordagem.

Nem todas as diretrizes clínicas e protocolos pós-operatórios normalmente utilizados enfocam ambientes de esportes de elite, nem todas as pesquisas envolvem populações de esportes de elite. Como resultado, nossa abordagem de reabilitação foi criada, aplicada e desenvolvida na união do rúgbi de elite e evoluiu amplamente com base na experiência clínica, com o apoio das melhores pesquisas disponíveis.

Modelo com base em tarefas/critérios

Embora seja necessário fornecer cronogramas precisos com base em experiências clínicas anteriores para trabalhar ao retornar de uma lesão, é essencial que tanto o jogador quanto a equipe técnica estejam cientes de que o processo de lesão é conduzido pelo jogador que cumpre os critérios de saída e marcos durante o processo do RAJ em vez de ditar prazos.

O jogador lesionado tem metas de progresso definidas ao longo do processo de reabilitação e deve cumpri-las para avançar para a próxima fase. O prazo de prognóstico dado é fluido e pode ser alterado dependendo de como o jogador progride na jornada de reabilitação. É importante garantir que o jogador saiba que este prazo também pode ser acelerado se estiver progredindo bem; por exemplo, se em todas as semanas de uma lesão de 14 semanas eles estiverem 1 dia à frente das metas planejadas, eles estarão 14 dias antes do planejado.

Rúgbi de 15 e suas demandas no ombro

A incidência de lesões no ombro no rúgbi de 15 é de 13 por 1.000 horas de jogo (Usman et al., 2014). Para entender como reabilitar um ombro com sucesso, é necessário entender as demandas globais que um ombro terá de tolerar durante o rúgbi de 15. Em média, 116 contatos de todos os tipos (*tackle*, colisão e queda) são observados em uma partida de rúgbi de 15 (Hendricks et al., 2014). Para cada grupo posicional, avançados ou recuados, cada indivíduo é submetido a 33 a 42 contatos como um avançado ou 10 e 23 contatos como um recuado (Reardon et al., 2017).

Em termos das forças exercidas no cenário de *tackle*, Seminati et al. (2016) observaram que forças entre 1,78 e 1,96 kN serão exercidas no atacante e no portador da bola, respectivamente. No campo, forças de até 2 kN serão experimentadas pelo jogador que realiza um *tackle* (Usman et al., 2014). Outro aspecto das demandas do jogo que é importante entender é o *scrum*. Quarrie e Wilson (2000) observaram forças entre 6.210 e 9.090 N produzidas coletivamente no *scrum*.

Também deve haver um bom entendimento das demandas posicionais de cada jogador, pois isso ditará como a reabilitação progredirá. Por exemplo, um talonador (*hooker*) precisará ter a habilidade de alcançar acima da cabeça para realizar um lançamento de alinhamento lateral, enquanto um jogador de linha traseira precisa garantir que eles tenham ombro e força de punho adequados nas distâncias externas, uma vez que uma grande proporção de suas situações de *tackle* provavelmente serão realizadas enquanto tenta agarrar um oponente que está tentando desviar para evitar o *tackle* em alta velocidade.

Ombros saudáveis

Para entender os ombros sintomáticos, devemos primeiro compreender como os ombros funcionam quando são assintomáticos. Sabemos por pesquisas anteriores (Escamilla et al., 2009) que o manguito rotador é o grande responsável por manter a estabilidade articular e controlar a translação da cabeça do úmero.

Manguito rotador

Wattanaprakornkul et al. (2011a,b) mostraram por meio de eletromiografia (EMG) que o manguito rotador é recrutado dependendo da direção do movimento do braço. Especificamente, durante os movimentos baseados na flexão do ombro, o manguito posterior (supraespinal, infraespinal, redondo menor) é mais ativo do que o manguito anterior (subescapular); durante os movimentos baseados na extensão do ombro, o manguito anterior é mais ativo; durante os movimentos de abdução do ombro, ocorre uma relativa cocontração entre os manguitos anterior e posterior (Tabela 22.1).

Tabela 22.1 Correlação entre o movimento do ombro e o viés do manguito rotador.

Movimento	Viés de manguito
Flexão	Manguito posterior
Extensão	Manguito anterior
Abdução	Cocontração

Avaliação

Não há evidência consistente de que qualquer procedimento de exame utilizado em avaliações de ombro tenha níveis aceitáveis de confiabilidade (May et al., 2010). Uma revisão sistemática em 2007 revelou que a precisão diagnóstica do teste de Neer para impacto, do teste de Hawkins-Kennedy para impacto e do teste de Speed para patologia labral é limitada (Hegedus et al., 2007).

Os testes de ombro podem mostrar benefícios quando aplicados em grupos ou na exclusão de certas patologias, mas há uma falta de especificidade e sensibilidade ao realizar esses testes de maneira isolada. Clinicamente, valorizamos os testes de instabilidade de agrupamento quando indicado pelo mecanismo de lesão. Um algoritmo de avaliação proposto é mostrado na Figura 22.1.

Sabendo que durante os movimentos baseados na flexão do ombro, o manguito posterior é mais ativo, o objetivo é fornecer um estímulo que aumente a atividade do manguito posterior para provocar mudanças positivas nos sintomas. Duas maneiras potenciais de aumentar a atividade do manguito posterior são por meio da preensão manual (Sporrong et al., 1995; 1996) ou pela adição de uma força de rotação externa isométrica resistida à tarefa sintomática ou significativa baseada em flexão.

Subsequentemente, durante os movimentos baseados na extensão do ombro, o manguito anterior é mais ativo; o objetivo é fornecer um estímulo que aumente a atividade do manguito anterior para causar mudanças positivas nos sintomas. Postulamos que isso pode ser alcançado pela adição de uma força de rotação interna isométrica resistida. Durante os movimentos baseados na abdução do ombro, há uma cocontração do manguito anterior e posterior (Wattanaprakornkul et al., 2011a,b). Esta cocontração fornece uma compressão da cabeça do úmero na glenoide (Reed et al., 2018) e reduz a translação da cabeça do úmero (Wattanaprakornkul et al., 2011a,b).

Isso pode ser reproduzido pela adição de uma força compressiva aplicada externamente, comprimindo a cabeça do úmero na glenoide durante a tarefa sintomática ou significativa. Esta força compressiva também pode ser alcançada realizando atividades de sustentação de peso por intermédio do membro superior (p. ex., posição ajoelhada de quatro pontos) e avaliando se isso afeta positivamente o movimento sintomático ou a tarefa significativa (Tabela 22.2).

Conforme descrito anteriormente, o uso de uma atividade adicional durante a avaliação pode ser complementado pela adição de qualquer quantidade de atividades acessórias que não são direcionalmente específicas aos movimentos do ombro.

Reduzir o comprimento da alavanca (p. ex., braço) mantendo a flexão do cotovelo durante um movimento sintomático ou tarefa significativa, quando possível, reduzirá a demanda colocada sobre o ombro e o manguito rotador. A adição de uma atividade em cadeia cinética, como adicionar um movimento dominante da parte inferior do corpo (p. ex., um afundo ou um *step-up*) durante o movimento sintomático ou tarefa significativa aumentará a atividade do manguito por meio de um mecanismo de *feedforward*. A aplicação manual de um teste de assistência escapular em toda a extensão ajudará na atividade do músculo escapular axial. O objetivo de adicionar essas atividades acessórias às atividades de adição é afetar ainda mais positivamente a mudança no movimento sintomático ou tarefa significativa (Tabela 22.3).

Com base nos resultados da avaliação, o atleta geralmente se enquadrará em uma das quatro grandes categorias mostradas na Tabela 22.4.

Papel da imagem no ombro esportivo

O uso de exames de imagem, analgésicos, anti-inflamatórios não esteroidais (AINEs), injeções de esteroides e locais no manejo de problemas no ombro no rúgbi profissional devem ser vistos como sendo distintos do manejo normal de uma população não esportiva, amadora ou semiprofissional. Existem alguns casos em que essas vias são utilizadas. Esses adjuvantes podem auxiliar no processo de tomada de decisão clínica, ajudando a fornecer um diagnóstico precoce. Além disso, eles também podem ser aplicados para ajudar a reduzir os prazos de reabilitação e permitir que os jogadores voltem a jogar o mais rapidamente, mas com a maior segurança possível. Se essas vias forem utilizadas, o jogador ainda precisará atender aos critérios de RAJ para estar disponível para treinar e jogar.

Do mesmo modo, podem ajudar nas decisões clínicas sobre se uma reabilitação conservadora ou não conservadora é a mais apropriada.

Em geral, a imagem é reservada para aqueles que têm uma etiologia traumática e apresentação clínica que sugere uma luxação ou subluxação. Para aquelas lesões com características clínicas principalmente em torno da dor, a ressonância magnética (RM)/artrografia por ressonância magnética (ARM) pode não

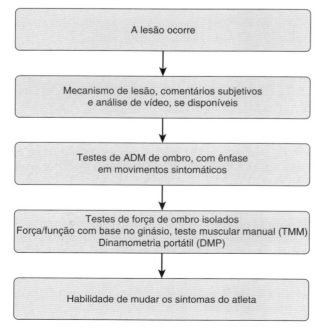

Figura 22.1 Algoritmo de avaliação para exame do ombro. *ADM*, amplitude de movimento.

Reabilitação do Ombro no Rúgbi: Proposta de Abordagem para o Manejo — **Capítulo** | 22 |

Tabela 22.2 **Atividades adicionais realizadas durante a avaliação clínica.**

Movimento sintomático	Atividade adicional	Ação
Flexão	Aperto de mão	Aumentar a atividade do manguito posterior
	Resistência de rotação externa	
Extensão	Resistência de rotação interna	Aumentar a atividade do manguito anterior
Abdução	Compressão	Replicação de cocontração por compressão
	Sustentação de peso	

Tabela 22.3 **Atividades acessórias realizadas durante a avaliação clínica.**

Movimento	Atividade acessória	Ação
Todos	Redução do comprimento da alavanca	Diminuir a carga de trabalho do manguito
	Atividade de cadeia cinética	Aumentar a atividade do manguito por meio do mecanismo de *feedforward*[a]
	Assistência escapular	Auxiliar a atividade do músculo escapular axial

[a]De McMullen, J., Uhl, T. L., 2000. A kinetic chain approach for shoulder rehabilitation. Journal of Athletic Training 35 (3), 329-337; Sciascia, A., Cromwell, R, 2012. Kinetic chain rehabilitation; a theoretical framework. Rehabilitation Research and Practise 1-9.

Tabela 22.4 **Quatro categorias amplas para classificar lesões esportivas no ombro.**

Categoria 1: "ombro machucado na manhã de segunda-feira"	
Mecanismo de lesão	Nenhum MDL claro. Provavelmente ter completado o jogo; apresenta pós-jogo/dia seguinte com dor/disfunção
Amplitude de movimento do ombro	ADM ativa (ADMA) > 70% com dor leve a moderada
Força isolada do ombro	Capacidade de fornecer um nível moderado a bom de resistência em testes com presença de dor e/ou fraqueza/inibição
Força funcional do ombro	Provavelmente será capaz de completar uma sessão de ginástica PSC modificada com o uso de levantamentos PSC regredidos (p. ex., flexão em vez de supino)
Capacidade de mudar os sintomas do atleta	O uso de uma atividade adicional e/ou uma atividade acessória fornece uma mudança positiva para seu movimento sintomático ou tarefa significativa
Prognóstico	Provavelmente completará o treinamento modificado ao longo da semana e estará disponível para jogar em 1 a 2 semanas. É improvável que tenha anormalidades estruturais; não requer investigação adicional (p. ex., ressonância magnética)
Categoria 2: lesões de curto a médio prazo	
Mecanismo de lesão	MDL claro e suspeito; imediatamente dolorido, provavelmente removido do jogo imediatamente ou dentro de alguns minutos se os sintomas não melhoraram
Amplitude de movimento do ombro	ADMA < 70% com dor moderada
Força isolada do ombro	Capacidade de fornecer nível baixo a moderado de resistência em testes com níveis moderados de dor e/ou fraqueza/inibição
Força funcional do ombro	Incapaz de concluir sessões de ginástica PSC modificadas com o uso de diminuições na carga de levantamento na PSC
Capacidade de mudar os sintomas do atleta	Mudanças fracas a mínimas no movimento sintomático ou tarefa significativa
Prognóstico	Incapaz de treinar. Provavelmente se tornará uma lesão de curto a médio prazo, com indisponibilidade para seleção de 2 a 8 semanas. Possíveis anormalidades estruturais; não requer mais investigação atualmente

(*continua*)

Tabela 22.4 Quatro categorias amplas para classificar lesões esportivas no ombro. (*Continuação*)

Categoria 3: falha na reabilitação de categoria 2	
Mecanismo de lesão	Como a categoria 2
Amplitude de movimento do ombro	
Força isolada do ombro	
Força funcional do ombro	
Capacidade de mudar os sintomas do atleta	
Prognóstico	O jogador pode ser manejado durante a temporada para permitir a disponibilidade para seleção, exigirá cirurgia pós-temporada. Isso exigirá semanas de treinamento altamente modificadas. Exigirá investigação adicional (p. ex., ressonância magnética, ARM, consulta ortopédica). Se não puder ser administrado durante a temporada, exigirá cirurgia o mais rápido possível. Vai se tornar um ombro de categoria 4

Categoria 4: reabilitação pós-operatória a longo prazo	
Mecanismo de lesão	MDL claro e suspeito – possível deslocamento/subluxação. Imediatamente doloroso e disfuncional; removido do jogo imediatamente
Amplitude de movimento do ombro	ADMA muito limitada, pode não estar disposto a tentar ADMA devido à dor ou apreensão
Força isolada do ombro	Pode não querer tentar o teste devido à dor ou apreensão. Provavelmente ficará muito fraco e dolorido se o teste for realizado
Força funcional do ombro	Não adequado para execução devido a dor, disfunção e/ou apreensão
Capacidade de mudar os sintomas do atleta	De nenhuma a pequenas mudanças no movimento sintomático ou na tarefa significativa. Pode não ser apropriado avaliar
Prognóstico	Alta indicação de uma anormalidade estrutural significativa; alta indicação para investigação posterior (p. ex., ressonância magnética, ARM, consulta cirúrgica) que exigirá intervenção cirúrgica

ADMA, amplitude de movimento ativa; *MDL*, mecanismo de lesão; *ARM*, artrografia por ressonância magnética; *PSC*, parte superior do corpo.

ser garantida, pois esses casos tendem a ser tratados de forma conservadora, independentemente da patologia subjacente, uma vez que geralmente respondem a AINEs e reabilitação de baixo nível.

O ombro do adolescente

Os jovens atletas que se enquadram na categoria 2 (ver Tabela 22.4) apresentam desafios distintos. Após a luxação, os atletas com menos de 18 anos têm alta incidência de recorrência após o tratamento conservador (Boileau et al., 2006). A cirurgia artroscópica para esses atletas também apresenta um desafio, com taxa de falha de até 70% em 31 meses após a lesão. Um estudo recente comparou as taxas de recorrência após estabilização artroscópica primária em jogadores de rúgbi agrupados em: < 16 anos, 16 a 17 anos e 25 anos. Ele mostrou porcentagens muito altas de falha em menores de 18 anos (Torrance et al., 2018). As decisões de manejo para esses atletas devem considerar:

1. Nível de participação: atleta recreativo ou de elite.
2. Lesão óssea: presença de lesão de Hill-Sachs (luxação anterior) e/ou perda da glenoide.
3. Quantidade e frequência das luxações anteriores: duas ou mais luxações anteriores do ombro podem ser uma indicação para cirurgia.

Esses casos devem ser avaliados individualmente antes de qualquer decisão ser tomada com o envolvimento sobretudo do jogador, pais/responsáveis, fisioterapeuta, médico e consultor.

Reabilitação do ombro lesionado

Após a avaliação e a categorização da pós-lesão, o caminho de reabilitação individual é dividido em camadas para se adequar às necessidades do atleta, sua lesão específica e quaisquer metas ou alvos adicionais. A seguir estão listados os pilares da reabilitação que consideramos importantes durante o processo de RAJ pós-lesão. Esses pilares permitem uma progressão lógica e estruturada ao longo do processo de RAJ e possibilitam uma exposição gradual e gradativa aos aspectos cada vez mais exigentes do rúgbi. Um aspecto importante desse processo no rúgbi de 15 de elite é garantir que a reabilitação seja abrangente.

Os pilares não se concentram apenas na reabilitação de uma lesão específica no ombro, mas também se dirigem ao atleta como um todo, para permitir que ele volte a jogar e atuar com as habilidades fisiológicas e psicológicas exigidas no rúgbi de 15 de elite. Isso garante que uma abordagem multidimensional e progressiva baseada em tarefas/critérios seja adotada por vários departamentos da organização (p. ex., fisioterapia, força e condicionamento, treinadores de rúgbi, nutrição).

Pilares de reabilitação

1. **Amplitude de movimento ativa assistida (ADMAA).** Geralmente, esses intervalos são utilizados principalmente em relação à flexão do ombro como um marcador para indicar quando a progressão pode ser apropriada.
2. **Amplitude de movimento ativa (ADMA).** Geralmente, esses intervalos são utilizados principalmente em relação à flexão do ombro como um marcador para indicar quando a progressão pode ser apropriada.
3. **Ativação isométrica do manguito rotador.** Produção de força por meio do manguito rotador sem que ocorra uma alteração no comprimento do músculo ou movimento do ombro (Mullaney et al., 2017).
4. **Condicionamento *off-feet*.** Treinamento aeróbico e anaeróbico sem sustentação de peso (p. ex., Wattbike).
5. **Exercícios de *endurance* do manguito rotador.** Exercícios que visam o manguito rotador com o objetivo de aumentar a capacidade de resistência.
6. **Condicionamento em pés.** Treinamento aeróbico e anaeróbico (p. ex., corrida) com sustentação de peso.
7. **Exercícios de cadeia cinética fechada (CCF).** Exercícios que são realizados enquanto os membros superiores ou inferiores estão em contato com um objeto fixo (De Mey et al., 2014).
8. **Exercícios de força excêntrica do manguito rotador.** Exercícios que visam especificamente o componente excêntrico da força do manguito rotador.
9. **Exercícios de cadeia cinética aberta (CCA).** Exercícios que são realizados enquanto os membros superiores ou inferiores não estão em contato com um objeto fixo e, portanto, estão livres para se mover (De Mey et al., 2014).
10. **Exercícios de força máxima da parte superior do corpo (PSC).** Programa de força com base no ginásio para atingir a força global da PSC.
11. **Força reativa do manguito rotador.** Exercícios que visam aumentar a velocidade na qual a musculatura do ombro pode mudar de absorver forças excentricamente para gerar forças concentricamente.
12. **Habilidades/reabilitação específicas do esporte/posição.** Exposição gradual e progressiva às habilidades baseadas no rúgbi.
13. **Habilidades de contato.** Exposição gradual e progressiva a habilidades baseadas em contato usadas para replicar as demandas do rúgbi de 15.
14. **Rúgbi.** Exposição gradual e progressiva às sessões de treinamento de rúgbi (Figura 22.2).

Lesões de categorias 3 e 4

A abordagem que geralmente adotamos com lesões no ombro das categorias 3 e 4 flui da esquerda para a direita do caminho de reabilitação do ombro (ver Figura 22.2). Isso permite o início da reabilitação de modo precoce, enquanto ainda estiver usando tipoia no pós-operatório. A progressão a partir desse ponto é guiada pelas amplitudes de movimento (ADM) assistida ativa e ativa, geralmente guiada pela flexão do ombro, e a progressão é determinada pela conclusão e competência de executar o pilar específico. Essa abordagem baseada em tarefa/critério permite um efeito cascata em direção aos pilares a serem empregados durante a recuperação do atleta. Um instantâneo de como os pilares de reabilitação interagem entre si é mostrado na Figura 22.3.

Por exemplo, quando a ADMAA está entre 60 e 90° de flexão do ombro, normalmente a ADMA estará entre 30 e 60° de flexão do ombro. Isso significa que podemos focar nossa ativação isométrica do manguito rotador em 90°, começando com o cotovelo apoiado. Nossa reabilitação de resistência do manguito rotador está focada em 45° de flexão, começamos os exercícios de CCF na ADMA disponível atualmente e nossa força excêntrica do manguito rotador a 0° flexão de ombro pode ser iniciada. Essencialmente, isso nos permite treinar a resistência, a força do manguito rotador e, posteriormente, a força reativa ao mesmo tempo, mas individualmente em faixas diferentes. Isso garante que estamos direcionando o ombro e o manguito rotador em vários intervalos, o mais cedo e com a maior segurança possível, com as seleções de exercícios adequadas.

Embora, para facilitar, as faixas tenham sido indicadas para permanecer em 0°, 45° e 90° ao exercitar o manguito rotador, na prática o ombro é colocado em várias faixas para garantir que seja treinado em toda a amplitude.

A Figura 22.4 é uma macro representação de como colocaríamos esse efeito cascata em camadas com relação a pilares de reabilitação baseados em exercícios específicos ao longo do caminho de reabilitação.

Lesões de categorias 1 e 2

O método de avaliação ditará onde o atleta iniciará o processo de reabilitação de lesões de ombro das categorias 1 e 2. O programa de cada atleta é projetado em conjunto com suas necessidades individuais.

O objetivo geral para a lesão de categoria 1 é minimizar o tempo perdido com a lesão. Como resultado, a reabilitação deve ser vista mais como uma abordagem baseada em regressão. O primeiro objetivo com uma lesão de categoria 1 é garantir a seleção para o rúgbi dentro de 1 a 2 semanas, colocando o rúgbi como prioridade.

Como segundo objetivo, a restauração da saúde e da função do ombro passa a ser o condutor que permitirá que o atleta volte com segurança ao treinamento completo e, portanto, esteja disponível para a seleção do jogo. Praticamente, isso faz com que todos os outros componentes da reabilitação se tornem modificáveis para atender a esses dois objetivos. Em teoria, isso é realizado regredindo do ponto final da via de reabilitação (*i. e.*, a partir da direita da via) até que o atleta possa tolerar e executar os componentes de um pilar de reabilitação específico com competência. Este então se torna o ponto de partida no processo de reabilitação e progride de volta para o rúgbi, conforme apropriado.

Como mencionado anteriormente, o ponto de partida para lesões da categoria 1 será ditado pela avaliação. Por exemplo, um atleta, com uma fixação completa, apresenta 1 dia pós-jogo sem nenhum mecanismo claro de lesão com dor durante toda a amplitude de movimento de flexão do ombro. A força isolada do seu ombro parece ser inibida pela dor. No entanto, funcionalmente, ele é capaz de realizar uma flexão de alcance total, mas com dor. O uso de uma atividade adicional e/ou uma atividade acessória fornece uma mudança positiva para sua apresentação.

Uma abordagem simples de três estágios é proposta:

1. **Integrar:** integrar atividades adicionais e/ou acessórias que se mostraram eficazes durante a avaliação de sua movimentação sintomática.
2. **Isolar:** isolar seus exercícios de manguito de direção específica. Por exemplo, este atleta apresentou dor à flexão do ombro. Atividades adicionais e/ou acessórias melhoraram o movimento sintomático (p. ex., redução da dor). Portanto, podemos postular que, desafiando ainda mais o manguito posterior com exercícios de reabilitação isolados, esperamos melhorar a apresentação do jogador (p. ex., reduzir a dor).
3. **Potencializar:** potencializa o complexo do ombro. As modificações do programa de ginástica da PSC podem ser usadas conforme apropriado para garantir que um estímulo de força seja mantido enquanto desafia o atleta.

Figura 22.2 Via de reabilitação do ombro.

ADMAA/ADMP (em flexão do ombro)	ADMA (flexão do ombro)	Ativação isométrica o manguito — RE (Amplitude externa RE Belly press)	Ativação isométrica o manguito — RI (Belly press)	Off-feet	Resistência muscular do manguito	Com os pés	Cadeia cinética fechada	Força do manguito — RE	Força do manguito — RI
0	0	Amplitude externa RE Belly press							
0 a 30	0	RE @ 0 / RE neutra / RE de amplitude interna	RI @ 0 / RI neutra / RI de amplitude externa	Roda de bicicleta					
30 a 60	0 a 30	RE @ 45 / RE neutra / RE de amplitude externa / RE de amplitude interna	RI @ 45 / RI neutra / RI de amplitude interna / RI de amplitude externa	Contrarrelógio para distância de duração mais longa / Sem esforços máximos / Sem andar de bicicleta	(Amplitude média, amplitude externa, amplitude interna, amplitude completa) RE @ 0 / Rotações externas em decúbito lateral 1.3×45 a 60 s / 2.3×10 a 12 / 3.3×8 a 10 — (Amplitude interna, aumento gradual para a amplitude externa completa) RI @ 0 / RI em pé com faixas / Cotovelo apoiado progredindo para o cotovelo sem apoio	Tecnologia de velocidade (sem uso de braço – mãos nos quadris/braços cruzados)	Mudanças de peso em pé (apoiado na mesa) / Rolar BG de pé com faixas e miniagachamento	RE @ 0 / RE excêntrica em decúbito lateral / Cotovelo apoiado progredindo para o cotovelo sem apoio	RI @ 0 / RI excêntrica em decúbito lateral/em pé
60 a 90	30 a 60	RE @ 90 / RI neutra / RI de amplitude interna / RI de amplitude externa	RI @ 90 / RI neutra / RI de amplitude interna / RI de amplitude externa	Distância média / Sem ficar em pé / Sem esforços de intensidade máximos	(Faixa média, faixa externa, faixa interna, faixa completa) RE @ 45 / 1.3×45 a 60 s / 2.3×10 a 12 / 3.3×8 a 10 — Amplitude interna, aumento gradual para a amplitude externa completa RI @ 45 / Cotovelo apoiado progredindo para o cotovelo sem apoio	Tecnologia de velocidade pliometria (sem uso do braço – mãos nos quadris/braços cruzados)	Progressão da amplitude do anterior / Belly press		
90 a 120	60 a 90			Qualquer sessão de bicicleta	(Amplitude média, amplitude externa, amplitude interna, amplitude completa) RE @ 45 / 1.3×45 a 60 s / 2.3×10 a 12 / 3.3×8 a 10 — Amplitude interna, aumento gradual para a amplitude externa completa RI @ 45 / Cotovelo apoiado progredindo para o cotovelo sem apoio	Introdução à corrida, caminhada/corrida leve / Tempo/corrida VAM / Introdução ao treinamento de velocidade e agilidade	Deslocamento de peso ajoelhado 4 apoios / Shoulder tap ajoelhado 4 apoios / Posição bear crawl / Posição bear crawl com shoulder tap / Bear crawl – linear / Bear crawl – linear + lateral / Rotações de bear crawl ± linear/lateral	RE @ 45	RI @ 45
120 a 150	90 a 120				RE @ 90 / RE prona / 1. Amplitude média a externa / RE supina / 1. Amplitude média a interna / 2. Aumente a amplitude externa conforme possível / RE em pé / 1. Amplitude média a interna / 2. Aumente a amplitude externa conforme possível	Condicionamento com corrida de velocidade e agilidade	Caminhada na parede / Movimento de "mexer na panela" na bola de pilates / Movimento walkout na bola de pilates / Exercício pike invertido / Movimento walkout em pike invertido	Cotovelo apoiado progredindo para o cotovelo sem apoio	
A partir de	120 a 150				RI @ 90 / RI prona / 1. Amplitude média a interna / RI supina / 1. Amplitude média a interna / 2. Aumente a amplitude externa conforme possível / RI em pé / 1. Amplitude externa ao máximo possível	Sessões de condicionamento específico de esporte/posição	BG pike / BG pike com shoulder tap ondulado	RE @ 90 / RE supina/prona excêntrica em decúbito lateral	RI @ 90 / RI supina/prona excêntrica
	A partir de				Cotovelo apoiado progredindo para o cotovelo sem apoio		Ponta-cabeça apoiado na parede / Ponta-cabeça apoiado na parede com elevações alternadas de mãos (e variações) / Ponta-cabeça / Caminhada em ponta-cabeça		Cotovelo apoiado progredindo para o cotovelo sem apoio

Figura 22.2 Via de reabilitação do ombro. ADMAA, amplitude de movimento assistida ativa; ADMA, amplitude de movimento ativa; ADMA, amplitude de movimento ativa; ADMP, amplitude de movimento passiva; BR, barra; BD, braço duplo; HT, halteres; RE, rotação externa; BG, bola de ginástica; RI, rotação interna; KB, Kettlebell; VAM, velocidade aeróbica máxima; CCA, cadeia cinética aberta; ADMP, amplitude de movimento passiva; BU, braço único; LT, levantamento turco; PSC, parte superior do corpo.

Força PSC

Cadeia cinética aberta	Horizontal — Empurrar	Horizontal — Puxar	Vertical — Empurrar	Vertical — Puxar	Força reativa do manguito	Habilidades específicas de esportes/reabilitação (atacantes) — Atacantes	Habilidades específicas de esportes/reabilitação (atacantes) — Defensores	Contato	Rúgbi
Levantamento turco rolamento corporal	**Nível 1 horizontal:** Flexões isométricas (vários graus de flexão do cotovelo)	**Nível 1 horizontal:** Puxar em aparelho com roldana BD / Puxar em aparelho com roldana BU / Aparelho com roldana para exercício horizontal			Bater na bola neutra / Bater na bola neutra para parar o lançamento/recepção da bola	Passando a bola para o fisioterapeuta / Técnica de *scrum* / Técnica de *tackle*	Passando a bola para o fisioterapeuta / Chutar/pegar com fisioterapeuta / Passar com treinador / Técnica de *tackle* chute/recepção com treinadores / Habilidades rúgbi/unidades sem contato	Padrões giratórios defendendo-se no combate corpo-a-corpo/luta corpo-a-corpo (controlado) / introdução de queda controlada / Contato de nível 1	Rúgbi sem contato / Rúgbi de contato com bolsa
1/4 LT / Exercício de CCA específico para a posição	**Nível 2 horizontal:** *Floor press* BR / *Floor press* HT / Supino HT / Flexão de BR (amplitude limitada)	**Nível 2 horizontal:** Remada BU KB/HT	**Nível 1 vertical:** Exercício do tipo *Jammer press*	**Nível 1 vertical:** Tração em aparelho com roldana BU de alto para baixo	45 batidas na bola / 45 batidas na bola para parar, pegar/devolver				
1/2 LT / Exercício de CCA específico para a posição			**Nível 2 vertical:** Desenvolvimento BU HT/KB	**Nível 2 vertical:** Cabo BU puxado para baixo / Cabo BD latido	90 batidas na bola / 90 batidas na bola para parar a bola em posição supina, pegar/devolver a bola / 1/2 ajoelhado, pegar/devolver a bola	Introdução ao levantamento de *line-out* (fisioterapeuta) / *Scrums* de nível 1 / Técnica de *Mauls*	Unidades sem contato / Rúgbi sem contato	Contato de nível 2	
LT completo / Exercício de CCA específico para a posição	**Nível 3 horizontal:** Flexão de braço compesso / Supino HT/KB / Supino BB	**Nível 3 horizontal:** Puxar pesos apoiado em mesa em pronação BR / Puxar peso apoiado em mesa em pronação KB/BR	**Nível 3 vertical:** Prensa militar BR	**Nível 3 vertical:** Barra fixa		Levantamento/recepção em *line-out* / Competição de *Line-out* / *Scrums* de nível 2 / *Mauls* reais / *Scrums* de nível 3 / Rúgbi completo	Rúgbi completo	Contato de nível 3	Rúgbi completo

Figura 22.2 (*Continuação*)

Parte | 2 | Aplicação Clínica

ADMA (flexão do ombro)	Ativação isométrica do manguito rotador		Condicionamento *off feet*	Exercícios de resistência para a musculatura do manguito rotador		Sentido de posição conjunta	Exercícios de força excêntrica do manguito rotador	
	Rotação externa	Rotação interna		Rotação externa	Rotação interna		Rotação externa	Rotação interna
30 a 60°	Iniciado em 90° de elevação do plano escapular 1. Segurar a rotação externa	Iniciado em 90° de elevação do plano escapular 1. Segurar a rotação interna	Sem esforços máximos Sem andar de bicicleta	Iniciado em 45° de elevação do plano escapular 1. Rotação de baixo para cima	Iniciado em 45° de elevação do plano escapular 1. Rotação de cima para baixo	1. Deslizar os braços no chão com direcionamento 2. RE/RI em abdução de 45° com *laser* 3. Exercícios gerais de CCA com direcionamento a *laser*	Iniciado em 45° de elevação do plano escapular 1. RE excêntrica em decúbito lateral/em pé	Iniciado em 45° de elevação do plano escapular 1. RI excêntrica em decúbito lateral/em pé

Figura 22.3 Pilares de reabilitação. *ADMA*, amplitude de movimento ativa; *RE*, rotação externa; *RI*, rotação interna; *CCA*, cadeia cinética aberta.

Pilar	Foco da reabilitação								
Ativação isométrica do manguito rotador	0°	45°	90°	Ativação pré-estimulação (se necessário)					
Resistência da musculatura do manguito rotador	Nada	0°	45°	90°	Ativação pré-estimulação				
Força excêntrica do manguito rotador	Nada	Nada	0°	45°	90°	Abordar déficits		Manutenção	Ganho
Pliometria/força reativa do manguito rotador	Nada	Nada	Nada	0°	45°	90°	90°/90°	Abordar déficits	
Parte superior do corpo (empurrar/puxar horizontalmente)	Nada	Nada	Nada	Introdução a	Hipertrofia	Força	Força máxima	Potência	Ganho
Parte superior do corpo (empurrar/puxar verticalmente)	Nada	Nada	Nada	Nada	Introdução a	Hipertrofia	Força	Força máxima	Potência

Figura 22.4 Tabela de treinamento simultâneo em cascata.

Para lesões de categoria 2, esta é essencialmente uma versão condensada da reabilitação das categorias 3 e 4. O atleta pode não precisar regredir totalmente para o início do caminho, uma vez que seu ponto de partida, semelhante às lesões de categoria 1, é específico para sua apresentação. A principal diferença com essas lesões é que, inicialmente, elas são incapazes de completar as sessões de rúgbi; portanto, a reabilitação torna-se o foco principal.

Ativação isométrica do manguito rotador

A ativação isométrica do manguito rotador pode começar desde o início do processo de reabilitação. Isso fornece um baixo nível de estímulo para a musculatura do manguito rotador (Figura 22.5).

No pós-operatório, ainda na tipoia, exercícios isométricos de rotação interna e externa podem ser concluídos com o lado contralateral fornecendo resistência de baixo nível. Como o exercício é ditado pelo esforço percebido e conforto do atleta, essa pode ser uma maneira segura de iniciar a reabilitação. Esse exercício pode progredir em vários intervalos, conforme apropriado. Isso se torna um precursor para iniciar a resistência do manguito rotador de baixo nível.

Exercícios de resistência da musculatura do manguito rotador

Conforme mencionado anteriormente, o manguito rotador desempenha um importante papel funcional e de estabilidade na articulação do ombro. Sem um manguito rotador que funcione

adequadamente e que possua as características de resistência, força e potência exigidas, é provável que ele seja exposto durante o esporte e o risco de lesões seja maior. Antes de desenvolver a força do manguito rotador e as características de potência, é importante primeiro garantir que ele tenha desenvolvido uma sólida capacidade de resistência. Essencialmente, esta capacidade de resistência é a pedra angular sobre a qual as características de desempenho do manguito rotador e força e potência globais serão construídas durante a reabilitação do atleta (Figura 22.6).

Ao planejar e realizar o exercício, é importante garantir que o atleta esteja ciente de que a área relevante é trabalhada; por exemplo, ao realizar um exercício de rotação externa, os motores primários devem ser o manguito posterior (redondo menor, supraespinal, infraespinal). Portanto, o indivíduo deve ser capaz de identificar uma queimação profunda na região posterior do manguito, em vez de sentir o deltoide posterior ou o trapézio superior principalmente em contato. Se o manguito posterior não for sentido, reorganizar a tarefa, reduzir a resistência ou minimizar a amplitude do movimento pode ser útil para envolver o manguito. É importante obter esse *feedback* do atleta, pois a falha em fazê-lo pode resultar em hiperatividade em outro grupo muscular, promoção de mais disfunção ou atraso no processo de RAJ. Além disso, qualquer combinação de atividades acessórias e/ou adicionais que tenham um efeito positivo no movimento sintomático do indivíduo ou na tarefa significativa pode ser adicionada, se necessário.

Em consonância com o objetivo de aumentar a resistência, a prescrição de exercícios exige que o atleta seja essencialmente capaz de realizar várias repetições de um exercício de baixa carga. Com o aumento da competência e com a resistência aprimorada, o intervalo de tempo será reduzido e substituído por faixas de

Reabilitação do Ombro no Rúgbi: Proposta de Abordagem para o Manejo — Capítulo | 22 |

Exercícios isométricos de ativação do manguito rotador							
0°Flexão/abdução do ombro		0° Flexão do ombro		45° de elevação do plano escapular		90° de elevação do plano escapular	
Rotação externa	Rotação interna	Rotação externa	Rotação interna	Rotação externa	Rotação interna	Rotação externa	Rotação interna
Seleção de exercícios							
1. RE amplitude externa iso	*Belly press* isométrica (RI amplitude interna)	1. Segurar a rotação externa	1. Segurar a rotação interna	1. Segurar a rotação externa	1. Segurar a rotação interna	1. Segurar a rotação externa	1. Segurar a rotação interna
Realizado com tipoia		Executado quando retirar a tipoia					
Progressão do exercício							
Não aplicável		1. RE de amplitude média 2. RE de amplitude interna Comece com o cotovelo apoiado, progredindo para cotovelo sem apoio	1. RI de amplitude média 2. RI de amplitude externa	1. RE de amplitude média 2. RE de amplitude interna 3. RE de amplitude externa Comece com o cotovelo apoiado, progredindo para cotovelo sem apoio, progrida para abdução/flexão do ombro a 45°		1. RE de amplitude média 2. RE de amplitude interna 3. RE de amplitude externa Comece com o cotovelo apoiado, progredindo para cotovelo sem apoio, progrida para abdução/flexão do ombro a 90°	
Prescrição de exercícios							
1. 3 × 10 s, manter 2. 3 × 20 s, manter 3. 3 × 30 s, manter Aumente a resistência conforme apropriado							
Qualquer combinação de atividades acessórias ou adicionais pode ser acrescentada, se necessário e apropriado, mas deve ser interrompida antes de progredir							

Figura 22.5 Exercícios isométricos de ativação do manguito rotador. *RE*, rotação externa; *RI*, rotação interna.

Exercícios de resistência do manguito rotador					
0° flexão do ombro		45° de elevação do plano escapular		90° de elevação do plano escapular	
Rotação externa	Rotação interna	Rotação externa	Rotação interna	Rotação externa	Rotação interna
Seleção de exercícios					
1. Rotações externas em decúbito lateral	1. Rotações internas em pé/decúbito lateral	1. Rotação de baixo para cima	1. Rotação de cima para baixo	1. Rotações supinas 2. Rotações pronas 3. Movimento de arqueiro 4. Rotações externas em pé	1. Rotações supinas 2. Rotações pronas 3. Rotações internas em pé
Progressão do exercício					
1. Amplitude média 2. Amplitude média a interna 3. Aumente a amplitude externa conforme possível Comece com o cotovelo apoiado, progredindo para cotovelo sem apoio		1. Amplitude média 2. Amplitude média a interna 3. Aumente a amplitude externa conforme possível Comece com o cotovelo apoiado, progredindo para cotovelo sem apoio; comece em 45° de elevação do plano escapular, progrida para a abdução horizontal		1. Amplitude média 2. Amplitude média a interna 3. Aumente a amplitude externa conforme possível Comece com o cotovelo apoiado, progredindo para cotovelo sem apoio, comece em 45° de elevação do plano escapular, progrida para a abdução horizontal	
Prescrição dos exercícios					
1. 3 × 20 a 30 s 2. 3 × 30 a 45 s 3. 3 × 15 a 20 repetições Aumente o peso/resistência conforme apropriado					
Qualquer combinação de atividades acessórias relevantes ou adicionais pode ser adicionada se necessário e apropriado, mas deve ser interrompida antes de progredir					

Figura 22.6 Exercícios de resistência do manguito rotador.

repetições específicas – normalmente, isso ocorre em linha com um aumento na carga levantada. Isso auxilia na transição e na mudança de foco para o desenvolvimento das características de força do manguito rotador durante o processo de reabilitação.

Sentido de posição articular (propriocepção)

Propriocepção é o sentido da posição relativa das partes do corpo de uma pessoa. A pesquisa e a experiência clínica sugerem que a sensação da posição da articulação do ombro (PAO) ou propriocepção é alterada em esportes de contato (Herrington et al., 2008; Morgan e Herrington, 2013). O contato resulta na redução do *feedback* dos mecanorreceptores em faixas externas após o ataque. Esses déficits sensorimotores aumentam potencialmente o risco de lesões em jogadores de rúgbi devido às repetidas demandas de contato do esporte. Durante o processo de reabilitação é necessário desenvolver essa característica desafiando os sistemas PAO a fim de ajudar a criar um atleta mais robusto (Figura 22.7).

Durante o processo de reabilitação, especialmente para aqueles com lesões de longa duração ou problemas crônicos contínuos, deve-se tomar cuidado para garantir que essa área não seja esquecida. A avaliação simples de PAO e propriocepção, como exercícios de direcionamento de rotação interna/externa, pode ser usada como uma ferramenta de avaliação e intervenção de tratamento. Esses exercícios são tipicamente introduzidos como um exercício de cadeia fechada em que o indivíduo deve mirar em certos marcadores, primeiro com os olhos abertos e, em seguida, após várias repetições, os olhos são fechados e é solicitado que movam a mão para um ponto específico. Isso pode ser medido objetivamente simplesmente medindo a distância do alvo até um determinado ponto em sua mão (p. ex., o segundo dedo). Da mesma maneira, durante os movimentos de rotação externa/rotação interna (RE/RI), um *laser* pode ser adicionado com o indivíduo sendo solicitado a realizar o movimento de rotação enquanto aponta o *laser* para um ponto fixo. Isso pode ser progredido pela adição de movimentos compostos do ombro em vários intervalos para desafiar ainda mais o atleta.

Exercícios de cadeia cinética fechada

Os exercícios em CCF ou em cadeia fechada são exercícios realizados em que a mão (para o movimento do braço) ou o pé (para o movimento da perna) está fixo no espaço e não pode se mover. A extremidade permanece em contato constante com a superfície imóvel, geralmente o solo ou a base de uma máquina. O oposto dos exercícios CCF são os exercícios de CCA.

Os exercícios de CCF são uma faceta vital da reabilitação do ombro do rúgbi. Isso é mais benéfico ao lidar com um ombro instável e pode progredir facilmente de CCF para CCA e para um treinamento específico para o esporte (Figura 22.8). Os exercícios de CCF aumentam as forças compressivas na articulação glenoumeral, o que por sua vez aumenta a propriocepção articular. Há também melhora na ativação muscular, principalmente na musculatura posterior do manguito rotador. Deve-se ter cuidado ao utilizar esses exercícios com atletas

que apresentam instabilidade posterior; no entanto, isso não é uma contraindicação.[1]

Os exercícios de CCF podem começar no estágio inicial de reabilitação quando o atleta tem ADMA mínima na flexão do ombro. As mudanças de peso em pé sobre uma cama (Figura 22.9 A) podem ser iniciadas e progredidas de acordo com a tabela a seguir. O treinamento no solo também é uma boa opção para a progressão quando o atleta tem 90° de ADMA na flexão do ombro. Para nós, o treino começa com exercícios de joelhos de quatro pontos e progride para posições de engatinhamento como *bear crawl* (Figura 22.9 B). A incorporação de mudanças de peso e variações de braço único (BU) ao *bear crawl* ajuda a melhorar o controle de BU na sustentação de peso. Adicionar tapinhas de ombro (Figura 22.9 C) e uma superfície instável para as pernas/pés do atleta (como uma bola de ginástica) são boas opções para aumentar a dificuldade do exercício. Os exercícios progredirão de posições estáticas de *bear crawl* para *bear crawl* em movimento linear e lateral e, eventualmente, para *bear crawl* multidirecional, incluindo rotações.

À medida que o alcance do atleta aumenta para > 120°, progredimos o atleta para posições invertidas, como uma posição carpada e, eventualmente, a parada de mão na parede com o objetivo de fazê-la sem sustentação total. Alguns atletas progredirão na caminhada em parada de mão. Essa é uma boa meta e um desafio para o atleta; afinal, embora ele nunca esteja nessa posição durante a competição, ela fornece confiança a ele, que sabe que pode apoiar e controlar seu peso corporal acima de sua cabeça em um exercício de caminhada em pé.

Força excêntrica do manguito rotador

Uma vez que a capacidade de resistência tenha progredido, o desenvolvimento da força é necessário para permitir que o ombro seja capaz de produzir e absorver as forças às quais será exposto durante um exigente jogo de alto contato de rúgbi de quinze. Essas características de força do manguito rotador aumentam a estabilidade do ombro, ao mesmo tempo em que fornecem a base na qual a força geral do ombro pode ser desenvolvida.

Ao evidenciar o fortalecimento do manguito rotador, focamos no componente excêntrico do movimento como um método mais rápido para desenvolver força. Ao realizar movimentos concêntricos/excêntricos padrão, o peso máximo levantado é sempre limitado pelo componente concêntrico, com as forças geradas pelo componente excêntrico de uma contração muscular sendo 50% maiores do que o componente concêntrico (Hortobágyi et al., 2001). Apenas o treinamento excêntrico fornece um caminho mais rápido para recuperar ou desenvolver a força concêntrica (Brandenburg e Docherty, 2000) (Figura 22.10).

Também observamos que o treinamento excêntrico reduz o potencial de ocorrência de estratégias compensatórias e melhora a adesão do desafio apresentado ao atleta. Esse é provavelmente o primeiro exercício desde o início da lesão em que o atleta sente que está sendo desafiado ao máximo. Como seria de se esperar, um jogador profissional de rúgbi adora ser desafiado, especialmente fisicamente, então a adição de força excêntrica fornece uma saída para isso.

---

[1] Comumente os exercícios em CCF são multiarticulares, tendo maior proximidade com funções diferenciadas, enquanto os exercícios em CCA são uniarticulares, trabalhando mais uma musculatura específica do que uma função.

Reabilitação do Ombro no Rúgbi: Proposta de Abordagem para o Manejo **Capítulo 22**

Sensação de posição articular		
ADMA 0 a 30°	ADMA 30 a 60°	ADMA 60 a 90° +
Seleção e progressão de exercícios		
1. Deslizamento do braço sobre a mesa com direcionamento	1. Deslizamento sobre o chão com direcionamento	1. Deslizamento na parede em pé com direcionamento
2. Exercícios de RE/RI a 0° com direcionamento com *laser*	2. Exercícios de RE/RI a 45° de abdução com direcionamento com *laser*	2. Exercícios de RE/RI a 90° de abdução/elevação do plano escapular com direcionamento com *laser*
3. Exercícios gerais de CCA com direcionamento a *laser*	3. Exercícios gerais de CCA com direcionamento a *laser*	3. Exercícios gerais de CCA com direcionamento a *laser*

Figura 22.7 Sensação de posição articular. *ADMA*, amplitude de movimento ativa; *RE*, rotação externa; *RI*, rotação interna; *CCA*, cadeia cinética aberta.

Exercícios de cadeia cinética fechada			
0 a 60° flexão do ombro	60 a 90° abdução do ombro	90 a 120° abdução do ombro	120° – ATDM flexão do ombro
Seleção de exercícios			Seleção e progressão de exercícios
1. Mudanças de peso em pé (apoiado na mesa)	1. Mudanças de peso ajoelhado de 4 apoios	1. Caminhada na parede e/ou 2. Rolar a bola de pilates com os joelhos	1. *Inchworm* pequeno 2. Exercício *pike* com bola de pilates 3. Exercício *pike* com bola de pilates tocando o ombro alternadamente 4. *Inchworm* completo
Progressões de exercícios			5. Manter a posição carpada 6. *Pike* com batidas de ombro alternadas 7. Flexão na posição carpada 8. Manter a posição de ponta-cabeça apoiando na parede 9. Manter a posição de ponta-cabeça apoiando na parede e alternando a mão no chão 10. Manter a posição de ponta-cabeça sem apoiar na parede 11. Caminhada de ponta-cabeça
1. Adicionar rolar na bola de pilates (aumentar ADM – ativamente) 2. Adicionar segurar a faixa isométrica (aumentar a atividade posterior do manguito) 3. Adicionar miniagachamento (aumentar ADM – passivamente) Aumente a amplitude/resistência conforme possível	1. Tocar os ombros alternadamente 2. Tocar no mostrador do relógio 3. Rastejamento linear 4. Rastejamento lateral 5. Rastejamentos multidirecionais 6. Rastejamentos reativos Posição inicial de joelhos, progrida para os dedos dos pés (posição *bear crawl*)	1. Adicionar segurar a faixa isométrica 2. a. Completar na ponta dos pés b. Adicionar segurar a faixa isométrica	
Prescrição de exercícios			
1. 3 × 10 a 20 s 2. 3 × 20 a 30 s 3. 3 × 30 a 45 s			Devido à variedade de progressões de exercícios utilizadas, é difícil de definir. Normalmente, os exercícios começam com durações fixas para manter as posições (p. ex., 10 segundos), intervalos de repetição específicos (p. ex., 6 a 8) para os toques/elevações e distância definida para a caminhada (p. ex., 5 metros). Estes são progredidos conforme apropriado.

Figura 22.8 Exercícios de cadeia cinética fechada. *ATDM*, amplitude total de movimento; *ADM*, amplitude de movimento.

O momento da sessão é uma consideração importante para o treinamento de força excêntrica. A introdução do reforço do manguito excêntrico é tipicamente introduzida em torno dos estágios de reabilitação, uma vez que é evidente a resistência suficiente do manguito. Nessa fase, o planejamento e a colocação são mais fáceis quando o treinamento de rúgbi não está envolvido: 2 dias por semana é normalmente um bom ponto de partida, como uma introdução ao treinamento de força do manguito com base excêntrica, para que o atleta se recupere entre as sessões. Assim que o atleta se acostumar ao desafio dos exercícios excêntricos, podem ser introduzidos dias alternados, o que permite 3 dias de treinamento de força por semana. Isso é importante por uma série de razões, mas principalmente para criar um atleta mais robusto e durável, pois reduz a probabilidade de novas lesões, e também auxilia na criação de um atleta mais dominante no campo de rúgbi.

A abordagem adotada e os exercícios que normalmente são utilizados complementam o trabalho de resistência do manguito. Tentamos não complicar as coisas e simplesmente carregar os exercícios de resistência do manguito e seguir os parâmetros padrão de treinamento de força e periodização. Isso é benéfico porque, após a conclusão do programa de resistência do manguito, sabemos que o atleta completou várias repetições do mesmo exercício ou de um exercício semelhante. Por causa dessa familiaridade, é possível ter certeza de que eles podem manter uma boa técnica, o exercício não agrava a lesão subjacente e, além disso, fornece uma medida para quantificar a progressão desde o início da reabilitação. Com essa abordagem, ao isolar o manguito enquanto adiciona carga pesada, estamos confiantes de que somos capazes de direcionar especificamente o manguito rotador mais do que os motores principais globais do ombro. No entanto, é importante garantir que você continue questionando o jogador "O que você acha que está funcionando?" ou "Onde está a queimação?", por exemplo, se ele estiver sentindo outras estruturas (p. ex., deltoide posterior) trabalhando mais do que o manguito posterior durante um exercício de rotação externa, a configuração do exercício deve ser alterada ou a carga modificada.

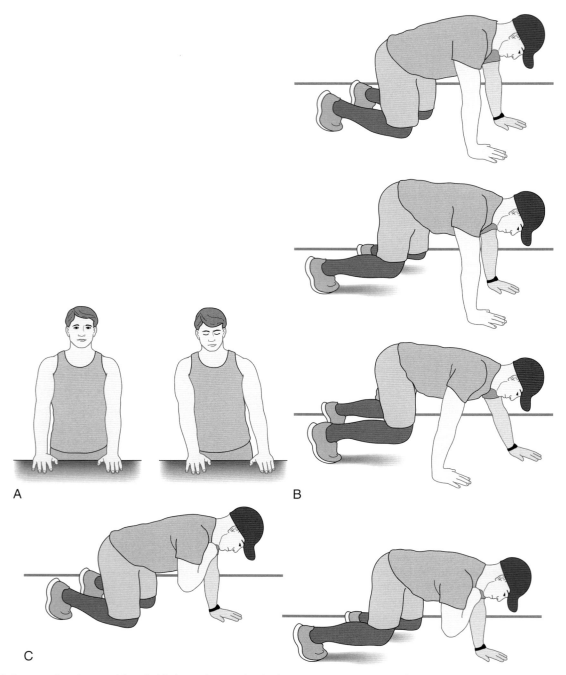

Figura 22.9 Progressões de exercícios. A. Mudança de peso de pé sobre uma cama. **B.** Posições de rastejamento de urso (*bear crawl*). **C.** Toques de ombro.

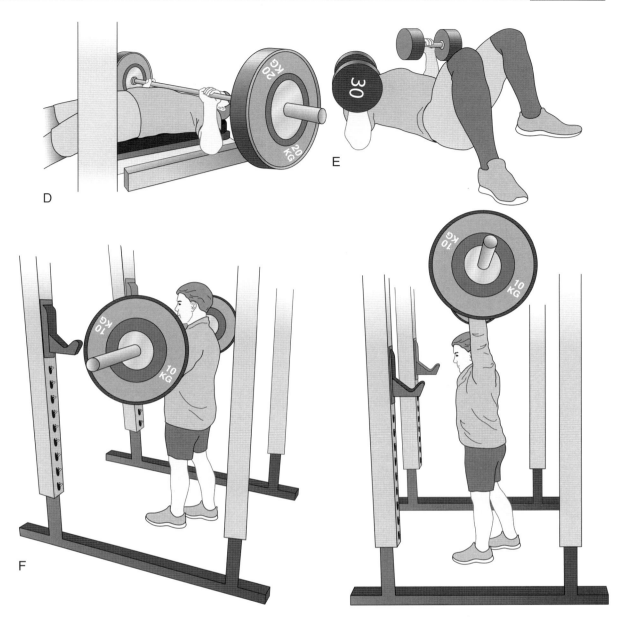

Figura 22.9 (*Continuação*) D. Posição inferior do supino. **E.** *Floor press.* **F.** *Military press.*

Conforme abordado, a seleção de exercícios excêntricos visa espelhar a seleção de exercícios de resistência. Deve-se tomar cuidado para garantir que toda a amplitude seja alcançada – que o atleta esteja trabalhando excentricamente desde a rotação externa completa até a rotação interna completa, enquanto controla a ação de abaixamento ou a ação excêntrica. Esse tempo de descanso pode ser usado de maneira produtiva, com o atleta completando outro exercício de reabilitação de ombro ou um exercício para a parte inferior do corpo. Isso ajuda na adesão pelo atleta, pois garante que a sessão de reabilitação não se torne proibitivamente longa.

Devido às demandas do exercício, o reabilitador deve funcionar como um motivador para estimular continuamente o atleta a controlar a fase excêntrica. Não é incomum trabalhar perto do fracasso com este tipo de treinamento, então o reabilitador deve avaliar a qualidade das repetições e responder adequadamente por:

1. Aumentar o incentivo ao atleta (intenção).
2. Reduzir as repetições solicitadas durante a série.
3. Selecionar um peso mais leve antes do início da próxima série.
4. Aumentar a carga.

Exercícios de cadeia cinética aberta

Embora uma grande proporção dos exercícios de reabilitação de ombro se concentre no desenvolvimento de resistência e força isoladamente, é importante incorporar os exercícios de CCA durante o processo de reabilitação. Este tipo de intervenção desafia a capacidade do jogador de controlar um peso não fixo durante o levantamento. Esses exercícios desafiam a integração do manguito rotador e a função global do ombro, o que auxilia na preparação do ombro do atleta para a natureza incontrolável do esporte (Figura 22.11).

Parte | 2 | Aplicação Clínica

Exercícios de força excêntrica do manguito rotador					
0° flexão/abdução do ombro		**45° de elevação do plano escapular**		**90° de elevação do plano escapular**	
Rotação externa	**Rotação interna**	**Rotação externa**	**Rotação interna**	**Rotação externa**	**Rotação interna**
Seleção de exercícios					
1. RE excêntrica decúbito lateral/em pé	1. RI excêntrica decúbito lateral/em pé	1. Rotação de baixo para cima	1. Rotação de cima para baixo	1. RE excêntrica em supino 2. RE excêntrica prona 3. RE excêntrica em pé 4. Posição de arqueiro excêntrico 5. Baixar o braço reto em decúbito lateral	1. RI excêntrica em supino 2. RI excêntrica prona 3. RI excêntrica em pé
Progressões de exercício					
1. Amplitude média 2. Amplitude interna a média 3. Aumente a amplitude externa conforme possível Cotovelo apoiado progredindo para o cotovelo sem apoio		1. Amplitude média 2. Amplitude interna a média 3. Aumente a amplitude externa conforme possível Cotovelo apoiado progredindo para o cotovelo sem apoio Comece o exercício com elevação do plano escapular, progrida para a abdução horizontal (45 ou 90°)			
Prescrição de exercícios					
1. 3 × 6 a 8 repetições 2. 3 × 4 a 6 repetições 3. 4 × 4 a 6 repetições 5 s mais baixo Começando 2 vezes/semana, aumentando para 3 vezes/semana		1. 3 × 6 a 8 repetições 2. 3 × 4 a 6 repetições 3. 4 × 4 a 6 repetições 5 s mais baixo Começando 2 vezes/semana, aumentando para 3 vezes/semana		1. 3 × 6 a 8 repetições 2. 3 × 4 a 6 repetições 3. 4 × 4 a 6 repetições 5 s mais baixo Começando 2 vezes/semana, aumentando para 3 vezes/semana	

Figura 22.10 Exercícios de força excêntrica do manguito rotador.

Exercícios de cadeia cinética aberta			
60 a 90° flexão do ombro	**90 a 120° flexão de ombro**	**120 a 150° flexão do ombro**	**Flexão do ombro com ATDM**
Seleção de exercícios e progressões			
1. Levantamento turco (LT) sem peso com *body roll* 2. LT com KB e *body roll* 3. LT com KB e *body roll* de baixo para cima	1. 1/4 de LT 2. Início de exercícios CCA específicos para a posição na amplitude disponível	1. 1/2 LT 2. Progressão de exercícios CCA específicos para a posição na amplitude disponível	1. LT completo 2. Progressão de exercícios CCA específicos para a posição na amplitude disponível

Figura 22.11 Exercícios de cadeia cinética aberta. *ATDM*, amplitude total de movimento; *KB*, *Kettlebell*; *CCA*, cadeia cinética aberta.

Praticamente, isso envolveria ter o jogador realizando uma atividade em um ambiente de reabilitação que espelha uma tarefa específica do rúgbi. A abordagem utilizada normalmente começa com um exercício simples de CCA e progride conforme apropriado para desafiar continuamente o atleta. O objetivo é expor de modo gradual e cada vez mais o jogador a uma tarefa específica do esporte em um ambiente altamente controlado como um precursor para realizar a atividade em um cenário controlado (p. ex., habilidades de rúgbi, retorno ao contato) antes de expor o jogador aos cenários caóticos incontroláveis que ocorrem durante o treinamento e os jogos de rúgbi.

A criação do exercício envolve a compreensão do papel e das demandas da posição em questão, um exemplo do qual é demonstrado na Tabela 22.5. A integração de exercícios de reabilitação que reproduzem uma tarefa do jogo permite que a intenção específica do esporte seja adicionada ao exercício.

Força da parte superior do corpo

Um dos principais objetivos de qualquer reabilitação é retornar o atleta às funções completas o mais rápido e de modo mais seguro possível. A força da PSC é vital no tratamento de lesões nos ombros, para permitir que resistam às demandas do jogo. Quando possível, é importante a reintegração imediata em um programa de ginástica modificado para a PSC, que então progride

Tabela 22.5 Posições de rúgbi, demandas relacionadas com o jogo e atividades de reabilitação e fortalecimento.

Posição	Demanda de jogo	Atividade de reabilitação
Pilar (prop)	Levantamento em *line-out*	Usando faixa elástica, realizar agachamento de desenvolvimento
Segunda linha/flanco	Recepção em *line-out*	Erguer o *kettlebell* acima da cabeça e caminhar
Scrum-half	Passe com a mão	Afundo lateral para arremesso de bola de pilates
Asa	*Hand-off* durante a quebra de linha	Afundo para frente em aparelho com cabos

236

Reabilitação do Ombro no Rúgbi: Proposta de Abordagem para o Manejo | Capítulo | 22 |

para retornar o atleta a um programa de ginástica completo. É aqui que uma boa colaboração multidisciplinar desempenha um papel fundamental.

Desde o início, uma vez que o atleta retorna à força da PSC, o objetivo deve ser devolvê-lo aos níveis de força pré-lesão, bem como aos levantamentos da PSC pré-lesão de escolha (p. ex., exercícios horizontais de afastar pesos da direção do torso do tipo *horizontal push* – supino, supino vertical sentado – barra, levantamento de peso do tipo *bench pull*). Isso pode ser alcançado seguindo o modelo de regressão/progressão (Tabela 22.6), normalmente começando com o exercício mais regressivo e progredindo na seleção de exercícios conforme apropriado.

Exercícios horizontais do tipo *horizontal push*

O supino continua sendo o principal exercício de levantamento horizontal na maioria dos programas de ginástica. Em termos de regressão desse exercício, o supino com halteres (HT) é considerado uma opção viável, pois mantém a resistência em toda a extensão, enquanto fornece ao jogador a capacidade de alterar a posição do braço para maior conforto. Como uma regressão, um exercício de CCF seria uma boa opção devido às demandas reduzidas de estabilidade exigidas, como uma flexão ponderada, novamente a posição e a largura da mão podem ser manipuladas para maior conforto. Em nossos atletas, uma flexão de peso corporal normalmente equivale a 55 a 60% do peso corporal, portanto, esse valor pode ser utilizado como um guia para prescrever cargas de resistência com segurança. Pode ser colocado peso adicional nas costas do indivíduo e, embora seja uma regressão do supino, ainda pode ser carregado com muito peso em toda a extensão do ombro.

Alguns jogadores sentirão dor na posição inferior do supino (ver Figura 22.9 D). Nesses casos, funciona bem reduzir o alcance de sua elevação. Inicialmente, gostaríamos de tentar o uso de um bloco sobre o tórax para reduzir a altura de modo que o alcance seja de aproximadamente três quartos do supino completo. No entanto, se mais restrição for necessária, uma *floor press* é uma boa opção (ver Figura 22.9 E). Em nossa experiência,

pouquíssimos jogadores, mesmo aqueles com ombros extremamente doloridos, são incapazes de tolerar uma *floor press* com braço duplo (BD). As opções BD e BU são outras opções viáveis na manipulação do estímulo, bem como no manejo de séries e repetições.

Pull up horizontal

Puxar tende a ser menos problemático para ombros gravemente feridos. Em termos de *pull up* horizontal, é importante garantir um exercício da PSC primário bilateral com tração na PSC acessório unilateral (ver Tabela 22.6).

Um *bench pull* com barra em posição prona continua sendo o principal levantamento para a maioria dos programas. Infelizmente, não é possível atingir a faixa completa devido ao posicionamento da barra de suporte da bancada. O uso de *kettlebells* (KB) é uma boa alternativa, devido à capacidade de puxar até a faixa final, enquanto uma pegada mais ampla garante conforto.

A remada curvada pode ser utilizada para atletas que têm dificuldade para deitar-se de bruços, como aqueles com lesões na articulação esternoclavicular, algumas lesões na parede torácica anterior ou entorses acromioclaviculares (EAC). Preferimos usar uma *pull up* horizontal baseada em cabo fixo; novamente, isso pode ser utilizado como BD/BU. Também é possível variar a altura da resistência do cabo para incorporar uma fileira alta a baixa e direcionar os afastadores escapulares inferiores. Uma remada na altura do peito ou uma puxada de baixo para cima fornece um estímulo semelhante a uma remada curvada para cima. O tipo e o posicionamento do punho podem ser alterados para maior conforto.

Exercícios verticais do tipo *vertical push*

Dadas as demandas do rúgbi de 15 profissional, as posições acima da linha horizontal do ombro representam o maior risco de desenvolver lesões graves no ombro (p. ex., posição de *tackle*). Portanto, é importante garantir que os atletas tenham

Tabela 22.6 **Modelo de regressão/progressão.**

Nível de dificuldade	Empurrão horizontal	Tração horizontal	Empurrão vertical	Tração vertical
Difícil	Supino com barra	*Bench pull* com KB	*Military press*	Tração na barra fixa com pegada supinada
	Supino HT	*Bench pull* com BR	Desenvolvimento de ombro BD HT/KB	Puxar cabo para baixo BD
	Flexão com peso	Remada BU HT/KB	Desenvolvimento de ombro BD HT/KB	Puxar cabo para baixo AS
	Flexão	Puxar cabo BU	*Jammer press*	Puxar cabo de cima para baixo BU
	Supino com barra e bloco sobre o peito	Remada BD		
	BR na *floor press*			
	HT/KB na *floor press*			
Fácil	Supino horizontal no cabo			

BR, barra; *BD*, braço duplo; *HT*, halteres; *KB*, *Kettlebell*; *BU*, braço único.

uma sobrecarga forte para suportar essas forças. Além disso, deve-se tomar cuidado para garantir que a elevação seja realizada com competência, dados os riscos envolvidos com a pressão acima da cabeça e o potencial para que estratégias compensatórias ocorram, causando estresse nas estruturas anatômicas (p. ex., coluna lombar).

O impulso vertical mais desafiador tecnicamente que utilizamos é o *military press* (ver Figura 22.9 F). É um movimento difícil devido aos riscos mencionados anteriormente; portanto, utilizamos uma prensa vertical BD/BU HT como uma alternativa prontamente disponível. Em vez de desafiar o atleta com um peso maior, uma prensa KB de baixo para cima desafiará o controle do ombro; isso pode ser feito em pé ou sentado. É apropriado alternar entre os levantamentos BD e BU semelhante aos movimentos horizontais.

Geralmente, descobrimos que um exercício de desenvolvimento de ombros do tipo *jammer press* é bem tolerado pela maioria dos atletas e é adequado para sessões de ginástica de equipe, potencialmente devido à sua natureza de cadeia fechada.

Pull-up vertical

Barras fixas continuam a ser o padrão-ouro para o desenvolvimento da força de tração vertical. No entanto, notamos que uma minoria do elenco não realiza este exercício devido a limitações estruturais subjacentes, histórico de lesões anteriores ou falha técnica.

Embora o desenvolvimento da força de puxada acima da cabeça seja uma boa opção, deve-se notar que o exercício é frequentemente realizado de maneira inadequada, a tal ponto que os indivíduos colocam um estresse adicional em outras estruturas anatômicas (p. ex., a região lombopélvica) e geram problemas de padrão muscular que pode causar lesões em outras áreas. No entanto, este é um ótimo exercício de força para a PSC quando executado com proficiência. Ao realizar este exercício, certifique-se de:
- Tornozelo em dorsiflexão
- Pelve neutra (evite inclinação anterior e posterior)
- Tronco em posição correta, ou seja, costelas para baixo, quadril fixo
- Extensão torácica mínima
- Coluna cervical/crânio mantendo-se neutra.

Como uma regressão, podem ser utilizados trações com BU em aparelhos de roldanas, com variações BD empregadas de acordo com a indicação. Conforme mencionado anteriormente, eles podem ser manipulados em termos de posição da parte inferior do corpo (em pé, sentado, ajoelhado, meio ajoelhado) e posição de preensão.

Força reativa do manguito rotador

Até este ponto na reabilitação do atleta, o manguito rotador foi priorizado como um rotador umeral e um estabilizador da articulação glenoumeral. A força reativa do manguito rotador é treinada para desafiar o ombro de uma maneira que replique as demandas do esporte, especificamente vistas em uma situação de *tackle*, onde o complexo do ombro é necessário para absorver grandes forças.

É importante que o manguito seja capaz de reagir de modo rápido e adequado, principalmente na absorção dessas forças, a fim de manter a integridade da articulação durante o ataque e a passagem, que são executados principalmente pelos músculos motores primários globais do complexo do ombro.

Nosso foco ao treinar a força reativa do manguito é predominantemente focado no manguito anterior, seu papel na desaceleração das forças rotacionais externas sobre a cabeça do úmero, especialmente na abdução. Isso ocorre porque a abdução forçada e a rotação externa são um dos mecanismos mais comuns de lesões estruturais graves no ombro (Hart e Funk, 2013). Esses exercícios são progredidos por meio de amplitudes quando apropriado, com o objetivo de melhorar a taxa de desenvolvimento de força (TDF), permitindo assim que o manguito absorva as forças de forma eficiente (Figura 22.12).

Retorno ao jogo

Habilidades específicas de esporte e posição

Da mesma maneira que sobrecarrega sistematicamente o programa de reabilitação de um atleta, deve ser tomado muito cuidado para expor gradualmente o atleta às demandas do esporte após seu retorno da lesão (Figura 22.13).

O processo de reabilitação existe para garantir principalmente que o atleta tenha as características fisiológicas básicas necessárias para participar do jogo. No entanto, sem a exposição gradativa às tarefas específicas do jogo e da posição, o atleta não será capaz de aumentar sua confiança nem de desenvolver mais essas habilidades. Do início ao meio, essas habilidades baseadas no jogo podem ser imitadas no ambiente de ginástica para permitir a exposição controlada e fornecer um estímulo de treinamento (p. ex., arremessos laterais de bola medicinal para replicar passes ou desenvolvimento de ombro com barra para replicar levantamento de linha). É importante ressaltar que um jogador precisa ser exposto a essas habilidades o mais rápido possível do ponto de vista médico. Afinal, durante uma reabilitação de médio a longo prazo, há tempo suficiente para desenvolver aspectos de

Exercícios de força reativa do manguito rotador		
0 a 30° flexão do ombro	30 a 90° flexão do ombro	90° + flexão do ombro
Seleção de exercícios e progressões		
1. Bater para parar a bola	1. Bater para parar a bola	1. Bater para parar a bola
2. Lançamento e recepção da bola	2. Pegar/arremessar bola com apoio para o cotovelo	2. Pegar/arremessar a bola meio ajoelhado
	3. Pegar/arremessar bola pesada sem apoio para o cotovelo	3. Pegar/arremessar a bola em supino
Aumente o peso/resistência conforme apropriado		

Figura 22.12 Exercícios de força reativa do manguito rotador.

Reabilitação do Ombro no Rúgbi: Proposta de Abordagem para o Manejo — Capítulo | 22 |

Habilidades específicas de esporte/posição									
30 a 60° flexão do ombro		60 a 90° flexão do ombro		90 a 120° flexão de ombro		120 a 150° flexão do ombro		ATDM flexão do ombro	
Atacantes	Defensores	Atacantes	Defensores	Atacantes	Atacantes	Atacantes	Defensores	Defensores	Atacantes
Análise de vídeo		Introdução à passagem com fisioterapeuta		Pode iniciar habilidades de contato + progressões		Habilidades de contato de nível 2		Habilidades de contato de nível 3	
Revise as próprias habilidades do jogo para destacar os pontos fortes/fracos		Passando com treinadores		Técnica de *scrum* com treinadores	Continue a desenvolver habilidades específicas/ relevantes conforme necessário	Introdução ao levantamento no alinhamento com controle por fisioterapia	Continue a desenvolver habilidades específicas/ relevantes conforme necessário	Competição em *Line-out*	Continue a desenvolver habilidades específicas/ relevantes conforme necessário
Revisão de habilidades com treinadores		Introdução ao chute/pega com fisioterapeuta		Técnica de *Maul*				*Scrum* completo	
Planejamento de desenvolvimento de habilidades com treinadores								*Mauls* reais	
Visualização de habilidade de jogo		Chute/pega com treinadores		Sessões de habilidades sem contato		Sessão de rúgbi modificada sem contato — *Mauls* e *scrums* controlados		Sessões completas de rúgbi	

Figura 22.13 Habilidades específicas do esporte/posição. *ATDM*, amplitude total de movimento.

seu próprio jogo que não sejam de alto risco, como passe, lançamento de alinhamento lateral ou chute.

Retorno às habilidades de contato

Deve-se ter cuidado para expor o atleta a cenários de contato graduados e controlados, progredindo para contato total controlado antes da reintegração no treinamento baseado em equipe. Muito provavelmente a lesão original foi resultado de um cenário de contato. Portanto, essa exposição progressiva ao contato permite não apenas o desenvolvimento da própria confiança do jogador, mas também a confiança de que seu ombro reabilitado pode suportar as demandas do esporte e permitir que ele domine o campo de jogo novamente.

A exposição a um retorno ao contato pode começar cedo. No entanto, é útil ter treinadores de rúgbi qualificados para discutir a técnica adequada, revisar o mecanismo de lesão do jogador e avaliar clipes de vídeo de suas técnicas de *tackle* ou contato durante um período de tempo para destacar quaisquer problemas, de modo que eles possam ser resolvidos durante a reabilitação. O uso de visualização e indicação nos estágios iniciais auxilia nessa exposição precoce e no desenvolvimento de uma técnica de contato aprimorada.

Assim que o atleta for capaz de reiniciar o contato, uma exposição gradativa pode começar, conforme destacado na Figura 22.14. Isso deve ser amplamente baseado em garantir que a técnica de contato e *tackle* seja desenvolvida de um nível corretivo a um alto nível com um técnico de rúgbi habilidoso, quando disponível. A importância do aprimoramento da técnica não deve ser subestimada. A técnica de ataque correta deve permitir que as forças sejam dissipadas por todo o corpo, em vez de isolar o ombro para absorver forças massivas que obviamente aumentarão o risco de nova lesão.

Antes de o atleta ser liberado para retornar ao treinamento de contato total e especialmente antes de ser liberado para retornar ao jogo, pode ser útil discutir abertamente se ele sente que há alguma área em que está inseguro. Abordar isso com antecedência dá tempo para que isso seja resolvido. O resultado dessas discussões pode incluir o aumento da força do manguito ou do ombro global, condicionamento ou confiança em situações de contato.

Apesar de gastar tempo criando critérios de RAJ estruturados e de liderança objetiva, há casos em que os atletas progridem com base na função, em vez de atingir as pontuações objetivas de força. Isso ocorre quando, devido à gravidade da lesão, é improvável que a função total do ombro retorne. Nestes casos, os critérios de RAJ são considerados flexíveis e as decisões são amplamente baseadas em função, desempenho e capacidade de tolerar as demandas do esporte.

Reintegração e retorno ao desempenho

Medidas de resultado

Os principais marcadores de resultados são utilizados para monitorar o progresso durante a reabilitação e fornecer uma medição objetiva sobre qualidades e atributos principais específicos. Na prática, são utilizados testes isolados de força e potência do manguito rotador, juntamente com o teste global de força do ombro. Esses são marcadores importantes para progressões e pontuações; isso será comparado a ambos os escores de força da linha de base e comparações entre os lados lesionados e não lesionados (Figura 22.15).

Um método de teste de força isolado é a dinamometria portátil (DMP). Isso vem com uma advertência: esse método é muito

Habilidades de contato		
Contato de nível 1	**Contato de nível 2**	**Contato de nível 3**
Técnica de queda/rolamento	Introdução aos cenários controlados de contato	Cenários de contato não controlados e ao vivo
Introdução à técnica de *tackle*	Começar a exposição à tomada de decisão/contato enquanto está cansado	Replicação de cenários de contato de jogo sob fadiga
Exposição a posições de desdobramento		Contato "osso com osso"
Contato com almofadas, sacos de espuma	Contato com almofadas, sacos de espuma	Focando em qualquer deficiência destacada na técnica de *tackle*
Construindo confiança e habilidade técnica	Continue a desenvolver confiança e habilidade técnica	
Intenção e intensidade mínimas	Intenção e intensidade crescentes	Intenção e intensidade máximas
Técnica de *scrum* com treinadores	*Scrum* controlado (p. ex., 1 contra 1, 2 contra 2)	*Scrum* completo
Técnica de *maul*	*Mauls* controlados	*Mauls* completos
Liderado por fisioterapeuta, supervisionado pelo técnico	Liderado pelo treinador, supervisionado pelo fisioterapeuta	Liderado pelo treinador, supervisionado pelo fisioterapeuta

Figura 22.14 Habilidades de contato.

239

Parte | 2 | Aplicação Clínica

Retorno a	Marco	Contato	Outras considerações
Habilidades estáticas	ATDM sem dor	Sessões de técnica de *tackle* submáxima de baixo nível, incluindo queda/rolamento. (Foco apenas na técnica)	Visualização do contato – explicação
	Atingindo resistência muscular do manguito a 90°		Avaliações de vídeo da técnica de *tackle* pré-lesão
	Atingindo força do manguito a 45°		Avaliações em vídeo das melhores práticas de técnica de *tackle* (individual/outro)
	Atingindo força reativa do manguito em 0°		Discussão com treinadores
Retorno ao contato nível 1	Força do manguito > 80% (DMP)	Sessões de técnica de *tackle* de baixo nível, incluindo queda/ rolamento. (Foco da técnica com progressão de forças e intenção)	Continue a visualização, revisão de vídeo e discussão com o treinador
	Força BD PSC > 80% da linha de base antes da lesão		Introdução às sessões de habilidades sem contato
	Força BU PSC > 80% do lado não lesionado		Revisão de vídeo de sessões concluídas de técnica de *tackle*
Retorno ao contato nível 2	Força do manguito > 85% (DMP)	Continuando as sessões de técnica de *tackle*. (Foco de competência, forças máximas e intenção. Abordar contatos de almofada/bolsa apenas)	Sessões específicas da posição sem contato (exercícios específicos para jogadores defensivos/ofensivos)
	Força BD PSC > 85% da linha de base pré-lesão		Treinamento de equipe sem contato
	Força BU PSC > 85% do lado não lesionado		
	Conclusão tecnicamente competente do RAC 1		
Retorno ao contato nível 3	Força do manguito > 85% (DMP)	Progressão das sessões de técnica de *tackle*. (Foco no resultado, forças e intenção máximas, cenários de contato total controlado progredindo para situações não controladas ao vivo)	Sessões de unidades sem contato (exercícios específicos para jogadores defensivos/ofensivos)
	Força BD PSC > 85% da linha de base pré-lesão		Treinamento de equipe sem contato
	Força BU PSC > 85% do lado não lesionado		Continue a construir confiança em cenários de contato
	Conclusão tecnicamente competente do RAC 2		Pode participar de exercícios de contato controlado no treinamento
Retorno ao treinamento completo	Força do manguito > 85%	Continuando as sessões de técnica de *tackle*. Conteúdo selecionado com base nas fraquezas ou necessidades do jogador	Participação total no treinamento
	Força BD PSC > 85% da linha de base pré-lesão		Crie confiança com cenários de contato não controlados e ao vivo
	Força BU PSC > 85% do lado não lesionado		Resolva quaisquer problemas/preocupações destacados pelo atleta
	Conclusão tecnicamente competente do RAC 3		
Retorno ao jogo	Força do manguito > 85%	Continuando as sessões de técnica de *tackle*. Conteúdo selecionado com base nas fraquezas ou necessidades do jogador	Considerações sobre o carregamento com o pé
	Força BD PSC > 85% da linha de base pré-lesão		Treinamento com equipe completa sem limitações
	Força BU PSC > 85% do lado não lesionado		Atleta se sente pronto para voltar a jogar
	Tecnicamente competente em cenários de contato ao vivo		
Retorno ao desempenho	Força do manguito > 90%	Continuando as sessões de técnica de *tackle*. Conteúdo selecionado com base nas fraquezas ou necessidades do jogador	Discussão e revisão com treinadores
	Força BD PSC > 90% da linha de base pré-lesão		Treinamento 1:1 com treinadores nos déficits de habilidade destacados
	Força BU PSC > 90% do lado não lesionado		Trabalhar para exceder as linhas de base anteriores (PSC, PIC, condicionamento, habilidades)
	Continue a abordar os déficits		

Figura 22.15 Tabela de reintegração. *BD*, braço duplo; *ATDM*, amplitude total de movimento; *DMP*, dinamometria portátil; *PIC*, parte inferior do corpo; *RAC*, retorno ao contato; *BU*, braço único; *PSC*, parte superior do corpo.

dependente do operador. Por esse motivo, protocolos e procedimentos para garantir que os testes permaneçam padronizados são importantes. Testamos as forças nas rotações interna e externa em três faixas: 0°, 45° e 90° de flexão/abdução do ombro, e no final do caminho também testamos a força nas faixas finais de abdução/rotação externa (90°/90°).

Lesões pós-operatórias no ombro também devem ser testadas com dinamometria isocinética por recomendação do consultor, comparando o pico de torque e a produção de força máxima, juntamente com a análise da curva de força do atleta para destacar quaisquer déficits.

Alternativamente, um esfigmômetro pode ser empregado como um método simples de monitorar os escores de força em termos de pressão (mmHg). Isso pode ser uma opção se os DMP não estiverem prontamente disponíveis.

O teste de força é apenas um componente das medidas de resultado e deve ser visto em conjunto com todos os outros pilares do processo de tomada de decisão. Deve-se ter cuidado para garantir que as decisões de RAJ não sejam baseadas apenas nesses resultados de teste, mas também levem em consideração uma visão holística do atleta (p. ex., competência técnica de *tackle*).

As sessões de técnica de *tackle* podem ser realizadas como sessões autônomas ou integradas a sessões de reabilitação conduzidas por fisioterapeutas. Tarefas simples, como queda ou rolamento controlados, podem ser realizadas em tapetes macios; outras tarefas como defesa, *tackle* controlado em uma espuma de *tackle* e exposição a outros cenários de contato podem ser realizadas. Essas tarefas são muito úteis para ajudar a construir confiança e reduzir a evitação por medo – já que a maioria desses jogadores se machucou em situações de *tackle*. Durante o estágio intermediário a tardio da reabilitação e no RAJ e no retorno

ao desempenho, o *feedback* e a experiência do treinador são um componente valioso. Quando a técnica de *tackle* é pobre, há um grande potencial de lesão, especialmente quando o ombro é colocado em posições de "risco", como as mencionadas anteriormente. Achamos que, se o jogador usar seu corpo de maneira eficaz durante as atividades de rúgbi, as forças às quais o ombro está exposto serão dissipadas por todo o corpo, em vez de se concentrarem em torno da própria articulação do ombro. Este processo é parte integrante do processo de reabilitação. Nenhuma quantidade de resistência do manguito, força do manguito ou força do ombro protegerá adequadamente o ombro quando a técnica de *tackle* é inadequada.

Manejo durante a temporada

Quando as sessões de rúgbi fazem parte da programação semanal de um atleta, o planejamento e a implementação da reabilitação se tornam mais difíceis. O mais desafiador é o manejo de lesões de categorias 2 e 3 durante o período da temporada, onde o objetivo é manejar os sintomas e a reabilitação do jogador, ao mesmo tempo que o torna disponível para seleção.

Esses casos são tratados individualmente, uma vez que nem todas as lesões poderão ser "manejadas" e podem exigir um tempo longe das demandas do rúgbi para permitir que um processo de reabilitação focado ocorra.

A decisão de tentar manejar a lesão de um atleta na temporada não deve ser tomada de modo leviano. O Departamento Médico funciona como uma única engrenagem em um sistema muito maior; por isso, é importante envolver e colaborar com outros departamentos nesse processo, especificamente o Departamento

Reabilitação do Ombro no Rúgbi: Proposta de Abordagem para o Manejo — Capítulo | 22 |

de Força e Condicionamento e a Comissão Técnica. Esta contribuição multidisciplinar garante que todas as partes envolvidas, incluindo o atleta, estejam cientes da lesão, do prognóstico e dos riscos envolvidos no manejo de um atleta durante a temporada.

Todas as partes devem contribuir para o processo de tomada de decisão e auxiliar na criação de uma estrutura para tentar permitir que o atleta seja administrado durante a temporada. Todas as partes devem estar cientes de que, ao administrar a temporada de um atleta, o principal objetivo do rúgbi é garantir a disponibilidade para seleção para os jogos. Consequentemente, deve-se entender que a disponibilidade para o treinamento de rúgbi provavelmente será modificada. Por exemplo, é improvável que um jogador participe de exercícios de treinamento de contato total, e suas sessões de ginástica da PSC serão modificadas para exercícios mais adequados para os ombros, com grande ênfase nos exercícios de reabilitação do ombro.

Fora dos jogos e do treinamento de rúgbi, a maior prioridade do atleta é reabilitar o ombro. Como resultado, isso tem prioridade sobre todos os outros aspectos do treinamento. Isso não quer dizer que o atleta não realize nenhum outro treinamento durante esse período, mas sim qualquer janela de oportunidade disponível para realizar a reabilitação. Na prática, é necessário adotar uma abordagem fluida com a reabilitação; o conteúdo geral do treinamento e as progressões dos exercícios, embora bem pensados e estruturados, frequentemente precisam ser modificados para permitir sua conclusão durante a semana de treinamento agitada. Fora das sessões de reabilitação e força da PSC, a microdosagem de exercícios selecionados pode ser benéfica. Essa é essencialmente uma abordagem "pequena e frequente" – por exemplo, fazer com que o atleta execute 2 a 3 exercícios específicos destinados a lidar com grandes déficits ao longo do dia ou da semana, como antes das sessões de mobilidade, de ginástica ou baseadas em arremesso.

Em última análise, apesar de o objetivo ser "manejar" o atleta, é importante revisar o processo regularmente. Por exemplo, ao tentar controlar a lesão, se o jogador não puder jogar em campo devido à natureza da lesão, então uma abordagem somente de reabilitação ou um contato com o cirurgião ortopédico para obter sua opinião médica pode ser mais adequado.

Conclusão

A estrutura apresentada é considerada útil na prática clínica. No entanto, é essencial que a lesão de cada jogador seja totalmente avaliada e compreendida para garantir que o caminho de reabilitação seguido seja específico para eles, suas lesões, seus déficits individuais, suas demandas esportivas e os recursos disponíveis. O raciocínio clínico e uma abordagem personalizada são sempre fundamentais no manejo de qualquer patologia; a estrutura que propomos não deve ser vista como uma panaceia universal para todos os problemas do ombro.

Referências bibliográficas

Boileau, P., Villalba, M., Hery, J., Balg, F., Ahrens, P., Neyton, L., 2006. Risk factors of shoulder instability after arthroscopic Bankart repair. Journal of Bone & Joint Surgery 88 (8), 1755-1763.

Brandenburg, J.P., Docherty, D., 2002. The effects of accentuated eccentric loading on strength, muscle hypertrophy, and neural adaptations in trained individuals. Journal of Strength and Conditioning Research 16 (1), 25-32.

De Mey, K., Danneels, L., Cagnie, B., Borms, D., T'Jonck, Z., Van Damme, E., et al., 2014. Shoulder muscle activation levels during four closed kinetic chain exercises with and without Redcord slings. Journal of Strength and Conditioning Research 28 (6), 1626-1635.

Escamilla, R.F., Yamashiro, K., Paulos, L., Andrews, J.R., 2009. Shoulder muscle activity and function in common shoulder rehabilitation exercises. Sports Medicine 39 (8), 663-685.

Hart, D., Funk, L., 2013. Serious shoulder injuries in professional soccer: return to participation after surgery. Knee Surgery, Sports Traumatology, Arthroscopy 23 (7), 2123-2129.

Hegedus, E.J., Goode, A., Campbell, S., Morin, A., Tamaddoni, M., Moorman, C.T., et al., 2007. Physical examination tests of the shoulder: a systematic review with meta-analysis of individual tests. British Journal of Sports Medicine 42 (2), 80-92.

Hendricks, S., Matthews, B., Roode, B., Lambert, M., 2014. Tackler characteristics associated with tackle performance in rugby union. European Journal of Sport Science 14, 753-762.

Herrington, L., Horslet, I., Whitaker, L., Rolf, C., 2008. Does a tackling task effect shoulder joint position sense in rugby players? Physical Therapy in Sport 9 (2), 67-71.

Hortobágyi, T., Devita, P., Money, J., Barrier, J., 2001. Effects of standard and eccentric overload strength training in young women. Med Sci Sports Exerc 33 (7), 1206-1212.

May, S., Chance-Larsen, K., Littlewood, C., Lomas, D., Saad, M., 2010. Reliability of physical examination tests used in the assessment of patients with shoulder problems: a systematic review. Physiotherapy 96 (3), 179-190.

McMullen, J., Uhl, T.L., 2000. A kinetic chain approach for shoulder rehabilitation. Journal of Athletic Training 35 (3), 329–337.

Morgan, R., Herrington, L., 2013. The effect of tackling on shoulder joint positioning sense in semi-professional rugby players. Physical Therapy in Sport 1-5.

Mullaney, M.J., Perkinson, C., Kremenic, I., Tyler, T.F., Orishimo, K., Johnson, C., 2017. EMG of shoulder muscles during reactive isometric elastic resistance exercises. The International Journal of Sports Physical Therapy 12 (3), 417-424.

Quarrie, K., Wilson, B., 2000. Force production in the rugby union scrum. Journal of Sports Sciences 18 (4), 237-246.

Reardon, C., Tobin, D.P., Tierney, P., Delahunt, E., 2017. Collision count in rugby union: A comparison of micro-technology and video analysis methods. Journal of Sports Sciences 35 (20), 2028-2034.

Reed, D., Cathers, I., Halaki, M., Ginn, K., 2018. Shoulder muscle activation patterns and levels differ between open and closed-chain abduction. Journal of Science and Medicine in Sport 21 (5), 462-466.

Sciascia, A., Cromwell, R., 2012. Kinetic chain rehabilitation; a theoretical framework. Rehabilitation Research and Practise 1-9.

Seminati, E., Cazzola, D., Preatoni, E., Trewartha, G., 2016. Specific tackling situations affect the biomechanical demands experienced by rugby union players. Journal of Sports Biomechanics 16 (1), 58-75.

Sporrong, H., Lamerud, G., Herberts, P., 1995. Influences on shoulder muscle activity. European Journal of Applied Physiology and Occupational Physiology 71 (6), 485-492.

Sporrong, H., Palmerud, G., Herberts, P., 1996. Hand grip increases shoulder muscle activity: an EMG analysis with static hand contractions in 9 subjects. Acta Orthopaedica Scandinavica 67 (5), 485-490.

Torrance, E., Clarek, C.J., Monga, P., Funk, L., Walton, M.J., 2018. Recurrence after arthroscopic labral repair for traumatic anterior instability in adolescent rugby and contact athletes. The American Journal of Sports Medicine 46 (12), 2969-2974.

Usman, J., McIntosh, A., Fréchède, B., 2014. An investigation of shoulder forces in active shoulder tackles in rugby union football. Journal of Science and Medicine in Sport 14 (6), 547-552.

Wattanaprakornkul, D., Cathers, I., Halaki, M., Ginn, K., 2011a. The rotator cuff muscles have a direction specific recruitment pattern during shoulder flexion and extension exercises. Journal of Science and Medicine in Sport 14 (5), 376-382.

Wattanaprakornkul, D., Halaki, M., Cathers, I., Ginn, K., 2011b. Direction-specific recruitment of rotator cuff muscles during bench press and row. Journal of Electromyography and Kinesiology 21 (6), 1041-1049.

Capítulo | 23 |

Avaliação do Ombro Esportivo

Marcus Bateman

Princípios

Filtro de diagnóstico

Como acontece com qualquer tipo de avaliação clínica, deve haver conhecimento prévio e compreensão do que estamos avaliando. Existe ampla variedade de patologias que podem afetar o ombro, e a nossa avaliação clínica deve ser um meio de estreitar as possibilidades de maneira fundamentada e sistemática para finalmente concluir um único diagnóstico preciso.

Identificação precoce de patologia grave

A primeira prioridade da avaliação deve ser sempre excluir patologias com potencial de perda de vida ou de membros, como infecção, trauma neurovascular grave ou malignidade. Embora essas apresentações, felizmente, sejam raras, as consequências de mudança de vida de diagnósticos perdidos ou atrasados significam que essas patologias devem estar sempre em primeiro plano em nossas mentes. Existem patologias menos graves, e também muito importantes, especificamente relacionadas à cintura escapular, que devem ser consideradas como requerendo intervenção urgente, como rupturas do tendão do peitoral maior e rupturas traumáticas do manguito rotador. Essas lesões requerem reparo cirúrgico precoce para facilitar a cura bem-sucedida e dar a maior chance de retorno ao jogo.

Na ausência de trauma, a primeira patologia a ser excluída é a artrite séptica aguda (infecção de uma articulação). Os pacientes geralmente apresentam um início recente de dor intensa, mesmo em repouso e com movimentos leves do ombro, sintomas de febre, sensação geral de mal-estar e sinais objetivos de inflamação das articulações, como inchaço, aumento do calor e vermelhidão da pele ao redor da articulação.

Histórico

Idade como preditor de patologia

A idade é um fator chave no processo de raciocínio clínico quando se considera a probabilidade de certas patologias. Por exemplo, a capsulite adesiva do ombro (ombro congelado), normalmente é vista em pessoas com idade entre 40 e 60 anos. Ocasionalmente, apresenta-se em indivíduos na faixa dos 30 anos, mas de modo geral está associada ao diabetes tipo 1. Nunca é vista em pessoas com menos de 30 anos; isso também é verdadeiro

para a osteoartrite primária da articulação glenoumeral. Portanto, pacientes jovens que apresentam rigidez e dor nos ombros devem ter um alto índice de suspeita de patologias mais graves, como artropatia inflamatória, artrite séptica ou malignidade. Enquanto a incidência da maioria dos cânceres aumenta com a idade, adolescentes e adultos na casa dos 20 anos têm a maior incidência de osteossarcoma.

O sintoma mais comum de dor no ombro é "impacto" – o paciente descreve uma dor aguda e mecânica durante certas atividades. Esses sintomas são geralmente um sinal de patologia degenerativa do manguito rotador em pacientes com mais de 40 anos, mas nos jovens deve ser considerado um possível sinal de instabilidade "subclínica".

Mecanismo de início

Provavelmente, a parte mais importante do histórico é o mecanismo de início. A ausência de trauma significativo obviamente exclui fraturas, luxação da articulação acromioclavicular (AC) e rupturas do manguito rotador em pacientes com menos de 40 anos. No caso de trauma, é importante determinar a posição do braço no impacto. Por exemplo, um golpe direto no acrômio, como cair de lado de uma bicicleta enquanto ainda segura o guidão ou cair de lado no chão enquanto segura uma bola de rúgbi contra o peito, levanta a suspeita de fratura da clavícula ou deslocamento da articulação AC. Um golpe direto ou queda com o ombro em posição de rotação externa abduzida levanta a suspeita de luxação anterior do ombro. Uma dor súbita e intensa ao levantar peso levanta a suspeita de ruptura do tendão, por exemplo, o peitoral maior ou o bíceps braquial.

Sintomas de instabilidade

É importante entender que instabilidade é diferente de frouxidão. A frouxidão é o movimento excessivo de uma articulação em comparação ao que é considerado normal, enquanto a instabilidade acontece quando essa frouxidão causa sintomas como dor, subluxação ou deslocamento descontrolado e perda de função. Os pacientes podem apresentar sintomas de "choque" de dor aguda em certos intervalos de movimento (geralmente acima da cabeça). Isso é comum a partir da meia-idade como um sintoma de degeneração do manguito rotador. No entanto, em jovens, em especial com menos de 25 anos, é mais provável que seja um sintoma precoce de instabilidade e deve ser correlacionado com achados de exame clínico de frouxidão ou provocação de instabilidade. Em contrapartida, a instabilidade pode ser subluxação ou luxação óbvia de uma articulação, que precisa ser correlacionada com qualquer trauma anterior, pois há um alto risco de lesão estrutural do complexo cápsula-ligamento, que resulta em alta taxa de novas lesões, principalmente em jovens após o trauma. O questionamento subjetivo é muito importante em pacientes com instabilidade significativa, pois a ausência de trauma orienta o caminho do tratamento para o manejo não operatório.

Ocupação (esporte) e risco potencial específico do esporte

Esportes de colisão claramente apresentam maior risco de lesões traumáticas do que esportes sem colisão, mas há outras questões específicas do esporte a serem consideradas. Esportes com alta demanda de ombro incluem aqueles que envolvem arremesso (p. ex., lançamento de dardo, críquete, beisebol, handebol, natação, esportes com raquete e voleibol). Esses esportes praticados repetidamente por anos podem levar a anormalidades adquiridas no ombro por meio de microtrauma ou aumento do risco de certas lesões. Por exemplo, as rupturas anteroposteriores do lábio superior (SLAP, do inglês *superior labrum anterior posterior*), são comumente vistas em esportes de arremesso com um fator subjetivo chave de perda da força/distância de arremesso ou dor ao arremessar. Outra adaptação comum em esportes aéreos é o ganho gradual da rotação externa do ombro com a correspondente perda da rotação interna, denominado déficit de rotação interna glenoumeral (GIRD, do inglês *glenohumeral internal rotation deficit*). Isso pode levar a um maior risco de sintomas de "impacto" no ombro, mas ao contrário daqueles pacientes com frouxidão subjacente, esses pacientes têm restrição à sua amplitude de movimento tanto na rotação interna quanto na amplitude total do arco de rotação.

Localização da dor

A localização da dor pode ser útil no direcionamento do exame clínico. A dor no trapézio superior e nas regiões da borda medial da escápula tem muito mais probabilidade de estar relacionada à coluna cervical do que ao ombro, portanto, o primeiro elemento objetivo do exame deve ser avaliar o pescoço. Às vezes, o paciente localizará a dor com muita precisão e isso é típico de patologia localizada na articulação AC ou no bíceps, quando o paciente aponta diretamente para a área com um dedo. Ocorre com maior frequência, embora a dor seja mais difusa: ou na região do deltoide, que é comum para dor relacionada com o manguito rotador, ou na região da inserção do deltoide no meio do úmero, comum para dor na articulação glenoumeral. Se o paciente descreve uma dor anterior profunda que não é palpável, especialmente com estalo durante o movimento ou uma vaga sensação de que algo está fora do lugar, isso deve levantar suspeitas de ruptura SLAP.

Fatores agravantes

A dor noturna é geralmente considerada um sinal de alerta de patologia grave, mas com relação ao ombro é uma queixa comum. Portanto, é importante esclarecer se isso é puramente posicional, ou seja, acordar ao rolar sobre o ombro afetado, ou se é persistente e não está relacionado com mudanças de posição. O último cenário é uma característica muito comum do ombro congelado, mas pode representar também infecção, tumor ou doença inflamatória das articulações.

Sintomas neurológicos

É raro que pacientes com patologia local do ombro se queixem de sintomas neurológicos. Dores lancinantes ou déficits sensoriais que se estendem abaixo do cotovelo em direção à mão geralmente estão relacionadas à coluna cervical. Uma patologia incomum, mas significativa, que pode atingir pessoas de qualquer idade é a neurite braquial (também conhecida como síndrome de Parsonage-Turner), que pode afetar qualquer um ou vários nervos do plexo braquial. Normalmente, se apresenta como dor nevrálgica intensa na ausência de trauma que pode afetar a cintura escapular ou todo o membro e é mal controlada com analgesia. A causa é incerta, mas ocorre geralmente durante períodos de estresse fisiológico no corpo, como durante uma doença, após uma cirurgia e no parto. A dor inicial é seguida por fraqueza muscular e distúrbios sensoriais dos nervos afetados.

Também é importante perguntar sobre os sintomas neurológicos após um trauma significativo, pois eles podem ser facilmente esquecidos. Isso é particularmente importante após a luxação do ombro (nervo axilar), fraturas da diáfise do úmero (nervo radial), fratura da clavícula e lesões por tração do braço (plexo braquial). Se o paciente reclamar de déficit sensorial ou fraqueza, o exame objetivo deve se concentrar em estabelecer o padrão de déficit neurológico e se isso se relaciona mais a uma radiculopatia cervical, neuropatia ou trauma por compressão de nervo periférico ou uma patologia no nível do plexo.

Exame clínico

Avaliação no campo

Isso deve ser o mais breve possível para evitar interrupções no esporte, mas sempre priorizando a saúde do indivíduo. A avaliação deve incluir a observação da integridade da pele ou perda de sangue direcionada pelo local da dor seguida pela avaliação da deformidade na estrutura óssea, como deslocamento da clavícula ou uma aparência quadrada do deltoide, o que pode indicar luxação da articulação glenoumeral (Figura 23.1). Quaisquer descobertas significativas devem resultar na saída do jogador do

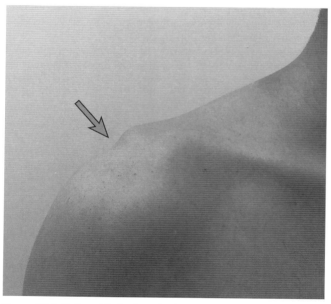

Figura 23.1 Deformidade da articulação acromioclavicular consistente com luxação.

campo para uma avaliação mais detalhada; da mesma maneira, se houver dor significativa com movimento passivo do ombro ou dor significativa à palpação firme da clavícula, escápula ou braço.

Avaliação fora do campo

Observação

No campo, muitas vezes não é possível expor o membro para uma avaliação visual completa, mas isso é obrigatório em qualquer exame fora do campo. Procure por:

Deformidade. O contorno do ombro parece arredondado como o ombro contralateral ou há uma aparência quadrada para indicar uma possível luxação da articulação glenoumeral? Se for quadrada, há uma proeminência anteroinferior ao coracoide ou posteriormente para indicar a direção da luxação (Figura 23.2)? A extremidade distal da clavícula parece mais alta que o acrômio de modo significativo e assimétrica em comparação com o lado contralateral para indicar uma luxação da articulação AC ou fratura da extremidade distal da clavícula? A clavícula parece encurtada ou bulbosa no meio, indicando uma possível fratura? Existe alagem considerável da escápula em repouso para levantar a suspeita de patologia do nervo torácico longo? A assimetria sutil ou pseudossulcos, onde apenas o ângulo inferior da escápula é proeminente, em oposição ao alado verdadeiro, onde toda a borda medial da escápula é proeminente (Figura 23.3), é comum e não é motivo de preocupação. Existe uma deformidade de Popeye do bíceps, seja com um deslocamento do ventre do músculo proximal para indicar uma ruptura do tendão distal, ou uma protuberância do ventre do músculo com cavidade perto da axila, indicando uma ruptura do tendão proximal da cabeça longa?

Hematomas. Hematomas e descoloração significativos imediatos após o trauma são indicativos de lesão óssea ou vascular; portanto, devem ser considerados uma emergência. Normalmente, hematomas são vistos 24 a 48 horas após a lesão e, se extensos ou presentes após um incidente que não envolveu trauma direto, por exemplo, ao levantar um peso pesado, devem ser considerados como um indicador de uma lesão significativa, como uma fratura ou ruptura de tendão.

Perda de massa muscular. A perda de massa muscular raramente é observada em pessoas com menos de 50 anos, portanto, deve ser considerada significativa. Pode representar as sequelas da patologia para o nervo que irriga o músculo afetado ou ruptura da inserção do tendão. No ombro, o deltoide deve ser inspecionado, principalmente após a instabilidade do ombro, pois o nervo axilar está sujeito a lesões. Os músculos supraespinal e infraespinal do manguito rotador podem ser facilmente examinados visualmente pela inspeção do volume muscular acima e abaixo da espinha da escápula. A perda do infraespinal isolado é rara e não deve ser confundida com um sinal de ruptura do manguito rotador, uma vez que as rupturas do manguito começam na parte superior da inserção do tendão (*i. e.*, a porção supraespinal) e se estendem para a porção infraespinal em rupturas maiores posteriormente. Portanto, a perda do infraespinal isolado não está relacionada à laceração, mas geralmente é um sinal de compressão do ramo inferior do nervo supraescapular. Os cistos paralabrais podem se formar após lesão labral no ombro, como após instabilidade ou com microtrauma repetido em esportes de arremesso, e têm o potencial de comprimir o nervo supraescapular. Essa compressão pode ser próxima à incisura supraescapular, caso em que ambos os ramos podem ser afetados, resultando em atrofia tanto do supraespinal quanto do infraespinal, ou próximo à incisura espinoglenoide, quando apenas o ramo inferior é afetado, resultando em atrofia isolada do infraespinal (Figura 23.4) (Moore e Hunter, 1996). Quando há perda do supraespinal e do infraespinal, é mais provável a ruptura do manguito rotador (dependendo do histórico subjetivo), mas a lesão do nervo supraescapular ou neurite braquial devem sempre ser considerados diagnósticos diferenciais.

Inchaço. O inchaço no ombro é raro e, quando presente, deve ser considerado um achado significativo. Após o trauma, pode indicar no geral uma alta probabilidade de fratura óssea. Na ausência de trauma, o inchaço da articulação glenoumeral pode ser um sinal de patologia grave, como infecção ou malignidade, exceto em idosos, quando é mais provável que esteja relacionado à artropatia degenerativa da ruptura do manguito rotador (artrite como resultado da migração superior do úmero contra o acrômio devido à ruptura maciça do manguito rotador). Da mesma maneira, o inchaço óbvio da articulação AC sem trauma deve ser

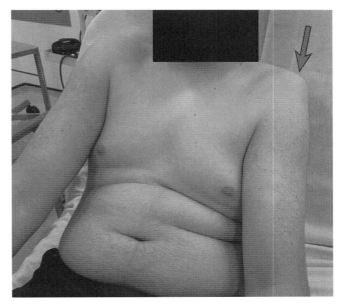

Figura 23.2 Comparação da aparência quadrada de um ombro deslocado anteriormente (*seta*) com a aparência arredondada do lado não afetado.

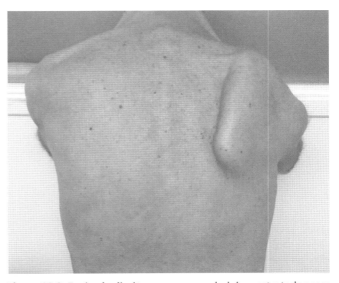

Figura 23.3 Escápula direita com asas verdadeiras retratadas com o paciente apoiado com as duas mãos contra a parede.

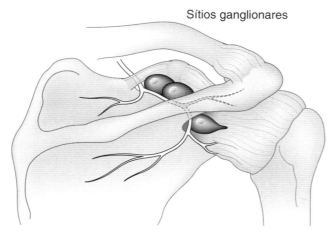

Figura 23.4 Diagrama mostrando como um gânglio pode comprimir o nervo supraescapular em diferentes sítios ao longo de seu curso. (Adaptada de Moore T. P., Hunter R. E., 1996. Suprascapular nerve entrapment. Operative Techniques in Sports Medicine 4 [1], 8-14.) (*Esta figura se encontra reproduzida em cores no Encarte.*)

considerado preocupante em pacientes mais jovens, ao passo que pode ser visto em pacientes mais idosos como consequência da artropatia por ruptura do manguito rotador.

Vermelhidão. A vermelhidão é um sinal chave de inflamação ativa, portanto, quando presente sobre uma articulação, deve levantar a suspeita imediata de infecção, a menos que seja causada por trauma na própria pele. Deve-se priorizar a exclusão de sepse e direcionar a avaliação de acordo com questionamentos subjetivos detalhados sobre sinais de alerta e exames de imagem e laboratoriais apropriados.

Palpação

Sensibilidade óssea. Isso deve ser avaliado após o trauma. Palpe o comprimento da clavícula, acrômio e espinha da escápula enquanto solicita ao paciente que relate qualquer sensibilidade significativa que possa indicar uma fratura. A palpação firme por meio dos músculos que recobrem o úmero também pode levantar a suspeita de uma fratura se estiver significativamente sensível. Se houver sensibilidade, tente avaliar se o osso é sólido durante o movimento ativo ou passivo do membro. Se houver movimento ou crepitação, então a imagem radiográfica é necessária.

Articulações. A articulação esternoclavicular (EC), AC e a glenoumeral devem ser palpadas para sensibilidade, calor excessivo, inchaço, crepitação durante o movimento e a estabilidade. As articulações EC e AC são muito superficiais e fáceis de palpar, enquanto a articulação glenoumeral pode ser difícil se houver tecido mole sobreposto significativo. Dor significativa provocada mesmo por um leve toque sobre uma articulação, especialmente quando associada a vermelhidão e calor, é uma preocupação significativa e deve ser considerada uma articulação séptica e assim investigada.

Amplitude de movimento

Em primeiro lugar, avalie a amplitude de movimento ativa de rotação externa em comparação com o lado não afetado. Se houver um déficit, reavalie passivamente. Uma restrição da rotação externa passiva indica rigidez da articulação glenoumeral, como o ombro congelado, artropatia, infecção ou luxação bloqueada. Nesse caso, espere que todos os outros movimentos do ombro também sejam restringidos. Isso pode limitar sua capacidade de realizar outros testes clínicos, e o foco da avaliação deve então mudar para a causa da restrição (ver seção *Imageamento*).

A rotação externa ativa restrita, mas com amplitude passiva completa, sugere fraqueza significativa do manguito rotador posterossuperior (supraespinal, redondo maior e infraespinal), conforme observado em rupturas do manguito rotador ou lesões do nervo supraescapular. Na presença de sepse articular significativa, é importante observar que mesmo movimentos sutis muito pequenos, como rotação do antebraço para longe do abdome, para menos do que o ponto neutro, são gravemente dolorosos. Além de avaliar os déficits de amplitude de movimento, também avalie a hipermobilidade. A maioria dos adultos tem uma faixa de rotação externa entre 50 e 80°. Se o paciente tem 90° ou mais, considere isso como hipermóvel; pode ser um fator predisponente para instabilidade.

Em seguida, avalie o movimento funcional atrás das costas medindo até que ponto o paciente pode estender a mão pela coluna e compare com o lado não afetado. Uma restrição dolorosa pode ser o resultado de uma série de patologias, mas uma gama completa de movimentos sem dor exclui a rigidez da articulação glenoumeral.

Avalie a amplitude total de flexão de ambos os ombros ao mesmo tempo, observando o movimento dinâmico das escápulas. Deve-se observar uma escápula alada significativa ou assimetria óbvia. Se normal, peça ao paciente para repetir o movimento de 10 a 20 vezes enquanto segura um peso de 1 kg em cada mão, para observar se qualquer asa ou simetria escapular dinâmica é perceptível com carga ou fadiga (*i. e.,* o movimento da escápula parece anormal após 10 a 20 repetições do movimento, ao passo que inicialmente parecia normal).

Avalie a abdução do ombro por meio de um arco de movimento completo, levando o paciente a relatar quaisquer sintomas de dor. Dor no arco médio, aproximadamente 60 a 120°, pode indicar manguito rotador ou dor relacionada à bursa. Dor extrema na abdução completa pode indicar dor na articulação AC. Novamente, avalie a hipermobilidade de abdução – considerada relevante se for alcançado um valor maior que 180° (*i. e.,* além da vertical, com o cotovelo atrás da cabeça).

Em atletas *overhead*, considere a avaliação específica da amplitude total do déficit de movimento (ATDM) ou GIRD. Isso é medido com o paciente deitado em decúbito dorsal para reduzir o movimento escapular. O braço do paciente é abduzido a 90° e a amplitude total de movimento é medida usando um goniômetro ou inclinômetro de rotação externa extrema a rotação interna extrema. A medição é então comparada ao lado não afetado. Um déficit de 20° (ATDM) foi relatado como clinicamente relevante (Kibler et al., 2012). O GIRD é medido de maneira semelhante com o paciente em decúbito dorsal, mas desta vez medindo a amplitude de movimento da rotação vertical à rotação interna extrema antes de comparar com o outro lado (Figura 23.5). Um GIRD de 8° foi relatado como clinicamente relevante (Kibler et al., 2012).

Testes clínicos

Os testes clínicos nunca devem ser interpretados isoladamente, pois nenhum dos testes "especiais" do ombro tem altas especificidade e sensibilidade. Os testes precisam sempre ser um complemento e os achados devem ser correlacionados ao histórico subjetivo.

Manguito rotador

O achado mais significativo do teste do manguito rotador é a fraqueza, pois isso pode indicar um defeito estrutural, como uma

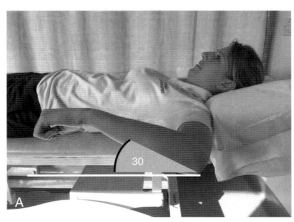
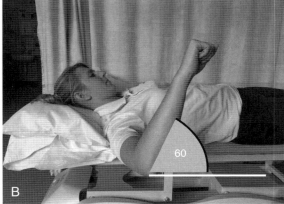

Figura 23.5 No exemplo, a medição da rotação interna em decúbito dorsal revela um déficit de rotação interna glenoumeral de 30° (GIRD) afetando o ombro direito do paciente (B) em comparação com o ombro esquerdo (A).

ruptura do tendão, ou ser resultado de um déficit neurológico. É muito comum que a dor seja provocada por esses testes e esses achados não são necessariamente atribuíveis apenas ao manguito rotador, portanto, devem ser considerados no contexto de toda a avaliação.

O subescapular pode ser testado de três maneiras (Pennock et al., 2011):

Teste belly press. O paciente coloca a mão na barriga com o cotovelo a 90° e à frente da linha média. O testador tenta puxar a mão da barriga enquanto o paciente resiste. Se a posição anterior do cotovelo for mantida, o teste é normal. Se o cotovelo se projetar para trás (i. e., o ombro se estende), isso destaca uma possível ruptura do subescapular.

Teste do abraço de urso. O paciente coloca a mão no ombro oposto com o cotovelo sem apoio no peito. O testador tenta puxar a mão do ombro. Se o paciente não conseguir manter a posição inicial, isso sugere uma possível ruptura do subescapular.

Teste de retirada, ou teste de Gerber. O paciente coloca a mão atrás das costas com o dorso da mão contra a coluna lombar. O testador aplica resistência enquanto o paciente tenta levantar a mão da coluna (posteriormente). Fraqueza significativa sugere uma possível ruptura do subescapular. Esse teste pode não ser possível, pois os pacientes com dor podem não conseguir colocar a mão na posição inicial.

O manguito rotador posterossuperior (supraespinal, infraespinal, redondo menor) pode ser testado de várias maneiras (Beaudreuil et al., 2009), incluindo:

Teste de rotação externa isométrica. O paciente fica em pé com os cotovelos flexionados a 90° e os ombros em rotação neutra. Ele é instruído a girar externamente os ombros, enquanto o testador resiste ao movimento com as duas mãos. A força pode então ser comparada ao lado não afetado.

Sinal de atraso da rotação externa. Se houver uma fraqueza considerável da rotação externa isométrica, gire passivamente o ombro até a rotação externa completa. Peça ao paciente para manter essa posição antes de soltar o braço. Um resultado positivo é quando o paciente não consegue manter a posição e o braço oscila de volta para a posição neutra. Isso sugere uma ruptura maciça do manguito ou lesão significativa do nervo supraescapular.

Teste de lata cheia. O braço é abduzido a 90° no plano da escápula com a mão orientada de modo que o polegar aponte para cima. O testador aplica uma força para baixo para avaliar a dor e a força em comparação com o lado não afetado. Alguns pacientes podem não tolerar abdução de 90°, então o teste pode ser modificado para uma posição mais baixa. Dor e fraqueza podem indicar ruptura do manguito rotador; no entanto, a bursite e a tendinite calcificada podem produzir achados semelhantes.

Teste de lata vazia (Jobe). Isso é semelhante ao teste de lata cheia, porém a mão é orientada de modo que o polegar aponte para o chão. Às vezes, os sintomas são provocados nesta posição quando o teste de lata cheia parece normal.

Dor e instabilidade nas articulações acromioclaviculares (Yewlett et al., 2012)

Palpação. A dor nas articulações AC é muito localizada e a articulação estará sensível à palpação.

Teste do cachecol (scarf test). O paciente flexiona o ombro em 90° e realiza uma adução com a mão em direção ao ombro oposto. Sobrepressão é aplicada. Um teste positivo reproduz a dor localmente na articulação AC.

Teste de instabilidade. Se houver um deslocamento da articulação AC, o testador deve descarregar o peso do braço e avaliar se a deformidade diminui. Em caso afirmativo, é menos provável que o paciente necessite de intervenção cirúrgica. Em seguida, avalie qualquer instabilidade sagital aplicando uma força anteroposterior e posteroanterior à clavícula. Se houver translação significativa, é mais provável que o paciente precise de estabilização cirúrgica, pois isso sugere que todos os três ligamentos estabilizadores se romperam.

Ruptura do peitoral maior

Método Bateman. Esse método de teste do peitoral maior envolve o testador ficar cara a cara com o paciente. Primeiro, o paciente coloca as duas mãos nos ombros do testador e aplica uma força para baixo (Figura 23.6 A). O testador tem então as duas mãos livres para palpar o contorno do ventre do músculo peitoral e a fixação do tendão para verificar a assimetria. Isso contrai as fibras inferiores (esternais). Em segundo lugar, o paciente coloca as mãos na face lateral dos deltoides do testador e aplica uma força de adução (i. e., tentando bater palmas) (Figura 23.6 B). Isso inclui as fibras superiores (claviculares) e as inferiores. Novamente, o

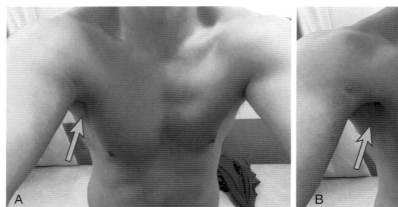
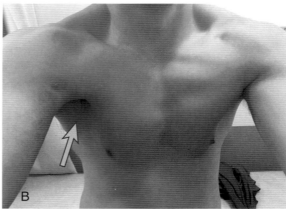

Figura 23.6 Contorno do músculo peitoral de um paciente com ruptura do tendão peitoral maior direito, enquanto aplica (A) uma pressão para baixo nos ombros do avaliador e (B) uma pressão de adução nos ombros do avaliador.

testador apalpa a simetria da barriga do músculo ou da inserção do tendão. Qualquer diferença significativa sugere uma possível ruptura e deve ser encaminhada para exames de imagem.

Ruptura do bíceps

Peça ao paciente para tensionar o bíceps e observar qualquer deformidade (como mencionado anteriormente). Este é o sinal diagnóstico mais óbvio. Se não tiver certeza, enquanto o bíceps permanece tenso, faça o teste do gancho.

***Teste de gancho* ou hook test (O'Driscoll et al., 2007).** É realizado colocando um dedo em forma de gancho atrás do tendão distal e puxando para frente. Um tendão intacto pode ser facilmente sentido como uma estrutura sólida, ao passo que um tendão rompido pode não ser palpável ou não oferecer resistência.

Teste o bíceps resistindo à supinação do antebraço para dor e fraqueza, enquanto observa qualquer deformidade na barriga do músculo.

Lesão SLAP e tendinopatia do bíceps proximal

O histórico subjetivo de dor anterior profunda, estalido, instabilidade vaga e um lançamento fraco são os fatores mais importantes, mas as suspeitas podem ser reforçadas por testes clínicos.

Palpação. A cabeça longa do tendão do bíceps pode estar dolorida proximalmente ao longo do sulco bicipital.

Teste de compressão ativa de O'Brien (O'Brien et al. 1998). O braço do paciente é flexionado a 90° e aduzido 30° com o polegar apontando para cima. O testador aplica uma força para baixo à qual o paciente deve resistir e observa a dor profunda no ombro na parte anterior. O polegar é então apontado para baixo e a mesma força para baixo é aplicada. Se a dor aumentar com o polegar apontando para baixo, isso pode indicar uma ruptura SLAP ou patologia do bíceps proximal. Um teste positivo também pode indicar patologia da articulação AC, portanto, o resultado deve ser considerado no contexto do histórico e de outros testes clínicos.

Lançamento resistido (Taylor et al., 2017). Para simular o sintoma do paciente de um arremesso fraco, peça ao paciente para colocar o braço em uma posição de arremesso enquanto o testador aplica uma força para resistir ao movimento. Avalie a presença de dor ou fraqueza que possa indicar uma ruptura SLAP ou patologia do bíceps proximal.

Frouxidão e instabilidade da articulação glenoumeral

A frouxidão da articulação glenoumeral é bastante subjetiva no que diz respeito à quantidade de translação que é significativa, e também depende do paciente estar suficientemente relaxado para ser testado completamente.

Sinal do sulco (Neer e Foster, 1980). O paciente senta-se com o braço relaxado ao lado do corpo. O testador aplica uma força de tração para baixo no úmero enquanto observa a translação inferior da cabeça do úmero. Esse teste também pode induzir apreensão de deslocamento – um achado de instabilidade.

Testes de apreensão e realocação (Farber et al., 2006). Com o paciente sentado ou deitado em decúbito dorsal, o braço é abduzido a 90° com o cotovelo flexionado a 90°. O testador coloca uma das mãos no ombro anterior e com a outra gira passivamente externamente o ombro. Se o paciente estiver apreensivo nesta posição de subluxação adicional do ombro, isso é um sinal de instabilidade anterior. Esse achado é reforçado se uma pressão anterior-posterior for aplicada ao ombro durante a repetição do teste e a sensação de apreensão diminuir.

Teste de jerk (Seung-Ho et al., 2004). Com o paciente sentado, o ombro é flexionado a 90° e aduzido com rotação interna. O testador aplica uma força no cotovelo flexionado para que a cabeça do úmero seja empurrada posteriormente na glenoide (Figura 23.7). Isso pode reproduzir apreensão ou um estalo doloroso no ombro, indicando instabilidade posterior.

Frouxidão generalizada: pontuação de Beighton

Na presença de sintomas de instabilidade ou dor sem trauma em atletas jovens, o rastreamento da mobilidade articular generalizada deve ser realizado. O escore Beighton avalia a hipermobilidade, com 4 pontos ou mais considerados relevantes (Grahame, 2007):
- 1 ponto cada para hiperextensão do cotovelo
- 1 ponto para cada extensão passiva do dedo mínimo de 90° ou mais

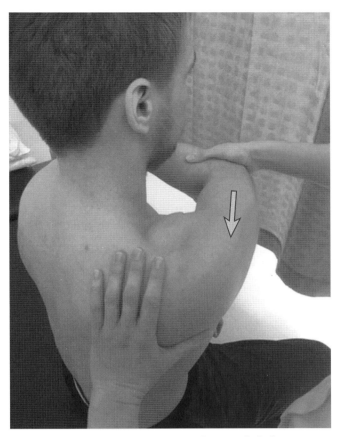

Figura 23.7 Demonstração do teste de *jerk*.

- 1 ponto para cada polegar paralelo ao antebraço em flexão passiva do punho
- 1 ponto cada para hiperextensão do joelho
- 1 ponto para tocar as palmas das mãos no chão em pé com os joelhos estendidos.

Testes diferenciais para o pescoço e triagem neurológica

Quando o distúrbio sensorial está presente no membro superior ou quando o padrão de dor inclui o pescoço/região do trapézio superior/região da borda medial da escápula, é necessária uma avaliação neurológica e da coluna cervical (ver Capítulo 26).

Avaliação funcional

Teste de estabilidade da extremidade superior de cadeia cinética fechada (Goldbeck e Davies, 2000). Isso pode ser utilizado como uma ferramenta de avaliação funcional, especialmente se uma pontuação de linha de base pré-lesão foi documentada para comparação. Essa avaliação funcional de alto nível pode medir se um atleta voltou à condição física anterior à lesão. Pacientes do sexo masculino adotam uma posição inicial de flexão total, enquanto as mulheres aderem uma posição inicial de flexão ajoelhada. As mãos são colocadas contra marcadores espaçados de 36 polegadas. O paciente é instruído a mover uma mão para tocar a outra e vice-versa. O teste mede a quantidade de toques em um período de 15 s. O teste é repetido três vezes e uma pontuação média é registrada. Pontuações de referência foram relatadas, no entanto existe variedade. Portanto, o teste é mais bem usado em comparação com as pontuações normais da linha de base do paciente individual.

Imageamento

Os exames de imagem devem ser utilizados para apoiar o diagnóstico com base no histórico e na apresentação clínica. Esteja sempre ciente de que os achados de imagem não são 100% precisos e podem gerar achados falso-negativos ou falso-positivos.

Radiografia simples. A radiografia do ombro tem baixa exposição à radiação e é uma opção de imagem barata e acessível. A radiografia simples é recomendada para pacientes com rigidez de ombro, aqueles com dor significativa e após trauma para excluir fratura, luxação, osteoartrite e tendinite calcificada. A radiografia simples também pode mostrar evidências de malignidade, infecção ou necrose avascular. Duas visualizações em planos diferentes são preferíveis em vez de uma.

Ultrassonografia. É frequentemente preferida à ressonância magnética (RM) para suspeita de patologia do manguito rotador, pois tem precisão semelhante, é mais barata e mais bem tolerada pelos pacientes. Também pode ser realizada diretamente na clínica. O benefício adicional é a capacidade de avaliar as estruturas dos tecidos moles durante o movimento para identificar patologias incomuns, como a subluxação do tendão da cabeça longa do bíceps.

Tomografia computadorizada (TC). Uma modalidade de imagem em corte transversal que usa uma alta dose de radiação principalmente para avaliar o osso. Raramente é utilizada no ombro, exceto após fraturas complexas, luxações quando há suspeita de lesão óssea ou no planejamento de uma cirurgia de artroplastia.

Ressonância magnética (RM). A imagem transversal de alta resolução é utilizada para identificar rupturas do manguito rotador/bíceps/tendão peitoral, cistos paralabrais, osteoartrite e tumores. No entanto, é mal tolerada pelos pacientes devido à claustrofobia e ao tempo necessário para a conclusão do exame. A qualidade da imagem também pode ser prejudicada por pequenos movimentos ou pela presença de implantes metálicos na área.

Artrograma por ressonância magnética (ARM). Semelhante à RM, mas com a adição de uma injeção de um agente de contraste líquido na articulação glenoumeral antes do exame. O contraste permite uma avaliação mais clara das rupturas labrais e capsulares. Essa é a modalidade preferida para pacientes com sintomas de instabilidade.

Testes laboratoriais

Sangue e aspiração. Se o paciente apresentar um início recente de uma articulação muito dolorida, vermelha, quente e inchada com características sistêmicas de mal-estar, deve ser realizada uma aspiração da articulação com microscopia, cultura e sensibilidade. Além disso, deve ser feita uma triagem de sangue urgente para avaliar marcadores inflamatórios elevados (taxa de hemossedimentação e proteína C reativa) e contagem de leucócitos. Em casos menos urgentes, onde o inchaço e a rigidez das articulações estão presentes sem dor intensa ou características sistêmicas, uma aspiração pode não ser necessária, mas o sangue deve ser rastreado primeiro para infecção e inflamação, juntamente com a função hepática de rotina, eletrólitos e possivelmente fator reumatoide e antígenos peptídicos citrulinados anti-cíclicos (anti-CCP) se houver suspeita de artrite inflamatória.

Neurofisiologia. O teste de condução nervosa periférica e o teste de eletromiografia (EMG) da cintura escapular podem ser úteis na diferenciação entre radiculopatia cervical e lesões de nervos periféricos. No ombro, pode ser um teste útil se houver suspeita de neurite braquial para avaliar quais nervos são afetados, ou após a luxação do ombro para avaliar a lesão do nervo axilar. Se repetido após 3 a 6 meses, pode medir os sinais de recuperação se o progresso clinicamente aparente for lento.

Conclusão

A avaliação precisa do ombro requer fundamentalmente uma base de conhecimento da patologia, etiologia e epidemiologia da área. A avaliação clínica deve usar todas as informações disponíveis – subjetivas e objetivas – para restringir a variedade de diagnósticos possíveis, idealmente para um ou uma pequena quantidade que pode então ser investigada com exames de imagem, se apropriado. Confiar puramente em testes clínicos objetivos sem compreensão suficiente da patologia e correlação com achados subjetivos leva a diagnósticos errados. Lembre-se de que o histórico é fundamental.

Referências bibliográficas

Beaudreuil, J., Nizard, R., Thomas, T., Peyre, M., Liotard, J.P., Boileau, P., et al., 2009. Contribution of clinical tests to the diagnosis of rotator cuff disease: a systematic literature review. Joint Bone Spine 76, 15-19.

Farber, A.J., Castillo, R., Clough, M., Bahk, M., Mcfarland, E.G., 2006. Clinical assessment of three common tests for traumatic anterior shoulder instability. Journal of Bone and Joint Surgery 88, 1467–1474.

Goldbeck, T.G., Davies, G.J., 2000. Test-retest reliability of the Closed Kinetic Chain upper extemity stability test: a clinical field test. Journal of Sport Rehabilitation 9, 35-45.

Grahame, R., 2007. The need to take a fresh look at criteria for hypermobility. Journal of Rheumatology 34, 664-665.

Kibler, W.B., Sciascia, A., Thomas, S.J., 2012. Glenohumeral internal rotation deficit: pathogenesis and response to acute throwing. Sports Medicine and Arthroscopy Review 20, 34-38.

Moore, T.P., Hunter, R.E., 1996. Suprascapular nerve entrapment. Operative Techniques in Sports Medicine 4, 8–14.

Neer, C.S.,2nd, Foster, C.R., 1980. Inferior capsular shift for involuntary inferior and multidirectional instability of the shoulder. A preliminary report. Journal of Bone and Joint Surgery. American Volume 62, 897-908.

O'Brien, S.J., Pagnani, M.J., Fealy, S., Mcglynn, S.R., Wilson, J.B., 1998. The active compression test: a new and effective test for diagnosing labral tears and acromioclavicular joint abnormality. The American Journal of Sports Medicine 26, 610-613.

O'Driscoll, S.W., Goncalves, L.B.J., Dietz, P., 2007. The hook test for distal biceps tendon avulsion. The American Journal of Sports Medicine 35, 1865-1869.

Pennock, A.T., Pennington, W.W., Torry, M.R., Decker, M.J., Vaishnav, S.B., Provencher, M.T., et al., 2011. The influence of arm and shoulder position on the bear-hug, belly-press, and lift-off tests: an electromyographic study. The American Journal of Sports Medicine 39, 2338-2346.

Seung-Ho, K., Jae-Chul, P., Jun-Sic, P., Irvin, O., 2004. Painful jerk test: a predictor of success in nonoperative treatment of posteroinferior instability of the shoulder. The American Journal of Sports Medicine 32, 1849-1855.

Taylor, S.A., Newman, A.M., Dawson, C., Gallagher, K.A., Bowers, A., Nguyen, J., et al., 2017. The "3-pack" examination is critical for comprehensive evaluation of the biceps–labrum complex and the bicipital tunnel: a prospective study. Arthroscopy 33, 28-38.

Yewlett, A., Dearden, P.M.C., Ferran, N.A., Evans, R.O., Kulkani, R., 2012. Acromioclavicula-86.

Capítulo | 24 |

Cotovelo Esportivo

Daniel Williams, Shivan Jassim e Ali Noorani

A finalidade deste capítulo é apresentar uma visão geral das condições comuns relacionadas com o cotovelo esportivo. Nossos objetivos são:
- Apresentar a anatomia da articulação do cotovelo, biomecânica da atividade normal e arremesso
- Apresentar perspectivas de instabilidade aguda e crônica do cotovelo, tendinopatias e rupturas de tendão
- Traçar planos de tratamento para essas condições.

Introdução

A função do cotovelo é posicionar a mão no espaço e atuar como fulcro para as atividades do antebraço e facilitar as atividades da vida diária. As demandas dos atletas vão além das funções normais do dia a dia; portanto, pequenas limitações na amplitude de movimento ou potência podem afetar significativamente o desempenho atlético.

As principais queixas do cotovelo estão relacionadas à dor, à instabilidade e à rigidez. Esses sintomas são o resultado de lesões agudas e sequelas de pequenos traumas crônicos ou repetitivos. A resolução de um desses sintomas pode levar à deterioração de outro.

O braço de arremesso pode ser o foco principal dos sintomas crônicos em um atleta. Altas tensões são aplicadas no cotovelo nas várias fases do arremesso, compostas pelos múltiplos ciclos que são realizados nos treinamentos e competições. Como tal, um treinamento cuidadoso para otimizar a técnica é vital para a prevenção e o manejo de lesões. Os melhores tratamentos para muitas doenças que afetam o cotovelo esportivo ainda estão em debate. A terapia, os tratamentos minimamente invasivos e a cirurgia têm papéis importantes na reabilitação para recuperar um cotovelo estável e sem dor com uma amplitude de movimento completa.

Anatomia do cotovelo

Osteologia

A articulação do cotovelo é composta por três articulações (Figura 24.1):

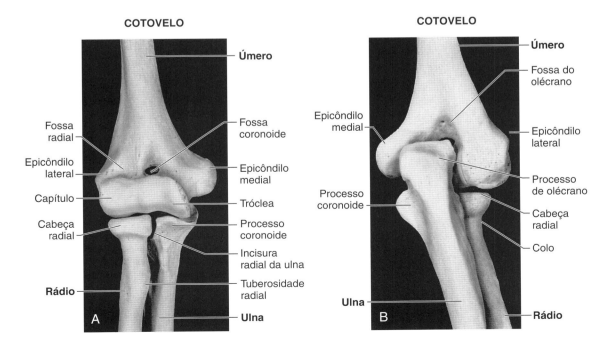

Figura 24.1 Ossos do cotovelo. **A.** Vista anterior. **B.** Vista posterior.

- A articulação ulno-umeral, que atua como uma dobradiça para flexão e extensão no cotovelo
- A articulação radiocapitelar, que atua como um pivô para pronação-supinação do antebraço
- A articulação radioulnar proximal, também envolvida na pronação-supinação do antebraço.

A articulação ulno-umeral pode ser considerada uma dobradiça uniaxial, exceto nos extremos do movimento. O eixo de rotação está no centro dos arcos formados pelo sulco troclear e pelo capítulo. A amplitude de movimento é geralmente em torno de 0 a 150° de flexão/extensão, embora a amplitude funcional para atividades da vida diária seja menor do que isso – 30 a 130° aproximadamente. O intervalo funcional para supinação é de 50° na articulação radiocapitelar. O esportista pode ter e exigir uma maior amplitude de movimento, como hiperextensão do cotovelo em atletas arremessadores.

Ligamentos

Os ligamentos do cotovelo (Figura 24.2) são estabilizadores primários importantes. O ligamento colateral ulnar (LCU) surge da posição anteroinferior do epicôndilo medial e se insere no tubérculo sublime do coronoide medial. O LCU oferece resistência às forças de valgo por meio de seus três componentes principais:
- Banda anterior (mais importante)
- Banda transversal
- Banda posterior, importante na flexão máxima do cotovelo.

O complexo do ligamento colateral lateral (LCL) é composto por:
- Ligamentos colaterais radiais (LCRs)
- Ligamento colateral ulnar lateral (LCUL)
- Ligamento colateral acessório
- Ligamento anular, estabilizando a articulação radioulnar proximal.

O LCUL é o estabilizador primário para varo e rotação externa. Ele se origina do ponto isométrico no epicôndilo lateral e se fixa na crista supinadora da ulna.

Músculos

Os músculos que cruzam a articulação do cotovelo desempenham papel na sua estabilidade dinâmica, bem como no controle motor do antebraço das seguintes maneiras:
- Extensão do cotovelo pelo tríceps e, em um grau muito menor, pelo ancôneo
- Flexão do cotovelo pelo braquial, braquiorradial e bíceps braquial
- Supinação do antebraço pelo bíceps braquial e supinador
- Pronação do antebraço pelo pronador redondo e pronador quadrado.

Biomecânica

A biomecânica do arremesso tem sido amplamente estudada, principalmente a dos arremessadores de beisebol. Forças extraordinárias são geradas, tornando o cotovelo vulnerável a lesões. O lançamento pode ser dividido em cinco fases distintas:

Fase I (preparação). Nesta fase preparatória, o cotovelo flexiona e o antebraço fica ligeiramente pronado.

Fase II (armação). O ombro abduz e se move em rotação externa máxima, o cotovelo flexiona entre 90 e 120° e o antebraço é totalmente pronado.

Fase III (aceleração). Uma grande força direcionada para a frente é gerada conforme a extremidade se move em rápida extensão do

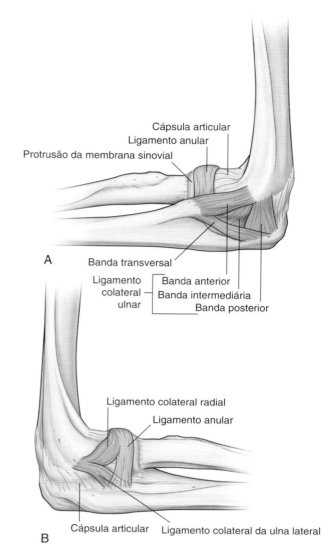

Figura 24.2 Aspectos medial (A) e lateral (B) do cotovelo esquerdo mostrando a cápsula articular e os ligamentos colaterais radial e ulnar. (*Esta figura se encontra reproduzida em cores no Encarte.*)

cotovelo. Estudos biomecânicos demonstram grandes forças de cisalhamento medial, forças compressivas laterais e estresse em valgo no cotovelo. A maior parte do estresse em valgo é transmitido ao feixe anterior do LCU. O restante do estresse é dissipado pelas estruturas de suporte secundárias, ou seja, a musculatura flexor-pronadora (Rossy e Oh, 2016).

Fase IV (desaceleração). A contração excêntrica ocorre em todos os músculos para desacelerar o braço. Alto torque é gerado durante esta fase, colocando o ombro e o bíceps em risco de lesão.

Fase V (finalização). Nesta fase final, as forças são dissipadas e o corpo se reequilibra para parar o movimento para a frente.

Instabilidade do cotovelo

A estabilidade do cotovelo é vital para o seu bom funcionamento e sem dor. A estabilidade depende da relação entre os estabilizadores estáticos das articulações articulares e as estruturas capsuloligamentares. A estabilidade dinâmica é conferida pelos músculos que cruzam a articulação. A instabilidade segue padrões mais bem definidos e pode ser resultado de uma lesão traumática ou secundária a síndromes de uso excessivo crônicas.

Em 2001, O'Driscoll et al. propuseram a "fortaleza da estabilidade do cotovelo", delineando estabilizadores primários e secundários do cotovelo (O'Driscoll et al., 2001). Os estabilizadores primários são a articulação umeral da ulna, que impede a translação posterior da ulna, a banda anterior do LCU, que resiste ao estresse em valgo, e o LCUL, que suporta a rotação externa e o estresse em varo. Os estabilizadores secundários são a articulação radioumeral e as origens flexora e extensora comuns. Esse sistema é comum de ser utilizado atualmente. No entanto, vale a pena reconhecer outras estruturas importantes para a estabilidade, principalmente a cápsula anterior e os estabilizadores dinâmicos, notadamente o bíceps braquial, o braquial e o tríceps.

Instabilidade aguda

O cotovelo é a segunda articulação mais frequentemente deslocada. Uma luxação simples do cotovelo é definida como uma lesão em que não há fraturas concomitantes além de pequenas avulsões periarticulares de 1 ou 2 mm (Josefsson et al., 1984). Não está dentro do escopo desse capítulo discutir luxações de fratura mais complexas. A maioria das luxações é posterior ou posterolateral (Figura 24.3). Há muito tempo é proposto que o mecanismo de deslocamento é o valgo e a rotação externa. Com o antebraço fixo, essa rotação posterolateral resulta em subluxação e deslocamento progressivos da cabeça do rádio (Osborne e Cotterill, 1966, O'Driscoll et al., 1992), que resulta em uma lesão de tecido mole lateral a medial descrita por O'Driscoll como o "círculo Horii" (O'Driscoll, 1999). A análise de vídeo mais recente de luxações de cotovelo registradas sugere um mecanismo de valgo hiperfisiológico em um cotovelo estendido (Schreiber et al., 2013). Isso resultaria no padrão reverso de lesão começando com as cápsulas anteriores e a banda anterior do LCU e progredindo lateralmente. Esse padrão de lesão tem sido apoiado por estudos de ressonância magnética (RM), que sugerem que as estruturas mediais são lesionadas mais comumente do que as estruturas laterais – essas últimas nunca são lesionadas isoladamente (Rhyou e Kim, 2012; Schreiber et al., 2014). Com isso em mente, Robinson et al. (2017) propuseram uma escala de instabilidade começando com o complexo ligamentar medial e progredindo para a origem flexora comum, cápsula anterior, complexo ligamentar lateral e finalmente a origem extensora comum.

Os algoritmos de investigação, imobilização e tratamento variam consideravelmente entre cirurgiões e unidades. O risco de necessitar de cirurgia para instabilidade recorrente após luxações simples administradas de maneira conservadora é de 2,3% (Modi et al., 2015). Como mencionado anteriormente, as imagens de RM mostram lesões ligamentares em todos os pacientes (Schreiber et al., 2014); portanto, o risco de tratamento excessivo após a RM é significativo. Os autores se perguntam se isso é verdade após o exame sob anestesia (ESA). Na verdade, Josefsson et al. (1987) realizaram um ensaio clínico randomizado (ECR) comparando o manejo operatório e não operatório de 30 pacientes com luxações agudas. Todos eles foram submetidos a um ESA antes da randomização. Sob anestesia, todos os pacientes apresentavam instabilidade medial e 16 dos 30 apresentavam instabilidade medial e lateral. Além disso, todos tiveram ruptura ou avulsão dos ligamentos medial e lateral na cirurgia. No entanto, os resultados não mostraram nenhuma diferença no desfecho em termos de amplitude de movimento ou instabilidade recorrente em 1 ano entre aqueles que se submeteram à cirurgia e tratamento conservador.

Um ECR de 100 pacientes comparando a imobilização em gesso longo por 3 semanas com a mobilização precoce (dentro de 2 dias) não mostra diferença na amplitude de movimento, escores de resultados, ossificação heterotópica ou instabilidade recorrente após as primeiras 6 semanas. No entanto, nas primeiras 6 semanas, os pacientes no grupo de mobilização precoce tiveram melhor desempenho em todas essas métricas (Iordens et al., 2015).

O autor principal prefere uma mobilização precoce e usa um protocolo de reabilitação *overhead*. O paciente começa cedo a amplitude de movimento do cotovelo (dentro de 1 semana) em uma posição supina com o ombro flexionado a 90°. Flexão e extensão controladas são realizadas com a mão e o antebraço

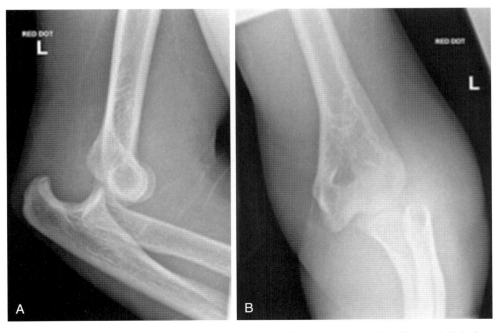

Figura 24.3 Radiografia demonstrando uma luxação posterolateral simples do cotovelo. **A.** Radiografia lateral. **B.** Radiografia anteroposterior.

mantidos acima da cabeça com o antebraço em pronação. Essa abordagem minimiza os efeitos da gravidade e das forças angulares. A rotação do antebraço é normalmente mantida em neutro durante o repouso, mas pode ser ajustada em padrões específicos de lesão. Por exemplo, a pronação estabiliza o cotovelo deficiente em LCL e a supinação estabiliza um cotovelo deficiente em LCU.

Embora a cirurgia para instabilidade recorrente seja rara após uma simples luxação do cotovelo, a condição não possui um prognóstico positivo. Em um estudo de 110 luxações simples de cotovelo em uma média de 88 meses após a lesão, 8% dos pacientes reclamaram de instabilidade subjetiva, 56% de rigidez e 62% de dor. Além disso, 19% dos atletas da coorte tiveram que desistir de seu esporte ou modificar sua técnica (Anakwe et al., 2011).

Instabilidade crônica

Instabilidade rotatória posterolateral

A instabilidade rotatória posterolateral (IRPL) é a maneira mais comum de instabilidade sintomática crônica do cotovelo. Isso ocorre por causa de falha no LCUL. A ruptura do LCUL causa rotação externa anormal do rádio e da ulna em relação ao úmero distal. Isso resulta no deslocamento posterior da cabeça do rádio em relação ao capítulo. Ocorre de modo mais comum após um trauma, mas pode ser secundário a um procedimento iatrogênico, como artroscopia, liberação do epicôndilo lateral ou após injeções de esteroides. Com a dor lateral do cotovelo, travamento e captação sendo a queixa predominante, costuma ser inicialmente diagnosticada como cotovelo de tenista, síndrome do túnel radial ou artrite radiocapitelar.

A IRPL é um diagnóstico clínico e pode ser facilmente esquecido se não houver suspeita. Um histórico cuidadoso e um exame detalhado são essenciais. Conforme descrito, a subluxação posterolateral da cabeça do rádio ocorre quando uma carga axial é aplicada a um braço posicionado em supinação e valgo, como empurrar para cima de uma cadeira de braços largos. O exame clínico e os testes de provocação são elaborados para simular essa posição. Já os exames específicos para um paciente com possível IRPL incluem o teste do *pivot-shift* lateral (Figura 24.4), o de tração posterolateral, e o de recolocação, o sinal da cadeira e a dor e instabilidade ao realizar uma flexão ativa no chão.

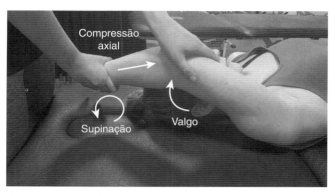

Figura 24.4 Teste do *pivot-shift* lateral. Em um paciente em decúbito dorsal com o antebraço hipersupinado, um estresse em valgo é aplicado junto com a carga axial. O cotovelo começa em extensão total e é flexionado lentamente. A instabilidade geralmente ocorre em torno de 30 a 45°.

As radiografias simples e a RM são úteis para excluir outros diagnósticos, como artrite da articulação radiocapitelar e epicondilite lateral (EL), mas têm pouco valor na confirmação de lesão ou dano ao LCUL. O'Driscoll et al. (1992) classificaram a IRPL em estágios distintos de 1 a 3 com base no grau de subluxação/luxação e lesão de tecidos moles. A Figura 24.5 é uma radiografia de um paciente com uma IRPL de grau 2 e uma luxação posterolateral de aspecto empoleirado.

Embora a modificação da atividade e a fisioterapia trabalhando nos estabilizadores dinâmicos do cotovelo possam ajudar, a cirurgia é frequentemente indicada em pacientes com instabilidade sintomática persistente. Nessa situação, a cirurgia é importante, não só para o alívio sintomático, como também para prevenir a alteração artrítica, que pode ocorrer rapidamente no cotovelo instável. A fisiologia avascular e hipocelular do tecido ligamentar significa que o reparo direto raramente é indicado na instabilidade crônica. Portanto, o objetivo da cirurgia é garantir um enxerto robusto, estável e durável do ponto isométrico no epicôndilo lateral até a crista supinadora. Vários autoenxertos, aloenxertos e ligamentos sintéticos têm sido utilizados e fixados de diferentes maneiras. Todas as séries são muito pequenas e heterogêneas para fazer comentários sobre a melhor técnica possível.

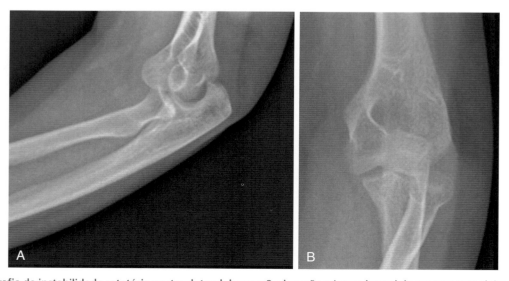

Figura 24.5 Radiografia de instabilidade rotatória posterolateral de grau 2 e luxação póstero lateral de aspecto empoleirado. **A.** Radiografia lateral. **B.** Radiografia anteroposterior.

Apesar disso, os resultados da reconstrução são muito bons. Uma revisão de Anakwenze et al. (2014) descobriu que 91% dos pacientes tiveram um resultado bom a excelente após a cirurgia com uma amplitude de movimento de aproximadamente 5 a 135°. Eles relataram uma taxa de complicações de 11% e uma taxa de recorrência de 8%. Outros estudos relataram que a taxa de instabilidade recorrente chega a 25% (Jones et al., 2012). Reuter et al. (2016) realizaram uma revisão retrospectiva de sete estudos contendo 148 pacientes que tiveram reparo ou reconstrução para IRPL. Eles descobriram que não havia consenso sobre imobilização ou reabilitação pós-operatória. A maioria dos casos teve um limite pós-operatório de extensão fixado em 30°, mas esse variou entre 1 dia e 6 semanas. No geral, os pacientes em sua série recuperaram resultados aceitáveis elevados após a reconstrução.

Instabilidade em valgo

A banda anterior do LCU é a restrição estática primária ao estresse em valgo. A banda anterior se estende em forma de leque desde a crista anteroinferior do epicôndilo medial até sua fixação no tubérculo sublime na ulna medial. A lesão pode ocorrer após trauma agudo, ser secundária a estresse repetitivo em valgo (microtrauma) ou iatrogênica, geralmente como resultado de liberação excessiva da ulna.

Atletas *overhead*, como arremessadores de beisebol e lançadores de dardo, não são apenas mais suscetíveis a essa lesão, como também têm maior probabilidade de se tornarem sintomáticos. Esses atletas se queixam de dor no cotovelo medial frequentemente e de perda de velocidade ou precisão no arremesso. Os sintomas geralmente desaparecem com repouso e modificação da atividade. A sobrecarga crônica da extensão em valgo pode causar impacto do olécrano posteromedial, compressão radiocapitelar e sintomas dos nervos ulnares no cotovelo.

Em casos crônicos, pode haver muito pouco para observar no exame. Pode haver sensibilidade do LCU e perda de extensão secundária ao estímulo do olécrano medial. Deve-se ter cuidado ao avaliar a função e a estabilidade do nervo ulnar. A estabilidade em valgo deve ser testada em toda a amplitude de movimento, mas é mais sensível a 20 a 30°. Testes específicos para instabilidade em valgo incluem a manobra de ordenha e o teste de esforço em valgo em movimento.

Devem ser feitas radiografias simples e, embora não sejam dignas de nota de um modo geral, podem revelar alterações degenerativas em casos crônicos, particularmente osteófitos do olécrano medial. As radiografias de estresse mostram lacunas ou assimetria lado-a-lado. O artrograma por RM é o padrão-ouro e pode revelar rupturas de espessura parcial ou abaixo da superfície.

A instabilidade medial crônica é incomum em quem não participa de esportes de arremesso acima da cabeça. Devem ser testados tratamentos conservadores na maioria dos casos, que incluem um período de descanso seguido de fortalecimento do pronador flexor e o desenvolvimento de uma técnica de arremesso melhor. Rettig et al. (2001) constataram que o tratamento conservador permitiu que apenas 42% dos atletas retornassem ao nível anterior de esporte e isso levou em média quase 6 meses. Eles não encontraram nenhuma maneira de prever quais pacientes evoluiriam bem com o tratamento não operatório (Rettig et al., 2001). Isso levou a um aumento da cirurgia para instabilidade em valgo. Foram descritas várias técnicas, enxertos e métodos de fixação. Em 1974, foi realizada uma reconstrução bem-sucedida do LCU medial em Tommy John, um arremessador da Liga Principal de Beisebol dos EUA. A reconstrução do LCU ainda é comumente referida como "procedimento Tommy John". A técnica foi publicada em 1986 (Jobe et al., 1986) e envolvia um enxerto de tendão livre em forma de oito por meio de túneis ósseos na ulna e no epicôndilo medial. Essa técnica foi adaptada e novas técnicas de ancoragem levaram a um maior retorno ao esporte e menores taxas de complicações (Watson et al., 2014a). Nessa revisão de 1.368 pacientes, a taxa geral de complicações foi de 12,9%, mais comumente uma neuropraxia do nervo ulnar e a taxa de retorno ao jogo foi de 78,9%.

Epicondilite lateral

A EL é uma lesão por uso excessivo que ocorre como consequência da sobrecarga na origem do extensor comum, especificamente no extensor radial curto do carpo (ERCC). Afeta com mais frequência o braço dominante e é mais frequente em pessoas que realizam atividades prolongadas e rápidas, como digitar, trabalhar manualmente e tocar piano. Até 50% dos jogadores de tênis desenvolvem EL durante suas carreiras e isso fez com que a condição fosse comumente referida como "cotovelo de tenista". Acredita-se que a extensão excêntrica recorrente do punho e a pronação do antebraço, sobretudo durante o golpe de *backhand*, sejam as responsáveis. E é agravado por uma técnica pobre, uma raquete pesada e tamanho de empunhadura abaixo do ideal.

Apesar da crença comum de que EL não é uma condição inflamatória, Cook e Purdam (2009) propuseram um modelo contínuo, incorporando informações clínicas, histológicas e de imagem. Eles descrevem um processo de microtrauma repetido, deterioração do tendão e, finalmente, degeneração. Microscopicamente, o aspecto no local de inserção é de hiperplasia angiofibroblástica e colágeno desorganizado, com ausência de células inflamatórias, ou seja, um processo degenerativo em vez de inflamatório.

O atleta apresentará dor lateral no cotovelo ao redor da proeminência óssea que se irradia para baixo no antebraço. Isso geralmente é associado e exacerbado pela preensão e uma contração repetitiva dos extensores do punho. Os pacientes se queixam de uma redução subjetiva na força de preensão com frequência.

O exame revela sensibilidade na origem do ERCC no (ou apenas distal ao) epicôndilo lateral. Existem vários testes de provocação para auxiliar no diagnóstico, todos com o objetivo de estimular a dor no epicôndilo lateral. Eles envolvem extensão resistida do punho (teste de Cozens; Figura 24.6) ou extensão do

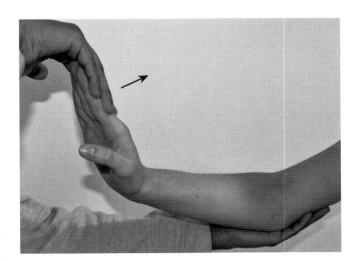

Figura 24.6 Teste de Cozens. Estabilize o cotovelo em 90° de flexão com uma das mãos enquanto apalpa o epicôndilo lateral. Posicione a mão do paciente em desvio radial, pronação do antebraço e extensão completa do punho. O paciente é solicitado a manter esta posição contra a força de flexão manual aplicada à mão e ao punho, fornecendo extensão resistida do punho. O teste é considerado positivo se produzir dor na área do epicôndilo lateral.

dedo (principalmente dedo médio) (teste de Maudsley; Figura 24.7). Além disso, pacientes que receberam tratamento prévio com injeções de corticosteroide no local podem apresentar sinais de lipoatrofia, como despigmentação ou adelgaçamento da pele ao redor do epicôndilo lateral.

O diagnóstico é principalmente clínico, baseado no histórico e no exame físico. As investigações podem ser úteis para excluir outras causas de dor no epicôndilo lateral. Os diagnósticos diferenciais comuns incluem radiculopatia cervical, alterações degenerativas ou síndrome do túnel radial, uma neuropatia de compressão do nervo interósseo posterior.

Geralmente, radiografias simples não apresentam nada digno de nota, embora revelem de modo ocasional calcificações menores na origem extensora comum; elas são úteis para excluir a artrite radiocapitelar. A ultrassonografia pode ser útil nas mãos de um operador experiente e pode demonstrar bem um tendão ERCC hipoecoico espessado. Além disso, as fases do Doppler podem detectar a neovascularização. A RM pode demonstrar espessamento ou ruptura da origem do ERCC com aumento da intensidade do sinal nas sequências ponderadas em T2. A RM também pode identificar uma ruptura sob a superfície do LCL. O autor principal sente que, quando presente, a ruptura pode resultar em microinstabilidade e um subsequente aumento na deformação na origem do extensor comum (estabilizador secundário). Isso pode contribuir para o cotovelo de tenista refratário.

A EL geralmente é autolimitada e remite em 12 a 18 meses. O objetivo do tratamento é controlar a dor, preservar a função e prevenir a deterioração, e permitir ao atleta retornar à função normal. A EL é uma condição que tende a responder favoravelmente a métodos não operatórios. Consequentemente, as injeções e a cirurgia devem ser reservadas para casos recalcitrantes.

Repousar e evitar o comportamento agravante pode levar à resolução dos sintomas, embora no atleta de elite essa não seja uma estratégia favorável. Portanto, além da correção da técnica, existem várias terapias para o tratamento da EL:

Fisioterapia

A fisioterapia é a base do tratamento para EL. Os regimes têm como objetivo manter a amplitude de movimento do cotovelo, além do fortalecimento excêntrico dos extensores comuns. Isso tem se mostrado superior ao repouso sozinho, embora nenhum regime seja superior a outro. Além disso, é vital para a reabilitação do cotovelo a estabilização da escápula recrutando os músculos periescapulares. A fisioterapia combinando a manipulação do cotovelo e os exercícios tem um benefício superior do que "esperar para ver" nas primeiras 12 semanas. Este benefício não é mais aparente em 26 semanas, ambos são superiores às injeções de esteroides (Bisset et al., 2006).

Agentes anti-inflamatórios

Os anti-inflamatórios não esteroidais e a analgesia podem ajudar a controlar os sintomas e permitir a terapia na fase inicial do processo da doença. As injeções de esteroides foram bem estudadas em EL. A ação dos esteroides é predominantemente anti-inflamatória e, portanto, seu mecanismo de ação é pouco compreendido. Existem boas evidências de que as injeções de esteroides, apesar de fornecerem um bom alívio da dor a curto prazo, são prejudiciais a médio e longo prazo para dor, força de preensão, gravidade dos sintomas e duração em comparação com nenhum tratamento (Coombes et al., 2010; Olaussen et al., 2013). Apesar dessa evidência de alto nível, não houve impacto sobre o uso disseminado de esteroides para tratar essa condição (Fujihara et al., 2018).

Órtese

Cintas de contraforça ampliam a área de estresse aplicado no músculo ERCC e reduzem a tensão na origem do extensor comum. Embora a maior alteração biomecânica na carga do tendão ERCC ocorra quando as órteses são colocadas sobre o ventre muscular, os melhores resultados clínicos ocorrem quando dispostas logo distalmente ao epicôndilo. Elas têm sido utilizadas com efeitos benéficos para reduzir os sintomas e têm se mostrado melhores do que a tala do punho. Na verdade, com efeito imediato, eles podem melhorar a força de preensão sem dor (Sadeghi-Demneh e Jafarian, 2013). Seu efeito a médio e longo prazo é menos claro, apesar da boa tolerância e do perfil de baixo risco.

Tratamentos biológicos

Estão disponíveis vários tratamentos biológicos e estão sendo investigados para o tratamento de EL, principalmente plasma rico em plaquetas (PRP). Variação na preparação, ativação e grupos de controle em ECRs têm dificultado tirar conclusões quanto à sua eficácia em comparação com os tratamentos mais tradicionais. Vários ECR mostraram eficácia do PRP em relação às injeções de esteroides, que agora sabemos ser prejudiciais na tendinopatia (Lebiedziński et al., 2015; Peerbooms et al., 2010). Peerbooms et al. (2010) mostraram uma taxa de sucesso de 73% em 52 semanas em comparação com 51% para injeções de esteroides. O PRP também demonstrou ser superior à injeção de anestésico local em 8 semanas (Mishra e Pavelko, 2006). No entanto, as evidências são conflitantes com alguns estudos que não mostram nenhuma diferença significativa (de Vos et al., 2014). No ombro, biopsias de tendões tendinopáticos do manguito rotador após PRP demonstraram características de tecido alteradas, incluindo celularidade reduzida, vascularidade e níveis aumentados de apoptose (Carr et al., 2015). Pela primeira vez a segurança do PRP foi questionada, embora não tenha tido efeitos clínicos deletérios.

Outros tratamentos não cirúrgicos foram descritos, como adesivos de nitrato, ablação térmica por radiofrequência, terapia por ondas de choque extracorpórea, terapia a *laser* e acupuntura. Embora cada uma dessas modalidades tenha algumas evidências de baixo nível para apoiá-las, seu papel nos algoritmos de tratamento de EL permanece obscuro. A literatura existente não fornece evidências conclusivas de que existe um método preferido de tratamento não cirúrgico para esta condição (Sims et al., 2014). A EL é uma condição geralmente autolimitada em 95%

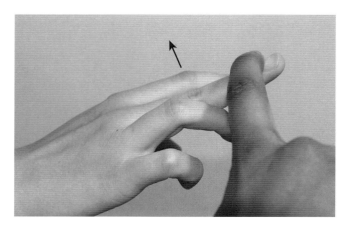

Figura 24.7 Teste de Maudsley. Estabilize o cotovelo em 90° de flexão com o punho em extensão neutra e a palma da mão paralela ao solo. Enquanto apalpa o epicôndilo lateral, peça ao paciente para estender o dedo médio contra sua forç a contrária. Um teste positivo é indicado por dor no epicôndilo lateral.

dos pacientes, com resolução em um período de 12 a 18 meses. Na verdade, existem poucas evidências de que, a longo prazo, qualquer intervenção não cirúrgica é melhor do que somente a observação (Sayegh e Strauch, 2015).

Tratamento cirúrgico

Existem várias técnicas cirúrgicas, todas com o objetivo de desbridar e ressecar o tecido tendinopático do tendão ERCC e descorticar o epicôndilo lateral. Todas as técnicas, sejam abertas, percutâneas ou artroscópicas, podem ser realizadas em regime diurno e permitem a reabilitação precoce.

Existem algumas variações de técnica, dentro de cada procedimento, como fechar ou não o tendão do ERCC ou recolocar o tendão na origem do extensor comum. As técnicas artroscópicas têm a vantagem de examinar o resto do cotovelo em busca de patologias alternativas, mas sem dúvida apresentam tempos cirúrgicos mais longos e maiores riscos em comparação com as técnicas abertas. Não há estudos que demonstrem uma vantagem clara de uma técnica sobre a outra, incluindo variações dentro da cirurgia aberta. Altos índices de satisfação foram relatados com cada técnica. As complicações da cirurgia incluem infecção, ossificação heterotópica, lesão do nervo e lesão iatrogênica de LCUL.

Um estudo comparando a cirurgia simulada com um desbridamento da porção doente do tendão não mostrou diferenças no resultado em 6 meses e 2,5 anos, embora limitado por um pequeno tamanho da amostra. Ambos os grupos mostraram melhora significativa nos sintomas (Kroslak e Murrell, 2018).

É opinião do autor principal que a cirurgia deve ser reservada para EL recalcitrante que passou por um período prolongado de tratamento não operatório. A RM deve ser realizada em um estabelecimento de cuidados secundários para excluir uma ruptura na origem do extensor comum ou LCL. Em casos recalcitrantes sem ruptura, também vale a pena considerar o PRP antes da cirurgia, pois, apesar da falta de consenso na literatura, é minimamente invasivo e há evidências de que 89% dos pacientes melhoraram a dor e 82% voltaram ao trabalho. Apenas 7% dos pacientes desta série foram convertidos para tratamento cirúrgico (Ford et al., 2015). O algoritmo do autor principal para o tratamento de EL é mostrado na Figura 24.8. Recomendamos encaminhamento para atenção secundária após falha do tratamento conservador por 3 meses. Nesse ponto, 70% dos pacientes melhoraram após a fisioterapia (Olaussen et al., 2013). Embora aumente para quase 90% em 6 meses, para evitar perder um diagnóstico mais sério e devido ao impacto prejudicial na qualidade de vida do paciente, acreditamos que 3 meses é razoável.

Epicondilite medial

A epicondilite medial (EM) tem muitas características semelhantes à EL, pois é uma lesão por uso excessivo que afeta a origem da massa do flexor/pronador comum, levando à tendinose degenerativa. Está associada a esportes que incluem pronação e flexão de punho repetitivas do antebraço. Ela é menos comum do que EL, mais difícil de tratar e tem uma base de evidências menos extensa para o tratamento.

Frequentemente, EM é referida como "cotovelo de jogador de golfe", como também é prevalente em levantadores de peso, arremessadores de beisebol, remadores e jogadores de críquete, todos submetidos à flexão repetitiva do punho/pronação do antebraço.

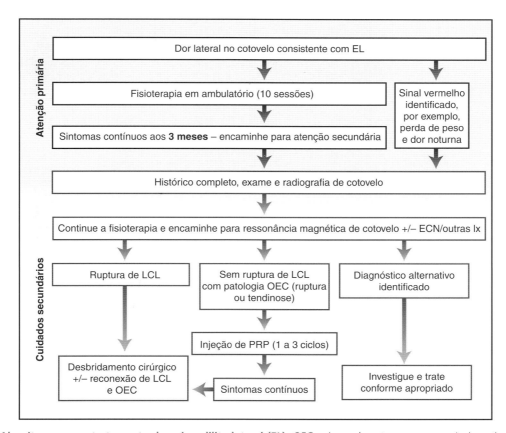

Figura 24.8 Algoritmo para o tratamento da epicondilite lateral (EL). *OEC*, origem do extensor comum; *Ix*, investigações; *LCL*, ligamento colateral lateral; *ECN*, estudos de condução nervosa; *PRP*, plasma rico em plaquetas.

Além disso, a EM pode se desenvolver como uma resposta secundária a uma única grande força em valgo ao longo do cotovelo, muitas vezes causando uma avulsão da origem do flexor pronador comum.

Pensou-se que as rupturas afetavam predominantemente as origens do tendão do pronador redondo e flexor radial do carpo; entretanto, estudos mais recentes mostram que todos os músculos da origem do flexor comum são afetados (com exceção do palmar longo). Microscopicamente é indistinguível de EL, mostrando tendinose angiofibroblástica.

Os pacientes apresentam dor localizada no epicôndilo medial, e pioram com a preensão. Há sensibilidade sobre o epicôndilo medial distal e dor com resistência à pronação/flexão do punho do antebraço. A EM coexiste comumente com uma neurite da ulna e acredita-se que seja uma consequência de tração, aprisionamento e compressão. Um exame cuidadoso para procurar sinais de instabilidade em valgo (insuficiência LCU) e compressão/neuropatia do nervo ulnar deve ser realizado para evitar diagnósticos incorretos.

Assim como acontece com EL, radiografias simples e RM podem mostrar calcificação intratendínea ou esporões de tração e podem ser úteis na exclusão de diagnósticos alternativos, como rupturas de LCU ou lesões osteocondrais que podem mimetizar EM.

As modalidades de tratamento descritas para EL são todas apropriadas no tratamento de EM. No entanto, como acontece com EL, a base de evidências não demonstra superioridade de uma técnica sobre a outra e, em muitos casos, são demonstrados apenas benefícios a curto prazo. Em termos de intervenção cirúrgica, o principal objetivo do tratamento é a excisão do tecido patológico na origem do flexor comum, com opções de liberação do túnel cubital nos casos de compressão do nervo ulnar. O perfil de complicações inclui lesão dos nervos cutâneos ulnar ou antebraquial medial e liberação inadvertida da origem do LCU. Os resultados da cirurgia são, mais uma vez, bons a excelentes em cerca de 90% dos pacientes. Resultados piores estão associados com sintomas do nervo ulnar (Gabel e Morrey, 1995).

Rupturas/avulsões de tendão

Ruptura do tendão do bíceps distal

As rupturas do tendão do bíceps distal ocorrem em homens de meia-idade, com poucos relatos na literatura de rupturas do bíceps distal em pacientes do sexo feminino. A história clássica é de uma força de extensão significativa aplicada ao cotovelo flexionado, seguida por uma contração excêntrica do bíceps e uma sensação de laceração na região da fossa cubital. O paciente descreverá um "estalo" ou uma sensação de "ceder" frequentemente. A ruptura pode ocorrer como resultado de uma laceração aguda ou em conjunto com degeneração crônica, geralmente assintomática.

A patologia da ruptura do tendão não é bem compreendida e tende a ocorrer na inserção na tuberosidade radial. Isso pode ser devido à relativa natureza hipovascular dessa área. Também se acredita que o impacto mecânico pode levar ao atrito quando o antebraço está pronado e o espaço entre a ulna e a tuberosidade radial é significativamente reduzido.

O histórico clínico e o quadro podem tornar o diagnóstico claro. Os pacientes apresentam com frequência equimose significativa da fossa cubital, contorno muscular anormal com dor e fraqueza na supinação e na flexão. O'Driscoll et al. (2007) descreveram o teste do gancho ou *Hook test* para rupturas do bíceps distal que tem uma sensibilidade e especificidade de 100%, melhor do que a RM. Com o cotovelo mantido a 90° de flexão, o antebraço é supinado e o ombro abduzido a 90° e girado internamente, o

examinador pode então enganchar a ponta do polegar em torno da borda lateral do tendão do bíceps na fossa cubital se o bíceps distal não estiver rompido.

Os pacientes podem ter uma ruptura parcial ou o exame pode ser confundido pela presença da aponeurose bicipital intacta. Esses pacientes devem ser submetidos a investigações adicionais. Geralmente, radiografias simples são normais, pois o tendão raramente avulsiona da tuberosidade. A modalidade de imagem de escolha é a RM. O cotovelo deve ser escaneado na chamada posição FAS (cotovelo flexionado, ombro abduzido, antebraço supinado). Isso cria tensão no tendão e minimiza sua obliquidade e rotação, resultando em uma visão longitudinal "verdadeira" do tendão (Chew e Giuffrè, 2005).

Estima-se que uma ruptura completa resulte em uma redução de 40% na potência de supinação e 30% na potência de flexão, embora uma abordagem não operatória possa ser feita. Isso é inaceitável para a maioria dos atletas (Morrey et al., 1985).

A técnica cirúrgica para reparar o tendão envolve, em grande parte, o reparo anatômico da tuberosidade radial. Ainda existe controvérsia quanto ao uso de uma técnica de uma ou duas incisões; a primeira está associada a maiores taxas de lesão nervosa e a última a maiores taxas de ossificação heterotópica. Além disso, o uso de diferentes técnicas de fixação é assunto de muito debate na literatura ortopédica. Opções que incluem fixação com âncoras de sutura, túneis ósseos, parafusos de interferência ou botões corticais suspensórios, já tiveram seus métodos descritos. Watson et al. (2014b) realizaram uma revisão dos métodos e técnicas de fixação. Eles observaram que a taxa de complicações não diferiu significativamente entre as abordagens de uma e duas incisões. Eles descobriram que o uso de um túnel ósseo e um botão cortical tinha taxas de complicações significativamente menores em comparação com outros métodos de fixação.

O ideal é que os reparos sejam realizados precocemente, antes que haja retração, adesão e degeneração significativa do tendão. No entanto, bons resultados foram obtidos com apresentação tardia. Mesmo quando a tensão criada pelo tendão do bíceps distal contraído é alta, ele pode ser reconectado de forma confiável à inserção anatômica com até 90° de flexão do cotovelo com resultados excelentes (Morrey et al., 2014). Os protocolos de reabilitação no pós-operatório podem utilizar atividades de amplitude de movimento anteriores com métodos de fixação progressivamente mais fortes.

Ruptura do tendão do tríceps

A lesão no tríceps distal é menos comum do que no bíceps distal, embora a demografia do paciente e os fatores de risco associados sejam semelhantes. O mecanismo de ruptura é geralmente uma forte contração muscular excêntrica contra uma grande carga. As rupturas tendem a ocorrer na inserção do tríceps na cabeça do olécrano, e não na junção musculotendínea.

Os pacientes reclamam de um estalo doloroso no cotovelo. Eles geralmente têm amplitude de movimento passiva completa com um óbvio atraso do extensor. A potência do tríceps deve ser testada contra a gravidade para evitar subestimar o grau de lesão. Devem ser feitas radiografias simples, pois elas podem mostrar uma fratura por avulsão da ponta do olécrano. A RM pode ocasionalmente ser útil se houver alguma incerteza diagnóstica e pode detectar ruptura incompleta.

Mais uma vez, o tratamento não operatório não tem papel no atleta, devido à redução da força na extensão do cotovelo. A imobilização do cotovelo é mal tolerada e a fixação cirúrgica precoce deve ter como objetivo ser robusta o suficiente para permitir o

Cotovelo Esportivo — Capítulo | 24 |

movimento precoce. O reparo cirúrgico geralmente é realizado por meio de uma única incisão posterior aberta e pode utilizar âncoras de sutura, túneis ósseos ou uma combinação deles.

A reabilitação tem como objetivo permitir o movimento passivo precoce e evitar a extensão ativa do cotovelo contra a gravidade durante a fase inicial da cura.

Pontos-chave

- A articulação do cotovelo no atleta pode ser afetada por dor, rigidez e instabilidade

- O objetivo de todos os tratamentos não operatórios e cirúrgicos é permitir a amplitude de movimento precoce. Deve-se evitar a imobilização em modelos de gesso
- As tendinopatias ao redor do cotovelo são comuns e geralmente autolimitadas. Há muita controvérsia quanto ao melhor tratamento. A cirurgia precoce deve ser evitada sempre que possível
- A instabilidade pode ocorrer após trauma agudo ou atenuação crônica. Uma investigação meticulosa é necessária para um diagnóstico preciso e um planejamento de tratamento
- O tratamento não operatório não tem papel nas rupturas agudas do tendão ao redor do cotovelo no atleta.

Referências bibliográficas

Anakwe, R.E., Middleton, S.D., Jenkins, P.J., McQueen, M.M., Court-Brown, C.M., 2011. Patient-reported outcomes after simple dislocation of the elbow. The Journal of Bone and Joint Surgery. American Volume 93 (13), 1220-1226.

Anakwenze, O.A., Kwon, D., O'Donnell, E., Levine, W.N., Ahmad, C.S., 2014. Surgical treatment of posterolateral rotatory instability of the elbow. Arthroscopy 30 (7), 866-871.

Bisset, L., Beller, E., Jull, G., Brooks, P., Darnell, R., Vicenzino, B., 2006. Mobilisation with movement and exercise, corticosteroid injection, or wait and see for tennis elbow: randomised trial. British Medical Journal 333, 939.

Carr, A.J., Murphy, R., Dakin, S.G., Rombach, I., Wheway, K., Watkins, B., et al., 2015. Platelet-rich plasma injection with arthroscopic Acromioplasty for chronic rotator cuff tendinopathy: a randomized controlled trial. The American Journal of Sports Medicine 43 (12), 2891-2897.

Chew, M.L., Giuffrè, B.M., 2005. Disorders of the distal biceps brachii tendon. RadioGraphics 25 (5), 1227-1237.

Cook, J.L., Purdam, C.R., 2009. Is tendon pathology a continuum? A pathology model to explain the clinical presentation of load-induced tendinopathy. British Journal of Sports Medicine 43, 409-416.

Coombes, B.K., Bisset, L., Vicenzino, B., 2010. Efficacy and safety of corticosteroid injections and other injections for management of tendinopathy: a systematic review of randomised controlled trials. Lancet 376, 1751-1767.

de Vos, R.J., Windt, J., Weir, A., 2014. Strong evidence against platelet-rich plasma injections for chronic lateral epicondylar tendinopathy: a systematic review. British Journal of Sports Medicine 48 (12), 952-956.

Ford, R.D., Schmitt, W.P., Lineberry, K., Luce, P., 2015. A retrospective comparison of the management of recalcitrant lateral elbow tendinosis: platelet-rich plasma injections versus surgery. Hand 10 (2), 285-291.

Fujihara, Y., Huetteman, H.E., Chung, T.T., Shauver, M.J., Chung, K.C., 2018. The effect of impactful articles on clinical practice in the United States: corticosteroid injection for patients with lateral epicondylitis. Plastic and Reconstructive Surgery 141 (5), 1183-1191.

Gabel, G.T., Morrey, B.F., 1995. Operative treatment of medial epicondylitis. Influence of concomitant ulnar neuropathy at the elbow. The Journal of Bone and Joint Surgery. American Volume 77 (7), 1065-1069.

Iordens, G.I., Van Lieshout, E.M., Schep, N.W., et al., 2015. Early mobilisation versus plaster immobilisation of simple elbow dislocations: results of the FuncSiE multicentre randomized clinical trial. British Journal of Sports Medicine 51 (6), 531-538.

Jobe, F.W., Stark, H., Lombardo, S.J., 1986. Reconstruction of the ulnar collateral ligament in athletes. The Journal of Bone and Joint Surgery. American Volume 68-A, 1158-1163.

Jones, K.J., Dodson, C.C., Osbahr, D.C., Parisien, R.L., Weiland, A.J., Altchek, D.W., et al., 2012. The docking technique for lateral ulnar collateral ligament reconstruction: surgical technique and clinical outcomes. Journal of Shoulder and Elbow Surgery 21 (3), 389-395.

Josefsson, P.O., Gentz, C.F., Johnell, O., Wendeberg, B., 1987. Surgical versus non-surgical treatment of ligamentous injuries following dislocation of the elbow joint. A prospective randomized study. The Journal of Bone and Joint Surgery. American Volume 69, 605-608.

Josefsson, P.O., Johnell, O., Gentz, C.F., 1984. Long-term sequelae of simple dislocation of the elbow. The Journal of Bone and Joint Surgery. American Volume 66, 927-930.

Kroslak, M., Murrell, G.A.C., 2018. Surgical treatment of lateral epicondylitis: a prospective, randomized, double-blinded, placebo-controlled clinical trial. The American Journal of Sports Medicine 46 (5), 1106-1113.

Lebiedziński, R., Synder, M., Buchcic, P., Polguj, M., Grzegorzewski, A., Sibiński, M., 2015. A randomized study of autologous conditioned plasma and steroid injections in the treatment of lateral epicondylitis. International Orthopaedics 39 (11), 2199-2203.

Mishra, A., Pavelko, T., 2006. Treatment of chronic elbow tendinosis with buffered platelet-rich plasma. The American Journal of Sports Medicine 34 (11), 1774-1778.

Modi, C.S., Wasserstein, D., Mayne, I.P., Henry, P.D., Mahomed, N., Veillette, C.J., 2015. The frequency and risk factors for subsequent surgery after a simple elbow dislocation. Injury 46, 1156-1160.

Morrey, B.F., Askew, L.J., An, K.N., Dobyns, J.H., 1985. Rupture of the distal tendon of the biceps brachii. A biomechanical study. The Journal of Bone and Joint Surgery. American Volume 67 (3), 418-421.

Morrey, M.E., Abdel, M.P., Sanchez-Sotelo, J., Morrey, B.F., 2014. Primary repair of retracted distal biceps tendon ruptures in extreme flexion. Journal of Shoulder and Elbow Surgery 23 (5), 679-685.

O'Driscoll, S.W., Goncalves, L.B., Dietz, P., 2007. The hook test for distal biceps tendon avulsion. The American Journal of Sports Medicine 35 (11), 1865-1869.

O'Driscoll, S.W., Morrey, B.F., Korinek, S., An, K.N., 1992. Elbow subluxation and dislocation. A spectrum of instability. Clinical Orthopaedics and Related Research 280, 186-197.

O'Driscoll, S.W., 1999. Elbow instability. Acta Orthopaedica Belgica 65 (4), 404-415.

O'Driscoll, S.W., Jupiter, J.B., King, G.J., Hotchkiss, R.N., Morrey, B.F., 2001. The unstable elbow. Instructional Course Lectures 50, 89-102.

Olaussen, M., Holmedal, O., Lindbaek, M., Brage, S., Solvang, H., 2013. Treating lateral epicondylitis with corticosteroid injections or non-electrotherapeutical physiotherapy: a systematic review. British Medical Journal Open 3,e003564.

Osborne, G., Cotterill, P., 1966. Recurrent dislocation of the elbow. The Journal of Bone and Joint Surgery. American Volume 48, 340-346.

Peerbooms, J.C., Sluimer, J., Bruijn, D.J., Gosens, T., 2010. Positive effect of an autologous platelet concentrate in lateral epicondylitis in a double-blind randomized controlled trial: platelet-rich plasma versus corticosteroid injection with a 1-year follow-up. The American Journal of Sports Medicine 38 (2), 255-262.

Rettig, A.C., Sherrill, C., Snead, D.S., Mendler, J.C., Mieling, P., 2001. Nonoperative treatment of ulnar collateral ligament injuries in throwing athletes. The American Journal of Sports Medicine 29, 15-17.

Reuter, S., Proier, P., Imhoff, A., Lenich, A., 2016. Rehabilitation, clinical outcome and return to sporting activities after posterolateral elbow instability: a systematic review. European Journal of Physical and Rehabilitation Medicine.

Rhyou, I.H., Kim, Y.S., 2012. New mechanism of the posterior elbow dislocation. Knee Surgery, Sports Traumatology, Arthroscopy 20 (12), 2535-2541.

Robinson, P.M., Griffiths, E., Watts, A.C., 2017. Simple elbow dislocation. Shoulder & Elbow 9 (3), 195-204.

Rossy, W.H., Oh, L.S., 2016. Pitcher's elbow: medial elbow pain in the overhead-throwing athlete. Current Reviews in Musculoskeletal Medicine 9 (2), 207-214.

Sadeghi-Demneh, E., Jafarian, F., 2013. The immediate effects of orthoses on pain in people with lateral epicondylalgia. Pain Research and Treatment 2013, 353597.

Sayegh, E.T., Strauch, R.J., 2015. Does nonsurgical treatment improve longitudinal outcomes of lateral epicondylitis over no treatment? A meta-analysis. Clinical Orthopaedics and Related Research 473 (3), 1093-1107.

Schreiber, J.J., Potter, H.G., Warren, R.F., Hotchkiss, R.N., Daluiski, A., 2014. Magnetic resonance imaging findings in acute elbow dislocation: insight into mechanism. The Journal of Hand Surgery 39, 199-205.

Schreiber, J.J., Warren, R.F., Hotchkiss, R.N., Daluiski, A., 2013. An on-line video investigation into the mechanism of elbow dislocation. The Journal of Hand Surgery 38, 488-494.

Sims, S.E., Miller, K., Elfar, J.C., Hammert, W.C., 2014. Non-surgical treatment of lateral epicondylitis: a systematic review of randomized controlled trials. Hand (N Y) 9 (4), 419-446.

Watson, J.N., McQueen, P., Hutchinson, M.R., 2014a. A systematic review of ulnar collateral ligament reconstruction techniques. The American Journal of Sports Medicine 42 (10), 2510-2516.

Watson, J.N., Moretti, V.M., Schwindel, L., Hutchinson, M.R., 2014b. Repair techniques for acute distal biceps tendon ruptures: a systematic review. The Journal of Bone and Joint Surgery. American Volume 96 (24), 2086-2090.

Capítulo | 25 |

Lesões nas Mãos e nos Punhos: Boxe em Foco

Ian Gatt

Introdução

A mão e o punho são os locais mais comuns de lesão no boxe. O autor trabalhou com o time nacional da Grã-Bretanha nos últimos três ciclos olímpicos: Londres 2012, Rio 2016, e Tóquio 2020, realizada em 2021. Depois de investir um tempo considerável no entendimento das principais lesões que ocorrem nesse esporte, várias abordagens de avaliação, técnicas terapêuticas e estratégias preventivas foram implementadas por meio de tentativa e erro. Pesquisas indicam que a incidência de lesões nessas áreas diminuiu, enquanto a disponibilidade geral de treinamento aumentou. Este capítulo fornecerá uma visão das principais lesões que ocorrem na mão e no punho nesse esporte.

Para entender as lesões que ocorrem na mão e no punho no boxe, é útil apreciar alguns aspectos técnicos. Os boxeadores podem adotar uma postura ortodoxa (liderando com o braço esquerdo e perna esquerda) ou uma postura canhota (liderando com o braço direito e perna direita); ocasionalmente, há também os *switchers*, que alternam entre as posições durante uma competição. Uma apreciação de diversas posturas e dominância pode impactar no manejo das lesões. Os tipos de socos desferidos em uma competição estão associados à postura. Eles são divididos principalmente em socos de braço reto ou dobrado. A mão inicial é usada predominantemente para:

- *Jabs* (socos de braço reto)
- Ganchos (socos de braço dobrado indo de fora para dentro)
- *Upper cuts* (braço dobrado de cima para baixo).
  A mão traseira é usada predominantemente para:
- Cruzado (soco direto)
- *Upper cuts*.

Ganchos não são comumente desferidos com a mão de trás devido a sua maior distância do oponente em comparação com a mão dianteira. No entanto, ganchos usando as costas da mão podem ser utilizados durante a luta curta (*i. e.*, quando os dois boxeadores estão próximos, *in-fighting*). Durante qualquer competição, os boxeadores podem desferir qualquer um desses socos, dependendo da tática. Os atletas podem desferir socos únicos ou múltiplos socos durante qualquer fase do ataque.

Como em qualquer esporte, entender as forças que são geradas e, por sua vez, absorvidas por um atleta é fundamental para entender as lesões. No boxe, a velocidade máxima de um único soco foi medida em 8,16 m/s para amadores (Walilko et al., 2005) e 8,9 m/s para boxeadores profissionais (Atha et al., 1985). Atha et al. (1985) relataram que para replicar uma força de soco equivalente de 4.096 N, conforme registrado em seu estudo, um martelo de madeira acolchoado de 6 kg teria que martelar a 32 km/h. O nível de especialização produzirá diferentes forças de soco. Em grupos de elite, intermediários e novatos, as forças máximas de soco para a mão traseira foram registradas em 4.800 N, 3.722 N e 2.381 N, respectivamente (Smith et al., 2000).

O tipo de soco também produzirá diferentes forças de soco. A maioria dos estudos que avaliam as forças no boxe concorda que o gancho do braço dominante produzirá mais força do que um *jab* do braço dominante, enquanto um soco cruzado de trás produzirá uma força maior do que o gancho do braço dominante (Lenetsky et al., 2013). Parece altamente plausível que as forças produzidas sejam absorvidas principalmente pelos nós dos dedos, ou seja, as articulações metacarpofalangianas (MCF), e isso se relaciona com as lesões nas mãos que foram relatadas em vários estudos (Hame e Malone, 2000; Loosemore et al., 2017). Isso também fez com que o termo "fratura do boxeador" se tornasse amplamente utilizado (Gladden, 1957). As forças também atingem o resto da mão e do punho, resultando em diversos ferimentos. Dignas de nota são as lesões articulares carpometacarpal (CMC) observadas em boxeadores amadores de elite, que podem impactar de modo significativo nos dias perdidos de treinamento (Loosemore et al., 2016).

Finalmente, os boxeadores passam por diferentes tipos de treinamento de boxe, variando de nenhum impacto até a maior quantidade de impacto na região da mão e punho. Eles vão na ordem: boxe sombra, golpe com vara, bolsas de água, bolsas macias, bolsas pesadas, almofadas, *sparring* técnico e *sparring* aberto. Essa informação é útil ao progredir um boxeador de nenhum impacto para o retorno total às atividades de boxe, com manipulação de variáveis de intensidade (porcentagem de soco desferido) e volume (número de rodadas, geralmente expresso em 3 minutos/rodada) possível. Portanto, a equipe de saúde deve ter pleno conhecimento das diversas atividades antes de projetar um programa conservador ou pós-operatório.

Principais lesões que ocorrem na mão e no punho no boxe

Os boxeadores sofrem lesões em todas as partes do corpo, o que está relacionado com a mecânica esportiva específica e com outras estratégias gerais de condicionamento, como correr. No entanto, lesões nas mãos e nos punhos são "o pão com manteiga" desse esporte. Em nível nacional olímpico, entre 2005 e 2009, as lesões de mão e punho foram responsáveis por aproximadamente

35% de todas as registradas em treinamento e competição para o time da GB (Loosemore et al., 2017). Além disso, o total de dias perdidos para o treinamento e a duração geral foi significativamente maior nessas áreas do que em qualquer outra parte do corpo. Lesões nas mãos e nos punhos também são um fardo nas fileiras profissionais, com muitos boxeadores precisando de tempo livre do treinamento e da competição. Logo, este capítulo terá enfoque em compreender e manejar as principais lesões sofridas no boxe que afetam a disponibilidade para treinamento (Figura 25.1), que são:
- Lesões de banda sagital nas articulações (articulações MCF)
- Instabilidade CMC no punho
- Lesões do ligamento colateral ulnar (LCU) na base do polegar.

Nós dos dedos: lesões na banda sagital

Os nós dos dedos (região demonstrada na imagem), também conhecidos como articulações MCF, apresentam a maior incidência de qualquer lesão na região da mão e do punho, embora o treinamento com essa lesão seja mais possível, mesmo quando os sintomas estão presentes. As lesões ocorrem de modo agudo ao bater uma região anatômica óssea em um oponente em um *sparring* ou competição; socos na testa do oponente com a mão dianteira ou com a mão traseira, ou no cotovelo ao lançar um *upper cut*. Isso pode resultar em rupturas de uma das bandas sagitais (também chamada de "capa extensora") da articulação (Figuras 25.1 e 25.2). Postula-se que, junto com o contato direto, também ocorre uma força de cisalhamento na articulação ao impactar um oponente. Isso criaria uma força de alongamento em um lado da articulação com uma força de encurtamento ocorrendo no outro, explicando por que apenas uma das duas bandas sagitais de ancoragem é comumente ferida. Esse cisalhamento é ainda mais reforçado por achados clínicos ao avaliar a mobilidade da articulação pós-trauma: aumento do deslizamento acessório transversal em uma direção (comumente direção ulnar), com diminuição da mobilidade na direção oposta (direção radial). Esses achados de mobilidade articular na articulação são observados de maneira semelhante ao avaliar clinicamente um polegar "em choque", pelo que comumente o LCU (um dos colaterais) é ferido resultante de uma força de cisalhamento ocorrendo em uma direção de abdução (valgo ou radial).

Os sintomas nos nós dos dedos também ocorrem de maneira insidiosa, principalmente relacionados com golpes repetidos de equipamentos de treinamento, como um saco de boxe. As articulações mais comumente lesionadas são a primeira e a segunda (i. e., dedos indicador e médio). Isso se deve ao contato no impacto que ocorre predominantemente nessas áreas, conforme observado pelo teste de impacto em um filme de pressão realizado na equipe de boxe da Grã-Bretanha. Ocasionalmente, a quarta articulação (i. e., o dedo mínimo) é ferida, no geral como resultado de uma lesão aguda. A articulação do dedo anular é ferida raramente.

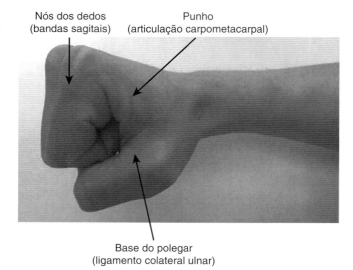

Figura 25.1 Locais das principais lesões ocorridas no boxe.

Apresentação/testagem para lesões da banda sagital

A apresentação e o teste de lesões da banda sagital são mostrados no Boxe 25.1.

Medidas objetivas

Medidas objetivas para qualquer lesão esportiva são importantes, pois vinculam as informações subjetivas à gravidade da lesão. As informações coletadas auxiliarão nas decisões clínicas e na disponibilidade do treinamento. No boxe, medidas objetivas para lesões nas mãos e nos punhos são fundamentais para fornecer o nível necessário de cuidado nesse esporte, protegendo os atletas. Isso também se aplica a outras lesões discutidas neste capítulo.

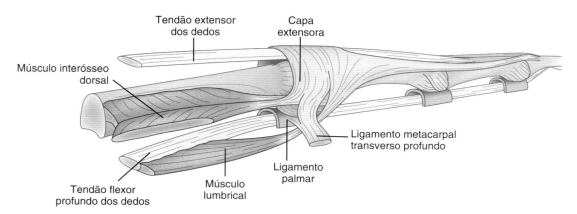

Figura 25.2 Anatomia do dedo com capa extensora (bandas sagitais) da articulação. (*Esta figura se encontra reproduzida em cores no Encarte.*)

> **Boxe 25.1 Lesões de banda sagital**
>
> **Mecanismo**
> - Impacto direto
> - Frequentemente devido à baixa qualidade do curativo ou da luva.
>
> **Exame**
> - O inchaço na articulação é comum
> - Dor à palpação em ambos os lados da capa extensora (um lado mais do que o outro)
> - Um defeito pode ser sentido (parece um orifício sem resistência do tecido), indicando um potencial rompimento das bandas sagitais ou da cápsula
> - Dor ocasional no aspecto volar (palma) da articulação MCF
> - Sensação da articulação rígida na flexão passiva da articulação MCF – às vezes pode ser esponjosa (inflamatória) ou vazia (nenhuma resistência sentida na flexão passiva – parece bastante hipermóvel)
> - Subluxação do tendão extensor na flexão – nem sempre e pode ocorrer em indivíduos normais – pode ser confirmada com ultrassom dinâmico.

MCF, metacarpofalangeana.

Amplitude de movimento

Fechar o punho pode ser doloroso tanto em condições agudas quanto crônicas, com redução da amplitude de movimento (ADM) visível ou medida. A ADM articular é melhor testada usando um goniômetro metálico de dedo, que é colocado diretamente sobre a articulação (Figura 25.3 A). O punho deve inicialmente ser colocado em extensão total para eliminar a musculatura extensora. O punho pode então ser colocado em flexão total para testar a flexibilidade muscular (extensores dos dedos). Identificar quais estruturas (músculo *versus* articulação) podem reduzir a ADM da articulação auxilia na escolha de estratégias apropriadas. A partir da triagem realizada na equipe de boxe da Grã-Bretanha pré-lesão, espera-se que a primeira articulação geralmente tenha menos ADM do que a segunda, e a segunda menos ADM do que a terceira e a quarta. Isso possivelmente se deve ao micro ou macrotrauma que ocorre ao longo dos anos nessas áreas. Obviamente, a comparação entre os lados é recomendada.

Força (função de mão)

A habilidade de fechar os punhos no boxe é importante, especialmente na fase final do soco. Nessa fase crucial do soco, o comprometimento pode resultar em perda potencial de energia do movimento dos tecidos moles ao tensionar os músculos no contato (Richards, 1997). Além da produção de energia reduzida, a incapacidade de cerrar o punho cria um punho menos estável no contato, o que coloca as estruturas de mão-punho em risco de lesão ou lesões adicionais.

A mão tem três padrões principais de preensão: preensão palmar, preensão em pinça e pinça lateral. O teste recomendado para força de preensão em lesões de articulação usa o dinamômetro de preensão de mão (ver Figura 25.3 B) e o procedimento discutido por Gatt et al. (2018): em pé, braços ao lado do corpo com extensão total do cotovelo, com todas as medidas realizadas alternadamente três vezes sem descanso. Para cada medição, o dinamômetro é pressionado por 3 segundos com o valor de pico de força registrado.

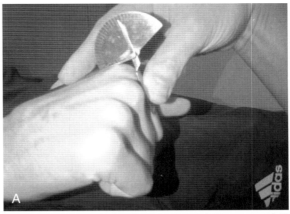

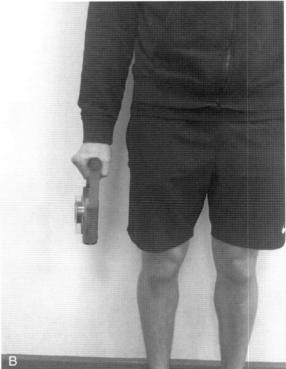

Figura 25.3 Medidas objetivas para os nós dos dedos. **A.** Goniômetro de dedo para amplitude de movimento. **B.** Dinamômetro de empunhadura para avaliação de empunhadura.

Trabalho diagnóstico (investigações)

A informação subjetiva, a avaliação objetiva e a reação ao tratamento inicial devem orientar os médicos profissionais de saúde sobre a melhor maneira de proceder. Se os sintomas forem bastante persistentes, ou com base na justificativa clínica, uma ultrassonografia deve ser considerada. Ela pode identificar danos estruturais à articulação, detectar uma sinovite crônica ou uma subluxação do tendão extensor sobre a face dorsal da articulação (ultrassom dinâmico mais apropriado), que na maioria dos casos pode ser observada no exame clínico, sem a necessidade de diagnóstico complementar por imagem, durante a flexão da articulação. Os resultados podem apoiar a abordagem de tratamento atual ou indicar a necessidade de abordagens mais invasivas, como terapia de injeção ou intervenções cirúrgicas. As informações de um exame de ultrassom não devem ser utilizadas para determinar se a cirurgia deve ocorrer, mas sim para aumentar o conhecimento para administrar o boxeador. Uma investigação

Parte | 2 | Aplicação Clínica

mais detalhada usando a ressonância magnética (RM) pode ser útil, em especial na identificação da integridade da cápsula.

Manejo conservador

Estratégias de proteção

A maioria dos boxeadores consegue manter o *status* de treinamento completo com uma lesão na articulação do dedo, se relativamente sem dor no impacto. Às vezes, essas articulações podem ficar sem dor por um período e, em seguida, agravar-se com base na competição ou nos requisitos de treinamento. Foi observado que a redução das forças que atuam na articulação pode manter o *status* de disponibilidade total enquanto permite que a área cicatrize durante os estágios iniciais de uma lesão. Da mesma maneira, pode ajudar a reduzir a probabilidade de recorrência ou cronicidade. As estratégias a serem consideradas são predominantemente luvas e técnicas de bandagem. A qualidade e o tamanho das luvas devem ser considerados, já que a maioria dos boxeadores usa luvas muito pequenas, com enchimento insuficiente ou simplesmente gastas. Os boxeadores devem considerar a aquisição de pelo menos dois pares de luvas: um para *sparring* e outro para o treino com sacos/almofadas. A proteção dos nós dos dedos começa enrolando a mão e o punho antes de colocar as luvas, levando em consideração as estratégias de descarga apropriadas. Isso inclui o uso de:

* Espuma de melhor qualidade cobrindo os quatro nós dos dedos
* Espuma "*donuts*" em qualquer nó do dedo afetado para descarregar áreas de sensibilidade (Figura 25.4 A)
* Dupla fita adesiva com o dedo adjacente para reduzir as forças em valgo (Figura 25.4 B)
* Bandagem em forma de oito no nó do dedo para reduzir a flexão do mesmo (Figura 25.4 C)
* Uma "barra" na palma da mão com os envoltórios (Figura 25.4 D)
* Considerar o uso de sacos mais macios (p. ex., sacos de água).

Gelo e compressão

Na fase aguda, o frio deve ser considerado com gelo picado, se disponível, com sacos de gelo tradicionais (com filme plástico para manter o saco firmemente no lugar). Isso deve ser seguido por compressão, usando uma bandagem coesa de 2,5 cm ao redor da articulação (abordagem em oito; Figura 25.4 C). Também existem equipamentos elétricos ou movidos a bateria que podem ser utilizados para fornecer frio (crioterapia) e compressão à área. Isso tem a vantagem adicional de usar abordagens de compressão contínuas *versus* sequenciais. Posteriormente, deve ser utilizado para auxiliar no controle da dor após quaisquer sessões de impacto durante o retorno precoce ao treinamento. Se for uma área que pode inflamar ocasionalmente, o uso regular de gelo ajudará no manejo a longo prazo. Como estratégia preventiva, as mãos podem ser imersas, após a sessão, em um balde de gelo e água (crioimersão) (sugerem-se 20 segundos dentro e 40 segundos fora × 5).

Terapia manual (mobilizações articulares)

A avaliação e o tratamento da terapia manual são aconselháveis nos estágios iniciais de qualquer lesão na mão e no punho. A ADM de flexão é comumente perdida devido ao choque articular. É recomendada a avaliação do deslizamento da articulação posteroanterior (PA) e qualquer disfunção restaurada para melhorar a ADM de flexão e a sensação final. Abdução e adução são outros movimentos disponíveis nos nós dos dedos ocorrendo no plano sagital. Como discutido anteriormente, os nós dos dedos podem ser forçados em uma direção mais ulnar. Isso pode prejudicar a quantidade de movimento do plano sagital que ocorre. A avaliação do deslizamento transversal da articulação é recomendada, pois, mesmo quando a ADM de flexão é restaurada, se houver uma disfunção do deslizamento transversal, ela pode prolongar os sintomas. Além da disfunção local, é importante avaliar o resto da mão, o punho e o antebraço, pois as limitações articulares nessas áreas podem afetar indiretamente os sintomas na articulação; logo, deve-se sempre pensar na osteocinemática, assim como na artrocinemática.

Modalidades de eletroterapia

Modalidades de eletroterapia como o *laser*, que na prática clínica apresentam resultados positivos em termos de dor, podem ser incluídas na abordagem terapêutica. Os *lasers* da classe IIIb são os modelos mais comumente utilizados e adequados para o uso terapêutico. Nos últimos anos, os *lasers* de classe IV foram introduzidos para lesões de mão e punho, com evidências anedóticas indicando que eles substituem os *lasers* de classe IIIb devido à maior intensidade gerada. São necessárias mais evidências, cuja discussão está além do escopo deste capítulo; porém, o autor utilizou a classe IIIb por vários anos com *feedback* positivo nessas áreas.

Acupuntura

A acupuntura tem um papel benéfico no controle dos sintomas e deve ser considerada com cuidado quando utilizada em torno dos requisitos de treinamento (i. e., é comum a hipersensibilização pós-tratamento). Ao considerar a lesão na articulação, vale a pena avaliar os músculos interósseos, bem como os músculos extrínsecos do antebraço, que podem proporcionar dor referida na mão e simular sintomas de articulação.

Mobilização de tecidos moles

A mobilização de estruturas de tecidos moles deve ser considerada por meio de técnicas de pressão positiva ou negativa (i. e., empurrar ou levantar a pele). A pressão positiva pode ser alcançada utilizando técnicas de massagem tradicionais ou com a ajuda de técnicas de massagem de tecidos moles assistida por instrumento (IASTM, do inglês *instrument-assisted soft tissue massage*). A pressão negativa pode ser alcançada por meio de técnicas de tecido conjuntivo, ventosas ou equipamentos elétricos que fornecem sucção. Todas essas técnicas podem ser consideradas para estruturas de tecidos moles na mão, punho e antebraço. Especificamente, para os nós dos dedos, as ferramentas IASTM podem ser utilizadas sobre a região lesionada para o controle da dor. Essas técnicas foram consideradas eficazes quando realizadas antes do início do treinamento, devido à sua capacidade de dessensibilizar (entorpecer) a área. Os boxeadores podem pensar em como auto-IASTM para maximizar o impacto a longo prazo dessa estratégia.

Reabilitação (terapia por exercícios)

A reabilitação é a base do tratamento de qualquer lesão na mão e no punho no boxe. Os principais objetivos dos exercícios nas articulações são manter uma boa ADM de flexão ao redor dessa articulação, condicionar os músculos/tendões ao redor dessa articulação e dessensibilizar a dor. Observou-se que realizando alguns exercícios principais (Figura 25.5) antes de iniciar o processo de enfaixar as mãos, as lesões nas mãos e nos punhos podem ser tratadas de maneira mais eficaz. Essas estratégias também foram

Lesões nas Mãos e nos Punhos: Boxe em Foco Capítulo | 25 |

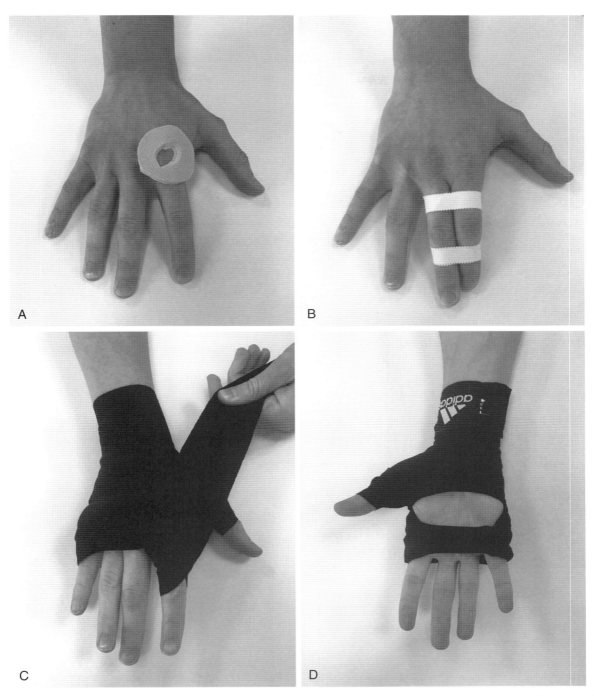

Figura 25.4 Estratégias de descarregamento para os nós dos dedos. **A.** "*Donut*" de espuma sendo usado para o primeiro nó do dedo. **B.** Bandagem dupla dos dedos indicador e médio. **C.** Técnica em oito no dedo indicador. **D.** Uma "barra" criada usando bandagem.

observadas para reduzir o risco de lesões, criando um aquecimento mais direto da região da mão-punho. Os exercícios também devem ser realizados após o treinamento, de preferência após a aplicação de gelo nos nós dos dedos, se houver uma lesão ativa, para maximizar o controle dessas condições.

O uso de bandas de resistência, barras de resistência e bolas com espinhos deve ser considerado para a maioria dos estágios de lesão nesta região (ver Figura 25.5). As bandas de resistência (Figura 25.5 A) são utilizadas para desenvolver a força/resistência dos extensores da mão, as barras de resistência (Figura 25.5 B) para desenvolver a força/resistência dos flexores-extensores do punho e dos pronadores-supinadores do antebraço e a bola com espinhos ou bola reflexa (Figura 25.5 C) visa dessensibilizar a articulação por meio de massagem vigorosa sobre a região sintomática. Essa técnica também pode ser utilizada para outras lesões de mão e punho, complementando as técnicas do IASTM voltadas para o controle da dor.

O alongamento dos extensores dos dedos também é importante, pois manter o punho fechado permite menos estresse sobre a articulação, reduzindo o alongamento do tendão extensor central nas bandas sagitais. Portanto, é uma estratégia muito útil esticar o punho fechado (em especial, garantindo que os nós dos dedos indicador e médio permaneçam fechados) em flexão, com o cotovelo em extensão total.

265

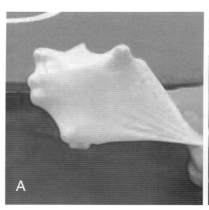 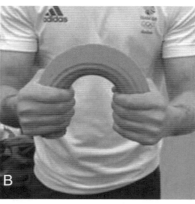 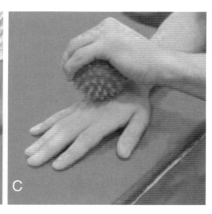

Figura 25.5 Reabilitação para os nós dos dedos. A. Abridores de banda de resistência para tendão extensor e condicionamento da articulação do nó do dedo. **B.** Regime de flexo-extensão do punho da barra de resistência e pronação-supinação do antebraço. **C.** Massagem com bola com espinhos para dessensibilização da dor.

Anti-inflamatórios e terapia de injeção

É melhor evitar os anti-inflamatórios, principalmente nas primeiras 72 horas de qualquer lesão aguda, pois podem interromper o processo de cicatrização e impactar na qualidade do colágeno, tornando o reparo mais fraco. Quando uma articulação é predominantemente inflamatória em vez de mecânica, e não está respondendo bem às estratégias de tratamento descritas até o momento, um curso de anti-inflamatórios guiados por um médico pode auxiliar na progressão dos sintomas. Isso deve ser combinado com estratégias de descarregamento apropriadas para maximizar o resultado.

Quando houver um componente inflamatório crônico na patologia e nenhuma mudança nos sintomas em resposta ao tratamento, considere uma injeção de esteroide nessa área seguida por uma descarga inicial por até 72 horas antes do retorno subsequente às estratégias de treinamento. As injeções não são a primeira linha de tratamento e as outras estratégias descritas anteriormente devem ser adequadamente consideradas em primeiro lugar.

Intervenção cirúrgica

As informações subjetivas e objetivas combinadas com a reação ao tratamento inicial devem orientar o médico sobre a melhor maneira de proceder. Os boxeadores com lesões agudas graves com bandas sagitais rompidas podem ser mantidos em treinamento e competição, conforme os sintomas permitirem. Deve ser considerado o ganho de desempenho de curto *versus* longo prazo. Uma intervenção cirúrgica pode ser justificada se os sintomas forem persistentes, afetarem a disponibilidade de treinamento ou desempenho de competição.

Os procedimentos cirúrgicos são bem-sucedidos na maioria dos casos e um protocolo de reabilitação pós-operatório sob medida pode aumentar o resultado da cirurgia (Boxe 25.2). A maioria dos boxeadores requer um período de 4 meses antes de retornar ao *status* de treinamento completo. Os estágios iniciais podem variar dependendo do cirurgião e do tipo de cirurgia. No entanto, é importante para um retorno seguro e oportuno ao treinamento e à competição uma carga ideal durante toda a fase de reabilitação.

> **Boxe 25.2 Protocolo pós-operatório para reparos da capa extensora**
>
> 1. Fase de imobilidade (0 a 4 semanas): atleta com tala removível para evitar flexão combinada excessiva da articulação e punho.
> 2. Fase de carregamento inicial (4 a 6 semanas): ADM/condicionamento inicial sem carregamento do tendão extensor.
> 3. Fase de carga progressiva (6 a 8 semanas): aumento no condicionamento com carga do tendão extensor.
> 4. Retorno à fase de boxe (8 a 14 semanas): retorno gradual ao boxe.
> 5. Fase de treinamento completo (14 a 16 semanas): monitoramento do boxeador em estado de treinamento completo.

ADM, amplitude de movimento.

Lesões da articulação carpometacarpal

A incidência de lesões nas articulações CMCs na equipe de boxe da Grã-Bretanha é menor do que nos nós dos dedos; no entanto, a gravidade e o impacto na disponibilidade de treinamento são maiores. O mecanismo comum de lesão é a flexão forçada do punho no impacto contra o oponente, durante o qual a mão é mantida em um punho consideravelmente fechado, o que força a(s) articulação(ões) CMCs a flexão. Como ocorre nos nós dos dedos, a segunda e/ou terceira articulações CMCs são feridas mais comumente devido ao contato no impacto que ocorre sobre suas respectivas articulações. Ao contrário de suas contrapartes ulnares (quarta e quinta articulações CMCs), a segunda e a terceira articulações CMCs não oferecem mobilidade articular, o que também as coloca em risco quando flexionadas com força.

A mão traseira é ferida mais comumente durante um soco cruzado ao atingir o oponente no topo da cabeça. Durante a parte final do soco, o oponente foi observado em uma análise retrospectiva de vídeo flexionando o pescoço para frente como um mecanismo de proteção, aumentando o torque de flexão no punho. Embora as técnicas de enfaixamento e luvas corretas possam reduzir a incidência, lesões ainda podem ocorrer e requerem tratamento adequado.

Apresentação/teste

A apresentação da lesão da articulação CMC é mostrada na Figura 25.6 e o Boxe 25.3 fornece um resumo da apresentação e dos testes para essas lesões.

Medidas objetivas

Amplitude de movimento

A ADM pode ser medida usando um inclinômetro ou um *smartphone* com o aplicativo apropriado. O antebraço deve ser colocado sobre uma superfície plana com o cotovelo dobrado e a mão pendurada para fora da mesa com a palma voltada para baixo (Figura 25.7 A). Para flexão e extensão, o dispositivo de medição deve ser colocado próximo ao terceiro nó do dedo sobre o osso metacarpo (MC). A flexão com o punho fechado e a extensão com a mão aberta medem a musculatura extensora e flexora, respectivamente. A flexão com o punho aberto e a extensão com o punho fechado medem a ADM da articulação do punho. Esses movimentos devem ser medidos e comparados com o lado oposto. Também é aconselhável medir o desvio radial e ulnar, pois esses movimentos são importantes para a biomecânica do punho. Para essas medidas, adota-se a mesma posição e método de flexão e extensão; no entanto, o antebraço deve estar voltado para a posição prona média (entre supinação total e pronação). A mão é mantida em punho. O dispositivo de medição deve ser colocado ao longo de uma linha imaginária entre a articulação interfalangiana proximal (IFP) do dedo indicador e o espaço da rede entre o polegar e o indicador (Figura 25.7 B). A quantidade de ADM e sintomas entre os lados podem ajudar a compreender a gravidade da lesão.

Força (função de mão)

Ao apresentar uma lesão na articulação CMC, o teste do dinamômetro de preensão manual deve ser considerado um dos primeiros testes, pois as informações obtidas guiarão o exame clínico e a tomada de decisão. Tal como acontece com as lesões dos dedos, o uso de um dinamômetro de preensão manual ajudará a compreender a capacidade funcional de fechar o punho nesse estágio (Gatt et al., 2018). De acordo com a experiência clínica, uma deficiência de 0 a 20% da preensão da mão com uma medida de dor de médio porte na preensão é considerada uma lesão leve a moderada, com possível tratamento conservador. Mais de 20%

> **Boxe 25.3 Lesões da articulação carpometacarpal**
>
> **Mecanismo**
> - Um golpe no topo da cabeça ou corpo do oponente, que resulta em flexão forçada no punho.
>
> **Exame**
> - O inchaço nas costas da mão é comum (ver Figura 25.6 A)
> - Efeito da tecla de piano se houver frouxidão na articulação CMC (ver Figura 25.6 B)
> - Saliência do carpo (protuberância óssea nas costas da mão) na articulação CMC (sinal tardio)
> - Sensibilidade à palpação da articulação CMC
> - Dor ao fechar o punho com frouxidão potencial da segunda e/ou terceira articulação CMC
> - Dor na carga axial (p. ex., aplicar força através do nó do dedo com uma pressão para cima)
> - Incapacidade de completar uma rosca direta invertida com barra ou halteres (i. e., palma voltada para baixo)
> - Muitas vezes pode ter > 20% de perda de força de preensão quando testado com dinamômetro de preensão manual em comparação com a linha de base (Gatt et al., 2018).

CMC, carpometacarpal. (Adaptado de Gatt, I., Smith-Moore, S., Steggles, C., Loosemore, M., 2018. The Takei handheld dynamometer: an effective clinical outcome measure too for hand and wrist function in boxing. Hand [NY] 13 (3), 319-324.)

de deficiência de preensão manual combinada com uma alta medida de dor indica um mau prognóstico e a cirurgia deve ser considerada. As medições da preensão manual devem ser um componente chave para auxiliar na progressão durante os estágios de carga dessa lesão. O teste isocinético é útil nessa situação, quando disponível. Pode melhorar tanto a avaliação quanto as estratégias terapêuticas.

Trabalho diagnóstico (investigações)

Com base no raciocínio clínico, deve ser considerada uma ultrassonografia dinâmica para avaliar a frouxidão ligamentar dessa articulação. Isso é mais bem suportado por meio de uma RM (é sugerida uma RM 3T), que pode fornecer informações mais detalhadas sobre as estruturas. Em alguns casos, avulsão do extensor radial curto do carpo (ERCC) na base do terceiro MC e/ou extensor radial longo do carpo (ERLC) no segundo MC pode ser observada, sendo o primeiro mais comum. Essas informações,

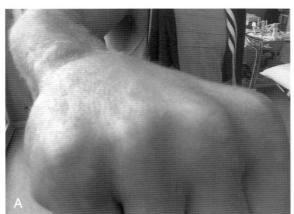 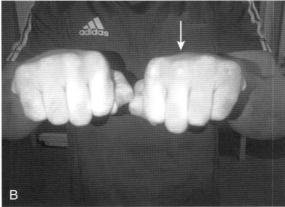

Figura 25.6 Apresentação da lesão carpometacarpal (CMC). **A.** Edema nas costas da mão. **B.** Efeito de tecla de piano ocorrendo no terceiro dedo ou CMC do dedo médio na mão esquerda (nó do dedo médio visto caindo com relação aos outros nós da mão). (*Esta figura se encontra reproduzida em cores no Encarte.*)

| Parte | 2 | Aplicação Clínica

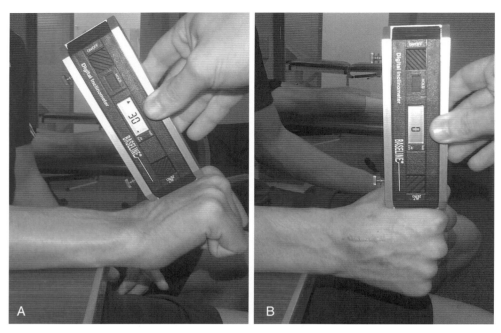

Figura 25.7 Medida da amplitude de movimento no punho usando um inclinômetro digital. **A.** Flexão-extensão. **B.** Desvio radial-ulnar.

juntamente com outras medidas objetivas de força de preensão manual, ADM e habilidades funcionais, combinadas com sintomas dentro e fora do boxe ajudarão a orientar o manejo. Uma radiografia simples deve ser considerado para descartar possíveis lesões ósseas. As fraturas não ocorrem comumente na haste longa do segundo e terceiro ossos MC, no entanto, as fraturas por avulsão que envolvem a inserção dos tendões ERLC e ERCC ocorrem na base do osso MC. Em contraste, mais fraturas foram registradas na haste longa do quinto osso MC. Isso possivelmente se deve ao maior movimento disponível na quinta articulação CMC, quando comparada à segunda e terceira articulações CMCs, afetando a torção que ocorre na haste longa do osso MC.

Manejo conservador

Estratégias de proteção

Para evitar a ocorrência de lesões, é importante reduzir o risco de ocorrência de flexão forçada no punho. Foram consideradas eficazes técnicas "cruzadas" (Figura 25.8 A) utilizando esparadrapo rígido sobre a parte de trás da região da mão e do punho. Nas categorias profissionais, essa abordagem pode ser continuada na competição. Nas fileiras dos amadores, como a fita tradicionalmente não é permitida, embora haja mudanças nas regras nos últimos anos para competidores de elite, é importante usar uma parte da bandagem para criar esses efeitos cruzados. Mais informações podem ser encontradas no YouTube (tutorial do canal *BOX Instructor* – Enfaixamento de mãos). Ao contrário dos nós dos dedos, pode ser difícil o treinamento contínuo com uma lesão nos CMCs.

Lesões leves podem ser mantidas em treinamento completo usando fita cruzada colocada sob a bandagem (*i. e.*, diretamente na pele) como um complemento para uma tala de proteção pronta para uso (Figura 25.8 B). Esta forma de órtese tem grande sucesso na redução da tensão nas articulações CMCs, pois diminui a flexão que ocorre no punho. Lesões moderadas devem ser tratadas com um período de descanso imediato. Sugere-se um mínimo de 3 semanas de repouso total na área, usando a tala durante todo o dia (e noite se tolerado). O teste de dinamometria de preensão manual deve ser realizado 1 vez/semana

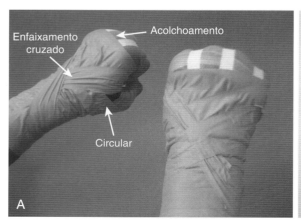
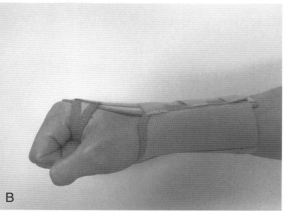

Figura 25.8 Proteção carpometacarpal com o objetivo de prevenir a flexão excessiva do punho. **A.** Uso de técnicas de bandagem circular e cruzada. **B.** Tala de punho pronta para uso.

Lesões nas Mãos e nos Punhos: Boxe em Foco **Capítulo** | **25** |

para avaliar a progressão. Se houver melhora, o prognóstico pode ser potencialmente favorável; caso contrário, a cirurgia deve ser considerada. Lesões graves devem ser consideradas para intervenção cirúrgica precoce, caso contrário, o resultado pode não ser bem-sucedido. Durante os estágios iniciais de retorno ao treinamento de lesões moderadas, o uso contínuo da tala durante o treinamento torna-se uma estratégia integral para prevenir novas lesões. Isso também é muito útil durante os estágios iniciais de retorno ao impacto no pós-operatório.

Gelo e compressão

Como acontece com uma lesão na articulação, o frio e a compressão devem ser considerados no estágio agudo desse tipo de lesão. Posteriormente, deve ser usado para auxiliar no controle da dor após quaisquer sessões de impacto durante o retorno precoce ao treinamento.

Terapia manual

Embora quase não haja movimento na segunda e terceira articulações CMCs, o jogo articular (especificamente o deslizamento AP) ainda pode ser afetado, influenciando os sintomas. Como essa articulação sofrerá um impacto em flexão, a mobilização usando um deslizamento AP pode restaurar a mobilidade acessória dessa articulação ajudando a aliviar os sintomas. Também é importante avaliar as articulações do carpo proximalmente, que podem ter sido afetadas pelo trauma inicial. Além disso, como os nós dos dedos, é importante avaliar o movimento do antebraço (supinação e pronação), pois as restrições podem afetar a posição do punho no impacto. Na prática clínica, garantir uma boa mobilidade em todas essas áreas melhora os resultados.

Eletroterapia

Assim como os ferimentos nos dedos, o *laser* pode ser um complemento útil para o processo de cicatrização. Além disso, o uso do ultrassom pulsado de baixa intensidade (LIPUS, do inglês *low-intensity pulsed ultrasound*) diretamente sobre a área tem apresentado bons resultados clínicos, amenizando os sintomas. Isso pode ser realizado como 20 minutos de tratamento contínuo, 1 vez/dia, 3 a 4 × semana, por um período de 3 a 4 semanas.

Acupuntura

Como nas lesões dos nós dos dedos, a acupuntura pode ser útil no tratamento dos sintomas para lesões CMCs leves a moderadas, onde nenhuma frouxidão ligamentar é observada. Deve-se ter cuidado, pois inicialmente pode tornar a área mais sensível antes de produzir qualquer resultado. Isso pode afetar a disponibilidade de treinamento; portanto, o momento e o tipo de abordagem requerem consideração cuidadosa.

Mobilização de tecidos moles

Intrinsecamente, a dessensibilização usando ferramentas IASTM localmente, reforçada por bola com espinhos é uma boa estratégia para o controle da dor. Extrinsecamente, é importante manter a musculatura do antebraço dorsal (extensores), pois eles podem influenciar o movimento miofascial e a ADM do punho. Um regime de alongamento automático e autoliberação

da musculatura extensora usando, por exemplo, um pequeno massageador vibratório ou rolar o antebraço diretamente em uma barra em uma prateleira pode melhorar os sintomas, porém de toda maneira será necessário a orientação prévia dos profissionais da saúde.

Reabilitação (terapia por exercícios)

A reabilitação é parte integrante do retorno seguro ao treinamento ou da manutenção do treinamento com essa lesão. Assim, é importante não sentir dor durante o impacto ou igualmente durante a reabilitação, pois pode afetar negativamente a progressão. O autor sugere para lesões leves a adoção de exercícios semelhantes descritos na seção de lesões da articulação para pré e pós-treinamento: faixas de resistência, barras de resistência e bolas com espinhos (ver Figura 25.5). Além disso, o uso pós-treinamento de rotações de resistência do antebraço (Figura 25.9 A) deve ser considerado para melhorar a mobilidade do antebraço por meio do controle do punho.

A terapia de vibração desempenha um papel significativo na resolução da dor. O uso de plataformas vibratórias (Figura 25.9 B) e bater nos pneus com uma barra de metal (Figura 25.9 C) pode fornecer maior estabilidade no punho por meio de *feedback* proprioceptivo. Outros exercícios que são altamente eficazes na estabilidade do punho são rosca bíceps reversa com halteres ou barra (palmas das mãos voltadas para baixo), que devem ser realizados com a deixa de manter o punho fixo durante todo o movimento. Em lesões moderadas, esses exercícios podem ser introduzidos se a área estiver relativamente livre de sintomas. No pós-operatório, esses exercícios ajudarão na progressão apropriada ao longo dos estágios. Se disponíveis, as máquinas isocinéticas devem ser consideradas para reabilitação, especialmente quando houver déficits de força.

Anti-inflamatórios e terapia de injeção

Idealmente, os anti-inflamatórios são evitados, pois tornam a área mais frouxa e, portanto, mais instável. Com lesões leves, esses medicamentos podem não ter um impacto muito negativo e podem ser clinicamente justificados. Para lesões moderadas, a escleroterapia (também chamada de proloterapia) deve ser considerada quando a tala estiver sendo utilizada durante o período da fase de repouso. Clinicamente, essa abordagem produziu resultados favoráveis e, se realizada, sugere-se repetir a injeção após 2 semanas para um resultado mais desejável. Nenhuma dessas estratégias deve ser considerada para lesões graves. Os anti-inflamatórios podem afetar negativamente o resultado da operação. A escleroterapia não afetará adversamente o resultado de uma operação e pode ser considerada na tentativa de levar um boxeador ao impacto total devido a uma grande luta ou competição antes da cirurgia.

Manejo cirúrgico

Na maioria dos casos, essas lesões resultam em cirurgia devido à perda de funcionalidade na região da mão e do punho e à incapacidade do boxeador de retornar às atividades de impacto. Os resultados ideais dependem da técnica cirúrgica correta, reabilitação adequada e progressão para estratégias de carga (Boxe 25.4 e Figura 25.10). A progressão do carregamento deve incluir o uso de uma tala, conforme discutido anteriormente, e a medição usando o dinamômetro de empunhadura é parte integrante do retorno seguro ao boxe.

269

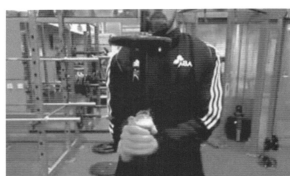
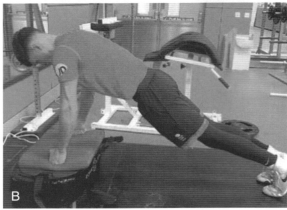
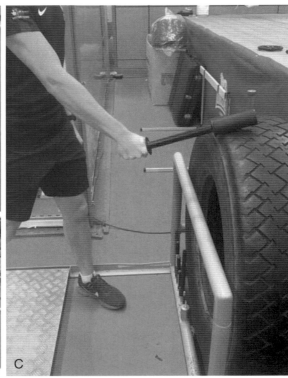

Figura 25.9 Exercícios de estabilidade mão-punho usando. **A.** Rotações do antebraço com uma barra "T" ponderada. **B.** Uma plataforma de vibração da placa de potência. **C.** Bater em um pneu com uma barra de metal.

Boxe 25.4 Protocolo pós-operatório para lesões da articulação carpometacarpal

1. Fase A de imobilidade (0 a 4 semanas): fios K presentes. Atleta engessado/tala removível. Sem atividades de suor devido ao risco de infecção.
2. Fase B de imobilidade (4 a 6 semanas): fios K removidos. Uso de tala removível. Atividades de suor são possíveis nesta fase.
3. Fase de carregamento inicial (6 a 8 semanas): ADM/condicionamento inicial usando adaptadores grossos de preensão.
4. Fase de carga progressiva (8 a 14 semanas): aumento no condicionamento com preensão completa.
5. Retorno à fase de boxe (14 a 18 semanas): retorno gradual ao boxe (uso estratégico de tala).
6. Fase de treinamento completo (18 a 20 semanas): monitoramento do boxeador em estado de treinamento completo (sem tala).

ADM, amplitude de movimento.

Lesão do ligamento colateral ulnar na base do polegar (articulação MCF)

Lesões no LCU não são tão comuns quanto lesões nos nós dos dedos e no CMC e os boxeadores geralmente são capazes de continuar o treinamento de boxe com este tipo de lesão. O mecanismo de lesão é uma força em valgo (abduzida) que ocorre na MCF do polegar, causando um grau de lesão ligamentar. Ao encaixar o desenho da luva e "dobrar o polegar" em direção ao punho (*i. e.*, manter o polegar mais perto do punho), o uso de técnicas de bandagem corretas contribui para estratégias de redução de lesões nesta região.

Apresentação/teste

A apresentação e o teste são mostrados no Boxe 25.5.

Medidas objetivas

Amplitude de movimento

Como os nós dos dedos, a ADM da articulação é mais bem testada usando um goniômetro metálico de dedo colocado diretamente

---

Boxe 25.5 Lesão do ligamento colateral ulnar

Mecanismo
- Uma força em valgo (abduzida) no polegar durante treino com aparador de espuma, *sparring* ou competição.

Exame
- Inchaço e falta de vontade de mover o polegar na articulação MCF
- Hipermobilidade/frouxidão com teste de estresse em valgo
- Hipomobilidade com teste de estresse em varo
- Dor sobre o lado ulnar (ligamento) e/ou lado radial (articulação) com teste em valgo
- Flexão reduzida com dor na faixa disponível (restrição da articulação MCF)
- Pontuação reduzida de preensão de pinça usando um dinamômetro portátil (DMP) ou *pinch hold* (Figura 25.11).

Lesões nas Mãos e nos Punhos: Boxe em Foco | Capítulo | 25

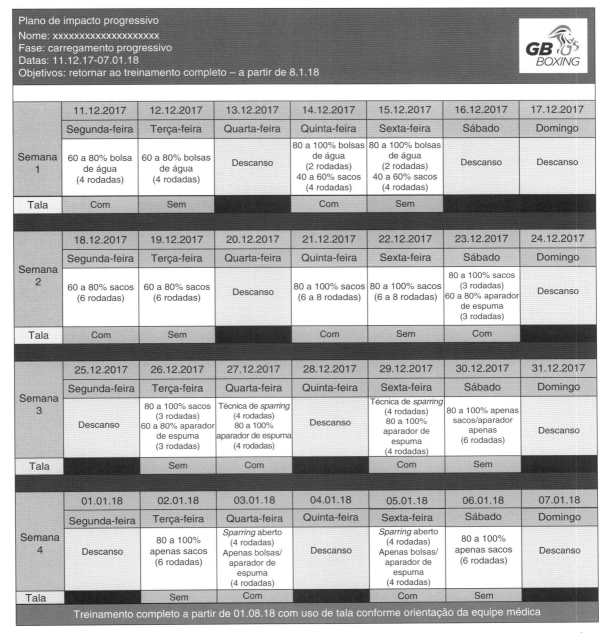

Figura 25.10 Plano de impacto progressivo para procedimentos pós-operatórios da articulação carpometacarpal.

sobre a articulação MCF. A flexão é geralmente mais afetada do que a extensão, sobretudo porque, junto com uma força de abdução, o polegar também é forçado a se estender. A flexão forçada será rígida e dolorosa na maioria das lesões.

Força (função de mão)

Como as lesões nas articulações dos dedos e CMC, as medidas de força ajudarão no raciocínio clínico e no manejo dessa lesão. No entanto, em contraste com as lesões da articulação dos nós dos dedos e da CMC, a dinamometria de preensão manual não parece ser uma ferramenta válida para lesões de LCU. Três ferramentas foram consideradas úteis: DMP, dinamômetro de aperto manual e placas ponderadas. Embora seja o dispositivo mais caro, a escolha preferida é o DMP (Figura 25.11 A), pois mantém o polegar em uma posição abduzida, enviesa o ligamento LCU e proporciona testes funcionais aprimorados para esse tipo de lesão. A metodologia sugerida é como a dinamometria de aperto de mão discutida para os nós dos dedos e CMC. O dinamômetro de preensão de pinça (Figura 25.11 B), como o DMP, é útil para avaliar clinicamente as lesões do LCU; no entanto, como o polegar é mantido em mais adução, os resultados podem ser errôneos (*i. e.*, eles podem indicar sintomas, mas não mostram a verdadeira gravidade da lesão). Além disso, esse dispositivo é mais adequado para testar uma pegada chave, que embora não pareça relevante para uma lesão LCU, pode ser útil em outros esportes que requerem este tipo de preensão (p. ex., tiro com arco). Na ausência desses dispositivos, podem ser consideradas placas ponderadas (Figura 25.11 C). Por exemplo, peça ao atleta para segurar placas de 10 kg com ambas as mãos utilizando uma pegada de aperto (*i. e.*, opondo a polpa do polegar em direção à polpa dos dedos) e tempo para falha de no máximo 2 minutos. A principal diferença entre os suportes da placa e o DMP é que o primeiro provavelmente testará

| Parte | 2 | Aplicação Clínica

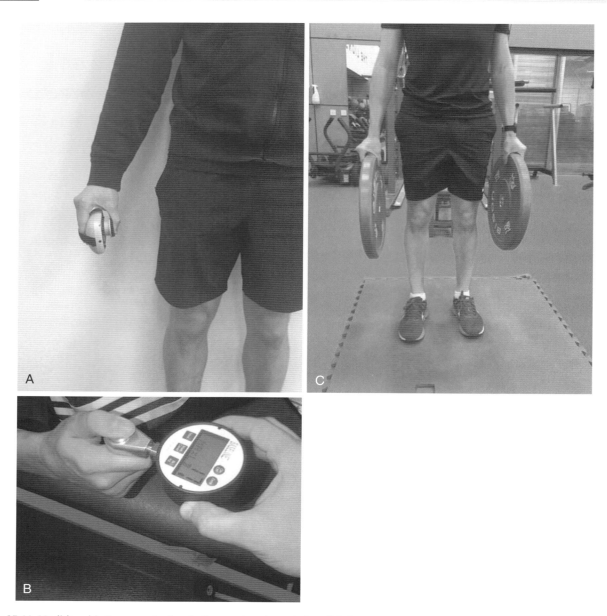

Figura 25.11 Medidas objetivas para lesões do ligamento colateral ulnar (LCU). **A.** Aperte o punho usando um dinamômetro portátil. **B.** Aperto de chave usando um dinamômetro de preensão. **C.** Aperte a pegada usando apoios de placa com peso (10 kg é sugerido usando apoios de 60 a 120 segundos para a maioria dos atletas).

o *endurance*, enquanto o último visa testar a força. No entanto, eles fornecem igualmente uma medida da diferença entre os dois lados, combinada com uma medida da dor, que pode ajudar a revelar a gravidade de uma lesão.

Trabalho diagnóstico (investigações)

Com base no raciocínio clínico, deve ser considerada uma ultrassonografia dinâmica para avaliar a frouxidão ligamentar dessa articulação. Isso será baseado nos sintomas relatados de modo predominante, medidas objetivas de força e na quantidade de flacidez encontrada clinicamente. O principal motivo para uma varredura é avaliar se uma lesão de Stener está presente. Isso ocorre quando a aponeurose do músculo adutor do polegar se interpõe entre o LCU rompido e seu local de inserção na base da falange proximal. Uma lesão de Stener não permite a cura adequada e, portanto, um procedimento cirúrgico é necessário.

Se nenhuma lesão de Stener estiver presente, os achados clínicos e a capacidade de continuar o treinamento devem orientar o processo de tomada de decisão.

Manejo conservador

Estratégias de proteção

Para evitar a ocorrência de lesões, é importante reduzir o risco de um episódio de extensão-abdução por flexão-adução do polegar enquanto se utiliza a bandagem. Isso pode ser reforçado com fita adesiva por meio de uma técnica de bandagem circular medial-lateral de dorsal-volar, de modo que encapsula a base do polegar e continua mais proximalmente ao longo do braço (ver Figura 25.8 A). Essa técnica também é útil para lesões CMCs, criando mais estabilidade estática no punho. Técnicas em "formato de oito" usando fita esportiva (Figura 25.12 A) são utilizadas de modo mais comum para proteção adicional no polegar na maioria das lesões LCU esportivas e podem ser consideradas antes de enfaixar a mão. Em competições essa estratégia é útil também para envolver boxeadores profissionais, bem como no estilo de competição amador, obviamente dentro das regras da competição específica. Para lesões mais moderadas, uma tala termoplástica sob medida (Figura 25.12 B) deve ser considerada, o que pode permitir a cura contínua de uma lesão enquanto mantém a disponibilidade de treinamento adequada.

Gelo e compressão

Assim como acontece com as lesões discutidas anteriormente, o frio e a compressão devem ser considerados na fase aguda de uma lesão. Em seguida, devem ser utilizados para o controle da dor após quaisquer sessões de impacto durante o retorno precoce ao treinamento.

Terapia manual

Da mesma maneira que para as lesões dos nós dos dedos, a terapia manual é um complemento útil na fase aguda das lesões do LCU para avaliar e controlar a lesão. As mobilizações em flexão ajudarão a restaurar a ADM completa, enquanto os deslizamentos ulnares transversais têm como objetivo restaurar a disfunção criada pela força de abdução. Um achado comum pós-tratamento pode ser que a frouxidão sentida ao fazer um teste em valgo foi reduzida; assim, a mobilidade reduzida sentida durante um teste de varo foi melhorada. É opinião do autor que a terapia manual realizada na fase aguda pode impactar positivamente nos resultados em lesões leves a moderadas.

Eletroterapia

Assim como nas lesões nos nós dos dedos, o *laser* pode ser um complemento útil para o processo de cicatrização. Isso não deve ser utilizado durante a fase de sangramento inicial de uma lesão LCU; é melhor considerá-lo após 24 horas.

Acupuntura

Da mesma maneira que as lesões da articulação dos nós dos dedos e CMCs, a acupuntura pode ser útil no tratamento dos sintomas para lesões de LCU leves a moderadas, na qual não é observada nenhuma frouxidão ligamentar. Essa modalidade é útil para pontos-gatilho da musculatura intrínseca do polegar (eminência tenar e primeiro interósseo dorsal) particularmente.

Mobilização de tecidos moles

O mesmo raciocínio para lesões nos nós dos dedos e CMCs se aplica às lesões LCUs. Uma vez que os ligamentos são as estruturas afetadas, a dessensibilização é uma boa estratégia para o controle da dor utilizando ferramentas IASTM reforçadas localmente por uma bola com espinhos. Extrinsecamente, é importante manter a musculatura do polegar (aspecto dorsal e volar). O alongamento também pode auxiliar os sintomas. Isso é mais bem realizado com o cotovelo reto, o polegar mantido dentro do punho fechado e o punho movido em direção ao desvio ulnar.

Reabilitação (terapia por exercícios)

Para lesões leves, os exercícios descritos para lesões nos nós dos dedos (ver Figura 25.5) são adequados para pré e pós-treinamento: bandas de resistência, barras de resistência e bolas com espinhos. Além disso, pode ser aplicado o uso pós-treinamento de sustentação de pegada de anilha em pinça (ver Figura 25.11 C). Esses podem ser progredidos com passagens de placa dinâmica (*i. e.*, passar uma placa ponderada de uma mão para outra utilizando os ombros como pêndulo) e quedas de placa dinâmica (*i. e.*, deixar uma placa ponderada cair e pegá-la com a outra mão). Ambos os exercícios devem ser realizados usando uma abordagem de *pinch hold*. Exercícios de empurrar com os dedos (Figura 25.13), com o objetivo de empurrar a parede e pousar na mesma mão apenas com polpas de todos os dedos e polegar tocando a parede, são bons para carregar o polegar, bem como outras estruturas na mão. Esse exercício pode ser progredido alternando-se de uma mão para a outra. O uso de vibração, conforme discutido nas articulações CMCs, também deve ser considerado para fornecer estabilidade no polegar com a posição da mão possivelmente mudando de sustentação de peso nas articulações na placa de força para sustentação de peso na polpa dos dedos e polegar.

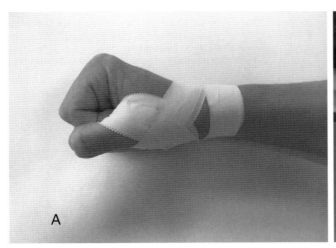 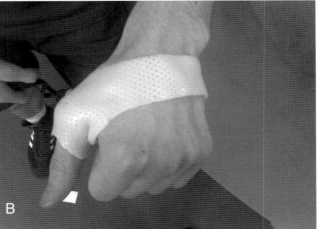

Figura 25.12 Técnicas de proteção do ligamento colateral ulnar. **A.** Cinta em formato de oito com fita esportiva. **B.** Tala termoplástica sob medida.

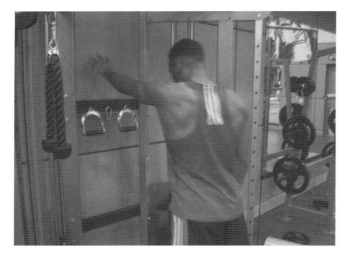

Figura 25.13 Exercício de empurrar contra a parede usado para reabilitação de lesões dos nós dos dedos, articulação carpometacarpal e ligamento colateral ulnar carregando essas estruturas de maneira controlada. Isso envolve a cadeia cinética: cotovelo, ombro, omoplata e tronco.

Anti-inflamatórios e terapia de injeção

Os anti-inflamatórios devem ser evitados idealmente; no entanto, com base na experiência clínica, as lesões do LCU costumam produzir melhores resultados com esses medicamentos em comparação com as lesões das articulações dos nós dos dedos e CMCs. Devido a um componente inflamatório crônico da patologia, e à ausência de alteração dos sintomas, pode-se considerar uma injeção de esteroide nessa área, quando aplicável, seguida de uma descarga inicial por até 72 horas e posterior retorno às estratégias de treinamento. As injeções tendem a ser menos utilizadas com essas lesões em comparação com lesões nos nós dos dedos e aplicadas com mais frequência quando comparadas com lesões CMCs (onde devem ser evitadas). Como mencionado anteriormente, as injeções não são um tratamento de primeira linha e as outras estratégias descritas devem ser consideradas em primeiro lugar adequadamente.

Manejo cirúrgico

Essas lesões podem ser tratadas de modo conservador na maioria dos casos, a menos que uma lesão de Stenor seja detectada na investigação diagnóstica. O resultado cirúrgico ideal depende da técnica cirúrgica correta, reabilitação apropriada e progressão para carga (Boxe 25.6). Ao contrário dos nós dos dedos e dos CMCs, o polegar não tem impacto em todos os socos e, portanto, a progressão para o carregamento não é tão direta. Logo, se os sintomas foram mínimos durante a o treinamento com sacos, é importante considerar inicialmente o uso de uma tala termoplástica sob medida (ver Figura 25.12 B) com progressão para fita em forma de oito (ver Figura 25.12 A) durante treinos com aparadores de espuma e atividades de *sparring* para evitar novas lesões. É importante força no polegar e, portanto, é sugerido o uso de um DMP para progressão da atividade.

> **Boxe 25.6 Protocolo pós-operatório para lesões do ligamento colateral ulnar do polegar**
>
> 1. Fase de imobilidade (0 a 4 semanas): atleta engessado/tala removível.
> 2. Fase de carregamento inicial (4 a 6 semanas): ADM/condicionamento inicial sem carregamento do tendão extensor. Uso de tala removível (principalmente para evitar "travamento")/tala noturna.
> 3. Fase de carregamento progressivo (6 a 8 semanas): aumento nas atividades de condicionamento.
> 4. Retorno à fase de boxe (8 a 12 semanas): retorno gradual ao boxe (uso de tala termoplástica sob medida para atividades de treinos com aparadores de espuma/*sparring*).
> 5. Fase de treinamento completo (12 a 14 semanas): monitoramento do boxeador em estado de treinamento completo (sem tala).

Conclusões

O nó do dedo, o punho e o polegar são as regiões anatômicas de maior risco no boxe. Essas lesões podem ocorrer igualmente, independentemente do boxeador ser um atleta amador ou profissional. Envolver as mãos de maneira adequada e usar a luva certa são os fatores mais importantes para ajudar a reduzir o risco de lesões. Em seguida, manter uma boa flexibilidade, em especial para os extensores do punho, com exercícios de condicionamento. É aconselhável realizar alguns exercícios específicos para as mãos e para os punhos antes de fazer o curativo, como parte de uma rotina de aquecimento correta. Após as sessões, também é aconselhável aplicar gelo rotineiramente na região da mão e do punho para evitar o acúmulo de microtrauma, que pode causar lesões.

O manejo conservador dessas lesões segue a ordem: LCU, nó do dedo e articulação CMC (ver Figura 25.13). Portanto, é importante ter uma abordagem metodológica ao exame clínico para decidir entre uma abordagem conservadora ou operatória. O manejo inicial adequado dessas lesões, em particular CMC, pode impactar na resolução dos sintomas. Logo, a educação deve fazer parte das estratégias de redução de lesões. Além disso, como as regiões da mão e do punho incorrem em entorses articulares predominantemente em vez de tensões musculares, a compreensão da complexa mecânica articular melhorará o desfecho dos sintomas. Qualquer modalidade de tratamento ou regime de exercícios também deve seguir uma abordagem personalizada e baseada em evidências clínicas, com uma justificativa clara.

Finalmente, se os sintomas não desaparecerem em tempo hábil ou se houver suspeita que o atleta pode ter sofrido uma lesão grave, é importante considerar exames de imagem ou encaminhamento a um cirurgião. Medidas subjetivas de dor ligadas a atividades funcionais no boxe (*i. e.*, acertar um saco ou um oponente no *sparring*), com medidas objetivas (principalmente força e mobilidade associada à dor na execução) devem orientar a escolha de qualquer tratamento e progressão.

Referências bibliográficas

Atha, J., Yeadon, M.R., Sandover, J., et al., 1985. The damaging punch. British Medical Journal (Clinical Research Edition) 291 (6511), 1756-1757.

Gatt, I., Smith-Moore, S., Steggles, C., Loosemore, M., 2018. The Takei handheld dynamometer: an effective clinical outcome measure too for hand and wrist function in boxing. Hand (N Y) 13 (3), 319-324.

Gladden, J.R., 1957. Boxer's knuckle; a preliminary report. The American Journal of Surgery 93 (3), 388-397.

Hame, S.L., Melone, C.P., 2000. Boxer's knuckle in the professional athlete. The American Journal of Sports Medicine 28 (6), 879-882.

Lenetsky, S., Harris, N., Brughelli, M., 2013. Assessment contributors of punching forces in combat sports athletes: implications for strength and conditioning. Strength & Conditioning Journal 35 (2), 1-7.

Loosemore, M., Lightfoot, J., Gatt, I., et al., 2016. Hand and wrist injuries in elite boxing: a longitudinal prospective study (2005-2012) of the Great Britain Olympic boxing squad. American Association of Hand Surgery 1-7.

Loosemore, M., Lightfoot, J., Palmergreen, D., et al., 2017. Boxing injury epidemiology in the great britain team: a 5-year surveillance study of medically diagnosed injury incidence and outcome. British Journal of Sports Medicine 49, 1100-1107.

Richards, L., 1997. Posture effects on grip strength. Archives of Physical Medicine and Rehabilitation 78 (10), 1154-1156.

Smith, M.S., Dyson, R.J., Hale, T., et al., 2000. Development of a boxing dynamometer and its punch force discrimination efficacy. Journal of Sports Science and Medicine 18 (6), 445-450.

Walilko, T.J., Viano, D.C., Bir, C.A., 2005. Biomechanics of the head for olympic boxer punches to the face. British Journal of Sports Medicine 39 (10), 710-719.

Capítulo | 26 |

Coluna Cervical: Avaliação de Risco e Reabilitação

Alan J. Taylor e Roger Kerry

Introdução

O pescoço é uma área frequentemente esquecida do corpo em termos de avaliação e tratamento (Figura 26.1). Em outras regiões anatômicas, os terapeutas se concentram em retornar os pacientes aos níveis anteriores à lesão. As estratégias de reabilitação visam aos déficits de força e resistência musculares identificados em programas de treinamento abrangentes que levam os pacientes a uma variedade de exercícios, desde isometria até pliometria, enquanto identificam e habilitam estratégias psicológicas concomitantemente. Todos os elementos são incorporados aos programas de reabilitação, à medida que os pacientes passam por um complexo cronograma de retorno ao condicionamento físico, que os preparam para as demandas de seu esporte, passatempo ou atividade física. No entanto, na região craniocervical os terapeutas têm oferecido historicamente pouco mais do que exercícios de amplitude de movimento e isométricos de flexores profundos do pescoço, talvez combinados com elementos de terapia manual e conselhos, antes de encorajar suas cargas a voltarem à ação. Essa estratégia geralmente tem sucesso limitado e muitos passam a sofrer cronicidade (Lamb et al., 2012). Este capítulo explora as razões subjacentes para essa aparente incompatibilidade e oferece orientação para terapeutas que reabilitam a coluna cervical no esporte ou em qualquer ambiente.

Avaliação de risco da coluna cervical em um contexto esportivo

A incidência de lesão cervical catastrófica e concussão diminuiu de modo significativo nos últimos 30 anos, pois as mudanças nas regras de vários esportes resultaram em menos colisões diretas ao pescoço ou traumatismo craniano. Apesar disso, bem mais da metade das lesões catastróficas no esporte são lesões no pescoço. Esse tipo de lesão é relatado em uma variedade de esportes de contato, como rúgbi, futebol, boxe e futebol americano, e se estende a uma ampla variedade de esportes sem contato, como esqui, ciclismo, hipismo, lacrosse (Petschauer et al., 2010), mergulho (Brajkovic et al., 2013) e surfe. As lesões são relatadas em todos os níveis, desde a escola (Olympia et al., 2007) e a recreação até o nível profissional (Rihn et al., 2009). Este capítulo abrange as lesões menores mais comuns da coluna cervical ou concussão que ocorrem secundariamente a lesões esportivas ou colisões diretas entre jogadores. Esse tipo de lesão pode causar traumas de aceleração e desaceleração (Langer et al., 2008) na cabeça ou no pescoço e resultar em apresentações complexas de

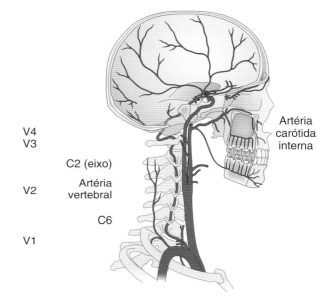

Figura 26.1 Anatomia normal dos vasos sanguíneos da cabeça e do pescoço. (Reproduzia com autorização de McCarthy, C. 2010. Combined Movement Theory. Churchill Livingstone, Edinburgh.) (*Esta figura se encontra reproduzida em cores no Encarte.*)

tontura, dor no pescoço e dores de cabeça, que são difíceis de avaliar e controlar com eficácia.

Dor de cabeça e tontura: perigo ou direção para o tratamento?

O paciente pós-trauma que apresenta uma combinação de dor no pescoço, dor de cabeça e tontura ou outros sintomas associados é um desafio para qualquer profissional da saúde. Pode ser que o espectro de uma possível patologia séria, como fratura ou disfunção arterial cervical (DAC) associada, seja um fator que explica porque os profissionais da saúde parecem relutantes em reabilitar a coluna cervical.

Como os médicos devem proceder?

No caso de trauma esportivo e a ausência evidenciada de fratura da coluna cervical por meio da regra 1da coluna C canadense (Stiell et al., 2001), há duas considerações principais para o clínico:
- DAC
- Lesão cerebral traumática (LCT).

Disfunção arterial cervical

O Quadro Internacional para Exame da Região Cervical para Potencial de Disfunção Arterial Cervical (IFOMPT, do inglês *International Framework for Examination of the Cervical Region for Potential of Cervical Arterial Dysfunction*; Rushton et al., 2014) oferece orientação aos profissionais da saúde para avaliação de risco segura por meio de raciocínio clínico sólido. DAC é um termo genérico que cobre uma variedade de patologias vasculares, desde aterosclerose até dissecção arterial (Tabela 26.1).

Em uma situação esportiva, com base na idade e na saúde do atleta, a doença vascular subjacente seria considerada menos provável, enquanto a dissecção arterial traumática, seria uma hipótese potencial, ainda que rara. Dissecção é conhecida por ocorrer como resultado de trauma contuso aos vasos devido ao impacto direto sobre os vasos (Degen et al., 2017) e/ou como resultado de mecanismos desconhecidos ligados a uma série de atividades, como *tackles* ou *scrums* no rúgbi e atividades sem contato, como a corrida (Fragaso et al., 2016; Suzuki et al., 2018).

Dissecção da artéria carótida interna

Crissey formulou, em 1974, a hipótese e descreveu quatro mecanismos que podem causar a lesão da artéria carótida (Crissey et al., 1974):
- Hiperextensão do pescoço associada à rotação
- Golpe direto no pescoço
- Trauma intraoral contuso
- Fratura da base do crânio envolvendo o canal carotídeo.

Apresentação clínica

Comumente, a apresentação da dissecção da artéria carótida envolve cefaleia de início agudo, o que torna difícil a diferenciação precoce com a concussão. A Figura 26.2 ilustra os locais comuns de dor. É sugerido que a dor ipsilateral pode afetar pescoço, face, região mandibular e cabeça simultaneamente. A detecção pode ser mais fácil em 50% ou mais que desenvolveram a síndrome de Horner. Isso ocorre devido à compressão, estiramento ou hipoperfusão das fibras simpáticas dentro da parede da artéria carótida. Uma síndrome de Horner de início agudo (tamanho da pupila diminuída, pálpebra caída e sudorese diminuída no lado afetado da face) associada com dor no pescoço na cabeça é quase patognomônica de dissecção da artéria carótida. Cerca de 10% dos pacientes podem sofrer paralisia dos nervos cranianos, geralmente afetando os níveis IX-XII. Além disso, alguns pacientes relatam zumbido pulsátil, provavelmente associado ao sopro da dissecção e estenose resultante.

Qualquer combinação dos sintomas mencionados anteriormente ou achados do exame deve aumentar o índice de suspeita do clínico de dissecção da carótida e o paciente deve ser encaminhado para investigação imediata. O exame ortopédico ou de terapia manual não é indicado e não deve ser realizado como rotina nesses casos. Em geral, o exame adicional para suspeita de lesão é realizado por meio de angiografia por ressonância magnética (ARM) ou angiografia por tomografia computadorizada (ATC). O ultrassom duplex é utilizado em alguns centros como uma investigação preliminar.

Manejo

Até o momento da publicação, não havia diretrizes baseadas em evidências para o manejo da dissecção carotídea. A maioria é considerada caso a caso, com pacientes sendo tratados de modo conservador por meio de tratamento antitrombótico ou terapia antiplaquetária ou ambos (Rao et al., 2011). Em casos selecionados, foi sugerida a colocação de *stent* endovascular como uma opção segura e eficaz para restaurar a integridade do lúmen do vaso e prevenir acidente vascular encefálico (AVE) (Martinelli et al., 2017).

Dissecção da artéria vertebral

A dissecção da artéria vertebral (DAV) foi relatada como uma das causas identificáveis mais comuns de AVE em pessoas com idade

Tabela 26.1 Variedade de patologias arteriais abrangidas pelo termo disfunção arterial cervical (DAC).

Estrutura/local	Patologia	Sintomas/apresentação
Artéria carótida	Aterosclerose • estenótica • trombótica • aneurismática	Comumente silencioso, possível carotidínia ou ataque isquêmico transitório (AIT), acidente vascular encefálico (AVE)
Artéria carótida	Hipoplasia	Normalmente silencioso
Artéria carótida	Dissecção	Dor, AIT, paralisia dos nervos cranianos, síndrome de Horner
Artéria vertebral	Aterosclerose	Raro. Normalmente silencioso, possível AIT, AVE
Artéria vertebral	Hipoplasia	Normalmente silencioso
Artéria vertebral	Dissecção	Dor, AIT, paralisia dos nervos cranianos
Artéria temporal	Arterite de células gigantes	Dor temporal (dor de cabeça), sensibilidade no couro cabeludo, claudicação da mandíbula e da língua, sintomas visuais (diplopia ou perda de visão – pode ser permanente)
Vasos cerebrais	Síndrome de vasoconstrição cerebral reversível	Fortes dores de cabeça como cefaleia em trovoada
Qualquer vaso cervicocraniano	Anomalia ou malformação vascular	Possível dor de cabeça/pescoço, ou seja, aneurisma carotídeo não rompido

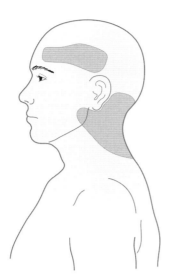

Figura 26.2 Distribuição somática típica da dor relacionada com a patologia e o trauma da artéria carótida interna. (Reproduzida, com autorização, de McCarthy C, 2010 Combined Movement Theory, Churchill Livingstone, Edinburgh.)

entre 18 e 45 anos (Kristensen et al., 1997). É reconhecido que a DAV é uma causa potencialmente tratável de ataque isquêmico transitório (AIT) e AVE (Beletsky et al., 2003). O diagnóstico imediato é essencial porque o maior risco de AVE em dissecções craniocervicais parece ocorrer nas primeiras semanas após a dissecção (Biousse et al., 1995). A DAV deve ser considerada no raciocínio clínico e na avaliação diagnóstica de pacientes que apresentam tontura ou dor craniocervical após trauma esportivo.

Apresentação clínica

É crucial que os profissionais da saúde estejam cientes de que a DAV pode se manifestar nos estágios iniciais como dor no pescoço ou dor de cabeça. Gottesman et al. (2012) em uma revisão sistemática relataram que 76% dos indivíduos estudados apresentaram dor no pescoço ou dor de cabeça "em algum momento durante sua apresentação" (Figura 26.3). Foram relatadas tontura ou vertigem em ~58% dos pacientes com DAV. Os esportes identificados especificamente neste estudo foram corrida, equitação, esqui, surfe e tênis. Há uma forte sugestão de que a DAV deva ser considerada como um diagnóstico diferencial em pacientes com dor no pescoço, cefaleia e tontura ainda que seja raro; isso parece particularmente pertinente em casos de trauma. Os autores afirmam que "isso é importante, sobretudo, para pacientes mais jovens, nos quais a combinação de tontura com dor craniofacial ou cervical pode ser confundida com um diagnóstico benigno, como enxaqueca vestibular".

As consequências neurológicas da DAV estão ligadas à isquemia cerebral pós-lesão associada a tromboembolismo, hipoperfusão, hemorragia ou uma combinação dessas condições.

Manejo

A DAV traumática pode ter complicações devastadoras, com relatos de taxa de AVE de 24% e mortalidade de 8% (Sanelli et al., 2002). É fundamental o reconhecimento precoce disso como uma emergência médica. Pacientes com diagnóstico de DAV que não desenvolveram sintomas isquêmicos são tratados com anticoagulação ou terapia antiplaquetária, dependendo do risco potencial de sangramento, localização da lesão e extensão da lesão (Simon e Mohseni, 2017). O reparo cirúrgico e a terapia endovascular são utilizados com lesões de alto grau e aquelas com contraindicações para anticoagulação ou terapia antiplaquetária que apresentam risco elevado de progressão. Atualmente, não há evidências que apoiem qualquer opção de tratamento e os pacientes diagnosticados parecem ser tratados caso a caso. Da mesma maneira, parece não haver uma rota evidenciada de volta ao esporte para aqueles que foram afetados por lesão vascular cervicocraniana.

Tontura contínua

Na ausência de fratura evidenciada ou DAC traumática, os clínicos ainda precisam manejar os casos pós-traumáticos em que a dor no pescoço e a tontura continuam sendo uma característica. Existem três considerações principais:
- LCT
- Tontura cervicogênica (TCG)
- Disfunção sensorimotora.

Lesão cerebral traumática

O leitor também pode consultar o Capítulo 27, que discute o tratamento de lesões na cabeça. A declaração de consenso de 2017 do Grupo de Concussão Esportiva (GCE) (McCrory et al., 2017) sugere que a concussão relacionada ao esporte (CRE) é "definida com frequência como representando os sintomas imediatos e transitórios de LCT". A LCT é utilizada de maneira intercambiável e regular com concussão e o painel de especialistas de Berlim, que elaborou esse documento de consenso, modificou a definição anterior da GCE para:
- CRE é uma LCT induzida por forças biomecânicas
- Várias características comuns podem ser utilizadas para definir clinicamente a natureza de um traumatismo cranioencefálico:
  - A CRE pode ser causada por um golpe direto na cabeça, rosto, pescoço ou em qualquer outra parte do corpo com uma força impulsiva transmitida à cabeça
  - A CRE resulta geralmente no início rápido de comprometimento de curta duração da função neurológica que se resolve de maneira espontânea. No entanto, em alguns casos, os sinais e sintomas evoluem ao longo de vários minutos a horas
  - A CRE pode resultar em alterações neuropatológicas, mas os sinais e sintomas clínicos agudos indicam um distúrbio

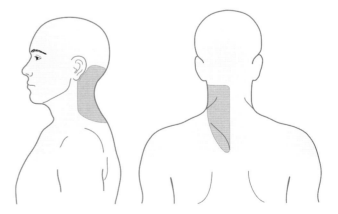

Figura 26.3 Distribuição somática típica da dor relacionada com a patologia e o trauma do sistema arterial vertebrobasilar. (Reproduzida, com autorização, de McCarthy C, 2010, Combined Movement Theory, Churchill Livingstone, Edinburgh.)

funcional em vez de uma lesão estrutural e, como tal, nenhuma anormalidade é observada em estudos de neuroimagem estrutural padrão

- A CRE resulta em uma variedade de sinais e sintomas clínicos que podem ou não envolver perda de consciência. A resolução das características clínicas e cognitivas segue um curso sequencial de um modo geral. No entanto, em alguns casos, os sintomas podem ser prolongados.

A declaração de consenso descreveu seis domínios clínicos específicos que podem ser incorporados a um diagnóstico específico de CRE da seguinte maneira:

1. Sintomas: somáticos (p. ex., dor de cabeça), cognitivos (p. ex., sensação de estar em uma névoa) e/ou sintomas emocionais (p. ex., instabilidade).
2. Sinais físicos (p. ex., perda de consciência, amnésia, déficit neurológico).
3. Comprometimento do equilíbrio (p. ex., instabilidade na marcha).
4. Mudanças comportamentais (p. ex., irritabilidade).
5. Comprometimento cognitivo (p. ex., tempos de reação retardados).
6. Distúrbios do sono/vigília (p. ex., sonolência).

Foi sugerido que, "se estiverem presentes sintomas ou sinais em qualquer um dos domínios clínicos, deve-se suspeitar de uma CRE e a estratégia de manejo adequada deve ser instituída".

Nesses casos, o raciocínio clínico avançado é a marca registrada da boa tomada de decisão. Recomenda-se que "todos os atletas devem passar por uma avaliação neurológica clínica (incluindo avaliação do estado mental/cognição, função oculomotora, sensorimotora geral, coordenação, marcha, função vestibular e equilíbrio) como parte de seu manejo geral" (McCrory et al., 2017). Os clínicos de terapia devem fazer a triagem para um médico ou neuropsicólogo se houver suspeita de CRE.

Sintomas persistentes

Sabe-se que, em alguns casos, os sintomas da CRE podem se tornar persistentes cuja definição padrão é "sintomas que persistem além dos prazos esperados (*i. e.*, > 10 a 14 dias em adultos e > 4 semanas em crianças)" (McCrory et al., 2017). O consenso de especialistas de Berlim sugere que "no mínimo, a avaliação deve incluir um histórico abrangente, exame físico focado e testes especiais onde indicado (p. ex., teste de exercício aeróbico graduado)". Eles continuam recomendando que "o tratamento deve ser individualizado e ter como alvo fatores de saúde, físicos e psicossociais específicos identificados na avaliação".

Manejo

Há evidências preliminares que apoiam o uso de:

1. Um programa individualizado de exercícios aeróbicos com sintomas limitados em pacientes com sinais pós-concussivos persistentes associados à instabilidade autonômica que induz anormalidades nos sistemas de órgãos e pode contribuir para a desregulação cardiovascular.
2. Um programa de fisioterapia direcionado em pacientes com disfunção na coluna cervical ou vestibular.
3. Uma abordagem colaborativa, incluindo terapia cognitivo-comportamental para lidar com qualquer humor persistente ou problemas comportamentais.

Os profissionais devem estar cientes de que há um crescente corpo de literatura indicando que os fatores psicológicos podem desempenhar um papel significativo na recuperação dos sintomas e contribuir para o risco de sintomas persistentes em alguns casos. A avaliação e o manejo de tais casos requerem uma anamnese cuidadosa e abrangente e um nível avançado de raciocínio clínico e tomada de decisão.

Tontura cervicogênica

A TCG se apresenta de maneira muito semelhante à DAC e aos elementos do LCT. A TCG é caracterizada por dor no pescoço com ou sem dor de cabeça, mas com descrições associadas de desequilíbrio, instabilidade, desorientação e redução da amplitude de movimento do pescoço (Reiley et al., 2017). A TCG é um diagnóstico de exclusão e não existe consenso na literatura quanto à testagem e diagnóstico resultante. Reiley et al. (2017) propuseram um processo gradual para o diagnóstico de TCG, que é detalhado na Figura 26.4.

Reiley et al. (2017) afirmam que "a TCG não deve ser considerada se o paciente não tem dor no pescoço", sugerindo que "a dor no pescoço pode ocorrer em repouso, com movimento ou com a palpação. Os sintomas causados por TCG devem ser exacerbados por movimentos que provocam dor no pescoço e diminuem com intervenções que aliviam a dor nessa região". No entanto, essas declarações parecem em grande parte não suportadas por estudos ou resultados de pesquisas.

A palavra "tonto" descreve uma gama de sensações. A prioridade do clínico é elucidar a natureza exata do relato de um paciente de "tontura" ou "vertigem", já que as duas podem ser utilizadas de modo errôneo e indistinto. Um método é pedir ao paciente para descrever a(s) sensação(ões) sem o uso da palavra "tontura". Quatro tipos subjetivos de tontura foram identificados: vertigem, desequilíbrio, pré-síncope e tontura (Reilly, 1990). O clínico deve ser capaz de diferenciar os tipos de tontura, pois o diagnóstico diferencial é peculiar a cada tipo.

Definições

A *vertigem* se refere à ilusão de movimento ambiental, classicamente descrita como "girando". Em geral, a sensação de movimento é rotatória, "como sair de um carrossel" ou "o solo se inclina para cima e para baixo, como se estivesse em um barco no mar" (Reilly, 1990). O *Dicionário Ilustrado de Medicina de Dorland* (Dorland, 2012) divide-o em dois tipos:

- Vertigem objetiva – sensação como se o mundo externo estivesse girando em torno do indivíduo
- Vertigem subjetiva – sensação como se o indivíduo estivesse girando no espaço.

Acredita-se que a vertigem verdadeira reflete geralmente uma disfunção em algum nível do sistema vestibular. A vertigem não é considerada um sintoma proveniente da coluna cervical, mas está mais relacionada com distúrbios vestibulares periféricos ou lesões nas vias vestibulares do sistema nervoso central (SNC).

O *desequilíbrio* é um distúrbio no equilíbrio ou coordenação que prejudica a deambulação. Os pacientes sugerem que "o problema está nas minhas pernas", mas outros sentem "tonturas da cabeça também". Como a deambulação agrava o problema, são essenciais a análise da marcha e o exame neurológico.

Pré-síncope significa que o paciente sente perda iminente de consciência. Nos casos em que o paciente de fato nunca perdeu a consciência, a reclamação "sinto que vou desmaiar" pode ser devido a uma série de explicações. No entanto, uma consideração de possível isquemia, que pode levar à síncope completa, deve ser investigada em conformidade.

A *tontura* se refere a uma sensação "na cabeça" que claramente não é vertiginosa ou pré-sincopal e que não está invariavelmente relacionada à deambulação. Alguns descrevem "flutuar" ou sentir "como se minha cabeça não estivesse presa ao meu corpo", estar "alto" ou "desorientado".

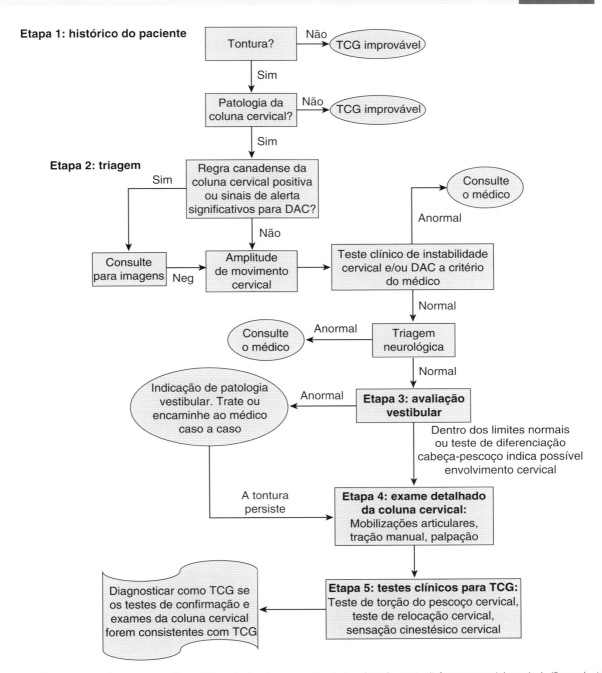

Figura 26.4 Algoritmo gradual para o diagnóstico de tontura cervicogênica (TCG). *DAC*, disfunção arterial cervical. (Reproduzida, com autorização, de Reiley, A.S., Vickory, F.M., Funderburg, S.E., Cesario, R.A., Clendaniel, RA., 2017. How to diagnose cervicogenic dizziness. Archives of Physiotherapy 7, 12.)

Os pacientes podem descrever alguns elementos de cada uma das categorias mencionadas anteriormente, o que torna a avaliação do trauma pós-esporte muito desafiadora (Reiley et al., 2017).

Disfunção sensorimotora

Uma triagem neurológica completa é indicada no trauma esportivo com tontura inexplicável prolongada, envolvendo a avaliação dos sintomas radiculares, miótomos, dermátomos, reflexos tendinosos profundos, sinais do neurônio motor superior e função do nervo craniano. A triagem apropriada deve ser feita na presença de achados neurológicos anormais. Na ausência de fratura, instabilidade cervical, DAC ou disfunção neurológica, é lógico considerar a avaliação sensorimotora.

Considerações sensorimotoras

O termo "sensorimotor" é utilizado para descrever a complexidade dos componentes de processamento aferente, eferente e central que fornecem e mantêm a estabilidade no sistema de controle postural (Kristjansson et al., 2009). Acredita-se que os déficits sensorimotores (Yu et al., 2011) sejam uma característica de lesão traumática no pescoço, como o trauma em chicote (TEC); portanto, pode haver considerações sensorimotoras no caso de trauma esportivo na região cervicocraniana. De fato, achados preliminares pós-concussão em 54 jogadores de elite do rúgbi de 15 sugerem estratégias de equilíbrio menores alteradas e controle do músculo do tronco alterado (Hides et al., 2017).

Distúrbios na entrada aferente do pescoço são postulados como causas de tontura, instabilidade, distúrbios visuais, estabilidade postural alterada e propriocepção cervical, que podem estar ligados ao controle do movimento da cabeça e dos olhos (Kristjansson et al., 2009). A Figura 26.5 ilustra os sistemas envolvidos nessa interação complexa. Está além do escopo desse capítulo abranger descrições fisiopatológicas detalhadas desse sistema. No entanto, sugere-se que as seguintes áreas sejam consideradas como parte da avaliação:

- Consciência cabeça-pescoço
- Controle de movimento do pescoço
- Habilidade postural: tontura e/ou instabilidade
- Distúrbios oculomotores.

A coluna cervical contribui para a consciência somatossensorial por meio de uma série de mecanismos.

Mecanorreceptores, reflexos e sistema nervoso simpático

Sabe-se que existe uma alta densidade de mecanorreceptores nos fusos musculares, articulações e ligamentos da coluna cervical alta. Acredita-se que essas aferências cervicais forneçam sentido proprioceptivo e informações ao SNC (Kristjansson et al., 2009). Essas mensagens viajam por vias sensoriais para o tálamo, cerebelo e córtex somatossensorial. Os aferentes cervicais também mediam informações e reflexos dos sistemas vestibular e visual e se comunicam com o sistema nervoso simpático (SNS) por meio de receptores beta bidirecionais nos tecidos musculares. Esse complexo sistema de comunicação desempenha um papel na atividade reflexa do pescoço, que interliga a orientação da cabeça, o movimento dos olhos e a estabilidade postural (Treleaven, 2008).

Possíveis mecanismos

A perturbação do controle sensorimotor pode resultar em uma sensação de *desequilíbrio* ou relatos de *tontura* por meio dos seguintes mecanismos:

- Por causa de trauma direto ou de alterações no *feedback* aferente devido à função muscular alterada
- Devido à irritação neural química de respostas inflamatórias locais nos tecidos circundantes
- Como parte de um efeito direto de mediadores orientados centralmente

- O SNS pode exercer um efeito na atividade do fuso muscular, resultando em alterações na função muscular.

Exame clínico

A avaliação da função oculomotora pode ser realizada examinando a qualidade dos movimentos e do controle ocular. O profissional também deve considerar qualquer reprodução dos sintomas durante o teste.

Avaliação do controle oculomotor

Movimento ocular de perseguição suave (posição neutra). O exame do controle oculomotor inclui a observação dos olhos seguindo um alvo em movimento (perseguição suave) enquanto mantém a cabeça imóvel. Os olhos devem se mover suavemente sem nistagmo.

Movimento sacádico dos olhos. O paciente é solicitado a mover os olhos rapidamente para fixar seu olhar entre vários alvos. Os alvos são colocados em várias direções de movimento diferentes. A incapacidade de se fixar no alvo, ultrapassá-lo ou fazer mais de dois movimentos com os olhos para alcançá-lo pode indicar um desempenho insatisfatório. Nesse caso, os olhos se moverão de maneira espasmódica ou saltitante, o que é normal.

Teste de torção do pescoço com perseguição suave (SPNT, do inglês smooth pursuit neck torsion test). O mesmo que o teste 1, mas com o tronco girado para atingir 45° de rotação cervical (a cabeça permanece parada). O desempenho prejudicado em torção em comparação com a posição neutra é sugestivo de uma influência aferente cervical. Essa manobra estimula os receptores cervicais, mas não os vestibulares, e mostrou potencial para identificar a entrada aferente cervical anormal, como uma causa subjacente de distúrbio sensorimotor (Tjell e Rosenhall, 1998; Williams et al., 2017; Yu et al., 2011).

Se a reprodução da tontura e/ou visão turva ocorrer durante os testes 1 e 2, o clínico fica imediatamente assegurado de que o espectro de DAC é muito menor no índice de suspeita, já que o sistema vascular não foi estressado durante nenhuma dessas manobras. Em outras palavras, os sintomas foram reproduzidos apenas pelos movimentos dos olhos.

O teste 3 deve ser realizado após uma verificação inicial de tontura em primeiro lugar (após a posição de torção de 45°), seguido por um movimento de perseguição suave. A reprodução

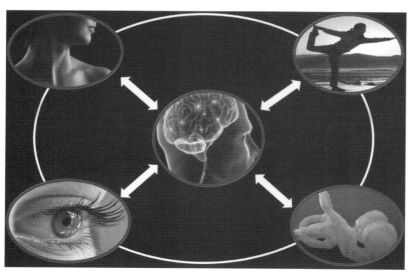

Figura 26.5 Entradas e saídas dos sistemas de propriocepção, visual, vestibular e de equilíbrio do pescoço que estão envolvidos na disfunção sensorimotora. (*Esta figura se encontra reproduzida em cores no Encarte.*)

da tontura após os movimentos dos olhos implicaria novamente na disfunção oculomotora relacionada ao distúrbio sensorimotor.

Testes adicionais

Uma vez que o clínico tenha certeza de que a DAC é improvável, testes adicionais do sistema sensorimotor podem ser realizados por meio da avaliação da estabilidade do olhar e da coordenação olho-cabeça.

Estabilidade do olhar. O paciente é solicitado a manter o foco visual em um alvo enquanto move a cabeça de maneira ativa e lenta em variações de rotação/flexão/extensão. O clínico deve observar a capacidade de manter o foco, movimentos suaves e/ou reprodução dos sintomas. A função prejudicada pode fornecer uma direção para a reabilitação.

Coordenação olho-cabeça. O paciente inicia o movimento dos olhos até um ponto a ser focalizado e então, enquanto mantém o foco, move a cabeça até esse ponto. Isso pode ser executado para a esquerda e a direita e para cima e para baixo. O clínico deve observar a incapacidade do paciente de manter a cabeça imóvel enquanto os olhos se movem, perda de foco durante os movimentos da cabeça e/ou reprodução dos sintomas. Essas descobertas apoiariam uma hipótese sensorimotora (Kristjansson e Treleaven, 2009) e forneceriam uma direção para a reabilitação.

Avaliação optocinética. O paciente é posicionado a 90 cm de uma parede com um apontador *laser* fixado em sua cabeça; é solicitado que ele gire a cabeça para a esquerda, direita ou em extensão e que mude para uma "posição normal da cabeça". A medição da posição final em comparação com a posição inicial é feita em milímetros, seja negativo, seja positivo, para indicar superação ou redução, respectivamente. O clínico deve observar qualquer reprodução de tontura, movimentos bruscos ou uma grande discrepância no erro de posição da articulação (de Vries et al., 2015) ao testar com os olhos abertos em comparação com os olhos fechados. Um achado de propriocepção prejudicada pode fornecer uma orientação para a reabilitação.

Dissociação cabeça-corpo. O paciente é solicitado a manter uma posição estável da cabeça, usando o *laser* como *feedback*, se necessário, enquanto movimenta o torso em uma série de atividades.

Sistema de controle postural. Isso inclui todos os elementos sensorimotores e musculoesqueléticos envolvidos no controle da orientação postural e do equilíbrio. O reflexo tônico do pescoço (RTP) é ativado pelos músculos da coluna cervical e ativa os músculos do corpo para criar uma base de suporte para equilíbrio e postura estável. A função do sistema pode ser avaliada indiretamente por meio de testes como o de Romberg ou o *Balance Error Scoring System* (BESS) (Iverson e Koehle, 2013) para avaliar as contribuições vestibulares, visuais e proprioceptivas para o equilíbrio. O equilíbrio prejudicado, em comparação com os dados normativos, pode ser uma direção para a reabilitação dos pacientes afetados.

Função motora

A musculatura do pescoço é responsável pela manutenção da postura cervicocraniana e por direcionar o movimento da cabeça. Como tal, tem sido usada como um indicador de disfunção do pescoço. No entanto, a incerteza permanece sobre a eficácia do exercício para dor no pescoço (Gross et al., 2015). Uma revisão sistemática em 2015 sugeriu que, apesar da escassez de evidências de alta qualidade, "Usar exercícios de fortalecimento específicos como parte da prática de rotina para dor cervicogênica crônica, cefaleia cervicogênica e radiculopatia pode ser benéfico" (Gross

et al., 2015). A publicação *The Neck Pain Guidelines: Revision 2017*, incorporou exercícios como parte do tratamento multimodal para dor no pescoço aguda e crônica. A controvérsia permanece quanto à dosagem ideal, o tipo e a frequência de exercício (Gross et al., 2015). Apesar da incerteza, há algumas pesquisas preliminares encorajadoras que sugerem que o fortalecimento do pescoço pode ter um papel na redução das taxas de lesão no pescoço (Naish et al., 2013) e pode de fato ser um fator de proteção para reduzir a concussão. Os músculos do pescoço são acessórios para a respiração (Axen et al., 1992) e os extensores cervicais mantêm a posição da cabeça por meio de uma função de resistência (Taylor et al., 2006), que é mínima durante a atividade normal, mas pode ser testada ao máximo em ambientes esportivos.

Estratégias de manejo clínico e reabilitação

Treinamento isométrico

O treinamento isométrico há muito é defendido no tratamento da dor e disfunção da coluna cervical (Jull et al., 2008). O uso do teste de flexão craniocervical (TFCC) como uma avaliação da função e da resistência dos flexores cervicais profundos (FCP) tem sido uma característica da prática fisioterapêutica por décadas. Os exercícios de FCP são prescritos como remédio para pacientes com dor e disfunção no pescoço. No entanto, os autores propõem que esse aparente foco excessivo nos flexores profundos do pescoço isométricos é semelhante a oferecer exercícios de quadríceps estáticos a um paciente com disfunção aguda ou crônica do joelho na vã esperança de que recuperem a função completa. Os profissionais da saúde devem considerar o exercício isométrico apenas como um ponto de partida no processo de reabilitação e incorporar programas de resistência progressiva que incluam todos os grupos musculares cervicais. Dito isso, o recrutamento de FCP é amplamente apoiado pela literatura (Jull et al., 2009) e pode ser considerado um ponto de partida razoável para a reabilitação neuromuscular após lesão esportiva. Porém, isso deve ser rapidamente seguido por um regime de exercícios que visa uma variedade de grupos musculares, uma vez que investigações preliminares descobriram que a força isométrica do pescoço e o treinamento estavam diretamente relacionados a lesões no pescoço e risco de concussão no esporte (Hrysomallis, 2016).

Treinamento de força global

O fortalecimento do pescoço tem sido associado a taxas reduzidas de lesões no rúgbi (Naish et al., 2013) e postulado como um fator protetor de redução do risco de concussão em esportes do ensino médio (Collins et al., 2014). Os déficits de força podem ser identificados por teste muscular manual, dinamômetro portátil (Versteegh et al., 2015) ou métodos mais sofisticados, como o sistema GS Gatherer (Barrett et al., 2015). Pesquisas preliminares sugerem que a força do pescoço, a amplitude de movimento e a suscetibilidade à fadiga podem ser influenciadas por regimes de treinamento focado no pescoço (Hrysomallis, 2016).

Uma variedade de exercícios de teste e reabilitação estão disponíveis para pacientes e clínicos com equipamentos básicos de ginástica. A Tabela 26.2 descreve uma série de progressões isométricas específicas do rúgbi. As Figuras 26.6 a 26.8 também ilustram as progressões de apoios isométricos até o treinamento de força com funções específicas. A abordagem do treinamento deve adotar o princípio do treinamento de resistência progressiva, em que a resistência é aumentada de maneira incremental quando o número de repetições prescrito é atingido (Minshull e Gleeson 2017).

Parte | 2 | Aplicação Clínica

Tabela 26.2 Exercícios usados no programa de intervenção de fortalecimento do pescoço para uma equipe profissional masculina de rúgbi de 15.

Nome do exercício	Descrição do exercício
Cabo isométrico – flexão do pescoço	Em pé, uma contenção de cabeça é colocada em volta da testa com o cabo no nível do occipital. O jogador fica de costas para a pilha de pesos e retrai o pescoço "encolhendo" o queixo. Ele pega o peso, dá um passo e se inclina para frente para levantar a carga utilizando os flexores do pescoço. O peso é mantido por 5 segundos
Cabo isométrico – extensão do pescoço	Em pé, um arnês de cabeça é colocado em volta da testa com um cabo na altura da testa. O jogador está voltado para a pilha de pesos e retrai o pescoço "encolhendo" o queixo. O jogador pega o peso, dá um passo e se inclina para trás para levantar a pilha de peso utilizando os extensores do pescoço. O peso é mantido por 5 segundos
Cabo isométrico – flexão lateral direita e esquerda	Em pé, um arnês de cabeça é colocado em volta da testa de modo que o cabo fique logo acima da orelha esquerda/direita. O jogador fica de frente para onde a pilha de pesos está localizada. O jogador então dá um passo lateral para longe da pilha de pesos e inclina-se lateralmente utilizando os músculos laterais do pescoço. O peso é mantido por 5 segundos
Cabo isométrico – flexão de pescoço de 45° à esquerda e à direita	Em pé, coloque o arnês de cabeça de modo que fique localizado entre o occipital e a orelha esquerda/direita. O jogador se afasta da pilha de pesos em um ângulo de maneira que a resistência estenda o pescoço de um lado (esquerdo ou direito) em um ângulo de 45°. O peso é mantido por 5 segundos
Cabo isométrico – extensão de pescoço com o corpo inclinado	Em uma posição agachada, quadris e joelhos são flexionados em aproximadamente 120°. O jogador fica de frente para a pilha de pesos e retrai o pescoço "dobrando" o queixo e, em seguida, pega o peso. O cabo é direcionado para o chão. O jogador então puxa para trás utilizando os extensores do pescoço. O peso é mantido por 5 segundos
Cabo isométrico – flexão lateral curvada	Em uma posição agachada, quadris e joelhos são flexionados em aproximadamente 120°. O jogador se agacha de lado na pilha de pesos e coloca o arnês de cabeça ao redor da cabeça de maneira que o cabo seja posicionado logo acima da orelha esquerda/direita. O jogador dá um passo lateral para longe da pilha de pesos e inclina-se para o lado usando os músculos laterais do pescoço. O peso é mantido por 5 segundos
Cabo isométrico com suporte de cabeça apertado – flexão lateral direita do pescoço com a escápula retraída	O exercício é realizado em uma máquina *crossover*. Em uma posição agachada, quadris e joelhos são flexionados em aproximadamente 120°. O arnês de cabeça é colocado em volta da testa de maneira que o cabo fique no nível da orelha esquerda. O jogador se posiciona de lado para a pilha de peso, em seguida, dá um passo lateral para a direita da pilha de peso e inclina-se lateralmente utilizando os músculos laterais direitos do pescoço. Ao mesmo tempo, o jogador usa o braço direito para puxar o outro cabo posicionado no chão até o peito. O peso é mantido por 5 segundos
Cabo isométrico com suporte de cabeça frouxo – flexão lateral do pescoço com *pull down* do músculo grande dorsal	O exercício é realizado em uma máquina *crossover*. Em uma posição recostada, quadris e joelhos são flexionados em aproximadamente 120°. O arnês de cabeça é colocado em volta da testa de modo que o cabo fique logo acima do nível da orelha esquerda. O jogador se posiciona de lado para a pilha de peso e dá um passo lateral para a direita da pilha de peso e inclina-se lateralmente usando os músculos laterais direitos do pescoço. Ao mesmo tempo, o jogador usa o braço esquerdo para puxar o outro cabo posicionado no chão para executar um *pulldown* horizontal do grande dorsal. O peso é mantido por 5 segundos
Simulação de *scrum* – flexores e extensores laterais do pescoço	O exercício é realizado na máquina de simulação de *scrum*. Ao carregar as almofadas com impulso de perna, os músculos do pescoço do jogador resistem a uma carga aplicada na cabeça pelo fisioterapeuta ou condicionador físico. Este exercício pode ser realizado em todos os ângulos com *feedback* fornecido por um esfigmomanômetro colocado entre as mãos da pessoa que está criando a carga e a cabeça do jogador. A carga isométrica é criada por 5 segundos

Adaptada de Naish, R., Burnett, A., Burrows, S., Andrews, W., Appleby, B., 2013. Can a specific neck strengthening program decrease cervical spine injuries in a men's professional rugby union team? A retrospective analysis. Journal of Sports Science and Medicine 12 (3), 542-550, with permission.

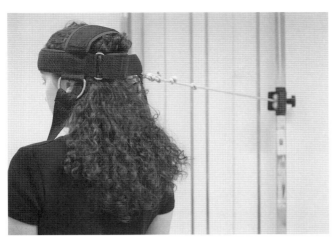

Figura 26.6 Cabo isométrico para flexão lateral.

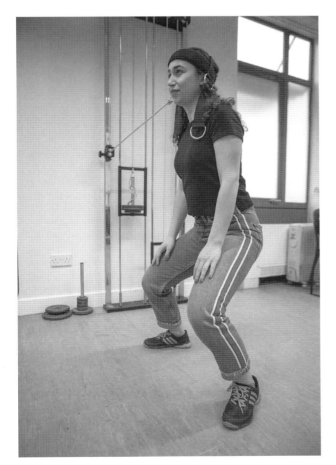

Figura 26.7 Cabo isométrico do pescoço durante a execução do agachamento.

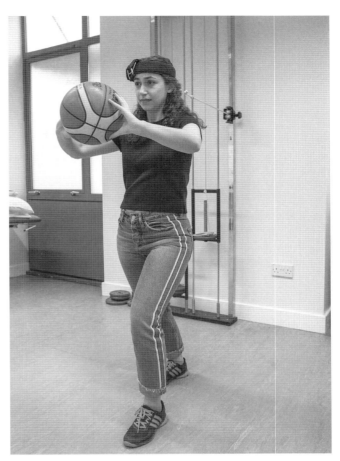

Figura 26.8 Cabo isométrico com atividade específica da tarefa.

Treinamento de resistência

Até o momento, dois artigos mostraram que tanto o treinamento de força quanto o de resistência foram eficazes no tratamento da dor no pescoço (Nikander 2006; Ylinen et al., 2007). No entanto, esses estudos foram em pacientes com dor cervical crônica e permanece desconhecido se isso pode ser extrapolado para uma população esportiva que provavelmente está em um ponto de partida muito mais elevado do ponto de vista de força e resistência. Nesse ponto, é razoável incluir o treinamento de resistência em um programa balanceado de retorno ao esporte.

Treinamento pliométrico

A eficácia do treinamento pliométrico e do treinamento de perturbação na aceleração da cabeça, rigidez cervical e risco de lesões permanece obscura. Embora essas técnicas sejam usadas como parte de programas de treinamento anedoticamente em esportes de alto nível, incluindo corrida de Fórmula 1, artes marciais, boxe e rúgbi, poucos estudos avaliaram sua eficácia. A Figura 26.9 demonstra um exemplo de exercícios pliométricos simples e específicos para o pescoço.

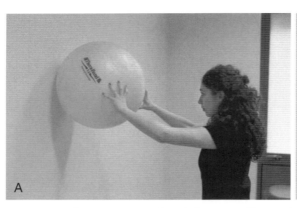 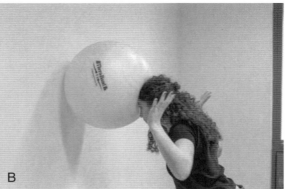

Figura 26.9 Impacto e direcionamento pliométricos específicos e simples para o pescoço. **A.** Estágio de preparação: segurar a bola a uma altura adequada para um alvo de cabeça. **B.** Soltar a bola com as mãos e mover a cabeça para a bola antes que ela caia.

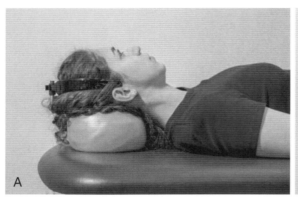 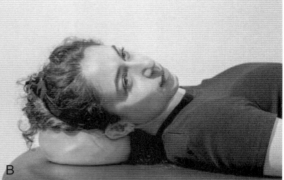

Figura 26.10 Atividade sensorimotora de estágio inicial com *laser*. De uma posição neutra (**A**), o paciente é instruído a mover o *laser* dentro de uma pequena área-alvo enquanto a cabeça está na bola desinflada (**B**).

Treinamento do sistema sensorimotor

O treinamento proprioceptivo do pescoço como parte de um programa de treinamento sensorimotor foi proposto como outra área de desenvolvimento, mas pode ser restrito devido à necessidade percebida de equipamentos sofisticados e caros (Alricsson et al., 2004). Os déficits identificados no sentido da posição da articulação da coluna cervical (propriocepção) podem ser retreinados simplesmente utilizando ponteiros *laser* montados em faixas de cabeça, conforme descrito a seguir (Figuras 26.10 a 26.12). Déficits de controle oculomotor identificados da mesma maneira podem ser divididos em exercícios realizados com a cabeça parada e enquanto a cabeça está em movimento. Isso imita atividades esportivas comuns. Os atletas precisam progredir para tarefas funcionais e dinâmicas, da caminhada para a corrida com a cabeça virada para a esquerda e para a direita ou para cima e para baixo, mantendo a direção e a velocidade (Figura 26.13). A introdução do trabalho com bola é particularmente relevante para esta área de treinamento para adicionar complexidade crescente. Os terapeutas devem se esforçar para introduzir os principais elementos funcionais do esporte em todas as tarefas de treinamento, a fim de manter o interesse e facilitar o retorno ao jogo.

Perspectivas de saúde mental

É bem conhecido que a prontidão física e psicológica para retornar ao esporte após uma lesão nem sempre coincidem (Clement et al., 2015; Podlog e Eklund, 2010). Andersen (2001) argumenta que o retorno de um atleta lesionado à atividade plena é um processo complicado e multifacetado. O processo é influenciado por uma infinidade de fatores, incluindo as características da lesão com variáveis biológicas, psicológicas e sociais. Esses fatores foram elencados como: características da lesão e fatores sociodemográficos, biológicos, psicológicos e sociais/contextuais (Brewer et al., 2002).

A coluna cervical é frequentemente considerada uma parte vulnerável da anatomia humana por atletas e profissionais da saúde. Normalmente, os atletas podem não revelar totalmente suas emoções relacionadas com as lesões; da mesma maneira, alguns profissionais podem relutar em progredir na reabilitação devido ao risco percebido. Estudos têm sugerido que em qualquer lesão deve haver uma consideração de estratégias para melhorar a integridade emocional de um atleta e monitorar regularmente os fatores psicossociais durante a reabilitação (Forsdyke et al., 2016). Considerações sobre a autoconfiança do atleta e emoções de ansiedade/medo aumentam a probabilidade de uma reabilitação bem-sucedida. A experiência da lesão pode ser enquadrada como uma oportunidade de crescimento e desenvolvimento. Os profissionais devem permitir, sempre que possível, que os atletas percebam uma experiência de lesão como positiva, pois sabe-se que isso está relacionado com resultados positivos. A recuperação física e psicossocial da lesão ocorre raramente no mesmo período. É essencial garantir que os atletas lesionados estejam física, psicológica, social, tática e tecnicamente prontos para retornar ao esporte (Forsdyke et al., 2016). Da mesma

Coluna Cervical: Avaliação de Risco e Reabilitação | Capítulo | 26 |

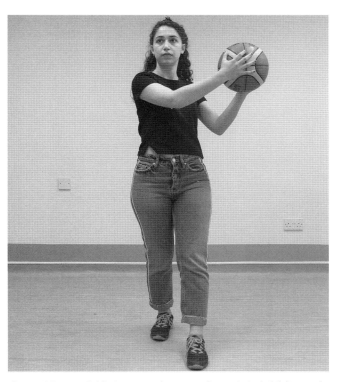

Figura 26.11 Atividade sensorimotora de estágio inicial com *laser*. O paciente gira a cabeça para atingir vários alvos de *laser* com a cabeça e a bola desinflada.

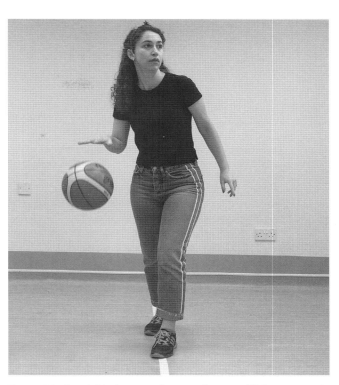

Figura 26.12 Atividade sensorimotora intermediária. Desassociação cabeça-corpo específica da tarefa com *feedback* a *laser*.

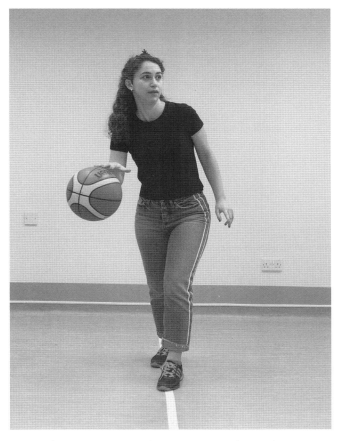

Figura 26.13 Atividade sensorimotora de estágio avançado. Treinamento de coordenação e controle cabeça-corpo-membro para tarefas específicas.

maneira, os profissionais devem ter conhecimento e habilidade para fornecer opções de manejo pragmáticas que são apoiadas pelas evidências atuais em uma região anatômica que infelizmente é negligenciada.

Resumo

- A coluna cervical costuma ser uma área do corpo sub-reabilitada
- Os profissionais da equipe de saúde devem ter uma abordagem sistemática para avaliação de risco que considere fratura potencial, instabilidade e/ou DAC em casos de trauma esportivo
- Tontura e sintomas associados podem estar ligados à disfunção benigna da coluna cervical ou síndromes pós-concussivas, que podem ter ligações com o sistema sensorimotor, os quais podem ser identificados e reabilitados com sucesso
- A reabilitação deve ter uma abordagem multifacetada, incorporando dimensões motoras, sensoriais e psicossociais
- Uma avaliação de risco e estratégia de reabilitação são resumidas na Figura 26.14.

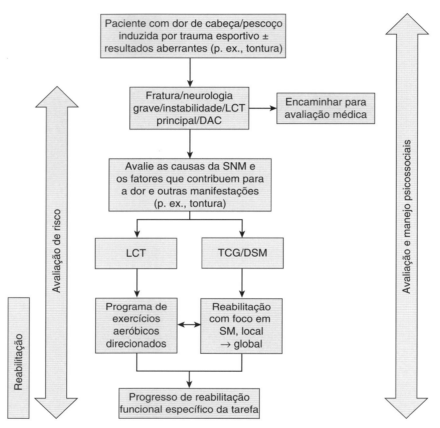

Figura 26.14 Algoritmo para avaliação de risco e reabilitação de pessoas com cervicalgia associada a trauma esportivo. *DAC*, disfunção da artéria cervical; *TCG*, tontura cervicogênica; *SNM*, sistema neuromuscular; *DSM*, disfunção sensorimotora; *LCT*, lesão cerebral traumática.

Referências bibliográficas

Alricsson, M., Harms-Ringdahl, K., Larsson, B., Linder, J., Werner, S., 2004. Neck muscle strength and endurance in fighter pilots: effects of a supervised training program. Aviation, Space, and Environmental Medicine. 75 (1), 23-28.

Andersen, M.B., Van Raalte, J.L., Brewer, B.W., 2001. Sport psychology service delivery: staying ethical while keeping loose. Psychology: Research and Practice. 32 (1), 12-18.

Axen, K., Haas, F., Schicchi, J., Merrick, J., 1992. Progressive resistance neck exercises using a compressible ball coupled with an air pressure gauge. Journal of Orthopaedic & Sports Physical Therapy. 16 (6), 275-280.

Barrett, M.D., McLoughlin, T.F., Gallagher, K.R., Gatherer, D., Parratt, M.T., Perera, J.R., et al., 2015. Effectiveness of a tailored neck training program on neck strength, movement, and fatigue in under-19 male rugby players: a randomized controlled pilot study. Open Access Journal of Sports Medicine. 6, 137-147.

Beletsky, V., Nadareishvili, Z., Lynch, J., Shuaib, A., Woolfenden, A., Norris, J.W., Canadian Stroke Consortium, 2003. Cervical arterial dissection: time for a therapeutic trial? Stroke 34 (12), 2856-2860.

Biousse, V., D'Anglejan-Chatillon, J., Touboul, P.J., Amarenco, P., Bousser, M.G., 1995. Time course of symptoms in extracranial carotid artery dissections. A series of 80 patients. Stroke 26 (2), 235-239.

Brajkovic, S., Riboldi, G., Govoni, A., Corti, S., Bresolin, N., Comi, G.P., 2013. Growing evidence about the relationship between vessel dissection and scuba diving. Case Reports in Neurology 5 (3), 155-161.

Brewer, B.W., Andersen, M.B., Van Raalte, J.L., 2002. Psychological aspects of sport injury rehabilitation: toward a biopsychosocial approach. In: Mostofsky, D.L., Zaichkowsky, L.D. (Eds.), Medical and Psychological Aspects of Sport and Exercise. Fitness Information Technology, Morgantown, WV, pp. 41-54.

Cantu, R.C., 2014. Neck strength: a protective factor reducing risk for concussion in high school sports. Journal of Primary Prevention. 35 (5), 309-319.

Clement, D., Arvinen-Barrow, M., Fetty, T., 2015. Psychosocial responses during different phases of sport-injury rehabilitation: a qualitative study. Journal of Athletic Training 50 (1), 95-104.

Collins CL, Fletcher EN, Fields SK, Kluchurosky L, Rohrkemper MK, Comstock RD, Crissey, M.M., Bernstein, E.F., 1974. Delayed presentation of carotid intimal tear following blunt craniocervical trauma. Surgery 75 (4), 543-549.

de Vries, J., Ischebeck, B.K., Voogt, L.P., van der Geest, J.N., Janssen, M., Frens, M.A., et al., 2015. Joint position sense error in people with neck pain: a systematic review. Manual Therapy 20 (6), 736-744.

Degen, R.M., Fink, M.E., Callahan, L., Fibel, K., Ramsay, J., Kelly, B.T., 2017. Internal carotid artery dissection after indirect blunt cervical trauma in an ice hockey goaltender. American Journal of Orthopedics 46 (3), E139-E143.

Dorland W.A.N. 2012. Dorland's Illustrated Medical Dictionary, thirty second ed. Saunders/Elsevier, Philadelphia, PA.

Forsdyke, D., Smith, A., Jones, M., Gledhill, A., 2016. Psychosocial factors associated with outcomes of sports injury rehabilitation in competitive athletes: a mixed studies systematic review. British Journal of Sports Medicine 50 (9), 537-544.

Fragoso, Y.D., Adoni, T., do Amaral, L.L., Braga, F.T., Brooks, J.B., Campos, C.S., et al., 2016. Cerebrum-cervical arterial dissection in adults during sports and recreation. Arquivos de Neuro-Psiquiatria 74 (4), 275-279.

Gottesman, R.F., Sharma, P., Robinson, K.A., Arnan, M., Tsui, M., Ladha, K., et al., 2012. Clinical characteristics of symptomatic vertebral artery dissection: a systematic review. Neurologist 18 (5), 245-254.

Gross, A., Kay, TM., Paquin, JP., Blanchette, S., Lalonde, P., Christie, T., et al. Cervical Overview Group. Exercises for mechanical neck disorders.

Hides, J.A., Franettovich Smith, M.M., Mendis, M.D., Smith, N.A., Cooper, A.J., Treleaven, J., et al., 2017. A prospective investigation of changes in the sensorimotor system following sports concussion. An exploratory study. Musculoskeletal Science & Practice 29, 7-19.

Hrysomallis, C., 2016. Neck muscular strength, training, performance and sport injury risk: a review. Sports Medicine 46 (8), 1111-1124.

Iverson, G.L., Koehle, M.S., 2013. Normative data for the balance error scoring system in adults. Rehabilitation Research and Practice 2013, 846418.

Jull, G.A., Falla, D., Vicenzino, B., Hodges, P.W., 2009. The effect of therapeutic exercise on activation of the deep cervical flexor muscles in people with chronic neck pain. Manual Therapy 14 (6), 696-701.

Jull, G.A., O'Leary, S.P., Falla, D.L., 2008. Clinical assessment of the deep cervical flexor muscles: the craniocervical flexion test. Journal of Manipulative and Physiological Therapeutics 31 (7), 525-533.

Kristensen, B., Malm, J., Carlberg, B., Stegmayr, B., Backman, C., Fagerlund, M., et al., 1997. Epidemiology and etiology of ischemic stroke in young adults aged 18 to 44 years in northern Sweden. Stroke 28 (9), 1702-1709.

Kristjansson, E., Treleaven, J., 2009. Sensorimotor function and dizziness in neck pain: implications for assessment and management. Journal of Orthopaedic & Sports Physical Therapy 39 (5), 364-377.

Lamb, S.E., Williams, M.A., Williamson, E.M., Gates, S., Withers, E.J., Mt-Isa, S., et al., 2012. Managing Injuries of the Neck Trial (MINT): a randomised controlled trial of treatments for whiplash injuries. Health Technology Assessment 16 (49), iii-iv, 1–141.

Langer, P.R., Fadale, P.D., Palumbo, M.A., 2008. Catastrophic neck injuries in the collision sport athlete. Sports Medicine and Arthroscopy Review 16 (1), 7-15.

Martinelli, O., Venosi, S., BenHamida, J., Malaj, A., Belli, C., Irace, F.G., et al., 2017. Therapeutical options in the management of carotid dissection. Vascular Surgery 41, 69-76.

McCrory, P., Meeuwisse, W., Dvořák, J., Aubry, M., Bailes, J., Broglio, S., et al., 2017. Consensus statement on concussion in sport – the 5th international conference on concussion in sport held in Berlin, October. British Journal of Sports Medicine 51 (11), 838-847.

Minshull, C., Gleeson, N., 2017. Considerations of the principles of resistance training in exercise studies for the management of knee osteoarthritis: a systematic review. Archives of Physical Medicine and Rehabilitation 98 (9), 1842-1851.

Naish, R., Burnett, A., Burrows, S., Andrews, W., Appleby, B., 2013. Can a specific neck strengthening program decrease cervical spine injuries in a men's professional rugby union team? a retrospective analysis. Journal of Sports Science and Medicine 12 (3), 542–550.

Neck pain guidelines: revision 2017: using the evidence to guide physical therapist practice. Journal of Orthopaedic & Sports Physical Therapy. 47 (7), 2017, 511-512.

Nikander, R., Mälkiä, E., Parkkari, J., Heinonen, A., Starck, H., Ylinen, J., 2006. Dose-response relationship of specific training to reduce chronic neck pain and disability. Medicine & Science in Sports & Exercise. 38 (12), 2068-2074.

Olympia, R.P., Dixon, T., Brady, J., Avner, J.R., 2007. Emergency planning in school-based athletics: a national survey of athletic trainers. Pediatric Emergency Care 23 (10), 703-708.

Petschauer, M.A., Schmitz, R., Gill, D.L., 2010. Helmet fit and cervical spine motion in collegiate men's lacrosse athletes secured to a spine board. Journal of Athletic Training 45 (3), 215-221.

Podlog, L., Eklund, R.C., 2010. Returning to competition after a serious injury: the role of self-determination. Journal of Sports Sciences. 28 (8), 819-831.

Rao, A.S., Makaroun, M.S., Marone, L.K., Cho, J.S., Rhee, R., Chaer, R.A., 2011. Long-term outcomes of internal carotid artery dissection. Journal of Vascular Surgery 54 (2), 370.

Reiley, A.S., Vickory, F.M., Funderburg, S.E., Cesario, R.A., Clendaniel, R.A., 2017. How to diagnose cervicogenic dizziness. Archives of Physiotherapy 7, 12. ; PubMed Central PMCID: PMC5759906.

Reilly, B.M., 1990. Dizziness. In: Walker, H.K., Hall, W.D., Hurst, J.W. (Eds.), Clinical Methods: The History, Physical, and Laboratory Examinations, third ed. Butterworths, Boston. Chapter 212.

Rihn, J.A., Anderson, D.T., Lamb, K., Deluca, P.F., Bata, A., Marchetto, P.A., et al., 2009. Cervical spine injuries in american football. Sports Medicine 39 (9), 697-708.

Rushton, A., Rivett, D., Carlesso, L., Flynn, T., Hing, W., Kerry, R., 2014. International framework for examination of the cervical region for potential of cervical arterial dysfunction prior to orthopaedic manual therapy intervention. Manual Therapy 19 (3), 222-228.

Sanelli, P.C., Tong, S., Gonzalez, R.G., Eskey, C.J., 2002. Normal variation of vertebral artery on CT angiography and its implications for diagnosis of acquired pathology. Journal of Computer Assisted Tomography. 26 (3), 462-470.

Simon, L.V., Mohseni, M., 2017. Vertebral Artery Injury. StatPearls Publishing, Treasure Island (FL).

Stiell, I.G., Wells, G.A., Vandemheen, K.L., Clement, C.M., Lesiuk, H., De Maio, V.J., et al., 2001. The Canadian C-spine rule for radiography in alert and stable trauma patients. JAMA 286 (15), 1841-1848.

Suzuki, S., Tsuchimochi, R., Abe, G., Yu, I., Inoue, T., Ishibashi, H., 2018. Traumatic vertebral artery dissection in high school rugby players: a report of two cases. Journal of Clinical Neuroscience 47, 137-139.

Taylor, M.K., Hodgdon, J.A., Griswold, L., Miller, A., Roberts, D.E., Escamilla, R.F., 2006. Cervical resistance training: effects on isometric and dynamic strength. Aviation, Space, and Environmental Medicine. 77 (11), 1131-1135.

Tjell, C., Rosenhall, U., 1998. Smooth pursuit neck torsion test: a specific test for cervical dizziness. American Journal of Otolaryngology 19 (1), 76-81.

Treleaven, J., 2008. Sensorimotor disturbances in neck disorders affecting postural stability, head and eye movement control. Manual Therapy 13 (1), 2-11.

Versteegh, T., Beaudet, D., Greenbaum, M., Hellyer, L., Tritton, A., Walton, D., 2015. Evaluating the reliability of a novel neck-strength assessment protocol for healthy adults using self-generated resistance with a hand-held dynamometer. Journal of Physiotherapy 67 (1), 58-64.

Williams, K., Tarmizi, A., Treleaven, J., 2017. Use of neck torsion as a specific test of neck related postural instability. Musculoskeletal Science & Practice 29, 115-119.

Ylinen, J., Häkkinen, A., Nykänen, M., Kautiainen, H., Takala, E.P., 2007. Neck muscle training in the treatment of chronic neck pain: a three-year follow-up study. Europa Medicophysica 43 (2), 161-169.

Yu, L.J., Stokell, R., Treleaven, J., 2011. The effect of neck torsion on postural stability in subjects with persistent whiplash. Manual Therapy 16 (4), 339–343.

Capítulo | 27 |

Manejo de Lesões na Cabeça

Etienne Laverse, Akbar de Medici, Richard Sylvester, Simon Kemp e Ademola Adejuwon

Introdução

A concussão, também conhecida como lesão cerebral traumática leve (LCTL), descreve uma síndrome clínica que se segue a um traumatismo cranioencefálico. É responsável por > 80% dos 1,4 milhão de casos estimados de lesão cerebral traumática (LCT) vistos em hospitais na Inglaterra e no País de Gales anualmente e afeta de 1,6 a 3,8 milhões de indivíduos nos EUA a cada ano (Cancelliere et al., 2014; Levin e Diaz-Arrastia, 2015). Esportes de contato e colisão apresentam vários graus de risco de causar traumatismo cranioencefálico. Exemplos de esportes de alto risco incluem hóquei, corrida de cavalos, rúgbi, futebol, basquete, futebol americano, críquete, *snowboard* e esqui (Giza et al., 2013).

Embora classificado como "leve", a LCTL repetida pode causar sequelas neurocognitivas significativas. Apesar de ser raro, a curto prazo (horas a semanas), pode resultar em uma "síndrome de segundo impacto" potencialmente fatal, em que um jogador com LCTL volta a jogar e, em seguida, sofre consequências catastróficas após um segundo impacto que está associado à autodisregulação e edema cerebral (Khong et al., 2016; Khurana e Kaye, 2012). As sequelas a longo prazo podem consistir em comprometimento cognitivo progressivo. Portanto, é essencial que todos os indivíduos envolvidos em esportes, incluindo técnicos, treinadores, pais e atletas, além da equipe de saúde, tenham uma compreensão prática do reconhecimento e do tratamento de lesões na cabeça de seus atletas.

Sintomas

A síndrome de LCTL compreende uma constelação de sintomas após a lesão biomecânica do cérebro. Os sintomas comumente relatados incluem dor de cabeça, distúrbios visuais, comprometimento da memória, desorientação e perda de consciência. A lesão cerebral ocorre como consequência de uma força aplicada diretamente na cabeça, rosto ou pescoço a partir do contato com um oponente, o solo ou outro objeto, ou de uma força aplicada em outra parte do corpo, com a força impulsiva transferida para a cabeça.

Diagnóstico e manejo

As diretrizes de manejo no esporte foram preparadas em grande parte a partir de processos de consenso reconhecidos, como a declaração de consenso do Grupo de Concussão Esportiva (CISG,

do inglês *Concussion Sport Group*) 2017 (McCrory et al., 2016), com o objetivo de prevenir mais lesões e limitar o impacto cumulativo de lesões repetidas na cabeça. Acredita-se que certos fatores contribuam para o risco de sustentar uma LCTL. Por exemplo, foi relatado que atletas do sexo feminino podem correr mais riscos em esportes como futebol ou basquete. O tipo de esporte praticado também terá um impacto no risco de contato com a cabeça/colisão, a frequência e a intensidade variam (Giza et al., 2013).

O primeiro passo no manejo de LCTL é o reconhecimento imediato de uma potencial LCTL. Os casos suspeitos devem ser avaliados por um membro da equipe médica ou profissional de saúde devidamente treinado para realizar tais avaliações. O cuidado padrão no local para traumas imediatos deve ser iniciado, incluindo o manejo apropriado de lesões potenciais da coluna cervical. A *Sport Concussion Assessment Tool* – 5ª edição (SCAT5) (2017) deve ser usada para apoiar a avaliação inicial pelos profissionais de saúde. Também é importante na fase inicial identificar sinais e sintomas que podem refletir uma lesão mais significativa, por exemplo, déficit focal persistente ou pontuação baixa na Escala de Coma de Glasgow (ECG). Esses indicadores sugerem lesões cerebrais moderadas a graves que requerem mais investigações e manejo adequado. Isso deve diminuir o limiar para o uso de imageamento cerebral, como tomografia computadorizada (TC) ou ressonância magnética (RM).

Qualquer atleta com suspeita de concussão deve ser retirado do jogo, avaliado clinicamente e monitorado quanto à deterioração. Nenhum atleta com diagnóstico de concussão deve voltar a jogar no dia da lesão.

As etapas subsequentes no manejo da LCTL compreendem um retorno gradativo aos estudos, trabalho e lazer que inclui avaliações regulares de sintomas e atividade física graduada, a fim de permitir a recuperação completa, boa forma física e segurança para futuras atividades esportivas.

A LCTL envolve processos fisiopatológicos complexos que afetam o cérebro após o impacto mecânico. A aceleração angular, rotacional ou linear do cérebro pode resultar em cisalhamento e disfunção neuronal. Apenas 10% desses casos apresentam perda de consciência associada; acredita-se que isso seja resultado de uma interrupção transitória no sistema de ativação reticular (Khurana e Kaye, 2012). Considera-se que uma evolução complexa dependente do tempo de patologias (uma cascata neurometabólica) ocorra após a lesão – isso é comprovado em modelos animais. A perturbação dos canais iônicos nas membranas neurais permite um efluxo de K^+ e um influxo de Ca^{2+}, e uma ativação das bombas de Na^+/K^+ na tentativa de restaurar o equilíbrio iônico. Este processo consome muita energia. As citocinas inflamatórias também são consideradas subjacentes à cascata molecular de eventos que seguem a LCTL e a inflamação pode desempenhar um papel fisiopatológico central (Khurana e Kaye, 2012).

O diagnóstico e o tratamento da LCT se baseiam amplamente na detecção e monitoramento de sinais e sintomas. É reconhecido que faltam marcadores objetivos para diagnosticar, classificar e prognosticar; pesquisas estão em andamento para explorar marcadores moleculares e de imagem cerebral para auxiliar no processo. É crucial o manejo ideal, pois também pode haver implicações escolares e financeiras, especialmente para atletas mais jovens (Hobbs et al., 2016).

Todos os esquemas diagnósticos atuais exigem que o atleta experimente uma força externa na cabeça seguida por alguma alteração na função cerebral. As diretrizes determinam que, em todos os casos suspeitos de LCTL, o indivíduo deve ser retirado do jogo e avaliado por um profissional de saúde licenciado. Portanto, a educação sobre a LCTL direcionada para atletas e treinadores é importante para encorajar o relato de sintomas e o reconhecimento imediato da lesão.

As características observadas com frequência após a LCTL incluem olhar vago, confusão, atrasos nas respostas motoras e verbais, desorientação, déficits de memória e falta de coordenação. A maioria dos pacientes adultos não complicados com um único episódio de LCT se recupera espontaneamente nos primeiros dias a semanas após a lesão, com 80 a 95% dos atletas retornando às medidas neurocognitivas basais entre 3 e 6 meses após a lesão. A disfunção cognitiva pode persistir por um período mais longo e a lesão axonal difusa (LAD) no cérebro (Figuras 27.1 e 27.2) é considerada a patologia primária (Kawata et al., 2016; Siman et al., 2015).

Reconhecimento imediato da lesão cerebral traumática leve ao lado do campo

O consenso atual é de que qualquer pessoa com suspeita de LCTL deve ser removida imediatamente do campo de jogo. Deve-se suspeitar de LCTL após um evento de traumatismo cranioencefálico se qualquer um dos sinais ou sintomas no Boxe 27.1 forem observados ou relatados.

Vários esportes profissionais introduziram triagens fora do campo para atletas com suspeita e possível LCTL. Esses protocolos de triagem são projetados para determinar se um jogador que sofreu um traumatismo craniano onde as consequências do impacto na cabeça não são claras precisa ser definitivamente removido do jogo; eles não são utilizados para fazer ou refutar um diagnóstico de concussão, a menos que sejam vistos sinais observáveis no momento do impacto na cabeça. Esses protocolos são aplicados apenas em esportes de elite para adultos, nos quais médicos treinados e experientes estão presentes. Em todas as outras configurações, deve ser utilizada a estratégia "reconhecer e remover".

Os principais elementos da *10-minute off-field World Rugby Head Injury Assessment* (HIA 1) são: revisão das imagens do jogo quanto à presença de sinais observáveis, questões de avaliação de memória, testes de memória imediata e atrasada, capacidade de reverter sequências de números, teste de equilíbrio de marcha/caminhada em tandem, verificação de sintomas de concussão, revisão por médico para outros sinais de concussão (Figura 27.3) e segunda revisão de imagens do jogo para presença de sinais observáveis.

Se forem encontrados sinais observáveis no vídeo, ou se o jogador cometer erros na avaliação, ou se, no julgamento do médico, o jogador estiver mostrando qualquer sinal de concussão, então o jogador não retornará para o jogo. Essa abordagem foi lançada pela primeira vez durante a Copa do Mundo de Rúgbi 2015 e reduziu o número de jogadores não removidos no momento da concussão de 50% para menos de 10%.

A adição de revisão de vídeo em tempo real lateral e da sala da equipe de saúde oferece identificação e avaliação aprimoradas de impactos na cabeça e permite uma revisão mais abrangente de todo o processo.

Sinais de alerta

Um sinal de alerta é um indicador potencial de patologia grave. Embora a LCTL geralmente tenha um curso benigno, a possibilidade de lesão mais grave deve ser considerada como parte do processo de avaliação, pois pode exigir etapas adicionais de manejo. Os sinais e sintomas que podem indicar lesão mais significativa e, portanto, levam a investigações adicionais, como imageamento cerebral (Figuras 27.4 e 27.5), são mostrados no Boxe 27.2.

Avaliação clínica

Atletas com suspeita de LCTL devem ser avaliados inicialmente por profissionais de saúde usando o SCAT5. O processo de diagnóstico compreende uma avaliação de vários domínios, incluindo:

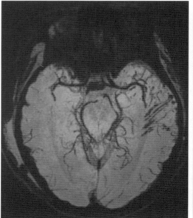 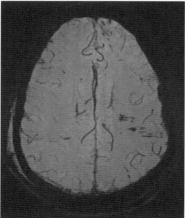 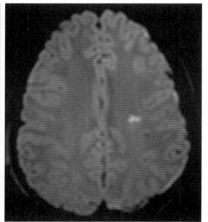

Figura 27.1 Ressonância magnética de lesão axonal difusa. Imagem ponderada em suscetibilidade magnética (IPSM) e de difusão mostrando microssangramentos e lesões por cisalhamento, respectivamente.

Manejo de Lesões na Cabeça **Capítulo | 27 |**

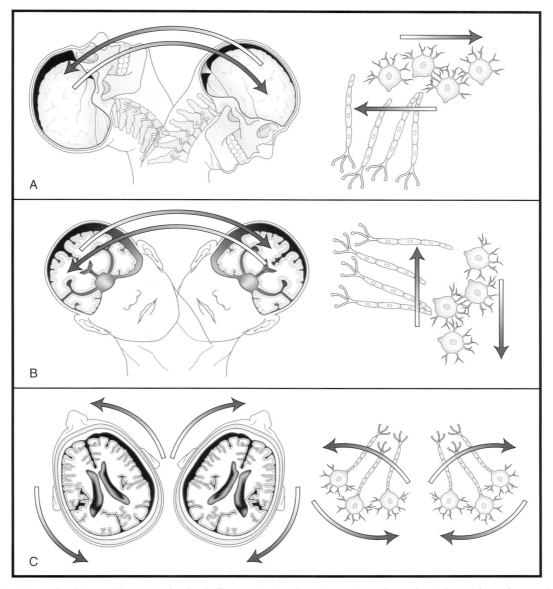

Figura 27.2 Lesão cerebral traumática: axonal e de cisalhamento. A aceleração angular ou linear do cérebro pode resultar em cisalhamento e disfunção neuronal. (*Esta figura se encontra reproduzida em cores no Encarte.*)

Boxe 27.1 Sinais e sintomas observáveis de lesão cerebral traumática leve

Sinais
- Perda de consciência
- Deitar-se imóvel no chão
- Problemas de lentidão para se levantar/instabilidade/falta de equilíbrio
- Segurar/apertar a cabeça
- Olhar atordoado/vazio.

Sintomas
- Dor de cabeça
- Tontura
- Fadiga/sonolência
- Náuseas/vômito
- Sentir ou demonstrar lentidão/embotamento mental, mudança emocional ou tristeza
- Visão embaçada.

Boxe 27.2 Lesão cerebral traumática leve: sinais e sintomas que podem indicar lesão mais significativa

Sinais
- Déficits focais, por exemplo, fraqueza dos membros ou distúrbio do campo visual
- Mais de um episódio de vômito
- Convulsão por impacto
- Fratura craniana aberta ou deprimida
- Deterioração da consciência
- Aumento da confusão ou irritabilidade
- Mudança de comportamento incomum.

Sintomas
- Dor de cabeça intensa ou crescente
- Dor forte no pescoço
- Visão dupla
- Deficiência auditiva.

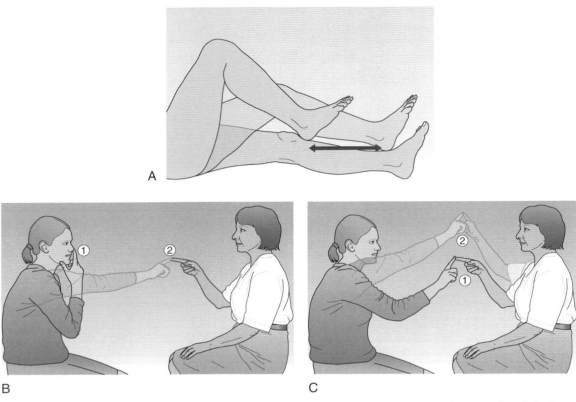

Figura 27.3 Testes de coordenação comuns: A. Calcanhar à canela. **B.** Teste dedo-nariz-dedo. **C.** Examinador movendo o dedo-alvo. *1*, cotovelo flexionado; *2*, cotovelo estendido.

- Avaliação dos sintomas (p. ex., dor de cabeça, náuseas, tontura, sensação de estar "em uma névoa", sensibilidade à luz/ruído)
- Testes de memória
- Testes de concentração
- Triagem neurológica
- Testes de coordenação
- Testes de equilíbrio.

O uso de escalas de sintomas LCTL SCAT5 ajuda a documentar a progressão dos sintomas em função do tempo. Uma carga maior de sintomas na apresentação inicial está associada a uma recuperação pior. O sintoma mais comum é a dor de cabeça, seguido por tontura.

Se um evento concussivo for testemunhado ou suspeito, e se qualquer um dos domínios mencionados anteriormente for considerado anormal, a LCTL deverá ser suspeitada, e o tratamento apropriado, instituído. Por exemplo, quando houver suspeita de lesão mais séria, com a identificação de sinais ou sintomas de alerta, os atletas deverão ser transferidos para o centro de emergência/traumatismo mais próximo para cuidados mais intensivos.

Investigações

LCTL é um diagnóstico clínico e as investigações são utilizadas quando há suspeita de lesão mais grave. Estas incluem imagens cerebrais de TC padrão e/ou RM. As sequências-padrão de varredura do cérebro são geralmente normais nas LCTL. A TC pode detectar sangramento agudo (p. ex., hemorragia subdural) e fraturas cranianas. No entanto, certas sequências de RM, como a imagem ponderada em suscetibilidade magnética (IPSM) (ver Figura 27.1), podem revelar alterações microvasculares associadas com a LCTL na forma de microssangramentos e a imagem do tensor de difusão pode fornecer informações sobre lesões axonais e vasculares difusas que as varreduras-padrão podem não detectar (Sharp et al., 2011; Sharp e Jenkins, 2015). O significado clínico desses achados não é totalmente compreendido. No entanto, alterações vasculares sutis ou outras alterações cerebrais podem não ser reveladas pelos exames-padrão usuais e, portanto, correlatos radiológicos não são observados rotineiramente.

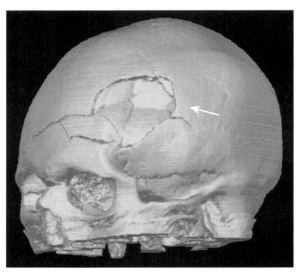

Figura 27.4 Fratura craniana deprimida.

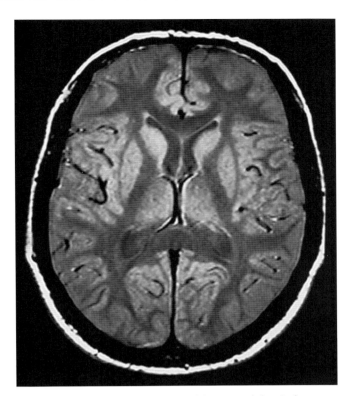

Figura 27.5 Ressonância magnética normal do cérebro.

Manejo agudo

O atleta com suspeita de LCTL deve ser retirado imediatamente do jogo e avaliado clinicamente no local por meio do atendimento pré-hospitalar de emergência padrão. Atenção especial deve ser dada à exclusão de lesões da coluna cervical. Se isso não puder ser excluído, o atleta deve ser imobilizado, deixando no local qualquer equipamento esportivo que não interfira no manejo clínico, como um capacete, e transferido para o hospital para posterior avaliação e imageamento.

Após a avaliação inicial e a exclusão de lesões traumáticas significativas, uma avaliação mais focada dos domínios afetados por LCTL deve ser examinada por meio das ferramentas de avaliação padronizadas, como o SCAT5.

A LCTL é uma lesão em evolução na fase aguda e o atleta deve ser observado durante as primeiras horas após a lesão para qualquer deterioração (p. ex., diminuição da pontuação ECG). A avaliação seriada de acompanhamento é recomendada, pois os sintomas podem evoluir ou ter um início tardio; uma lista de verificação de sintomas é útil para rastrear a recuperação.

É importante observar que os sintomas podem se desenvolver ao longo de várias horas e a extensão da lesão pode não ser imediatamente aparente. Portanto, os atletas não devem ter permissão para voltar a jogar no dia da lesão. Um hematoma epidural em expansão pode ser a causa de deterioração neurológica após um período de melhora aparente e em uma minoria de casos; contusão cerebral e hematomas subdurais também podem ser responsáveis por um intervalo lúcido.

Tratamento de lesão cerebral traumática leve

O objetivo principal é limitar mais lesões. As atividades cognitivas e físicas devem ser ajustadas de acordo com os sintomas. A quantidade de exercício e repouso após uma lesão deve ser proporcional e o repouso prolongado completo não é considerado a melhor abordagem. No entanto, atividades que requerem concentração, ou seja, tarefas cognitivamente exigentes (p. ex., jogar videogame) podem exacerbar os sintomas e o exercício físico prematuro pode intensificar os sintomas pós-concussão e deve ser evitado por 24 a 48 horas. Após um período inicial de descanso, o atleta deve retornar às atividades da vida diária normalmente. Se os sintomas ainda estiverem presentes, essas atividades devem estar abaixo do nível que agrava os sintomas (atividade limitada pelos sintomas ou repouso relativo). Há evidências limitadas para apoiar o uso de farmacoterapia na fase aguda do manejo de LCTL.

O atleta pode iniciar um retorno gradual ao jogo, de preferência sob supervisão da equipe de saúde, após a resolução completa dos sintomas e o período mínimo de descanso estipulado pelo esporte (14 dias para rúgbi de 15 e futebol). Existem vários protocolos específicos para esportes, que compreendem normalmente níveis distintos (Tabela 27.1). Atletas adultos podem progredir a cada dia para o próximo nível se forem capazes de completar o nível atual sem provocar sintomas (Hobbs et al., 2016; McCrory et al., 2016); no entanto, recomenda-se que aqueles com 19 anos ou menos levem 48 horas, em vez de 24, para concluir cada estágio. Assim, o atleta adulto pode concluir o protocolo completo em 1 semana se permanecer assintomático o tempo todo. Se os sintomas ocorrerem novamente, é aconselhável que o atleta volte ao nível anterior e tente a atividade física após um período de 24 horas de descanso. Recomenda-se a revisão com a equipe de saúde antes de retomar o treinamento de contato completo. Os testes neuropsicológicos podem ajudar a fornecer medidas objetivas da função cognitiva e reduzir a dependência no relato subjetivo de sintomas pelo atleta ao aconselhar sobre o retorno ao jogo. A recuperação do desempenho cognitivo ao nível da pré-temporada faz parte dos critérios usados para decidir quando o atleta pode voltar a jogar. No entanto, essa abordagem em si não é infalível e há uma necessidade definitiva de marcadores mais objetivos para auxiliar na avaliação.

Sintomas crônicos/persistentes

Os atletas se recuperam geralmente dentro de dias a semanas. Os fatores de risco para recuperação atrasada incluem:
- Pouca idade (< 16 anos)
- Início agudo de dores de cabeça do tipo enxaqueca
- Déficit de memória
- Histórico recente de LCTL.

O indicador mais forte de recuperação mais lenta de LCTL é a gravidade dos sintomas iniciais de uma pessoa nos primeiros dias após a lesão. Notavelmente, um baixo nível de sintomas no primeiro dia após a lesão é um indicador de prognóstico favorável. Estudos indicaram que um transtorno neuropsiquiátrico pré-lesão está relacionado à persistência dos sintomas por 3 meses ou mais após a LCTL. Quando os sintomas se estendem além dos habituais 10 a 14 dias em adultos (> 4 semanas em crianças), podem ser úteis mais informações de especialistas, como de neurologistas ou médicos do esporte com experiência em manejo de LCTL. Isso pode ser no ambiente de uma clínica dedicada à concussão (p. ex., o Instituto de Saúde do Esporte e Exercício, Londres, Reino Unido), onde investigações adicionais, como testes neuropsicológicos mais detalhados e neuroimagem avançada (p. ex., IPSM, recuperação de inversão atenuada por fluido ou sequências ponderadas T2*) podem ser consideradas em um ambiente multidisciplinar.

Parte | 2 | Aplicação Clínica

Tabela 27.1 Protocolo graduado de retorno ao jogo em atletas com lesão cerebral traumática leve.

Estágio de reabilitação	Exercício funcional em cada estágio da reabilitação	Objetivo para cada etapa
1. Sem atividade	Repouso físico e cognitivo	Recuperação
2a. Se os sintomas persistirem em 24 horas: atividade limitada pelos sintomas	Inicialmente atividades da vida diária que não provocam sintomas. Considere folga ou adaptação de trabalho ou estudo	Retorno às atividades normais (conforme os sintomas permitirem)
2b. Exercício aeróbico leve	Caminhada, natação ou ciclismo estacionário, mantendo intensidade < 70% da frequência cardíaca máxima prevista; sem treinamento de resistência	Aumento da frequência cardíaca
3. Exercícios específicos para esportes	Exercícios de patinação no hóquei no gelo, exercícios de corrida no futebol. Sem atividades de impacto na cabeça	Adição de movimento
4. Exercícios de treinamento sem contato	Progressão para exercícios de treinamento mais complexos, por exemplo, exercícios de passagem em futebol e hóquei no gelo; pode iniciar resistência progressiva	Exercício, coordenação e carga cognitiva
5. Prática de contato total	Após a liberação médica, participação das atividades normais de treinamento	Restauração da confiança e avaliação das habilidades funcionais pela equipe de treinamento
6. Retorno ao jogo	Jogo normal	

Sintomas como tontura e dificuldade de equilíbrio podem ser resultado de anormalidades vestibulares e a contribuição de um especialista no manejo dessas pode ser tratada em tais clínicas especializadas. Podem ser benéficas as intervenções, incluindo reabilitação psicológica, cervical e vestibular. O tratamento farmacológico da cefaleia (em particular com características de enxaqueca) pode ser útil se esses sintomas persistirem além do primeiro mês após a LCTL.

O caso ilustrativo no Boxe 27.3 destaca as complexidades potenciais da LCTL e ressalta o benefício de buscar contribuições de especialistas para casos complexos.

Há um interesse crescente nos efeitos a longo prazo do traumatismo craniano em esportes, principalmente as anormalidades neurocognitivas que podem ter um impacto significativo no bem-estar dos jogadores (inclusive aposentados) e consequências psicossociais importantes. Tudo isso tem levado a uma crescente preocupação pública sobre os efeitos das lesões cerebrais traumáticas nos esportes de contato. Pensa-se que LCT repetitiva, incluindo golpes subconcussivos na cabeça, pode estar associada a uma taupatia neurodegenerativa – encefalopatia traumática crônica (ETC) com acúmulo de proteína tau em espaços perivasculares em sulcos corticais profundos – em atletas (Ling et al., 2017).

Assim, a LCTL inócua pode estar associada a uma patologia cerebral funcional significativa. Como consequência desse maior reconhecimento, as entidades desportivas tomaram medidas para minimizar e, sempre que possível, prevenir o risco de LCTL. Por exemplo, a aplicação de regras mais rígidas de cartões vermelhos para cotovelos altos em duelos de cabeça no futebol profissional é apoiada por evidências de menor risco de contatos de cabeça e LCTL com tais aplicações.

Um histórico de LCTL é conhecido por aumentar o risco de lesões futuras e sintomas basais, bem como desregulação cognitiva e psiquiátrica a longo prazo em atletas. Também é difícil prever quais atletas sofrerão a longo prazo, pois a resolução dos sintomas não indica automaticamente a recuperação total do evento traumático.

A abordagem atual para diagnosticar LCTL depende dos sintomas relatados pelo paciente e de um exame neurológico para avaliar a extensão da lesão. No entanto, os atletas são conhecidos por subnotificar os sintomas e isso pode afetar de modo negativo o processo de diagnóstico. Os testes neuropsicológicos são úteis e as imagens cerebrais, em certos casos, podem fornecer informações clínicas adicionais. No entanto, a avaliação clínica permanece limitada, uma vez que a extensão da lesão no cérebro, em particular as alterações microestruturais que resultam da LCTL, permanece desconhecida. O protocolo de retorno gradual ao jogo é um guia útil para permitir um retorno seguro – embora não seja eficaz para todos os casos. Definir a recuperação por estar livre de sintomas potencialmente traz o risco de um retorno prematuro ao jogo, colocando os atletas em risco de mais traumas.

A pesquisa para avaliar a validade dos biomarcadores de fluido na avaliação de LCTL está em andamento, a fim de adicionar outras medidas objetivas à avaliação atual. No entanto, ainda não foram incorporados à prática clínica (Mercier et al., 2013). A maioria dos estudos de biomarcadores LCTL é conduzido geralmente por hipóteses. É hipotetizado que o dano à unidade neurovascular, que consiste em células endoteliais microvasculares cerebrais e neurônios, pode permitir que algumas moléculas cruzem a barreira hematencefálica (Kawata et al., 2016). O desenvolvimento de métodos para detectar esses marcadores pode ajudar a diagnosticar LCTL com rapidez e precisão e, logo, a mitigar os efeitos neurológicos a longo prazo. A necessidade de biomarcadores diagnósticos como um meio mais objetivo de avaliar LCTL em atletas e para auxiliar no prognóstico também é destacada na recente declaração de consenso da 5th International Conference on Concussion in Sport, realizada em Berlim em 2016 (McCrory et al., 2017).

Eletroencefalograma (EEG), técnicas avançadas de neuroimagem, testes genéticos e biomarcadores de fluido são algumas

Manejo de Lesões na Cabeça **Capítulo** |27|

Boxe 27.3 Estudo de caso

Sintomas persistentes após LCTL

Um jogador universitário de rúgbi de 21 anos apresenta-se 4 meses após a lesão, jogando rúgbi sustentado. Ele não tem marcadores de LCT grave e uma TC de crânio normal.

Sintomas persistentes

O paciente não consegue retornar aos estudos ou à atividade física devido a fortes cefaleias com características de enxaqueca, faz uso de analgesia diariamente, apresenta desequilíbrio e tontura, vertigem visual, fadiga, falta de concentração e comprometimento da memória subjetiva, mau humor e ansiedade.

Resultados do exame

Exame neurológico e vestibular normal

Descobertas da investigação

A RM do cérebro com sequências de imagem ponderadas por suscetibilidade é normal, sem evidência de LAD. A avaliação vestibular mostra evidências de disfunção vestibular periférica unilateral. Neuropsicologia – comprometimento global leve em grande parte devido a dificuldades de atenção sentidas para refletir a influência do mau humor, em vez de função cerebral prejudicada.

Abordagem de manejo

A enxaqueca pós-traumática complicada por uso excessivo de analgesia é tratada reduzindo a ingestão de analgesia para < 2 dias/semana e iniciando amitriptilina 10 mg (dose aumentando gradualmente para 40 mg). Disfunção vestibular tratada com reabilitação vestibular dirigida por fisioterapeuta especialista. Transtorno de humor tratado com terapia cognitivo-comportamental.

Resultado

Resolução gradual dos sintomas ao longo de 3 meses, permitindo o retorno aos estudos acadêmicos e plena atividade física.

das modalidades que estão sendo estudadas no ambiente de pesquisa e podem adicionar outros componentes objetivos às nossas etapas de investigação e manejo de LCTL no futuro.

Prevê-se que os biomarcadores de fluido, incluindo proteínas neuronais do sangue, que refletem de maneira confiável a extensão da lesão neuronal, possam diagnosticar e antever a recuperação clínica e/ou determinar o risco de potenciais deficiências cumulativas após a lesão. O polipeptídeo leve do neurofilamento (NF-L), encontrado em axônios mielinizados de grande calibre, é um exemplo de um biomarcador que foi encontrado elevado no soro e no líquido cefalorraquidiano (LCR) após a LCT. Estudos com boxeadores mostraram uma correlação positiva entre golpes de cabeça e níveis de NF-L no LCR, bem como com a carga de sintomas e a recuperação (Roy, 2017).

Embora não exista um padrão-ouro para o diagnóstico de LCTL, espera-se que os marcadores moleculares e de imagem possam, melhorar a precisão da avaliação da gravidade da lesão e ajudar no prognóstico e orientação para o retorno ao jogo futuramente. No momento, é importante que as diretrizes estabelecidas sejam seguidas, de modo que o reconhecimento aprimorado da síndrome possa permitir que o tratamento ideal seja instituído precocemente, a fim de mitigar as consequências a longo prazo de repetidas LCTL.

Pontos-chave

- Atletas com suspeita de concussão devem ser retirados de imediato do campo de jogo
- O tratamento padrão para traumas deve ser aplicado de maneira aguda, incluindo o exame de lesão da coluna cervical
- O processo de diagnóstico de concussão aguda envolve um exame clínico apoiado pela ferramenta de avaliação SCAT5
- A base do tratamento é o manejo sintomático seguido por um programa gradativo de exercícios antes do retorno total ao jogo
- Podem ser necessárias modificações nos programas escolares ou de trabalho
- Atletas com 19 anos ou menos devem ser tratados de modo mais conservador
- Atletas com sintomas persistentes devem ser encaminhados para avaliações especializadas por neurologistas ou médicos do esporte, por exemplo, em uma clínica de concussão
- Episódios repetidos ou únicos de LCTL podem estar associados a comprometimento neurocognitivo a longo prazo e ETC
- A pesquisa de biomarcadores radiológicos e moleculares está em andamento e pode contribuir com outras ferramentas objetivas para auxiliar no manejo geral da LCTL.

Referências bibliográficas

Cancelliere, C., Hincapié, C.A., Keightley, M., Godbolt, A.K., Côté, P., Kristman, V.L., et al., 2014. Systematic review of prognosis and return to play after sport concussion: results of the international collaboration on mild traumatic brain injury prognosis. Archives of Physical Medicine and Rehabilitation 95, S210-S229.

Giza, C.C., Kutcher, J.S., Ashwal, S., Barth, J., Getchius, T.S.D., Gioia, G.A., et al., 2013. Summary of evidence-based guideline update: evaluation and management of concussion in sports: report of the Guideline Development Subcommittee of the American Academy of Neurology. Neurology 80, 2250-2257.

Hobbs, J.G., Young, J.S., Bailes, J.E., 2016. Sports-related concussions: diagnosis, complications, and current management strategies. Neurosurgery Focus 40, E5.

Kawata, K., Liu, C.Y., Merkel, S.F., Ramirez, S.H., Tierney, R.T., Langford, D., 2016. Blood biomarkers for brain injury: what are we measuring? Neuroscience and Biobehavioral Reviews. 68, 460-473.

Khong, E., Odenwald, N., Hashim, E., Cusimano, M.D., 2016. Diffusion tensor imaging findings in post-concussion syndrome patients after mild traumatic brain injury: a systematic review. Front Neurology 7, 156.

Khurana, V.G., Kaye, A.H., 2012. An overview of concussion in sport. Journal of Clinical Neuroscience 19, 1–11.

Levin, H.S., Diaz-Arrastia, R.R., 2015. Diagnosis, prognosis, and clinical management of mild traumatic brain injury. The Lancet Global Health 4422, 1–12.

Ling, H., Morris, H.R., Neal, J.W., Lees, A.J., Hardy, J., Holton, J.L., et al., 2017. Mixed pathologies including chronic traumatic encephalopathy account for dementia in retired association football (soccer) players. Acta Neuropathology 133, 337–352.

McCrory, P., Meeuwisse, W., Dvorak, J., Aubry, M., Bailes, J., Broglio, S., et al., 2017. Consensus statement on concussion in sport — the 5th international conference on concussion in sport held in Berlin, October 2016. British Journal of Sports Medicine 51 (11), 838–847.

Mercier, E., Boutin, A., Lauzier, F., Fergusson, D.A., Simard, J.-F., Zarychanski, R., et al., 2013. Predictive value of S-100β protein for prognosis in patients with moderate and severe traumatic brain injury: systematic review and meta-analysis. British Medical Journal 346, 1–16, f1757.

Roy, P., 2017. A blood test for concussion? Neurology 1780–1781.

Sharp, D.J., Jenkins, P.O., 2015. Concussion is confusing us all. Practical Neurology 15, 172–186.

Sharp, D.J., Beckmann, C.F., Greenwood, R., Kinnunen, K.M., Bonnelle, V., De Boissezon, X., et al., 2011. Default mode network functional and structural connectivity after traumatic brain injury. Brain 134, 2233–2247.

Siman, R., Shahim, P., Tegner, Y., Blennow, K., Zetterberg, H., Smith, D.H., 2015. Serum SNTF increases in concussed professional ice hockey players and relates to the severity of postconcussion symptoms. Journal of Neurotrauma. 32, 1294–1300

Sport concussion assessment tool, 2017. Fifth ed. British Journal of Sports Medicine 51, 851–858. Chapter .

Capítulo | 28 |

Abordagem de Alto Desempenho para Otimizar uma Pré-Temporada da Liga Principal de Futebol

David McKay

Introdução

Antes da temporada competitiva de qualquer equipe, é altamente recomendável ter um período preparatório produtivo. Essa etapa é conhecida como pré-temporada, dura geralmente de 3 a 12 semanas e prepara os jogadores, física e taticamente, para as demandas da temporada de competição. Uma variedade de aspectos não modificáveis deve ser considerada, incluindo vários jogos com tempos de resposta curtos, viagens extensas, fatores ambientais exclusivos, demandas da filosofia do treinador principal e estilo de jogo desejado. A maior parte do tempo gasto será dedicada à construção dos níveis de preparação dos jogadores além dos níveis da temporada anterior, com o ensino de conceitos táticos muito específicos no treinamento e dentro de uma progressão de jogos de pré-temporada programada.

A pré-temporada acontece quando os padrões físicos são estabelecidos e reforçados. Eles definem as expectativas para toda a temporada. É indiscutível que um dos dois maiores objetivos da equipe de desempenho, com a comissão técnica, é melhorar o atletismo específico do futebol dos jogadores. O outro é ter todos os jogadores do elenco disponíveis para seleção e prontos para disputar o primeiro jogo da temporada competitiva.

O futebol profissional está se tornando mais rápido e mais exigente fisicamente; portanto, ampliou-se a importância da pré-temporada de maneira considerável para preparar os jogadores e atender às demandas desse esporte explosivo (Bush et al., 2015). Com isso, os jogadores devem retornar ao treinamento da pré-temporada com uma base respeitável de condicionamento físico e força para reduzir o risco de lesões e maximizar as melhorias de desempenho (Gabbett et al., 2016). Portanto, a implementação de um programa individualizado fora da temporada pode otimizar a prontidão para a pré-temporada.

A seguir, é descrito como chegar, planejar e entregar uma pré-temporada ideal para se preparar para a rotina de uma temporada de futebol.

A base: fora da temporada

O período fora da temporada costuma variar de 3 a 12 semanas no futebol profissional. A implementação de um programa de baixo volume fora da temporada aumenta de modo significativo o risco de lesões ao retornar ao treinamento competitivo (Blanch e Gabbett, 2015). Por isso, é vital garantir um equilíbrio entre a recuperação passiva/ativa e o treinamento fora de temporada. A parte inicial do período fora de temporada apresenta uma oportunidade de recuperação completa e ativa (treinamento cruzado, tênis etc.) na tentativa de se recuperar física e mentalmente do desgaste da competição durante a temporada (Malone et al., 2015). Após esse período de recuperação prescrita, é implementado um programa individualizado, específico para esporte, com foco em indicadores-chave de desempenho, tais como:

1. Desenvolvimento de força/potência.
2. Volumes e intensidades de corrida.
3. Condicionamento específico do futebol.

Desenvolvimento de força/potência

Demonstrou-se que ter a quantidade adequada de força e potência aumenta a resiliência de um indivíduo às demandas competitivas do jogo e reduz a probabilidade de lesões. Além disso, pode melhorar os principais componentes físicos, como velocidade de *sprint*, altura de salto e eficiência de corrida (Suchomel et al., 2016). Pode ser desafiador desenvolver essas qualidades durante a pré-temporada e a temporada, devido às listas de jogos congestionadas e ao alto volume de sessões de treinamento em campo. Portanto, é essencial desenvolver essas qualidades dentro do programa de treinamento fora de temporada. A Tabela 28.1 oferece uma visão geral do modelo do programa fora de temporada.

O objetivo desse treinamento de força e potência é estressar os músculos e tendões para permitir que eles se adaptem em preparação para a próxima temporada. Os isquiotibiais desempenham um papel importante nos movimentos de alta velocidade, que estão se tornando mais frequentes no jogo moderno. A força excêntrica dos isquiotibiais recebe muito interesse por causa de seu efeito protetor sugerido nas lesões por distensão dos isquiotibiais (Opar et al., 2015). Um protocolo de treinamento de força excêntrico (como os exercícios nórdicos para os isquiotibiais) pode produzir dor muscular de início tardio (DMIT) significativa e, sem uma exposição progressiva, pode afetar negativamente o desempenho e aumentar o risco de lesões.

Incluir um volume maior de exercícios nórdicos para os isquiotibiais fora da temporada permitirá uma dose de manutenção eficaz mínima (Presland et al., 2018) na pré-temporada e na temporada para evitar DMIT, enquanto minimiza o risco de lesão de isquiotibiais (Bourne et al., 2016).

A Tabela 28.2 apresenta o programa de treinamento excêntrico para os isquiotibiais fora da temporada. Esse protocolo é

Parte | 2 | Aplicação Clínica

Tabela 28.1 **Programa de treinamento fora de temporada.**

Semana	Foco	Séries/repetições	Frequência
1	Introdução de força de base	3 × 8	2, parte superior do corpo 2, parte inferior do corpo
2	Força de base + introdução de carga excêntrica	3 a 4 × 5 a 6	2, parte superior do corpo 2, parte inferior do corpo
3	Força submáxima + carga excêntrica + introduzir potência	3 a 4 × 5 a 6	2, parte superior do corpo 2, parte inferior do corpo
4	Força/potência máxima + sobrecarga excêntrica	3 a 4 × 5 a 6	1, parte superior do corpo 1, parte inferior do corpo 1, corpo inteiro
5	Força/potência máxima	3 a 5 × 4 a 5	1, parte superior do corpo 1, parte inferior do corpo 1, corpo inteiro
6	Força/potência máxima (estreitamento)	3 × 4 a 5	1, parte superior do corpo 1, parte inferior do corpo 1, corpo inteiro

Tabela 28.2 **Programa excêntrico de isquiotibiais fora da temporada.**

Semana	Exercício	Séries/repetições	Andamento	Frequência
1	Ponte para glúteos com deslizamento excêntrico de isquiotibiais	3 × 5	Excêntrico de 5 segundos	2 sessões
2	Exercícios nórdicos para isquiotibiais com auxílio de faixa	3 × 4		2 sessões
3	Exercícios nórdicos para isquiotibiais com/sem auxílio de faixa	3 × 3/1 repetições (3 assistidas/ 1 não assistida)		2 sessões
4	Exercícios nórdicos para isquiotibiais com/sem auxílio de faixa	3 × 2/2 repetições (2 assistidas/ 2 não assistidas)		2 sessões
5	Exercícios nórdicos para isquiotibiais	3 × 3		2 sessões
6	Exercícios nórdicos para isquiotibiais	3 × 4		1 sessão

uma parte de um programa de fortalecimento dos isquiotibiais; para mitigar o risco de lesões também é essencial incluir exercícios unilaterais e bilaterais de quadril e isquiotibiais dominantes (Bourne et al., 2016). Outro fator importante é a exposição em corrida em alta velocidade de mais de 90% da velocidade máxima de um jogador (Malone et al., 2017).

Volumes e intensidades de corrida

Depois de um período significativo de descanso, a condição física básica do jogador acumulada ao longo do tempo por meio de uma carga de treinamento crônica será reduzida de modo considerável. Para esportes de campo predominantemente baseados na corrida, como o futebol, é vital reconstruir essa carga crônica de treinamento no período fora da temporada, a fim de aumentar a tolerância dos tecidos e a resistência cardiovascular para o início da pré-temporada (Kelly e Coutts, 2007). Isso também é feito com um plano de treinamento progressivo que aumenta os volumes e as intensidades de corrida.

O plano semanal fora de temporada é composto por duas classificações de sessões: trabalho linear e multidirecional. Ambas consistem em variáveis alternadas, incluindo volume e intensidade. Há 4 dias dentro do programa semanal: volume linear, intensidade multidirecional, intensidade linear e volume multidirecional. Os volumes e as intensidades das sessões aumentarão de modo progressivo até a última semana fora da temporada. Durante a última semana fora da temporada, os jogadores completarão apenas três sessões na tentativa de diminuir o ritmo para a primeira semana de treinamento da pré-temporada.

A manipulação de intensidades e volumes pode ser realizada de várias maneiras. Algumas variáveis modificáveis comuns incluem distância total percorrida, distância percorrida em altas velocidades, porcentagem de velocidade máxima alcançada, quantidade de acelerações e desacelerações e quantidade de mudanças controladas e aleatórias na direção (Russell et al., 2016). É vital monitorar e progredir nas exposições de corrida de alta velocidade variando de 60% a mais de 90% da velocidade máxima de um indivíduo, pois parece estressar significativamente a musculatura da cadeia posterior e mitigar o risco de lesões (Malone et al., 2017). Portanto, é recomendado alcançar

Abordagem de Alto Desempenho para Otimizar uma Pré-Temporada da Liga Principal de Futebol **Capítulo | 28 |**

essas velocidades desde o início do período fora da temporada, com as exposições à velocidade máxima ocorrendo nas últimas 1 a 2 semanas em preparação para o início da pré-temporada. A inclusão da corrida de alta velocidade é sobretudo importante para os atletas que participarão dos testes de velocidade ao chegarem à concentração da pré-temporada. Expor os jogadores a altas velocidades antes da pré-temporada permite à equipe técnica mais liberdade para planejar as sessões de treinamento no que diz respeito ao tamanho das áreas de jogo.

Condicionamento específico do futebol

A última parte do programa fora de temporada é a integração do treinamento específico do futebol, que muitas vezes é negligenciado, pois não está diretamente sob o escopo de prática da equipe de desempenho. Isso pode ser alcançado por meio da colaboração com a equipe técnica. Ao integrar o trabalho específico do futebol com o trabalho físico, os jogadores podem realizar o desenvolvimento técnico e físico. Por exemplo, um jogador de campo pode trabalhar nos aspectos técnicos do cruzamento de uma bola, seguido por uma corrida de recuperação de alta intensidade no dia de corrida de qualidade linear. Da mesma maneira, esse mesmo jogador de campo poderia trabalhar nos aspectos técnicos de defesa em uma situação 1 contra 1 no dia de quantidade multidirecional. O condicionamento específico do futebol não apenas refina a técnica, como também expõe progressivamente um jogador a demandas técnicas de "alto risco", como chutar a bola, o que pode aumentar o risco de lesão se sobrecarregado incorretamente (Charnock et al., 2009). Essas sessões também expõem os atletas a padrões de movimento, processos cognitivos, calçados e superfícies de solo específicos aos quais eles serão expostos durante o treinamento da pré-temporada.

O Boxe 28.1 descreve as estratégias utilizadas para conectar os três componentes fora da temporada.

A estrutura: pré-temporada

Os principais objetivos da nossa equipe de alto desempenho no treinamento de pré-temporada são os seguintes:
1. Avaliar o estado de preparação inicial dos jogadores na chegada.
2. Trabalhar em colaboração com a equipe técnica para planejar, progredir e monitorar as cargas de treinamento para melhorar os níveis de preparação física do time.
3. Desenvolver força/potência.

Testagem

Nossa bateria de teste é dividida em três fases. A fase 1 começa antes da primeira sessão de treinamento. Um exame físico e sanguíneo completo é administrado pelos médicos da equipe, além do teste de composição corporal de sete dobras cutâneas realizado por um nutricionista especializado. O objetivo do exame físico completo é garantir que nenhum problema tenha ocorrido fora da temporada e que todas as novas contratações tenham permissão médica para treinar sem restrições. As principais áreas de enfoque em relação ao painel de sangue são os níveis de vitamina D e ferro. Os achados desse teste permitem que o nutricionista de alto desempenho prescreva suplementação e planos dietéticos individualizados. Os resultados da composição corporal são um dos nossos padrões de profissionalismo físico. Todos os jogadores de linha devem retornar ao início da pré-temporada com 10% de gordura corporal ou menos e os goleiros com 13% de gordura

---

Boxe 28.1 Estratégias para conectar os componentes do treinamento fora de temporada

- As sessões sempre começam com uma preparação geral (aquecimento) específico para as demandas futuras
- O condicionamento em campo e o treinamento específico do futebol precedem as sessões de força/potência da parte inferior do corpo para minimizar o risco de lesões
- Os dias de corrida linear são combinados com sessões de força/potência da parte inferior do corpo para manter as tensões da cadeia posterior no mesmo dia para minimizar o acúmulo de fadiga ao longo da semana
- 1 ou 2 dias de folga após os dias com foco na corrida linear e força/potência da parte inferior do corpo
- Os primeiros dias de volta à academia após 1 dia de folga consistem em força da parte superior do corpo e trabalho de potência.

---

corporal ou menos (esses padrões estão na extremidade superior e podem variar em diferentes níveis de jogo). Caso esses padrões não sejam atendidos, os jogadores em questão terão sessões de treinamento adicionais e intervenções nutricionais para melhorar sua composição corporal.

A fase 2 é baseada em ginástica e mede a força/potência dos membros inferiores, resistência e assimetrias. É prescrito um protocolo de teste muscular isocinético na máquina Biodex e um teste de uma repetição no Nordbord para cada jogador. Consideramos um desequilíbrio de 15% ou mais para colocar um jogador em risco maior de lesão e ele será obrigado a realizar trabalho de força adicional dentro do seu programa de força/potência (van Dyk et al., 2016). Em referência ao Nordbord, uma pontuação de 337 N ou abaixo indica baixa força excêntrica dos flexores do joelho e esses jogadores requerem trabalho de força adicional em suas sessões semanais (Timmins et al., 2015).

A fase 3 e última fase de nossa bateria de testes ocorre na primeira semana da pré-temporada e é composta de testes de desempenho em campo. Esses testes são projetados para se concentrar na recuperação da frequência cardíaca, capacidade aeróbica máxima e velocidade linear máxima. Nosso primeiro dia de volta ao treinamento envolve um aquecimento genérico seguido por 4 minutos do teste de recuperação intermitente yoyo nível 2 (submáx yoyo) seguido por 3 minutos de repouso. O objetivo desse teste é alcançar aproximadamente 80 a 85% da frequência cardíaca máxima de um jogador e, em seguida, avaliar o quão bem eles podem se recuperar no período subsequente de 3 minutos. Foi demonstrado que a recuperação da frequência cardíaca (eficiência) está correlacionado ao *status* da aptidão aeróbica do jogador e, portanto, quantifica a condição aeróbica na qual os jogadores retornam ao treinamento (Veugelers et al., 2016). Em nosso segundo dia de treinamento, os jogadores realizam um aquecimento genérico com um foco maior na mudança de direção e nos movimentos de corte. O teste de *endurance* de yoyo nível 2 é utilizado para avaliar tanto a capacidade aeróbica ($\dot{V}O_{2máx}$) quanto a frequência cardíaca máxima. Um objetivo secundário desse teste de campo máximo é criar um ambiente competitivo entre os indivíduos. Nossos padrões para esse teste são os seguintes (goleiros não participam):
- Nível 14,9 e acima: apto para treinar sem restrição
- Nível 13,6 a 14,8: apto para treinar, mas será necessário completar o treinamento de condicionamento físico adicional
- Nível 13,5 e abaixo: não apto para treinar e será necessário treinar separadamente da equipe até que as melhorias necessárias sejam feitas.

O teste final dessa fase, velocidade linear máxima, ocorre no final da primeira semana da pré-temporada. Nesse dia, o

301

aquecimento contém várias atividades de preparação de velocidade linear. Por exemplo, variações de marcha, pulos e salto com mudança de direção progredindo para exercícios preso a um parceiro – marcha/salto/corrida resistidos seguidos por repetições de aceleração e terminando com "acúmulos" de 18/27/36/45 metros em intensidades crescentes. Após um descanso completo (> 3 minutos), os jogadores são obrigados a realizar duas corridas cumulativas de 45 metros terminando em 100% de intensidade.

As corridas cumulativas consistem em:

- 0 a 7 metros a 50% da velocidade máxima
- 7 a 18 metros a 50 a 80% da velocidade máxima
- 18 a 45 metros a 80 a 100% da velocidade máxima.

Os resultados desse teste são capturados com nosso sistema de posicionamento global (GPS, do inglês *global positioning system*) e apresentados em metros por segundo ($m.s^{-1}$). Esse teste captura as velocidades máximas do jogador para monitorar suas exposições semanais de alta velocidade e velocidade de *sprint* ao longo da temporada. O momento do teste é muito importante, pois expor os jogadores à velocidade máxima nos primeiros dias pode colocá-los em maior risco de lesão (Higashihara et al., 2018). Essa é uma preocupação específica para novas contratações que podem não ter concluído nosso programa fora da temporada e chegar no dia 1 despreparados. Portanto, programamos esse teste para o final da primeira semana de treinamento, o que permite que os jogadores sejam expostos gradualmente a velocidades crescentes dentro das sessões de treinamento.

No início da pré-temporada, esses testes ajudam a traçar um quadro do estado físico do time. A próxima etapa é testar novamente durante a pré-temporada e a temporada para quantificar a melhoria. A Tabela 28.3 descreve nossa abordagem para retestar.

Planejando e progredindo cargas de treinamento

Transição da fase fora da temporada para a pré-temporada

Um dos principais objetivos da equipe de desempenho, com a comissão técnica, é ter todos os jogadores de uma equipe disponíveis e prontos para a seleção e para o primeiro jogo da temporada competitiva. Para atingir a disponibilidade máxima, deve haver um plano seguro e progressivo em vigor, enquanto também sobrecarrega os jogadores para melhorar sua capacidade física. Porém, fazer isso muito rápido ou de maneira agressiva pode ser prejudicial para o time. A carga de treinamento a que todos os jogadores foram expostos durante a fase fora da temporada deve ser entendida e utilizada para evitar grandes picos de volume e/ou intensidade (Hulin et al., 2013) para minimizar o risco de lesões durante a pré-temporada.

A Tabela 28.4 mostra um exemplo de como construímos as cargas de treinamento semanais (agudas) dos jogadores fora da temporada a partir de um ponto de vista de volume (distância total percorrida em quilômetros) e intensidade (distância de corrida de alta velocidade coberta em metros) (Blanch e Gabbett, 2015; Bowen et al., 2016). Observe que utilizamos duas métricas para simplificar o processo de prescrição e monitoramento.

Uma vez definida uma distância inicial, nesse caso 16 km de distância total percorrida e 700 m de corrida em alta velocidade, é recomendado ficar abaixo de um aumento de 15% na carga ao progredir na semana seguinte (Blanch e Gabbett, 2015; Gabbett, 2016). Portanto, a prioridade fora da temporada é avançar de modo suave para a pré-temporada. Por exemplo, se a meta da primeira semana da pré-temporada é atingir 35 km de distância total, então a meta da última semana fora da temporada é cobrir aproximadamente 30 a 32 km (ou 10 a 15% de 35 km). É importante notar que esse aumento de 10 a 15% na carga de treinamento serve como um guia e não uma regra rígida. Ao usar essa faixa de porcentagem como um guia, é importante considerar a conformidade de cada indivíduo durante a fase fora da temporada. Devido a uma série de fatores, como acesso às instalações, condições climáticas e compromissos pessoais, a carga alcançada pode variar dentro de uma equipe. Portanto, a bateria de testes fornece uma visão importante da condição física do time no dia 1 da pré-temporada.

Pré-temporada: planejamento do quadro geral

A pré-temporada é dividida em três fases principais e começa com uma fase de sobrecarga de treinamento, que consiste nas semanas 1, 2 e 3. A fase 2 é classificada como a fase de sobrecarga

Tabela 28.3 **Abordagem para retestar a aptidão física.**

Protocolo de teste	Frequência	Observações
Composição do corpo	A cada 4 a 6 semanas no mesmo dia da semana, ao mesmo tempo	
Trabalho sanguíneo	Pré-temporada/meio da temporada	
Biodex		Apenas retestado dentro de um protocolo de retorno ao jogo para um jogador lesionado
Nordbord	Semanal ou quinzenalmente em nossas sessões de treinamento de força/potência da parte inferior do corpo	
Teste yoyo Submáx	A cada 4 a 6 semanas no multidirecional + 3 dentro do aquecimento	
Yoyo TEN2	Apenas retestado dentro de um protocolo de retorno ao jogo para um jogador lesionado	
Velocidade máxima linear	Rastreado semanalmente ao longo da temporada para novas velocidades máximas, mas não retestado	

TEN2, teste de *endurance* yoyo nível 2.

Abordagem de Alto Desempenho para Otimizar uma Pré-Temporada da Liga Principal de Futebol — Capítulo 28

Tabela 28.4 Exemplo de construção de cargas de treinamento semanais dos jogadores fora da temporada.

Semana	Distância total (km)	Corrida total de alta velocidade (m)
1	16 km	700 m
2	18 km	800 m
3	20 km	950 m
4	23 km	1.100 m
5	25 km	1.300 m
6	30 km	1.500 m

do jogo e ocorre durante as semanas 4 e 5. As fases 1 e 2 são seguidas pela fase 3, uma fase de subcarga ou redução gradual de 1 semana.

Fase 1: fase de sobrecarga de treinamento

A fase 1 visa sobrecarregar os jogadores fisicamente por meio de sessões de treinamento técnico e físico. As cargas de treinamento-alvo são determinadas a partir do plano fora da temporada, embora o objetivo seja atingir cargas semanais excessivas da semana média da temporada (25 a 30 km) para gerar adaptações de treinamento e aumentar a tolerância de carga. A semana 1 é utilizada para sobrecarregar os jogadores sem especificar uma qualidade física. Limitamos as oportunidades de obter corridas em alta velocidade e podemos esperar quantidades moderadas de acelerações e desacelerações com equipes moderadas (5 contra 5 a 7 contra 7) e dimensões de jogo de tamanho moderado (29 metros de largura × 36 metros de comprimento a 45 metros de largura × 54 metros de comprimento). Durante esta semana, os esforços de corrida de alta velocidade são controlados em exercícios de corrida separados das sessões específicas de futebol (p. ex., uma corrida entre as duas grandes áreas em 12 segundos seguida por 24 segundos de recuperação ativa para 2 séries de 6 repetições). A parte final da semana 1 é um amistoso de 30 minutos (2 × 15 minutos) para aumentar a tolerância ao jogo. Durante as semanas 2 e 3, sobrecarregamos os jogadores por meio de sessões técnicas e táticas com a ênfase na alternância entre carregamento multidirecional e de velocidade com sessões de recuperação. O carregamento multidirecional é obtido por meio de uma grande quantidade de acelerações e desacelerações com mudanças multiplanares de direção. A maioria é obtida em treinos utilizando equipes 1 contra 1 a 5 contra 5 em uma área de jogo pequena a moderada (13 metros de largura × 18 metros de comprimento a 29 metros de largura × 36 metros de comprimento). Durante as sessões de carga multidirecional, o quadríceps, os adutores e os glúteos são os grupos musculares predominantemente estressados. A comissão técnica pode utilizar esses exercícios para introduzir temas táticos como pressão, organização defensiva e transições em ritmo acelerado. O carregamento de velocidade é então alcançado por meio da exposição a altas velocidades lineares (> 5,5 m.s^{-1}) para volumes moderados (400 a 600 m) e velocidades de *sprint* (> 7 m.s^{-1}) para volumes baixos (100 a 200 m). Eles ocorrem durante jogos de equipe de 9 contra 9 a 11 contra 11 usando grandes áreas (68 metros de largura × 77 metros de comprimento a 68 metros de largura × 109 metros de comprimento). A comissão técnica pode utilizar esses exercícios para introduzir estilos táticos, como contra-ataques

e recuperação defensiva. Durante as sessões de carga de velocidade, os isquiotibiais são o grupo de músculos predominantemente estressados. A semana 2 termina com o primeiro amistoso em que todos os jogadores jogam por 45 minutos. A semana 3 termina com um amistoso de 60 minutos.

Fase 2: fase de sobrecarga do jogo

A fase 2 envolve sobrecarregar os jogadores por meio de partidas competitivas, em vez de sessões de treinamento tático. No entanto, o volume total da distância diminui em até 20%. Essa fase é a mais exigente de toda a pré-temporada. A semana 4 consiste em duas exposições de jogo de 75 minutos separadas por um tempo de intervalo de 3 dias. Os dias anteriores e posteriores aos jogos consistem em sessões de treinamento baseadas em recuperação e envolvem exercícios táticos de baixa intensidade. Essa programação expõe os jogadores a vários jogos com intervalos curtos entre eles. A semana 5 envolve 1 semana de treinamento tático com um amistoso de 90 minutos em preparação para a temporada competitiva. O objetivo é reduzir a carga da semana 4 em 5% para a semana 5.

Fase 3: subcarga ou fase de redução

A fase final é uma fase de subcarga. A semana 6 é a última semana de treinamento que leva ao primeiro jogo competitivo da temporada. O objetivo é reduzir a carga de treinamento em 10% da semana 5. Isso é conseguido por meio da redução dos tempos de treinamento e da limitação de sessões adicionais. Se feito corretamente, os jogadores serão física e mentalmente revigorados antes do importantíssimo primeiro jogo da temporada.

Progressão do jogo dentro do planejamento de "visão geral"

Ter todos os jogadores física, mental e taticamente preparados para o primeiro jogo da temporada competitiva exige que eles sejam expostos a vários jogos na pré-temporada. Os jogos de pré-temporada fornecem intensidades, ambientes competitivos e pressões que são impossíveis de replicar apenas com o treinamento. A quantidade de jogos disputados normalmente dependerá da duração da pré-temporada, mas como nossa pré-temporada dura 6 semanas, as equipes jogam de 4 a 6 jogos no geral. Nossos jogos de pré-temporada são progredidos pelo número de minutos jogados e o objetivo é atingir cerca de 375 minutos de futebol competitivo por jogador por meio de um modelo de progressão de 30/45/60/75/75/90 minutos. Nossa progressão de minutos de jogo da pré-temporada tem como objetivo aumentar de modo gradual a tolerância às demandas do jogo competitivo. Para que cada jogador consiga uma exposição igual aos minutos de jogo disputados, a equipe técnica deve ser criativa com sua programação. Programamos o primeiro jogo como um jogo intratime composto frequentemente por períodos de 2 ou 3 × 15 minutos (dependendo da quantidade) e garantimos que todos os jogadores tenham 30 minutos de tempo de jogo. Após o jogo intratime, um jogo regular de 90 minutos é agendado e o time compõe duas formações diferentes de 11 jogadores para cada período de 45 minutos. Para as exposições de 60 e 75 minutos, implementamos dois arranjos distintos no mesmo dia. Uma equipe utiliza os 11 jogadores iniciais planejados para a equipe titular. A outra equipe é composta por jogadores reservas. O jogo final é um jogo de 90 minutos. Esse jogo é agendado 1 semana

Parte | 2 | Aplicação Clínica

antes do início da temporada e ocorre normalmente em um estádio. Com isso em mente, um outro jogo com os reservas é organizado no dia seguinte para garantir que os jogadores reservas acumulem o tempo de jogo relevante.

Monitoramento

É vital a implementação de um sistema de monitoramento objetivo e subjetivo de qualidade para maximizar a eficiência do planejamento e manipulação das cargas de treinamento. Nossa equipe de desempenho utiliza GPS em tempo real para cada sessão de jogo para quantificar o volume e a intensidade de exercícios e sessões individuais. A partir do *feedback* do GPS ao vivo, é possível adicionar ou reduzir a carga de treinamento para atingir as metas diárias e semanais. As principais métricas que priorizamos durante a pré-temporada são: distância total, distância de corrida de alta velocidade (CAV) (55 a 70% da velocidade máxima), distância de *sprint* (DS) (> 70% da velocidade máxima), velocidade máxima (m.s^{-1}) e total combinado de acelerações e desacelerações (quantidade de esforços > 3 m.s^{-2}).

A distância total é um medidor do volume absoluto ao qual um jogador é exposto. A distância total quando dividida pela duração da sessão também pode ser utilizada para exibir metros por minuto (m min^{-1}) e é um medidor da intensidade do exercício ou da sessão. Metros por minuto podem mostrar diferenças posicionais em certos exercícios, que podem então ser considerados para planejamento futuro.

As seguintes métricas são utilizadas para monitorar o carregamento de velocidade. CAV, DS e velocidade de pico são medidos em metros por segundo. CAV pode ser individualizada por meio da obtenção de > 55% da velocidade máxima de um indivíduo (alcançada durante o teste) ou um valor absoluto de > 5,5 m.s^{-1} mantido por pelo menos 1 segundo. A DS é então classificada como > 70% da velocidade máxima de um indivíduo ou um valor absoluto de > 7 m.s^{-1} mantido por pelo menos 1 segundo. A distâncias de CAV e de *sprint* são exibidas como um acúmulo de distância dentro de um exercício ou sessão. As métricas de velocidade são monitoradas para garantir que os jogadores sejam expostos de modo progressivo a volumes maiores, sem criar um pico desnecessário. As métricas de velocidade também podem ser utilizadas para identificar jogadores com carga insuficiente, o que se mostrou associado ao aumento do risco de lesões (Hulin et al., 2015; Hulin et al., 2016).

Monitoramos de perto as medidas de intensidade, incluindo velocidades relativas de corrida, para garantir que nossos jogadores atinjam > 90% de sua velocidade máxima em dias de carregamento de velocidade. É vital que os jogadores sejam expostos a > 90% de sua velocidade máxima em um período de 7 a 10 dias. A velocidade de pico também é monitorada para garantir que não ocorra superexposição (Malone et al., 2017).

A métrica final que requer atenção avalia o carregamento multidirecional e é a quantidade total de acelerações e desacelerações (m.s^{-2}) executadas. É importante monitorar as métricas de carregamento multidirecional para evitar a monotonia do treinamento e possíveis problemas de uso excessivo. O objetivo é diminuir as exposições de ações de alta aceleração e desaceleração (m.s^{-2}) nos 2 dias anteriores ao dia do jogo, devido ao estresse biomecânico do movimento (Higashihara et al., 2018; Varley e Aughey, 2013).

Como uma equipe de desempenho, as métricas mencionadas anteriormente são monitoradas em uma base diária, semanal e rotativa de 4 semanas. É utilizado o modelo de carga de trabalho aguda:crônica para criar uma imagem das cargas físicas externas aplicadas nos jogadores individuais (Hulin et al., 2013; Hulin et al., 2015). O modelo de carga de trabalho aguda:crônica é utilizado como um guia objetivo para monitorar potenciais picos ou quedas na carga de treinamento, pois ambos têm uma associação com risco aumentado de lesão (Gabbett et al., 2016). A principal limitação do uso da razão agudo:crônico é o intervalo de tempo necessário para desenvolver o denominador, tornando a razão inválida durante o primeiro mês da pré-temporada.

Para garantir que as prescrições de treinamento estejam alinhadas com o quadro geral da pré-temporada, é essencial receber informações subjetivas dos jogadores sobre a preparação física antes do treinamento e a taxa de esforço percebido (TEP) após o treinamento (Borg, 1970; Hooper et al., 1995).

Na manhã de cada dia de treinamento, os jogadores avaliam a qualidade do sono, dores musculares e fadiga geral em uma escala de 1 a 5 (Hooper et al., 1995). Essa informação subjetiva fornece à equipe de desempenho uma visão de como eles responderam à sessão anterior. Elas também podem atuar como um sistema de alerta para destacar quaisquer respostas inesperadas que possam exigir atenção adicional. Além disso, pode permitir pequenos ajustes em uma sessão, como implementar um jogador extra na equipe sem responsabilidade defensiva, o que limitará sua carga de treinamento. Além dessas três áreas de investigação, obtemos *feedback* subjetivo da equipe em uma escala de TEP de 1 a 10 após cada sessão de treinamento (Borg, 1970). O *feedback* do jogador nos permite avaliar o sucesso de nossa prescrição de treinamento e pode ser utilizado para mostrar como os jogadores estão respondendo às prescrições de intensidade de treinamento. Ambos os métodos de receber *feedback* do jogador requerem uma compreensão das escalas aplicadas e honestidade dos jogadores para garantir que eles não exagerem ou diluam as informações que nós, como equipe de desempenho, exigimos para um monitoramento eficiente.

Conforme mencionado anteriormente, também utilizamos monitores de frequência cardíaca para testar o *status* de recuperação da frequência cardíaca a cada 4 a 6 semanas. O rastreamento diário da frequência cardíaca pode ser utilizado para quantificar a resposta interna ao treinamento. Monitorar as respostas da frequência cardíaca é importante para entender as demandas que diferentes atividades impõem aos jogadores. Conhecer as demandas específicas que diferentes atividades colocam nos jogadores é vital no planejamento geral e na progressão de uma pré-temporada.

Desenvolvimento de força/potência

Durante o período fora da temporada, um jogador sobrecarrega suas qualidades de força e potência, o que deve ser continuado na pré-temporada, pois essas qualidades são fundamentais para aspectos-chave de desempenho no futebol e na mitigação do risco de lesões (Stølen et al., 2005). O planejamento de sessões de força/potência pode ser difícil, devido ao grande volume de sessões táticas e jogadores disponíveis. As sessões de força/potência são agendadas para 1 dia antes de uma recuperação ou dia de folga para permitir uma recuperação adicional antes da próxima sessão em campo. Sessões de força/potência não são agendadas dentro de 72 horas de um jogo competitivo, pois podem induzir níveis prejudiciais de fadiga. Nos estágios iniciais da pré-temporada, muitas vezes implementamos sessões de força/potência imediatamente após as exposições de jogo de 30 e 45 minutos, pois esses jogos ocorrem geralmente antes de 1 dia de descanso/recuperação. As sessões de força/potência ocorrem sobretudo na academia; no entanto, às vezes os conduzimos em campo quando as instalações e as circunstâncias permitem.

Para garantir a carga adequada de trabalho de força/potência, muitas vezes dividimos o time em três grupos. O primeiro grupo consiste nos jogadores que completaram o programa de fora da temporada, aumentando a probabilidade de sustentar uma base de força suficiente. O segundo grupo consiste naqueles que podem não ter completado o plano fora de temporada completo, mas têm mais de 5 anos de experiência em treinamento de força/potência. Finalmente, o terceiro grupo consiste em novas contratações que também não completaram um cronograma de treinamento fora de temporada e têm menos de 5 anos de experiência em treinamento de força/potência. O conteúdo de cada grupo muda ligeiramente para aplicar os exercícios apropriados. As repetições e séries também são prescritas dependendo dos objetivos do grupo e das sessões. A Tabela 28.5 demonstra como agrupamos uma sessão básica de força/potência da parte inferior do corpo para o time.

Também há oportunidades nas sessões de treinamento em campo para treinar qualidades de força ou potência. Em dias de treinamento apropriados, a implementação de uma minissessão de potência (microdosagem) dentro do aquecimento pode fornecer a oportunidade perfeita para desenvolver qualidades explosivas por meio do uso de variações de salto com obstáculos e saltos horizontais. O foco nessas minissessões de potência não está no volume, mas sim na intensidade e na taxa de desenvolvimento de força. Esses tipos de exercícios de potência não são utilizados apenas em aquecimentos, mas também em treinos competitivos, como 1 contra 1 ou 2 contra 2. Por exemplo, um exercício começa com uma quantidade especificada de saltos com barreiras seguidos por uma corrida rápida para a bola, que o técnico joga da linha lateral, seguido por um ataque à baliza. Outra oportunidade de fazer sessões de força ou potência em campo surge quando os jogadores são divididos em três equipes dentro da sessão. Nesse cenário, duas equipes estão jogando jogos com campo reduzido (JCR) enquanto a outra equipe está descansando. A equipe que está descansando pode usar o tempo livre para uma minissessão de força ou potência. Essa minissessão de força e potência pode incluir exercícios de peso corporal ou força com carga, variações de salto, arremessos de *medicine ball* e arrastões de trenó com pesos.

Resumo

A pré-temporada de uma equipe é utilizada para construir uma plataforma física sólida que leva à temporada competitiva. Essa plataforma física não começa somente quando os jogadores voltam aos treinos. Um plano deve estar em vigor desde o último dia da temporada anterior. Esse plano é específico fora de temporada que se concentra sobretudo na recuperação antes de sobrecarregar as qualidades de força e potência e aumentar de modo progressivo a distância e a intensidade da corrida. Esses volumes e intensidades de corrida devem garantir uma base de exposições à CAV antes do retorno dos jogadores ao treinamento, mitigando o risco de lesões associadas a grandes picos na carga de treinamento. A pré-temporada deve, então, continuar a construir tolerância progressivamente às demandas do treinamento de futebol e partidas competitivas. Por meio de um planejamento cuidadoso, o desempenho e a equipe técnica podem fornecer janelas de oportunidade para sessões de desenvolvimento tático, de força, potência, aeróbico e anaeróbico, além de equipes competitivas e uma boa recuperação. O monitoramento contínuo durante a pré-temporada permite que ajustes sejam feitos para minimizar picos ou quedas desnecessárias na carga de treinamento. A pré-temporada determinará a robustez do time, e pode ser vital para estabelecer padrões físicos a serem mantidos ao longo da temporada.

Tabela 28.5 **Sessão de força/potência básica da parte inferior do corpo.**

Bloco	Exercício	Séries/repetições
Grupo 1	**Foco: força máxima/potência reativa**	
A1	Levantamento terra com barra sextavada	3 × 5
A2	Salto em profundidade	3 × 3
B1	Exercícios nórdicos para isquiotibial inferior	3 × 3
B2	Exercício de resistência total antiextensão do core	3 × 8
Grupo 2	**Foco: força/potência de base**	
A1	Levantamento terra com *kettlebell*	3 × 6
A2	Salto de contramovimento	3 × 4
B1	Exercícios nórdicos para isquiotibiais	3 × 2/2
B2	Exercício de resistência total antiextensão do core (ajoelhado)	3 × 8
Grupo 3	**Foco: fundamentos de força de base/desenvolvimento de potência**	
A1	Padrão de *hip hinge* com o peso corporal	3 × 8 a 10
A2	Salto sem contramovimento	3 × 5
B1	Slide excêntrico de isquiotibiais (5 segundos excêntrico)	3 × 5
B2	Posição de prancha abdominal frontal	3 × 8 a 10

Referências bibliográficas

Blanch, P., Gabbett, T.J., 2015. Has the athlete trained enough to return to play safely? The acute: chronic workload ratio permits clinicians to quantify a player's risk of subsequent injury. British Journal of Sports Medicine 50 (8), 471-475.

Borg, G., 1970. Perceived exertion as an indicator of somatic stress. Scandinavian Journal of Rehabilitation Medicine 2, 92-98.

Bourne, M.N., Duhig, S.J., Timmins, R.G., Williams, M.D., Opar, D.A., Al Najjar, A., et al., 2016. Impact of the Nordic hamstring and hip extension exercises on hamstring architecture and morphology: implications for injury prevention. British Journal of Sports Medicine 51 (5), 469-477.

Bowen, L., Gross, A.S., Gimpel, M., Li, F.-X., 2016. Accumulated workloads and the acute: chronic workload ratio relate to injury risk in elite youth football players. British Journal of Sports Medicine 51 (5), 452-459.

Bush, M., Barnes, C., Archer, D.T., Hogg, B., Bradley, P.S., 2015. Evolution of match performance parameters for various playing positions in the English Premier League. Human Movement Science 39, 1-11.

Charnock, B.L., Lewis, C.L., Garrett Jr., W.E., Queen, R.M., 2009. Adductor longus mechanics during the maximal effort soccer kick. Sports Biomechanics 8, 223-234.

Gabbett, T.J., Hulin, B.T., Blanch, P., Whiteley, R., 2016. High training workloads alone do not cause sports injuries: how you get there is the real issue. British Journal of Sports Medicine 50 (8), 444-445.

Gabbett, T.J., 2016. The training-injury prevention paradox: should athletes be training smarter and harder? British Journal of Sports Medicine 50 (5), 273-280.

Higashihara, A., Nagano, Y., Ono, T., Fukubayashi, T., 2018. Differences in hamstring activation characteristics between the acceleration and maximum-speed phases of sprinting. Journal of Sports Sciences 36, 1313-1318.

Hooper, S.L., Mackinnon, L.T., Howard, A., Gordon, R.D., Bachmann, A.W., 1995. Markers for monitoring overtraining and recovery. Medicine & Science in Sports & Exercise 27, 106.

Hulin, B.T., Gabbett, T.J., Blanch, P., Chapman, P., Bailey, D., Orchard, J.W., 2013. Spikes in acute workload are associated with increased injury risk in elite cricket fast bowlers. British Journal of Sports Medicine 48 (8), 708-712.

Hulin, B.T., Gabbett, T.J., Caputi, P., Lawson, D.W., Sampson, J.A., 2016. Low chronic workload and the acute: chronic workload ratio are more predictive of injury than between-match recovery time: a two-season prospective cohort study in elite rugby league players. British Journal of Sports Medicine 50 (16), 1008-1012.

Hulin, B.T., Gabbett, T.J., Lawson, D.W., Caputi, P., Sampson, J.A., 2015. The acute: chronic workload ratio predicts injury: high chronic worklo-ad may decrease injury risk in elite rugby league players. British Journal of Sports Medicine 50 (4), 231-236.

Kelly, V.G., Coutts, A.J., 2007. Planning and monitoring training loads during the competition phase in team sports. Strength and Conditioning Journal 29, 32.

Malone, J.J., Di Michele, R., Morgans, R., Burgess, D., Morton, J.P., Drust, B., 2015. Seasonal training-load quantification in elite English premier league soccer players. International Journal of Sports Physiology and Performance 10, 489-497.

Malone, S., Roe, M., Doran, D.A., Gabbett, T.J., Collins, K., 2017. High chronic training loads and exposure to bouts of maximal velocity running reduce injury risk in elite Gaelic football. Journal of Science and Medicine in Sport 20, 250-254.

Opar, A.D., Williams, D.M., Timmins, G.R., Hickey, J.J., Duhig, J.S., Shield, J.A., 2015. Eccentric hamstring strength and hamstring injury risk in Australian Footballers. Medicine & Science in Sports & Exercise 47, 857-865.

Presland, J.D., Timmins, R.G., Bourne, M.N., Williams, M.D., Opar, D.A., 2018. The effect of Nordic hamstring exercise training volume on biceps femoris long head architectural adaptation. Scandinavian Journal of Medicine & Science in Sports.

Russell, M., Sparkes, W., Northeast, J., Cook, C.J., Love, T.D., Bracken, R.M., et al., 2016. Changes in acceleration and deceleration capacity throughout professional soccer match-play. The Journal of Strength & Conditioning Research 30, 2839-2844.

Stølen, T., Chamari, K., Castagna, C., Wisløff, U., 2005. Physiology of soccer. Sports Medicine 35, 501-536.

Suchomel, T.J., Nimphius, S., Stone, M.H., 2016. The importance of muscular strength in athletic performance. Sports Medicine 46, 1419-1449.

Timmins, R.G., Bourne, M.N., Shield, A.J., Williams, M.D., Lorenzen, C., Opar, D.A., 2015. Short biceps femoris fascicles and eccentric knee flexor weakness increase the risk of hamstring injury in elite football (soccer): a prospective cohort study. British Journal of Sports Medicine 50 (24), 1524-1535.

van Dyk, N., Bahr, R., Whiteley, R., Tol, J.L., Kumar, B.D., Hamilton, B., et al., 2016. Hamstring and quadriceps isokinetic strength deficits are weak risk factors for hamstring strain injuries: a 4-year cohort study. The American Journal of Sports Medicine 44, 1789-1795.

Varley, M.C., Aughey, R.J., 2013. Acceleration profiles in elite Australian soccer. International Journal of Sports Medicine 34, 34-39.

Veugelers, K.R., Naughton, G.A., Duncan, C.S., Burgess, D.J., Graham, S.R., 2016. Validity and reliability of a submaximal intermittent running test in elite Australian football players. The Journal of Strength & Conditioning Research 30, 3347-3353.

Capítulo | 29 |

Introdução ao Trabalho em uma Academia de Futebol de Elite

Diane Ryding

Introdução

Este capítulo apresenta conceitos gerais sobre como trabalhar com o atleta em desenvolvimento em uma academia de futebol de elite. A abordagem centrada no atleta e o trabalho multidisciplinar são apresentados junto com aspectos próprios do trabalho com crianças, sobretudo aqueles ligados ao crescimento e à maturação. Muitos fisioterapeutas iniciam suas carreiras esportivas trabalhando com equipes de jovens ou academias; existem diferenças inerentes às práticas de trabalho com crianças e adolescentes em comparação com os adultos.

Equipe multiprofissional e abordagem centrada no atleta

As academias de futebol empregam equipes de várias profissões para se envolver no desenvolvimento do futebolista juvenil (Figura 29.1), com o objetivo final de produzir jogadores que estejam em um nível de desempenho para a equipe profissional desse clube.

Uma academia de futebol moderna adota uma abordagem centrada no atleta, na qual as necessidades de desenvolvimento do jogador são a principal preocupação e há uma conduta colaborativa e multidisciplinar para desenvolvê-lo. Ao trabalhar com o atleta jovem, o responsável também é um membro importante dessa equipe. A abordagem centrada no atleta capacita o jogador a se engajar em seu próprio desenvolvimento e o encoraja a se responsabilizar pela sua jornada de desenvolvimento. Ele tem oportunidades de autoavaliação, reflexão e definição de metas. A equipe multiprofissional facilita ao jogador o desenvolvimento de habilidades de resolução de problemas e tomada de decisões, que visa aprimorar seu desempenho individual e o da equipe. Em última análise, a abordagem centrada no atleta envolve planejamento a longo prazo, mesmo que isso signifique aceitar contratempos a curto prazo (Kidman et al., 2010).

O papel da equipe multiprofissional é apoiar a evolução das necessidades do jogador em cada estágio do seu desenvolvimento e ajudá-lo a alcançar seu potencial máximo, embora, em última análise, esse "potencial" varie entre os jogadores. Durante as reuniões regulares dessa equipe, as áreas para melhora e enriquecimento do jogador serão identificadas, as intervenções são planejadas, as metas e um cronograma para reavaliação serão documentados. A equipe multiprofissional seleciona os membros mais adequados para trabalhar com o jogador, já que nem todas as profissões são exigidas em todas as fases do processo de desenvolvimento. É importante que qualquer discussão de natureza sensível ou confidencial ocorra apenas com a presença das pessoas apropriadas; o sigilo médico ainda se aplica em um ambiente esportivo.

Cada membro da equipe multiprofissional deve ter uma função definida e também uma avaliação sobre quando o conhecimento e as habilidades de outros profissionais podem ser utilizados, com vias de encaminhamento multidisciplinares identificadas. Também haverá "subequipes" que trabalham juntas, como a equipe de ciência do esporte e medicina (Figura 29.2) dentro da equipe maior. A integração intradepartamental, a consciência do que outros membros da equipe multiprofissional podem oferecer, com canais claros de comunicação entre os departamentos são cruciais para garantir que ocorra uma contribuição apropriada e oportuna. Para desenvolver o jogador da academia ao máximo, a própria equipe multiprofissional deve se tornar eficaz.

Desenvolver pessoas, não apenas jogadores de futebol

A infância é um período fugaz na vida de alguém. Quem trabalha com crianças tem o privilégio de fazer parte desse momento

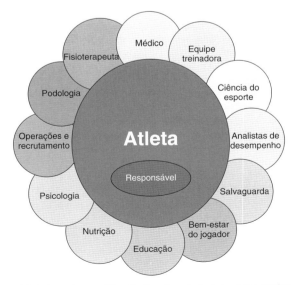

Figura 29.1 A equipe multiprofissional pode incluir várias profissões.

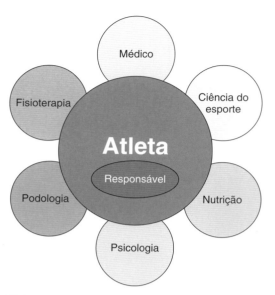

Figura 29.2 Departamento de ciência e medicina do esporte. Dentro da equipe multiprofissional, haverá subequipes menores que trabalharão em conjunto de maneira eficaz, como a equipe médica ou a de medicina e ciência do esporte.

definidor e memorável, mas isso vem com responsabilidade. Uma alta porcentagem de crianças envolvidas em academias não progredirá para as categorias profissionais; portanto, é responsabilidade de todos os colaboradores da academia garantir que o tempo despendido seja agregado ao desenvolvimento de habilidades para a vida para além do futebol. A equipe multiprofissional garantirá que ocorra o desenvolvimento pessoal e social da criança em aspectos que incluem trabalho em equipe, organização e habilidades de gerenciamento de tempo, resolução de problemas, resiliência, respeito, jogo limpo e a importância de trabalhar duro. Quanto aos princípios do futebol, a ênfase nas faixas etárias mais jovens está no desenvolvimento do jogador e em "aprender a treinar", enquanto nas faixas etárias mais velhas a ênfase é em "aprender a competir".

Guardiões da cultura e valores do clube

Todos os membros da equipe multiprofissional serão os guardiões da cultura e dos valores do clube e terão um papel fundamental na manutenção das expectativas e padrões estabelecidos pelo clube. Como alguns jogadores da academia não partem da mesma compreensão básica do que constitui um comportamento socialmente aceitável, é importante que o clube tenha uma filosofia clara que defina os padrões e valores esperados. Os jogadores e a equipe devem garantir que os valores sejam mantidos ao representar o clube, tanto dentro quanto fora do campo. Os jogadores aprendem filosofias do clube, como respeitar os outros, ser gracioso na vitória e mostrar respeito na derrota.

Avaliação clínica e planejamento de tratamento no jovem jogador de futebol

Ambiente

É crucial ter um ambiente adequado e amigável para aliviar o estresse do jovem jogador. Citações motivacionais e mensagens positivas podem ser exibidas, com conselhos de outros membros da equipe multiprofissional ou de jogadores profissionais experientes. Antes de uma avaliação clínica, os pais da criança ou um adulto apropriado devem estar presentes como acompanhante. O procedimento de avaliação deve ser claramente explicado – pôsteres e modelos anatômicos ajudarão a ilustrar os diagnósticos.

Avaliação subjetiva

Se um adulto for solicitado a explicar a história de uma lesão durante uma avaliação, ele pode fornecer informações sobre o mecanismo inicial da lesão junto com a duração e a apresentação atual dos sintomas. As crianças podem não fornecer a informação tão facilmente. Logo, o questionamento do jogador infantojuvenil pode precisar ser mais investigativo, a fim de descobrir informações pertinentes. O terapeuta também pode considerar fatores externos e quaisquer atividades não relacionadas ao futebol. Por exemplo, a criança tem um novo jogo de computador que passou horas jogando? Viajou com os amigos para a praia, jogaram bola por muito tempo? O jogador se machucou praticando outro esporte ou atuando por outra equipe que ele pode estar relutante em revelar? Crianças e adolescentes podem ficar apreensivos em oferecer certas informações por medo de causar problemas; assegure-os de que, quando crianças, é esperado que participem de outras atividades.

Escalas de dor

Várias escalas subjetivas estão disponíveis ao avaliar a dor no jogador pediátrico. Tanto a escala de avaliação de dor FACES, de Wong-Baker (Wong e Baker, 1988), quanto a FACES de dor revisada (FPS-R) (Hicks et al., 2001) usam seis faces representadas graficamente ou em desenho animado com expressões faciais diversas. Eles estão bem estabelecidos e são recomendados para o uso em crianças de 5 a 12 anos e de 3 a 18 anos, respectivamente, com evidências de validade, confiabilidade e capacidade de detectar mudanças (Stinson et al., 2006). A Escala Numérica de Dor (END) utiliza uma gama de números, de 0 a 10 ou de 0 a 100, em formato falado ou gráfico. O menor número representa nenhuma dor e o maior número representa a maior dor possível e foi considerado confiável em crianças com mais de 8 anos para dor aguda (Pagé et al., 2012). A Escala Visual Analógica (EVA) é recomendada para crianças com mais de 8 anos de idade (Stinson et al., 2006).

Avaliação objetiva, observacional e comportamental

Observe o jovem jogador durante a avaliação objetiva quando ele entra na sala e ainda não tem consciência de estar sendo observado. Sinais indicadores, como joelhos enlameados, machucados ou calça rasgada, podem indicar que o jogador está praticando esportes na escola ou jogando com os amigos. O profissional de saúde deve determinar se a avaliação subjetiva e objetiva se correlacionam (ver *Salvaguarda*).

Após a avaliação clínica, a explicação do diagnóstico e do plano de tratamento, peça ao jogador para repetir o que foi discutido, pois isso fornecerá ao médico avaliador uma boa indicação do entendimento do atleta.

Uma avaliação clínica completa determinará se outras investigações são apropriadas e/ou necessárias. Mesmo os profissionais de saúde em um clube com bons recursos devem usar suas habilidades de raciocínio clínico e garantir que as ferramentas de diagnóstico adicionais (como a ressonância magnética) sejam utilizadas apenas quando indicado clinicamente. É inadequado o encaminhamento desnecessário para novas investigações apenas porque são recursos acessíveis para o clube de futebol.

O uso excessivo dessas modalidades de diagnóstico pode afetar de modo negativo o jovem jogador em uma perspectiva psicológica, criando falsas expectativas de como as lesões são avaliadas e diagnosticadas. Isso tem o potencial de aumentar as expectativas ou criar ansiedade durante a fase de avaliação de lesões futuras, se o jogador não for encaminhado para mais testes de diagnósticos.

Planejamento da reabilitação

Os conceitos da abordagem centrada no atleta devem ser incorporados ao longo do processo de reabilitação. O objetivo é que o jogador se aproprie da sua recuperação e se sinta fortalecido durante todo o processo. O fisioterapeuta deve ajudar o jogador a aprender sobre o seu próprio corpo e sempre estimular o questionamento (Figura 29.3). Para envolver o jogador no próprio estabelecimento de metas, uma "lista de problemas" pode ser reinventada como uma "folha de desafio", para provocar um maior apelo aos atletas pediátricos.

A reabilitação é planejada frequentemente como um modelo com base em critérios (em vez de um modelo de escala de tempo), em que o objetivo é atingir os critérios documentados desejados antes de avançar para a próxima fase. Para manter a motivação, o jogador deve receber uma justificativa para os exercícios/fases. Eles devem ter um bom entendimento do processo de reabilitação e dos objetivos a serem alcançados antes de retornar ao futebol. Ao longo do processo de reabilitação, o fisioterapeuta fornecerá ao jogador oportunidades de trabalho de modo independente e garantirá exercícios apropriados para a sua idade, que não devem estar além das capacidades da criança para parecerem mais emocionantes. Deve ser fornecido *feedback* regular com o jogador envolvido na revisão de seu progresso e reavaliação dos seus objetivos.

Durante a reabilitação, é imperativo considerar o jovem jogador em sua totalidade, e não apenas a articulação ou membro lesionado. O tempo deve ser utilizado de modo eficaz para desenvolver outros aspectos do jogador de futebol, como aptidão cardiovascular, ganho de força e potência. A fase de reabilitação é a oportunidade perfeita para o jogador ter informações adicionais de outros membros da equipe multiprofissional. O fisioterapeuta pode coordenar sessões de ginástica ou de campo com o cientista do esporte. As vias de encaminhamento ao nutricionista ou ao psicólogo do clube devem ser ativadas assim que o jogador sofrer uma lesão de longa duração. Incentive o jogador a compreender que é fundamental para o seu sucesso manter uma atitude positiva durante a fase de reabilitação. Em última análise, eles não podem mudar o que aconteceu com eles, mas podem controlar a sua atitude.

Como evitar a medicalização excessiva

Ao tratar crianças e adolescentes jogadores de futebol, a ênfase é na educação e em uma abordagem de tratamento com base em exercícios. As mobilizações articulares ou técnicas de tecidos moles ainda podem ser utilizadas, mas é importante evitar a criação de dependência envolvendo técnicas manuais, bandagem ou mesmo tratamento por um membro da equipe. O objetivo é estimular um ambiente de tratamento adequado, onde o jovem aprenda sobre o seu corpo e como cuidar dele.

Bandagem

Um tratamento controverso no jogador adolescente é o uso de fitas esportivas. A fita é aplicada para controlar o edema, apoiar uma articulação lesionada ou limitar o movimento em uma direção específica, a fim de proteger uma articulação/estrutura ligamentar em cicatrização ou previamente lesionada. Uma fita rígida é utilizada para restringir o movimento das articulações e uma fita adesiva elástica ou fita elástica coesiva (que se cola a si mesma e não à pele) é usada para compressão e para apoiar as articulações ou músculos.

Deve haver uma compreensão clara do objetivo da fita, antes da aplicação, qual a fita mais apropriada a ser utilizada e a técnica de aplicação. Uma abordagem consistente entre os fisioterapeutas do clube em relação à indicação de uso e aplicação da fita ajudará a manter a continuidade. Jogadores adultos podem, às vezes, receber mais apoio psicológico do que físico com as técnicas de bandagem. Evite criar dependência desnecessária da fita ao trabalhar com pediatria.

Desenvolvimento atlético a longo prazo

Ao trabalhar com atletas profissionais seniores, frequentemente há pressão para voltar de uma lesão de fontes externas, como equipe técnica, pressão dos colegas ou mesmo por motivos financeiros. Também pode haver pressão interna dos próprios atletas. Ao trabalhar com futebolistas infantojuvenis, a equipe de saúde deve garantir que o desenvolvimento a longo prazo do jogador tenha precedência sobre quaisquer pressões externas ou internas e ganhos a curto prazo.

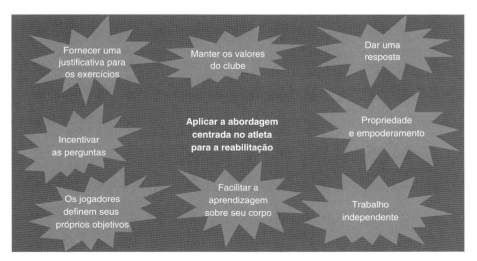

Figura 29.3 Aplicação da abordagem centrada no atleta para a reabilitação.

Parte | 2 | Aplicação Clínica

Crescimento e maturação

Crescimento e maturação são termos utilizados frequentemente como sinônimos. O crescimento ocorre de modo predominante durante as primeiras duas décadas de vida e é um aumento no tamanho do corpo como um todo ou de partes específicas. Maturação é o processo de progredir em direção à maturidade ou à estatura adulta (Malina et al., 2004a). A maturação é considerada em termos de estágio e tempo, ou seja, taxa de maturação e tempo (Cumming et al., 2018). Para distinguir ainda mais, "a maturação é um processo e a maturidade é um estado", (Malina et al., 2004a). Um exemplo dessas diferenças é que as crianças podem ter a mesma altura, mas em vários estágios de maturidade esquelética em relação à porcentagem de altura final atingida (i. e., altura adulta).

O esporão de crescimento na adolescência nas mulheres começa por volta dos 9 ou 10 anos de idade, atinge o pico por volta dos 12 anos e termina por volta dos 16. No sexo masculino, a aceleração começa aos 10 ou 11 anos, atinge o pico por volta dos 14 e para em torno dos 18 anos de idade (Malina et al., 2004a). O pico de velocidade de crescimento (PVC) é o período em que ocorre a taxa máxima de crescimento e o deslocamento de maturidade previsto é definido como a quantidade de tempo antes ou depois do PVC (Kozieł e Malina, 2018).

Qual é a "idade" do jogador?

Uma criança é definida como sendo "um ser humano com menos de 18 anos" (Assembleia Geral da ONU, 1989), embora essa definição possa variar entre os países. No entanto, uma criança pode ter várias "idades" simultaneamente, considerando sua idade cronológica, biológica e psicológica.

Idade cronológica

A idade cronológica é a idade de uma pessoa medida em anos, meses e dias a partir da data de nascimento.

"Idade" biológica ou esquelética

A "idade" biológica ou esquelética ou o estado de maturação da criança é um conceito dinâmico e não estático e pode diferir da idade cronológica dessa pessoa. O estado de maturação pode ser estimado por métodos que comparam o estado de maturação do indivíduo com dados populacionais normativos em relação à idade cronológica (Johnson et al., 2017). O estado de maturidade indica o progresso que o indivíduo está passando para atingir a maturidade biológica (Malina, 1971) e a maturidade pode ser definida pela diferença entre a idade cronológica e a idade esquelética (Johnson et al., 2009). Existem técnicas invasivas e não invasivas disponíveis para estimar a maturação.

Avaliação da maturidade biológica: métodos invasivos

Radiografias de punho e mão. A idade esquelética é considerada o método mais preciso de avaliação da maturidade biológica, sendo as radiografias da mão e do punho esquerdos o padrão-ouro (Engebretsen et al., 2010). Esse método avalia as mudanças e fornece um registro objetivo do *status* de maturidade do esqueleto em desenvolvimento em um único ponto no tempo. Isso é possível porque a ossificação epifisária e a fusão de ossos individuais ocorrem em vários momentos durante o processo de maturação.

Os três métodos utilizados mais frequentemente para avaliar a maturidade esquelética de acordo com Engebretsen et al. (2010) são o método Greulich-Pyle (Greulich e Pyle, 1959), o Tanner-Whitehouse (Tanner et al., 1962, 1983, 2001) e o Fels (Roach et al., 1988). O método Greulich-Pyle compara as radiografias de mão-punho com imagens em um atlas e o método Tanner-Whitehouse (agora em sua terceira edição; TW3) atribui uma pontuação numérica com base na avaliação de 20 ossos, dependendo do aparecimento de indicadores de maturidade. Finalmente, o método de Fels considera uma quantidade maior de indicadores de maturidade do que o método TW3 e inclui avaliação de cada osso do carpo, as epífises e diáfises do rádio, ulna e dos metacarpos e falanges de primeiro, terceiro e quinto dígitos (Malina et al., 2004a). Ao utilizar esses métodos, as crianças são classificadas como na média, maduras tardias ou precoces, subtraindo a idade esquelética da idade cronológica. As crianças são classificadas como maturadoras precoces ou maturadoras tardias se sua idade esquelética for 1 ano mais velha ou mais jovem, respectivamente, do que sua idade cronológica. Os maturadores normais têm uma idade esquelética que está dentro de 1 ano de sua idade cronológica (Johnson et al., 2009; Malina et al., 2004b). Deve-se ter cuidado ao interpretar os dados da radiografia de punho e mão, pois há uma grande variação na maturidade biológica de jogadores com idades cronológicas semelhantes. Johnson et al. (2009) demonstraram que um terço dos jogadores estão fora da categoria de maturidade "normal". Existem também diferentes taxas de maturidade em diferentes origens étnicas (Malina et al., 2004a) e maturidade óssea precoce em adolescentes do sexo feminino (Engebretsen et al., 2010). Isso tem implicações quando se considera que é provável que haja uma ampla gama de idades biológicas em crianças agrupadas para a prática de esportes em faixas de idade cronológica.

O uso de radiografias de mão e punho para determinar a idade esquelética pode não ser ético no ambiente esportivo (Dvorak et al., 2007a), e as radiografias para determinar a idade em crianças e adolescentes saudáveis não podem ser endossadas por comitês éticos em muitos países (Engebretsen et al., 2010).

Avaliação do desenvolvimento dos pelos genitais/púbicos. A Escala de Maturidade Sexual de Tanner foi concebida para avaliar o desenvolvimento físico em crianças, adolescentes e adultos e é utilizada para determinar o estado de maturação (Marshall e Tanner, 1969, 1970). Isso requer avaliação clínica por um profissional médico ou uma autoavaliação das características sexuais secundárias para determinar o estágio de maturação da mama, genital ou testicular. Durante a autoavaliação, os adolescentes recebem desenhos de figuras que representam a Escala de Maturidade Sexual de Tanner e são solicitados a selecionar o desenho/estágio que melhor indica seu próprio estágio de desenvolvimento. Schlossberger et al. (1992) descobriram que havia uma tendência de os indivíduos superestimarem seu desenvolvimento durante os estágios iniciais de maturação e subestimarem seu desenvolvimento em estágios posteriores. Os pesquisadores também descobriram que um exame iminente pode induzir o adolescente a ser mais preciso sobre a autoavaliação.

Essa técnica é considerada invasiva em relação ao espaço pessoal do indivíduo e não é utilizada no futebol rotineiramente. Se empregada, essa técnica seria limitada ao uso na puberdade (Malina et al., 2012).

Avaliação da maturidade biológica: métodos não invasivos

Métodos que utilizam medidas antropométricas. Métodos que utilizam dados antropométricos em vez de avaliação esquelética são considerados indicadores não invasivos da maturação biológica do adolescente e são utilizados frequentemente em academias de futebol.

Os métodos Khamis e Roche (1994) e Mirwald et al. (2002) usam equações de predição para determinar a estatura (altura) adulta final da criança. A idade cronológica, a altura em pé atual (estatura de alongamento) e o peso da criança estão incluídos nas equações para ambos os modelos de previsão. Além desses parâmetros, o método de Khamis e Roche (1994) também inclui a altura mediana dos pais autorreferida nos cálculos e o método Mirwald et al. (2002) leva em consideração a altura sentada. Ambos os métodos têm como objetivo predizer quando uma criança passará pelo PVC, permitindo ao clínico avaliar a que distância uma criança está do PVC e predizer o quanto ela está distante do pico de crescimento (valor de deslocamento). O valor de deslocamento de maturidade é calculado subtraindo a idade cronológica na previsão do tempo previsto em que ocorre o PVC. Este pode ser um valor negativo se a criança estiver antes do PVC, um valor zero se estiver próximo do PVC ou um valor positivo se a criança tiver passado do PVC.

Essas técnicas antropométricas são eficientes em termos de tempo, requerem equipamento barato e não necessitam de um treinamento extensivo para serem realizadas. Consequentemente, são comumente utilizadas no futebol. No entanto, existem limitações para esses modelos de previsão. Malina e Kozieł (2014) descobriram que a previsão de "idade em PVC" (IPVC) tem aplicabilidade entre meninos de maturação média de 12 a 16 anos em contraste com meninos de maturação precoce e tardia. Descobriu-se que a equação de Mirwald subestima a IPVC real em idades mais jovens e nos primeiros anos de vida e a superestima em idades mais avançadas e em maturadores tardios. Kozieł e Malina (2018) também observaram que as equações não eram úteis para meninas de maturação precoce e tardia, com uma janela para a avaliação de meninas com maturidade média não sendo aparente. O uso da altura parental mediana autodeterminada no método de Khamis e Roche (1994) é uma limitação devido ao risco de informações incorretas serem fornecidas. Muitos desses estudos também se baseiam em participantes caucasianos de origens socioeconômicas de classe média, enquanto no futebol esses modelos são aplicados a várias origens étnicas e socioeconômicas.

Imageamento por ressonância magnética. O uso da ressonância magnética oferece a possibilidade de estimar a maturidade biológica/cronológica sem a necessidade de radiação ionizante, mas ainda não substituiu o uso de radiografias de mão e punho.

Dvorak et al. (2007a,b) tentaram usar ressonâncias magnéticas de punho esquerdo para determinar a idade cronológica em uma tentativa de garantir a participação cronológica apropriada em jogadores de futebol do sexo masculino. Com base nessas duas investigações, Engebretsen et al. (2010) concluíram que a ressonância magnética era uma ferramenta viável para a triagem de jogadores do sexo masculino nos grupos Sub-16 e Sub-17, mas na época não havia evidências para apoiar o uso da ressonância magnética de punho para determinação da idade em atletas do sexo masculino abaixo de 14 anos e acima de 17 anos de idade. Em 2016, Tscholl et al. determinaram que, devido à maturidade óssea precoce em adolescentes do sexo feminino, o grau de fusão da epífise radial distal na ressonância magnética não é recomendado para determinação da idade pré-torneio em participantes do sexo feminino de Sub-17 e mais jovens. Durante esse estudo, a fusão completa da epífise radial distal foi observada em meninas de 14 e 15 anos de idade.

Mais recentemente, um atlas de estudos de ressonância magnética do joelho abrangendo os anos pediátrico e adolescente foi criado e validado por Pennock et al. (2018). Eles encontraram uma forte correlação entre a idade cronológica e a idade óssea com excelente confiabilidade interobservador e intraobservador demonstrada. Estudos em menor escala examinaram a viabilidade de avaliação da idade esquelética em ressonâncias magnéticas da mão esquerda, com Hojreh et al. (2018) e Serinelli et al. (2015) encontrando boa correlação com a idade cronológica estimada. Estudos futuros são necessários para avaliar os resultados desses estudos de punho em amostras maiores que incluem indivíduos de uma variedade de etnias e origens socioeconômicas.

Naqueles com mais de 18 anos, a clavícula é utilizada para avaliação da maturidade, pois é o último osso do corpo humano a completar a fusão (Buckley e Clark, 2017). Um estudo piloto de Schmidt et al. (2015) investigou o uso de ressonância magnética para verificar a idade de jogadores em torneios de futebol Sub-20 e descobriram que a presença de uma placa epifisária clavicular totalmente ossificada parece fornecer evidências de completamento do vigésimo ano de vida. No entanto, isso também requer um estudo mais aprofundado, incluindo uma maior quantidade de participantes.

Idade psicológica

O termo "idade psicológica" refere-se ao desenvolvimento emocional/cognitivo/psicológico de uma criança. A correlação entre a idade física e psicológica de uma criança não é necessariamente linear. Um jogador pode atingir a altura de um adulto na metade da adolescência, mas isso não significa que tenha a maturidade emocional e cognitiva de um adulto. O estado de maturidade cognitiva e emocional da criança deve ser considerado na avaliação e tratamento do jogador. Por exemplo, um jogador de 14 anos pode ter 182 cm de altura e parecer fisicamente um adulto, mas isso não significa que a sua mente seja capaz de processar informações como um adulto.

Efeito da idade relativa e *biobanding*

O *efeito da idade relativa* é um fenômeno que sugere que há assimetrias nas distribuições de datas de nascimento em jogadores de futebol profissional sênior e juvenil (Vaeyens et al., 2005). Os jogadores nascidos no início do ano de seleção são favorecidos e os nascidos no final do ano são discriminados (Helsen et al., 2012). Isso geralmente se deve à seleção associada à maturação.

No Reino Unido, o calendário acadêmico e esportivo vai de 1º de setembro a 31 de agosto e agrupa as crianças com base na idade cronológica. Consequentemente, as crianças do Reino Unido nascidas nos meses de setembro a dezembro podem ter uma vantagem na seleção em comparação com jogadores mais jovens nascidos no final desse ano de seleção. Essas datas para a faixa etária cronológica podem variar internacionalmente, com muitos países usando 1º de janeiro a 31 de dezembro para agrupar as crianças cronologicamente. Logo, nesses países, as crianças nascidas entre janeiro e março podem ter a vantagem de seleção. Musch e Hay (1999) determinaram que o efeito da idade relativa se mostrou presente independentemente da variação na data de corte.

Com relação à seleção de jogadores da academia, Johnson et al. (2017) sugerem que o estado de maturação esquelética está mais associado à seleção esportiva do que o quadrimestre de nascimento. Esse estudo sugere que as academias tendem a favorecer aqueles nascidos no início do ano de seleção em um grau relativamente pequeno; em contraste, favorecem muito mais os atletas que amadurecem mais cedo. Conforme discutido por Musch e Hay (1999), a discriminação contra os jogadores menores e esqueleticamente menos maduros pode limitar suas oportunidades e eles podem abandonar o esporte mais cedo, em vez de

Parte |2| Aplicação Clínica

continuar até atingir a maturidade, quando a desvantagem da idade é superada. Na verdade, se os jogadores qualificados estão dispersos proporcionalmente pela população, então é uma estratégia falha selecionar jogadores apenas do grupo de maturadores precoces, pois o talento potencial no grupo de maturadores tardios e normais será excluído ou perdido (Johnson et al. 2017). As diferenças nos *status* de maturação também têm o potencial de funcionar adversamente contra os maturadores precoces, pois eles podem usar sua fisicalidade durante o jogo em vez de desenvolver suas habilidades técnicas nos primeiros anos da adolescência. Isso pode ter consequências negativas quando os outros jogadores alcançam o mesmo *status* de maturação e diz-se que "recuperaram o atraso".

Para neutralizar o efeito da idade relativa, os treinadores de futebol costumam levar em consideração a data de nascimento do jogador no que diz respeito à identificação do talento e à seleção do jogador. No entanto, comparar jogadores com outros de idades cronológicas semelhantes não leva em conta as diferenças de maturação; consequentemente, o *biobanding* foi sugerido. *Biobanding* é o processo de agrupar atletas com base em atributos associados ao crescimento ou maturação, em vez da idade cronológica (Cumming et al., 2017) em uma tentativa de "nivelar o campo de jogo".

Aspectos práticos do trabalho na academia

Salvaguarda

Salvaguarda é o processo de proteger crianças e adultos em risco. Muitas academias terão um oficial de proteção designado, mas todos os membros da equipe multiprofissional têm a responsabilidade de aderir às políticas de proteção a fim de proteger as crianças com quem trabalham e a si próprios. Sempre siga o código de conduta e ética de sua profissão e trabalhe dentro das diretrizes de proteção do empregador.

É importante observar que a criança pode usar a fisioterapia ou a sala de tratamento como saída do campo de futebol. Use habilidades de raciocínio clínico para determinar o seguinte:

- O mecanismo de lesão se encaixa na apresentação?
- O histórico subjetivo e os achados da avaliação objetiva se correlacionam?
- O jogador foi ao fisioterapeuta repetidamente para incidentes/lesões relativamente leves?
- Ao falar sobre o retorno do jogador ao treinamento, o jogador parece apreensivo?
- Existem hematomas que causam preocupação ou estão em áreas anatômicas que não são comumente causadas pelo esporte, por exemplo, peito/tórax/braço/ombro em futebolistas?
- Alguma preocupação foi levada ao conhecimento da equipe médica anteriormente?

Se surgirem dúvidas após a avaliação, considere se algum dos seguintes fatores pode estar influenciando a apresentação do jogador:

- O jogador está sofrendo *bullying*? Isso pode ser por outro jogador, um membro da equipe ou até mesmo por seus pais após o treinamento
- O jogador está lutando dentro do grupo e achando o treinamento difícil? Qualquer lesão leve pode ser catastrofizada por uma criança que não está apreciando o futebol
- O jogador parece ansioso ou tem medo de falhar?
- Há evidência de expectativa excessiva por parte dos pais?
- O jogador está sendo submetido à pressão do grupo de pares?

Criação de um ambiente seguro

Considere as medidas de proteção adequadas dentro do ambiente de trabalho em mudança, na sala de fisioterapia, na academia, na área da piscina ou no hotel. A melhor prática seria que os membros da equipe não fiquem sem supervisão em áreas confinadas com crianças da academia. Isso promove um ambiente seguro para a criança e para o funcionário. Reporte qualquer prática ou comportamento inadequado imediatamente de acordo com as diretrizes do empregador. Certifique-se sempre de que fatores culturais e religiosos sejam considerados ao tratar qualquer paciente.

Se o clube ou empregador não tiver uma política de proteção, é possível encontrar mais informações no site da Federação Inglesa de Futebol no documento intitulado Mantendo o Futebol Seguro e Agradável (The Football Association, 2017).

Viagem com crianças em idade escolar

Preparação pré-torneio

Para todos os torneios e turnês, o clube deve realizar avaliações de risco pré-competição. Essas avaliações de risco incluirão informações sobre os jogadores e os locais, incluindo o hotel e os estádios. É importante estar familiarizado com isso e sempre trabalhar dentro das políticas e procedimentos da organização.

Transporte

Se o *kit* médico principal estiver guardado no porão da aeronave ou do ônibus, uma pequena maleta médica pode ser transportada como bagagem de mão para lidar com ferimentos leves ou incidentes durante o trajeto. Considere o que seria necessário para lidar com uma criança com sangramento nasal ou enjoo de viagem. Certifique-se de que os jogadores tenham todos os medicamentos essenciais na bagagem de mão.

Volta à rotina

Incentive uma dieta equilibrada e tente manter os conselhos dietéticos consistentes, simples e compreensíveis para jogadores jovens. Durante a competição, a comida costuma ser rica em carboidratos e é consumida pelo menos 2 horas antes do início dos jogos. O nutricionista do clube pode liderar a estratégia alimentar, mas no nível da academia, o técnico e a equipe médica do torneio costumam supervisionar as necessidades alimentares dos jogadores.

Certifique-se de que os jogadores e a equipe lavem as mãos com sabão ou use álcool gel regularmente para reduzir o risco de propagação de doenças infecciosas dentro da equipe.

Fatores ambientais a considerar

- Hidratação: os jogadores podem beber água da torneira? Quanto eles precisarão beber devido à duração e a frequência das partidas e fatores ambientais como temperatura, umidade ou altitude?
- Quais equipamentos e roupas são necessários para o clima? O protetor solar será necessário?
- Leve em consideração que muitas crianças podem nunca ter viajado para fora de sua área local
- A saudade de casa pode ser um fator que contribui para a apresentação de um jogador.

Múltiplas funções de membros da equipe multiprofissional

Apenas uma seleção do quadro total da equipe multiprofissional viajará com uma equipe da academia; consequentemente, para o bem-estar dos jogadores, os membros assumem aspectos de papéis normalmente desempenhados por outros profissionais. Todos os funcionários serão os pais naquele local e exercerão a função de pastoral infantil; eles cuidarão das necessidades nutricionais e de hidratação e garantirão que os procedimentos de proteção sejam cumpridos.

Primeiros socorros

Fisioterapeutas que trabalham no esporte são solicitados frequentemente a fornecer atendimento de emergência durante as partidas. É importante que qualquer pessoa que aceitar essa responsabilidade tenha realizado um curso de primeiros socorros esportivos apropriado e que essas habilidades sejam praticadas regularmente para manter a competência. Planos de ação de emergência devem estar em vigor para todos os locais de treinamento e jogo.

Resumo

A atuação do fisioterapeuta no esporte é multifacetada e vai além de trabalhar apenas em uma sala de tratamento. Qualquer fisioterapeuta ou terapeuta esportivo que trabalhe em um sistema de academia deve estar ciente de suas funções e responsabilidades, tanto em casa quanto no exterior. Eles devem ser capazes de adaptar suas estratégias de avaliação e tratamento para a população pediátrica e compreender os aspectos de crescimento e maturação.

Referências bibliográficas

Buckley, M.B., Clark, K.R., 2017. Forensic age estimation using the medial clavicular epiphysis: a study review. Radiologic Technology 88 (5), 482-498.

Cumming, S.P., Lloyd, R.S., Oliver, J.L., Eisenmann, J.C., Malina, R.M., 2017. Bio-banding in sport: applications to competition, talent identification, and strength and conditioning of youth athletes. Strength and Conditioning Journal 39 (2), 34-47.

Cumming, S.P., Brown, D.J., Mitchell, S., Bunce, J., Hunt, D., Hedges, C., et al., 2018. Premier League academy soccer players' experiences of competing in a tournament bio-banded for biological maturation. Journal of Sports Sciences 36 (7), 757-765.

Dvorak, J., George, J., Junge, A., Hodler, J., 2007a. Age determination by magnetic resonance imaging of the wrist in adolescent male football players. British Journal of Sports Medicine. 41 (1), 45-52.

Dvorak, J., George, J., Junge, A., Hodler, J., 2007b. Application of MRI of the wrist for age determination in international U-17 soccer competitions. British Journal of Sports Medicine 41 (8), 497-500.

Engebretsen, L., Steffen, K., Bahr, R., Broderick, C., Dvorak, J., Janarv, P.-M., et al., 2010. The International Olympic Committee Consensus Statement on age determination in high-level young athletes. British Journal of Sports Medicine 44 (7), 476-484.

Greulich, W.W., Pyle, S.I., 1959. Radiographic atlas of skeletal development of the hand and wrist. The American Journal of the Medical Sciences 238 (3), 393.

Helsen, W.F., Baker, J., Michiels, S., Schorer, J., Van Winckel, J., Williams, A.M., 2012. The relative age effect in European professional soccer: did ten years of research make any difference? Journal of Sports Sciences 30 (15), 1665-1671.

Hicks, C., Baeyer, C., Spafford, P., van Korlaar, I., Goodenough, B., 2001. The Faces Pain Scale-Revised: toward a common metric in pediatric pain measurement. Pain 93 (2), 173-183.

Hojreh, A., Gamper, J., Schmook, M.T., Weber, M., Prayer, D., Herold, C.J., et al., 2018. Hand MRI and the Greulich-Pyle atlas in skeletal age estimation in adolescents. Skeletal Radiology 47, 963-971.

Johnson, A., Doherty, P.J., Freemont, A., 2009. Investigation of growth, development, and factors associated with injury in elite schoolboy footballers: prospective study. The British Medical Journal 338, b490.

Johnson, A., Farooq, A., Whiteley, R., 2017. Skeletal maturation status is more strongly associated with academy selection than birth quarter. Science and Medicine in Football 1 (2), 157-163.

Khamis, H.J., Roche, A.F., 1994. Predicting adult stature without using skeletal age: the Khamis-Roche method. Pediatrics 94 (4), 504-507.

Kidman, L., Lombardo, B.J., 2010. Athlete-centred Coaching: Developing Decision Makers, second ed. IPC Print Resources, Worcester, UK.

Kozieł, S.M., Malina, R.M., 2018. Modified maturity offset prediction equations: validation in independent longitudinal samples of boys and girls. Sports Medicine 48, 221-236.

Malina, R.M., 1971. A consideration of factors underlying the selection of methods in the assessment of skeletal maturity. American Journal of Physical Anthropology 35 (3), 341-346.

Malina, R.M., Kozieł, S.M., 2014. Validation of maturity offset in a longitudinal sample of Polish boys. Journal of Sports Sciences 32 (5), 424-437.

Malina, R., Eisenmann, J., Cumming, S., Ribeiro, B., Aroso, J., 2004b. Maturity-associated variation in the growth and functional capacities of youth football (soccer) players 13-15 years. European Journal of Applied Physiology 91 (5-6), 555-562.

Malina, R.M., Coelho, E., Silva, M.J., Figueiredo, A.J., Carling, C., Beunen, G.P., 2012. Interrelationships among invasive and non-invasive indicators of biological maturation in adolescent male soccer players. Journal of Sports Sciences 30 (15), 1705-1717.

Malina, R.M., Bouchard, C., Bar-Or, O., 2004a. Growth, Maturation, and Physical Activity. Human Kinetics, Champaign, IL.

Marshall, W.A., Tanner, J.M., 1969. Variations in pattern of pubertal changes in girls. Archives of Disease in Childhood 44 (235), 291-303.

Marshall, W.A., Tanner, J.M., 1970. Variations in the pattern of pubertal changes in boys. Archives of Disease in Childhood 45 (239), 13-23.

Mirwald, R.L., Baxter-Jones, A.D., Bailey, D.A., Beunen, G.P., 2002. An assessment of maturity from anthropometric measurements. Medicine & Science in Sports & Exercise 34 (4), 689-694.

Musch, J., Hay, R., 1999. The relative age effect in soccer: cross-cultural evidence for a systematic discrimination against children born late in the competition year. Sociology of Sport Journal 16 (1), 54-64.

Pagé, M.G., Katz, J., Stinson, J., Isaac, L., Martin-Pichora, A.L., Campbell, F., 2012. Validation of the numerical rating scale for pain intensity and unpleasantness in pediatric acute postoperative pain: sensitivity to change over time. The Journal of Pain 13 (4), 359-369.

Pennock, A.T., Bomar, J.D., Manning, J.D., 2018. The creation and validation of a knee bone age atlas utilizing MRI. The Journal of Bone and Joint Surgery 100 (4), e20.

Roche, A.F., Chumlea, W.C., Thissen, D., 1988. Assessing the skeletal maturity of the hand-wrist: FELS Method. Charles C. Thomas; Springfield, IL.

Schlossberger, N.M., Turner, R.A., Irwin, C.E., 1992. Validity of self-report of pubertal maturation in early adolescents. Journal of Adolescent Health 13 (2), 109-113.

Schmidt, S., Vieth, V., Timme, M., Dvorak, J., Schmeling, A., 2015. Examination of ossification of the distal radial epiphysis using magnetic resonance imaging. New insights for age estimation in young footballers in FIFA tournaments. Science & Justice 55, 139-144.

Serinelli, S., Panebianco, V., Martino, M., Battisti, S., Rodacki, K., Marinelli, E., et al., 2015. Accuracy of MRI skeletal age estimation for subjects 12-19. Potential use for subjects of unknown age. International Journal of Legal Medicine 129 (3), 609-617.

Stinson, J.N., Kavanagh, T., Yamada, J., Gill, N., Stevens, B., 2006. Systematic review of the psychometric properties, interpretability and feasibility of self-report pain intensity measures for use in clinical trials in children and adolescents. Pain 125 (1-2), 143-157.

Tanner, J.M., Whitehouse, R.H., Cameron, N., Marshall, W.A., Healy, M.J.R., Goldstein, H., 1983. Assessment of Skeletal Maturity and Prediction of Adult Height (TW2 Method), second ed. Academic Press, London, UK.

Tanner, J.M., Healy, M.J.R., Goldstein, H., Cameron, N., 2001. Assessment of Skeletal Maturity and Prediction of Adult Height (TW3 Method), third ed. Saunders, London.

Tanner, J.M., Whitehouse, R.H., 1962. Growth at Adolescence, second ed. Blackwell Scientific Publications, Springfield, Illinois, USA.

The Football Association, 2017. Keeping Football Safe and Enjoyable. Available from: Keeping Football Safe and Enjoyable (2017). Available at: http://www.thefa.com/-/media/thefacom-new/files/about-the-fa/2017/keeping-football-safe-enjoyable.ashx?la=en.

Tscholl, P.M., Junge, A., Dvorak, J., Zubler, V., 2016. MRI of the wrist is not recommended for age determination in female football players of U-16/U-17 competitions. Scandinavian Journal of Medicine & Science in Sports 26 (3), 324-328.

UN General Assembly, 20 November 1989. Convention on the Rights of the Child, vol. 1577. United Nations, Treaty Series, p. 3, available at: http://www.refworld.org/docid/3ae6b38f0.html. [Accessed January 2018].

Vaeyens, R., Philippaerts, R.M., Malina, R.M., 2005. The relative age effect in soccer: a match-related perspective. Journal of Sports Sciences 23 (7), 747-756.

Wong, D.L., Baker, C.M., 1988. Pain in children: comparison of assessment scales. Pediatric Nursing 14 (1), 9-17.

Capítulo | 30 |

Ossos em Crescimento: Anatomia e Fraturas

Diane Ryding

Introdução

Em medicina e reabilitação pediátricas, frequentemente surge a afirmação de que "crianças não são miniadultos", mas o que isso significa? Como as lesões diferem em um atleta com esqueleto imaturo? Para compreender as lesões musculoesqueléticas pediátricas, os médicos devem estar cientes das variações anatômicas entre esqueletos maduros e imaturos, que causam um conjunto único de lesões na população pediátrica. As epífises, as placas epifisárias (de crescimento) e as apófises de um esqueleto em desenvolvimento correm o risco de sofrer lesões.

Esse capítulo discutirá a anatomia dos ossos longos pediátricos, o crescimento ósseo e as fraturas que podem ocorrer no esqueleto em desenvolvimento. Está além do escopo deste capítulo discutir todas as fraturas pediátricas, mas estão incluídas aquelas que podem ser vistas em um ambiente de academia de futebol de elite junto com uma visão geral de tratamento.

Anatomia dos ossos longos pediátricos

Com base em Malina et al. (2004):
- A *diáfise* é a haste do osso. Ela contém o centro de ossificação primário, que é o local de deposição do osso no modelo de cartilagem, transformando cartilagem em osso. Em ossos longos, ela está localizada na porção média do osso
- O *periósteo* é uma membrana que cobre a superfície externa da diáfise. Essa camada tem a capacidade de produzir osteoblastos
- A *epífise* é a extremidade arredondada dos ossos longos que contribui para uma articulação. Ela se desenvolve a partir de um centro de ossificação secundário formado na cartilagem no final da diáfise. Os ossos longos dos braços e pernas têm centros de ossificação em ambas as extremidades. Ossos curtos da mão e do pé têm apenas centros de ossificação secundários em uma das extremidades
- A *fise/placa epifisária* é o nome dado à cartilagem epifisária/placa de crescimento
- A *metáfise* é a região onde ocorre a ossificação. É a porção estreita de um osso longo entre a epífise e a diáfise que contém a placa de crescimento
- A *apófise* é uma excrescência óssea normal que é o centro de ossificação secundário. A unidade musculotendínea se liga à apófise, que se funde com o osso ao longo do tempo.

Ponto-chave

A epífise contribui para uma articulação e a apófise para uma fixação teno-óssea.

Crescimento ósseo

No período pré-natal, as crianças começam com um esqueleto de cartilagem que é substituído por osso à medida que a criança cresce. No final de cada osso existe um centro de ossificação (epífise) com uma fise aderente (placa de crescimento), que é perpendicular ao eixo longo do osso (Engebretsen et al., 2010). O osso cresce em comprimento na direção da epífise pela proliferação de células da cartilagem e matriz intercelular na metáfise (Malina et al., 2004). As células da cartilagem da fise se multiplicam e se transformam com a mineralização e um novo osso é produzido; isso contribui para o crescimento diafisário (Engebretsen et al., 2010). Em outras palavras, a cartilagem calcifica eventualmente e é substituída por osso (Figura 30.1). O osso cresce em largura ao se depositar tecido ósseo na superfície externa ou subperiosteal. O osso na superfície interna (endosteal) é reabsorvido (Malina et al., 2004).[1]

Os ossos param de crescer quando a proliferação das células da cartilagem diminui e a ossificação ocorre em um ritmo mais rápido. Há união epifisária eventualmente onde a epífise e a metáfise se fundem; nesse momento, a maturidade esquelética ocorre e a fise (placa de crescimento) desaparece. As mulheres, em média, completam o processo de ossificação dos centros secundários mais cedo do que os homens (Malina et al., 2004).

Classificação de Salter-Harris de fraturas fisárias

Podem ocorrer fraturas que afetam a fise (placa de crescimento) devido às variações anatômicas nos ossos em crescimento. Esses tipos de fraturas são comumente descritos por meio da classificação Salter-Harris I-IV (Salter e Harris, 1963) (Boxe 30.1) e podem ser lembrados utilizando o mnemônico "Salter" (Figura 30.2).

Sinais e sintomas

Fraturas fisárias, como outras fraturas, podem se apresentar com dor, inchaço, deformidade, movimento limitado, sensibilidade óssea ou capacidade reduzida ou total de suportar peso no membro inferior.

---

[1] N.R.T.: processo de metabolismo e catabolismo ósseo, influenciado por diferentes fatores como a lei de WOLF (crescimento relacionado com as linhas de tensão e tração).

| Parte | 2 | Aplicação Clínica

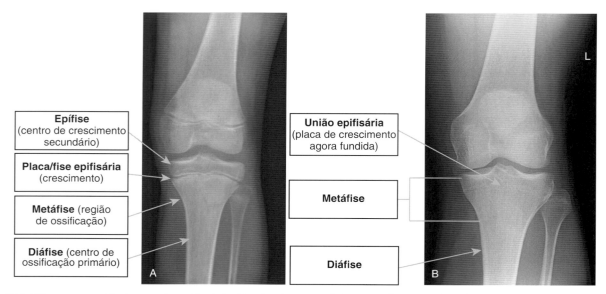

Figura 30.1 Diferenças anatômicas: radiografia de joelho de criança e adulto. **A.** Joelho esquerdo pediátrico: esqueleto imaturo/em desenvolvimento. **B.** Joelho esquerdo adulto: esqueleto maduro/desenvolvido.

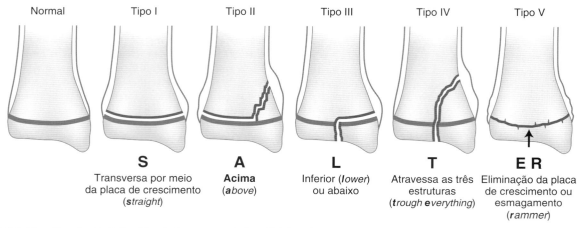

Figura 30.2 Classificação de Salter-Harris das características fisárias. O mnemônico "Salter" pode ser útil para lembrar os diferentes tipos.

Boxe 30.1 Classificação de Salter-Harris das características fisárias

- Uma fratura do tipo I é uma separação por meio da fise. É mais comum em pacientes mais jovens com uma fise mais espessa
- Uma fratura do tipo II entra pelo plano da fise e sai pela metáfise. O fragmento metafisário separado é conhecido como fragmento de Thurston Holland. O tipo II é responsável por 74% das fraturas fisárias
- Uma fratura do tipo III entra no plano da fise e sai pela epífise. Esse é um tipo de fratura menos comum, mas apresenta o risco adicional de artrite pós-traumática e parada de crescimento
- Uma fratura do tipo IV cruza a fise, estendendo-se da metáfise à epífise. Esse tipo de fratura possui um elemento de instabilidade longitudinal. Existe o risco de parada fisária completa ou crescimento assimétrico ou deformidade
- Um tipo V é uma lesão por esmagamento que resulta em lesão da fise, muitas vezes devido a forças compressivas.

Adaptado de Cepela, D.J., Tartaglione, J.P., Dooley, T.P., Patel, P.N., 2016. Classifications in brief: Salter-Harris classification of pediatric physeal fractures. Clinical Orthopaedics and Related Research 474 (11), 2531-2537.

Diagnóstico e tratamento

Fraturas fisárias podem resultar em distúrbios de crescimento; portanto, para evitar potenciais consequências adversas a longo prazo, é imperativo que qualquer jogador pediátrico com suspeita de fratura seja encaminhado para uma radiografia. Qualquer fratura fisária significativa será acompanhada por cerca de 1 ano após a lesão no ambulatório de ortopedia para monitorar qualquer complicação de crescimento.

Pontos-chave

Uma crença comum é que os médicos do pronto-socorro "apenas enfaixam" fraturas menores nos dedos e alguns pais relutam em passar horas esperando com seus filhos por isso, mas o risco de tratamento incorreto de uma fratura fisária do dedo pode ter implicações a longo prazo para a função da mão.

Tome cuidado com o atleta pediátrico que se apresenta com uma deformidade articular traumática, pois ela pode não ser decorrente de luxação da articulação, mas sim de fratura intra-articular. Por exemplo, uma aparente "luxação da patela" pode ser, na verdade, uma fratura fisária do fêmur distal.

Fraturas incompletas

Os ossos das crianças apresentam maior grau de elasticidade quando comparados aos ossos dos adultos, o que os torna suscetíveis a fraturas incompletas. Existem três tipos comuns.

Fraturas em galho verde

As fraturas em galho verde são transversais por meio do córtex, onde um lado do osso é quebrado e o outro apenas dobrado e a quebra não perturba o córtex oposto, ou seja, o osso dobra e se quebra como um galho verde. Ting et al. (2016) constataram que ocorrem na faixa etária de 2 a 15 anos, com média de idade de 6,9 anos.

Fratura em fivela (*torus*)

As fraturas em fivela (*torus*) são incompletas da diáfise de um osso longo, caracterizadas por abaulamento do córtex, e envolvem frequentemente a junção metafisária e diáfise (Figura 30.3). Elas ocorrem durante uma força de carregamento axial, no rádio distal. As fraturas em fivela do rádio distal costumam ser tratadas com uma tala em vez de gesso; esse é um tipo de fratura estável inerente ao baixo risco de deslocamento (Williams et al., 2013). Eles ocorrem em pré-adolescentes, mas Ling e Cleary (2018) descobriram que também há ocorrência na faixa etária de 0 a 16 anos, com idade média de 9 anos.

Deformidade plástica

As deformidades plásticas afetam os ossos longos, mais comumente o rádio e a ulna, seguidos pela fíbula. O osso dobra ou se curva ao longo de seu eixo longitudinal seguindo uma força de carga, mas não há ruptura distinta do córtex. Em uma revisão em pequena escala, Vorlat e De Boeck (2003) descobriram que a idade média das fraturas do arco radial era de 7 anos e 5 meses.

Ferramentas de decisão clínica de fratura

As ferramentas de decisão clínica utilizadas na avaliação de lesões de membros inferiores servem como diretrizes para a solicitação de exames radiográficos, com o objetivo de evitar exames desnecessários em serviços de emergência (Figura 30.4). Essas ferramentas podem ser úteis para profissionais de saúde que trabalham no cenário de esportes agudos.

Regras de pé e tornozelo de Ottawa

Uma meta-análise de Dowling et al. (2009) sugere que essas regras parecem ser uma ferramenta confiável para excluir fraturas em crianças com mais de 5 anos de idade quando apresentam lesões no tornozelo e mediopé. A sensibilidade combinada foi de 98,5% (IC 95%, 97,3 a 99,2%), o que significa que 1,5% das fraturas podem ser perdidas usando as regras.

Regras do joelho de Ottawa

Em 2003, Bulloch et al. validaram as regras de Ottawa do joelho em crianças acima de 5 anos, determinando que o uso dessas regras pode reduzir com segurança a necessidade de radiografias de joelho. No entanto, os médicos devem ter um alto índice de suspeição e baixo limiar para investigações adicionais (ressonância magnética [RM]) se um jogador pediátrico apresentar um grande derrame no joelho, como Pennock et al. (2017) sugerem que as fraturas intra-articulares podem não ser vistas nas radiografias simples de atletas com esqueleto imaturo.

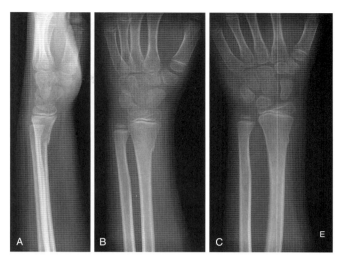

Figura 30.3 Fratura em fivela. **A.** Vista lateral. **B.** Vista oblíqua. **C.** Vista posteroanterior. *E*, esquerda.

Tratamento de fratura

A equipe de saúde da academia deve seguir as orientações ortopédicas sobre a imobilização da fratura na fase pós-fratura imediata. Se a fratura estiver estável e for seguro fazê-lo, a equipe médica trabalhará com o jogador em outras áreas do corpo enquanto protege a estrutura de cicatrização durante a fase de imobilização. Uma vez que a fratura tenha cicatrizado, a reabilitação consistirá em recuperar a amplitude de movimento, força funcional, propriocepção e capacidade pliométrica, com a construção do condicionamento cardiovascular e voltar para a atividade de estágio final específica da posição. Um retorno em fases ao treinamento com manejo de carga será utilizado conforme necessário. O fisioterapeuta garantirá que o jogador esteja confortável e confiante no treinamento antes de devolvê-lo aos jogos competitivos.

Fraturas crônicas que afetam a placa de crescimento

Além das lesões fisárias agudas, Caine et al. (2006) sugerem que lesões fisárias crônicas podem ocorrer se o treinamento esportivo tiver duração e intensidade suficientes. Em casos extremos, isso pode levar a distúrbios do crescimento ósseo.

Fraturas por avulsão apofisária

A apófise surge durante a puberdade, como centro de ossificação secundário, e não se funde até o final da adolescência (Gidwani et al., 2004). Durante esse tempo, é a parte mais fraca da junção musculotendínea, razão pela qual ocorre uma avulsão apofisária em vez de uma lesão muscular (Lozano-Berges et al., 2017;

Pontos-chave

No futebol, essas fraturas costumam manifestar-se em um jovem goleiro que se queixa de dor no punho após parar um chute (geralmente relatada como hiperextensão do punho). Elas também podem ocorrer após uma queda com a mão estendida.

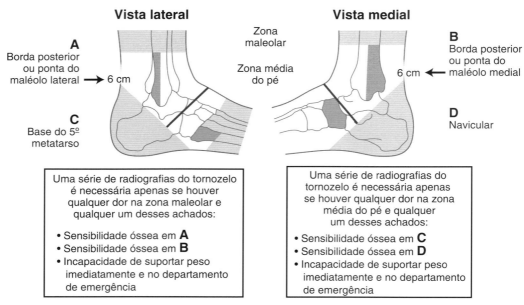

Figura 30.4 Regras do tornozelo de Ottawa, um auxílio à decisão para excluir fraturas do tornozelo e da porção média do pé. (Adaptada de Bachman et al., 2003.)

Schiller et al., 2017). Em outras palavras, a apófise é o elo mais fraco da cadeia de músculo, tendão e osso (Gidwani et al., 2004).

Durante uma fratura por avulsão apofisária, um fragmento de osso é puxado para fora da massa óssea principal como resultado de uma força de tração repentina aplicada devido a uma poderosa contração muscular (Porr et al., 2011). As fraturas por avulsão apofisária ocorrem nas inserções apofisárias de grandes unidades musculotendíneas, e também podem acontecer nas inserções dos ligamentos, por exemplo, na origem do ligamento talofibular anterior.

A cartilagem em crescimento ossifica no fim da adolescência e a conexão entre a apófise e o corpo do osso se fortalece. Nesse ponto, a unidade musculotendínea passa a ser a estrutura mais fraca na transferência de força entre músculo e osso (Porr et al., 2011), explicando porque as lesões mudam quando se trabalha com atletas esqueleticamente maduros.

Fraturas por avulsão apofisária pélvica

Existem vários locais na pelve do adolescente que podem suportar uma lesão por avulsão (Figura 30.5). A Tabela 30.1 demonstra esse tipo de fratura por avulsão, o músculo correspondente criando a tração e a ação muscular potencial durante o mecanismo de lesão. A Tabela 30.2 mostra os resultados de dois estudos sobre fraturas apofisárias pélvicas.

Sinais e sintomas

Os sinais e sintomas de fraturas por avulsão da apófise pélvica incluem:
- Início súbito e agudo de dor precedido por uma forte contração muscular. Uma sensação de estalo é relatada frequentemente
- Dificuldade de locomoção e dor limitadora de atividade
- Pode-se observar inchaço e/ou hematoma
- Dor e fraqueza na avaliação do grupo muscular correspondente
- Dor localizada, sensibilidade à palpação do local da avulsão.

Clinicamente, um atleta com avulsão da espinha ilíaca anteroinferior (EIAI) pode ser incapaz de erguer a perna reta, ao passo que a avulsão da tuberosidade isquiática pode causar dor ao sentar-se.

Diagnóstico/imagem

Em um ambiente de academia de elite, a RM é a primeira escolha de investigação para identificar uma avulsão apofisária. A radiografia simples ou a tomografia computadorizada (TC) também podem ser utilizadas, embora a dosagem de radiação ionizante deva ser levada em consideração. Uma tomografia computadorizada pode ser necessária se a cirurgia for necessária; a cirurgia é reservada para grandes fraturas principalmente ou quando a fratura está deslocada de modo considerável (> 20 mm).

Tratamento

- O tratamento inicial inclui proteção e descarregamento da área lesionada, com a capacidade de sustentação de carga sendo parcial ou ausente, com o uso de muletas canadense, dependendo do índice de suspeita e da apresentação da lesão
- O gelo pode ser aplicado durante os primeiros 2 a 3 dias regularmente para aliviar a dor e a inflamação. O gelo deve ser aplicado por um mínimo de 10 minutos, mas não mais do que 20 a 30 minutos. O tempo ideal entre as aplicações deve ser pautado pela dor e desconforto (ACPSEM, 2010)
- Durante esse período de descarga inicial, é mantida a amplitude de movimento nas articulações não afetadas e as atividades de condicionamento geral são continuadas, embora não comprometam/estressem o local da avulsão
- Após a fase inicial de cicatrização da fratura, um programa de carga gradual é iniciado, levando em consideração as tensões aplicadas nos tecidos afetados
- Um programa de reabilitação graduado terá como objetivo recuperar toda a amplitude de movimento da articulação afetada e daqueles ao seu redor (p. ex., coluna lombar). O jogador deve recuperar boa força, potência e flexibilidade muscular do membro como um todo, bem como o comprimento neural, capacidade cardiovascular e habilidade pliométrica antes de progredir para atividades esportivas específicas
- É utilizado um retorno ao jogo em fases (ver seção *Retorno ao treinamento e retorno ao jogo adiante*).

Ossos em Crescimento: Anatomia e Fraturas Capítulo | 30 |

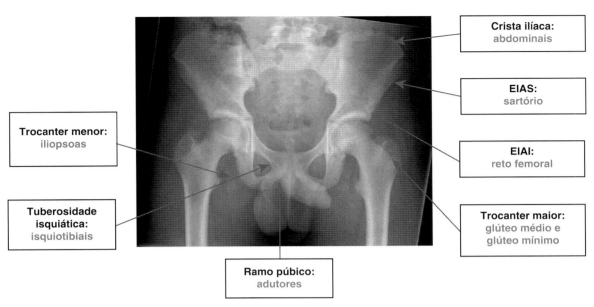

Figura 30.5 Radiografia pélvica pediátrica demonstrando locais de avulsões pélvicas e músculos envolvidos. *EIAI*, espinha ilíaca anteroinferior; *EIAS*, espinha ilíaca anterossuperior.

Tabela 30.1 Fraturas por avulsão.

Tipo de avulsão pélvica	Músculo	Ação potencial durante a avulsão
Avulsão da espinha ilíaca anterior inferior (EIAI)	Origem do reto femoral	Pode ocorrer após a contração do reto femoral. 50% das avulsões EIAI são causadas por chutes (Schuett et al., 2015)
Avulsão da espinha ilíaca anterior superior (EIAS)	Origem do sartório	Ocorre durante a contração repentina do músculo sartório quando o quadril é estendido com o joelho flexionado (Schuett et al., 2015)
Tuberosidade isquiática	Origem dos isquiotibiais	Causada por uma carga excêntrica súbita nos isquiotibiais proximais, como ocorre no chute (Schuett et al., 2015). Pode ser diagnosticada como uma distensão do tendão da coxa erroneamente e o manejo inadequado pode levar a complicações com a não união (Gidwani et al., 2004)
Crista ilíaca	Inserção de abdominais	Ocorre com a forte contração muscular dos oblíquos internos/externos e do músculo transverso do abdome. Pode acontecer em atividades de rotação ou mudança de direção repentinas e pode incluir as que incluem balanço do braço e contração oposta do glúteo médio e tensor da fáscia lata
Trocanter menor	Inserção de iliopsoas	Contração repentina dos flexores do quadril
Ramo púbico	Origem dos adutores	Contração repentina dos adutores. Isso pode incluir mudança repentina de direção
Trocânter maior	Inserção do glúteo médio e do glúteo mínimo	Raro em pediatria, mas pode ocorrer com uma contração repentina dos rotadores laterais, por exemplo, glúteo médio/mínimo

EIAI, espinha ilíaca anteroinferior; *EIAS*, espinha ilíaca anterossuperior. (Adaptada de Gidwani, S., Jagiello, J., Bircher, M., 2004. Avulsion fracture of the ischial tuberosity in adolescents – an easily missed diagnosis, British Medical Journal 329 [7457], 99-100; Schuett, D.J., Bomar, J.D., Pennock, A.T., 2015. Pelvic apophyseal avulsion fractures: a retrospective review of 228 cases. Journal of Pediatric Orthopedics 35 [6], 617-623.)

Parte | 2 | Aplicação Clínica

Tabela 30.2 Os resultados de dois estudos em grande escala sobre fraturas apofisárias pélvicas.

Schuett et al., 2015	Rossi e Dragoni, 2001
228 casos de fraturas apofisárias pélvicas em 225 pacientes	203 casos de fraturas apofisárias pélvicas em 198 atletas adolescentes (vários esportes)
Faixa etária: 10,7 a 18,2 anos	Faixa etária: 11 a 17 anos
Idade média: 14,5 anos ± 1,4 anos nos homens; 14 anos ± 1,2 anos nas mulheres	Idade média: 13,8 anos
Homens > mulheres (76% homens *versus* 24% mulheres)	Homens > mulheres (68,5% homens *versus* 31,5% mulheres)
Avulsões apofisárias em ordem de frequência	
EIAI (49%) EIAS (30%) Tuberosidade isquiática (11%) Crista ilíaca (10%) O mecanismo de lesão mais comum foi *sprint*/corrida (39%) seguido de chute (29%) A cirurgia foi indicada em apenas 3% dos casos, o deslocamento da fratura > 20 mm aumentou o risco de não união em 26 vezes	Tuberosidade isquiática (109 casos; 54%*) EIAI (45 casos; 22%*) EIAS (39 casos; 19%*) Canto superior da sínfise púbica (7 casos; 3%*) Crista ilíaca (3 casos; 1,5%*)

*As porcentagens foram adicionadas para permitir ao leitor comparar os estudos facilmente. *EIAI*, espinha ilíaca anteroinferior; *EIAS*, espinha ilíaca anterossuperior. (Adaptada de Rossi, F., Dragoni, S., 2001. Acute avulsion fractures of the pelvis in adolescent competitive athletes: prevalence, location and sports distribution of 203 cases collected. Skeletal Radiology 30 [3], 127-131; Schuett, D.J., Bomar, J.D., Pennock, A.T., 2015. Pelvic apophyseal avulsion fractures: a retrospective review of 228 cases. Journal of Pediatric Orthopaedics 35 [6], 617-623.)

Conselhos gerais para ausências prolongadas do futebol devido a lesões

- Definir "desafios" e metas de curto e longo prazo ajudará a envolver o jovem jogador em sua reabilitação
- Incluir os pais/responsáveis no plano de manejo os ajuda a apoiar a criança. Outros membros da equipe multiprofissional, como psicólogos e equipe técnica, podem ajudar a manter a motivação do jogador durante longos períodos de lesão. O jogador também pode achar benéfico falar com outras pessoas que passaram por experiências semelhantes
- O conselho nutricional pode ser útil durante esse período, enquanto eles não são tão ativos
- Os pais podem relatar que o jogador está demonstrando problemas comportamentais/alterações de humor em casa durante um período prolongado de lesão. Tranquilize o jogador que a frustração é uma resposta comum após uma lesão significativa, mas explique que embora eles não possam controlar o que aconteceu com eles, eles podem manter uma atitude positiva e um comportamento apropriado.

Retorno ao treinamento e retorno ao jogo

Podem ser feitas alterações na intensidade, duração ou frequência do treinamento quando um jogador está retornando após uma ausência prolongada devido a uma lesão. O jogador pode participar em um regresso ao jogo em fases, com meias sessões ou trabalhos técnicos ligeiros a serem realizados inicialmente, de forma a reduzir o tempo de exposição e a carga no regresso ao treinamento.

Os atletas pediátricos devem retornar ao treinamento e completar as sessões totalmente sem problemas antes de serem expostos à intensidade e carga de uma situação de jogo ao "retornar ao jogo".

Avulsão da espinha tibial (fraturas da eminência tibial)

Essa é uma avulsão óssea do ligamento cruzado anterior (LCA) de sua inserção na eminência intercondilar. É relativamente rara e é o equivalente funcional a uma ruptura do LCA em um atleta adolescente ou adulto. Scrimshire et al. (2018) encontraram a média de idade de 11,8 anos.

Sinais e sintomas

As fraturas da eminência tibial podem mimetizar uma lesão do LCA clinicamente, com o jogador apresentando dor no joelho, hemartrose, diminuição da amplitude de movimento e dificuldade para sustentar o peso.

Tratamento

É necessária uma investigação mais aprofundada e uma revisão ortopédica. O tipo de fratura determinará se uma abordagem conservadora ou cirúrgica é apropriada.

Avulsão do tubérculo tibial

O tubérculo tibial se desenvolve a partir de um centro de ossificação secundário na tíbia proximal e se desenvolve devido à tração (Frey et al., 2009). Fraturas por avulsão são ocorrências relativamente raras e a avulsão ocorre no geral durante atividades de corrida ou salto. Frey et al. (2009) afirmam que o período mecanicamente vulnerável nos homens é de aproximadamente 13 a 16 anos de idade; idade média de 13,7 anos (variação de 11 anos e 5 meses a 17 anos e 6 meses). Pretell-Mazzini et al. (2016) encontraram que a média de idade no momento da cirurgia era de 14,6 anos; eles afirmam que devido ao fechamento da fise tibial proximal de posterior para anterior, o padrão de

320

Ossos em Crescimento: Anatomia e Fraturas — Capítulo 30

fratura depende da quantidade de fechamento da fise quando a lesão ocorre. Essas fraturas podem ser classificadas usando as classificações de Watson-Jones (Watson-Jones, 1955) ou Ogden (Ogden et al., 1980).

Frey et al. (2009) encontraram uma forte predominância de homens com essa lesão e sugerem que maiores tensões de tração são colocadas no tubérculo tibial devido ao fato de os homens geralmente serem fisicamente maiores com quadríceps mais fortes. A fise tibial também se fecha mais tarde nos homens do que nas mulheres.

Nenhuma correlação definitiva foi encontrada entre a doença de Osgood-Schlatter (DOS) e fraturas por avulsão da tíbia, mas Pretell-Mazzini et al. (2016) relataram que um histórico prévio de DOS está associado a fraturas por avulsão da tíbia em 23% dos casos nos artigos que revisaram. No entanto, eles afirmam que ainda não está claro qual a porcentagem de pacientes com DOS que desenvolverá uma fratura.

Sinais e sintomas

- Início súbito de dor na região do tubérculo tibial durante atividades de salto ou corrida
- O jogador apresenta inchaço/hemartrose no joelho, amplitude de movimento reduzida, atraso extensor e patela alta com avulsões mais significativas. A palpação do tubérculo tibial é dolorosa e pode haver um fragmento ósseo ou deformidade identificável
- A síndrome compartimental é uma complicação potencialmente grave que deve ser considerada na apresentação inicial dessa lesão (Frey et al., 2009).

Diagnóstico/imageamento

A radiografia simples ou RM são utilizadas para exames de imagem e diagnóstico.

Tratamento

O manejo da fratura depende do grau de avulsão. Esses casos podem ser tratados de maneira conservadora com imobilização por gesso ou tratados cirurgicamente com redução aberta ou artroscópica e fixação interna/fixação percutânea com parafuso.

Fraturas por avulsão do calcâneo

Avulsões do tendão de Aquiles são lesões pediátricas raras, mas Yu e Yu (2015) descrevem cargas crônicas resultando em fraturas por estresse que são diagnosticadas erroneamente como doença de Sever.

Visão geral esquemática

Uma visão geral diagramática das fraturas pediátricas e outras condições musculoesqueléticas pediátricas que podem afetar jovens atletas pode ser encontrada no Capítulo 31 (ver Figura 31.1).

Resumo

É importante para aqueles que trabalham com atletas com esqueleto imaturo estarem totalmente cientes das diferenças esqueléticas entre adultos e crianças e os tipos de fratura correspondentes. Os profissionais da saúde devem ter um baixo limiar para encaminhamento ortopédico, se houver qualquer suspeita de fratura. Isso pode ajudar no diagnóstico precoce ou até mesmo evitar a não detecção de uma fratura da placa epifisária ou avulsão do tendão/ligamento. Essas condições têm o potencial de levar a distúrbios de crescimento e podem ter implicações funcionais a longo prazo se mal manejadas.

Referências bibliográficas

ACPSEM, 2010. Acute Management of Soft Tissue Injuries. ACPSEM, Sheffield, UK.

Bachmann, L.M., Kolb, E., Koller, M.T., Steurer, J., ter Riet, G., 2003. Accuracy of Ottawa ankle rules to exclude fractures of the ankle and midfoot: systematic review. British Medical Journal 326, 417.

Bulloch, B., Neto, G., Plint, A., Lim, R., Lidman, P., Reed, M., et al., 2003. Validation of the Ottawa knee rule in children: a multicenter study. Annals of Emergency Medicine 42 (1), 48-55.

Caine, D., DiFiori, J., Maffulli, N., 2006. Physeal injuries in children's and youth sports: reasons for concern? British Journal of Sports Medicine 40 (9), 749-760.

Cepela, D.J., Tartaglione, J.P., Dooley, T.P., Patel, P.N., 2016. Classifications in brief: Salter-Harris classification of pediatric physeal fractures. Clinical Orthopaedics and Related Research 474 (11), 2531-2537.

Dowling, S., Spooner, C.H., Liang, Y., Dryden, D.M., Friesen, C., Klassen, T.P., et al., 2009. Accuracy of Ottawa Ankle Rules to exclude fractures of the ankle and midfoot in children: a meta-analysis. Academic Emergency Medicine 16 (4), 277-287.

Engebretsen, L., Steffen, K., Bahr, R., Broderick, C., Dvorak, J., Janarv, P.-M., et al., 2010. The International Olympic Committee Consensus Statement on age determination in high-level young athletes. British Journal of Sports Medicine 44 (7), 476-484.

Frey, S., Hosalkar, H., Cameron, D.B., Heath, A., Horn, B.D., Ganley, T.J., 2009. Tibial tuberosity fractures in adolescents. Journal of Children's Orthopaedics 2 (6), 469-474.

Gidwani, S., Jagiello, J., Bircher, M., 2004. Avulsion fracture of the ischial tuberosity in adolescents--an easily missed diagnosis. British Medical Journal 329 (7457), 99-100.

Ling, S.-N.J., Cleary, A.J., 2018. Are unnecessary serial radiographs being ordered in children with distal radius buckle fractures? Radiology Research and Practice 2018, 5143639.

Lozano-Berges, G., Matute-Llorente, Á., González-Agüero, A., Gómez-Bruton, A., Gómez-Cabello, A., Vicente-Rodríguez, G., et al., 2017. Soccer helps build strong bones during growth: a systematic review and meta-analysis. European Journal of Pediatrics 177, 295-310.

Malina, R.M., Bouchard, C., Bar-Or, O., 2004. Growth, Maturation, and Physical Activity. Human Kinetics, Champaign, IL.

Ogden, J.A., Tross, R.B., Murphy, M.J., 1980. Fractures of the tibial tuberosity in adolescents. The Journal of Bone and Joint Surgery. American Volume 62 (2), 205-215.

Pennock, A.T., Ellis, H.B., Willimon, S.C., Wyatt, C., Broida, S.E., Dennis, M.M., et al., 2017. Intra-articular physeal fractures of the distal femur: a frequently missed diagnosis in adolescent athletes. Orthopaedic Journal of Sports Medicine 5 (10), 2325967117731567.

Porr, J., Lucaciu, C., Birkett, S., 2011. Avulsion fractures of the pelvis – a qualitative systematic review of the literature. Journal of the Canadian Chiropractic Association 55 (4), 247-255.

Pretell-Mazzini, J., Kelly, D.M., Sawyer, J.R., Esteban, E.M.A., Spence, D.D., Warner, W.C., et al., 2016. Outcomes and complications of tibial tubercle fractures in pediatric patients: a systematic review of the literature. Journal of Pediatric Orthopedics 36 (5), 440-446.

Rossi, F., Dragoni, S., 2001. Acute avulsion fractures of the pelvis in adolescent competitive athletes: prevalence, location and sports distribution of 203 cases collected. Skeletal Radiology 30 (3), 127-131.

Salter, R.B., Harris, W.R., 1963. Injuries involving the epiphyseal plate. Journal of Bone and Joint Surgery 45 (3), 587-622.

Schiller, J., DeFroda, S., Blood, T., 2017. Lower Extremity avulsion fractures in the Pediatric and adolescent athlete. Journal of the American Academy of Orthopaedic Surgeons 25 (4), 251-259.

Schuett, D.J., Bomar, J.D., Pennock, A.T., 2015. Pelvic apophyseal avulsion fractures: a retrospective review of 228 cases. Journal of Pediatric Orthopedics 35 (6), 617-623.

Scrimshire, A.B., Gawad, M., Davies, R., George, H., 2018. Management and outcomes of isolated paediatric tibial spine fractures. Injury 49 (2), 437-442.

Ting, B.L., Kalish, L.A., Waters, P.M., Bae, D.S., 2016. Reducing cost and radiation exposure during the treatment of pediatric greenstick fractures of the forearm. Journal of Pediatric Orthopedics 36 (8), 816-820.

Vorlat, P., De Boeck, H., 2003. Bowing fractures of the forearm in children. Clinical Orthopaedics and Related Research 413, 233-237.

Watson-Jones, R., 1955. Fractures and Joint Injuries, vol. 2, fourth ed. Lippincott Williams & Wilkins, Baltimore.

Williams, K.G., Smith, G., Luhmann, S.J., Mao, J., Gunn 3rd, J.D., Luhmann, J.D., 2013. A randomized controlled trial of cast versus splint for distal radial buckle fracture. Pediatric Emergency Care 29 (5), 555-559.

Yu, S.M., Yu, J.S., 2015. Calcaneal avulsion fractures: an often forgotten diagnosis. American Journal of Roentgenology 205 (5), 1061-1067.

Capítulo | 31 |

Ossos em Crescimento: Osteocondroses e Condições Pediátricas Graves

Diane Ryding

Introdução

Este capítulo apresenta uma visão geral das osteocondroses articulares e não articulares, com seus princípios de manejo relativos a um ambiente de academia de futebol de elite. Ele também aborda condições graves e sinistras nas quais o diagnóstico pode perder-se, além de processos de doenças, como infecções e tumores nos ossos ou nas articulações.

No fim deste capítulo, há uma seção de resumo com a visão geral da faixa etária de ocorrências das doenças abrangidas por este e pelo Capítulo 30.

Osteocondroses

Osteocondrose é o termo utilizado para descrever um grupo de doenças autolimitadas que afetam o esqueleto em crescimento. Elas são classificadas como *apofisite não articular* ou *de tração* se afetarem os centros de ossificação secundários, *intra-articulares* caso atinjam uma articulação (causando necrose) ou *fisária* como na doença de Sheuermann. Elas resultam de um período de crescimento, lesão ou uso excessivo da placa de crescimento em desenvolvimento e centros de ossificação circundantes (Atanda et al., 2011).

Osteocondroses não articulares: apofisite de tração

- Apofisite do tubérculo tibial (doença de Osgood-Schlatter [DOS])
- Apofisite do polo da patela (síndrome de Sinding-Larsen Johansson)
- Apofisite do calcâneo (doença de Sever)
- Apofisite da cabeça do quinto metatarso (MT) (doença de Iselin).

Tratamento de apofisite e princípios de manejo

A apofisite não articular é comumente referida como "dores de crescimento", é induzida por sintomas, é de natureza autolimitada e se resolve com o fechamento da fise. A explicação da condição reduzirá as preocupações do jogador e dos pais e irá tranquilizá-los de que a dor não se deve a nenhuma patologia desconhecida ou extremamente grave.

Avaliação

Avalie e resolva qualquer tensão na musculatura dos membros inferiores, incluindo iliopsoas, quadríceps, isquiotibiais, gastrocnêmico e sóleo, que pode demonstrar rigidez após períodos de rápido crescimento. Da mesma maneira, avalie se há fraqueza na musculatura dos membros inferiores (incluindo os músculos glúteos). Identifique quaisquer anomalias biomecânicas e encaminhe para podologia, conforme apropriado.

Modificação de atividade

O manejo de carga pode ser adotado para gerenciar os sintomas e permitir que os níveis de dor permaneçam dentro dos limites aceitáveis para o jogador. Podem ser feitas alterações na intensidade, duração ou frequência dos treinos, com a utilização de meias-sessões ou trabalhos técnicos ligeiros de modo a reduzir a carga. Considere a carga combinada de outras atividades ou esportes dos quais a criança participa fora do futebol.

Estratégias de autogestão

A aplicação de gelo após o treino pode aliviar a dor.

Reabilitação

Um período de reabilitação pode ser necessário se o jogador estiver lutando para lidar com a carga de treinamento modificada. Durante esse tempo, outros aspectos do desenvolvimento físico do jogador também podem ser abordados, por exemplo, força funcional da parte superior/inferior do corpo, controle neuromuscular e flexibilidade. O jogador pode trabalhar para manter sua capacidade cardiovascular por meio de atividades cardiovasculares de baixa carga, mas de alta intensidade. Se o jogador for incapaz de completar os exercícios de reabilitação devido à dor, um breve período de descanso pode ser benéfico.

Retorno gradual ao jogo

Se um jogador não estiver jogando devido a sintomas, um retorno gradual ao jogo pode ser adotado com o uso de meias-sessões ou gerenciamento de carga por modificação da duração ou intensidade das sessões.

Apofisite de tração do tubérculo tibial (doença de Osgood-Schlatter)

A DOS é uma apofisite de tração do tubérculo tibial causada por esforço repetitivo no tendão do quadríceps (Circi et al., 2017). Apresenta-se em crianças em crescimento (meninos, 12 a 15 anos; meninas, 8 a 12 anos), é devido à tensão repetitiva no centro de ossificação secundário do tubérculo tibial e os sintomas são exacerbados com frequência por atividades de corrida ou salto ou por contato direto, como ajoelhar (Gholve et al., 2007). As alterações radiográficas incluem irregularidade da apófise com separação do tubérculo tibial nos estágios iniciais devido a microavulsões que ocorrem no tubérculo tibial condrofibro-ósseo; a fragmentação pode ocorrer em estágios posteriores (Circi et al., 2017; Gholve et al., 2007). A condição pode reaparecer por 12 a 18 meses antes que o jogador atinja a maturidade esquelética nessa região e haja o fechamento da apófise (Circi et al., 2017).

Sinais e sintomas

- Pode manifestar-se unilateral ou bilateralmente
- A dor aumenta durante ou após a atividade esportiva (correr/pular)
- A dor costuma ser exacerbada pelo teste resistido do quadríceps
- É provável que haja tensão nos membros inferiores, de maneira específica (mas não exclusivamente) envolvendo o quadríceps. O jogador demonstra com frequência uma redução na medida do calcanhar às nádegas no teste de flexão do joelho em pronação devido a um surto de crescimento
- A dor é relatada no tubérculo tibial no quadríceps resistido ou ao agachar ou realizar afundo
- Há dor à palpação do tubérculo tibial
- Avalie biomecânica alterada, pronação excessiva/varo da porção traseira do pé
- A longo prazo, o jogador pode desenvolver uma proeminência óssea permanente e indolor sobre o tubérculo tibial.

Diagnóstico

Normalmente, o diagnóstico é feito pela avaliação clínica, mas as alterações podem ser observadas na radiografia simples, na ultrassonografia ou na ressonância magnética (RM).

Plano de tratamento e manejo

Consulte os princípios de tratamento e manejo da apofisite, com atenção específica aos alongamentos do quadríceps.

Apofisite do polo inferior da patela (síndrome de Sinding-Larsen Johansson)

Esse tipo de apofisite afeta o tendão proximal da patela em sua inserção no polo inferior da patela. É uma condição autolimitada, ocorrendo entre 10 e 14 anos de idade (Carr et al., 2001).

Sinais e sintomas

- Pode manifestar-se unilateral ou bilateralmente
- A dor aumenta durante ou após a atividade esportiva
- A dor costuma ser exacerbada pelo teste resistido do quadríceps
- Há dor e sensibilidade pontual à palpação do polo da patela com possível edema dos tecidos moles
- Há tensão/fraqueza nos membros inferiores envolvendo especificamente o quadríceps assim como a DOS.

Diagnóstico, tratamento e plano de manejo

A doença de Sinding-Larsen Johansson costuma ser um diagnóstico clínico, mas as alterações podem ser observadas por meio de ultrassonografia, radiografias ou RM. O manejo é semelhante ao dado nos princípios de tratamento e manejo da apofisite, com atenção específica aos alongamentos do quadríceps.

Apofisite do calcâneo (doença de Sever)

A apofisite calcânea provoca dor no calcanhar relacionada à placa de crescimento apofisária do calcâneo. Ocorre entre as idades de 8 e 15 anos (James et al., 2013), com a média de idade na apresentação sendo de 10 a 10,8 anos (Davison et al., 2016; Rachel et al., 2011). Sua etiologia é desconhecida, mas o aumento da tensão no tendão de Aquiles (TA) devido ao crescimento rápido pode criar tração na placa de crescimento da apófise do calcâneo. Anormalidades biomecânicas também podem contribuir para a dor no calcanhar.

Sinais e sintomas

Com base em Scharfbillig et al. (2008) a apofisite do calcâneo se apresenta da seguinte maneira:

- Pode ser unilateral ou bilateral e presente após um período de rápido crescimento
- Não há histórico de trauma
- A dor piora durante/após a atividade esportiva, mas melhora com o repouso e melhora pela manhã
- Há dor e sensibilidade na inserção do TA no calcâneo ou a dor pode se estender ao redor dos lados do calcâneo ou por baixo
- Há um teste de compressão positivo, em que a compressão médio-lateral da área apofisária do calcâneo provoca dor na ausência de trauma sério
- Provoca dor ao ficar na ponta dos pés ou na dorsiflexão passiva
- Tensão no gastrocnêmio/sóleo está presente frequentemente.

Diagnóstico/imageamento

Este é um diagnóstico clínico; imagens costumam ser necessárias, a menos que haja suspeita de avulsão.

Plano de tratamento e manejo

A abordagem do tratamento é fundamentada em uma combinação de fisioterapia (com atenção específica aos alongamentos do gastrocnêmio e sóleo), avaliação biomecânica, uso de elevação do calcanhar e modificação da carga. Consulte também o tratamento da apofisite e os princípios de manejo.

As considerações biomecânicas (James et al., 2013) podem ser resumidas da seguinte maneira:

- Uma posição valgo da porção traseira do pé pode afetar o mecanismo do molinete (windlass) e alterar a força necessária no TA
- Se forças de impacto repetitivas forem consideradas causadoras de trauma na apofisite, o uso de uma órtese com calcanhar ou elevação com propriedades de absorção de choque pode ser útil para amortecimento e alívio da dor dos tecidos moles do calcâneo
- Uma elevação precoce do calcanhar ou discrepância no comprimento da perna pode aumentar a carga do TA. Um salto alto pode ser utilizado para corrigir esses problemas, mas deve ser inserido em cada troca de sapato.

Wiegerinck et al. (2016) compararam uma abordagem "esperar para ver" com elevação do calcanhar ou exercício excêntrico em uma escala de tempo de 6 semanas e 3 meses; cada um

Ossos em Crescimento: Osteocondroses e Condições Pediátricas Graves **Capítulo** |31|

resultou em uma redução clinicamente relevante e estatisticamente significativa da dor no calcanhar devido à apofisite do calcâneo. De uma perspectiva relatada pela criança, no estágio de 6 semanas, o grupo de aumento do calcanhar melhorou mais do que o de "esperar para ver", e de uma perspectiva parental, os exercícios excêntricos melhoraram mais do que o grupo de "esperar para ver". O autor conclui que os pacientes e pais devem ser consultados sobre sua opção de tratamento preferida.

James et al. (2016) encontraram uma vantagem relativa no uso de levantamentos de calcanhar com relação às órteses préfabricadas na escala de tempo de 1 e 2 meses. No entanto, no estágio de 6 e 12 meses, eles não encontraram nenhuma vantagem relativa de nenhuma das abordagens de tratamento. Isso sugere que a elevação do calcanhar nos estágios iniciais da terapia pode ajudar as crianças com a doença de Sever a permanecerem fisicamente ativas.

Dicas clínicas

Revise o calçado que a criança está utilizando (tênis/tênis escolares); desencoraje-os a optar por tênis planos sem amortecimento suficiente para o calcanhar ou apoio da porção medial do pé. Aconselhe o jogador a usar tênis em casa, em vez de pés descalços, se estiver lutando com os sintomas. Se a elevação do calcanhar for fornecida como parte do plano de manejo, explique à criança a importância crescente do alongamento dos músculos gastrocnêmio e sóleo.

Apofisite da base do quinto metatarso (doença de Iselin)

A doença de Iselin é uma osteocondrose ou apofisite de tração na base do quinto MT. A radiografia pode mostrar uma aparência fragmentada da apófise com crescimento ósseo excessivo (Gillespie, 2010). A doença de Iselin é causada por pequenos traumas repetitivos devido à força no tendão fibular curto. Afeta homens e mulheres e aparece pela primeira vez em radiografias aproximadamente aos 8 a 11 anos de idade em meninos e 11 a 14 anos em meninas (Forrester et al., 2017). A fusão da apófise geralmente está completa aos 17 a 18 anos de idade (Gillespie, 2010).

Sinais e sintomas

- Pode haver causa não traumática (início insidioso) ou traumática (lesão por inversão do tornozelo)
- Dor e aumento da sensibilidade são encontrados na palpação até a quinta base do MT na inserção do fibular curto
- Pode haver inchaço observável na face lateral do pé e o jogador pode estar mancando devido à dor.

Diagnóstico/imageamento

Este é um diagnóstico clínico, mas a radiografia pode ser necessária para descartar uma fratura ou um osso acessório, como o os vesalianum, que pode causar dor.

Plano de tratamento e manejo

Consulte os princípios de tratamento e manejo da apofisite. Um período de imobilização pode ser necessário em casos mais graves e a excisão cirúrgica ou fixação ocasional é necessária se houver dor contínua ou não união.

Osteocondrose articular

Este grupo inclui o seguinte:
- Doença de Legg-Calvé-Perthes (DLCP)
- Osteocondrite dissecante (OCD)
- Doença de Köhler
- Doença de Freiberg.

Doença de Legg-Calvé-Perthes

A DLCP é uma necrose avascular (NAV) idiopática da epífise proximal do fêmur. É comumente observada em crianças com idades entre 4 e 8 anos, com um viés masculino (proporção masculino/feminino de 4:1); é bilateral em 10 a 13% dos casos (Ramachandran e Reed, 2016).

A DLCP é considerada um processo patogênico multifatorial. Leroux et al. (2017) afirmam que a DLCP se desenvolve após dois episódios de isquemia (duplo insulto) pelo menos, mas o possível envolvimento de microtrauma, agressões ambientais, condições pré-natais, fatores genéticos ou hipercoagulabilidade permanece controverso.

Sinais e sintomas

- A criança está mancando. Dor referida na virilha, coxa ou joelho pode estar presente sem qualquer histórico de trauma. No entanto, a dor pode não ser intensa e a claudicação pode ser o achado significativo
- Redução da abdução e rotação interna do quadril no exame.

Diagnóstico e tratamento

A radiografia simples e/ou exames de RM são utilizados para confirmar o diagnóstico. Embora não seja indicada em todos os casos, uma abordagem cirúrgica (comumente osteotomia) visa prevenir a perda de congruência articular, restaurando a epífise à sua posição central dentro do copo acetabular. Como consequência, isso orienta o processo de remodelamento (Leroux et al., 2017). A reabilitação pós-operatória dependerá da cirurgia. Na faixa etária mais jovem, repouso (cargas na região específica) e anti-inflamatórios podem ser aconselhados como uma abordagem não operatória.

Osteocondrite dissecante

A OCD é uma alteração idiopática focal do osso subcondral com risco de instabilidade e ruptura da cartilagem articular adjacente que pode resultar em osteoartrite prematura (Edmonds e Shea, 2013). A etiologia não é completamente compreendida, mas trauma agudo, microtrauma repetitivo, insuficiência vascular local e fatores genéticos foram propostos como causas potenciais. Launay (2015) sugere um viés masculino com uma proporção masculino:feminino de 4:1 e uma prevalência entre as idades de 10 e 13 anos. O Grupo de Estudo Pesquisa sobre OCD do Joelho (ROCK, do inglês *Research on Osteochondritis Dissecans of the Knee*) sugere que os jovens de 12 a 19 anos são os mais afetados (ROCK, 2018).

Sinais e sintomas

O histórico e os achados clínicos podem ser vagos e o diagnóstico pode se basear em radiografias simples ou diagnóstico de RM (Bauer e Polousky, 2017). Os itens a seguir são típicos na apresentação:
- Dor articular inespecífica exacerbada pela atividade
- Dor vaga e mal localizada

Parte |2| Aplicação Clínica

- Sintomas mecânicos, como bloqueio articular, podem indicar a presença de um corpo solto
- Derrame articular
- Amplitude limitada de movimento da articulação
- Ponto de sensibilidade sobre o côndilo femoral afetado
- A atrofia do quadríceps pode ser um achado tardio.

Diagnóstico e tratamento

Radiografias simples podem ser úteis, mas a RM é recomendada para estadiamento (*i. e.*, determinar a estabilidade da lesão) (DiFiori et al., 2014), muitas vezes utilizando o Sistema de Classificação de Lesão de Cartilagem da International Cartilage Repair Society (ICRS). Os fatores que determinam se a intervenção cirúrgica é indicada incluem o estado fisário, a estabilidade do fragmento, a presença de um corpo solto, os requisitos funcionais do paciente junto com o tamanho, estágio e profundidade da lesão (Erickson et al., 2013).

Lesões semelhantes a cistos juvenis estáveis de < 1,3 mm de comprimento na RM têm a maior validade preditiva para o potencial de cura com tratamento não operatório (Krause et al., 2013). O objetivo de uma abordagem conservadora é permitir o reparo do osso subcondral ao mesmo tempo em que se obtém uma articulação funcional sem dor. Repouso e restrição de atividades físicas que causam estresse compressivo excessivo e repetitivo no joelho afetado são frequentemente aconselhados até que os sintomas desapareçam e a lesão esteja progredindo para a cura (Andriolo et al., 2018). As características da lesão, localização, envolvimento e estabilidade da cartilagem articular, maturidade esquelética e sintomatologia devem ser considerados ao planejar as progressões da reabilitação (Paterno et al., 2014; Yang et al., 2014). A fisioterapia visa proteger o tecido em cicatrização ao mesmo tempo em que busca reduzir o derrame articular, recuperar a amplitude de movimento (ADM) articular e fortalecer a musculatura dos membros inferiores. No final das contas, um retorno gradual ao jogo e uma modificação de carga são implementados. No entanto, Krause et al. (2013) sugerem que o manejo conservador pode falhar em até 50% dos casos. Fatores prognósticos negativos incluem tamanho de lesão maior, estágios de lesão mais graves e maior maturidade esquelética, com edema ou bloqueio (Andriolo et al., 2018).

Doença de Köhler

A doença de Köhler é uma rara osteocondrose idiopática do osso navicular do tarso, com a National Organization for Rare Disorders (NORD, 2004) sugerindo que pode ser o resultado de compressão relacionada ao estresse em um momento crítico durante o período de crescimento.

Sinais e sintomas

- É geralmente unilateral na apresentação
- Apresenta-se em crianças de 5 a 6 anos, mas foram relatados casos em crianças de 2 a 11 anos; tem um viés masculino (Sharp et al., 2003)
- A dor aumenta com a descarga de peso e a criança caminha na face lateral do pé. Dor e inchaço na porção medial do pé e na borda medial estão presentes na avaliação (Gillespie, 2010).

Diagnóstico e tratamento

As radiografias simples podem excluir uma fratura, mas mostram fragmentação, esclerose e estreitamento ou achatamento do osso navicular do tarso. A doença de Köhler também pode ser um achado radiográfico incidental sem dor e sensibilidade (Gillespie, 2010).

A condição em si é autolimitada por natureza e, portanto, manejada de acordo com os sintomas. O tratamento pode variar de uma "espera vigilante" a um período de imobilização. Analgésicos e órteses para os pés também podem ajudar os sintomas, que geralmente remitem em 1 ano, mas podem persistir por até 2 anos.

Doença de Freiberg

A doença de Freiberg é uma osteocondrose/osteonecrose da cabeça do MT. Ocorre geralmente na segunda cabeça do MT (68%), mas pode ocorrer nos outros MTs menores, de maneira mais comum no terceiro (27%) e, em seguida, no quarto (3%) (Carmont et al., 2009).

A etiologia é desconhecida, mas acredita-se que seja multifatorial. Trauma e problemas circulatórios (levando à NAV) desempenham um papel importante, mas não único. A idade de início varia na literatura, mas parece ocorrer em todas as idades após a adolescência. Al-Ashhab et al. (2013) encontraram que a média de idade era de 18,3 anos (variação de 14 a 24 anos) em 10 pacientes do sexo feminino. Há uma tendência de mulher para homem de 5:1 de acordo com Katcherian (1994).

Sinais e sintomas

A doença de Freiberg normalmente se apresenta com:
- Dor (e possivelmente inchaço) na cabeça do segundo MT (ou menor cabeça do MT)
- Marcha antálgica, dor ou rigidez na mobilização
- A dor aumenta com a atividade
- A dor aumenta ao aumentar a carga de peso no antepé, como em calçados de salto alto
- Um pequeno derrame pode ser palpável e um calo pode ser visto abaixo da cabeça afetada do MT (Lin e Liu, 2013).

Diagnóstico e tratamento

Radiograficamente, a segunda cabeça (ou afetada) do MT pode parecer achatada, com áreas de esclerose aumentada e fragmentação (Lin e Liu, 2013).

O tratamento conservador com foco na descarga e alívio do estresse é uniformemente aceito como o manejo inicial adequado (Cerrato, 2011). A redução ou modificação da atividade é recomendada e Schade (2015) sugere medicação anti-inflamatória não esteroide, preenchimento (sob a cabeça do MT), órteses ou imobilização como opções de tratamento conservador.

Se o tratamento conservador falhar, existe uma grande variedade de procedimentos cirúrgicos, mas Schade (2015) sugere que o procedimento ideal é desconhecido.

Osteocondrose fisária

Doença de Scheuermann

Na doença de Scheuermann, há um desenvolvimento anormal da coluna torácica, onde o aspecto anterior da vértebra não se desenvolve tão rapidamente quanto o aspecto posterior; isso

Ossos em Crescimento: Osteocondroses e Condições Pediátricas Graves **Capítulo** | **31** |

produz uma deformidade em forma de cunha característica vista nas radiografias e, como consequência, causa a hipercifose característica. Outros sinais radiográficos incluem nódulos de *Schmorl*, achatamento anterior da placa terminal vertebral e descolamento anterior de uma apófise do anel. Essa osteocondrose se desenvolve antes da puberdade e é mais proeminente durante o estirão de crescimento na adolescência (Fotiadis et al., 2008), com Gokce e Beyhan (2016) sugerindo que o início típico da apresentação é de 13 a 16 anos de idade. Ainda não está claro se existe um viés de gênero.

A etiologia da cifose de Scheuermann permanece obscura, sendo condição idiopática; é considerada multifatorial com influências mecânicas, metabólicas e endócrinas sendo postuladas (Bezalel et al., 2014; Ristolainen et al., 2012). Essa é uma condição autolimitante, com a progressão da doença cessando assim que o indivíduo atinge a maturidade esquelética.

Sintomas e diagnóstico

Esse é um diagnóstico predominantemente radiográfico, mas a apresentação inicial incluirá uma cifose torácica estrutural, que o paciente não consegue corrigir de maneira consciente. Essa cifose pode parecer mais óbvia na posição flexionada para frente. O movimento da coluna é reduzido e pode haver dor associada, embora ela não seja a apresentação predominante. A definição geralmente aceita, publicada por Sørensen, é que pelo menos três corpos vertebrais consecutivos com um mínimo de 5° de acunhamento devem estar presentes na radiografia para justificar o diagnóstico (Sørensen, 1964).

Tratamento

Faltam evidências de alta qualidade para o manejo conservador da doença de Scheuermann na literatura; assim, o gerenciamento dependerá do grau de cifose. Em 2010, o artigo de consenso da 7th Society on Scoliosis Orthopaedic and Rehabilitation Treatment (SOSORT) foi publicado sobre o tratamento conservador da cifose idiopática e de Scheuermann (de Mauroy et al., 2010). O consenso considerou que a rigidez da curva, localização anatômica e dor local são informações essenciais antes de decidir sobre os métodos de tratamento. O consenso concorda com a utilidade da fisioterapia e das órteses rígidas no objetivo de corrigir a hipercifose torácica durante a adolescência, com muitos optando pela fisioterapia antes da órtese. Os principais objetivos terapêuticos do exercício físico em pacientes com risco de necessitar de órtese são o autocontrole postural, o autoalongamento e o treinamento de propriocepção. Resistência muscular, exercícios de fortalecimento, alongamento (peitorais e isquiotibiais) e técnicas de respiração também estão incluídos, sendo a média de 20 minutos de exercícios em casa. O principal objetivo da órtese é evitar a hiperflexão na parede anterior. A finalidade da órtese é restaurar o alinhamento das forças musculares, reduzir a carga contínua e fornecer espaço para o desenvolvimento adequado dos discos toracolombares. A rigidez da órtese foi sugerida como a principal razão para o tratamento malsucedido.

Em termos de opções cirúrgicas, Riouallon et al. (2018) sugerem que a cirurgia de fusão primária apenas posterior e anterior/posterior (AP) combinada para cifose de Scheuermann fornece resultados funcionais e radiológicos estáveis; portanto, a técnica de fusão AP deve ser reservada para grandes deformações. A idade média na época da cirurgia era de 23 anos e a cifose média era de 77°. Um acompanhamento a longo prazo mostrou que não houve correlação entre o grau de cifose e a qualidade de vida ou a saúde autorreferida ou dor nas costas (Ristolainen et al., 2012).

Outras apresentações pediátricas cujo diagnóstico não pode ser perdido

Epífise femoral superior desviada

Uma epífise femoral superior (ou capital) desviada (EFSD/EFCD) ocorre quando há ruptura anatômica através da fise femoral proximal e deslocamento do colo femoral com relação à cabeça do fêmur. A cabeça femoral permanece posicionada anatomicamente no acetábulo enquanto a metáfise se move anterior e superiormente com relação à epífise. A EFSD pode se manifestar após um pequeno trauma, mas geralmente seu início é insidioso por natureza. A causa exata dessa condição é desconhecida, mas Alshryda et al. (2018) sugerem que o aumento das forças de cisalhamento e fraqueza da fise durante a adolescência podem ser fatores contribuintes. Fatores hormonais e o excesso de peso da criança também foram propostos.

Naseem et al. (2017) sugerem uma incidência de 1 a 10/100.000. Boles e El-Khoury (1997) sugerem que os homens são mais afetados do que as mulheres, com o pico de idade de ocorrência de EFSD sendo ligeiramente maior para meninos (variação de 10 a 17 anos; média de 13 a 14 anos) do que para meninas (variação de 8 a 15 anos; média de 11 a 12 anos). Os desvios são classificados com frequência como estáveis se o paciente for capaz de suportar peso (com ou sem muletas) ou instáveis se o suporte de peso não for possível (Loder et al., 1993). No entanto, Alshryda et al. (2018) sugerem que os pesquisadores estão desafiando essa definição. A identificação imediata de EFSD é crucial, pois o manejo subótimo pode levar a incapacidades substanciais.

Sinais e sintomas

Os sinais e sintomas de EFSD incluem:

- Dor no quadril/coxa e/ou joelho. Pode ser um início súbito (não traumático) ou gradual ao longo de um período de meses. A dor no quadril pode ser referida ao joelho por meio do nervo obturador medial; portanto, qualquer criança com dor no joelho também deve ser submetida a um exame de quadril
- Andar claudicante, antálgico ou rotacionado externamente com possíveis sinais de Trendelenburg
- A rotação externa da perna afetada e uma discrepância no comprimento da perna podem ser aparentes
- Reduzida ADM do quadril, sobretudo rotação interna com dor e proteção.

Diagnóstico e tratamento

Na suspeita do jogador ter EFSD, forneça-o muletas (sem suporte de peso, ou seja, sem apoio no membro em questão) e providencie o encaminhamento imediato a um pronto-socorro para avaliação médica. Uma radiografia simples costuma ser a investigação diagnóstica primária.

Uma EFSD exigirá pinagem cirúrgica, para manter os ossos no lugar até que a placa epifisária se funda. O tipo de fixação dependerá da distância que a cabeça do fêmur deslocou. Alguns cirurgiões podem defender a fixação do lado não afetado para evitar futuros desvios, pois aproximadamente 20% dos pacientes apresentam desvios bilaterais, mas isso é controverso. As complicações a longo prazo incluem osteoartrite, condrólise e NAV, com um estudo de Loder et al. (1993) encontrando NAV desenvolvida em 47% dos desvios instáveis (14 de 30 quadris), mas em

327

nenhum dos desvios estáveis (0 de 25). O processo de reabilitação é orientado pelo cirurgião ortopédico.

Impacto femoroacetabular

O consenso de Warwick de 2016 definiu a síndrome do impacto femoroacetabular (IFA) como "um distúrbio clínico do quadril relacionado ao movimento com uma tríade de sintomas, sinais clínicos e achados de imagem. Representa o contato prematuro sintomático entre o fêmur proximal e o acetábulo" (Griffin et al., 2016, p. 1170).

Existem dois tipos de morfologia de IFA, *cam* ou *came* e *em pinça*, os quais podem ocorrer de maneira independente ou simultânea. No entanto, a presença de morfologia came e/ou pinça nem sempre leva ao IFA (van Klij et al., 2018).

Morfologia de came ou cam. É mais prevalente em homens do que mulheres (23,9 *versus* 9,9%) (*Pf* < 0,001) (Li et al., 2017). Também é mais prevalente em adultos do que em adolescentes, mas demonstrou aumentar gradualmente durante o crescimento do esqueleto (van Klij et al., 2018). A morfologia de came foi observada a partir dos 10 anos de idade (Palmer et al., 2018).

Morfologia em pinça. Igualmente comum em homens e mulheres (29,7 *versus* 35,1%) (Li et al., 2017), com morfologia em pinça sendo observada a partir dos 12 anos de idade (Li et al., 2017; Monazzam et al., 2013).

Ross et al. (2017) revisaram a cirurgia para IFA em 39 pacientes com esqueleto imaturo e determinaram uma idade média de 15,8 anos (intervalo de 12,8 a 19,3 anos).

Sintomas e diagnóstico

As informações a seguir baseiam-se no consenso de Warwick por Griffin et al. (2016):

Os sintomas, sinais clínicos e achados de imagem devem estar presentes para diagnosticar a síndrome IFA:
- Dor no quadril, estalidos, travamento, rigidez ou fraqueza
- Dor no quadril/virilha relacionada ao movimento; também pode ser relatada dor nas costas, nádegas ou coxa
- Teste de ADM restrita do quadril, teste FARI positivo (flexão, adução e rotação interna) – que é sensível, mas não específico
- Achados radiológicos de morfologia came ou pinça. A tomografia computadorizada (TC), RM ou injeções intra-articulares no quadril também podem auxiliar no diagnóstico.

Tratamento

A abordagem conservadora inclui educação do paciente, modificação da atividade e analgesia. A fisioterapia inclui ADM do quadril, estabilidade do quadril (ativação glútea), controle neuromuscular e dissociação lombopélvica.

A abordagem cirúrgica tem como objetivo corrigir a morfologia do quadril. A fisioterapia pós-operatória é uma abordagem geralmente com base em critérios conduzida pelo protocolo pós-operatório (que é específico do cirurgião/cirurgia).

Espondilólise e espondilolistese lombar

A dor lombar no adolescente (DLA) é comum na população de atletas, mas o conhecimento da apresentação da espondilólise e espondilolistese no atleta adolescente é importante para que os resultados ideais sejam alcançados.

Espondilólise

A espondilólise é um defeito ósseo ou fratura por estresse que se desenvolve por meio da *pars interarticularis* ou arco vertebral como a parte mais fraca da vértebra; pode ocorrer unilateral ou bilateralmente. Uma fratura é "completa" se passar pela *pars* ou "incompleta" se aparecer em um lado do córtex e não no outro (Gregory et al., 2004).

A espondilólise pode ocorrer em qualquer idade ou em qualquer nível, mas a grande maioria ocorre em L5 (85 a 95%), seguida por L4 (5 a 15%), com a incidência parecendo ser maior na população atlética jovem (Standaert e Herring, 2000). Em um estudo com jogadores de críquete e jogadores de futebol, Gregory et al. (2004) descobriram que a idade mediana de início da dor lombar foi de 17,5 anos (intervalo de 11,5 a 44 anos) com a maioria das fraturas completas sendo identificadas em L5 (66,7%), seguido por L3 (15,7%), depois L4 (6,9%). As fraturas incompletas distribuíram-se de maneira mais uniforme nos três níveis lombares inferiores, predominando L5 (41,7%), seguido de L4 (37,5%) e L3 (20,8%).

Acredita-se que a espondilólise seja de desenvolvimento ou adquirida secundariamente a trauma crônico de baixo grau (Leone et al., 2011). No desenvolvimento, o processo de ossificação *pars interarticularis* ocorre de posterior para anterior e a incompletude congênita pode predispor a fraturas por estresse (Lawrence et al., 2016; Purcell e Micheli, 2009). Acredita-se que a espondilólise ou espondilolistese seja adquirida devido a fatores mecânicos, pois nenhum caso foi detectado em pacientes não ambulatoriais em comparação com a incidência de 5,8% na população geral (*P* < 0,001) (Rosenberg et al., 1981). A hiperextensão e a rotação repetidas da coluna lombar são propostas como fatores predisponentes (Gregory et al., 2004).

Espondilolistese

A espondilolistese pode ser definida como o deslocamento anterior do corpo vertebral em referência aos corpos vertebrais limítrofes (Gagnet et al., 2018). Uma classificação etiológica de espondilólise e espondilolistese foi apresentada por Wiltse et al. em 1976 e inclui cinco tipos: displásico (defeito congênito), ístmica (fadiga da *pars* após múltiplas fraturas por estresse cicatrizadas, alongamento da *pars* ou uma fratura aguda da *pars*), degenerativa, traumática ou neoplásica. Em jovens atletas, a espondilolitese ístmica é o tipo predominante identificado, onde ocorreu uma fratura da *pars* bilateral, levando ao desvio da vértebra. Isso ocorre com frequência (mas não de maneira exclusiva) em uma direção para frente e é comum um desvio de L5 em S1. Em um acompanhamento a longo prazo (45 anos) Beutler et al. (2003) descobriram que apenas os pacientes que tinham defeito na *pars* bilateral progrediram para espondilolistese.

Um método adotado para classificar a gravidade da espondilolistese é a classificação de Meyerding (Meyerding, 1932), que considera a gravidade da espondilolitese com base na porcentagem que um corpo vertebral deslizou para a frente sobre o corpo vertebral abaixo:
- Grau 1: 0 a 25%
- Grau 2: 26 a 50%
- Grau 3: 51 a 75%
- Grau 4: 76 a 99%
- Grau 5: 100%.

Capítulo | 31 |

Ossos em Crescimento: Osteocondroses e Condições Pediátricas Graves

Sintomas e diagnóstico de espondilólise

Nenhum teste clínico, sozinho ou combinado, pode distinguir entre espondilólise e outros tipos de DLA (Sundell et al., 2013), com Alqarni et al. (2015) sugerindo que o teste de hiperextensão unipodal utilizado ("teste de cegonha" em pé) não tem virtualmente valor no diagnóstico de pacientes com espondilólise. Consequentemente, Gregory et al. (2004) sugerem que todos os atletas que apresentam dor lombar relacionada à atividade que aumenta com a extensão lombar devem ser investigados para espondilólise.

A espondilólise também pode ser assintomática, mas pode ser uma causa de instabilidade da coluna, dor nas costas e radiculopatia (Leone et al., 2011) com dor irradiando para a região das nádegas ou parte posterior da coxa. Os achados clínicos podem incluir rigidez dos flexores e isquiotibiais do quadril, fraqueza dos abdominais e glúteos e uma postura lordótica excessiva (Lawrence et al., 2016).

É possível diagnosticar espondilólise por TC, RM ou por uma radiografia simples oblíqua. Embora, a TC seja mais sensível para visualizar as alterações degenerativas regionais e esclerose associada aos defeitos da *pars*, a RM é capaz de detectar edema de medula óssea precoce, o que pode sugerir uma resposta ao estresse sem uma linha de fratura visível (Leone et al., 2011). Em uma radiografia oblíqua, o "sinal do cão escocês" identificará uma espondilólise, onde um defeito/quebra na *pars interarticularis* aparece como uma coleira no "cão escocês". Em comparação com os outros dois métodos, a RM não emite radiação ionizante e, portanto, é a investigação primária preferida em atletas adolescentes com suspeita de espondilólise. É importante observar que a espondilólise pode ser um achado incidental na RM em um paciente assintomático.

Tratamento de espondilólise

Há falta de grandes ensaios clínicos controlados no manejo fisioterapêutico da espondilólise e o próprio tratamento pode depender dos achados da RM. É elaborado um programa de reabilitação com base em critérios e em torno do grau de espondilólise (unilateral/bilateral ou alto sinal e linha de fratura visível), cronogramas de cicatrização biológica e, em última análise, sintomatologia.

Na fase inicial, o jogador recebe conselhos sobre a postura e se absterá de qualquer atividade esportiva até que os sintomas se acalmem/resolvam, a fim de permitir a cicatrização óssea. Nessa fase de cura, a reabilitação pode incluir exercícios de estabilidade central estática de baixa carga e sem dor em posições apoiadas. Ocasionalmente, os cirurgiões defendem o uso de órtese espinal durante a fase de cura. Embora sejam necessários estudos maiores adicionais, há algumas evidências de que o ultrassom pulsado de baixa intensidade (UPBI) possa ser benéfico no tratamento da espondilólise lombar em estágio inicial, para melhorar os prazos de cicatrização de fraturas (Busse et al., 2002) e de retorno ao jogo (Tsukada et al., 2017).

Os exercícios progredirão à medida que os sintomas diminuírem, com a inclusão de alongamentos para os músculos isquiotibiais, glúteos ou flexores do quadril, conforme apropriado, com exercícios de mobilidade lombar/torácica e trabalho progressivo de estabilidade funcional do núcleo. Assim que os sintomas iniciais forem resolvidos, haverá uma fase de carregamento progressivo que permite escalas de tempo de cura da fratura. O jogador começará o trabalho cardiovascular de baixa carga, progredindo de volta para corrida, corrida rápida, trabalho multidirecional

e treinamento específico do esporte e um programa gradual de retorno ao jogo.

Se as lesões da *pars* lombar permanecerem sintomáticas após um longo período de tratamento conservador, pode ser necessária uma abordagem cirúrgica, como a fixação do parafuso espinal.

Sintomas e diagnóstico de espondilolistese

Pacientes com escorregamento de grau 1 ou 2 podem não apresentar sintomas e, portanto, uma abordagem conservadora será selecionada. Um jogador com espondilolistese lombar que causa compressão da raiz nervosa pode apresentar radiculopatia ou relatar "dores de pontaria" nos membros inferiores na extensão lombar. Eles podem adotar uma postura lombar cifótica para reduzir os sintomas e aliviar a pressão das raízes nervosas (Gagnet et al., 2018). Uma revisão sistemática de Alqarni et al. (2015) sugere que parece haver utilidade na palpação dos processos da coluna lombar para o diagnóstico de espondilolistese lombar. Pode haver um degrau visível ou palpável no nível do deslizamento com anormalidades dos tecidos moles associadas. Imageamento com RM, radiografia ou TC podem confirmar o diagnóstico.

Tratamento de espondilolistese

Lundine et al. (2014) descobriram que o manejo não operatório da criança minimamente sintomática ou assintomática com espondilolistese de alto grau não leva a problemas significativos.

Aqueles que não respondem ao tratamento conservador (alívio da dor, órteses e fisioterapia) ou com graus maiores de escorregamento (grau 3 e acima) podem precisar de fixação cirúrgica. Bouras e Korovessis (2015) sugerem que se um jogador for submetido a uma cirurgia (reparo da *pars* e fusão curta), o retorno ao jogo dependerá da modalidade e varia de 6 a 12 meses, com proibição em esportes de colisão.

Dica clínica

Embora o passo clássico ou palpável descrito possa estar presente em alguém com espondilolistese de alto grau, a capacidade de detectar um escorregamento de baixo grau depende do grau de escorregamento e dos tecidos moles circundantes, portanto, pode não ser perceptível. Se houver suspeita, deve ser investigado!

Infecções ósseas e articulares: artrite séptica e osteomielite aguda

A artrite séptica e a osteomielite afetam as articulações sinoviais e os ossos, respectivamente. A artrite séptica pode ocorrer de maneira isolada ou como um processo secundário relacionado à osteomielite subjacente (Monsalve et al., 2015). A artrite séptica afeta as articulações sinoviais e pode ser causada por infiltração bacteriana, viral ou fúngica. Qualquer articulação pode ser afetada, mas as infecções bacterianas afetam geralmente as articulações maiores, sobretudo joelhos, tornozelos, ombros, quadris, cotovelos ou punhos (NORD, 2009). A osteomielite costuma ser de origem bacteriana e, entre crianças e adolescentes, os ossos longos das pernas e braços são os mais afetados, especialmente a epífise (NORD, 2005). Uma infecção pode entrar na articulação por meio da corrente sanguínea por uma ferida ou lesão próxima, com infecções bacterianas que progridem com rapidez.

329

Sintomas

Um jogador com artrite séptica ou osteomielite costuma apresentar um início agudo de dor com uma articulação/membro edematoso, quente e sensível com ADM restrita e incapacidade de suportar peso. O jogador pode estar com febre, sistematicamente indisposto ou ter um histórico recente de infecção local ou trauma (incluindo escoriações simples).

Diagnóstico e tratamento

Essa é uma emergência ortopédica. É necessário o encaminhamento urgente para o setor de acidentes e emergências para investigações adicionais que podem incluir exame de sangue (hemograma completo, proteína C reativa, taxa de hemossedimentação), ultrassonografia e aspiração articular ou radiografias. Manz et al. (2018) defendem o uso de RM e detecção sistemática de patógenos, incluindo testes de ácido nucleico para limitar o uso de antibióticos de amplo espectro com a duração do tratamento. As articulações sépticas podem exigir artrotomia e lavagem na cirurgia.

Dica clínica

Se um jogador recebeu prescrição de antibióticos para uma infecção recente, eles podem mascarar os sintomas de artrite séptica e osteomielite e a apresentação pode ser mais sutil. Esteja ciente do relato de "pista falsa" de uma lesão incerta com o objetivo de explicar a apresentação.

Tumores diagnosticados erroneamente como lesões musculoesqueléticas

A mensagem importante é que a apresentação clínica de um tumor musculoesquelético pode imitar a de uma lesão esportiva. Um estudo de Muscolo et al. (2003) descobriu que, "radiografias de baixa qualidade e um diagnóstico original inquestionável, apesar dos sintomas persistentes, foram as causas mais frequentes de um diagnóstico errôneo". Toda a equipe médica que trabalha com jogadores pediátricos deve permanecer consciente dos potenciais sinais de alerta no atleta pediátrico, incluindo dor em repouso, dor noturna ou quaisquer sintomas que não se enquadrem no padrão normal ou que estejam piorando com o tempo. Deve ocorrer o encaminhamento médico imediato se o médico tiver quaisquer suspeitas.

Sarcomas são cânceres que começam nos tecidos conjuntivos, como músculos, ossos ou células de gordura. Os cânceres ósseos primários podem ocorrer em qualquer idade, mas geralmente são diagnosticados em crianças mais velhas e adolescentes (American Cancer Society, 2016) (Tabela 31.1).

Saúde óssea, crescimento, maturação e lesões

Mesmo com todo o potencial para lesões ósseas, uma revisão sistemática e meta-análise feita por Lozano-Berges et al., 2017, sugere que começar a jogar futebol na fase pré-púbere e continuar até a puberdade parece ser apropriado para melhorar a saúde óssea durante esses períodos de desenvolvimento e estágios futuros.

Enquanto a relação entre maturação, crescimento e condições musculoesqueléticas permanece plausível, Swain et al. (2018) descobriram que o corpo de conhecimento atual está sob alto risco de viés, impedindo a capacidade de estabelecer se a maturidade biológica e o crescimento são fatores de risco independentes para condições musculoesqueléticas.

Resumo

Qualquer terapeuta que trabalha com um público pediátrico deve estar ciente das lesões específicas e processos de doença que podem se apresentar no esqueleto em desenvolvimento, desde os tipos mais comuns de osteocondroses até patologias mais graves e sérias, onde o risco de diagnóstico incorreto pode ser prejudicial para uma carreira ou mesmo a vida de um jovem (Figura 31.1). Na verdade, a declaração de que "crianças não são miniadultos" não poderia ser mais precisa.

Tabela 31.1 **Sarcomas (cânceres de ossos e tecidos moles).**

Sarcoma	Locais mais comuns	Apresentação potencial
Osteosarcoma	Fêmur (42%, com 75% desses no fêmur distal) Tíbia (19%, com 80% desses na tíbia proximal) Úmero (10%, com 90% desses proximais) Crânio ou mandíbula (8%) Pelve (8%)	Distribuição bimodal da idade: primeiro pico entre 10 e 14 anos, sugerem uma relação com o estirão de crescimento do adolescente; segundo pico em adultos > 65 anos de idade Os sintomas podem incluir dor nos ossos que piora à noite ou com atividade. Inchaço ao redor do osso
Sarcoma de Ewing	Pelve, fêmur e tíbia com a parede torácica/escápula	Adolescentes e adultos jovens Sintomas de acordo com o osteossarcoma
Rabdomiossarcoma	Células do músculo esquelético	Pode ocorrer em adolescentes e adultos, mas é comumente encontrado em crianças menores de 10 anos de idade Os sintomas podem incluir caroços (dolorosos/não dolorosos), inchaço ou problemas intestinais

Adaptada de American Cancer Society, 2016. Tipos de cânceres que se desenvolvem em adolescentes. Disponível em: https://www.cancer.org/cancer/cancer-inadolescents/what-are-cancers-in-adolescents.html; Ottaviani, G., Jaffe, N., 2009. The epidemiology of osteosarcoma. Cancer Treatment and Research 152, 3-13. https://doi.org/10.1007/978-1-4419-0284-9_1.

Ossos em Crescimento: Osteocondroses e Condições Pediátricas Graves — Capítulo | 31 |

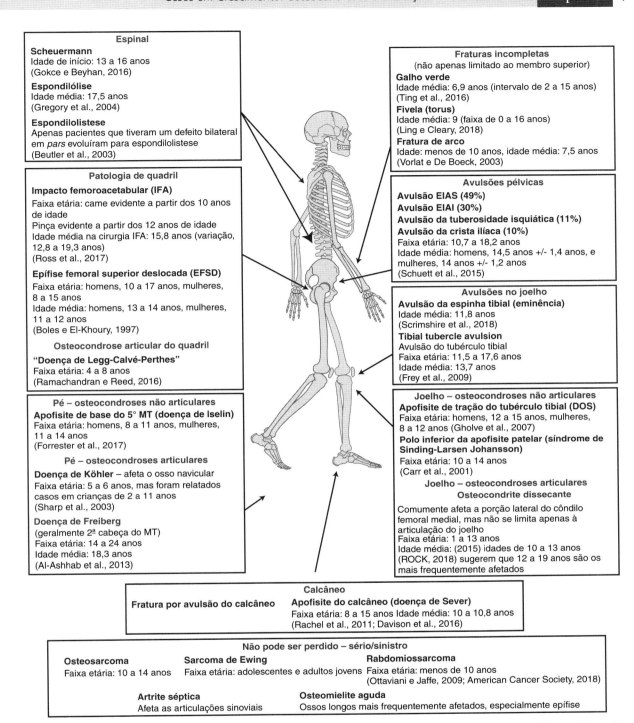

Figura 31.1 Visão geral das condições e lesões musculoesqueléticas pediátricas que podem afetar jovens atletas. *EIAI*, espinha ilíaca anteroinferior; *EIAS*, espinha ilíaca anterossuperior; *MT*, metatarso.

Referências bibliográficas

Al-Ashhab, M.E.A., Kandel, W.A., Rizk, A.S., 2013. A simple surgical technique for treatment of Freiberg's disease. The Foot 23 (1), 29-33.

Alqarni, A.M., Schneiders, A.G., Cook, C.E., Hendrick, P.A., 2015. Clinical tests to diagnose lumbar spondylolysis and spondylolisthesis: a systematic review. Physical Therapy in Sport 16, 268-275.

Alshryda, S., Tsang, K., Chytas, A., Chaudhry, M., Sacchi, K., Ahmad, M., et al., 2018. Evidence based treatment for unstable slipped upper femoral epiphysis: systematic review and exploratory patient level analysis. Surgeon 16 (1), 46-54.

American Cancer Society, 2016. Types of cancers that develop in adolescents. Available at: https://www.cancer.org/cancer/cancer-in-adolescents/what-are-cancers-in-adolescents.html.

Andriolo, L., Candrian, C., Papio, T., Cavicchioli, A., Perdisa, F., Filardo, G., 2018. Osteochondritis dissecans of the knee - conservative treatment strategies: a systematic review. Cartilage 10 (3), 267-277.

Atanda Jr., A., Shah, S.A., O'Brien, K., 2011. Osteochondrosis: common causes of pain in growing bones. American Family Physician 83 (3), 285-291.

Bauer, K.L., Polousky, J.D., 2017. Management of osteochondritis dissecans lesions of the knee, Elbow and Ankle. Clinics in Sports Medicine 36 (3), 469-487.

Beutler, W., Fredrickson, B., Murtland, A., Sweeney, C., Grant, W., Baker, D., 2003. The natural history of spondylolysis and spondylolisthesis: 45-year follow-up evaluation. Spine 28 (10), 1027-1035. discussion 1035.

Bezalel, T., Carmeli, E., Been, E., Kalichman, L., 2014. Scheuermann's disease: current diagnosis and treatment approach. Journal of Back and Musculoskeletal Rehabilitation 27 (4), 383-390.

Boles, C., El-Khoury, G.Y., 1997. Slipped capital femoral epiphysis1. Radiographics 17 (4), 809-823. Available at: https://pubs.rsna.org/doi/pdf/10.1148/radiographics.17.4.9225384.

Bouras, T., Korovessis, P., 2015. Management of spondylolysis and low-grade spondylolisthesis in fine athletes. A comprehensive review. European Journal Of Orthopaedic Surgery & Traumatology : Orthopedie Traumatologie 25 (Suppl. 1(S1)), S167-S175.

Busse, J.W., Bhandari, M., Kulkarni, A.V., Tunks, E., 2002. The effect of low-intensity pulsed ultrasound therapy on time to fracture healing: a meta-analysis. CMAJ : Canadian Medical Association Journal 166 (4), 437-441. Available at: http://www.ncbi.nlm.nih.gov/pubmed/11873920. [Accessed 19 June 2018].

Carmont, M.R., Rees, R.J., Blundell, C.M., 2009. Current concepts review: Freiberg's disease. Foot & Ankle International 30 (2), 167-176.

Carr, J.C., Hanly, S., Griffin, J., Gibney, R., 2001. Sonography of the patellar tendon and adjacent structures in pediatric and adult patients. American Journal of Roentgenology 176 (6), 1535-1539.

Cerrato, R.A., 2011. Freiberg's disease. Foot and Ankle Clinics 16 (4), 647-658.

Circi, E., Atalay, Y., Beyzadeoglu, T., 2017. Treatment of Osgood–Schlatter disease: review of the literature. Musculoskeletal Surgery 101 (3), 195-200.

Davison, M.J., David-West, S.K., Duncan, R., 2016. Careful assessment the key to diagnosing adolescent heel pain. The Practitioner 260 (1793), 30-32. 3 Available at: http://www.ncbi.nlm.nih.gov/pubmed/27382917. [Accessed 26 May 2018].

de Mauroy, J., Weiss, H., Aulisa, A., Aulisa, L., Brox, J., Durmala, J., et al., 2010. 7th SOSORT consensus paper: conservative treatment of idiopathic Scheuermann's kyphosis. Scoliosis 5 (9), 1-15. Available at: http://www.scoliosisjournal.com/content/5/1/9. [Accessed 1 June 2018].

DiFiori, J.P., Benjamin, H.J., Brenner, J.S., Gregory, A., Jayanthi, N., Landry, G.L., et al., 2014. Overuse injuries and burnout in youth sports: a position statement from the American Medical Society for Sports Medicine. British Journal of Sports Medicine 48 (4), 287-288.

Edmonds, E.W., Shea, K.G., 2013. Osteochondritis dissecans: editorial comment. Clinical orthopaedics and related research. Association of Bone and Joint Surgeons 471 (4), 1105-1106.

Erickson, B.J., Chalmers, P.N., Yanke, A.B., Cole, B.J., 2013. Surgical management of osteochondritis dissecans of the knee. Current Reviews in Musculoskeletal Medicine 6, 102-114.

Forrester, R.A., Eyre-Brook, A.I., Mannan, K., 2017. Iselin's disease: a systematic review. Journal of Foot & Ankle Surgery 56 (5), 1065-1069. 2017/08/27.

Fotiadis, E., Kenanidis, E., Samoladas, E., Christodoulou, A., Akritopoulos, P., Akritopoulou, K., 2008. Scheuermann's disease: focus on weight and height role. European Spine Journal 17 (5), 673-678.

Frey, S., Hosalkar, H., Cameron, D.B., Heath, A., David Horn, B., Ganley, T.J., 2008. Tibial tuberosity fractures in adolescents. Journal of Paediatric Orthopaedics 2 (6), 469-474.

Gagnet, P., Kern, K., Andrews, K., Elgafy, H., Ebraheim, N., 2018. Spondylolysis and spondylolisthesis: a review of the literature. Journal of Orthopaedics 15 (2), 404-407.

Gholve, P.A., Scher, D.M., Khakharia, S., Widmann, R.F., Green, D.W., 2007. Osgood Schlatter syndrome. Current Opinion in Pediatrics 19 (1), 44-50.

Gillespie, H., 2010. Osteochondroses and apophyseal injuries of the foot in the young athlete. Current Sports Medicine Reports 9 (5), 265-268.

Gokce, E., Beyhan, M., 2016. Radiological imaging findings of scheuermann disease. World Journal of Radiology 8 (11), 895-901. Baishideng Publishing Group Inc.

Gregory, P.L., Batt, M.E., Kerslake, R.W., 2004. Comparing spondylolysis in cricketers and soccer players. British Journal of Sports Medicine 38, 737-742.

Griffin, D.R., Dickenson, E.J., O'Donnell, J., Agricola, R., Awan, T., Beck, M., et al., 2016. The Warwick Agreement on femoroacetabular impingement syndrome (FAI syndrome): an international consensus statement. British Journal of Sports Medicine 50 (19), 1169-1176. 2016/09/16.

James, A.M., Williams, C.M., Haines, T.P., 2013. Effectiveness of interventions in reducing pain and maintaining physical activity in children and adolescents with calcaneal apophysitis (Sever's disease): a systematic review. Journal of Foot and Ankle Research 6 (1), 16. 2013/05/07.

James, A.M., Williams, C.M., Haines, T.P., 2016. Effectiveness of footwear and foot orthoses for calcaneal apophysitis: a 12-month factorial randomised trial. British Journal of Sports Medicine 50 (20), 1268-1275. 2016/02/27.

Katcherian, D.A., 1994. Treatment of Freiberg's disease. The Orthopedic Clinics of North America 25 (1), 69-81. Available at: http://www.ncbi.nlm.nih.gov/pubmed/8290232. [Accessed 25 June 2018].

Krause, M., Hapfelmeier, A., Möller, M., Amling, M., Bohndorf, K., Meenen, N.M., 2013. Healing predictors of stable juvenile osteochondritis dissecans knee lesions after 6 and 12 months of nonoperative treatment. The American Journal of Sports Medicine, 41(10). SAGE PublicationsSage CA, Los Angeles, CA, pp. 2384-2391.

Launay, F., 2015. Sports-related overuse injuries in children. Orthopaedics & Traumatology: Surgery & Research 101 (1), S139-S147.

Lawrence, K.J., Elser, T., Stromberg, R., 2016. Lumbar spondylolysis in the adolescent athlete. Physical Therapy in Sport, 20. Elsevier, pp. 56-60.

Leone, A., Cianfoni, A., Cerase, A., Magarelli, N., Bonomo, L., 2011. Lumbar spondylolysis: a review. Skeletal Radiology, 40(6). Springer-Verlag, pp. 683-700.

Leroux, J., Abu Amara, S., Lechevallier, J., 2017. Legg-Calve-Perthes disease. Orthopaedics & Traumatology: Surgery Research. 2017/11/21.

Li, Y., Helvie, P., Mead, M., Gagnier, J., Hammer, M.R., Jong, N., 2017. Prevalence of femoroacetabular impingement morphology in asymptomatic adolescents. Journal of Pediatric Orthopedics 37 (2), 121-126.

Lin, H.-T., Liu, A.L.-J., 2013. Freiberg's infraction. Case Reports 2013 (jun18 1). p. bcr2013010121-bcr2013010121.

Ling, S.-N.J., Cleary, A.J., 2018. Are unnecessary serial radiographs being ordered in children with distal radius buckle fractures? Radiology Research and Practice 5143639.

Loder, R.T., Richards, B.S., Shapiro, P.S., Reznick, L.R., Aronson, D.D., 1993. Acute slipped capital femoral epiphysis: the importance of physeal stability. The Journal of Bone and Joint Surgery. American Volume 75 (8), 1134-1140. Available at: http://www.ncbi.nlm.nih.gov/pubmed/8354671. [Accessed 28 May 2018].

Lozano-Berges, G., Matute-Llorente, A., González-Agüero, A., Gómez-Bruton, A., Gómez-Cabello, A., Vicente-Rodríguez, G., et al. 2018. Soccer helps build strong bones during growth: a systematic review and meta-analysis. European Journal of Pediatrics 177, 295-310.

Lundine, K.M., Lewis, S.J., Al-Aubaidi, Z., Alman, B., Howard, A.W., 2014. Patient outcomes in the operative and nonoperative management of high-grade spondylolisthesis in children. Journal of Pediatric Orthopedics 34 (5), 483-489.

Manz, N., Krieg, A.H., Heininger, U., Ritz, N., 2018. Evaluation of the current use of imaging modalities and pathogen detection in children

Ossos em Crescimento: Osteocondroses e Condições Pediátricas Graves

with acute osteomyelitis and septic arthritis. European Journal of Pediatrics 177 (7), 1071-1080.

Meyerding, H.W., 1932. 'Spondyloptosis. Surgery, Gynecology & Obstetrics 54, 371-377.

Monazzam, S., Bomar, J.D., Dwek, J.R., Hosalkar, H.S., Pennock, A.T., 2013. Development and prevalence of femoroacetabular impingement-associated morphology in a paediatric and adolescent population. The Bone & Joint Journal 95–B (5), 598-604.

Monsalve, J., Kan, J.H., Schallert, E.K., Bisset, G.S., Zhang, W., Rosenfeld, S.B., 2015. Septic arthritis in children: frequency of coexisting unsuspected osteomyelitis and implications on imaging work-up and management. American Journal of Roentgenology 204 (6), 1289-1295.

Muscolo, D.L., Ayerza, M.A., Makino, A., Costa-Paz, M., Aponte-Tinao, L.A., 2003. Tumors about the knee misdiagnosed as athletic injuries. The Journal of Bone and Joint Surgery. American Volume 85–A (7), 1209-1214. Available at: http://www.ncbi.nlm.nih.gov/pubmed/12851344. [Accessed 25 February 2018].

Naseem, H., Chatterji, S., Tsang, K., Hakimi, M., Chytas, A., Alshryda, S., 2017. Treatment of stable slipped capital femoral epiphysis: systematic review and exploratory patient level analysis. Journal of Orthopaedics and Traumatology 18 (4), 379-394.

NORD (National Organization for Rare Disorders), 2004. Köhler Disease [online] Available at: https://rarediseases.org/rare-diseases/kohler-disease/ [Accessed 8th April 2018].

NORD (National Organization for Rare Disorders), 2005. Osteomyelitis [online] Available at: https://rarediseases.org/rare-diseases/osteomyelitis/ [Accessed 10th April 2018].

NORD (National Organization for Rare Disorders), 2009. Arthritis, Infectious [online] Available at: https://rarediseases.org/rare-diseases/arthritis-infectious/ [Accessed 9th April 2018].

Ottaviani, G., Jaffe, N., 2009. The epidemiology of osteosarcoma. Cancer Treatment and Research 152, 3-13.

Palmer, A., et al., 2018. Physical activity during adolescence and the development of cam morphology: a cross-sectional cohort study of 210 individuals. British Journal of Sports Medicine 52, 601-610.

Paterno, M.V., Prokop, T.R., Schmitt, L.C., 2014. Physical therapy management of patients with osteochondritis dissecans: a comprehensive review. Clinics in Sports Medicine 33 (2), 353-374.

Purcell, L., Micheli, L., 2009. Low back pain in young athletes. Sports Health 1(3), 212-222.

Rachel, J.N., Williams, J.B., Sawyer, J.R., Warner, W.C., Kelly, D.M., 2011. Is radiographic evaluation necessary in children with a clinical diagnosis of calcaneal apophysitis (Sever disease)? Journal of Pediatric Orthopaedics 31 (5), 548-550.

Ramachandran, M., Reed, D.W., 2016. Legg–Calvé–perthes disease of the hip. Orthopaedics and Trauma 30 (6), 461-470.

Riouallon, G., Morin, C., Charles, Y.-P., Roussouly, P., Kreichati, G., Obeid, I., et al., 2018. Posterior-only versus combined anterior/posterior fusion in Scheuermann disease: a large retrospective study. European Spine Journal 27 (9), 2322-2330.

Ristolainen, L., Kettunen, J.A., Heliövaara, M., Kujala, U.M., Heinonen, A., Schlenzka, D., 2012. Untreated Scheuermann's disease: a 37-year follow-up study. European Spine Journal 21 (5), 819-824.

ROCK (Research in Osteochondritis of the Knee), 2018. Patient Education. [online] Available at: https://kneeocd.org/patient-education/#1492949877752-4d44c196-4604 [Accessed 5th March. 2018].

Rosenberg, N.J., Bargar, W.L., Friedman, B., 1981. The incidence of spondylolysis and spondylolisthesis in nonambulatory patients. Spine 6 (1), 35-38. Available at: http://www.ncbi.nlm.nih.gov/pubmed/7209672. [Accessed 19 June 2018].

Ross, J.R., Stone, R.M., Ramos, N.M., Bedi, A., Larson, C.M., 2017. Surgery for femoroacetabular impingement in skeletally immature patients: radiographic and clinical analysis. Orthopaedic Journal of Sports Medicine 5 (7_Suppl. 6). 2325967117S0025.

Schade, V.L., 2015. Surgical management of Freiberg's infraction. Foot & Ankle Specialist 8 (6), 498-519.

Scharfbillig, R.W., Jones, S., Scutter, S.D., 2008. Sever's disease: what does the literature really tell us? Journal of the American Podiatric Medical Association 98 (3), 212-223. Available at: http://www.ncbi.nlm.nih.gov/pubmed/18487595. [Accessed 26 May 2018].

Schuett, D.J., Bomar, J.D., Pennock, A.T., 2015. Pelvic apophyseal avulsion fractures: a retrospective review of 228 cases. Journal of Pediatric Orthopaedics 35 (6), 617-623.

Scrimshire, A.B., Gawad, M., Davies, R., George, H., 2018. Management and outcomes of isolated paediatric tibial spine fractures. Injury 49 (2), 437-442.

Sharp, R.J., Calder, J.D.F., Saxby, T.S., 2003. Osteochondritis of the navicular: a case report. Foot & Ankle International 24(6), 509-513.

Sørensen, K.H., 1964. Scheuermann's Juvenile Kyphosis: Clinical Appearances, Radiography, Aetiology, and Prognosis. Munksgaard, Copenhagen.

Standaert, C.J., Herring, S.A., 2000. Spondylolysis: a critical review. British Journal of Sports Medicine 34, 415-422.

Sundell, C.G., Jonsson, H., Ådin, L., Larsén, K.H., 2013. Clinical examination, spondylolysis and adolescent athletes. International Journal of Sports Medicine 34 (3), 263-267.

Swain, M., Kamper, S.J., Maher, C.G., Broderick, C., McKay, D., Henschke, N., 2018. Relationship between growth, maturation and musculoskeletal conditions in adolescents: a systematic review. British Journal of Sports Medicine 52, 1246-1252.

Ting, B.L., Kalish, L.A., Waters, P.M., Bae, D.S., 2016. Reducing cost and radiation exposure during the treatment of pediatric greenstick fractures of the forearm. Journal of Pediatric Orthopaedics 36 (8), 816-820.

Tsukada, M., Takiuchi, T., Watanabe, K., 2017. Low-intensity pulsed ultrasound for early-stage lumbar spondylolysis in young athletes. Clinical Journal of Sport Medicine 1.

van Klij, P., Heerey, J., Waarsing, J.H., Agricola, R., 2018. The prevalence of cam and pincer morphology and its association with development of hip osteoarthritis. Journal of Orthopaedic & Sports Physical Therapy 48 (4), 230-238.

Vorlat, P., De Boeck, H., 2003. Bowing fractures of the forearm in children. Clinical Orthopaedics and Related Research 413 (413), 233-237.

Wiegerinck, J.I., Zwiers, R., Sierevelt, I.N., van Weert, H.C., van Dijk, C.N., Struijs, P.A., 2016. Treatment of calcaneal apophysitis. Journal of Pediatric Orthopaedics 36 (2), 152-157.

Wiltse, L.L., Newman, P.H., Macnab, I., 1976. Classification of spondylolisis and spondylolisthesis. Clinical Orthopaedics and Related Research (117), 23-29. Available at: http://www.ncbi.nlm.nih.gov/pubmed/1277669. [Accessed 20 June 2018].

Yang, J.S., Bogunovic, L., Wright, R.W., 2014. Nonoperative treatment of osteochondritis dissecans of the knee. Clinics in Sports Medicine 33 (2), 295–304.

Capítulo | 32 |

Evento Cardíaco no Atleta Jovem

Dean Chatterjee, Nikhil Ahluwalia e Aneil Malhotra

Introdução

A morte súbita cardíaca (MSC) em atleta jovem é um evento raro; no entanto, no esporte é vital estar ciente desse evento devastador e das suas consequências. A MSC é definida como "[...] um evento não traumático, não violento, inesperado e resultante de parada cardíaca súbita dentro de seis horas de saúde normal previamente testemunhada" (Sharma et al., 1997). A MSC é a falha inesperada da função cardíaca durante o exercício ou esporte ou imediatamente após o exercício sem trauma. O coração para de bombear de modo adequado e, portanto, o atleta perde a consciência, desmaia e morre inevitavelmente, a menos que o ritmo cardíaco normal possa ser restaurado.

Para compreender a gravidade da situação, é importante conhecer os números gerais de MSC em atletas (Harmon et al., 2015a):

- A incidência é de aproximadamente 1/50 mil
- A idade média de morte em atletas é 23 anos
- 40% das mortes em atletas são de < 18 anos de idade
- É mais comum em homens do que em mulheres (9:1)
- 90% das mortes ocorrem durante ou imediatamente após o esforço.

Analisando os dados epidemiológicos, fica claro o quão vital é estar ciente da condição. Existem várias causas de MSC, incluindo anormalidades congênitas e anatômicas, cardiomiopatias, arritmias, causas indeterminadas e adquiridas. As manifestações clínicas podem variar de dor no peito, dispneia e palpitações até tontura de esforço e síncope. Os atletas também podem ser assintomáticos.

O atendimento médico das equipes esportivas pode ser agitado e frenético, na melhor das hipóteses. São componentes essenciais para o manejo de risco para atletas (Shah et al., 2018) uma política de triagem clara para patologia cardíaca, conforme discutido adiante, e a preparação completa da equipe interdisciplinar para parada cardíaca súbita e MSC (Boxe 32.1). O leitor também pode consultar o Capítulo 42 sobre preparação para ajuda de emergência.

A triagem cardíaca pré-participação (TCP) em atletas tem como premissa a detecção de doenças cardíacas associadas à MSC. A justaposição de patologia trágica em um histórico de estado de saúde exemplar de atletas jovens tem um impacto emocional significativo e apresenta uma preocupação de saúde que salta aos olhos do público. Consequentemente, é compreensível o desejo de identificar aqueles que correm maior risco por meio de um processo de triagem. No entanto, a implementação prática de um programa robusto e eficaz é complexa. As controvérsias contemporâneas a respeito da TCP giram em torno da relação custo-efetividade, protocolo de triagem e casos falso-positivos no contexto de remodelamento cardíaco induzido por exercício.

A patologia associada à MSC pode manifestar de modo ocasional sintomas de advertência que levam ao diagnóstico por

---

> **Boxe 32.1 Preparação para o dia do jogo**
>
> Os dias de jogos costumam ser caóticos para os departamentos de medicina esportiva e, muitas vezes, combinados com as pressões do jogador e dos dirigentes. A disponibilidade da equipe também pode variar nas ligas inferiores, levando a vários aspectos de um protocolo de ação de emergência sendo executado pelo mesmo provedor (p. ex., o fisioterapeuta ou médico da equipe). Dado que a maioria dos eventos esportivos são altamente visíveis e divulgados, a gestão de cada incidente está sob escrutínio. As falhas são frequentemente enfatizadas na mídia, destacando-se a necessidade de lidar com as emergências de maneira sistemática e eficiente.
>
> Nesse ambiente, é fundamental ser sistemático e seguro ao abordar eventos como MSC. Os clínicos esportivos não lidam com lesões com risco de vida diariamente; portanto, a preparação é a chave. Uma equipe médica na jornada deve estar preparada para qualquer evento possível e a prática de cenários é fundamental. São fornecidos um resumo dos pontos-chave e uma discussão mais detalhada desse tópico (Shah et al., 2018).
>
> Embora seja útil o aumento da conscientização sobre comorbidades cardíacas em atletas por meio de triagem, são cruciais as intervenções urgentes. No caso de um colapso não traumático, deve-se presumir uma parada cardíaca súbita. É essencial que todos os membros da equipe no dia da partida estejam prontos e preparados para isso. O líder da equipe deve permanecer calmo o tempo todo e cada membro precisa conhecer o seu papel e todos devem se esforçar para alcançar o resultado ideal para o atleta. Uma abordagem sistemática deve ser seguida e revisada durante todo o evento.
>
> É essencial estar em contato regular com a equipe de gestão durante todo o evento. Será preocupante e perturbador para todos os envolvidos. A vítima não é apenas mais um atleta, mas um participante e amigo de muitos dos membros da equipe. Atualizações regulares são vitais para garantir que todos estejam informados sobre a condição do jogador e saibam os próximos passos. Os familiares do jogador podem estar no público e é vital que eles sejam mantidos avisados o tempo todo.

Adaptado de Corrado, D., Basso, C., Pavei, A., Michieli, P., Schiavon, M., Thiene, G., 2006. Trends in sudden cardiovascular death in young competitive athletes after implementation of a preparticipation screening program. JAMA 296 (13), 1593-1601.

Parte | 2 | Aplicação Clínica

meio de métodos tradicionais de saúde. Porém, muitos casos permanecem clinicamente indolentes até que um evento índice significativo, muitas vezes fatal, e a análise do eletrocardiograma (ECG) possam melhorar drasticamente a sensibilidade. A detecção precoce por meio da TCP pode mitigar o risco de MSC por meio da estratificação de risco, prevenção primária e facilitar recomendações de atividades com base em evidências (Corrado et al., 2006).

Morte súbita cardíaca em atletas

As estimativas de MSC na população jovem obtidas por meio de dados de atestados de óbito sugerem a existência de pelo menos 8 mortes por semana na Inglaterra e no País de Gales (Papadakis et al., 2009). Os enormes benefícios multissistêmicos para a saúde associados à prática regular de exercícios são vistos em nível populacional. No entanto, o risco de MSC é quase 3 vezes mais provável em atletas do que em indivíduos sedentários (Corrado et al., 2003). Isso é conhecido como o "paradoxo do exercício" e pode ser uma tragédia altamente visível, bem como uma perda significativa de anos de vida. A MSC é a causa mais comum de morte em atletas jovens no Reino Unido, durante a atividade, e também fora do campo (Wasfy et al., 2016). A fisiopatologia responsável não é clara, mas a exposição recorrente às catecolaminas associada ao exercício intenso e crônico pode induzir a manifestação fenotípica de distúrbios cardíacos subjacentes, como arritmia fatal.

A incidência de MSC em atletas é estimada em 0,3 a 8 por 100 mil atletas (Harmon et al., 2015a). Os esportes com maior incidência de MSC em atletas jovens parecem ser futebol e basquete (Harmon et al., 2011). Essa tendência pode ser decorrente de popularidade e alta aceitação desses esportes, como também das paradas repentinas e dos movimentos dinâmicos envolvidos que podem causar surtos adrenérgicos em atletas com predisposição à MSC.

Uma incidência muito maior é observada em atletas do sexo masculino em comparação com atletas do sexo feminino com uma razão de 9:1. Essa proporção chega a 19:1 entre atletas de elite (Harmon et al., 2011). Embora isso, em parte, possa ser devido à prática historicamente maior do esporte entre os homens, não explica completamente esse viés. Além disso, foi observada uma maior incidência em atletas negros do que em atletas brancos (Harmon et al., 2011).

É importante esclarecer a distinção entre MSC durante o exercício e MSC no atleta que realiza grandes volumes de exercício atlético. Estudos em nível populacional sugerem que, embora a MSC possa ocorrer durante ou logo após o exercício, sua incidência na população em geral é baixa (Papadakis et al., 2009). A triagem pré-participação é projetada para abordar a última coorte de MSC e ocorre a qualquer momento, em um indivíduo atlético. A MSC em atletas jovens e competitivos pode ocorrer fora do contexto de exercícios e até mesmo durante o sono. Isso sugere uma relação alternativa ou indireta entre surtos de catecolaminas induzidos por exercício e MSC.

Condições cardíacas relacionadas

Os primeiros programas de triagem de atletas foram estabelecidos para identificar distúrbios cardíacos subjacentes associados a arritmias ventriculares fatais. É importante direcionar um programa de rastreamento para as causas subjacentes mais importantes. No contexto da MSC, isso requer consideração da idade e do *status* atlético, pois a distribuição etiológica pode variar de acordo com essas variáveis fixas. Enquanto a doença aterosclerótica e anomalias da artéria coronariana são as causas mais prevalentes em populações não atléticas e atletas mais velhos, as cardiomiopatias hereditárias predominam em atletas jovens (Chugh e Weiss, 2015).

No geral, a doença coronariana aterosclerótica é a causa mais comum de MSC em todos os atletas. No entanto, sua patogênese não se adapta bem às tecnologias de triagem existentes. A previsão da carga de doença aterosclerótica em indivíduos assintomáticos não é recomendada devido ao custo, aos efeitos adversos das ferramentas de rastreamento e às taxas historicamente altas de falso-positivo. O foco das ferramentas de triagem existentes, sobretudo em grupos de atletas, é identificar os distúrbios cardíacos hereditários, estruturais e elétricos associados à MSC.

A avaliação clínica direcionada desta coorte pode destacar sintomas de advertência e foram relatados em 30% dos sobreviventes (Vettor et al., 2015). Esses sintomas podem incluir síncope, tontura, dor no peito, dispneia e palpitações. Isso pode ser negligenciado pelo atleta ou mesmo pelos métodos tradicionais de saúde. No entanto, é necessária a análise crítica desses sintomas para conservar o valor ou arriscar diluir de modo significativo o valor preditivo positivo.

As cardiomiopatias clinicamente quiescentes frequentemente se manifestam como anormalidades eletrocardiográficas. A cardiomiopatia hipertrófica (CMH) é mais associada à MSC na literatura americana contemporânea. O desarranjo característico dos miócitos cardíacos que é o substrato arritmogênico na CMH, com a hipertrofia ventricular, produz anormalidades no ECG em 95% dos casos. A cardiomiopatia arritmogênica ventricular direita, mais precisamente conhecida como cardiomiopatia ventricular arritmogênica (CVA), é a condição culpada mais frequente em alguns estudos europeus. Apresenta-se com alterações da onda T anterior em 80% dos casos. Também podem ser detectadas outras cardiomiopatias, como a cardiomiopatia dilatada, embora a sua sensibilidade pelo ECG seja menor. Canalopatias como a síndrome do QT longo congênito, a síndrome de Brugada e a síndrome de Wolff-Parkinson-White (WPW) também podem ser demonstradas por meio de anormalidades características dessa modalidade. No entanto, a penetrância dessas condições é incompleta e inespecífica e é importante lembrar que a triagem não é uma ferramenta de estratificação de risco, mas sim um teste diagnóstico.

A evolução do processo de triagem permitiu a expansão para detectar doenças cardíacas adicionais em uma população jovem que, se diagnosticada posteriormente, pode ter um benefício de morbidade de intervenção precoce ou vigilância, incluindo para condições como doença cardíaca valvular e aortopatias.

Anormalidades coronarianas congênitas são outra causa comumente citada de MSC, embora a anormalidade anatômica seja difícil de prever sem ferramentas de imagem cardíaca, como a ecocardiografia em primeira instância e as técnicas mais detalhadas, como a tomografia computadorizada (TC) cardíaca.

A necropsia cardíaca em indivíduos falecidos levou ao reconhecimento de uma contribuição etiológica distinta da síndrome da morte súbita por arritmia (SMSA) (Behr et al., 2007). O diagnóstico de exclusão é feito após morte súbita no contexto de exame toxicológico e coração histopatologicamente normais na necropsia. A natureza dessa condição significa que ela não é receptiva às ferramentas de diagnóstico existentes e mais estudos são necessários para caracterizá-la. Também é essencial uma avaliação familiar adicional de parentes de primeiro grau.

336

Evento Cardíaco no Atleta Jovem **Capítulo** | **32** |

Quem avaliar

O estudo da MSC e da literatura existente tende a se concentrar em atletas jovens. Isso se deve em parte à sua predisposição fisiológica ao *status* de atleta de elite e, portanto, eles são o maior foco da regulamentação do esporte e da ciência do esporte.

A implementação anterior da TCP possibilita a detecção precoce de patologias antes dos sintomas e, portanto, maior redução da população de MSC. No entanto, as características fenotípicas das quais as ferramentas de triagem dependem para detecção podem não estar presentes em jovens, e a implementação prematura pode reduzir a sensibilidade. As características de ECG que seriam consideradas anormais em adultos podem representar o "padrão de ECG juvenil" em desenvolvimento, que se resolvem de maneira espontânea e são benignas (Basu et al., 2018). A triagem com base no ECG prematuro pode interpretar erroneamente isso como doença e levar a ansiedade e subsequente investigação desnecessária. O padrão de ECG juvenil tende a se resolver por volta dos 16 anos de idade; logo, seria prudente fazer a triagem de indivíduos com idade superior (Figura 32.1).

Em contraste, o surgimento de atletas recreativos de meia-idade e atletas veteranos deve chamar a atenção para uma coorte menos estudada e que não deve ser ignorada. Nesse grupo, a distribuição relacionada à idade das etiologias da MSC significa que o foco patológico se afasta da cardiomiopatia e se direciona à doença aterosclerótica. Por isso, testar todos com os mesmos critérios não é uma opção. Pode ser necessária uma abordagem modificada para essa população, e o valor das vias tradicionais de triagem é menos claro.

A implementação de uma política nacional de rastreio cardiovascular de atletas é explorada no boxe *Estudo de caso*.

Estudo de caso

Experiência italiana

A Itália reconheceu o papel do médico do esporte e a necessidade de avaliação médica antes da participação nos esportes desde a década de 1950. Um programa patrocinado foi estabelecido nacionalmente em 1982 para fornecer atenção médica especializada e fornecer cuidados preventivos a uma população que sentia ter maior necessidade de cuidados médicos do que a população em geral. O fato de o direcionamento ser clínico, em vez de socioeconômico, possibilitou a implementação de um programa obrigatório de triagem pré-participação, incluindo avaliação cardíaca, para todos os atletas competitivos.

A triagem inicial para todos os atletas inclui ECG, avaliação física e histórico pelo custo de € 50. Dos atletas amadores selecionados, descobriu-se que 9% justificam uma investigação mais aprofundada com base na suspeita do médico; 2% apresentam anormalidades cardíacas subjacentes – entretanto, nem todos requerem tratamento ou intervenção. Os atletas olímpicos são submetidos a um programa de triagem mais intensivo, incluindo ecocardiograma e teste de esforço.

Esse programa permitiu a coleta de dados mais robustos. A análise de tendência de tempo durante um período de 26 anos após a implementação do programa de triagem demonstrou uma redução acentuada na incidência anual de MSC em atletas rastreados, com a redução do valor de pico inicial de 3,6 por 100 mil para 0,4 por 100 mil (Corrado et al., 2006). Em contraste, a incidência na população não atlética não rastreada permaneceu em 0,7 a 0,8 por 100 mil no mesmo período. Assim, o programa de triagem diminuiu a incidência de MSC em atletas para valores menores do que na população em geral.

Adaptado de Corrado, D., Basso, C., Pavei, A., Michieli, P., Schiavon, M., Thiene, G., 2006. Trends in sudden cardiovascular death in young competitive athletes after implementation of a preparticipation screening program. JAMA 296 (13), 1593-1601.

Desenho do programa de triagem

O valor preditivo positivo de um teste diagnóstico se correlaciona com a probabilidade pré-teste do indivíduo avaliado. Um resultado positivo em uma coorte não estratificada e não selecionada tem mais probabilidade de representar um falso-positivo. Portanto, o valor de um teste de rastreamento é estratificar e selecionar positivamente aqueles indivíduos com alta probabilidade de doença de base para serem submetidos ao teste diagnóstico subsequente.

Foi estabelecida pela Organização Mundial da Saúde (OMS) uma série de medidas de triagem de saúde pública como o padrão para auditar os programas de triagem propostos. Os critérios de rastreamento de Wilson e Jungner (1968) determinam que a condição rastreada deve ser: (1) um problema de saúde significativo, (2) que pode ser detectado suficientemente cedo, (3) para permitir a intervenção terapêutica; deve haver (4) uma compreensão clara da fisiopatologia, (5) o teste em si deve ser economicamente justificável e (6) deve ser aceito pela população em geral.

Com relação ao rastreamento cardíaco em atletas, os critérios (3) e (4) estão bem estabelecidos e são relacionados diretamente com a doença de base. Temos uma boa compreensão das causas mais prevalentes de MSC como resultado do estudo translacional e da pesquisa básica. Além disso, intervenções médicas e de estilo de vida eficazes existem para nos permitir alterar a progressão da doença e reduzir o risco de MSC. Estes são amplamente independentes da modalidade de rastreamento e, portanto, não dependem da ferramenta de rastreamento. Os critérios (2), (5) e (6) dependem da estrutura e dos componentes do programa. O critério (1) é ambíguo e, embora a grande tragédia da MSC seja reconhecida universalmente, a incidência geral de MSC é baixa e deve ser considerada contra os danos atribuídos à triagem da população, bem como os casos de falso-positivos submetidos a investigações em cascata e ansiedade desnecessária. De modo indireto, isso é um reflexo da especificidade dos testes de rastreamento. As ferramentas mais estabelecidas para triagem cardíaca são:

- Histórico médico e exame físico
- ECG de repouso de 12 derivações
- Ecocardiografia.

Uma combinação entre essas ferramentas tende a formar a base da maioria dos programas de TCP.

Histórico médico e exame físico

O papel inicial do histórico médico é determinar a probabilidade de pré-triagem de base de um indivíduo. O rastreamento é uma ferramenta de estratificação de risco; caso um atleta tenha alta probabilidade de doença cardíaca subjacente, como um histórico familiar de cardiomiopatia hereditária, deve ser redirecionado para avaliação de especialista apropriado.

A avaliação direta do paciente por meio de anamnese e exame físico deve ser realizada com a intenção de identificar sintomas suspeitos no atleta. No entanto, a dificuldade está em atribuir valor aos sintomas inespecíficos. A American Heart Association (AHA) defende fortemente o valor dessa avaliação e delineia um questionário de 12 pontos de alto rendimento para discriminar de maneira mais eficaz as características significativas (Maron et al., 2007).

Uma questão fundamental de custo é se um médico especialista da linha de frente é necessário para realizar esse questionamento e exame. Comparações retrospectivas de protocolos com e sem especialistas experientes sugerem que o valor inferido por

337

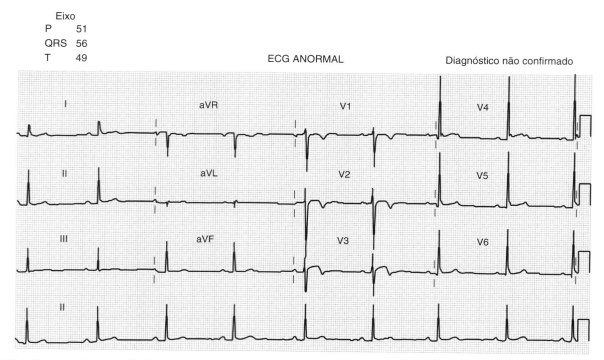

Figura 32.1 Eletrocardiograma (ECG) demonstrando um padrão juvenil típico em um atleta de 14 anos de idade. Observe a inversão da onda T anterior em V1-V2 e uma onda T bifásica em V3. Esses achados estão presentes em até 10% dos menores de 15 anos de idade e remitem na grande maioria dos casos aos 16 anos. A inversão da onda T anterior está associada à cardiomiopatia.

uma capacidade de avaliar os verdadeiros sintomas contra sintomas não relacionados, como dor torácica atípica isolada, se traduz em uma diminuição significativa na quantidade de atletas encaminhados para testes posteriores e menor custo geral (Drezner et al., 2016).

No entanto, a estratificação depende totalmente dos sintomas preexistentes no atleta ou do reconhecimento da importância das características em sua família. Isso demonstra baixa sensibilidade para detectar doenças cardíacas (Harmon et al., 2015b). Uma avaliação física completa pode permitir a identificação de valvopatias e aortopatias; no entanto, isso pode não se traduzir em uma redução na MSC.

Portanto, embora a avaliação de um médico possa satisfazer o critério (6), na população em geral, a sensibilidade é baixa e limita (2) a detecção precoce.

O papel do eletrocardiograma de repouso de 12 derivações

As limitações do rastreamento de ECG para detectar doença arterial coronariana são reconhecidas e o foco dessa modalidade é a detecção de cardiomiopatias hereditárias e canalopatias iônicas que se manifestam como anormalidades no ECG. No entanto, uma avaliação da anormalidade requer um entendimento profundo do ECG normal de 12 derivações em repouso e isso é significativamente mais complicado em um atleta.

O exercício a longo prazo pode conferir adaptações cardíacas fisiológicas, estruturais e eletrocardiográficas. Essas características reconhecidas são chamadas de "coração de atleta" – um fenômeno benigno (Baggish e Wood, 2011). A dificuldade surge porque algumas características podem se sobrepor aos achados eco e eletrocardiográficos iniciais de processos cardiomiopáticos patológicos, muitas vezes referidos como características de "zona cinzenta". Pode ser um processo desafiador atribuir sua etiologia a um atleta.

Foi emitida orientação especializada para delinear os limites aceitos de adaptações suprafisiológicas de exercício daqueles que podem representar patologia e requerem caracterização adicional. A declaração de consenso internacional mais recente foi publicada em 2017 para ajudar a orientar o médico por intermédio do ECG do atleta (Figura 32.2) (Drezner et al., 2017).

Análises retrospectivas de protocolos de triagem que empregam triagem de ECG com a avaliação do médico reconheceram a sensibilidade superior do ECG na identificação de casos com cardiomiopatias e canalopatias subjacentes. Também é observado o valor clínico adjuvante da identificação de WPW.

A triagem de ECG é tão amplamente reconhecida como fundamental que levou especialistas em cardiologia do esporte a solicitar uma reconsideração e revisão dos protocolos que excluem o ECG, para incorporá-la (Harmon et al., 2015b).

Custos de infraestrutura e cursos de treinamento para a triagem pré-participação também devem ser levados em consideração no cálculo do custo total da triagem, assim como os recursos ao considerar o papel do ecocardiograma; o potencial para visualizar o miocárdio, bem como defeitos valvares, congênitos e septais melhora a taxa de detecção de certas patologias, mas pode parecer normal quando o defeito primário é elétrico.

Consenso ESC e AHA para triagem cardíaca pré-participação em atletas

As recomendações contemporâneas dos comitês de especialistas em cardiologia europeus e americanos defendem fortemente a adoção da TCP (Maron et al., 2007; Mont et al., 2017). Elas foram adotadas por órgãos reguladores que supervisionam os esportes. Os mais proeminentes incluem o Comitê Olímpico Internacional (COI) e a FIFA, que sugerem um ECG de 12 derivações,

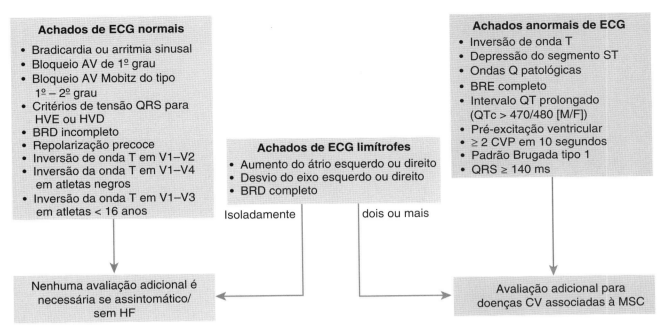

Figura 32.2 Recomendações internacionais para a interpretação do eletrocardiograma (ECG) de um atleta. *AV*, atrioventricular; *CV*, cardiovascular; *HF*, histórico familiar; *BRE*, bloqueio de ramo esquerdo; *HVE*, hipertrofia ventricular esquerda; *CVP*, contrações ventriculares prematuras; *BRD*, bloqueio de ramo direito; *HVD*, hipertrofia ventricular direita; *MSC*, morte súbita cardíaca.

histórico médico e exame físico como o padrão básico. No Reino Unido, a Federação Inglesa de Futebol, a Rugby Football Union (RFU) e a Lawn Tennis Association implementaram programas em todo o país de acordo com essas recomendações.

Embora existam diretrizes consensuais de manejo, o papel da equipe multiprofissional é fornecer ao atleta informações e estratificação de risco para apoiar a tomada de decisão autônoma.

Perspectiva ética

A via de TCP está repleta de questões éticas. Desde o início, submeter um indivíduo assintomático e saudável a um teste que pode mudar sua vida deve ser considerado e aconselhado ativamente. Junto com as dificuldades que envolvem o manejo de atletas com distúrbios cardíacos quiescentes, a ansiedade pela incerteza do processo diagnóstico a todos os atletas submetidos a testes de triagem adjuvante e o potencial de casos falso-positivos devem ser considerados. A incorporação de TCP deve ser parte do dever de cuidado de um profissional de saúde por meio do seu objetivo de reduzir a incidência de MSC. O fornecimento de aconselhamento sobre estilo de vida e terapia pode ser ainda mais complicado pela incerteza do diagnóstico e da penetrância sintomática da cardiomiopatia quiescente.

O processo de consentimento antes da triagem deve cobrir os componentes do teste de primeira linha e suas implicações, incluindo informar o paciente sobre as implicações médicas de um possível diagnóstico positivo, bem como o impacto potencial na participação competitiva. Essa informação deve ser transmitida com sensibilidade para refletir o valor positivo do teste.

A intenção do teste de triagem é identificar atletas assintomáticos com uma condição cardíaca subjacente significativa. No entanto, o tratamento subsequente de um atleta saudável baseia-se no estilo de vida e nas recomendações terapêuticas na ausência de sintomas patológicos. Essas preocupações influenciam os componentes do teste e a necessidade de caminhos de manejo claros para os vários resultados em cada estágio do processo de triagem. O ideal é a integração com serviços de apoio, exames e especialistas em cardiologia esportiva secundária.

Como para todos os indivíduos que recebem um diagnóstico de cardiomiopatia ou distúrbio arritmogênico, os atletas de maior risco podem exigir estratégias preventivas invasivas, como desfibrilação implantável ou intervenção cirúrgica.

Conclusão

A TCP é recomendada pela ESC e pela AHA, endossada por uma série de organizações esportivas, incluindo COI, FA e RFU. Nenhum protocolo atingirá 100% de sensibilidade devido à incidência inerente de SMSA e às dificuldades de identificação de doença arterial coronariana aterosclerótica significativa. No entanto, as cardiomiopatias são as causas mais comuns de MSC em atletas jovens e podem ser detectadas de maneira eficaz com a triagem de ECG.

A TCP robusta de atletas com histórico médico, avaliação clínica e ECG de 12 derivações em repouso está associada a uma redução na prevalência de MSC. À medida que o processo de avaliação se torna mais eficiente e padronizado, os custos associados reduzem e promovem ainda mais a adoção.

Referências bibliográficas

Baggish, A.L., Wood, M.J., 2011. Athlete's heart and cardiovascular care of the athlete: scientific and clinical update. Circulation 123 (23), 2723-2735.

Basu, J., Malhotra, A., Styliandis, V., Miles, H.D., Parry-Williams, G., Tome, M., et al., 2018. 71 Prevalence and progression of the juvenile pattern in the electrocardiogram of adolescents. Heart 104, A63-A63.

Behr, E.R., Casey, A., Sheppard, M., Wright, M., Bowker, T.J., Davies, M.J., et al., 2007. Sudden arrhythmic death syndrome: a national survey of sudden unexplained cardiac death. Heart 93, 601-605.

Chugh, S.S., Weiss, J.B., 2015. Sudden cardiac death in the older athlete. Journal of the American College of Cardiology 65 (5), 493-502.

Corrado, D., Basso, C., Rizzoli, G., Schiavon, M., Thiene, G., 2003. Does sports activity enhance the risk of sudden death in adolescents and young adults? Journal of the American College of Cardiology 42 (11), 1959-1963.

Corrado, D., Basso, C., Pavei, A., Michieli, P., Schiavon, M., Thiene, G., 2006. Trends in sudden cardiovascular death in young competitive athletes after implementation of a preparticipation screening program. JAMA 296 (13), 1593-1601.

Drezner, J.A., Sharma, S., Baggish, A., Papadakis, M., Wilson, M.G., Prutkin, J.M., et al., 2017. International criteria for electrocardiographic interpretation in athletes: consensus statement. British Journal of Sports Medicine 51, 704-731.

Drezner, J.A., Harmon, K.G., Asif, I.M., Marek, J.C., 2016. Why cardiovascular screening in young athletes can save lives: a critical review. British Journal of Sports Medicine 50, 1376-1378.

Harmon, K.G., Asif, I.M., Klossner, D., Drezner, J.A., 2011. Incidence of sudden cardiac death in National Collegiate Athletic Association athletes. Circulation 123 (15), 1594-1600.

Harmon, K.G., Asif, I.M., Maleszewski, J.J., Owens, D.S., Prutkin, J.M., Salerno, J.C., et al., 2015a. Incidence, etiology, and comparative frequency of sudden cardiac death in National Collegiate Athletic Association athletes: a decade in review. Circulation 132, 10-19.

Harmon, K.G., Zigman, M., Drezner, J.A., 2015b. The effectiveness of screening history, physical exam, and ECG to detect potentially lethal cardiac disorders in athletes: a systematic review/meta-analysis. Journal of Electrocardiology 48 (3), 329-338.

Maron, B.J., Thompson, P.D., Ackerman, M.J., Balady, G., Berger, S., Cohen, D., et al., 2007. Recommendations and considerations related to preparticipation screening for cardiovascular abnormalities in competitive athletes: 2007 update: a scientific statement from the American Heart Association council on nutrition, physical activity, and metabolism: endorsed by the American College of Cardiology Foundation. Circulation 115 (12), 1643-1655.

Mont, L., Pelliccia, A., Sharma, S., Biffi, A., Borjesson, M., Terradellas, J.B., et al., 2017. Pre-participation cardiovascular evaluation for athletic participants to prevent sudden death: position paper from the EHRA and the EACPR, branches of the ESC. Endorsed by APHRS, HRS, and SOLAECE. Europace 19 (1), 139-163.

Papadakis, M., Sharma, S., Cox, S., Sheppard, M.N., Panoulas, V.F., Behr, E.R., 2009. The magnitude of sudden cardiac death in the young: a death certificate-based review in England and Wales. Europace 11 (10), 1353-1358.

Shah, R., Chatterjee, A.D., Wilson, J., 2018. Creating a model of best practice: the match day emergency action protocol. British Journal of Sports Medicine 52, 1535-1536.

Sharma, S., Whyte, G., McKenna, W.J., 1997. Sudden death from cardiovascular disease in young athletes: fact or fiction? British Journal of Sports Medicine 31 (4), 269-276.

Vettor, G., Zorzi, A., Basso, C., Thiene, G., Corrado, D., 2015. Syncope as a warning symptom of sudden cardiac death in athletes. Cardiology Clinics 33 (3), 423-432.

Wasfy, M.M., Hutter, A.M., Weiner, R.B., 2016. Sudden cardiac death in athletes. Methodist DeBakey Cardiovascular Journal 12 (2), 76-80.

Wilson, J.M., Jungner, Y.G., 1968. Principles and practice of mass screening for disease. Boletin de la Oficina Sanitaria Panamericana Pan American Sanitary Bureau 65 (4), 281-393.

Capítulo | 33 |

Como Desenvolver Qualidades de Velocidade em Atletas Jovens

Johnny Wilson, Michael Sup, Mark Wilson, Marc-André Maillet e Said Mekary

Introdução

Velocidade é a distância percorrida por unidade de tempo (Elert, 2017). Com velocidades mais altas, um atleta está se movendo mais rápido, independentemente da direção. Os exercícios puros de treinamento de *sprint*, que se concentram no estilo e na eficiência, são unidimensionais e sem função específica para o esporte e estão fora do escopo deste capítulo. Em vez disso, nosso interesse está nas vantagens particulares do treinamento de velocidade para esportes de invasão (futebol, rúgbi, hóquei, basquete etc.) em jovens atletas. Este capítulo se concentrará em como desenvolver qualidades motoras, cognitivas e de velocidade perceptual em crianças entre as idades de 5 e 16 anos. Balyi e Hamilton (2004) separam a maturação em três estágios distintos: anos de amostragem (idades de 5 a 11 anos), de especialização (10 a 16 anos) e de investimento (15 a 18 anos). Neste capítulo, os autores se concentram nos primeiros dois estágios de treinabilidade acelerada.

O treinamento de velocidade hábil em atletas jovens pode ser planejado, reativo ou ambos, mas todos devem ser em referência a movimentos dinâmicos, padrões motores complexos, eficiência neuromuscular e proprioceptiva (Mulvany e Wilson, 2018). Neste capítulo, discutiremos:

- Quando as crianças podem começar a desenvolver sua capacidade de velocidade funcional
- As influências da natureza (o biológico inerente) e da criação (treinamento e efeitos psicossociais)
- As janelas aceleradas de treinabilidade e como treinar velocidade ultraespecificamente nos estágios de maturação distintos, mas sobrepostos (Ericsson, 2008).

Quando é possível desenvolver qualidades de velocidade em crianças?

Para construir qualidades de velocidade nas crianças, elas precisam ser expostas a intervenções de velocidade rotineiramente ao longo da infância. De acordo com o American College of Sports Medicine (Faigenbaum e Chu, 2017), movimentos explosivos críticos podem ser introduzidos a partir dos 5 anos de idade. No entanto, Avery Faigenbaum (2002) fornece algumas estipulações, afirmando que:

> *Embora não haja exigência de idade mínima para participação em um programa de treinamento de jovens, todos os participantes devem ter maturidade emocional para aceitar e seguir as orientações e apreciar genuinamente os benefícios e riscos potenciais associados ao treinamento.*

Faigenbaum, 2002, p. 32

Portanto, se uma criança tem inteligência emocional e está pronta para participar de esportes organizados e estruturados, como vôlei, futebol, rúgbi ou basquete, ela geralmente está pronta para realizar um programa de treinamento supervisionado.

Uma criança tem que possuir o "gene de desempenho/velocidade"?

Qualquer noção de que uma criança nasce rápida ou lenta parece ser um argumento fundamentalmente falho. Essa mentalidade atende apenas à *natureza* (que nascemos de uma determinada maneira e isso não pode ser mudado) e exclui o enorme potencial que a *criação* pode fornecer (o resultado da prática deliberada) (Ericsson, 1993). Embora todos nós tenhamos uma composição genética única como seres humanos, é um mito a ideia de que existe um único "gene de velocidade/desempenho" ou "gene do atleta", ou mesmo um conjunto de genes (Tucker et al., 2012). Apesar de ser verdade que todos temos um limite de desempenho genético, ele só pode ser percebido por meio do processo de prática deliberada e específica que visa melhorar qualquer aspecto do desempenho que desejamos, nesse caso a velocidade (Ericsson, 1993). Em outras palavras, a visão que os treinadores podem adotar é que é a interação entre a natureza e a criação que determina o resultado da capacidade de uma criança de alcançar seu potencial de velocidade fisiológica e psicológica (Tucker et al., 2012; Vaeyens et al., 2008).

Está além do escopo deste capítulo discutir genética, epigenética e os avanços mais recentes nas tecnologias de edição de genes e sua influência na otimização de velocidade na população de jovens atletas. No entanto, o leitor deve estar ciente do progresso nesses campos um tanto embrionários e das vantagens que eles podem trazer em breve.

Fases de treinabilidade acelerada

As crianças podem ser treinadas estrategicamente em velocidade durante três períodos distintos de maturação. Cientes desses momentos diferentes, os treinadores podem utilizá-los para integrar exercícios simples específicos do esporte que ajudarão a desenvolver qualidades essenciais de velocidade e reduzir o risco

341

Parte | 2 | Aplicação Clínica

de lesões e as taxas de abandono (Balyi e Way, 2005). Os treinadores também podem ser mais específicos para as demandas do jogo e as necessidades de seus jogadores, dependendo da janela de treinamento maturacional em que se encontram. Conforme estabelecido por Balyi e Hamilton (2004), essas três janelas são:
- Anos de amostragem: 5 a 11 anos de idade
- Anos de especialização: 10 a 16 anos de idade
- Anos de investimento: 15 a 18 anos de idade.

Para os fins deste capítulo, trataremos apenas das duas primeiras etapas.

Anos de amostragem: 5 a 11 anos de idade

Foco na velocidade para os anos de amostragem

Agilidade: uma habilidade física que permite aos atletas desacelerar, mudar de direção ou acelerar em resposta a um sinal relevante para a tarefa.

Fase de diversão e de aprender a treinar

Existem vários termos que podem ser utilizados para descrever esse período: pré-pubescente, meia-infância, pré-adolescência etc. No entanto, esses autores acreditam que a taxonomia de "amostragem" reflete melhor o propósito desse período fugaz da vida de uma criança (Balyi e Hamilton, 2004). A *amostragem* se presta naturalmente à ideia de que as crianças devem experimentar tantos esportes diferentes e ambientes de aprendizagem quanto possível para construir padrões de movimento físico básicos sólidos. O futebol, ao contrário da ginástica, é um esporte de especialização tardia e, portanto, a denominação de Balyi do termo "amostragem" para descrever esse período parece muito adequado.

Essa fase deve sempre se concentrar na diversão, com ênfase no desenvolvimento das habilidades fundamentais de movimento da criança, como parar, começar, mudar de direção, pular, pousar e equilibrar uma perna (Balyi e Hamilton, 2004). De uma perspectiva psicossocial, devemos ter um viés para oferecer sessões que promovam a motivação intrínseca, centrando-se nos próprios significados e objetivos do jovem.

Mesmo nessa idade, as crianças ainda têm necessidades básicas que precisam ser consideradas ao desenvolver qualidades atléticas:
- *Competência,* a necessidade de acreditar que eles são bons em uma tarefa (reforço positivo do treinador ao entrar e sair de um exercício de escada)
- *Autonomia,* que existe um grau de controle (capacidade de tomar decisões na sessão de treinamento, como durante cenários 1 contra 1 ou 2 contra 2)
- *Identificação,* a necessidade de significado e propósito (a criança entende porque está realizando um determinado exercício ou jogo e como isso pode ajudá-la a melhorar seu esporte).

Teoriza-se que todos estão correlacionados e as necessidades devem ser satisfeitas a fim de otimizar a motivação intrínseca e o resultado de desempenho ideal (Reinboth et al., 2004; Ryan e Deci, 2000). Além disso, do ponto de vista neurológico, a área do cérebro conhecida como sistema de ativação reticular (SAR) é extremamente sensível a novidades e atividades que despertam curiosidade (Steriade, 1996). Assim, sempre que um jovem atleta encontra um exercício que seja novo, agradável e sem estresse, o SAR é alertado para dar mais atenção à tarefa, o que auxilia no aprendizado de novas habilidades.

Durante essa janela de treinabilidade acelerada, a pesquisa sugere que as tarefas devem ter como alvo o sistema neural para melhorar a coordenação, eficácia e velocidade do movimento para desenvolver altos níveis de agilidade (Figura 33.1) (Van Praagh, 1998).

O que é agilidade?

Tecnicamente, é difícil definir agilidade. Alguns a definem tradicionalmente como a ação física de mudar de direção, parar e começar – sem qualquer reconhecimento do papel integral de como o cérebro e a natureza dinâmica em constante mudança do futebol podem afetar o desempenho de agilidade. Embora existam várias definições para agilidade, gostamos da maneira como Verstegen et al. (2001) a definem, como "uma habilidade física na qual os jogadores podem desacelerar, mudar de direção ou acelerar em resposta a um sinal relevante para a tarefa, como um oponente ou antecipação de um passe de um companheiro de equipe".

O que não é agilidade

Uma simples busca por exemplos de exercícios de agilidade na internet produzirá uma série de clipes divertidos de jogadores realizando diferentes movimentos em ritmo e com coordenação excepcional por meio de escadas, cones, postes, pistas de obstáculos etc. Embora esses exercícios sejam excelentes para desenvolver a coordenação e qualidades como melhorar a frequência da passada (pés rápidos), eles não ajudam a melhorar necessariamente o desempenho de agilidade do jogador. Isso não quer dizer que esses exercícios práticos devam ser removidos das sessões de treinamento. Longe disso, eles devem ser abraçados, pois certamente ajudam os jogadores a desenvolver qualidades fundamentais de movimento que os capacitarão a se destacar no esporte. No entanto, movimentos pré-planejados, como virar em um cone ou arrastar os pés lateralmente em uma escada, ocorrem muito raramente durante o jogo.

Por que treinar agilidade?

No futebol, as mudanças de direção, paradas e largadas são no geral em resposta a um estímulo externo – esses movimentos não são planejados, são caóticos e podem ocorrer em um instante, por exemplo, tentando escapar ou vencer um oponente em uma situação 1 contra 1, 2 contra 1 ou 1 contra 2. Nesses cenários, os jogadores precisam processar uma série de informações e então decifrar qual opção levará ao resultado desejado. Porém, mais do que isso, eles precisam tomar essa decisão mais rápido do que o seu oponente; eles precisam desenvolver a capacidade de pensar e agir rapidamente.

Portanto, se realmente desejamos melhorar o desempenho de agilidade de um jogador, devemos incluir atividades que o obriguem a reconhecer e reagir de maneira adequada a cenários não planejados, replicando o jogo tanto quanto possível, como exercícios reativos e jogos em campo reduzido (Sheppard e Young, 2006).

Prática de agilidade para ajudar a reduzir a incidência de lesões

A pesquisa indica que se os treinadores incluem atividades para as quais os jogadores não são capazes de se planejar e, em vez disso, têm que reagir, isso não só melhora sua agilidade, mas também reduz a probabilidade de se machucar, já que movimentos não planejados são um fator de risco de lesão conhecido no futebol (Besier et al., 2001). Portanto, o desempenho da agilidade no treinamento em crianças é a chave para o sucesso no futebol.

Como Desenvolver Qualidades de Velocidade em Atletas Jovens

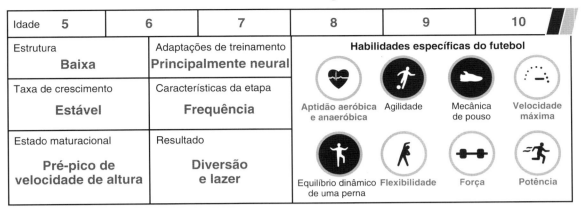

Figura 33.1 Anos de amostragem. (Adaptada de Balyi, I., Hamilton, A., 2004. Long-Term Athlete Development: Trainability in Childhood and Adolescence: Windows of Opportunity, Optimal Trainability. National Coaching Institute British Columbia and Advanced Training and Performance Ltd, Victoria, Canada.)

Como treinar agilidade

Uma maneira simples de incorporar atividades de agilidade em sessões práticas é dividir as atividades em três estágios durante os anos de amostragem: pliometria.

Estágio 1: movimentos planejados

- Mudança de direção/aceleração/desaceleração
- Pliometria submáxima:
  - Atividades de salto e pouso submáximos: essas atividades podem ser introduzidas com segurança, garantindo que todos os saltos sejam submáximos em esforço, com ênfase na aterrissagem "silenciosa" (com bom controle). Esses exercícios pliométricos de *baixo limiar* (submáximos) podem ajudar a melhorar o perfil de potência de uma criança (imperativo para agilidade), bem como reduzir o risco de lesão sem contato, especialmente ao pousar de uma altura em uma única perna
- Concentre-se na frequência da passada, ou seja, o tempo que o pé fica em contato com o solo (pés rápidos)
- Uso de cones/postes/escadas/instrução/apito etc.
- Dois a quatro exercícios por sessão
- Uma ou duas repetições por exercício
- 2 a 10 segundos por exercício
- 5 a 15 segundos de descanso entre cada exercício
- Tempo total de aplicação prática do estágio 1: 2 a 3 minutos.

Estágio 2: movimentos reativos

- Exercícios competitivos: espelhar/pique-pega/sombra e atividades de esquiva
- Um a três exercícios por sessão
- Uma a três repetições por exercício
- 10 a 20 segundos por exercício
- 10 a 30 segundos de descanso entre cada exercício
- Tempo total de aplicação prática do estágio 2: 2 a 4 minutos.

Estágio 3: jogos em campo reduzido

- 1 contra 1/2 contra 2/3 contra 2/5 contra 5 etc. (tamanho do campo adequado ao número de jogadores)
- 5 a 10 exercícios por sessão
- 1 a 3 repetições por exercício
- 20 segundos a 4 minutos por jogo em campo reduzido.

Exemplos de atividades de treinamento de agilidade nos anos de amostragem

Estágio 1: movimentos físicos planejados

Mudando de direção

- Passe por 4 cones/postes/portões o mais rápido possível
- Repita 3 vezes
- 5 segundos de descanso entre cada repetição

Estágio 2: movimentos físicos reativos

Atividade de agilidade reativa com parceiro

Esse exercício reforça a capacidade psicológica e a estrutura física, expondo a criança a vários cortes de alta velocidade, freios, desacelerações, acelerações, movimentos laterais, retrocesso, viradas e *sprints* curtos. Múltiplos cones coloridos são espalhados de modo aleatório em torno de uma área de 9 × 9 m ou área de 6 × 6 m com um cone central no meio da área. Uma criança anda pela área de trabalho e nomeia uma cor. A criança que realiza a atividade reage à cor convocada e corre para o cone, toca o cone com a mão e corre de volta para o cone central e aguarda a chamada de outra cor.

Progressões/regressões: um mundo de oportunidades infinitas

- Múltiplas dicas:
  - Nomeie três cores e veja se a pessoa que está realizando a atividade consegue lembrar a sequência de cores chamada enquanto participa
  - Chame o vermelho e o jogador deve ir para o azul etc.

Estágio 3: jogos em campo reduzido

O jogo em campo reduzido combina uma infinidade de tarefas com base na agilidade por meio de jogos divertidos que são cognitiva e fisicamente desafiadores. Os exemplos podem incluir *tag* rúgbi, jogos de marcação e 1 contra 1, 2 contra 2 com e sem bola. Esses jogos em campo reduzido podem ser realizados como parte do aquecimento, no corpo de uma sessão de treino ou durante o resfriamento. O treinador pode ajustar a complexidade dos jogos dependendo da capacidade da criança de entender o que está sendo pedido a ela, tornando mais simples se ela não entender ou aumentando o desafio cognitivo se ela achar que é muito fácil. Todos os exercícios/jogos podem ser adaptados à capacidade de coordenação das crianças e devem, sempre que possível, ser realizados a toda velocidade.

Prescrição de exercícios

Em geral, bem pouca periodização precisa ocorrer durante essa fase de treinabilidade. No entanto, todos os programas ainda devem ser estruturados e monitorados. De acordo com o Departamento de Saúde dos EUA (2018), crianças com idades entre 5 e 11 anos devem acumular pelo menos 60 minutos de atividade física moderada a vigorosa diariamente, incluindo atividades vigorosas pelo menos 3 dias por semana, a fim de obter benefícios para a saúde. Com relação às tarefas baseadas na agilidade, elas devem durar de modo ideal entre 5 e 10 segundos para garantir repetições de alta qualidade e que o foco esteja na construção da conexão mente-corpo em vez de uma base aeróbica ou anaeróbica. Em termos de relação entre treino e competição, pesquisadores eminentes nessa área como Faigenbaum (2002) e Balyi (2005) sugerem uma divisão de 70% treino e 30% competição.

Medida de resposta da frequência cardíaca durante os anos de amostragem

Esses autores acreditam que o uso da frequência cardíaca para monitorar a intensidade do exercício não é necessário para crianças entre 5 e 10 anos de idade, uma vez que um treinamento altamente estruturado pode não ser necessário durante os anos de amostragem devido à imaturidade do sistema cardiovascular.

Medida de participação ativa durante os anos de amostragem

Durante os anos de amostragem, a diversão e o prazer devem estar na vanguarda de qualquer resultado da sessão. Embora isso seja mais bem medido por meio de diálogo e *feedback* auditivo entre jogadores e treinadores, há potencial para correlacionar essas experiências de jogo divertidas e agradáveis com certas medições de dados quantitativos.

A participação ativa é uma métrica que fornece um meio de analisar quantitativamente o gasto de energia pela medição do equivalente metabólico de tarefas (MET) por meio de tecnologia vestível. Um MET é registrado continuamente ao longo da sessão. O MET é categorizado em três zonas de participação ativa: (1) baixa (1 a 3 METs), (2) moderada (3 a 6 METs) e (3) vigorosa (6+ METs) (Haskell et al., 2007). Essa métrica fornece aos treinadores uma porcentagem de quão ativas as crianças foram durante uma sessão de treinamento e quão intensa foi a sessão, destacando quanto tempo é gasto operando nas zonas de atividade física baixa, moderada e vigorosa. Por exemplo, se uma criança está em movimento por 75% da sessão treinamento, então sua porcentagem de PA é de 75%. Esses 75% serão então divididos para mostrar qual a porcentagem de atividade baixa, média e vigorosa. Porém, se a criança só se mexesse metade da sessão, a PA seria de 50% e novamente se divide em atividades baixas, moderadas e vigorosas.

Anos de especialização: 10 a 16 anos de idade

Foco na velocidade para os anos de especialização

- Velocidade máxima
- Aceleração
- Desaceleração
- Desempenho de *sprint* repetido.

Treinamento para a fase de treinamento

Essa fase foi denominada "anos de especialização", pois representa um período em que as crianças podem se concentrar na prática deliberada para melhorar as habilidades específicas do futebol, já que a maioria está preparada para adquirir essas habilidades específicas do esporte (Balyi e Hamilton, 2004). Trata-se de um período-chave, pois também marca o início do desenvolvimento de força e potência nas crianças. Isso ocorre devido a alterações fisiológicas significativas nos sistemas musculoesquelético e neuromuscular, sobretudo devido a influências maturacionais (aumento dos níveis de hormônio do crescimento associado à puberdade) (Beunen e Malina, 1988; Venturelli et al., 2008). Durante essa fase, as crianças experimentarão ganhos rápidos de massa óssea, massa muscular e estatura física (altura) (Bass et al., 1999). Portanto, a pesquisa postula que o foco do treinamento de velocidade para essa faixa etária deve ser em torno de uma intervenção de força para capitalizar sobre esse aumento natural dos hormônios de crescimento (Balyi e Hamilton, 2004). Observe que as crianças também podem ser introduzidas ao treinamento aeróbico com o início do pico de velocidade de crescimento (PVC; um grande surto de crescimento) (Balyi e Way, 2005). No entanto, isso está fora do escopo deste capítulo.

Desenvolvimento de qualidades de velocidade em meninos e meninas

Durante esta fase, meninos e meninas geralmente seguem taxas comparáveis de desenvolvimento em crescimento e maturação, bem como taxas semelhantes de força, potência, velocidade, resistência aeróbica e controle neuromuscular (Beunen e Malina, 2005). Como resultado, de uma perspectiva de treinamento, eles podem seguir programas de treinamento semelhantes durante essa janela de treinabilidade (Lloyd et al., 2011). Normalmente, o início do surto de crescimento do adolescente ocorre cerca de 2 anos antes nas meninas do que nos meninos (~10 anos nas meninas *versus* ~12 anos nos meninos). As meninas também terão PVC mais cedo do que os meninos (12 anos *versus* 14 anos) (Beunen e Malina, 1988; 2005).

Características da passada para desenvolver velocidade

Enquanto os anos de amostragem se concentraram no desenvolvimento da *frequência da passada* por meio de uma intervenção neural, atividades para melhorar o *comprimento da passada* (distância entre a saída do dedão e a aterrissagem do pé) também são adicionadas nessa fase de treinamento acelerado, com foco em um estímulo de força e potência (Figura 33.2) (Cavanagh et al., 1989). Esses autores acreditam que é fundamental desenvolver essas características em jogadores de futebol juvenil para que eles possam utilizar a frequência de passada para atividades com base na agilidade, como fugir de um oponente, e utilizar o comprimento da passada para atividades mais longas e lineares, como um contra-ataque acima de 40 m (Rompotti et al., 1975). Aumentos no comprimento da passada ocorrerão de maneira natural conforme a massa muscular do atleta aumenta durante a fase puberal. Isso se correlaciona com um aumento na produção de força e o aumento resultante na distância entre a saída do dedão e a aterrissagem do pé (Hunter e Smith, 2007). No entanto, os atletas jovens podem melhorar ainda mais o comprimento da passada por meio da prática deliberada durante os anos de especialização e das intervenções a seguir (Tucker et al., 2012).

Treinamento de resistência

A pesquisa sugere que, como o perfil de força de uma criança atleta se desenvolve rapidamente durante a puberdade, isso terá uma influência natural e positiva na velocidade máxima. No entanto, também adverte que os treinadores não devem confiar no crescimento e maturação apenas para melhorar as qualidades que se baseiam na velocidade durante essa janela de treinabilidade acelerada (Faigenbaum et al., 2016; Lesinski et al., 2015; Rumpf et al., 2012). Em vez disso, os treinadores devem incorporar o treinamento de resistência como parte de suas sessões de treinamento para melhorar a produção de força, que está associada a um melhor desempenho de *sprint* em atletas jovens (Christou et al., 2006). Um modelo de regressão sugere que uma melhora modesta de 10% na força em meninos pode resultar em um aumento de até 4,2% no desempenho de *sprint* (Faigenbaum et al., 2016). Enquanto isso, Meylan (2014) ilustrou que uma melhoria de 10% na altura do salto pode provocar uma melhoria de 2% no desempenho de *sprint* em atletas jovens, destacando assim o impacto positivo que um programa de força e potência pode ter no desempenho de *sprint* em jovens. Foi demonstrado que a pliometria melhora os perfis de força e potência de atletas jovens. São atividades relativamente seguras e convenientes que podem ser realizadas no final do aquecimento durante as sessões de treinamento. A pliometria pode ajudar a melhorar as qualidades de velocidade, como agilidade, velocidade linear e velocidade máxima em atletas jovens da seguinte maneira:

Pliometria. Os exercícios de salto multidirecional, também conhecidos como pliometria, são uma maneira excelente para desenvolver agilidade e promover familiarização com mudanças inesperadas de direção, bem como melhorar a velocidade máxima em crianças (Besier et al., 2001). Ao incorporar exercícios pliométricos simples no final do aquecimento em sessões de treinamento 2 vezes/semana durante um período curto de 6 semanas, foi demonstrado que a altura do salto, velocidade de aceleração acima de 5 m, velocidade máxima acima de 20 m, desempenho de agilidade com e sem a bola e a habilidade máxima de golpear a bola podem ser melhoradas significativamente (Villarreal et al., 2015). A pliometria ponderada (uso de *medicine ball*) também demonstrou melhorar o desempenho de velocidade (Faigenbaum, 2002).

Corrida de alta velocidade

Para melhorar o desempenho de *sprint* em jovens atletas, é imperativo expô-los a atividades de corrida de alta velocidade, como corrida máxima ou corridas resistidas para promover uma resposta anabólica para ajudar a aumentar a potência (Rumpf et al., 2012). Ao incorporar atividades com base em *sprints* no aquecimento e no corpo da sessão de treinamento, as crianças constroem elementos fisiológicos essenciais para o desenvolvimento do desempenho de velocidade.

Prescrição de exercícios

Os anos de especialização, sobretudo de 14 a 16 anos, são caracterizados por uma grande quantidade de prática deliberada (Cotê e Vierimaa, 2014). Nessa fase, o monitoramento da carga começa a se tornar um componente importante na periodização do atleta – monitorando a intensidade e o volume do exercício a fim de prevenir sobretreinamento e lesões.

Exemplos de atividades de treinamento de desempenho de velocidade para os anos de especialização

- Melhorar o desempenho da *aceleração* pela prática da corrida com esforço máximo ao longo de 5 m e realizando saltos pliométricos horizontais de esforço máximo com peso corporal
- Melhorar a *velocidade máxima* correndo o mais rápido possível ao longo de 20 a 30 m e por meio do peso corporal vertical máximo e de saltos pliométricos ponderados (10 a 30% de 1 repetição máxima)
- Melhorar o desempenho da *agilidade* introduzindo atividades que exigem que os jogadores pensem e se movam rapidamente, obrigando-os a reagirem a um estímulo externo não planejado
- Melhorar a *habilidade* de *sprints* repetidos (potência anaeróbica) aumentando a duração das atividades baseadas em *sprints* (até 20 segundos) para começar a construir capacidade anaeróbica em jogadores de futebol juvenil de 15 a 16 anos de idade (maturidades média e precoce).

Para uma discussão mais aprofundada sobre o mecanismo e a aplicação prática das atividades baseadas em *sprint*, consulte o Capítulo 18.

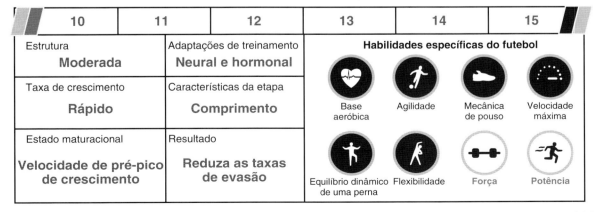

Figura 33.2 Anos de especialização. (Adaptada de Balyi, I., Hamilton, A., 2004. Long-Term Athlete Development: Trainability in Childhood and Adolescence: Windows of Opportunity, Optimal Trainability. National Coaching Institute British Columbia and Advanced Training and Performance Ltd, Victoria, Canada.)

Parte | 2 | Aplicação Clínica

Ao apresentar os atletas jovens a atividades com o objetivo de melhorar as qualidades físicas atléticas, como a velocidade, é sempre melhor subestimar suas capacidades físicas e aumentar gradualmente o volume e a intensidade da intervenção, em vez de superestimar suas habilidades e aumentar potencialmente o risco de lesões. Um ponto inicial sensato seria 1 a 3 séries de 6 a 10 repetições em um exercício da parte inferior do corpo 2 vezes/semana em dias não consecutivos, um exemplo sendo 1 série de 6 repetições de saltos de agachamento no final do aquecimento.

Também é importante notar que pode ser necessário diminuir o volume e a intensidade das sessões de treinamento durante os períodos de crescimento rápido para reduzir o risco de lesões relacionadas ao crescimento, como lesões apofisárias (p. ex., doença de Osgood-Schlatter, doença de Sever, síndrome de Sinding-Larsen Johansson). Portanto, expor as crianças a programas de exercícios planejados apropriadamente em termos de intensidade de carga moderada a alta, que se adaptam ao estado maturacional da criança e com competência técnica apropriada, pode ajudar muito a melhorar seu perfil físico atlético (Kelly et al., 1990; Nelson et al., 1994).

Para benefícios à saúde, as crianças devem acumular nessa fase pelo menos 60 minutos diários de atividade física moderada a vigorosa, que também deve incluir atividades de intensidade vigorosa pelo menos 3 vezes/semana (Pescatello, 2014). Recomenda-se que a proporção de treinamento para competição seja de 60% de treinamento *versus* 40% de competição e treinamento específico de competição (Balyi e Hamilton, 2004).

Acompanhamento durante os anos de especialização

Monitoramento da resposta da frequência cardíaca

O sistema circulatório é vital para a função humana em repouso, além de ser parte integrante da capacidade de se ajustar às demandas de exercícios agudos e crônicos. Com o sistema respiratório, o sistema cardiovascular é responsável, pelo fornecimento de oxigênio e nutrientes aos tecidos ativos por meio da corrente sanguínea (Stanfield, 2012). Durante uma sessão aguda de exercícios, o sistema cardiovascular aumentará o fornecimento de oxigênio e substrato aos músculos em atividade, a fim de atender aos requisitos de trifosfato de adenosina (ATP) do exercício (Stanfield, 2012). Existe uma relação linear entre a intensidade do exercício e a frequência cardíaca. À medida que a carga de trabalho do exercício aumenta, também aumenta a resposta da frequência cardíaca (Pescatello, 2014). A resistência cardiovascular reflete a capacidade de sustentar uma atividade vigorosa. É importante por duas razões: (1) a participação em muitas atividades físicas exige esforço vigoroso sustentado e (2) a saúde dos sistemas cardíaco e respiratório está relacionada aos níveis de resistência a fadiga, em grande parte porque o treinamento que melhora a aptidão torna esses sistemas mais eficientes.

Uso da frequência cardíaca para ajudar a prescrever sessões de treinamento

Os níveis de intensidade de atividade física no laboratório de pesquisa são expressos frequentemente com relação ao consumo máximo de oxigênio ($\dot{V}O_{2máx}$). No entanto, essa medida é cara e nem sempre viável ou prática fora do laboratório (Warburton et al., 2006). Métodos alternativos de cálculo da intensidade ideal do exercício em crianças estão disponíveis. A frequência cardíaca (FC) é uma medida prática, objetiva e válida da taxa de trabalho do exercício. A fórmula para adultos "220 – idade" é utilizada de modo frequente para prescrever a intensidade do exercício para crianças. No entanto, como afirma Rowland (1990), a $FC_{máx}$ determinada pelo teste máximo em esteira e cicloergômetro máximo permanece constante ao longo dos anos pediátricos. Logo, o uso de uma fórmula para adultos fortemente dependente da idade pode não ser apropriado. Embora o exercício seja fundamental para a saúde das crianças, medir a $FC_{máx}$ para crianças da mesma maneira que medimos para adultos pode colocar as crianças em risco de sobretreinamento e outros efeitos negativos, como dispneia e tonturas (Alleyne, 1998). Outra equação utilizada para prever a $FC_{máx}$ em uma população é 208 – (0,7 × idade) proposta por Tanaka et al. (2001). Dado que essa fórmula é ligeiramente menos dependente da idade, mostrou-se mais confiável ao medir a frequência cardíaca máxima em crianças (Mahon et al., 2010; Verschuren et al., 2011).

Ao utilizar a frequência cardíaca para medir a intensidade do exercício em atividades que desenvolvem capacidades físicas e mentais durante a fase final do grupo de especialização, existem alguns pontos a serem considerados. A intensidade e a duração das atividades físicas precisam ser baseadas na maturidade da criança, na formação médica e em experiências anteriores com exercícios. Além disso, independentemente da idade, a intensidade do exercício deve sempre começar baixa e progredir gradualmente.

As diretrizes para medir a intensidade do exercício em crianças durante a fase final de especialização são as seguintes:
- Atividade física de intensidade moderada: 55 a 69% da $FC_{máx}$ e 40 a 59% da reserva de frequência cardíaca
- Atividade física de intensidade vigorosa: > 70% da $FC_{máx}$ e > 60% da frequência cardíaca de reserva.

Desafios

Uma das dificuldades nessa área é que ainda se desconhece muito sobre o crescimento humano, sobretudo nos anos de formação. As crianças não são miniadultos e os princípios que dizem respeito aos adultos para desenvolver qualidades de velocidade podem não ser apropriados para o grupo infantil. Devemos ser cautelosos ao aplicar às crianças quaisquer princípios científicos baseados na população adulta. O desenvolvimento de qualidades de velocidade em crianças deve ser encarado de um ponto de vista a longo prazo, relacionado com um período de anos, em vez de semanas e meses. Portanto, é importante que todas as intervenções de velocidade sejam rastreadas, registradas e monitoradas para garantir a continuidade e a progressão. O desafio é que as crianças podem deixar de amar o esporte por um tempo, ou mudar de escola, clube ou esporte, fazendo com que nem sempre seja possível manter um registro contínuo. Uma solução pode ser a aplicação de tecnologia vestível que acompanha a criança, independentemente das mudanças que ela enfrente, de modo que todas as intervenções possam ser registradas e baixadas para um banco de dados central. Isso pode então ser acessado pela criança, o treinador, os pais etc., para garantir que a exposição da criança a um estímulo de velocidade e qualquer outra atividade física seja contínua e progressiva.

Conclusão

Embora o tema central desse capítulo seja o desenvolvimento de qualidades de velocidade em crianças, os autores reconhecem que o bem-estar da criança é o fator mais importante e defendem

Como Desenvolver Qualidades de Velocidade em Atletas Jovens — Capítulo | 33 |

fortemente o desenvolvimento saudável da criança acima dos resultados de desempenho.

Este capítulo tem como objetivo assegurar aos técnicos e aos médicos que é possível treinar qualidades de velocidade em crianças a partir dos 5 anos de idade. A chave é desenvolver essas qualidades ao longo de todo o período da infância e da adolescência, com uma compreensão sólida do estado de maturação da criança e combiná-lo com um estímulo de treinamento apropriado.

Talvez então, ao planejar atividades de velocidade, devamos considerar várias abordagens de aprendizagem e uma solução mais heurística centrada no atleta. A seleção dos exercícios deve ser baseada na capacidade da criança, tanto física quanto mental, e também nas demandas funcionais do esporte em um ambiente criativo e agradável. Para desenvolver qualidades de velocidade específicas do esporte, como agilidade, devemos buscar ativamente os cenários mais aleatórios e imprevisíveis e ter como objetivo sustentar a ativação e a aquisição de habilidades complexas dentro deles. Ao adotar essa metodologia, o jovem atleta estará preparado para se adaptar aos inesperados estressores do esporte.

Referências bibliográficas

Alleyne, J.M., 1998. Safe exercise prescription for children and adolescents. Paediatrics and Child Health 3 (5), 337-342.

Balyi, I., Hamilton, A., 2004. Long-Term Athlete Development: Trainability in Childhood and Adolescence—Windows of Opportunity—Optimal Trainability. National Coaching Institute British Columbia and Advanced Training and Performance Ltd, Victoria, Canada.

Balyi, I., Way, R., 2005. The role of monitoring growth in the long-term athlete development. Canadian Sport for Life.

Bass, S., Delmas, P.D., Pearce, G., Hendrich, E., Tabensky, A., Seeman, E., 1999. The differing tempo of growth in bone size, mass and density in girls is region-specific. Journal of Clinical Investigation 104, 795-804.

Besier, T.F., Lloyd, D.G., Ackland, T.R., Cochrane, J.L., 2001. Anticipatory effects on knee joint loading during running and cutting manoeuvres. Medicine & Science in Sports & Exercise 33, 1176-1181.

Beunen, G.P., Malina, R.M., 1988. Growth and physical performance relative to the timing of the adolescent spurt. Exercise and Sport Sciences Reviews 16, 503-540.

Beunen, G.P., Malina, R.M., 2005. Growth and biological maturation: relevance to athletic performance. In: Bar-Or, O. (Ed.), The Child and Adolescent Athlete. Blackwell Publishing, Oxford, pp. 3-17.

Cavanagh, P., Kram, R., 1989. Stride length in distance running: velocity, body dimensions, and added mass effects. Medicine & Science in Sports & Exercise 21, 467-479.

Christou, M., Smilios, I., Sotiropoulos, K., Volaklis, K., Pilianidis, T., Tokmakidis, S.P., 2006. Effects of resistance training on the physical capacities of adolescent soccer players. Journal of Strength and Conditioning Research 20, 783-791.

Côté, J., Vierimaa, M., 2014. The developmental model of sport participation: 15 years after its first conceptualization. Science & Sports Volume 29, Supplement, S63-S69.

Elert, G., 2017. Speed and velocity. The Physics Hypertextbook. Available at: https://physics.info/velocity/.

Ericsson, K.A., 2008. Deliberate practice and acquisition of expert performance: A general overview. Academic Emergency Medicine 15 (11), 988-994.

Ericsson, K.A., Krampe, R. Th., Tesch-Romer, C., 1993. The role of deliberate practice in the acquisition of expert performance. Psychological Review 100, 363-406.

Faigenbaum, A., Chu, D., 2017. Plyometric training for children and adolescents. In: American College of Sports Medicine, Indianapolis.

Faigenbaum, A., 2002. Resistance training for adolescent athletes. Athletic Therapy Today 7 (6), 30-35.

Faigenbaum, A.D., Lloyd, R.S., MacDonald, J., Myer, G.D., 2016. Citius, altius, fortius: beneficial effects of resistance training for young athletes. British Journal of Sports Medicine 50, 3-7.

Haskell, W.L., Lee, I.M., Pate, R.R., Powell, K.E., Blair, S.N., Franklin, B.A., et al., 2007. Physical activity and public health: updated recommendation for adults from the American College of Sports Medicine and the American Heart Association. Medicine and Science in Sports and Exercise 39 (8), 1423-1434.

Hunter, I., Smith, G.A., 2007. Preferred and optimal stride frequency, stiffness and economy: Changes with fatigue during a 1-h high-intensity run. European Journal of Applied Physiology 100, 653-661.

Kelly, P.J., Twomey, L., Sambrook, P.N., Eisman, J.A., 1990. Sex differences in peak adult bone mineral density. Journal of Bone and Mineral Research 5, 1169-1175.

Lesinski, M., Prieske, O., Granacher, U., 2015. Effects and dose–response relationships of resistance training on physical performance in youth athletes: a systematic review and meta-analysis. British Journal of Sports Medicine 1-17.

Lloyd, R.S., Oliver, J.L., Hughes, M.G., Williams, C.A., 2011. The influence of chronological age on periods of accelerated adaptation of stretch-shortening cycle performance in pre-and postpubescent boys. Journal of Strength and Conditioning Research 25, 1889-1897.

Mahon, A.D., Marjerrison, A.D., Lee, J.D., Woodruff, M.E., Hanna, L.E., 2010. Evaluating the prediction of maximal heart rate in children and adolescents. Research Quarterly for Exercise and Sport 365 (81), 466-471.

Meylan, C.M.P., Cronin, J., Oliver, J.L., Hopkins, W.G., Pinder, S., 2014. Contribution of vertical strength and power in sprint performance in young male athletes. International Journal of Sports Medicine 35, 749-754.

Mulvany, S., Wilson, J., 2018. Complex Adaptive Modelling in Sport Science and Sports Medicine. Available at: https://wilsonmulvany.wordpress.com/2018/10/18/model-number-1-neuromuscular-systems-conditioning-nsc-advantaged-stacked-over-preparedness-for-sport-specific-demand/.

Nelson, M.E., Fiatarone, M.A., Morganti, C.M., Trice, I., Greenberg, R.A., Evans, W.J., 1994. Effects of high-intensity strength training on multiple risk factors for osteoporotic fractures. Journal of American Medical Association 272, 1909-1914.

Pescatello, L.S., 2014. ACSM's Guidelines for Exercise Testing and Prescription, ninth ed. Wolters Kluwer/Lippincott Williams & Wilkins Health, Philadelphia.

Reinboth, M., Duda, J.L., Ntoumanis, N., 2004. Dimensions of coaching behavior, need satisfaction and the psychological and physical welfare of young athletes. Motivation and Emotion 28, 297.

Rompotti, K., 1975. A study of stride length in running. In: Canham, D., Diamond, P. (Eds.), International Track and Field Digest. Champions on Film, 1975, Ann Arbor, MI, pp. 249-256.

Rowland, T.W., 1990. Exercise and Children's Health. Human Kinetics, Champaign, IL, pp. 27-83.

Rumpf, M.C., Cronin, J.B., Pinder, S.D., Oliver, J., Hughes, M., 2012. Effect of different training methods on running sprint times in male youth. Pediatric Exercise Science 24, 170-186.

Ryan, R.M., Deci, E.L., 2000. Intrinsic and extrinsic motivations: classic definitions and new directions. Contemporary Educational Psychology 25, 54-67.

Sheppard, J.M., Young, W.B., 2006. Agility literature review: classifications, training and testing. Journal of Sports Sciences 24, 919-932.

Stanfield, C.L., 2012. Principles of Human Physiology, fifth ed. Benjamin Cummings, San Francisco, CA.

Steriade, M., 1996. Arousal: revisiting the reticular activating system. Science 272 (5259), 225.

Tanaka, H., Monahan, K.D., Seals, D.R., 2001. Age-predicted maximal heart rate revisited. Journal of the American College of Cardiology 37, 153-156.

Tucker, R., Collins, M., 2012. What makes champions? A review of the relative contribution of genes and training to sporting success. British Journal of Sports Medicine 46, 555-561.

US Department of Health and Human Services, 2018. Physical Activity Guidelines for Americans, 2nd edition. Washington, DC: US Department of Health and Human Services.

Vaeyens, R., Lenoir, M., Williams, A.M., et al., 2008. Talent identification and development programmes in sport: current models and future directions. Sports Medicine 38, 703-714.

van Praagh, E., 1998. Paediatric Anaerobic Performance. Human Kinetics Publisher, Inc, Champaign, IL.

Venturelli, M., Bishop, D., Pettene, L., 2008. Sprint training in preadolescent soccer players. International Journal of Sports Physiology and Performance 3, 558-562.

Verschuren, O., Maltais, D.B., Takken, T., 2011. The 220-age equation does not predict maximum heart rate in children and adolescents. Developmental Medicine & Child Neurology 53, 861-864.

Verstegen, M., Marcello, B., 2001. Agility and coordination. In: Foran, B. (Ed.), High Performance Sports Conditioning. Human Kinetics, Champaign, IL, pp. 139-165.

Villarreal, E., et al., 2015. Effects of plyometric and sprint training on physical and technical skill performance in adolescent soccer players. Journal of Strength and Conditioning Research 29 (7), 1894-1903.

Warburton, D.E., Nicol, C.W., Bredin, S.S., 2006. Prescribing exercise as preventive therapy. Canadian Medical Association Journal 174 (7), 961-974.

Capítulo | 34 |

Condicionamento para a Batalha do Momentum: Uso Prático da Tecnologia GPS para Estratégias de Condicionamento

Adam Sheehan

Introdução

Momentum é algo engraçado em um jogo de rúgbi. São momentos que até o torcedor mais novato pode perceber com a mesma precisão que o treinador mais sábio. Os momentos de ímpeto no rúgbi costumam ser grandes batalhas físicas e psicológicas de vontade, aquelas passagens do jogo que chegam às últimas páginas dos jornais de domingo. São os momentos que podem surgir de uma defesa à prova d'água que faz com que uma equipe se levante e afaste um oponente dominante, ou podem ser momentos de ataque em que gigantes desferem um golpe esmagador em um peixinho por meio de um contra-ataque letal.

Este capítulo explicará como as equipes desenvolvem as qualidades físicas não apenas para sobreviver a essas batalhas, como também vencê-las. Será explorado o uso e a implementação de tecnologia de sistemas de posicionamento global (GPS, do inglês *global position systems*) para maximizar o desenvolvimento físico dos jogadores para os atributos dessa equipe específica.

Introdução ao GPS

O avanço da tecnologia GPS, com a facilidade de visualização de dados por meio de plataformas personalizadas, causou uma proliferação de usos para essa ferramenta. Ele é utilizado por uma grande quantidade de equipes em esportes profissionais e de elite (Cummins et al., 2013). As equipes normalmente recorrem ao GPS para auxiliar no monitoramento e na compreensão das demandas de seu esporte. A facilidade de utilização e a grande quantidade de pontos de dados coletados são fundamentais para fornecer um entendimento mais profundo de todos os esportes. Assim como em muitas jornadas de descoberta, no início examina-se apenas o mapa antes de começar a tomar decisões sobre para onde ir, antes de finalmente calcular quanto tempo levará para chegar a certos pontos do mapa. Uma visão geral dos grandes marcos ao longo da jornada do GPS é fornecida a seguir.

1. Estágio de coleta de dados. A introdução inicial de qualquer nova tecnologia naturalmente permitirá um período de aclimatação em que o objetivo principal da nova tecnologia é a coleta de dados. A tecnologia GPS não é diferente. Os usuários podem avaliar pesquisas publicadas dentro de um determinado esporte, mas o benefício da coleta de GPS dentro de uma equipe é a entrega de uma perspectiva que é única para aquela equipe específica. Essa fase inicial se correlaciona com a identificação das bordas do mapa, e fornece uma visão geral das demandas das fases de treinamento, demandas semanais, tipos de sessão e demandas de exercícios específicos.

2. Estágio de comparação. Esse estágio utiliza os dados que foram coletados para fazer comparações entre os tipos de treino, comparar treinos *versus* jogos e diferenças posicionais de grupo ou discrepâncias ou características do jogador/atleta.

3. Estágio de implementação. A informação recolhida é extrapolada para tirar conclusões significativas sobre treino ou jogos. Isso pode ser tão simples quanto comparar a eficácia de sessões semelhantes ou utilizar o jogo como uma referência e, em seguida, basear o treinamento nessas demandas. Também pode ser utilizado para verificar a carga semanal total ao longo das semanas com relação ao ciclo (dias entre os jogos – e o efeito dos dias de recuperação disponíveis) desse treinamento.

4. Estágio de previsão. Se essa fase é realmente atingida é um ponto de discórdia devido ao ambiente caótico imprevisível do esporte; certamente é o mais difícil dos estágios. A previsão das demandas de treinamento é óbvia em sua utilidade, mas difícil em sua implementação. Basear o treinamento semanal em um histórico contextual das semanas anteriores – utilizando esses dados para destacar a necessidade de sessões de alta ou baixa carga – pode ajudar na construção de 1 semana de treinamento eficaz. Esses dados podem ser refinados ainda mais pela identificação de quais indivíduos estão sendo sobrecarregados ou insuficientes, o que é importante no manejo de um time de jogo e não apenas de um conjunto de pessoas que jogam juntas. Finalmente, as informações de GPS podem ser utilizadas para focar com precisão o desenvolvimento físico, por exemplo, onde um jogador é deficiente ou para ajudar a avaliar a carga de trabalho de um indivíduo com base em sua capacidade para esse trabalho naquele ponto de tempo específico; isso utiliza alguns dos trabalhos de Gabbett sobre razões agudas:crônicas (Gabbett, 2012). Ele reduz o risco de lesões, ajuda a fornecer um nível saudável de disponibilidade do jogador para auxiliar na competição de times e nas escolhas dos treinadores para otimizar o desempenho geral da equipe.

Muito desse trabalho pode ser executado com algumas das métricas *plug-and-play* básicas comuns em todas as plataformas GPS. O manejo de plataformas GPS muitas vezes se desenvolve com a familiaridade da equipe e dos profissionais com ele e a utilização das informações. Portanto, tende a surgir a necessidade de responder a perguntas cada vez mais específicas ou detalhadas. Os sistemas GPS de elite de primeira linha permitem uma personalização muito maior, o que permite mais controle e autonomia ao usuário final para interpretar e inferir significado a partir de um escopo maior de métricas. A configuração é altamente dependente do sistema escolhido, mas todos os sistemas operarão com algumas categorias gerais. Dependendo do seu esporte, a prioridade desses parâmetros mudará; porém, todos os esportes terão uma combinação e sub-bandas de categorias que, quando configuradas, podem dar uma visão significativa do esporte em questão e desenvolver uma imagem contextual melhor para aquele esporte.

Todos os sistemas têm as três categorias básicas de informação:
- *Velocidade* – demandas com base em corrida
- *Aceleração* – mudança de demandas de velocidade
- *Impacto* – medição da força G dos impactos.

Ao utilizar esses parâmetros, a maioria dos sistemas permite a configuração de várias bandas dentro dessas categorias. Isso possibilita uma avaliação mais aprofundada e enquadrar parte da natureza contextual das informações. Já existe um corpo de pesquisa que identifica bandas para cada uma das categorias de parâmetros listadas anteriormente. A Figura 34.1 mostra algumas bandas típicas vistas nas diferentes categorias dentro da configuração do autor, as razões para definir as bandas dessa maneira e também a aplicação potencial dessas bandas.

Velocidade

A categoria de velocidade abrangerá todos os movimentos com base em corrida por meio de GPS. Algumas das métricas simples utilizadas com mais frequência são "distância", "metros por minuto" ou "corrida em alta velocidade". A capacidade de personalizar as bandas em diferentes velocidades permite um maior entendimento das demandas e dos esforços de corrida para qualquer sessão. As bandas de velocidade eram aplicadas anteriormente como um método de banda absoluto ou relativo. Isso significa que as equipes podem decidir qualificar todos os indivíduos por faixas absolutas, avaliá-los pela mesma velocidade máxima absoluta, ou podem escolher observá-los com relação a uma porcentagem individual da velocidade máxima. A maioria dos sistemas de elite tem a capacidade de realizar ambas as avaliações e é um excelente método não apenas para avaliar o desempenho de um indivíduo por meio da velocidade absoluta, como também para analisá-lo com relação à sua própria velocidade máxima individual.

Aceleração

A categoria de aceleração abrangerá todas as mudanças de movimentos de velocidade registrados por meio do acelerômetro, incluindo eventos de aceleração e desaceleração. Ao utilizar essa categoria, os treinadores podem identificar as demandas de mudança de direção, não apenas a quantidade total de acelerações e desacelerações, como também a distância para cada um desses eventos e, por meio do uso das bandas de intensidade, detalhará a gravidade dos eventos de mudança de direção. Essas informações podem ser aplicadas para determinar demandas típicas, bem como destacar diferenças significativas entre grupos posicionais e até mesmo distinções dentro do grupo para frequência de esforços ou em distâncias percorridas em zonas de aceleração ou desaceleração.

Impacto

Os impactos são registrados por meio do acelerômetro integrado e medidos em força G. Essa função está disponível na maioria dos dispositivos de nível elite. Essa informação é de importância particular no rúgbi de 15 ou em outros esportes com base em contato, visto que o único fator determinante na intensidade do jogo é a gravidade e a frequência dos eventos de impacto. A maioria dos sistemas de elite também executa algoritmos com os dados de impacto para identificar mais eventos de colisão. Esses eventos de colisão são detectados por meio de uma combinação dos dados do acelerômetro, a orientação do giroscópio e o impacto registrado nos dados da força G, e fornece critérios mais rigorosos para a detecção de colisão.

Demandas

Demandas gerais

O rúgbi é um jogo simples independentemente do seu nível. As demandas físicas gerais para todos os jogadores são correr, pular, fugir e evitar ou fazer um *tackle*. Como um jogo de ataque de 80 minutos baseado em campo, as demandas gerais também são simples. Durante a partida, o jogador busca expor o espaço no ataque e reduzi-lo na defesa. Essas demandas são como as de muitos outros esportes de campo. O rúgbi difere de outros esportes na natureza física e de confronto das colisões e batalhas de bola parada (Tabela 34.1). Ao desenvolver as demandas físicas necessárias para jogar, podemos categorizá-las em três grupos genéricos.

Corrida. A necessidade de ter uma habilidade altamente desenvolvida para atingir a velocidade máxima e repetir isso com frequência; a necessidade de correr normalmente 6 km ao longo de um jogo e ter uma proporção dessa distância em alta velocidade.

Mudança de direção. A capacidade de acelerar e desacelerar com frequência e em altas velocidades. De um modo geral, esses eventos de aceleração e desaceleração são altamente específicos de posição em relação à intensidade e frequência dos esforços.

Colisões. As colisões são parte integrante do rúgbi de 15. A natureza de contato do jogo é um atributo chave em seu espetáculo. Um jogador de rúgbi precisa produzir esforços de colisão para parar um oponente na defesa, e ser robusto o suficiente para entrar em esforços de colisão no ataque. Existem perfis perceptíveis para as demandas de colisão das diferentes posições de uma equipe de rúgbi e não há dúvida de que isso manteve a diversidade da forma atlética jogando em um campo de rúgbi. As posições avançadas têm uma quantidade maior de colisões quando comparadas às posições recuadas. De maneira curiosa, e como um subproduto de como as colisões são avaliadas, muitas vezes são os recuados que têm uma proporção maior de suas colisões nas zonas de alta aceleração. Isso se deve principalmente à velocidade de entrada em eventos de colisão.

Demandas específicas

A especificidade é uma variável chave do treinamento e um princípio central da melhoria do desempenho (Gabbett et al., 2012). A necessidade de treinamento para alcançar altos níveis de especificidade aumenta de acordo com o nível de jogo. No nível superior, a especificidade e a capacidade de transferência do condicionamento físico são de suma importância para o sucesso em um determinado esporte. A ênfase nisso é ainda mais exagerada pela contínua "corrida armamentista" figurativa em

Condicionamento para a Batalha do Momentum: Uso Prático da Tecnologia GPS para Estratégias... | Capítulo | 34 |

Velocidade

Banda	Banda 1	Banda 2	Banda 3	Banda 4	Banda 5	Banda 6	Banda 7
Absoluto	0 a 2,2 m/s	2,2 a 4,4 m/s	4,4 a 5,5 m/s	5,5 a 7 m/s	7 a 8 m/s	8 a 9 m/s	9 a 11 m/s
Racional	Andar	Corrida leve	Corrida	Corrida de alta velocidade	Muita CAV	Distância do *sprint*	Velocidade máxima
Relativo	0 a 20%	20 a 40%	40 a 55%	55 a 70%	70 a 85%	85 a 90%	90 a 110%
Racional	Zona de corrida de baixo nível		Condicionamento da zona de corrida	Zonas de corrida de alta intensidade		Zona de *sprint*	*Sprint* máximo

CAV, corrida de alta velocidade.

Aceleração

	Desaceleração			Ponto médio	Aceleração		
Banda	Banda 1	Banda 2	Banda 3	Banda 4	Banda 5	Banda 6	Banda 7
Absoluto	−10 m/s a −6 m/s	−6 m/s a −4 m/s	−4 m/s a −2 m/s	−2 m/s a 2 m/s	2 m/s a 4 m/s	4 m/s a 6 m/s	6 m/s a 10 m/s
Racional	Desaceleração grave	Alta desaceleração	Desaceleração moderada	Baixa celeração e desaceleração	Aceleração moderada	Alta aceleração	Aceleração grave

Impactos

Banda	Banda 1	Banda 2	Banda 3	Banda 4	Banda 5	Banda 6	Banda 7	Banda 8
Força G	1 a 2 g	2 a 4 g	4 a 5 g	5 a 6 g	6 a 7 g	7 a 8 g	8 a 9 g	9 a 15 g
Racional	Micro impactos	Impacto e baixo grau	Impactos moderados		Impactos pesados		Impactos graves	

Figura 34.1 Algumas faixas típicas de velocidade, aceleração e impacto vistas em sistemas GPS.

Tabela 34.1 Comparação de métricas de distância, velocidade, carga e esforços para diferentes posições de rúgbi. Os números apresentados são médias por sessão (*i. e.*, jogo)

Posição	Dist. med. (m)	Metragem por minuto (m/min)	PL med.	PL med. (sessão lenta)	Dist. cob. med. (m)	CAV med. (m/s)	MDD tot. med.	Colisões médias	Esf. tot. med.	ERAI
Pilar	4.282	63	463	250	181	38	45	31	93	2
Avante de segunda linha	4.905	65	546	265	361	67	64	45	140	4
Talonador	5.074	68	529	247	431	112	56	38	131	6
Linha de *back*	5.842	68	644	307	576	163	79	55	185	9
Abertura	5.125	75	481	199	605	199	47	24	118	9
Centro	5.784	73	571	235	855	346	55	33	158	16
Meio *scrum*	6.269	74	625	248	1158	422	68	35	183	16
Back 3	6.006	71	543	230	918	471	49	28	153	17

Dist. med., distância percorrida na sessão em metros; *metragem por minuto*, distância total dividida pelo tempo; *PL med.*, *PlayerLoad* médio da sessão (*PlayerLoad* é uma métrica personalizada do *Catapult* para avaliar a demanda de sobrecarga); *dist. cob. med.*, métrica personalizada da distância total coberta a ≥ 4,4 m/s; *CAV med.*, distância total percorrida a ≥ 5,5 m/s (*i. e.*, corrida em alta velocidade); *MDD tot. med.*, quantidade total de esforços de mudança de direção/eventos de aceleração e desaceleração; *colisões médias*, quantidade total de eventos de colisão maior que 4 G; *Esf. tot. med.*, combinação de todos os esforços de corrida de alta intensidade, mudança de direção e colisão; *ERAI*, quantidade total de esforços repetidos de alta intensidade para a sessão.

351

termos de melhoria de desempenho. A tecnologia GPS pode ajudar ao destacar as demandas físicas específicas dos jogos de uma equipe e fornecer um meio de avaliar o treinamento adequado. O nível geral de preparação física é desenvolvido à medida que o jogador sobe de posição no esporte profissional; e o principal fator de distinção em todos os níveis é a sua habilidade técnica. No entanto, como existem muitas estruturas para o desenvolvimento físico ao longo das idades, no nível superior o condicionamento físico é específico e exclusivo para a equipe em questão.

A aptidão aeróbica geral é desenvolvida desde tenra idade, com aperfeiçoamento de força adicional e de potência à medida que o jogador fica mais velho. No nível universitário do rúgbi, entre as idades de 18 e 22 anos, o desenvolvimento máximo de força e potência são combinados com a capacidade anaeróbica como qualidades físicas essenciais para vir à tona. O desenvolvimento da potência máxima e da velocidade máxima são essenciais em um nível sênior, antes da evolução da capacidade anaeróbica. A nível internacional, todas essas qualidades já estão normalmente no seu pico e por isso o foco está na otimização de maneiras de reduzir a fadiga que permitem um desempenho de pico. Isso reflete o fato de que a maioria dos jogadores internacionais são bem desenvolvidos fisicamente e possuem habilidades técnicas e táticas de alto nível. A mitigação da fadiga em benefício do "sentir-se apto" é mais importante do que um maior desenvolvimento físico, pois já é alta e as janelas de competição costumam ser muito curtas para que o verdadeiro desenvolvimento físico seja o foco principal.

As necessidades posicionais diferem quanto mais especializado for o nível de jogo. Em um ambiente de equipe de elite, muitas vezes é possível ter algumas diferenças entre os jogadores, mesmo entre aqueles que jogam na mesma posição. Isso pode produzir um nível de complexidade e tomada de decisão urgente com relação a quais características priorizar e quais qualidades de aptidão focar. É importante ter uma compreensão profunda das demandas do dia de treinamento e jogos e facilitar o desenvolvimento de qualidades de condicionamento físico suplementares dentro ou ao redor das demandas de treinamento. Essa compreensão profundamente enraizada das demandas de treinamento proporcionará maior precisão e especificidade para a entrega de melhorias físicas essenciais e quando abordá-las.

Atualmente, a tecnologia GPS é o único meio prático de determinar esse nível granular de aptidão individual. O tempo é um recurso limitado no nível de elite devido ao "congestionamento" das atividades da temporada e à alta prioridade dada à recuperação destaca a necessidade de um alto grau de especificidade. Ter focos específicos em diferentes momentos ao longo do ano é essencial devido à natureza semana a semana de uma temporada de quase 1 ano em conjunto com o impacto físico sobre os jogadores devido à natureza exigente e conflituosa do jogo. Nesse contexto, o GPS pode ser utilizado como uma ferramenta para avaliar as demandas contínuas da equipe durante a temporada, podendo focar nas demandas do cronograma geral de treinamento, bem como nas demandas de treinamento em uma determinada semana. Ao utilizar esses dados, aumentos apropriados no volume de treinamento, intensidade ou densidade de trabalho podem ser planejados e implementados na semana da temporada competitiva e aumentados ainda mais nas semanas em que não há jogo. Ênfase deve ser dada ao tempo necessário para o treinamento de uma equipe para fornecer o estímulo físico para a sustentabilidade a longo prazo na temporada.

Ao compreender a padronização típica das demandas físicas em jogos, o treinamento de uma equipe pode ser projetado para simular esses eventos, permitindo que uma qualidade de condicionamento físico detalhada seja derivada do planejamento técnico e tático da semana. Alavancar a qualidade da aptidão física para um exercício técnico específico resultará no seu desenvolvimento desde a execução meramente técnica até a capacidade de realizar essas habilidades técnicas sob fadiga.

GPS: papel no planejamento

O planejamento da semana de treinamento é uma das principais áreas onde o GPS pode ser utilizado com a taxa de percepção de esforço (TPE) dos jogadores, dados e informações coletadas por meio de questionários de monitoramento e bem-estar. Isso fornece a trindade de informações sobre o estado atual de fadiga e preparação. Enquanto lida com o caos e o congestionamento das partidas semanais, são disponibilizados *insights* rápidos e úteis sobre a prontidão da equipe.

Existem três maneiras simples para lidar com uma temporada de até 32 jogos competitivos, excluindo as janelas internacionais para as partidas de teste.

1. *Planejar a carga semanal com base nas demandas semanais médias e no retorno disponível antes do próximo jogo competitivo.* Isso pode ser feito por meio de medidas de volume, intensidade e densidade tomadas diretamente do GPS. Exemplos disso podem ser: carga média total do jogador/carga dinâmica de estresse (ambas as métricas de prateleira com *Catapult* e *Statsports*, respectivamente) para cada sessão da semana, incluindo o jogo. Esse método permite equilibrar os dias de treino disponíveis contra a fadiga, otimizando assim o treinamento dentro de uma determinada semana. Uma divisão simples da carga de trabalho concluída para o período de retorno típico do dia de jogo (*i. e.,* 7 dias de intervalo durante a semana da temporada) pode permitir a realização de modificações adequadas, por exemplo, reduzindo a carga de trabalho em semanas com retorno mais curto ou aumentando as demandas de treinamento em semanas com um maior tempo de retorno. A decisão também pode ser tomada para aumentar o tempo de recuperação por meio de dias de descanso adicionais, quando aplicável.

2. *Usar razões agudas:crônicas (A:C) para entender as flutuações nas demandas de treinamento em um determinado momento dentro de uma equipe.* As proporções A:C, conforme popularizado por Hulin et al., 2016, podem ser utilizadas em conjunto com as informações de monitoramento de uma equipe para avaliar o risco de lesão de um determinado jogador dentro da equipe. Embora o risco relativo proposto por Gabbett não seja comprovado, os princípios básicos desse trabalho são a pedra angular de qualquer tipo de treinamento físico; ou seja, pouquíssimo treinamento ou treinamento em excesso é prejudicial e qualquer mudança rápida resulta em dores físicas e diminuição do desempenho. Uma advertência é que se deve comparar continuamente a proporção A:C com a quantidade absoluta de trabalho concluído.

3. *Médias e variação percentual.* Em nível de equipe ou individual, essas métricas podem ser utilizadas como um sistema de semáforo para fornecer algumas informações rápidas e acionáveis sobre as demandas de treinamento da equipe em qualquer nível de análise. Isso pode ser em um nível semanal, por sessão ou dia de treinamento, ou com informações suficientes, tempo de treinamento consistente e exercícios específicos. Conjuntos médios podem ser utilizados em algumas métricas principais para determinar a demanda de treinamento e a sua flutuação natural, mas quando combinados

GPS: papel no condicionamento

O surgimento e a facilidade de uso da tecnologia de monitoramento permitiram um nível sem precedentes de análise e interpretação das demandas de jogo e treinamento. Essas informações estão cada vez mais sendo utilizadas para desenvolver estratégias globais de condicionamento para o time, e para os grupos posicionais, diferenças de jogo, treinamento *versus* demanda de jogo e momentos críticos dentro dos jogos. Essa facilidade de uso e a proliferação do GPS tem permitido que uma dose de condicionamento cada vez mais detalhada e específica seja dada à equipe e modelada em função das demandas de agendamento e de treinamento, conforme mencionado anteriormente.

Essa capacidade de aumentar a especificidade do volume, intensidade e densidade do treinamento e alinhar isso com as demandas do jogo e o contexto no qual elas ocorrem forneceu um direcionamento para permitir o desenvolvimento de algumas qualidades físicas essenciais que melhoram o desempenho da equipe. A tecnologia GPS pode fornecer algumas das informações mais detalhadas que temos sobre as qualidades físicas necessárias ao nível de elite. Ela pode, muitas vezes, ser mal interpretada como sendo apenas uma ferramenta de monitoramento, e temos que lembrar que também deve ser utilizada para aprimoramento de desempenho. O *kit* de ferramentas GPS permitiu a integração de vários pontos de informação para ajudar a criar uma imagem contextual completa. Além de combinar informações sobre as demandas específicas e gerais para criar os cenários em que o aprimoramento físico e das habilidades se cruzam, ele também pode fornecer informações ao atleta e ao técnico com relação ao desempenho.

A utilização do GPS para avaliar o desempenho pode ser feita de várias maneiras. Normalmente, os treinadores gostam de entender as demandas do jogo em todos os níveis, a partir de uma "visão de ângulo amplo" e aprofundando nos mínimos detalhes de cada passagem ou jogo. Essa abordagem telescópica funciona melhor ao avaliar as demandas (Tabela 34.2). Cada nível convida a uma análise e interpretação adicionais com relação ao contexto específico etc.

Piores cenários

Os piores cenários (PC) foram destacados por Tim Gabbett (Austin et al., 2011a; Delaney et al., 2017). PC são passagens específicas do jogo que identificam o teto para o modelo de preparação física de um treinador de condicionamento. Elas são, por definição, eventos de jogo onde demandas de pico/máximas são colocadas sobre a equipe ou grupo. Também são excelentes para definir os limites superiores para a estrutura de condicionamento de alguém e podem ser facilmente categorizados com base na qualidade física (corrida, aceleração ou colisões), duração ou tipo de esforço. Isso permite que o técnico adapte o condicionamento a cenários de oposição realistas.

Como qualquer evento de treinamento máximo, é melhor utilizá-los com moderação. Os PC são sessões de trabalho extremamente fatigantes, exigidas com regularidade de uma sessão de treinamento da equipe. O uso de sessões de PC não é adequado como um meio de desenvolver a aptidão da mesma maneira que o treino de força máxima absoluta não é um meio razoável de melhora gradual; fadiga extrema é inerente a esses métodos. Ainda assim, com a base necessária de preparação física, o PC é um meio de sobrecarregar os jogadores de maneira supramáxima e pode ser um ingrediente chave para o planejamento da pré-temporada.

Passagens de significância

As passagens de jogo de significância (PdS) são maiores em duração ou intensidade do que aquelas que normalmente ocorrem dentro de um jogo. Elas podem ser utilizadas em conjunto com o maior valor discrepante de dados – o PC. Um exemplo pode ser a utilização de uma passagem artificialmente estendida de treinamento que imita as demandas do jogo até o ponto em que os níveis de aptidão podem tolerar a única passagem maior, o PC (Austin et al., 2011b). A PdS pode ser subdividida para destacar as tendências dentro de padrões específicos de jogo ou para uma avaliação simples de ataque-contradefesa de alta intensidade. Como a PdS acumula continuamente, também é possível destacar a diferença entre um nível de equipe e adversário ou seu próprio treinamento *versus* as demandas do jogo. Isso fornece uma visão sobre as passagens específicas do jogo que constituem uma partida. Assim, a PdS destaca efetivamente a necessidade de ter passagens no treinamento que imitem não apenas o tempo e a intensidade típicos, como também a frequência dessas passagens mais longas nos jogos contra adversários de primeira linha.

A premissa para usar a PdS para auxiliar no condicionamento está relacionada à ideia de que, conforme o nível de habilidade de uma equipe aumenta, os membros da equipe se tornam mais confortáveis dentro dos sistemas e táticas que mobilizam contra uma equipe adversária no ataque ou na defesa. Isso também está atrelado a um padrão de jogador mais elevado e a um grande contingente desses jogadores na mesma equipe. Além disso, conforme a capacidade de uma equipe de atacar e defender por mais tempo e com mais precisão aumenta, também ocorre:

- A necessidade de capacidade para tolerar o aumento da demanda física de cada passagem
- A necessidade de fazer *backup* e replicar esses tipos de passagens com tempo de descanso reduzido.

Essas passagens podem ser agregadas para destacar as diferenças nas tendências entre os times, competições e estilos de jogo. É difícil para as equipes não ter uma impressão digital do estilo de jogo que afeta essas passagens. O modo como jogam é também como treinam, refletindo o ditado de treinamento de que uma equipe fica melhor no que faz com frequência. Se uma equipe se sentir desconfortável com a duração, frequência ou intensidade dessas passagens, na maioria das vezes ela tentará retornar às suas próprias normas específicas quando estiver com a posse de

Tabela 34.2 **Níveis de granularidade em que o jogo no rúgbi pode ser avaliado com GPS.**

Jogo	Treinamento
Meio a meio	Exercício a exercício
Análise de tempo segmentar: blocos de 10, 5 ou 3 min	Variantes de exercício
Passagens multifásicas	Passagens simultâneas
PdS/PC	Bola
Análise minuto a minuto	

PdS, passagens de significância; *PC*, pior cenário.

bola. Muitas vezes, isso é o que as pessoas percebem como diferentes estilos de jogo, como:
- Posição tática e ataque estruturado
- Contra-ataque
- Continuidade e ataque não estruturado.

Criação dessas passagens

Ao utilizar as plataformas GPS atuais, os treinadores de condicionamento agora têm alguns meios eficazes de avaliar a PdS em jogos e treinamentos. Um jogo ou sessão de treinamento pode ser visto como um todo ou dividido em segmentos cada vez menores para analisar mais detalhes (Figura 34.2). Essa abordagem granular permite um melhor entendimento quanto à composição constituinte de qualquer jogo.

Um jogo pode ser dividido em metades ou quartos, que são compostos de momentos de jogo. O tempo da bola em jogo é meramente a remoção do tempo de transição ou tempo morto na metade. Ao observar todas essas passagens do tempo de jogo da bola, um esboço da demanda de passagem pode ser feito para um jogo inteiro. As passagens de significância são aquelas que são mais longas do que o comprimento médio da passagem. Frequentemente, são essas passagens de maior duração que estressam fisicamente o jogador. O pior cenário é apenas a maior passagem única de um jogo ou, como descrito anteriormente, de uma temporada de jogos.

A criação de bancos de dados comparativos dessas informações para análise pode orientar o treinador de condicionamento no que diz respeito à eficácia ou nível de intensidade de um exercício de treinamento em sua replicação da intensidade do jogo. Uma expansão posterior disso pode olhar para a replicação de passagens que ocorrem no jogo dentro do treinamento. Ter este tipo de simulação de jogo dentro do treinamento, ao mesmo tempo em que conecta o elemento técnico do jogo, é o objetivo eterno na criação de informações que não sejam apenas fisicamente relevantes, mas contextualmente relevantes para o jogo de um ponto de vista técnico e tático.

Os dados podem ser divididos ainda mais para avaliar grupos posicionais e até mesmo características individuais dos jogadores. Essas informações podem ser usadas em combinação com medidas de análise de desempenho (precisão do passe, conclusão do *tackle*, número de carregamentos etc.) para fornecer uma visão holística das demandas, ações e esforço dos indivíduos dentro de passagens específicas do jogo.

Esforços repetidos de alta intensidade

Esforços repetidos de alta intensidade (ERAI) são outro meio excelente de avaliar onde ocorrem os picos de demanda física.

Esforços repetidos de alta intensidade

Definição

Uma sessão que envolve três ou mais esforços de contato, aceleração ou corrida em alta velocidade com menos de 21 segundos entre cada esforço.

Adaptado de Austin, D., Gabbett, T., Jenkins, D., 2011c. The physical demands of Super 14 rugby union. Journal of Science and Medicine in Sport, 14 (3), 259-263.

O ERAI pode ser uma mistura desses três componentes ou compreender apenas corrida, aceleração ou impacto; no entanto, uma mistura é mais comum devido à natureza do jogo (Austin et al., 2011c). O nível de esforço é normalmente definido de modo que apenas grandes esforços sejam registrados. Em um jogo, tendências e diferenças podem ser vistas com relação à oposição, resultado, meio a meio, posição ou até mesmo indivíduos dentro de grupos posicionais semelhantes.

ERAI foi descrito na literatura de pesquisa como sendo crítico para o desempenho e o sucesso da equipe (Austin et al., 2011a). ERAI leva em consideração as três ações de esforço primárias do rúgbi de 15, os esforços de alta intensidade de corrida, mudança de direção e/ou colisões. Esses esforços compreendem a base fisiológica geral de todas as ações que ocorrem dentro de um jogo de rúgbi, excluindo eventos que se baseiam em estática, como *mauls* ou *scrums*. As demandas típicas de jogos como um todo podem ser avaliadas pela compreensão do tipo de esforço típico e da frequência desses esforços de alta intensidade em vários níveis, incluindo:
- As demandas da equipe como um todo, por sessão de treinamento ou jogo
- Diferenças posicionais de grupo, geralmente encontradas entre atacantes e recuados, e em um nível por posição
- Para atletas individuais em posições semelhantes e/ou por indivíduo.

Um exemplo disso pode ser uma análise detalhada da composição do ERAI das parcerias centrais no rúgbi de 15. Frequentemente, o 12 (primeiro centro) é mais focado na colisão, tanto no ataque quanto na defesa, e então pode ter um perfil de colisão muito diferente do 13 (segundo centro), que muitas vezes é mais um atacante e leitor defensivo do jogo, e, portanto, pode ter mais esforços de aceleração e esforços de corrida em comparação com o 12.

Uma análise dessas informações pode destacar as diferenças entre jogadores individuais em uma posição semelhante. No rúgbi, um treinador pode intencionalmente ter uma variedade de características aparentes em suas escolhas de seleção. Isso é visto com frequência na composição da última fileira. O perfil ERAI de cada um dos três jogadores pode ser marcadamente diferente com base nas características de habilidade e composição física dos jogadores individuais, por exemplo, um número 8 carregando a bola, uma ameaça de caça furtiva 7 e um focado no alinhamento lateral 6. A composição do ERAI será fortemente influenciada pela missão que cada um desses jogadores tem a tarefa de completar. Um entendimento quanto à demanda física e perfil de esforço combinado com o plano de jogo contextual pode auxiliar na entrega de estratégias de condicionamento para cada uma dessas subposições.

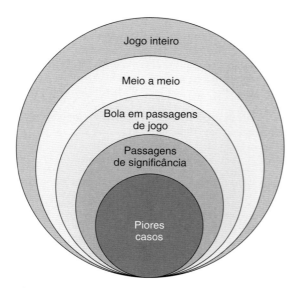

Figura 34.2 Meio visual de compreender a abordagem telescópica das demandas granulares do jogo.

Condicionamento para a Batalha do Momentum: Uso Prático da Tecnologia GPS para Estratégias... Capítulo | 34 |

Não há limite máximo para o número de esforços envolvidos ou período de tempo contido em uma única sessão, desde que cada esforço esteja conectado ao esforço anterior dentro de uma janela de 21 segundos. Por causa disso, ERAI pode ser extremamente relevante para o jogo, já que essa demanda básica de esforço é muitas vezes tecida diretamente em todas as ações de jogo, e a duração de uma passagem de jogo pode abrir a oportunidade para um atleta produzir momentos de alto esforço também como episódios de maior duração. O contrário também pode ser verdadeiro quando a falta de habilidade de um atleta em produzir esforços contínuos de alta intensidade resulta em erros técnicos que fazem o jogo parar.

Normalmente, a quantidade média de momentos ERAI dentro de um jogo é 17 ± 7. As diferenças podem ser vistas nos dados devido aos papéis táticos variáveis dentro das posições e às características físicas variáveis atribuídas a essas posições. Essas variações podem ser vistas na quantidade total de sessões, média de esforços por sessão e duração máxima do esforço.

O grupo posicional recuado geralmente tem mais episódios de ERAI quando comparado aos atacantes (Tabela 34.3), embora a quantidade média de esforços não difira significativamente. As diferenças são que os recuados pegam sessão de menor esforço em uma breve contestação do jogo, mas em passagens de longa duração, todas as posições são obrigadas a repetir os esforços no ataque ou na defesa. Isso explica, em parte, como os atacantes podem reunir uma quantidade semelhante de esforços quando chamados. A sessão típica de um ataque também tende a ser mais curta em duração e frequentemente o tempo entre os esforços é maior do que aquele visto pelas costas com relação aos esforços de aceleração e velocidade. No entanto, os impactos muitas vezes representam uma contribuição maior das sessões dos atacantes em comparação com os recuados, que podem ter uma grande quantidade de sessões, mas sem esforços de impacto registrados. Esses são normalmente vistos no apoio ao jogo de ataque.

Considerações

A tecnologia GPS tem suas falhas. Existem vários graus de erro, dependendo de quais parâmetros se escolheu para utilizar como seus principais determinantes de avaliação. Como todos os sistemas GPS, a precisão dos dados é pautada na qualidade do sinal recebido. Parâmetros simples são bastante precisos, como distância percorrida e detalhamento de tempo dos parâmetros de distância. No entanto, quanto maior a velocidade com que o parâmetro é medido, maior a oportunidade de erro na coleta de dados. Portanto, métricas como distância total e percorrida em zonas de baixa velocidade são bastante precisas, mas as acelerações em zonas altas são mais sujeitas a erros.

Os sistemas de nível de elite têm a capacidade de processamento de *hardware* e *software* para detectar com mais precisão micromovimentos, como mudança de direção e grandes mudanças na velocidade. Eles também têm a etiqueta de preço para acompanhar isso. Os dados de impacto e colisão requerem análise pós-*download* adicional e estão disponíveis apenas em sistemas de nível de elite que têm o acelerômetro de alta amostragem e *hardware* de giroscópio a bordo e os algoritmos para avaliar a precisão e validade dos dados coletados.

Seu esporte será uma consideração importante ao escolher um fornecedor de plataforma GPS, já que as principais plataformas vêm com algoritmos específicos para o esporte, por exemplo:

- *Catapult* tem quantidade de saltos do goleiro em direção à bola, análise de *scrum* para rúgbi, ERAI específico para hóquei ou eventos de salto
- *Statsport* tem contagem de chutes, *scrum* e análise de colisão para rúgbi de 15.

O aprendizado de máquina é a próxima fronteira para a geração de algoritmos e análises mais específicos para esportes. Os exemplos aqui incluem detecção automática de exercícios ou análise de marcha de jogadores individuais, onde o algoritmo pode fazer inferências com base em dados históricos exclusivos para aquele jogador em questão.

Um dos benefícios de ponta que a tecnologia GPS está começando a oferecer é a capacidade de combinar marcadores de desempenho específicos do esporte com a capacidade de contextualizar o desempenho por meio da integração de múltiplas fontes de informação. Essa capacidade de vincular várias camadas de informações – que vão desde informações subjetivas de bem-estar fornecidas pelos atletas, à resposta objetiva interna e externa ao treinamento obtido por GPS e frequência cardíaca, à avaliação do desempenho obtido por meio de análises de desempenho e *insights* de treinamento – é fundamental. É essa sinergia de informações que fornecerá alguns dos principais caminhos para progressão no futuro próximo.

Tabela 34.3 Comparação de ERAI e métricas de esforço para diferentes posições de rúgbi. Os números apresentados são por sessão (*i. e.*, jogo)

Posição	Max. sessões ERAI	Qtd. max. esf.	Med. qtd. esf.	Duração máxima do esforço	Duração média do esforço
Pilar	7	8	6	00:00:17	00:00:03
Talonador	11	9	7	00:00:11	00:00:03
Avante de segunda linha	12	9	7	00:00:09	00:00:03
Linha de *back*	20	11	7	00:00:12	00:00:04
Meio *scrum*	23	14	9	00:00:16	00:00:05
Abertura	18	15	6	00:00:11	00:00:02
Centro	26	14	8	00:00:21	00:00:02
Back 3	24	14	6	00:00:13	00:00:02

ERAI, esforços repetidos de alta intensidade; *qtd. max. esf.*, quantidade máxima de esforços por cada ERAI; *med. qtd. esf.*, quantidade média de esforços por cada sessão ERAI.

Conclusão

O objetivo deste capítulo foi fornecer uma visão sobre a aplicação prática do GPS, como uma ferramenta de monitoramento, e também como uma plataforma de aprimoramento de desempenho. O GPS ganhou destaque devido à sua capacidade de reunir percepções físicas sobre o mundo cativante do esporte. A informação apresentada nesse capítulo é esperançosamente um meio pelo qual um treinador de condicionamento pode utilizar GPS para monitorar como uma equipe está treinando e se desempenhando em comparação com os resultados e para avaliar a contribuição individual para esses desempenhos. Isso pode ser realizado por meio de uma análise das demandas de esforço e da produção dos indivíduos, conforme avaliado por esforços de alta intensidade ou sessões de ERAI.

O GPS também pode ser utilizado como uma plataforma compartilhada para avaliar o projeto e o resultado do treinamento em uma equipe interprofissional, por meio da replicação das passagens de intensidade do jogo para tornar o treinamento o mais específico possível ao contexto do jogo. Isso garante a entrega de um treinamento no qual o desenvolvimento físico, técnico e tático ocorre em uma intensidade relevante. Espera-se que as técnicas apresentadas ajudem a maximizar o desempenho naqueles momentos ocasionais, mas recompensadores, em jogos em que momento de grande intensidade ganha o dia.

Referências bibliográficas

Austin, D.J., Gabbett, T.J., Jenkins, D.J., 2011a. Repeated high-intensity exercise in a professional rugby league. The Journal of Strength and Conditioning Research 25 (7), 1898-1904.

Austin, D.J., Gabbett, T.J., Jenkins, D.J., 2011b. Repeated high-intensity exercise in professional rugby union. Journal of Sports Sciences 29 (10), 1105-1112.

Austin, D., Gabbett, T., Jenkins, D., 2011c. The physical demands of Super 14 rugby union. Journal of Science and Medicine in Sport, 14 (3), 259–263.

Cummins, C., Orr, R., O'Connor, H., West, C., 2013. Global positioning systems (GPS) and microtechnology sensors in team sports: a systematic review. Sports Medicine 43 (10), 1025-1042.

Delaney, J.A., Thornton, H.R., Pryor, J.F., Stewart, A.M., Dascombe, B.J., Duthie, G.M., 2017. Peak running intensity of international rugby: implications for training prescription. International Journal of Sports Physiology and Performance 12 (8), 1039-1045.

Gabbett, T.J., 2012. Sprinting patterns of national rugby league competition. The Journal of Strength and Conditioning Research 26 (1), 121-130.

Gabbett, T.J., Jenkins, D.G., Abernethy, B., 2012. Physical demands of professional rugby league training and competition using microtechnology. Journal of Science and Medicine in Sport 15 (1), 80-86.

Hulin, B.T., Gabbett, T.J., Lawson, D.W., Caputi, P., Sampson, J.A., 2016. The acute: chronic workload ratio predicts injury: high chronic workload may decrease injury risk in elite rugby league players. British Journal of Sports Medicine 50 (4), 231-236.

Capítulo | 35 |

Gerenciamento do Atleta *Overhead*

Steve McCaig

Introdução: o que é "o atleta *overhead*"?

Esportes como beisebol, tênis, *softball*, críquete, vôlei, handebol e polo aquático podem ser considerados esportes *overhead*. Todos eles envolvem atividades em que uma das mãos arremessa ou bate a bola acima da cabeça, com ou sem complemento, como uma raquete, na mão. Embora haja muitas diferenças entre esses esportes, o movimento que ocorre no membro superior durante essas tarefas é amplamente semelhante (Fleisig et al., 1996; Wagner et al., 2014), assim como as lesões sofridas nos membros superiores (McCaig e Young, 2016). Portanto, princípios semelhantes podem ser aplicados ao gerenciar as condições de saúde desses atletas.

Dor no braço de arremesso

A dor no braço de arremesso (DBA) tem sido utilizada para descrever o conjunto de condições de ombro e cotovelo relatadas em esportes *overhead* (McCaig e Young, 2016). Essas atividades causam condições semelhantes nos membros superiores por apresentarem fatores intrínsecos e extrínsecos semelhantes, como técnica, carga de trabalho, fatores físicos e psicossociais, que contribuem para as lesões. É vital compreender a biomecânica da atividade *overhead*, incluindo a patomecânica e as adaptações físicas associadas para gerenciar o atleta.

Biomecânica da atividade *overhead*

A biomecânica de um lançamento de beisebol e de um saque de tênis foi bem descrita, assim como outras atividades *overhead* (Cook e Strike, 2000; Fleisig et al., 1996; Kovacs e Ellenbecker, 2011; Wagner et al., 2014). Todos eles têm uma fase de preparação, aceleração e desaceleração (Tabela 35.1). Embora existam muitas diferenças entre esses esportes, os movimentos do membro superior variam pouco (Fleisig et al., 1996; Wagner et al., 2014). As qualidades físicas necessárias para cada fase da atividade *overhead* são descritas na Tabela 35.2 e os fatores-chave no desempenho de arremesso e risco de lesão são descritos na Tabela 35.3.

Fase de preparação

A fase de preparação inclui todas as ações realizadas para colocar o corpo em posição para atingir a rotação externa máxima (REM) do ombro durante a fase de elevação do braço (Fleisig, 2010).

Os estágios envolvidos durante a etapa de preparação variam entre os esportes, mas todos terminam em um estágio de elevação do braço. Em alguns cenários, o atleta começará com a bola na mão, como em um campo de beisebol ou saque de tênis, enquanto em outros o jogador deve se mover para a posição para pegar ou bater na bola, como um jogador externo de beisebol ou um rebatedor externo em voleibol. É importante reconhecer que outros fatores, como a base de suporte, por exemplo, polo aquático *versus* lançamento de beisebol, tempo e restrições de tomada de decisão, como saque de tênis *versus* zagueiro prestes a ser derrubado, também influenciarão a fase de preparação.

Fase de elevação do braço

Durante a fase de elevação, o ombro dominante se move para REM, que é crítico para o desempenho (Fortenbaugh et al., 2009; Whiteley, 2007). A pelve, seguida rapidamente pelo tronco, gira em direção ao alvo, o que força o membro superior em REM, que pode atingir até 200° (Werner et al., 1993). A REM é uma combinação de rotação externa (RE) da articulação glenoumeral (AGU), inclinação posterior da escápula e RE, extensão do tronco e valgo do cotovelo (Miyashita et al., 2010).

Fase de aceleração

Essa fase começa após a REM e termina no lançamento da bola ou contato com a bola e é o movimento articular mais rápido em todos os esportes, com o ombro girando a até 7.000°/s, que é o equivalente ao ombro completando cerca de 18 rotações completas por segundo, e o cotovelo se estende a 2.500°/s (Fleisig et al., 1995).

Fase de desaceleração

Essa fase tem início após o lançamento ou contato da bola e termina quando a próxima habilidade motora começa. Trata-se de uma etapa crucial para dissipar as forças geradas durante a aceleração. No entanto, cada esporte terá restrições variáveis que a afetam, como a rede de voleibol durante um ataque.

Patomecânica da atividade *overhead*

Acredita-se que o desenvolvimento da DBA esteja relacionado às tensões experimentadas no membro superior durante as principais fases e estágios da atividade *overhead* (Fleisig et al., 1995; Fortenbaugh et al., 2009; Wassinger e Myers, 2011).

Tabela 35.1 **Comparação entre as fases biomecânicas do lançamento de beisebol e serviço de tênis.**

Fases das atividades esportivas *overhead*		Estágios de arremesso de beisebol		Estágios de saque de tênis	
1. Fase de preparação	Começa com o primeiro movimento e termina na rotação externa máxima (REM) do ombro	1. Preparação	Começa quando o arremessador levanta a perna dianteira do chão e termina na flexão máxima do quadril da perna dianteira	1. Início	A bola e a raquete estão em repouso
		2. Passada	Começa quando a perna dianteira começa a se mover para a frente e termina quando entra em contato com o solo (contato do pé; CP)	2. Liberação da bola	Começa com o movimento inicial da bola e da raquete até que a bola seja liberada da mão que não saca
		3. Elevação do braço	Começa com CP e termina com REM	3. Carregamento	Desde a liberação até que a parte inferior do corpo esteja totalmente carregada em flexão máxima do joelho
				4. Elevação do braço	Começa no final da fase de carregamento e termina com REM, o que resulta na ponta da raquete em direção ao solo
2. Fase de aceleração	Começa com REM e termina no impacto ou lançamento da bola	4. Aceleração	De REM até que a bola seja lançada	5. Aceleração	De REM até o contato com a bola
				6. Contato	O breve período em que a raquete está em contato com a bola
3. Fase de desaceleração	Começa imediatamente após o lançamento da bola ou impactos e termina quando a próxima habilidade motora começa	5. Desaceleração	Seguindo o contato até a rotação interna máxima (RIM) do ombro	7. Desaceleração	Contato seguinte até RIM
		6. Execução	Qualquer movimento contínuo após RIM até que a próxima habilidade motora comece	8. Execução	Qualquer movimento contínuo após RIM até que a próxima habilidade motora comece

Adaptada de Kovacs, M., Ellenbecker, T., 2011. An 8-stage model for evaluating the tennis serve: implications for performance enhancement and injury prevention. Sports Health 3, 504-513.

Gerenciamento do Atleta *Overhead* — Capítulo | 35 |

Tabela 35.2 **Principais qualidades físicas necessárias para arremessos *overhead*.**

Fase de ação *overhead*	Região	Amplitude de movimento	Comprimento do tecido mole	Atividade muscular
Preparação	Membro inferior	Extensão do quadril da perna LD e abd.	Comprimento do flexor do quadril da perna LD	Perna LD con. ext. triplo
		Perna LD e LND e RE quadril	Comprimento do adutor de quadril de perna LD	Perna LD conc. quadril abd.
				Extensão tripla da perna LND rigidez
	Tronco	Rot. lateral torácica LD		Exc. então con. atividade abdominal oblíqua
		Torácica ext.		Exc. então con. flexores do tronco
	Membro superior	RE ombro LD	Comprimento menor do peitoral	RI exc. ombro LD e flex. hor.
		Ret. escápula LD		Exc. Músculos OCF
Aceleração	Membro inferior	RE e RI quadril LD		Extensão tripla da perna LND rigidez
				Extensão concêntrica de joelho LND
	Tronco			Atividade abdominal oblíqua con.
				Flexores do tronco con.
	Membro superior			Con. rápida RI ombro LD e flex. hor.
				Extensores concêntricos da escápula LD
Desaceleração	Membro inferior	RI e flex. do quadril LND	Comprimento do isquiotibial LND	Extensores de quadril exc. LND e RE
		RI quadril LD e abd.		Rigidez do joelho LND
	Tronco	Rot. torácica LND		Exc. extensores toracolombares
		Flex. tronco		
	Membro superior	RI ombro LD e flex. hor.		RE excêntrica ombro LD e hor. ext.
		Prot. escápula LD		Exc. Retratores de escápula LD
		Ext. e pron. do cotovelo LD		Exc. Flexores e supinadores de cotovelo LD
				Exc. Bíceps LD LH

abd., abdução; *OCF*, origem comum do flexor; *con.*, atividade muscular concêntrica; *LD*, lado dominante; *exc.*, atividade muscular excêntrica; *RE*, rotação externa; *ext.*, extensão; *flex.*, flexão; *hor.*, horizontal; *RI*, rotação interna; *LND*, lado não dominante; *pron.*, pronação; *prot.*, protração; *ret.*, retração; *rot.*, rotação.

Tabela 35.3 Fatores principais para desempenho de arremesso e risco de lesão.

Fatores principais para desempenho (velocidade e precisão)	Fatores principais para risco de lesão (redução das cargas articulares)
Maior comprimento da passada	Comprimento da passada
Pé no alvo no contato do pé	Pé no alvo no contato do pé
Sincronismo entre a rotação da pelve e do tronco durante a fase de elevação	Sincronismo entre a rotação da pelve e do tronco durante a fase de elevação
Faixa de rotação externa máxima no final da fase de elevação	Abdução do ombro durante o levantamento e aceleração
Flexão do tronco durante a aceleração	Flexão do cotovelo durante a fase de elevação
Ligeira extensão do joelho durante a aceleração	Extensão horizontal durante a fase de elevação
Siga em direção ao alvo	Rotação externa do ombro no contato do pé
	Flexão lateral do tronco
	Siga em direção ao alvo

Adaptada de Fleisig, G.S., 2010. Biomechanics of overhand throwing: implications for injury and performance. In: Portus, M. (Ed.) Conference of Science, Medicine and Coaching in Cricket. Conference Proceedings. Brisbane: Cricket Australia; Fortenbaugh, D., Fleisig, G.S., Andrews, J.R., 2009. Baseball pitching biomechanics in relation to risk and performance. Sport Health 1, 314-320; Whitelety, R., 2007. Baseball throwing mechanics as they relate to pathology and performance: a review. Journal of Sport Science and Medicine 6, 1-20.

Fase de elevação/aceleração

Faixas extremas de REM podem contribuir para o desenvolvimento de DBA por meio de choque interno e do fenômeno de "descascar" (Wassinger e Myers, 2011). O impacto interno é onde a superfície articular do manguito rotador posterossuperior e lábio glenoidal é comprimida entre a tuberosidade maior do úmero e a fossa glenoide (Burkhart et al., 2003a; Edelson e Teitz, 2000; Walch et al., 1992) (Figura 35.1 B). Embora esse seja um fenômeno normal que ocorre durante a RE na amplitude final em abdução (Edelson e Teitz, 2000), o estresse repetitivo de altas forças que ocorrem durante esportes *overhead* pode resultar em alterações patológicas no manguito rotador e lábio glenoide. O fenômeno de descascar acontece quando o tendão da cabeça longa do bíceps torce durante a REM; quando combinado com a atividade muscular, isso resulta no lábio sendo "descascado" da glenoide (Burkhart et al., 2003b). Acredita-se que isso contribua para o desenvolvimento de tendinopatias do bíceps e lesões labrais superiores (p. ex., LSAP, laceração labral superior de anterior para posterior) (Burkhart et al., 2003b) (Figura 35.1 C).

Durante a REM, as forças em valgo podem ultrapassar a resistência à tração do ligamento colateral ulnar (LCU) (Fleisig et al., 1995), o que pode levar à atenuação ou lesões agudas do LCU. A frouxidão resultante no LCU pode ocasionar a compressão da cabeça do rádio contra o capítulo e o olécrano, que impactam a fossa do olécrano medialmente durante o estresse em valgo. Esse processo e as patologias a ele associadas são conhecidos como sobrecarga de extensão em valgo (SEV) (Cain et al., 2003) (Figura 35.2). Os músculos da origem flexora comum (OFC) atuam como estabilizadores secundários ao estresse em valgo (An et al., 1981; Davidson et al., 1995) e o aumento da carga na OFC devido à frouxidão do LCU pode levar à tendinopatia da OFC. A frouxidão do valgo também pode comprimir o nervo ulnar em seu sulco posterior ao côndilo medial, resultando em irritação do nervo ulnar e neuropatia, podendo causar alterações na funcionalidade e dor neuropática (Cain et al., 2003).

Fase de desaceleração

Altos níveis de atividade muscular excêntrica ocorrem no manguito posterior e bíceps para controlar o movimento do ombro e do cotovelo durante a desaceleração, embora toda a cadeia cinética deva funcionar para absorver essas forças (Chu et al., 2016). A flexão de tronco e rotação contralateral inadequadas, e a flexão de quadril e rotação interna (RI) durante a desaceleração aumentam o estresse no ombro e cotovelo, o que pode levar ao desenvolvimento de DBA (Chu et al., 2016).

Adaptações para esportes *overhead*

As adaptações musculoesqueléticas ao esporte *overhead* são bem documentadas e provavelmente são necessárias para um alto desempenho. No entanto, elas também podem levar ao aumento do risco de lesões (Borsa et al., 2008; Whiteley et al., 2012). Essas adaptações incluem mudanças específicas de postura, mobilidade e força no membro superior dominante (Borsa et al., 2008; Forthomme et al., 2008; Whiteley et al., 2012). Ao avaliar o atleta *overhead*, é importante estar ciente de que esses achados são comuns em atletas assintomáticos.

Escápula

A escápula dominante comumente fica em depressão, rotação para baixo e interna (protração) com relação ao LND em atletas *overhead* (Forthomme et al., 2008; Oyama et al., 2008). Isso se deve ao aumento do volume muscular e à rigidez no peitoral menor e maior e no grande dorsal. A discinesia da escápula é encontrada em atletas *overhead* (Burn et al., 2016) e foi proposta como um fator de risco para DBA. No entanto, há evidências conflitantes para apoiar isso (Hickey et al., 2017; Myers et al., 2013; Struyf et al., 2013).

Amplitude de movimento de rotação na articulação glenoumeral

No atleta *overhead* assintomático, o ombro dominante geralmente exibe ganho na amplitude de movimento (ADM) da RE e diminuição na ADM da RI (déficit de RI glenoumeral [DRIG]) quando medido em abdução de 90°. A ADM de rotação total (ADMRT) (ADMRT = RE + RI) sendo semelhante nos lados dominante (LD) e não dominante (LND) (Borsa et al., 2008; Whiteley e Oceguera, 2016). O aumento na ADM da RE é considerado crucial para o desempenho da velocidade de lançamento, pois pode permitir uma maior REM (Fortenbaugh et al., 2009; Whiteley, 2007).

Acredita-se que essas mudanças na ADM ocorram devido a alterações nos tecidos moles ou ósseos (Borsa et al., 2008). As modificações dos tecidos moles incluem flacidez adquirida na cápsula anterior e rigidez na cápsula posterior do ombro e acredita-se que contribuam para o desenvolvimento de ganho na rotação externa (GRE) e DRIG, respectivamente (Borsa et al., 2008). Alterações no grau de torção umeral, que é o grau de torção no eixo longo do úmero, têm sido observadas de maneira consistente em atletas *overhead* (Whiteley et al., 2009; Yamamoto et al., 2006). O úmero do LD exibe retroversão humana aumentada em comparação com o LND e essas mudanças seriam responsáveis por qualquer GRE e DRIG observado em atletas *overhead* (Chant et al., 2007; Crockett et al., 2002; Whiteley e Oceguera, 2016). Acredita-se que o aumento da retroversão umeral melhora o desempenho e reduz o risco de dor no ombro, uma

Gerenciamento do Atleta *Overhead* | Capítulo | 35 |

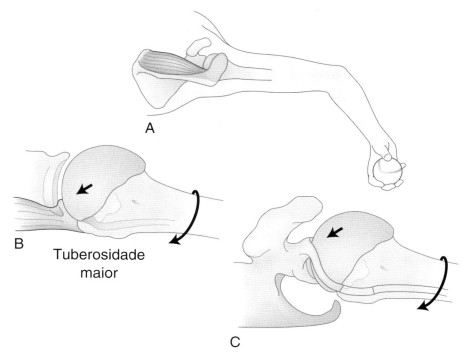

Figura 35.1 Impacto interno e o fenômeno de "descascar". A. Ombro em rotação externa máxima durante a fase de elevação **B.** Choque interno. **C.** Fenômeno de "descascar". (Adaptada de Chang, I.Y., Polster, J.M., 2016. Pathomechanics and magnetic resonance imaging of the thrower's shoulder. Radiologic Clinics of North America 54 [5], 801-815.) (*Esta figura se encontra reproduzida em cores no Encarte.*)

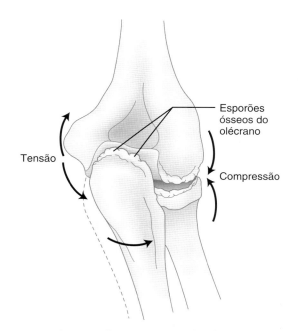

Figura 35.2 Sobrecarga de extensão em valgo. (Adaptada de Abrams, G., Safran, M., 2011. Valgus extension overload. In: Miller, M.D., Sanders, T.G. (Eds.), Presentation, Imaging and Treatment of Common Musculoskeletal Conditions: MRI – Arthroscopy Correlation. Elsevier Saunders, Philadelphia, PA.)

vez que menos estresse será colocado nos tecidos moles à medida que mais faixa de RE é permitida devido à geometria óssea (Whiteley et al., 2009).

Vários estudos descobriram que DRIG aumentado, falta de GRE, ADMRT reduzida e flexão do ombro foram associados à DBA (Camp et al., 2017; Clarsen et al., 2014; Shanley et al., 2011; Wilk et al., 2014; Wilk et al., 2015a, b), embora outros não tenham encontrado associação (Oyama et al., 2017). A medição precisa da ADM do ombro é crucial ao avaliar atletas *overhead*, e existem muitos métodos. No entanto, a amplitude do ombro medida variará significativamente dependendo do método utilizado, seja ele ativo ou passivo, e com ou sem estabilização da escápula (Wilk et al., 2009). Para um único profissional da saúde, descobrimos que medir a ADM de rotação da AGU passivamente com estabilização da escápula com um inclinômetro é um método confiável (Figuras 35.3 e 35.4).

Força da articulação glenoumeral

Atletas com sobrecarga demonstram consistentemente maior força de RI no ombro do LD e razão de força RI:RE aumentada, enquanto os rotadores externos não apresentam nenhuma mudança na força ou podem ter uma redução na força em comparação com o ombro do LND (Whiteley et al., 2012). Os rotadores internos contribuem significativamente para a velocidade de lançamento (Roach e Lieberman, 2014); no entanto, a fraqueza na RE e aumentos marcantes na razão RI:RE (> 1,5) foram associados ao aumento do risco de desenvolver DBA (Byram et al., 2010; Clarsen et al., 2014). O aumento da relação RI:RE pode fazer com que os rotadores externos sejam incapazes de controlar as forças de aceleração geradas pelos rotadores internos durante a fase de desaceleração, o que aumenta o risco de DBA (Whiteley et al., 2012).

Embora o teste isocinético seja considerado o padrão-ouro para avaliar a força do manguito rotador (Whiteley et al., 2012), consideramos a dinamometria manual útil para o clínico devido à sua facilidade de uso, natureza portátil e relativa economia. O teste de força de rotação da AGU pode ser concluído como um teste de "fazer" ou "quebrar". Em um teste de "fazer", o sujeito é solicitado a empurrar o mais forte possível para o terapeuta que corresponde a sua força e o dinamômetro mede sua contração isométrica máxima. Em um teste de "quebrar", o terapeuta pede ao sujeito para ficar parado e então aumenta

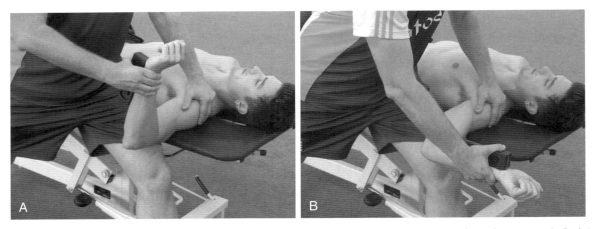

Figura 35.3 Medição da amplitude de movimento de rotação externa da articulação glenoumeral passivamente. **A.** Posição inicial. **B.** Posição final.

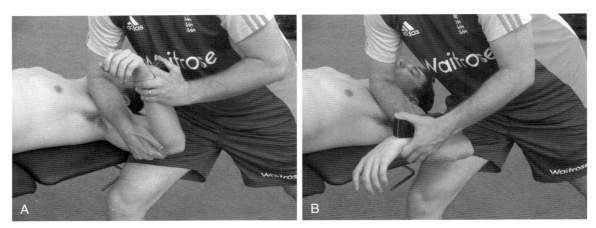

Figura 35.4 Medição da amplitude de movimento de rotação interna da articulação glenoumeral passivamente. **A.** Posição inicial. **B.** Posição final.

gradualmente sua força até que ele não seja mais capaz de manter essa posição. Isso mede sua contração excêntrica máxima e pode ser provocativo em ombros irritados. Testar a força do ombro em 90° de abdução é uma posição mais funcional para o atleta *overhead* (Figuras 35.5 e 35.6); pode ser provocativo para alguns atletas que precisem ser avaliados em 0° de abdução.

Amplitude de movimento do cotovelo

Não é incomum que atletas *overhead* tenham uma extensão reduzida do cotovelo e um ângulo de carregamento aumentado (Chang et al., 2010; Wright et al., 2006). No entanto, poucos estudos investigaram qualquer risco de lesão com essa associação.

Cadeia cinética (tronco e membro inferior)

Toda a cadeia cinética é utilizada durante as atividades *overhead* e sua função efetiva é crucial para o desempenho e redução do risco de lesões (Chu et al., 2016; Fortenbaugh et al., 2009). O papel da cadeia cinética é canalizar as forças geradas do membro inferior e tronco para o membro superior para aumentar a velocidade de RI do ombro, bem como absorver essas forças. Vários testes de desempenho dos músculos do membro inferior e do tronco se correlacionam com a velocidade de lançamento, como um salto lateral e um lançamento lateral de *medicine ball* (Freeston et al., 2016; Lehman et al., 2013).

Gerenciamento total do atleta *overhead*

O gerenciamento total é o processo contínuo de "planejar, fazer, revisar" aplicado a todos os aspectos do atleta para otimizar o desempenho e minimizar o risco de lesões. Encoraja os profissionais da saúde a serem proativos em vez de reativos a lesões (Newton et al., 2011). É importante que o praticante considere todos os fatores que podem afetar a capacidade do atleta de treinar e competir. O plano de gerenciamento total do atleta deve ser ajustado de acordo com as demandas do treinamento específico ou da fase competitiva.

Gestão entre temporadas

Todos os atletas precisam de uma fase de recuperação no final da temporada competitiva; entretanto, a duração desse período depende da intensidade e duração da temporada anterior e do tempo de preparação necessário para a próxima temporada. Embora, um período de folga das atividades *overhead* seja crucial para a recuperação física e psicológica, é importante que o atleta mantenha as qualidades físicas necessárias para a atividade durante essa fase. Se ficarem descondicionados, ficarão vulneráveis a lesões, pois pode haver tempo insuficiente para prepará-los para as demandas da próxima temporada competitiva.

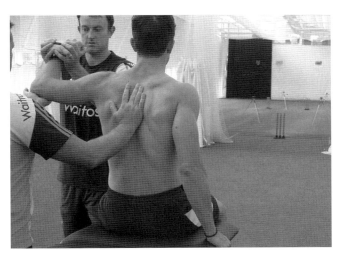

Figura 35.5 Medição da força de rotação externa com dinamômetro portátil.

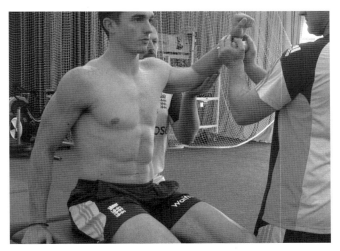

Figura 35.6 Medição da força de rotação interna com dinamômetro portátil.

O histórico pregresso de lesão é um fator de risco significativo, pode ocorrer porque ela nunca foi totalmente resolvida ou os fatores que contribuíram para a lesão não foram abordados (Finch e Cook, 2014). Distúrbios de membros inferiores e coluna podem afetar a função da cadeia cinética, o que pode aumentar a carga no membro superior durante o arremesso, aumentando o risco de DBA (Chu et al., 2016). A verificação de saúde periódica antes da temporada deve envolver uma revisão completa de quaisquer distúrbios musculoesqueléticos anteriores e quaisquer condições identificadas devem ser tratadas de maneira adequada durante o período entre temporadas.

O valor da triagem pré-temporada foi questionado (Bahr, 2016; Whiteley, 2016), particularmente no que diz respeito à previsão de lesões. Preferimos o termo "perfil", que descreve o processo de coleta de informações para entender melhor o atleta para informar seu manejo. Essa informação é utilizada para ajudar a informar o programa de preparação de cada jogador, estabelecer referências para a equipe e determinar linhas de base clínicas e funcionais, que podem ser manejadas para ajudar a determinar a prontidão para voltar a jogar após a lesão. O perfil do atleta *overhead* deve incluir uma avaliação de todos os requisitos físicos essenciais para o arremesso, bem como os requisitos de capacidade de trabalho específicos do esporte, usando testes com confiabilidade e validade estabelecidas. Após a conclusão do perfil, a equipe de suporte deve desenvolver um programa de preparação individualizado com base nesses resultados, em consulta com o atleta e a equipe técnica, pois isso melhorará a conformidade.

Quaisquer deficiências técnicas identificadas devem ser tratadas durante o período entre as temporadas, com foco em exercícios que abordem os fatores técnicos relacionados ao desempenho e ao risco de lesões (ver Tabela 35.3). Embora a análise de movimento em 3D seja o padrão-ouro para avaliar a biomecânica do arremesso, ela não é prática para a maioria dos esportes, pois requer equipamentos caros e consome muito tempo (McCaig e Young, 2016). Filmagens de alta velocidade podem ser utilizadas pelos treinadores e pela equipe de suporte para identificar áreas de desenvolvimento com base em um entendimento sólido de um modelo técnico ideal. Qualquer trabalho técnico deve ser concluído como parte de um retorno gradativo à atividade *overhead*, com base na preparação do atleta para as demandas da temporada competitiva. É fundamental que ele desenvolva a capacidade física para suportar a carga de trabalho de seu esporte; a fadiga pode resultar em alterações técnicas que podem aumentar o estresse no membro superior, aumentando a suscetibilidade a lesões (Erickson et al., 2016; Gabbett, 2016).

Gestão durante a temporada

Durante a temporada competitiva, é importante que os praticantes monitorem a carga de trabalho do atleta arremessador (carga externa) e a sua resposta a essa carga (carga interna). A relação entre a carga de trabalho do arremesso e o aumento do risco de lesões em esportes *overhead* está bem estabelecida (Black et al., 2016). Volumes mais altos de arremesso em uma base diária e semanal, dias de descanso reduzidos e aumentos na razão de carga de trabalho aguda:crônica (RTAC) aumentam o risco de desenvolver DBA (Black et al., 2016). A quantidade de arremessos que o atleta realiza deve ser registrado sempre que possível, assim como quaisquer outros esportes e cargas de treinamento. Infelizmente, monitorar a carga de trabalho de lançamento pode ser um desafio; os jogadores não conseguem se lembrar com precisão de quantos arremessos fizeram em cada sessão, nem a intensidade de cada arremesso pode ser quantificada. Avanços na tecnologia, como sistemas de posicionamento global (GPS) e unidades de medida inercial (UMI), facilitam o monitoramento de cargas de arremesso (Murray et al., 2017). Embora os custos sejam altos, podem ocorrer problemas tecnológicos, que requerem recursos humanos significativos e alguns atletas podem não querer utilizar as unidades (Warren et al., 2018). Descobrimos que o cálculo de unidades arbitrárias (UA) multiplicando as classificações de esforço percebido (CEP) da sessão e a duração da sessão é uma maneira prática de monitorar a carga de trabalho. Além disso, encontramos um aumento do risco de lesões e doenças em atletas de arremesso com cargas diárias e semanais mais altas e maior RTAC.

Questionários diários de bem-estar podem ser utilizados para monitorar a resposta do atleta à carga de trabalho e devem coletar informações como duração e qualidade do sono, dor muscular, sintomas de resfriado, humor e níveis de estresse, com as pontuações com base no que é normal para aquele indivíduo (Saw et al., 2017). Essas informações podem ser coletadas manualmente do atleta ou por meio de mensagens de texto ou aplicativos. Dor e fadiga podem frequentemente preceder a DBA; portanto, qualquer desvio das respostas normais do atleta deve ser discutido com ele e o manejo implementado conforme indicado.

Parte | 2 | Aplicação Clínica

As sessões agudas e crônicas de arremesso resultam em alterações no perfil musculoesquelético do arremessador. Essas mudanças incluem reduções na RI do ombro e da ADM do cotovelo (Dwelly et al., 2009; Kibler et al., 2012; Laudner et al., 2013; Reinold et al., 2008) e reduções na força de RE do ombro (Whiteley, 2010). Atletas com risco de desenvolver DBA devem ser monitorados para mudanças na função dos membros superiores regularmente ao longo de uma temporada (Whiteley, 2010). Como a força dos membros inferiores é crucial para o arremesso, isso também deve ser monitorado e pode ser feito por meio de um salto com contramovimento em um tapete de salto ou plataforma de força (Cormack et al., 2006; Laffaye et al., 2014). Se os recursos forem limitados, os atletas podem aprender uma rotina de autoverificação que pode incluir exercícios de mobilidade específicos, como alongamento em flexão horizontal, rotação torácica, agachamento com levantamento de barra acima da cabeça, agachamento parcial e agachamento parcial lateral. Elas podem ser realizadas diariamente como parte do aquecimento para outras atividades.

Qualquer monitoramento físico deve ser feito de maneira consistente no mesmo estágio da competição, seja após 1 dia de descanso antes de iniciar o treinamento naquele dia ou no dia seguinte a uma partida, dependendo da fase competitiva do esporte (Whiteley, 2010). O monitoramento regular permite que o praticante entenda o que é normal para aquele atleta, o que pode então ser utilizado para identificar quando essas mudanças excedem a variação normal. Os atletas devem receber *feedback* regular sobre qualquer informação que compartilhem, o que é crucial para obter sua "adesão". Se qualquer mudança significativa for observada, o praticante deve procurar modificar o treinamento do atleta ou a carga de trabalho competitiva, adicionar métodos de recuperação específicos, como terapia de tecido mole ou sessões de mobilidade extra, ou adicionar sessões de força quando apropriado (Gabbett et al., 2017). No entanto, quaisquer mudanças no programa do atleta, sobretudo durante sua programação competitiva, devem ser feitas em consulta cuidadosa com o atleta e o técnico e informadas pelas melhores evidências disponíveis do monitoramento do atleta (Gabbett et al., 2017).

Durante a temporada competitiva é importante que o atleta continue treinando para manter as qualidades físicas necessárias para um ótimo desempenho e para manter a robustez. Esse treinamento deve ser semelhante ao seu programa entre temporadas, mas o volume de séries e cargas é reduzido de acordo com as outras demandas de seu esporte. As sessões devem ser programadas como parte da programação semanal do atleta, levando em consideração sua programação de jogo e treinamento. Uma maneira fácil de implementá-los é incluir alguns desses exercícios como parte das sessões de aquecimento e recuperação.

Avaliação do atleta *overhead* lesionado

Qualquer atleta *overhead* com DBA deve ser avaliado cuidadosamente e o praticante deve ter um entendimento completo da apresentação da dor antes de iniciar um plano de tratamento. As seguintes questões são cruciais para isso:

1. Há algum sinal de alerta presente?
2. A apresentação é consistente com um distúrbio específico ou inespecífico?
3. Qual é o estágio do distúrbio? Agudo, persistente, agudo sobre persistente?
4. A apresentação da dor é mecânica, não mecânica ou mista?
5. A apresentação da dor responde ao teste de melhoria?
6. Quais são os fatores contribuintes (intrínsecos e extrínsecos) e eles são modificáveis?

Sinais de alerta

Embora incomum, a presença de sinais de alerta deve ser rastreada em todos os pacientes, incluindo atletas *overhead*, e o profissional da saúde deve continuar vigilante durante o processo de tratamento. A presença de sinais de alerta deve resultar em encaminhamento médico imediato para investigações adicionais (Lewis et al., 2015). É importante procurar um histórico de trauma no ombro ao avaliar o atleta *overhead*, principalmente por mergulho ou contato com um oponente, antes de desenvolver a DBA.

Dor específica *versus* dor inespecífica

O achado de anormalidades durante as investigações de atletas *overhead* assintomáticos é muito comum (Connor et al., 2003; Jost et al., 2005; Miniaci et al., 2002) e isso pode dificultar a interpretação dos resultados de qualquer investigação no atleta com DBA desafiante. Esse fenômeno também é comum em outras áreas do corpo e levou ao conceito de condições específicas e inespecíficas (O'Sullivan et al., 2015). Condições específicas são aquelas em que a apresentação da dor é consistente com a patologia encontrada na investigação. Condições específicas de ombro e cotovelo incluem luxações e subluxações na AGU, rupturas agudas no LCU, fraturas do membro superior, rupturas maciças do manguito rotador, lesões labrais-capsulares agudas no ombro e lesões ligamentares no cotovelo; essas condições podem exigir tratamento médico específico. No atleta *overhead* mais jovem, essas condições específicas são geralmente o resultado de trauma. No entanto, rupturas parciais do manguito rotador e tendinopatias, bursite do ombro, tenossinovite da cabeça longa do bíceps e lesões LSAP são comumente encontradas em atletas *overhead* assintomáticos (Connor et al., 2003; Jost et al., 2005; Miniaci et al., 2002) e esses podem ser considerados inespecíficos. Nessas condições, o manejo deve se basear na abordagem das disfunções de apresentação e nos fatores contribuintes, não no diagnóstico.

Apresentação da dor e estágio do distúrbio

A maioria das apresentações da DBA são mecânicas. No entanto, alterações na sensibilidade central podem ocorrer em atletas com histórico prolongado de DBA ou outras condições musculoesqueléticas e foram observadas em tendinopatias (Lewis et al., 2015). A presença de sintomas generalizados, hiperalgesia mecânica e alodinia deve alertar o clínico para a possibilidade de alterações centrais. Fatores psicossociais, como hipervigilância, medo e ansiedade e questões em torno da seleção podem influenciar a apresentação da dor e devem ser considerados como um fator potencial na apresentação da dor de cada atleta (Mitchell et al., 2015; Puentedura e Louw, 2012).

Teste de melhoria

O teste de melhoria envolve a aplicação de forças externas ou autoaplicadas no tórax, escápula, cabeça do úmero, cotovelo ou coluna cervicotorácica durante uma atividade agravante e observação dos efeitos dessa força (Lewis, 2009; Lewis et al., 2015). Muitas vezes, pode resultar em melhora imediata dos sintomas

Gerenciamento do Atleta *Overhead* | Capítulo | 35 |

e, caso isso ocorra, a intervenção pode ser incluída em um plano de manejo. Devido às velocidades de movimento durante esportes *overhead*, muitas vezes é difícil conduzir testes de melhoria durante as tarefas esportivas reais. No entanto, pode ser aplicado a componentes da tarefa ou outras atividades agravantes, por exemplo, alterar manualmente a posição da escápula ou da cabeça do úmero durante RE resistida a 90° de abdução.

Fatores contribuintes

Todas as apresentações de dor estão associadas a uma variedade de fatores contribuintes exclusivos para aquele indivíduo e condição (Lewis et al., 2015; Mitchell et al., 2015; O'Sullivan et al., 2015). Alguns deles são descritos na Tabela 35.4. Durante o exame, o profissional da saúde deve considerar a relevância e a importância desses fatores com relação à condição desse indivíduo e determinar quais são potencialmente modificáveis, pois isso orientará o manejo.

Gerenciamento do atleta *overhead* lesionado

Se algum sinal de alerta for identificado ou se o atleta tiver uma apresentação específica de dor, ele deve ser encaminhado a um profissional da saúde competente, de preferência um que esteja familiarizado com atletas *overhead*, para investigação adicional. Na ausência de sinais de alerta ou distúrbios específicos, um caminho de manejo para o atleta *overhead* é descrito na Figura 35.7.

A via é semelhante para distúrbios específicos, mas irá variar dependendo do manejo médico específico necessário. Os componentes desse plano de manejo não devem ser considerados como entidades separadas, pois há uma sobreposição considerável entre cada componente. É crucial que o atleta esteja no centro doplano e o compreenda e que todas as outras partes interessadas (treinadores, outra equipe de apoio, agentes) apoiem o plano. Isso é essencial para que qualquer plano de manejo seja eficaz. É importante que a linguagem utilizada para explicar a condição do atleta não contribua para crenças inúteis sobre lesões, pois isso pode ser prejudicial ao resultado (Saw et al., 2017).

Manejo da dor

A maior parte da DBA é dolorosa apenas durante a atividade *overhead* e geralmente se acomoda rapidamente com a modificação da carga. Alguns atletas podem continuar jogando apesar da DBA e podem exigir intervenções médicas, como medicamentos ou injeções para controlar os sintomas. Se o teste de melhoria for eficaz, essas técnicas podem ser integradas ao manejo para ajudar a controlar os sintomas; além disso, a gravação que replica essas técnicas também pode ser eficaz (Lewis, 2009; Lewis et al., 2015).

Abordagem dos fatores contribuintes e retorno ao carregamento

Devem ser introduzidas de imediato intervenções direcionadas que abordam os fatores contribuintes relevantes para a

Tabela 35.4 **Potenciais fatores que contribuem para a dor no braço de arremesso.**

Fatores intrínsecos	
Não modificáveis	
Geral	Sexo, idade, estado de maturação, genética, histórico de lesões, estrutura anatômica
Potencialmente modificável	
Controle motor	Atividades e técnicas específicas do esporte, arremessar, sacar, bater; posturas habituais e padrões de movimento
Mobilidade e flexibilidade	ADM específica de membro superior, tronco e membro inferior e comprimento muscular necessário para a tarefa
Condicionamento	Qualidades de força exigidas: força máxima, TDF, capacidade de trabalho; resistência muscular aeróbica geral e local, condicionamento específico do esporte
Fisiológico	Saúde geral, outras condições médicas, fadiga, sono
Psicológico	Crenças sobre lesões e doenças, medo e ansiedade, estratégias de enfrentamento, autoeficácia, depressão e estresse
Fatores extrínsecos	
Relacionado com o treinamento	Volume, intensidade, frequência e tipo de treinamento; competição e cronograma de treinamento; descanso e recuperação
Ambiental	Treinadores, companheiros de equipe, equipe de apoio, especialistas médicos, família, seleção de equipe e questões contratuais, trabalho, outras atividades, viagens, patrocinadores
Fatores sociais	Colegas de equipe, treinadores, famílias, agentes, trabalho
Outros	Tratamentos anteriores, dieta, suplementos, medicamentos

TDF, taxa de desenvolvimento de força; *ADM*, amplitude de movimento. (Adaptada de Mitchell, T., Burnett, A., O'Sullivan, P., 2015. The athletic spine. In: Joyce, D., Lewindon, D. [Eds.], Sports Injury Prevention and Rehabilitation: Integrating Medicine and Science for Performance Solutions. Routledge, Oxon, UK.)

365

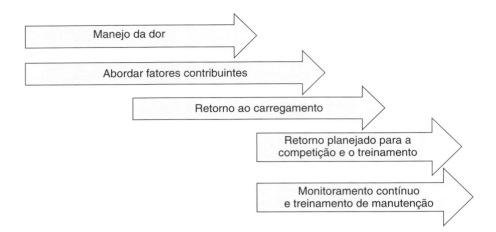

Figura 35.7 Caminho de manejo para o atleta *overhead* lesionado.

apresentação específica do atleta (Lewis, 2009). Exercícios de mobilidade específicos e terapia manual, como a de tecidos moles devem ter como alvo quaisquer restrições de movimento identificadas. O retreinamento motor deve ser introduzido para tratar quaisquer deficiências de controle específicas e exercícios de fortalecimento específicos devem abordar quaisquer déficits de força do manguito rotador ou da força muscular da escápula (Lewis, 2009; Lewis et al., 2015; Mitchell et al., 2015; O'Sullivan et al., 2015). Quaisquer exercícios relevantes para melhorar o movimento e controlar deficiências e déficits de força no tronco e membros inferiores devem ser introduzidos de imediato, independentemente da gravidade da DBA, assim como os exercícios de condicionamento geral e específico. É vital que o atleta tenha as qualidades físicas necessárias antes de retomar o programa de retorno ao arremesso. Educação e, às vezes, apoio psicológico podem ser necessários para lidar com quaisquer pensamentos, crenças e sentimentos inúteis que podem influenciar a apresentação da dor (Mitchell et al., 2015; O'Sullivan et al., 2015; Saw et al., 2017).

Retorno planejado para a competição e o treinamento

Um programa gradativo de retorno ao arremesso deve ser iniciado quando, de acordo com o exame clínico, os sintomas do atleta se acalmaram e ele recuperou as qualidades físicas necessárias para o arremesso. Esse programa deve seguir uma estrutura semelhante ao de lançamento de pré-temporada. No entanto, o atleta pode precisar progredir mais lentamente. Se a técnica foi considerada um fator contribuinte significativo, intervenções específicas para lidar com isso devem ser incluídas como parte desse programa, mas apenas em consulta com a equipe técnica. É importante que a distância arremessada seja gradualmente aumentada e, em seguida, a intensidade seja adicionada em distâncias mais curtas quando o atleta pode arremessar perto de sua distância máxima (Ax et al., 2009; Reinold et al., 2002). O volume dos arremessos deve refletir as demandas de competição e treinamento normais, mas o atleta deve ser monitorado para sinais de fadiga, como alterações na técnica, durante cada sessão (Ax et al., 2009; Reinold et al., 2002). Os sinais clínicos devem continuar normais à medida que o programa avança. A presença de qualquer dor ou desconforto é uma indicação de que o programa está progredindo muito rapidamente e deve ser ajustado de acordo (Ax et al., 2009; Reinold et al., 2002).

Monitoramento contínuo e reabilitação de manutenção

Uma vez que o atleta tenha retornado ao pleno treinamento e competição, ele deve continuar a ser observado de perto, pois são comuns episódios recorrentes de DBA. O arremesso e a carga de trabalho geral devem ser monitorados, assim como a resposta do atleta a esta carga (Gabbett et al., 2017; Whiteley, 2010). A presença de fadiga, dor, reduções na ADM e força da AGU podem indicar que o atleta não está lidando com essa carga de trabalho e pode estar em risco de recorrência da DBA (Whiteley, 2010). O atleta deve continuar com os principais aspectos de seu programa de reabilitação para manter as qualidades físicas exigidas para o arremesso e alguns atletas podem se beneficiar de uma terapia manual ou de tecido mole para lidar com quaisquer restrições de movimento ou dores musculares.

Conclusão

Para gerenciar qualquer atleta *overhead*, independentemente de seu esporte, é fundamental que o praticante tenha um conhecimento completo da biomecânica específica daquele esporte e patomecânica associada, bem como das qualidades físicas e adaptações associadas que ocorrem no atleta. O clínico precisa garantir que ele esteja preparado para as demandas competitivas e de treinamento específicas de seu esporte, incluindo atividades *overhead* e geral. Anormalidades são comumente encontradas no membro superior em atletas de arremesso assintomáticos durante as investigações, o que pode tornar a interpretação dessas varreduras em um atleta com DBA um desafio. O manejo de um atleta *overhead* com DBA deve abordar os fatores contribuintes específicos para a apresentação da dor desse atleta. Quando esses fatores forem resolvidos e sua dor estiver sob controle, eles devem ser reintroduzidos na atividade *overhead* de maneira planejada e gradativa, com monitoramento contínuo ao longo desse processo.

Referências bibliográficas

An, K.N., Fui, H.C., Morrey, B.F., 1981. Muscles that cross the elbow joint: a biomechanical analysis. Journal of Biomechanics 14, 659-669.

Axe, M., Hurd, W., Synder-Mackler, L., 2009. Data based interval throwing programs for baseball players. Sport Health 1, 145-153.

Bahr, R., 2016. Why screening tests to predict injury do not work – and probably never will …: A critical review. British Journal of Sports Medicine 50, 776-780.

Black, G.M., Gabbett, T.J., Cole, M.H., Naughton, G., 2016. Monitoring workload in throwing dominant sports: a systematic review. Sports Medicine 46, 1503-1516.

Borsa, P.A., Laudner, K.G., Sauers, E.L., 2008. Mobility and stability adaptations in the shoulder of the overhead athletes. a theoretical and evidence-based perspective. Sports Medicine 38, 17-36.

Burkhart, S.S., Morgan, C.D., Kibler, W.B., 2003a. The disabled shoulder: spectrum of pathology. part I: patho-anatomy and biomechanics. Arthroscopy 19, 404-420.

Burkhart, S.S., Morgan, C.D., Kibler, W.B., 2003b. The disabled shoulder: spectrum of pathology. part II: evaluation and treatment of SLAP lesions in throwers. Arthroscopy 19, 531-539.

Burn, M., McCulloch, P.C., Lintner, D.M., Liberman, S.R., Harris, J.D., 2016. Prevalence of scapula dyskinesis in overhead and nonoverhead athletes. a systematic review. The Orthopaedic Journal of Sports Medicine 4 (2), 2325967115627608.

Byram, I.R., Bushnell, B.D., Dugger, K., Charron, K., Harrell Jr., F.E., Noonan, T.J., 2010. Preseasons shoulder strength measurements in professional baseball pitchers: identifying players at risk for injury. American Journal of Sports Medicine 38, 1375-1382.

Cain, E.L., Dugas, J.R., Wolf, R.S., Andrews, J.R., 2003. Elbow injuries in throwing athletes: a current concepts review. American Journal of Sports Medicine 31, 621-635.

Camp, C.L., Zajac, J.M., Pearson, D.B., Sinator, A.M., Spiker, A.M., Werner, B.C.,et al., 2017. Decreased shoulder external rotation and flexion are greater predictors of injury than internal rotation deficits: analysis of 132 pitcher-seasons in professional baseball. Arthroscopy 33, 1629-1636.

Chang, H.Y., Chang, B.F., Jong, Y.J., 2010. Characteristics of elbow range of motions and dependent position comparison in high school baseball players. Formosan Journal of Physical Therapy 35, 284-291.

Chant, C.B., Litchfield, R., Griffin, S., et al., 2007. Humeral head retroversion in competitive baseball players and its relationship to glenohumeral rotation range of motion. Journal of Orthopaedic and Sports Physical Therapy 37, 514-520.

Chu, S.K., Jayabalan, P., Kibler, W.B., Press, J., 2016. The kinetic chain revisited: new concepts on throwing mechanics and injury. Physical Medicine and Rehabilitation 8, S69-S77.

Clarsen, B., Bahr, R., Haugsboe Ndersson, S., Munk, R., Myklebust, G., 2014. Reduced glenohumersal rotation, external rotation weakness and scapula dyskinesis are risk factors for shoulder injuries among elite male handball players: a prospective cohort study. British Journal of Sports Medicine 48, 1327-1333.

Connor, P.M., Banks, D.M., Tyson, A.B., Coumas, J.S., D'Alessandro, D.F., 2003. Magnetic resonance imaging of the asymptomatic shoulder in overhead athletes. American Journal of Sports Medicine 31, 724-727.

Cook, D.P., Strike, S.C., 2000. Throwing in cricket. Journal of Sport Sciences 18, 965-973.

Cormack, S.J., Newton, R.U., McGuigan, 2006. Neuromuscular and endocrine responses of elite players to an Australian rules football match. International Journal of Sports Physiology and Performance 3, 359-374.

Crockett, H.C., Gross, L.B., Wilk, K.E., et al., 2002. Osseous adaptation and range of motion at the glenohumeral joint in professional baseball pitchers. American Journal of Sports Medicine 30, 20-26.

Davidson, P.A., Pink, M., Perry, J., et al., 1995. Functional anatomy of the flexor pronator muscle group in relation to the medial collateral ligament of the elbow. American Journal of Sports Medicine 23, 245-250.

Dwelly, P.M., Tripp, B.S., Tripp, P.A., Eberman, L.E., Gorin, S., 2009. Glenohumeral rotational range of motion in collegiate overhead-throwing athletes during an athletic season. Journal of Athletic Training 44, 611-616.

Edelson, G., Teitz, C., 2000. Internal impingement in the shoulder. Journal of Shoulder and Elbow Surgery 9, 308-315.

Erickson, E.J., Sgori, T., Chalmers, P.N., Vignona, P., Lesniak, M., Bush-Joseph, C.A., et al., 2016. The impact of fatigue on baseball pitching mechanics in adolescent male baseballers. Arthroscopy 32, 762-771.

Finch, C.F., Cook, J., 2014. Categorising sports injuries in epidemiological studies: the subsequent injury categorisation (SIC) model to address multiple, recurrent and exacerbation of injuries. British Journal of Sports Medicine 48, 1276-1280.

Fleisig, G.S., 2010. Biomechanics of overhead throwing: Implications for injury and performance. In: Portus, M. (Ed.), Conference of Science, Medicine and Coaching in Cricket. Conference Proceedings. Brisbane, Cricket Australia.

Fleisig, G.S., Andrews, J.R., Dillman, C.J., Escamilla, R.F., 1995. Kinetics of baseball pitching with implications for injury mechanisms. American Journal of Sports Medicine 23, 233-239.

Fleisig, G.S., Escamilla, R.F., Andrews, J.R., Tomoyuki, M., Satterwhite, Y., Barrentine, S.W., 1996. Kinematic and kinetic comparison of baseball pitching and football passing. Journal of Applied Biomechanics 12, 207-224.

Fortenbaugh, D., Fleisig, G.S., Andrews, J.R., 2009. Baseball pitching biomechanics in relation to risk and performance. Sport Health 1, 314-320.

Forthomme, B., Crielaard, J.M., Crosier, J.L., 2008. Scapula positioning in athlete's shoulder: particularities, clinical measurements and implications. Sports Medicine 38, 369-386.

Freeston, J.L., Carter, T., Whitaker, G., Nicholls, O., Rooney, K.B., 2016. Strength and power correlates of throwing velocity in sub-elite male cricket players. Journal of Strength and Conditioning Research 30, 1646-1651.

Gabbett, T.J., 2016. The training–injury prevention paradox: shoulder athletes be training smarter and harder? British Journal of Sports Medicine 50, 273-280.

Gabbett, T.J., Nassis, G.P., Oetter, E., Pretorius, J., Johnston, N., Medina, D., et al., 2017. The athlete monitoring cycle: a practical guide to interpreting and applying training monitoring data. British Journal of Sports Medicine 51, 1451-1452.

Hickey, D., Solvig, V., Cavalheri, V., Harrold, M., McKenna, L., 2017. Scapula dyskinesis increases the risk of future shoulder pain by 43% in asymptomatic athletes: a systematic review and meta-analysis. British Journal of Sports Medicine 52, 102-110.

Jost, B., Zumstein, M., Pfirrmann, C.W., Zanetti, M., Gerber, C., 2005. MRI findings in throwing shoulders: abnormalities in professional handball players. Current Orthopaedic Practice 434, 130-137.

Kibler, W.B., Sciascia, A., Moore, S., 2012. An acute throwing episode decreases shoulder internal rotation. Clinical Orthopaedics and Related Research 470, 1545-1551.

Kovacs, M., Ellenbecker, T., 2011. An 8-stage model for evaluating the tennis serve: implications for performance enhancement and injury prevention. Sports Health 3, 504-513.

Laffaye, G., Wagner, P., Tombleson, Y., 2014. Countermovement jump height: gender and sport-specific differences in the force–time variables. Journal of Strength and Conditioning Research 28, 1096-1105.

Laudner, K., Lynall, R., Meister, K., 2013. Shoulder adaptations among pitchers and position players over the course of a competitive baseball season. Clinical Journal of Sports Medicine 23, 184-189.

Lehman, G., Drinkwater, E.J., Behm, D.G., 2013. Correlation of throwing velocity to lower body field tests in male college baseball players. Journal of Strength and Conditioning Research 27, 902-908.

Lewis, J., McCreesh, K., Jean-Sebastien, R., Ginn, K., 2015. Rotator cuff tendinopathy: navigating the diagnosis management conundrum. Journal of Orthopaedic and Sports Physical Therapy 45, 923-937.

Lewis, J.S., 2009. Rotator cuff tendinopathy/subacromial impingement syndrome: is it time for a new method of assessment? British Journal of Sports Medicine 43, 259-264.

McCaig, S., Young, M., 2016. Throwing mechanics in injury prevention and performance rehabilitation. In: Joyce, D., Lewindon, D. (Eds.), Sports Injury Prevention and Rehabilitation: Integrating Medicine and Science for Performance Solutions. Routledge, Oxon, UK.

Miniaci, A., Mascia, A.T., Salonen, D.C., Becker, E.J., 2002. Magnetic resonance imaging of the shoulder in asymptomatic professional baseball players. Journal of Sports Medicine 30, 66-73.

Mitchell, T., Burnett, A., O'Sullivan, K., 2015. The athletic spine. In: Joyce, D., Lewindon, D. (Eds.), Sports Injury Prevention and Rehabilitation: Integrating Medicine and Science for Performance Solutions. Routledge, Oxon, UK.

Miyashita, K., Kobayasi, H., Koshida, S., Urabe, Y., 2010. Glenohumeral, scapular, and thoracic angles at maximum shoulder external rotation in throwing. American Journal of Sports Medicine 38, 363-368.

Murray, N.B., Black, G.M., Whiteley, R.J., Gahan, P., Cole, M.H., Utting, A., et al., 2017. Automatic detection of pitching and throwing events in baseball with inertial measurements sensors. International Journal of Sports Physiology and Performance 12, 533-537.

Myers, J.B., Oyama, S., Hibberd, E.E., 2013. Scapular dysfunction in high school baseball players sustaining throwing-related upper extremity injury: a prospective study. Journal of Shoulder and Elbow Surgery 22, 1154-1159.

Newton, R.U., Cardinale, M., Nosaka, K., 2011. Total athlete management (TAM) and performance diagnosis. In: Strength and Conditioning – Biological Principles and Applications. Wiley-Blackwell, Oxford, UK.

O'Sullivan, P., Dankaets, W., O'Sullivan, K., Fersum, K., 2015. Multidimensional approach for the targeted management of low back pain. In: Jull, G., Moore, A., Falla, D., Lewis, J., McCarthy, C., Sterling, M. (Eds.), Grieve's Modern Musculoskeletal Physiotherapy, fourth ed. Elsevier Ltd, Oxford.

Oyama, S., Hibberd, E.E., Myers, J.B., 2017. Preseasons screening of shoulder range of motion and humeral retrotorsion does not predict injury in high school baseball players. Journal of Shoulder and Elbow Surgery 26, 1182-1189.

Oyama, S., Myers, J.B., Wassinger, C.A., Ricci, D., Lephart, S.M., 2008. Asymmetric resting scapula posture in healthy overhead athletes. Journal of Athletic training 43, 565-570.

Puentedura, E.J., Louw, A., 2012. A neuroscience approach to managing athletes with low back pain. Physical Therapy in Sport 13, 123-133.

Reinold, M.M., Wilk, K.E., Macrina, L.C., Shehane, C., Dun, S., Fleisig, G.S., et al., 2008. Changes in shoulder and elbow passive range of motion after pitching in professional baseball players. American Journal of Sports Medicine 36, 523-527.

Reinold, M.M., Wilk, K.E., Reed, J., Crenshaw, K., Andrews, J.R., 2002. Interval sport programs: guidelines for baseball, tennis, and golf. Journal of Orthopaedic and Sports Physical Therapy 32, 293-298.

Roach, N.T., Lieberman, D.E., 2014. Upper body contributions to power generation during rapid, overhead throwing in humans. Journal of Experimental Biology 217, 2139-2149.

Saw, A., Kellmann, M., Main, L.C., Gastin, P.B., 2017. Athlete self-report measures in research and practice: considerations for the discerning reader and fastidious practitioner. International Journal of Sports Physiology and Performance 12, S127-135.

Shanley, E., Rauh, M.J., Michener, L.A., Ellenbecker, T.S., 2011. Shoulder range of motion measures as risk factors for shoulder and elbow injuries in high school softball and baseball players. American Journal of Sports Medicine 39, 1997-2006.

Struyf, F., Nijs, J., Roussel, N.A., Mottram, S., Truijen, S., Meeusen, R., 2013. Does scapular positioning predict shoulder pain in recreational overhead athletes? International Journal of Sports Medicine 35, 75-82.

Wagner, H., Pfusterschmied, J., Tilp, M., Landlinger, J., von Duvillard, S.P., Muller, E., 2014. Upper-body kinematics in team-handball throw, tennis serve, and volleyball spike. Scandinavian Journal of Medicine and Science in Sports and Exercise 24, 345-354.

Walch, G., Boileau, P., Noel, E., Donnell, S., 1992. Impingement of the deep surface of the supraspinatus tendon on the posterior superior glenoid rim: an arthroscopic study. Journal of Shoulder and Elbow Surgery 1, 238-245.

Warren, A., Williams, S., McCaig, S., Trewartha, G., 2018. High acute:-chronic workloads are associated with injury in England & Wales cricket board development programme fast bowlers. Journal of Science and Medicine in Sport 21, 40-45.

Wassinger, C.A., Myers, J.B., 2011. Reported mechanism of shoulder injury during the baseball throw. Physical Therapy Reviews 16, 305-309.

Werner, S.L., Fleisig, G.S., Dillman, C.J., Escamilla, R.F., 1993. Biomechanics of the elbow during pitching. Journal of Orthopaedic and Sports Physical Therapy 17, 274-278.

Whiteley, R., 2010. Throwing mechanics, load monitoring and injury: perspective from physiotherapy and baseball as they relate to cricket. In: Portus, M. (Ed.), Conference of Science, Medicine and Coaching in Cricket. Conference Proceedings. Brisbane, Cricket Australia, pp. 21-24.

Whiteley, R., 2007. Baseball throwing mechanics as they relate to pathology and performance – a review. Journal of Sport Science and Medicine 6, 1-20.

Whiteley, R., 2016. 'Moneyball' and time to be honest about preseason screening: it is a sham making no inroads on the 1 billion dollar injury costs in baseball. British Journal of Sports Medicine 50 (14), 835-836.

Whiteley, R., Oceguera, M., 2016. GIRD, TRROM and humeral torsion-based classification of shoulder risk in throwing athletes are not in agreement and shoulder be used interchangeably. Journal of Science and Medicine in Sport 19, 816-819.

Whiteley, R., Oceguera, M.V., Valencia, E.B., Mitchell, T., 2012. Adaptations at the shoulder of the throwing athlete and implications for the clinicians. Techniques in Shoulder and Elbow Surgery 13, 36-44.

Whiteley, R.J., Ginn, K.A., Nicholson, L.L., et al., 2009. Sports participation and humeral torsion. Journal of Orthopaedic and Sports Physical Therapy 39, 256-263.

Wilk, K.E., Macrina, L.C., Fleisig, G.S., Aune, K.T., Porterfield, R.A., Harker, P., et al., 2014. Deficits in glenohumeral passive range of motion increase risk of elbow injury in professional baseball pitchers. American Journal of Sports Medicine 42, 2075-2081.

Wilk, K.E., Macrina, L.C., Fleisig, G.S., Aune, K.T., Porterfield, R.A., Harker, P., et al., 2015a. Deficits in glenohumeral passive range of motion increase risk of shoulder injury in professional baseball pitchers. American Journal of Sports Medicine 43, 2379-2385.

Wilk, K.E., Macrina, L.C., Fleisig, G.S., Porterfield, R.A., Simpson II, C.D., Harker, P., et al., 2015b. Correlation of glenohumeral internal rotation deficit and total rotational range of motion to shoulder injuries in professional baseball pitchers. American Journal of Sports Medicine 39, 329-335.

Wilk, K.E., Reinold, M.M., Macrina, L.C., et al., 2009. Glenohumeral internal rotation measurements differ depending on stabilization techniques. Sports Health 1, 131-136.

Wright, R.W., Steger-May, K., Wasserlauf, B.L., O'Neal, M.E., Weinberg, B.W., Paletta, G.A., 2006. Elbow range of motion in professional baseball pitchers. American Journal of Sports Medicine 34, 190-193.

Yamamoto, N., Itoi, E., Minagawa, H., et al., 2006. Why is the humeral retroversion of throwing athletes greater in dominant shoulder than in nondominant shoulders? Journal of Shoulder and Elbow Surgery 15, 571-575.

Capítulo | 36 |

Tratamento e Manejo de Lesões em Tecidos Moles

Graham Smith

Introdução

Todos os que praticam esportes correm o risco de sofrer lesão nos tecidos moles, e o modo como ela é tratada determina seu resultado. Os objetivos deste capítulo são dar uma visão geral dos princípios que, segundo o autor, devem ser seguidos para o tratamento de lesões de tecidos moles e dissipar muitos dos mitos e equívocos que se acumularam nos últimos anos com relação a esse aspecto extremamente importante da área da medicina musculoesquelética.

Classificação de lesões

Nos últimos anos, muitos artigos foram publicados com foco em encontrar "o Santo Graal" para o tratamento e manejo de lesões em tecidos moles. Consequentemente, há uma proliferação de opções de tratamento disponíveis, todas com o objetivo de acelerar o processo de cicatrização e retorno posterior às atividades. Sem querer criticar essa pesquisa, não há nada que possa alterar de modo realístico as respostas fisiopatológicas básicas que ocorrerão após uma lesão em tecido mole. Por isso, a compreensão dessas respostas é parte integrante do tratamento e manejo bem-sucedidos dessas lesões. Essas informações são ensinadas a todos os profissionais de saúde e médicos durante seu treinamento, mas geralmente em um momento em que suas implicações clínicas e funcionais não são totalmente compreendidas. Supõe-se também que, uma vez ensinado, não há motivos para revisitá-lo. No entanto, uma compreensão dessas respostas fisiopatológicas e de sua apresentação clínica é imperativa para qualquer pessoa responsável pelo tratamento e manejo de lesões em tecidos moles, não importa o nível em que trabalhe no campo da medicina esportiva.

Essas respostas fisiopatológicas à lesão são inerentes e o paciente se apresentará em um dos três estágios claramente definidos:
1. Fase aguda (inflamatória).
2. Fase subaguda (remodelamento).
3. Fase crônica (trauma não resolvido e/ou repetitivo).

Na ocasião que esse material é ensinado, cronogramas específicos de quando o paciente se apresentará em cada fase são frequentemente fornecidos. Isso pode levar a um mal-entendido sobre em que fase específica o paciente se encontra; consequentemente, medidas inadequadas são tomadas durante o manejo. É a resposta clínica e funcional em cada fase fisiopatológica e a maneira como ela se apresenta que deve ser determinada e tratada, em vez do tempo desde a lesão.

Fase aguda

Uma inflamação aguda é um estímulo único que tem uma resposta fisiopatológica claramente definida por seus sinais flogísticos: calor, inchaço, dor, descoloração (descrita como vermelhidão com frequência) e uma redução na amplitude de movimento/função. A resposta também será limitada no tempo, que geralmente é de 36 a 48 horas. Esse cronograma deve ser desconsiderado, pois dependerá totalmente do tamanho e da área afetada. Por exemplo, se a articulação interfalangiana de um dedo for lesionada, a resposta inflamatória aguda provavelmente será de 2 a 3 horas. No entanto, estudos evidenciam que, quando há trauma em uma articulação muito maior, como o joelho ou um golpe direto na face anterior da coxa, a fase aguda pode durar de 72 a 90 horas. Isso é feito com a condição de que não haja mais traumas na área e também é importante para a compreensão da inflamação aguda – não apenas como ela se apresenta, mas como deve ser tratada.

Para esclarecimento, uma inflamação aguda é uma resposta fisiopatológica a um estímulo ou lesão *única* e qualquer outro trauma que possa ocorrer durante essa fase alterará a resposta fisiopatológica. Esse assunto será discutido mais adiante, assim como o tratamento de lesões agudas.

Fase subaguda

Supondo que não haja mais trauma, o próximo estágio para o qual a lesão progredirá é uma fase subaguda ou de remodelamento. Acontece quando o tecido em cicatrização de estrutura semelhante à que foi traumatizado é depositado, mas dentro de uma estrutura colagenosa. Embora esse tecido possa ser de natureza semelhante, não terá a resistência das estruturas originais. Também foi hipotetizado que a força máxima será 80% do que era antes (Lin et al., 2004; Mercandetti e Cohen, 2017; Watson, 2016). Consequentemente, isso deve ser sempre considerado tanto na reabilitação quanto no retorno às atividades funcionais. É também uma das principais razões para programas de "manutenção", mesmo quando o paciente retorna às atividades esportivas. Isso também explica por que muitos atletas sofrem novas lesões, não necessariamente quando retornam ao esporte, mas na temporada seguinte, quando interrompem o programa de reabilitação que lhes permitiu fazê-lo.

O outro equívoco sobre essa fase é que ela é limitada a um período de 7 a 10 dias. Essa informação deve ser desconsiderada imediatamente, pois o processo de cicatrização pode continuar por até 120 dias ou mais (Gillquist, 1993; Hardy, 1989; Watson, 2016).

A apresentação clínica do paciente, em vez do tempo desde a lesão, confirma se ele ainda está na fase subaguda. Os pacientes nessa fase têm uma apresentação claramente definida. Eles têm uma facilidade de movimento dentro da amplitude disponível com desconforto e restrição em seus limites. Essa facilidade de movimento está sempre baseada nas seguintes condições:

- Os movimentos são realizados em direções anatômicas
- Não há mais trauma.

Consequentemente, os pacientes subagudos devem ser aconselhados a mover sua articulação/membro em uma direção anatômica de maneira repetitiva, mas sem forçar seus limites (Brukner e Khan, 2017; Smith, 1998). Eles também devem ser informados de que esse é o seu indicador clínico para determinar como estão progredindo. A amplitude de movimento, a força e a função devem melhorar à medida que o tecido em cicatrização é estabelecido em um alinhamento anatômico provocado por padrões corretos de movimento. Esses princípios devem ser aplicados até que o movimento anatômico completo, normal e comparativo seja obtido, sem dor, desconforto ou restrição, e independentemente do tempo decorrido desde o trauma único original.

Fase crônica

A inflamação crônica é definida como uma inflamação subaguda não resolvida ou que foi submetida a pequenos traumas repetitivos (Hurley, 1985; Smith, 1999; Watson, 2016). Essa fase é caracterizada por uma resposta colagenosa excessiva em que o colágeno é depositado em uma formação aleatória para proteger e fortalecer as estruturas que estão sendo traumatizadas repetidamente ou não estão sendo submetidas a movimentos em direções anatômicas para promover a cura.

Nessa fase, os pacientes queixam-se de rigidez e desconforto após períodos de inatividade que depois se amenizam com o movimento. Por exemplo, pacientes com problemas crônicos no tornozelo relatam rigidez pela manhã e sinais de melhora após uma caminhada leve. Consequentemente, a atividade que dá a redução da rigidez é também a agravante subjacente que provoca o trauma repetitivo menor. Daí a razão para determinar a atividade agravante o mais rápido possível para que ela possa ser modificada em conformidade.

Existem três fases fisiopatológicas da inflamação claramente definidas, cada uma com sua apresentação clínica específica. Cada etapa tem seu próprio regime de manejo específico, que se aplicado incorretamente ou no momento errado tem implicações que podem atrasar o retorno às funções normais ou esportivas. Esses problemas geralmente surgem quando as medidas de tratamento e reabilitação são aplicadas com relação apenas a períodos de tempo, em vez da fase inflamatória específica. A mensagem para levar para casa é concentrar-se na apresentação clínica e dar menos importância ao cronograma.

Um estudo de caso é apresentado a seguir para ilustrar. Embora seja um exemplo hipotético e simplista, ele mostra muitos dos problemas que podem ocorrer se as respostas fisiopatológicas normais não forem compreendidas e regimes de manejo inadequados forem aplicados. No entanto, é reconhecido que no esporte competitivo não é viável para todos os jogadores deixarem o campo de jogo se sofrerem uma lesão leve.

Determinação da fase

As perguntas a seguir devem ser feitas como algo normal na apresentação inicial:

1. O que aconteceu? O paciente pode explicar o mecanismo da lesão, o que ajudará a determinar estruturas que podem ter sido danificadas.

Estudo de caso

Dois jogadores de hóquei sofrem lesões de inversão idênticas no tornozelo aos 10 minutos de jogo. Nenhum deles teve lesões anteriormente e, desse modo, podem ser identificados como problemas pontuais na primeira vez. Um dos jogadores deixa o campo de jogo imediatamente, já o segundo permanece no campo pelo resto da partida.

Ambos os jogadores estão na sala de tratamento em pedestais adjacentes 10 minutos após o jogo. Em que estágio fisiopatológico está o jogador que saiu de campo agora? Da mesma maneira, em que fase está o jogador que permaneceu no campo?

As respostas para ambas as perguntas são simples e lógicas: o jogador que deixou o campo de jogo imediatamente estará na fase aguda de inflamação por ter sofrido uma lesão pontual, e o que permaneceu estará na fase crônica. Este último está na fase crônica porque provocou traumas repetitivos menores à lesão inicial, ocasionando uma resposta colagenosa, independentemente de terem se passado apenas 90 minutos desde o trauma inicial.

Ambos os jogadores são tratados, orientados sobre o que devem fazer durante a noite e são instruídos a apresentarem um relatório no dia seguinte.

Na manhã seguinte, os dois jogadores são reavaliados. A correia e o suporte são removidos do tornozelo do jogador que foi retirado do campo de jogo imediatamente e ele é solicitado a mover o tornozelo para cima e para baixo. Embora inicialmente relutante, ele é capaz de mover a articulação de maneira confortável sem qualquer dor ou desconforto, mas com uma restrição de amplitude. Também há uma ausência perceptível de inchaço. Consequentemente, a lesão está avançando para a fase subaguda e terá sintomas agudos mínimos.

O tornozelo do jogador que permaneceu em campo apresenta um pequeno edema de depressões nas margens articulares e quando solicitado a movimentar-se, apresenta rigidez e desconforto, que diminuem com a repetição. O jogador encontra-se na fase crônica de inflamação, embora tenham se passado menos de 24 horas desde o incidente. Portanto, se essa lesão fosse tratada como se estivesse na fase inflamatória aguda, o paciente seria aconselhado a descansar e não se mover por 36 a 48 horas. Isso pode levar a um edema altamente organizado (inchaço) com uma articulação extremamente rígida, os quais exigiriam tempo para serem tratados e resolvidos antes que o jogador pudesse pensar em retornar ao hóquei. Em contrapartida, o jogador que deixou o campo e está subagudo terá um regime de manejo completamente diferente, o que lhe dará uma chance muito melhor de um retorno mais cedo ao esporte.

O tratamento de lesões inflamatórias subagudas e crônicas é significativamente diferente das estruturas de tecidos moles com lesão aguda. Portanto, apesar de demorar menos de 24 horas após a lesão, os dois jogadores precisarão de um regime diferente.

---

2. O que você fez imediatamente após a lesão? O paciente conseguiu continuar as atividades ou foi forçado a parar? Isso determinará se foi um trauma isolado imediatamente protegido de novas lesões ou algo que foi submetido a um trauma repetitivo contínuo. Isso ajudará a determinar a fase fisiopatológica da lesão.

3. Houve inchaço e quando foi percebido pela primeira vez? Se o paciente sentiu latejamento e percebeu inchaço imediato, se a área lesionada estava quente e tensa ao toque, o médico deve suspeitar de sangramento. Se for uma lesão articular, é provável que tenha sido uma hemartrose (sangramento no espaço articular) e deve ser considerada uma emergência clínica. Ele terá um alto componente celular com aumento da atividade metabólica dentro da articulação, o que provocará calor. Um alto componente celular em qualquer espaço confinado também causa dor. No entanto, se o paciente não notou nenhum inchaço significativo

Tratamento e Manejo de Lesões em Tecidos Moles **Capítulo** | 36 |

até várias horas após a lesão e não houve relato de calor ou de dor, é provável que ele tenha um derrame sinovial se for um problema de articulação ou fluido tecidual se em tecido mole.

4. O que aconteceu imediatamente após a lesão? O que o paciente fez imediatamente após a lesão? Ele recebeu algum tratamento? Ele tomou algum medicamento? Todos esses fatores determinam onde o paciente se encontra dentro do espectro inflamatório para que as medidas de tratamento adequadas possam ser planejadas.

5. Como ele está agora e quais são os seus problemas? Nesse ponto, é necessário determinar o grau de incapacidade que o paciente possui na apresentação, independentemente do tempo decorrido desde a ocorrência da lesão. É essa determinação que ajudará a classificar a fase de inflamação e, posteriormente, a de reabilitação. Isso garantirá que as medidas de tratamento adequadas para a inflamação sejam aplicadas e os exercícios corretos sejam iniciados.

O conhecimento das respostas fisiopatológicas à lesão permite que o médico siga os seguintes objetivos específicos para cada estágio inflamatório:

Inflamação aguda. As estratégias de manejo serão abordadas com mais detalhes após as duas seções a seguir.

Inflamação subaguda. Os principais objetivos nessa fase de inflamação são:
1. Aumentar a amplitude de movimento dentro dos limites da dor e desconforto por meio das direções anatômicas normais.
2. Aumentar a força dos músculos que atuam sobre a área lesionada dentro dos limites da dor e desconforto e sem aplicar forças excessivas sobre eles. Os movimentos devem ser direcionados anatomicamente.
3. Restaurar e melhorar a propriocepção dentro dos limites da dor e do desconforto. Propriocepção é consciência articular e é imperativo reeducá-la o mais cedo possível, mesmo em uma posição sem sustentação de peso.

Inflamação crônica. Os objetivos nessa fase da inflamação são:
1. Identificar e interromper/minimizar as atividades agravantes. Se o paciente não for capaz de interromper a atividade agravante, é melhor aconselhá-lo sobre como administrar as respostas ao agravamento. São necessárias orientações sobre como se preparar para as atividades e minimizar a cronicidade.
2. Manter a amplitude de movimento disponível sem agravar ou provocar outros traumas menores.
3. Reduzir qualquer inchaço crônico nas áreas circundantes, utilizando medidas de fisioterapia que podem incluir massagem e mobilizações de tecidos moles. Aumenta a amplitude de movimento, força e propriocepção sem provocar mais traumas e sempre dentro dos padrões de movimento anatômicos.

Finalmente, o que pode se apresentar em uma fase inflamatória em um ponto pode logo se mover para outro. Não apenas os médicos devem estar cientes disso, como também os pacientes. Quando os pacientes recebem programas de exercícios, eles também devem ser instruídos sobre como avaliar se houve alguma alteração em seu estado inflamatório. Por exemplo, se em 1 dia o paciente faz exercícios apropriados para o estágio subagudo, mas na manhã seguinte acorda com rigidez e desconforto, ele já passou para o estágio crônico. Consequentemente, é importante que o paciente saiba o que fazer se isso ocorrer, para que possa manejá-lo corretamente, sem provocar mais traumas, até que possa ser reavaliado e devidamente orientado. Eles também devem ser aconselhados sobre a frequência com que isso ocorre e que isso não é incomum. Assim, é fácil avaliar como os problemas ocorrem quando a fisiopatologia não é totalmente compreendida e as medidas de tratamento são aplicadas de maneira inadequada.

Tratamento e manejo de lesões agudas

Essa é uma das áreas mais mal compreendidas do tratamento de lesões. Apesar de pesquisas significativas nesse campo, princípios que se mostraram ineficazes ainda estão sendo ensinados e aplicados. Mais preocupantes, os princípios fisiopatológicos básicos, incluindo as respostas dos tecidos ao trauma, são ignorados com frequência, com muitas das estratégias de tratamento ensinadas sendo anedóticas e desatualizadas.

Como afirmado anteriormente, a inflamação aguda é uma resposta fisiopatológica a um estímulo único ou trauma que resulta na área ficar quente, dolorida, descolorida (vermelha), inchada e, com isso, há perda de função. Essa resposta começa imediatamente.

Inchaço. Danos às membranas semipermeáveis dos tecidos dentro da área permitirão que o exsudado fluido e, em alguns casos, o sangue entre nos espaços dos tecidos. Esse fluido terá um alto componente celular que inclui células sanguíneas e plaquetas.

Calor. A liberação de células no espaço do tecido promove a atividade celular e o metabolismo, incluindo a coagulação e a deposição de colágeno na área. Esse metabolismo também gera calor.

Dor. À medida que o inchaço progride e o conteúdo celular aumenta, a pressão exercida aumenta e a dor e o desconforto são provocados.

Descoloração (vermelhidão). O metabolismo e o calor aumentados também elevam a circulação para os vasos periféricos, causando assim uma reação eritematosa na superfície da pele, que pode ser observada como vermelhidão ou descoloração, dependendo do tom da pele.

Perda de função. À medida que a dor e o inchaço aumentam, o movimento dentro da área fica prejudicado e, desse modo, a função fica comprometida.

Embora as informações anteriores sejam ensinadas na maioria dos cursos, elas são frequentemente ignoradas ao aplicar estratégias de tratamento durante esse estágio de inflamação. Consequentemente, se o exsudado nos espaços teciduais for o principal responsável por todos os itens mencionados anteriormente, isso deve ser interrompido ou minimizado. É importante ressaltar que, se o inchaço se estabelecer, não só causará dor, como também impedirá a progressão da reabilitação. Como afirmam Brukner e Khan (2017), "o processo de reabilitação começa imediatamente para controlar, minimizar e aliviar o inchaço". A prioridade do tratamento deve ser:
1. Compressão.
2. Elevação.
3. Resfriamento.
4. Redução da atividade.

Compressão

Deve-se priorizar a aplicação da compressão o mais cedo possível para minimizar o espaço disponível à entrada do líquido e para que ele possa absorver a pressão externa que será exercida por ele quando tentar entrar nos espaços do tecido. A compressão aplicada deve ser mantida enquanto houver potencial para ocorrer inchaço. Em uma grande área, como o quadríceps ou a articulação do joelho, a compressão deve ser mantida, sempre que possível, por até 90 horas após a lesão. Esse princípio é controverso, mas tem evidências para apoiar sua aplicação (Schröder e Pässler, 1994; Shelbourne et al., 1994) e se baseia nas indicações relacionadas aos cuidados pós-operatórios para reconstrução do LCA. Além disso, as respostas fisiopatológicas não param à noite;

371

elas continuam ao longo do ciclo de 24 horas. Os seguintes pontos-chave devem ser considerados:
- A compressão deve ser aplicada para cobrir toda a área que foi ferida com uma sobreposição. Por exemplo, com a articulação do joelho, a compressão deve estender-se de 2,5 cm acima da bursa suprapatelar até abaixo da tuberosidade tibial. Como uma diretriz, deve estender-se por pelo menos 2,5 cm acima e abaixo da parte afetada
- A compressão deve ser aplicada com algo que absorva a pressão externa de dentro da área lesionada. Dois exemplos de equipamentos que aplicam esses princípios incluem o *Cryocuff* e o *Game Ready*. No entanto, se esses equipamentos não estiverem disponíveis, enrolar a parte lesionada em uma toalha e, em seguida, prendê-la no lugar com uma bandagem de fita crepe será suficiente. Essa é uma bandagem de compressão que segue os princípios de Robert Jones e que eram utilizadas há muitos anos. A aplicação direta de fita elástica adesiva não é apropriada, pois é provável que enrugue e permita áreas onde o inchaço pode passar. Isso torna-se extremamente doloroso para o paciente e não atinge o efeito desejado. Da mesma maneira, o uso de bandagens tipo meia também não é adequado, pois elas ainda permitem que ocorra o inchaço e, se dobradas, a dobra tem o potencial de atuar como um torniquete. São mostrados exemplos de uma bandagem de compressão sendo aplicada utilizando uma toalha (Figura 36.1) e um *Cryocuff* (Figura 36.2).

A aplicação de compressão para minimizar o inchaço é uma prioridade. Não se deve permitir que o inchaço se estabeleça, pois causa dor, o que adiciona os seguintes problemas associados:
- Inibição neuromuscular local
- Movimento reduzido
- Força reduzida
- Padrões de movimento compensatórios
- A área não parece "normal" para o paciente.

Quanto mais cedo a compressão for aplicada, melhor. Porém, se após dias, semanas ou mesmo meses da lesão inicial o paciente for avaliado pela primeira vez e ainda apresentar edema, é provável que seja muito crônico, e a sua redução permanece como prioridade. No manejo de todos os tecidos moles e problemas relacionados às articulações, lembre-se: o inchaço é o inimigo do profissional da saúde!

Elevação

Depois de aplicada a compressão, a parte lesionada deve ser elevada. Idealmente, essa elevação deve ser acima do coração ou o mais alto possível, pois ela reduz a pressão hidrostática do fluxo sanguíneo na área. A produção e reabsorção normais de fluido tecidual dependem da razão entre as pressões hidrostática e osmótica e isso é comprometido quando as membranas semipermeáveis são rompidas com trauma. Qualquer medida que reduza a pressão hidrostática, como a elevação, ajudará a minimizar o exsudato inflamatório que entra nos espaços do tecido. Se a elevação for alta o suficiente, também é um dos principais fatores que permitem que a compressão seja sustentada.

Resfriamento

A aplicação de gelo na pele não para o inchaço! Os efeitos do gelo são extremamente superficiais e não têm efeito imediato nas membranas semipermeáveis que foram danificadas. A aplicação direta de gelo com o objetivo de parar o inchaço é ineficaz e inadequada.

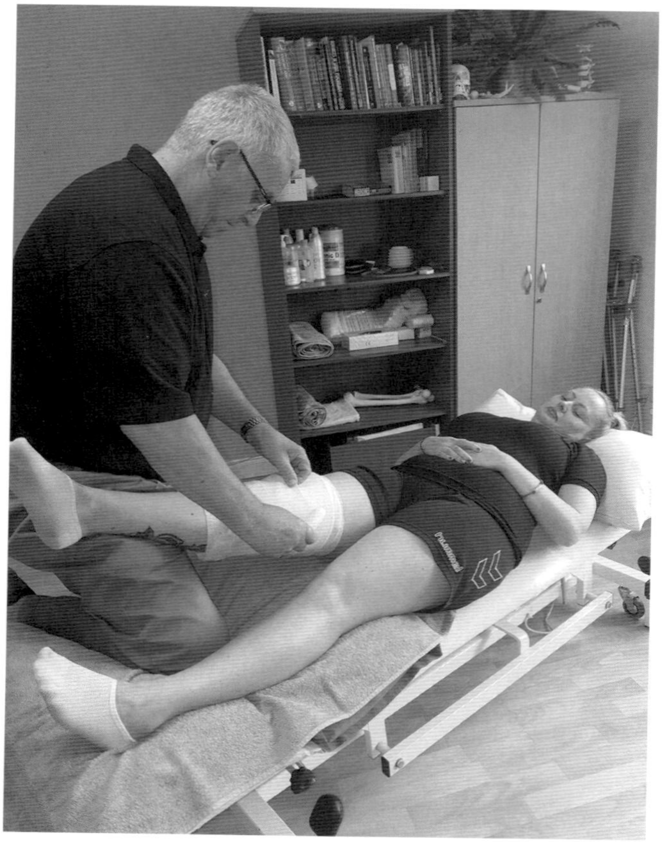

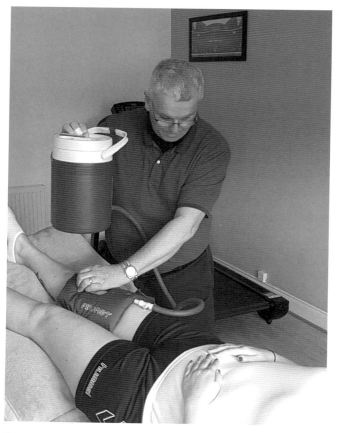

Figura 36.1 Aplicação de compressão (a prioridade) com algodão ou toalha e bandagem.

Figura 36.2 Compressão (prioridade), elevação (secundária) e resfriamento via *Cryocuff* ou produto similar.

Tratamento e Manejo de Lesões em Tecidos Moles **Capítulo** | 36 |

No entanto, resfriar a área por um período prolongado tem um efeito benéfico e, sempre que possível, deve ser aplicado. É importante ressaltar que a compressão não deve ser removida para permitir que o resfriamento seja aplicado. Equipamentos como as máquinas *Cryocuff* e *Game Ready* permitem que a água fria seja contida ou passada por meio da roupa de compressão, resfriando gradualmente as estruturas subjacentes. Isso significa que não há resposta vascular nos vasos sanguíneos periféricos, frequentemente descrita como um efeito de vasoconstrição e vasodilatação. Se a parte lesionada tiver uma bandagem de compressão, ela pode ser molhada com água fria para aplicar os mesmos princípios. Não é aconselhável colocar uma bolsa de gelo por baixo da roupa de compressão, pois isso permite que áreas potenciais para o inchaço ocorram.

O resfriamento sustentado reduzirá, por um período de tempo, a atividade metabólica dentro dos tecidos, diminuindo o fluxo sanguíneo para a área e, como consequência, o inchaço. Há também o benefício suplementar de reduzir os riscos de hipoxia secundária. Portanto, a aplicação de frio tem um efeito benéfico, mas resulta de um resfriamento gradual e não da intensidade associada à aplicação direta de pacotes de gelo. No entanto, o resfriamento não é uma grande prioridade e não deve ser aplicado antes da compressão e elevação.

Redução da atividade

As diretrizes geralmente descrevem isso como "repouso". Embora seja importante parar de mover a área e agravá-la, também é aconselhável que os pacientes tentem mover suavemente a parte lesionada por meio de outra área sem dor que esteja disponível pelo menos 1 vez a cada hora. Isso requer que a compressão seja retirada por um curto período de modo que o paciente possa fazer dois a três movimentos ativos suaves e sem dor. A compressão deve então ser reaplicada de imediato junto com a elevação. Se a parte lesionada for anatomicamente muito pequena, o período de tempo em que a compressão deve ser aplicada será menor do que se fosse uma área maior. Consequentemente, o repouso modificado, também conhecido como "repouso ativo" é o princípio a ser seguido, em vez da inatividade completa.

Os outros princípios-chave a serem considerados com relação ao tratamento de lesões agudas são proteger e prevenir. Portanto, a parte lesionada deve ser protegida, para evitar que o paciente realize atividades que possam causar mais traumas.

Compreender as respostas fisiopatológicas da inflamação ajudará significativamente o médico a aplicar estratégias de manejo adequadas para lesões em tecidos moles. É importante que o paciente seja classificado no estágio adequado de inflamação, não apenas no primeiro atendimento, mas a cada consulta subsequente. Da mesma maneira, também é necessário classificar em qual estágio da reabilitação o paciente deve estar trabalhando, para garantir um bom resultado.

Embora este capítulo não se concentre extensivamente na reabilitação, uma breve visão geral dos estágios da reabilitação e dos critérios que determinam o nível e as atividades que o paciente deve realizar são fornecidos a seguir. Também ajuda a entender quando os pacientes devem progredir para o próximo estágio.

Estágios de reabilitação

Existem quatro estágios principais de reabilitação após a lesão em tecidos moles, cada um com seus próprios critérios e atividades específicas. Esses são:

Reabilitação em estágio inicial

Descrito como o estágio de não sustentação de peso, os principais objetivos são:
- Aumentar a amplitude de movimento sem dor
- Aumentar a força e a propriocepção dentro dos limites da dor e do desconforto.

Esses princípios devem ser aplicados ao membro lesionado nas fases aguda e subaguda da inflamação.

Os pacientes não devem progredir para a descarga de peso total até que tenham alcançado os critérios necessários para avançar ao estágio intermediário de reabilitação. Estes são o estabelecimento de:
- Pelo menos dois terços da amplitude de movimento ativa anatômica normal (*i. e.*, em comparação com o outro membro)
- Controle excêntrico e concêntrico em toda a amplitude disponível
- Movimento totalmente indolor
- Nenhum ou mínimo inchaço.

Se o paciente atender a todos esses critérios, ele poderá passar para o próximo estágio.

Reabilitação de estágio intermediário

Descrito como o estágio progressivo de reabilitação, ele começa com um membro deficiente, mas progride até o ponto em que os membros do paciente são considerados entidades bilaterais. É a fase em que, se a lesão for no membro inferior, a reeducação da marcha torna-se parte integrante das atividades desenvolvidas. Da mesma maneira, como no estágio inicial, nenhuma força rotacional deve ser aplicada ao membro lesionado. Nenhuma corrida deve ser realizada durante esse estágio. A corrida pode ser introduzida apenas quando o paciente progrediu para o "estágio tardio" e isso só pode ocorrer quando o seguinte for alcançado:
- Amplitude ativa completa indolor em comparação com o lado oposto
- Capacidade de controlar o movimento tanto excêntrica quanto concentricamente
- Nenhum ou mínimo inchaço
- Marcha normal (apenas lesão nos membros inferiores); se o paciente puder progredir com um padrão de caminhada anormal, isso será exagerado quando a corrida começar.

Durante esse estágio, os pacientes podem estar nas fases subaguda ou crônica da inflamação, mas não na aguda. O paciente pode então progredir para o estágio tardio de reabilitação, uma vez que os critérios mencionados anteriormente tenham sido alcançados.

Reabilitação em estágio tardio

Descrito como o estágio dinâmico da reabilitação, em que o paciente deve realizar atividades bilaterais dinâmicas. As forças de corrida, salto, torção, rotação e giro podem começar durante essa fase. É também o estágio em que todos os exercícios e atividades realizados devem ser funcionais e adequados a qualquer atividade à qual o paciente espera retornar.

Os pacientes reaprenderão os padrões de movimento durante esse estágio. Sempre que possível, esses padrões de movimento devem estar dentro do ambiente para o qual o paciente está retornando ou o mais próximo possível dele. É também o estágio em que os pacientes não deveriam apresentar nenhuma resposta inflamatória e nem de natureza crônica. Se um paciente se queixa de rigidez e desconforto na manhã após a realização de exercícios de reabilitação tardia, então ele está trabalhando em um nível inadequado e submetendo a lesão a pequenos traumas repetitivos. É por isso que os pacientes devem ser reavaliados e classificados *diariamente*.

373

Estágio de reabilitação de pré-alta

O estágio final é o de pré-alta. O objetivo é identificar especificamente quaisquer deficiências no final do processo de reabilitação. Embora os estágios da reabilitação inicial, intermediário e tardio sejam progressivos e de natureza "cuidadosa", o estágio de pré-alta deve ser muito mais agressivo. Consequentemente, ele é aplicável apenas a certos pacientes – aqueles que sofreram lesões por um período de tempo razoável e que se espera que retornem às atividades dinâmicas ou a altos níveis de aptidão ocupacional.

Importância da classificação

As fases da inflamação e suas respostas fisiopatológicas, junto com o uso das etapas relevantes de reabilitação, são essenciais para o manejo eficaz de qualquer tecido mole ou problema relacionado com as articulações. Portanto, a classificação da fase fisiopatológica de um paciente deve ser feita toda vez que o paciente é visto por um médico ou diariamente pelo próprio indivíduo. Essa análise evitará problemas com o tratamento, a esclarecer por que as coisas podem estar dando errado ou por que não estão respondendo conforme o esperado. Por exemplo, se o paciente não atingiu os critérios exigidos para estar no estágio tardio de reabilitação, mas ele continua correndo e relata rigidez no tornozelo todas as manhãs, então ele está realizando atividades que são inadequadas para sua fase fisiopatológica. Eles estão provocando um estado inflamatório crônico por meio de traumas repetitivos.

Pontos importantes

Compreender os processos fisiopatológicos relacionados às três fases principais da inflamação é fundamental para permitir que o médico avalie as lesões dos tecidos moles de maneira adequada e aplique estratégias de manejo eficazes.

Ter uma compreensão dos estágios de reabilitação e dos critérios necessários para progredir em cada estágio ajudará a esclarecer por que alguns regimes de manejo falham.

A classificação da fase inflamatória e do estágio de reabilitação de um paciente – independentemente do tempo desde a lesão ou intervenções anteriores – deve ser realizada pelo paciente diariamente e em cada ocasião. Eles são vistos pelo médico para garantir um resultado bem-sucedido.

Em resumo, o manejo geral de lesões em tecidos moles deve ser baseado nos seguintes seis princípios:

1. Minimizar a extensão do dano inicial e do inchaço sempre que possível.
2. Reduzir e controlar qualquer inflamação e dor associadas.
3. Promover a cura do tecido danificado.
4. Manter, ou restaurar, amplitude de movimento, força, propriocepção e aptidão geral, especialmente durante a fase de cura (subaguda).
5. Reabilitar funcionalmente o paciente ferido para permitir que ele tenha um retorno seguro ao esporte.
6. Avaliar e corrigir quaisquer fatores predisponentes para reduzir o risco de recorrência.

Referências bibliográficas

Brukner, P., Khan, K., 2017. Brukner & Khan's Clinical Sports Medicine, fifth ed. McGraw-Hill, New York.

Gillquist, J., 1993. iii. Principles of repair. Current Orthopaedics 7 (3), 90-93.

Hardy, M.A., 1989. The biology of scar formation. Physical Therapy 69 (12), 1014-1024.

Hurley, J., 1985. Inflammation. In: Anderson, J.R. (Ed.), Muir's Textbook of Pathology, twelfth ed. Edward Arnold, London.

Lin, T.W.T., Cardenas, L., Soslowsky, L.J.L., 2004. Biomechanics of tendon injury and repair. Journal of Biomechanics 37 (6), 865-877.

Mercandetti, M., Cohen, A.J., 2017. Wound healing and repair (update). Medscape.

Schröder, D., Pässler, H.H., 1994. Combination of cold and compression after knee surgery. A prospective randomized study. Knee Surgery, Sports Traumatology, Arthroscopy 2 (3), 158-165.

Shelbourne, K.D., Rubenstein, R.A., McCarroll, J.R., Weaver, J., 1994. Postoperative cryotherapy for the knee in ACL reconstructive surgery. Orthopaedics International 2 (2), 165-170.

Smith, G.N., 1999. Sports Medicine – Clinical Update Royal College of General Practitioners Members Reference Book (1999–2000). Camden Publishing, London.

Smith, G.N., 1998. Return to fitness. In: Tidswell, M. (Ed.), Orthopaedic Physiotherapy. Churchill Livingstone, Edinburgh.

Watson, T., 2016. Soft Tissue Repair and Healing Review. Available at: http://www.electrotherapy.org/modality/soft-tissue-repair-and-healing-review.

Capítulo | 37 |

Programa de Força Durante a Temporada: Uma Perspectiva Profissional do Rúgbi – Programação ao Longo da Temporada

Aidan O'Connell

Introdução

O rúgbi profissional é um ambiente de pressão e de alto risco, no qual a otimização de força, potência e velocidade fornece uma vantagem de desempenho definitiva. Desenvolver e manter essas qualidades durante a pré-temporada pode ser simples. No entanto, a imprevisibilidade e a volatilidade inerentes a uma temporada de 40 jogos, combinada com respostas individuais não lineares transitórias a esse ambiente, cria um dos maiores desafios para a equipe técnica. Este capítulo examina como enfrentamos esse problema em uma equipe profissional de rúgbi e trabalhamos a força ao longo da temporada.

O organismo humano não foi projetado para jogar rúgbi.

Craig White

O rúgbi é um jogo físico e, taticamente, pode ser tão sutil quanto um jogo de xadrez e até explodir em vida com grandes jogadas que mudam o ímpeto. Esses momentos de virada de jogo, de um desvio explosivo a um bloqueio feroz, exigem que os jogadores estejam técnica, tática, mental e fisicamente aptos. É função dos treinadores de força e condicionamento trabalhar com os treinadores de rúgbi e a equipe médica para preparar os jogadores para operarem com sucesso nesse ambiente. De modo mais específico, os treinadores de força e condicionamento desenvolvem a força, a velocidade e a potência do jogador para virar o jogo e sua capacidade de fazer isso repetidamente durante a partida. Otimizar essas características físicas permite ao jogador não apenas sobreviver na zona de combate, mas também dominá-la.

Jogadores maiores, mais fortes e mais poderosos se recuperam mais rápido entre os jogos e agudamente entre as colisões, melhorando seu perfil de preparação física. Do ponto de vista psicológico, os níveis maiores de força aumentam a confiança em sua fisicalidade. Além disso, e crucialmente no esporte profissional, jogadores mais fortes se machucam com menos frequência, o que, por sua vez, tem um efeito positivo na disponibilidade do jogador. A correlação entre essa disponibilidade e a proporção de vitórias/derrotas no esporte está bem estabelecida. Criar um ambiente em que os jogadores treinem e joguem mais é um dos principais fatores de desempenho no esporte profissional.

O treinamento de força, o perfil de risco de lesões, um programa de recuperação/estilo de vida e um sistema de monitoramento de treinamento sensível são armas potentes na guerra de disponibilidade. O treinamento de força serve, sobretudo, para proteger melhor os jogadores contra a natureza violenta do jogo. Ele também cria robustez, aumentando a tolerância ao estresse do sistema musculoesquelético à carga. Além disso, os ganhos de força melhoram a eficiência do movimento, corrigindo perdas de energia causadas por músculos estabilizadores lentos e instabilidade articular. Esse mecanismo não apenas protege o corpo contra o risco de lesões, como também minimiza os padrões inadequados de movimento que roubam a força, a potência, a velocidade e a resistência dos jogadores.

A maior janela de oportunidade para os jogadores profissionais de rúgbi ficarem fortes é durante os anos maleáveis da adolescência por meio do sistema escolar e do sistema acadêmico subsequente. Os ganhos acentuados de força na adolescência diminuem à medida que os jogadores fazem a transição em suas carreiras profissionais, nas quais as janelas de oportunidade para o desenvolvimento de força são poucas e distantes entre si. No entanto, em uma base anual, a pré-temporada de 6 a 8 semanas oferece uma oportunidade de ouro para se fortalecerem. Os ganhos de força e a pré-temporada andam de mãos dadas, pois esse ambiente estável foi projetado para isso. A intensidade, o volume e a dosagem da sessão podem ser manipulados em conjunto com o processo de treinamento mais amplo para aumentar o tamanho, a força, a potência e a velocidade. A temporada de desenvolvimento de força tem, no entanto, uma proposta diferente.

Desde o pontapé inicial do jogo de abertura da temporada, uma batalha acontece durante todas as 40 semanas. Os treinadores são lançados de um ambiente estável de pré-temporada para o ambiente VICA (volátil, incerto, complexo, ambíguo) (Figura 37.1) durante a temporada. A precisão e a exatidão da prescrição do treinamento de força são muito difíceis nessas condições. Por exemplo, em qualquer semana, pode-se preparar os jogadores do time para até três competições: competição europeia ou da liga, competição por equipes B e competição nacional de segundo nível. Logisticamente, esses jogos podem ser em casa ou fora, o que pode envolver muitas viagens. O tempo de retorno entre os jogos pode variar de 5 a 8 dias. De uma perspectiva de desempenho bruto, a equipe deve atingir o pico ou operar próximo ao pico todas as semanas. Esses planos precisam ser ainda mais individualizados com base na seleção, idade, *status* da lesão, *status* de monitoramento e análise de necessidades individuais. Adicione os fatores emocionais causados por seleção, vitória ou derrota, lesão, fadiga física e mental e outros estressores externos

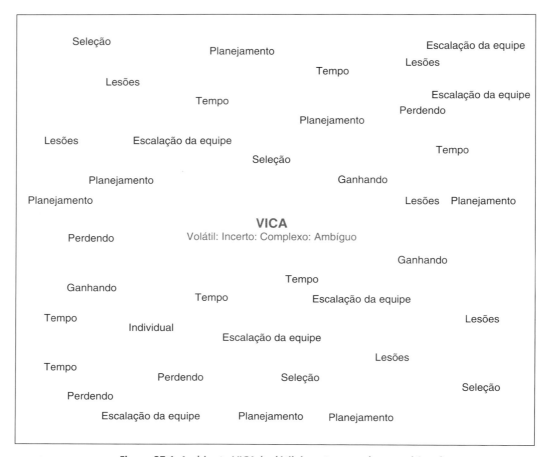

Figura 37.1 Ambiente VICA (volátil, incerto, complexo, ambíguo).

à equação e você terá uma mistura potente que, se não for gerenciada, tem o potencial de prejudicar uma temporada.

No entanto, em cada dificuldade existe uma oportunidade. O desempenho máximo em um ambiente de alto risco é estar no limite, reconhecendo a incerteza, antecipando problemas, assumindo riscos calculados, pensando nas possibilidades e encontrando soluções eficazes em meio à neblina. O gerenciamento do ambiente VICA com sucesso pode dar à equipe uma vantagem competitiva significativa sobre o oponente. A seção a seguir examinará soluções que podem otimizar o processo de treinamento de força durante a temporada.

Modelo de periodização adaptativa

Um processo de treinamento eficaz de força durante a temporada precisa ser baseado em uma plataforma filosófica e estratégica estável, embora tenha a flexibilidade e a adaptabilidade para entregar o programa com precisão. O alinhamento filosófico com o treinador de rúgbi e da operação com todos os departamentos para formar equipes de desempenho integradas, bem como a sensibilidade ao ambiente, são fundamentais para sua eficácia. Um plano de treinamento adaptativo fornece agilidade embutida sistemática no programa de treinamento para que ele possa se adaptar com mais rapidez e responder apropriadamente aos cenários em constante mudança que são apresentados. Esse processo adaptativo permite gerir em um ambiente complexo e imprevisível.

A periodização adaptativa é baseada na premissa de que cada jogador terá uma resposta biológica única ao processo de treinamento, e que o programa de força deve responder a essas mudanças e às condições ambientais atuais. Cada indivíduo, cada equipe e cada ambiente são únicos, assim como suas interações. A periodização adaptativa é caracterizada por:

1. Planejamento de cenário.
2. Ciclos de planejamento curtos.
3. Análise "e se".
4. Flexibilidade inerente.
5. Teste incorporado.
6. Múltiplos ciclos de *feedback*.
7. Tomada de decisão informada.
8. Revisão habitual.
9. "Soluções de desempenho multidepartamental".

Existem cinco estágios no modelo de periodização adaptativa (Figura 37.2). Cada um complementa e se baseia no anterior. A otimização de cada estágio regula positivamente todo o processo.

Estágio 1: estratégia geral – processo de alinhamento

A adaptabilidade e a habilidade de responder às mudanças são de suma importância ao se planejar em um ambiente VICA. No entanto, a eficácia desse processo dependerá da força da estrutura na qual ele é construído. As estratégias gerais que estabilizam esse ambiente não apenas incluem filosofia e modelo de treinamento de força fortes e resolutos durante a temporada, mas também se alinham e se integram com a filosofia de treinamento de rúgbi do técnico principal e com o processo de treinamento mais amplo. O programa de treinamento de força deve complementar o programa de rúgbi, em vez de tentar *ser o programa*.

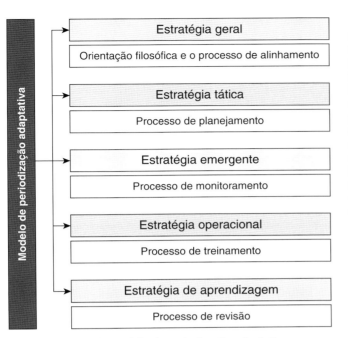

Figura 37.2 Modelo de periodização adaptativa.

Filosofia de treinamento de força

O primeiro passo na construção de um programa de força eficaz e no reforço da estabilidade do ambiente é ter uma filosofia inabalável de treinamento de força durante a temporada. Para o autor, essa filosofia é simplesmente otimizar a disponibilidade dos jogadores e construir confiança, tornando-os fortes e robustos o suficiente para atenderem às intensas demandas físicas do jogo. A confiança é a moeda do esporte de alto desempenho e as sessões de força são projetadas para inflar essa mercadoria valiosa.

Central a essa filosofia é o mantra de que estamos ficando maiores, mais fortes, mais rápidos e mais poderosos durante a temporada. Não estamos apenas mantendo os níveis de desempenho. Uma mentalidade de manutenção ao longo de uma temporada de 40 semanas não só levará à estagnação mental e à desmotivação, mas também ao descondicionamento físico e à degradação ao longo do tempo. É importante ressaltar que o programa reconhece que esse desenvolvimento deve agregar valor ao processo de treinamento mais amplo de rúgbi. Encontrar um equilíbrio entre o desenvolvimento sustentado na academia, enquanto guarda energia suficiente para treinar e jogar, é um equilíbrio complicado. Todos os jogadores têm tempo limitado para treinar e se recuperar. Portanto, devemos gastar nosso precioso tempo de treinamento de força com sabedoria, focando no que os jogadores precisam e no que dá o melhor retorno.

Modelo de treinamento de força

O modelo de treinamento de força durante a temporada é um modelo de força baseado em corrida por contato (Figura 37.3). Baseia-se na premissa de que melhorar essas características de força melhorará o desempenho direta e indiretamente, por meio da redução de lesões. O grau em que um jogador é exposto a requisitos de força com base no contato ou na corrida, e se essa exposição visa o desempenho ou a redução de lesões, dependerá de seu perfil de força, histórico de lesões, posição de jogo etc. O modelo tem três correntes distintas; elas se complementam e preparam o jogador para o próximo nível, passando do geral para o específico e do simples para o complexo. Além disso, dentro de cada fluxo, o jogador progride, em termos de velocidade, de lento para rápido, e de força baixa para força alta.

Fluxo de força fundamental

O fluxo de força fundamental ou de movimento serve para estabelecer uma força fundamental sólida para reconfigurar, ativar e estimular o corpo antes de exercícios mais extenuantes. Ele

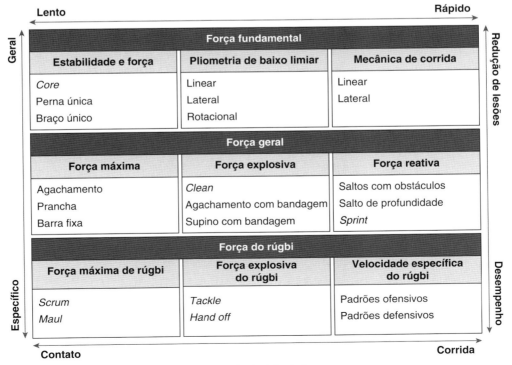

Figura 37.3 Modelo de força.

Parte | 2 | Aplicação Clínica

prepara o corpo para produzir e reduzir as forças elevadas de forma mais eficaz. Esse fluxo de movimento é subdividido em três seções:

- O papel dos exercícios de força central e de membro único é amenizar perdas de energia e padrões de movimento ineficientes, corrigindo desequilíbrios musculares e ativando estabilizadores lentos, principalmente no quadril lateral e no manguito rotador, contribuindo para a biomecânica adequada. A qualidade do tecido mole também é reforçada, maximizando a tolerância ao estresse da cadeia cinética
- A pliometria de baixo limiar ou a mecânica de pouso de membro único também melhoram os padrões de movimento ineficientes por meio do mecanismo de melhoria do controle e absorção de força
- A mecânica da corrida melhora a força específica da corrida diretamente, visando a força e a rigidez no tornozelo, no quadril lateral e no *core*. Como um subproduto, esses exercícios também podem reduzir o potencial de lesões e melhorar o desempenho na corrida, ensinando a postura correta, altura do quadril, posicionamento do pé, coordenação e ritmo de corrida.

Os exercícios de força de movimento juntamente com os exercícios de mobilidade formam o sistema de movimento no *Munster Rugby*. Esses exercícios são sistematicamente programados em sessões de preparação de movimento no início de cada dia de treinamento ou em aquecimentos de movimento antes das sessões de força e de campo. Os exercícios de *core* e de membro único também podem estar incluídos no programa de treinamento de força principal. Essa distribuição de trabalho em várias plataformas de treinamento permite que todos os aspectos da força sejam cobertos de forma abrangente durante o período da temporada mais ocupado e de pouco tempo.

Fluxo de força geral

Este fluxo visa construir força por meio de métodos de força máxima, força explosiva e força reativa:

- A força máxima é construída a partir dos três exercícios angulares de: agachamento, prancha, barra fixa e seus derivados. Esses exercícios são escolhidos por causa de sua capacidade de "retorno para o investimento" de desenvolver não apenas força, mas, com manipulação, potência e massa magra. A duração da largura de banda operacional é definida entre 75 e 90% da intensidade máxima
- A força explosiva é desenvolvida principalmente por meio do *clean* e suas variantes ou, alternativamente, por meio do agachamento dinâmico. Esses exercícios de força explosiva são programados com base na intenção e na qualidade da velocidade de movimento, com intensidade variando de 60 a 80% do máximo
- A força reativa é exercitada principalmente por meio do treinamento de rúgbi, com gestos específicos do esporte, e exercícios especialmente projetados para exporem os jogadores a

corridas de velocidade máxima. O trabalho de corrida de alta velocidade extra é dado aos jogadores que não têm exposição, conforme destacado por meio do sistema de posicionamento global (GPS) ou *feedback* subjetivo de um técnico ou do próprio jogador. Os jogadores recuados também são programados com pliometria reativa periodicamente durante a temporada, tanto para alimentar sua necessidade psicológica de velocidade, quanto para aumentar a rigidez do tornozelo conforme os arremessos ficam mais fracos durante os meses de inverno.

Fluxo de força de rúgbi

O fluxo de força do rúgbi (Figura 37.4) reconhece que treinar ou jogar o esporte fornece um estímulo de força inerente durante a temporada. Capacidades de geração e redução de força específicas significativas são treinadas semana após semana. Embora seja difícil quantificar a extensão e magnitude dessa exposição, o monitoramento cuidadoso da carga de treinamento, os dados de GPS e a análise de desempenho do rúgbi podem ajudar a lançar alguma luz. Essa informação é então usada para influenciar ainda mais o desenho do programa de força, pois destaca as qualidades de força que são super ou subexpostas durante o treinamento e as partidas de rúgbi.

Alinhamento filosófico e de treinamento

Uma estratégia central para moldar e dar vida ao modelo de força é alinhá-lo com a filosofia de treinamento de rúgbi do técnico principal. Por exemplo, informações táticas relacionadas ao estilo do esporte, ou se o técnico tem uma filosofia baseada em corrida ou contato, acrescentam profundidade ao programa de força, pois iluminam as características de força que irão complementar e agregar valor ao plano de jogo. O tempo que a equipe técnica leva para promover esse alinhamento no mundo volátil do esporte profissional também é extremamente importante. Uma configuração de treinamento estável não apenas fornece uma espinha dorsal forte para proteger contra essa turbulência, mas também permite que relacionamentos, sistemas e processos cresçam, se desenvolvam e evoluam junto com o tempo.

A próxima etapa no processo de alinhamento é gerenciar e estabilizar o processo de treinamento de rúgbi mais amplo e encontrar dentro dele um lar consistentemente seguro para lançar o programa todas as semanas. Nesse sentido, utilizamos a *periodização tática*, modelo de periodização desenvolvido para o futebol por Vítor Frade, docente da Universidade do Porto. A periodização tática reconhece que o desempenho é uma função da preparação tática, técnica, psicológica e física, e que, para otimizar esses componentes na época limitada pelo tempo, é melhor integrar e treinar todos os componentes juntos. Esse processo de sincronização da carga de trabalho reduz a complexidade, mas não a intensidade do treinamento.

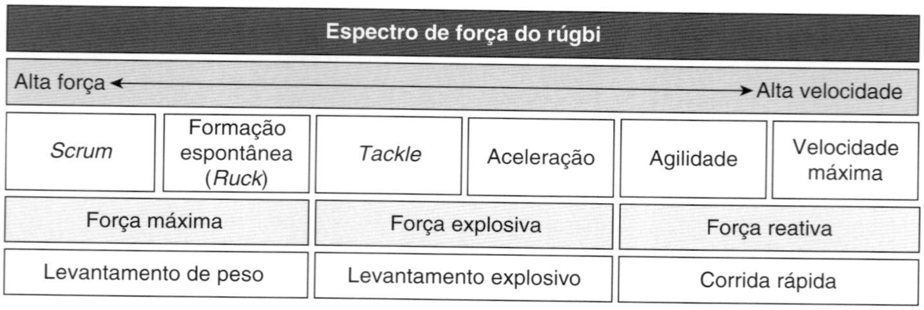

Espectro de força do rúgbi					
Alta força ←					→ Alta velocidade
Scrum	Formação espontânea (Ruck)	Tackle	Aceleração	Agilidade	Velocidade máxima
Força máxima		Força explosiva		Força reativa	
Levantamento de peso		Levantamento explosivo		Corrida rápida	

Figura 37.4 Espectro de força do rúgbi.

A periodização tática utiliza a filosofia tática do treinador principal como a plataforma de planejamento para a semana de treinamento. Por exemplo, os elementos táticos centrais de ataque, defesa e transições podem ser sobrecarregados e testados contra estresse em dias específicos da semana. Essas sessões são caracterizadas por uma intensidade que aumenta a capacidade de tomada de decisão dos jogadores, os níveis de concentração, as habilidades táticas e a preparação física. Embora a prática de alongamento promova a qualidade da sessão, o botão de estresse do treinamento pode ser aumentado ou diminuído por sessão, ou por semana, por meio da manipulação do volume. Essa manipulação e a estabilidade proporcionada por 1 semana de treinamento fixa criam um modelo de treinamento de rúgbi que facilita a consistência de desempenho ao longo de uma temporada de 40 semanas. Ele também fornece uma estrutura sólida na qual o programa de força pode ser consistentemente realizado todas as semanas. Além disso, as sessões de força podem ser planejadas para complementar as sessões de rúgbi que estão sendo treinadas em qualquer dia.

Em uma semana típica (Figura 37.5), com um jogo de sábado a sábado, o treinamento de força é programado no máximo 2 vezes/semana. As sessões são incorporadas à estrutura semanal no dia do jogo + 2 e no dia do jogo + 3. As sessões de força têm um planejamento vertical integrado visando múltiplas qualidades de força em uma única sessão. No momento em que este artigo foi escrito, nossa semana de treinamento é a seguinte:

Sessão de força 1: dia de força total do corpo

Tem como alvo a força de perna dupla e única, força de tração da parte superior do corpo e tamanho de tração da parte superior do corpo. Do ponto de vista do treinamento de rúgbi, o dia de jogo + 2 é um dia pesado em termos de aprendizado, mas um dia leve em termos de contato específico para o rúgbi e carga de corrida, com a restauração física na ordem do dia. Na maioria dos programas, colocar o trabalho da perna de maneira adequada no programa é um dos maiores enigmas. Colocamos neste dia porque é o dia mais leve em termos de carga de rúgbi. Além disso, a evidência anedótica sugere que esse dia com a perna dominante acelera o processo de recuperação, ajudando o corpo a reiniciar e recalibrar pós-jogo. Esse dia também tem a predominância de puxadas, principalmente para equilibrar o domínio do padrão de flexão de jogos e treinamento, e porque as estruturas anteriores do ombro ainda podem estar "danificadas" ou em processo de reparo após o jogo.

Sessão de força 2: dia de força total e da parte superior do corpo

O foco é mais especificamente na força explosiva, na força de impulso da parte superior do corpo e no *push/pull* com a parte superior do corpo. O dia de jogo + 3 é o principal dia de treinamento de rúgbi. É mental e fisicamente desgastante em todas as frentes, especialmente no que diz respeito ao contato e aos parâmetros de funcionamento extensivos. Consequentemente, as pernas são poupadas e a força de impulso da parte superior do corpo é priorizada. O dia de jogo + 3 também pode fornecer uma janela de oportunidade para treinar força explosiva, já que os jogadores estão em sua prontidão ideal para este estímulo. Além disso, esse estímulo os ativa para o grande dia que se avizinha, sem que o cansaço debilitante transborde para o campo.

Como mencionado anteriormente, podemos ajustar essas sessões dependendo de como os jogadores ou o ambiente estão se apresentando. As sessões podem alternar facilmente entre foco em redefinição, construção ou estímulo, dependendo do cenário emergente. É importante ressaltar que nos dias do jogo + 2 e do jogo + 3 as sessões de força, ou partes delas, podem ser trocadas e "misturadas e combinadas" para atender às necessidades de um indivíduo. Essa agilidade ou flexibilidade é um componente vital da temporada de programação e exploraremos isso com mais detalhes na próxima seção.

Estágio 2: estratégia tática – otimização do processo de planejamento

O período durante a temporada é o período de treinamento dominante para o rúgbi profissional. Nosso foco é desenvolver e preservar força, potência e tamanho durante toda a temporada e de uma à outra. Desenvolver e proteger o estímulo de força na temporada é realmente um processo desafiador, dado o fato de que os jogadores têm uma quantidade finita de tempo e energia para treinar a força. Portanto, precisamos maximizar o resultado a partir dos esforços empregados.

Nossa principal razão tática é que nós "planejamos resumidamente e frequentemente" em mini blocos de três a quatro jogos. Planejamos conforme necessário em ciclos curtos, dadas as imprecisões da previsão além desse período em um ambiente imprevisível. Em segundo lugar, as qualidades fundamentais de força, potência e tamanho são treinadas constantemente em todos esses blocos. Os exercícios usados para impulsionar essas qualidades também são mantidos consistentes na temporada com pouquíssima variabilidade. Essa consistência facilita

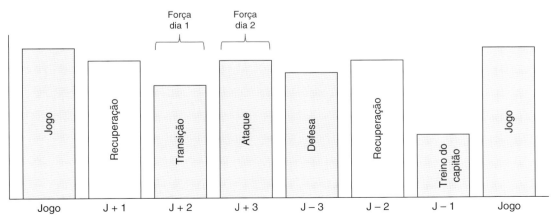

Figura 37.5 Agenda semanal.

a melhoria estreitando o foco e evita o estresse causado por mudanças e perturbações contínuas.

A consistência no programa não se expressa apenas por meio da seleção de exercícios, mas também por meio da intensidade. A intensidade é mantida consistentemente alta durante a temporada. Isso é possível trabalhando com larguras de banda operacionais restritas. Por exemplo, nossas faixas de intensidade para treinamento de força máxima são mantidas entre uma largura de banda estreita de 75 a 90% do máximo. Esse "ponto ideal" de força nos dá a capacidade de manobra para desenvolver força semana após semana. É importante ressaltar que ele adiciona mais eficiência ao programa porque evita as zonas mortas do treinamento muito leve ou muito pesado. Este último diminui o desempenho técnico e pode levar a uma possível hemorragia neural, superando, assim, quaisquer benefícios potenciais. Portanto, planejamos nossos programas dentro de uma largura de banda operacional muito estável em termos de seleção e intensidade de exercícios. No entanto, esse espaço tem variabilidade suficiente para simular a adaptação ao longo da temporada.

Nosso programa de força durante a temporada ideal, conforme mostrado na Figura 37.6, tem dois blocos ou ciclos de força complementares de três a quatro jogos que acontecem consecutivamente ao longo da temporada. A intensidade também é ciclada em forma de onda dentro de um bloco e de bloco a bloco. O primeiro bloco de força (bloco A) sobrecarrega o estímulo por meio de exercícios de resistência com barra de alta força, enquanto o segundo (bloco B) visa ao estímulo de força por meio de força explosiva, utilizando resistência de acomodação. A principal diferença entre eles é que o bloco B é direcionado para a potência. Por exemplo, no bloco de força, um agachamento com barra pode ser usado para promover a força máxima das pernas, enquanto na fase de força explosiva uma variação em faixas pode ser utilizada. A resistência de acomodação fornecida pela banda não só sobrecarregará o estímulo de força na extremidade superior, mas fornecerá maior potência de saída durante a porção inicial concêntrica do levantamento.

A próxima camada no processo de planejamento é decidir se o bloco, seja de força ou dominante de força explosiva, é uma oportunidade para desenvolver força ou um momento para ser mais conservador e se acomodar para preservar. O exame de fatores como a lista de jogos, oponentes, fase da competição, local do jogo etc., orienta esta importante decisão. Os níveis e tendências de força atuais também são considerados na equação. Podemos girar o *dial* para cima ou para baixo para um bloco de treinamento por meio da seleção de exercícios, manipulação de volume e utilizando intensidades relativas. A seleção de exercícios, um método sutil, mas eficaz, funciona escolhendo um exercício de orientação concêntrica menos desgastante em vez de um excêntrico-dominante. O volume pode ser manipulado em repetições, séries, sessões e blocos. Finalmente, a aplicação de intensidades relativas também nos dá grande flexibilidade operacional. Por exemplo, na fase de força, podemos manter a intensidade alta em 85% e proteger o estímulo atacando e desenvolvendo-o com quatro a cinco repetições ou preservando-o com duas a três repetições.

> *Se você tem que planejar um futuro além do horizonte de previsão, planeje a surpresa.*
>
> Philip Tetlock

Embora seja importante moldar o programa com base na previsão a curto prazo, a precisão da prescrição para um indivíduo em um determinado dia pode ser aumentada incorporando flexibilidade ao programa por meio de planejamento de contingência – em outras palavras, "imprevisibilidade planejada". Esse planejamento promove a autorregulação, fornecendo aos jogadores opções como séries abertas, mais séries, séries extras opcionais, escolha de exercícios, faixas de repetições e faixas de intensidade para escolher, dependendo de sua prontidão (Figura 37.7). Essa flexibilidade está no cerne do conceito de periodização adaptativa.

Programa de força durante a temporada													
Fase		Bloco A						Bloco B					
Foco 1		Força máxima						Força explosiva					
		Leve		Médio		Pesado		Leve		Médio		Pesado	
Agachamento		Regular						Regular + 25% do peso da banda					
	% 1RM/V(m/s)	75 a 80%	0,55 a 0,6 m/s	80 a 85%	0,5 a 0,55 m/s	85 a 90%	0,45 a 0,5 m/s	60 a 65%	0,7 a 0,75 m/s	65 a 70%	0,65 a 0,7 m/s	70 a 75%	0,6 a 0,65 m/s
	Reps	3 a 4		2 a 3		1 a 2		3 a 4		2 a 3		1 a 2	
	Séries	2 a 4		3 a 5		4 a 6		2 a 4		3 a 5		4 a 6	
Prancha		Regular						Regular + 10% do peso da banda					
	% 1RM/V(m/s)	75 a 80%	0,55 a 0,65 m/s	80 a 85%	0,45 a 0,55 m/s	85 a 90%	0,35 a 0,45 m/s	65 a 70%	0,65 a 0,7 m/s	70 a 75%	0,6 a 0,65 m/s	75 a 80%	0,55 a 0,6 m/s
	Reps	5 a 6		4 a 5		2 a 3		4 a 5		3 a 4		1 a 2	
	Séries	2 a 3		3 a 4		4 a 5		2 a 3		3 a 4		4 a 5	
Barra fixa		Regular						Regular + 5% do peso da banda					
	% 1RM	75 a 80%		80 a 85%		85 a 90%		65 a 70%		70 a 75%		75 a 80%	
	Reps	5 a 6		4 a 5		2 a 3		4 a 5		3 a 4		1 a 2	
	Séries	2 a 3		3 a 4		4 a 5		2 a 3		3 a 4		4 a 5	
Clean		*Clean*						*Jump shrug*					
	% 1RM	70 a 75%		75 a 80%		80 a 85%		55 a 60%		60 a 65%		65 a 70%	
	Reps	3 a 4		2 a 3		1 a 2		3 a 4		2 a 3		1 a 2	
	Séries	2 a 3		3 a 4		4 a 5		2 a 3		3 a 4		4 a 5	

Figura 37.6 Programa de força durante a temporada. *1RM*, 1 repetição máxima; *V*, velocidade.

Programa de força explosiva

		Velocidade de execução	Relógio	Reps	Série 1	Série 2	Série 3	Série 4	Série 5
1a	Jump shrug/agachamento com salto	2–0–X	3 min	3	2 @55%	2 @60%	2 @65%	2 @65%	
1b	Salto em profundidade/saltos com obstáculos	X			3	2	2	2	
2a	Agachamento com bandagem/barra hexagonal com bandagem	2–0–1	3 min	2	3 @55%	2 @60%	2 @65%	2 @70%	2 @>70%
2b	SCM/salto de caixa	X							
3a	Supino com bandagem/supino barra de supino	2–0–1	3 min	2	5 @65%	4 @70%	3 @75%	3+ @75%	
3b	Remada com HT/levantamento de peso do tipo bench pull	2–0–1			5 a 8	5 a 8	5 a 8		
4a	Inclinação com HT/jammer press	3–0–1	3 min	2	8 a 12	8 a 12	8 a 12		
4b	Tração de cabo/tração de faixa na altura do rosto	3–0–1			8a 12	8 a 12	8 a 12		

Figura 37.7 Programa ágil de força de resistência. Conjuntos em cinza-claro são conjuntos opcionais a serem concluídos com base na prontidão. SCM, salto de contramovimento; HT, haltere.

Estágio 3: estratégia emergente – otimização do processo de monitoramento

O que é certo durante as provações e tribulações durante a temporada é que as condições vão evoluir além das suposições feitas no processo de planejamento. O planejamento baseado na previsibilidade em um ambiente VICA normalmente dá errado devido à natureza dinâmica do ambiente e à variabilidade na resposta individual ao treinamento. Por exemplo, eventos agudos que podem redirecionar seu programa podem incluir sinais de alerta de marcadores objetivos e subjetivos de "prontidão para treinar", bem como dados de monitoramento de carga. A modificação do programa também pode ser garantida com base nas informações do departamento de saúde. De uma perspectiva mais geral, uma mudança de plano para a programação de treinamento de rúgbi na forma de, por exemplo, uma sessão de *scrum* improvisada também terá um efeito indireto no programa de força.

A capacidade do programa de força de mudar e se ajustar a novas circunstâncias reside na sensibilidade a esses eventos que se desenrolam. Um sistema de monitoramento multidepartamento abrangente, impulsionado por ciclos de *feedback* eficazes e canais de comunicação fluida, aumenta essa sensibilidade. Os sistemas de fluxo de trabalho rápidos e adaptáveis que alimentam os dados e informações pertinentes ao programa de força podem ser tão simples quanto realizar reuniões curtas diárias com vários departamentos que identificam desvios mais amplos do programa ou mudanças individuais à medida que ocorrem em tempo real. Essas trocas de informação ocorrem no início e no final de cada dia, bem como precedem todas as sessões de treinamento de força e arremesso. Esse processo aumenta a precisão da prescrição de treinamento, garantindo que as informações e os dados de todos os departamentos sejam atualizados, circulem com fluidez e entrem em ação.

Os ciclos formais de monitoramento e comunicação (Figura 37.8) são vitais ao gerenciar o ambiente emergente. No entanto, a imagem está incompleta sem *feedback* e entrada do jogador. Os próprios jogadores são uma fonte poderosa de conhecimento. Uma cultura de respeito e confiança entre os jogadores e o treinador garantirá que os jogadores forneçam informações voluntárias sobre suas necessidades de treinamento e prontidão, o mesmo ocorre com demais membros da equipe. A adaptação do programa com base em suas contribuições fortalecerá ainda mais esse vínculo.

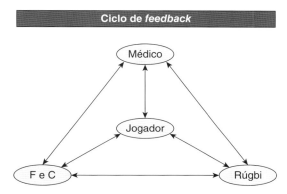

Figura 37.8 Ciclo de *feedback*. Comunicação recíproca entre treinadores de força e condicionamento (F e C), jogadores, treinadores de rúgbi e equipe médica.

Como treinadores, devemos falar com eles, ouvi-los e observá-los. Podemos obter informações importantes dos jogadores observando como eles interagem entre si e com os treinadores. Eles são mais silenciosos ou mais barulhentos do que o normal? Observar como eles estão se movendo na sessão de aquecimento/movimento antes da sessão de ginástica também irá esclarecer se quaisquer mudanças de última hora são justificadas.

Adaptar o programa de força a circunstâncias novas e emergentes durante a temporada requer uma tomada de decisão informada com base em fatos "concretos" e na intuição "instintiva".

Estágio 4: estratégia operacional – otimização do processo de treinamento

A eficácia do processo de fortalecimento durante a temporada depende da otimização do processo de treinamento. O planejamento e as estratégias emergentes devem ser complementados com sessões de treinamento de força que traduzam ou concretizem a programação em ação eficaz. Um ponto central para aumentar esse processo é uma forte cultura de desempenho que impulsiona a implementação do plano de ação. Uma cultura de desempenho pode ser definida como um conjunto de comportamentos esperados que emula do grupo durante cada sessão. Promovemos uma forte cultura de desempenho positivo, estabelecendo altos padrões de comportamento e desempenho, criando um ambiente competitivo e capacitando os jogadores por meio da autonomia dirigida (Figura 37.9).

Altos padrões de comportamento são definidos por meio de um código de conduta não escrito. Treine forte, mas com inteligência, concentre-se no processo e execute a sessão com intenção e excelência técnica. Alvos claros e transparentes (Figura 37.10) orientam os padrões de desempenho nas qualidades essenciais de força, potência e velocidade. Essas metas são baseadas nas melhores práticas internacionais por posição e os padrões mínimos são definidos para desafiar o jogador. Este processo fornece aos jogadores e treinadores uma bússola de desempenho e combustível para acender seu espírito competitivo. Tabelas de classificação, prêmios de desempenho e definição de metas específicas adicionam tempero. Os jogadores são, por natureza, animais competitivos e esse instinto pode ser ainda mais alimentado agrupando os jogadores com base na posição ou na proficiência em um determinado exercício. Além disso, quadros de líderes ao vivo durante a sessão, que fornecem *feedback* sobre pontuações de treinamento com base na velocidade ou esforços máximos, podem ajudar a eletrificar a atmosfera. A competição é saudável. No entanto, existem sessões e blocos onde a intensidade que a competição gera organicamente precisa ser moderada. Esta valiosa mercadoria pode ser de maior valor em outra parte do processo de treinamento.

A escolha é fundamental para um programa adaptativo de treinamento de força. As opções são oferecidas aos jogadores em torno do tipo de sessão, exercícios, faixas de intensidade e volume. Boas escolhas são feitas por jogadores bem-educados e informados que entendem o porquê ou a lógica por trás do programa. Escolher o caminho certo para o dia certo é um processo colaborativo de confiança mútua entre treinadores e jogadores. Este processo de autonomia dirigida capacita e motiva os jogadores, permitindo-lhes moldar seu próprio programa. Este canal de comunicação fluido e bidirecional também facilita o *feedback* e a tomada de decisões "em tempo real" durante a sessão. Por exemplo, uma sessão pode ser encerrada mais cedo se um jogador comunicar um problema; em contrapartida, as sessões podem ser estendidas se um jogador relatar que está "se sentindo ótimo" e deseja tentar novamente. No entanto, deve-se notar que a autonomia dirigida deve ser um espectro em que jogadores mais jovens, recém-recrutados ou menos afinados são mais fortemente orientados em comparação com a abordagem mais autônoma dada a profissionais experientes.

A cultura de desempenho fornece a estrutura na qual treinar. A essência do nosso trabalho como treinadores de campo é ajudar a orientar e facilitar os jogadores durante a implementação do programa. Fazemos isso por:

- Falar com os jogadores antes da sessão para explicar "o porquê" do programa; uma vez que eles entendem isso, sua intenção aumenta
- Explicar e demonstrar "o quê" para que os jogadores entendam a tarefa em mãos
- Destacar os mantras centrais de "intenção" e "execução técnica de qualidade"
- Entregar a sessão de treinamento com paixão e energia
- Treinar a sessão com foco e fornecer instrução de qualidade e *feedback* com base no que você pode ver, sentir e ouvir dos jogadores.

Para obter o melhor de cada sessão, nosso estado de preparação de treinamento, prontidão e entrega subsequente deve ser de alta qualidade inabalável. Essa consistência dá o tom aos jogadores, uma vez que se alimentam do nosso profissionalismo e energia. Assim que a sessão começa, estar mentalmente em um estado de "alerta alto" de atenção concentrada aumenta nossa sensibilidade em relação ao desempenho dos jogadores. A capacidade de mudar a atenção constantemente de um foco individual estreito para "pairar sobre a cabeça" e mergulhar na visão mais ampla nos permite treinar de forma mais eficaz. Combinar o *feedback* sensorial do que podemos ver, ouvir e sentir com nossa intuição e instinto orienta nossa tomada de decisão e nos permite programar e reprogramar individualmente à medida que avançamos.

Estágio 5: estratégia de aprendizagem – otimização do processo de revisão

A única maneira de vencer é aprender mais rápido do que qualquer outra pessoa.

Eric Ries

O ciclo de planejamento-execução-revisão nos dá uma estrutura de desempenho e tomada de decisão que nos ajuda a operar na incerteza da temporada. Como treinadores, amamos planejar e amamos a atmosfera inebriante de liderar uma sessão de treinamento. Fechar o ciclo e revisar geralmente é menos atraente.

Autonomia dirigida		
Jovem profissional fortemente orientado	⟷	Profissional autônomo experiente

Figura 37.9 Autonomia dirigida.

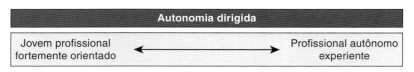

Figura 37.10 Alvos de força. *PC*, peso corporal.

Ou ficamos sem tempo ou fugimos de comentários críticos que esgotam o ego. Refletir sobre o desempenho e verificar nossas crenças e suposições de maneira rotineira e regular é um trabalho de amor que precisa ser exercitado.

O "hábito da revisão" nos dará a vantagem competitiva que desejamos, mas, como treinadores, podemos ser lentos para cultivar seus poderes inegáveis. Regulamentar positivamente essa parte do processo de treinamento e dessensibilizar o medo por meio de exposições frequentes requer revisões operacionais formalizadas e sistematizadas implantadas em todo o processo. Nosso método de revisão é caracterizado por uma análise pós-sessão simples e curta, no estilo lista de verificação, e revisões mais abrangentes que ocorrem no final de um ciclo de três a quatro jogos.

As sessões de treinamento de força podem ser vistas como um gigantesco laboratório de monitoramento no qual o treinamento é teste e o teste é treinamento. A análise de tendência simples de sessão para sessão e bloco para bloco nos permitirá analisar se os índices de força estão no caminho certo para o grupo e para o indivíduo. As metas podem ser reavaliadas e o programa redirecionado quando necessário. No entanto, não é apenas importante revisar os números; imediatamente após a sessão, formulários de *feedback* de verificação simples de 5 minutos para o treinador e o jogador são preenchidos (Figuras 37.11 e 37.12). Do ponto de vista do treinamento, uma escala móvel simples é usada para refletir sobre a organização, o planejamento, o fluxo e a entrega da sessão. Esse documento de verificação de saída também contém uma lista de jogadores que nos permite revisar rapidamente o desempenho de cada um após a sessão. Notas breves são feitas e todos os "sinais de alerta" ou informações relativas à participação do jogador nas sessões subsequentes são imediatamente distribuídos para a equipe de desempenho mais ampla.

Uma força formal viva ou revisão/previsão ocorre todos os meses. O objetivo principal dessa revisão é fornecer um fórum para explicar e examinar os dados de força de mês a mês. Ele também fornece uma plataforma para jogar "todas as cartas na mesa" para defender o programa anterior e delinear e defender o próximo programa para treinar colegas e a equipe médica. Esse processo permite que o programa seja submetido a um teste de resistência antes do lançamento, por meio da auditoria de erros e do destaque dos pontos fortes. Reunir e sintetizar outras perspectivas agrega valor ao programa, não apenas incorporando sua perícia técnica, mas também protegendo-o contra preconceitos cognitivos, como "viés de confirmação" e "pensamento de grupo". Esse processo de revisão de mente aberta e alerta a vieses facilita o crescimento e o desenvolvimento do programa perpétuo no mundo VICA, ajudando-nos a reconhecer no que erramos, superar a nós mesmos rapidamente, aprender e redirecionar.

Conclusão

O modelo de periodização adaptável fornece uma plataforma filosófica e estratégica estável para lançar o programa de força enquanto fornece a agilidade para operar com sucesso no ambiente VICA. A força motriz por trás do modelo é um grande conhecimento técnico, interpessoal e mental. A proficiência técnica garante que os processos de planejamento, programação, treinamento e revisão tenham o conhecimento metodológico necessário para o sucesso. As habilidades interpessoais garantem que as redes de comunicação e *feedback* estejam alinhadas e fluam livremente. Fortes habilidades mentais não só lhe dão a resiliência para treinar durante toda a temporada, mas também o equipam com a dose correta de prontidão cognitiva enquanto a guerra grassa ao seu redor. A prontidão cognitiva fornece a preparação e a agilidade necessárias para sustentar o desempenho do treinamento em um ambiente complexo e imprevisível.

A programação bem-sucedida durante a temporada requer programas inteligentes, ágeis e ricos em contingências, guiados pela reflexão e impulsionados pela prática deliberada de "desafios". A vitória por meio da névoa da guerra é uma ciência engenhosa que exige um questionamento profundo tanto do processo, quanto da direção tomada em cada conjuntura. A capacidade do programa de treinamento de força de esperar, adaptar-se e prosperar na imprevisibilidade pode ser uma vantagem competitiva real. No esporte profissional, essa pode ser a diferença entre ganhar e perder.

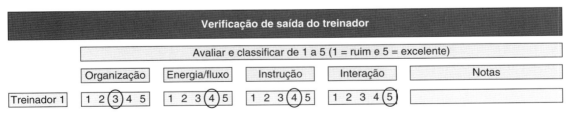

Figura 37.11 Verificação de saída dos treinadores.

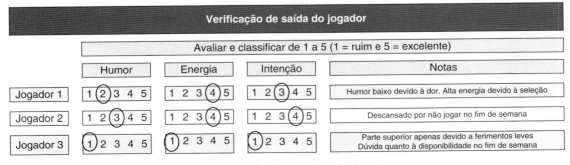

Figura 37.12 Verificação de saída dos jogadores.

Capítulo | 38 |

Análise de Movimento: a Ciência Encontra a Prática

David M. Clancy

Nada é mais revelador do que o movimento.

Martha Graham (1894-1991), dançarina e coreógrafa
norte-americana de dança moderna

Introdução

Este capítulo destacará a importância da análise do movimento para alcançar melhores resultados nos estágios iniciais de reabilitação, melhorias no desempenho e estratégias de prevenção de novas lesões.

Por que a análise de movimento é importante?

De acordo com a literatura, "[...] 35% dos pacientes não retornam aos níveis pré-lesão e 45% não retornam ao esporte competitivo" (Ardern et al., 2014). Esses números surpreendentes são relativos aos retornos do ligamento cruzado anterior (LCA); exemplos como esse tornaram a compreensão dos princípios do movimento, da neurofisiologia e da biomecânica da maior importância. Isso mostra que nós, como profissionais da saúde, podemos aprimorar nossas abordagens e melhorar nossos resultados clínicos.

Achamos que estamos fazendo um bom trabalho. No entanto, o trabalho publicado por Ardern et al. destaca que precisamos direcionar as deficiências em um grau maior para efetuar uma mudança significativa e fazer os atletas voltarem ao seu nível de jogo e/ou desempenho "esperado" pré-lesão.

O movimento é fundamental para toda a biologia, desde o movimento das células sanguíneas no sistema circulatório, passando pelo movimento dos íons por meio da membrana plasmática, até a imunidade, quando um fagócito se move em direção a um patógeno invasor. Em um nível macro, quando o movimento fica prejudicado após uma lesão, muitos aspectos fundamentais da vida podem ser afetados.

É vital incluir a análise do movimento na reabilitação, visto que a disfunção do movimento costuma ser um fator-chave nas lesões: pode ter contribuído para a lesão original ou pode ter se desenvolvido devido à lesão. Como exemplo, a disfunção do movimento, como valgo dinâmico do joelho, é o principal mecanismo de lesão do LCA (Hewett et al., 2005) – uma lesão esportiva catastrófica que pode arruinar a carreira do atleta. É preciso entender os fatores-chave que alimentam um momento valgo do joelho para que possam ser tratados especificamente.

A análise do movimento pode ser um elo entre as fases iniciais da reabilitação e os estágios finais da preparação em campo para um retorno ao jogo (RAJ) seguro. O objetivo da análise do movimento é identificar e corrigir a disfunção do movimento, restaurar a função neuromuscular (conexão cérebro-músculo) e melhorar a coordenação do movimento. Parece ser parte integrante do desenvolvimento de padrões de movimento seguros antes de direcionar as habilidades específicas do esporte na preparação para o RAJ completo e para reduzir estrategicamente os fatores de risco de novas lesões.

O que é análise de movimento?

O movimento é tanto a meta quanto a conclusão do sistema nervoso, que atua pelos ossos, articulações e músculos, terminando em uma posição predeterminada no espaço. Analisar o movimento, portanto, é o processo de avaliar a qualidade de um movimento no que se refere a uma tarefa, com a intenção de otimizar a facilidade e a eficiência dele. Existem várias maneiras de avaliar o movimento, desde o uso do olho treinado, a um telefone com câmera, a placas de força, até a implementação muito complexa de captura de movimento tridimensional. Todos os métodos têm o mesmo objetivo: identificar a disfunção e, em seguida, resolvê-la por meio de um retreinamento de movimento direcionado.

Termos empregados durante a análise do movimento

Uma análise detalhada do movimento é uma atividade complexa e deve envolver:
1. Descrição dos movimentos que ocorrem nas articulações envolvidas (detalhada e específica).
2. Plano(s) e eixo(s) em que ocorre o movimento.
3. Músculos que produzem o movimento.

Descrição dos movimentos envolvidos

> **Exemplo: análise de um agachamento de perna dupla**
>
> Isso envolve a compreensão de que o agachamento é um exercício composto de múltiplas articulações, projetado para atingir muitos músculos do membro inferior e do complexo lombopélvico-quadril (pelve, região lombar e abdominais). Ocorre nos planos sagital e frontal em cadeia cinética fechada (Figura 38.1).

Parte | 2 | Aplicação Clínica

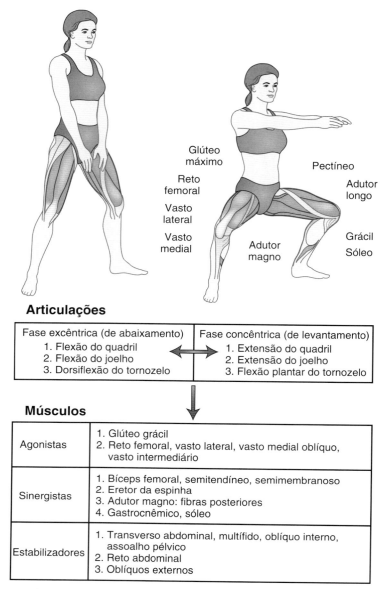

Figura 38.1 Ações articulares e musculares que ocorrem durante o agachamento. (*Esta figura se encontra reproduzida em cores no Encarte.*)

Planos e eixos em que o movimento ocorre

Todos os movimentos corporais ocorrem em planos diferentes e em torno de eixos diferentes (Figura 38.2). Um plano é uma superfície plana bidimensional imaginária que percorre o corpo. Um eixo é uma linha imaginária perpendicular ao plano, em torno da qual o corpo gira (Hamill et al., 2015).

Existem três planos de movimento:
1. *Plano sagital* – um plano vertical que passa pelo centro do corpo e o divide em lados esquerdo e direito. Os tipos de movimento de flexão e extensão ocorrem neste plano (p. ex., chutar uma bola de futebol, passe de peito no basquete, caminhar, pular, agachar).
2. *Plano frontal* – passa de um lado para o outro e divide o corpo na frente e nas costas. Os movimentos de abdução e adução ocorrem neste plano (p. ex., exercícios de salto, levantar e abaixar braços e pernas para os lados, "estrela" na ginástica artística).
3. *Plano horizontal ou transversal* – passa pelo centro do corpo e divide o corpo horizontalmente em uma metade superior e outra inferior. Os tipos de movimento de rotação ocorrem neste plano (p. ex., rotação do quadril em um *swing* de golfe, torção em um lançamento de disco, giro no basquete).

Existem três eixos de movimento em torno dos quais o corpo ou partes do corpo giram:
1. *Eixo transversal ou horizontal sagital* – essa linha corre da esquerda para a direita pelo centro do corpo (p. ex., quando uma pessoa dá uma cambalhota, ela gira em torno deste eixo).
2. *Eixo frontal ou anteroposterior* – essa linha vai da frente para trás por meio do centro do corpo (p. ex., quando uma pessoa dá uma estrela, ela está girando em torno do eixo frontal).
3. *Eixo vertical ou longitudinal* – essa linha vai de cima para baixo pelo centro do corpo (p. ex., quando um patinador dá um giro, eles estão girando em torno do eixo longitudinal).

Músculos que produzem o movimento

Ao analisar o movimento devemos considerar o tipo de contração (concêntrica, excêntrica ou isométrica) e a função dos músculos envolvidos – quais são os agonistas e antagonistas, sinergistas e estabilizadores? O Boxe 38.1 fornece definições dos termos-chave.

Análise de Movimento: a Ciência Encontra a Prática **Capítulo** | 38 |

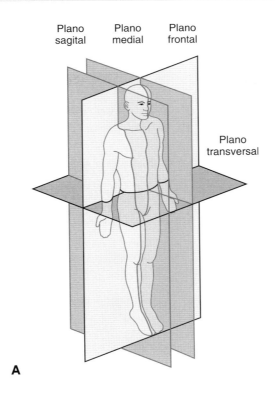

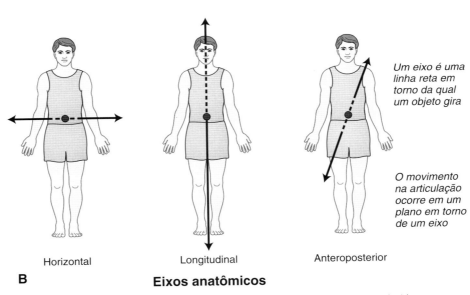

Figura 38.2 A. Planos do movimento. B. Eixos do movimento. (*Esta figura se encontra reproduzida em cores no Encarte.*)

Modelos de análise

Os três principais métodos de análise da biomecânica dos movimentos esportivos são:
- Fases do movimento
- Diagramas de corpo livre
- Modelos determinísticos.

Fases do movimento e diagramas de corpo livre são comumente usados por treinadores e cientistas do esporte, enquanto modelos determinísticos são usados em análises de movimento mais complexas e, portanto, com mais frequência em pesquisas esportivas.

Fases do movimento

Um movimento esportivo, especialmente para ações balísticas, como bater, arremessar e chutar, geralmente contém três fases principais:

1. A *preparação* contém todos os movimentos que preparam um atleta para o desempenho da habilidade, como o *back-swing*

387

Boxe 38.1 Glossário de termos de trabalho muscular

Insuficiência ativa

A incapacidade de um músculo que se estende por duas articulações para se contrair ao máximo em ambas ao mesmo tempo. Por exemplo, um soco poderoso ocorre com o pulso estendido, caso contrário, os flexores dos dedos não podem se contrair em todas as articulações interfalangianas do dedo e na articulação do punho ao mesmo tempo.

Antagonistas

Os músculos antagonistas são os músculos que produzem um torque articular oposto aos músculos agonistas. O antagonismo é apenas o papel que um músculo desempenha, dependendo de qual músculo é o agonista atualmente. Por exemplo, o bíceps às vezes atua como um agonista e outras vezes como um antagonista.

Agonistas

Os músculos agonistas fazem com que um movimento ocorra por meio de sua própria ativação; também referidos como "motores primários", uma vez que são os músculos considerados os principais responsáveis por gerar ou controlar um movimento específico.

Coativação/cocontração

Às vezes, durante uma ação conjunta controlada por um músculo agonista, o antagonista será ativado simultaneamente, naturalmente.

Contração concêntrica

O músculo está encurtando ativamente.

Contração excêntrica

O músculo está se alongando ativamente.

Contração isométrica

O músculo gera tensão, mas não muda em comprimento, por exemplo, segurando um peso com o braço estendido.

Relação comprimento-tensão

A observação de que a força isométrica exercida por um músculo depende de seu comprimento quando testado.

Desequilíbrio muscular

A respectiva igualdade entre o antagonista e o agonista, necessária para o movimento e a função musculares normais.

Insuficiência passiva

A incapacidade de um músculo que se estende por duas articulações para se alongar ao máximo em ambas ao mesmo tempo. Por exemplo, a dorsiflexão máxima não pode ser atingida com um joelho estendido quando o gastrocnêmio é alongado.

Inibição recíproca

O processo dos músculos de um lado de uma articulação relaxando para acomodar a contração do outro lado dessa articulação.

Ação sinérgica

Os sinergistas são às vezes chamados de "neutralizadores" porque ajudam a cancelar ou neutralizar o movimento extra dos agonistas para garantir que a força gerada funcione dentro do plano de movimento desejado. Por exemplo, ao fechar o punho, os extensores do punho se contraem para permitir flexão dos dedos mais forte nas articulações interfalangianas.

Domínio sinérgico

Processo pelo qual o principal músculo agonista de um movimento é inibido ou enfraquecido e o sinergista (um músculo auxiliar) se torna o principal contribuinte para o movimento.

---

durante uma tacada de golfe e a subida em um salto em distância. Deve-se analisar esporte por esporte, posição e função do jogador, além do estilo

2. A *execução* é o desempenho do movimento real que geralmente inclui um ponto de contato com um objeto (p. ex., contato entre o taco de golfe e a bola), a liberação de um objeto (p. ex., disco) ou uma fase de voo (p. ex., salto em distância)

3. O *acompanhamento* refere-se a todos os movimentos que ocorrem após a fase de execução (p. ex., levantamento da perna após chutar uma bola de futebol) que desaceleram o impulso do corpo para evitar lesões, preparar-se para outro movimento ou ambos.

É importante compreender essas três fases distintas do movimento. Se o atleta puder melhorar sua eficiência durante cada uma delas, pode haver uma melhora cumulativa dos gestos como um todo, de modo que ele seja realizado com menor gasto energético e melhor resultado.

Diagramas de corpo livre

Um diagrama de corpo livre é um diagrama visual do padrão de movimento esperado ou previsto. Isso geralmente é desenhado como um boneco simples. Treinadores e pesquisadores costumam usar a técnica para descrever uma subfase ou ponto de interesse em um padrão de movimento. Os treinadores costumam usá-los como auxiliares de dica para seus atletas. A Figura 38.3 é um exemplo simples de um diagrama de corpo livre de agachamento.

Modelos determinísticos

Um modelo determinístico é um paradigma de modelagem que descreve os fatores biomecânicos que determinam um movimento. Este modelo começa com o(s) fator(es) de desempenho primário (p. ex., deslocamento do salto para salto em distância, tempo de corrida em *sprint*), seguido por uma divisão em fatores secundários (elementos que contribuem para o fator de desempenho).

As relações entre uma medida de resultado de movimento e todos esses fatores são consideradas. Isso permite examinar a importância relativa de vários fatores que influenciam o resultado de um movimento (Peh et al., 2011). A Figura 38.4 examina a distância de voo como o fator de desempenho primário, com os fatores secundários sendo altura de decolagem, velocidade horizontal de decolagem e velocidade vertical de decolagem (Bartlett, 2007).

Independentemente da técnica empregada, a análise do movimento requer um planejamento cuidadoso. Essas técnicas também podem se adequar a análises qualitativas ou quantitativas de movimento. A análise qualitativa avalia a qualidade técnica do movimento (p. ex., ritmo, postura), enquanto as técnicas quantitativas avaliam o movimento utilizando números (p. ex., ângulos, distância, velocidade, força) e normalmente demandam maior tecnologia.

Modelos de análise de movimento

Ter um modelo utilizável para avaliar e treinar o movimento é importante para avaliar e melhorar a qualidade do movimento.

Análise de Movimento: a Ciência Encontra a Prática **Capítulo** | 38 |

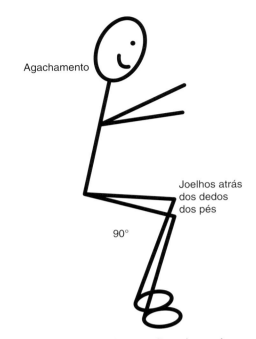

Figura 38.3 Diagrama de corpo livre de agachamento.

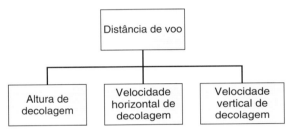

Figura 38.4 Fatores de distância de voo. (Adaptada de Bartlett, R., 2007. Introduction to Sports Biomechanics. Routledge, London.)

Disfunção do movimento

É imperativo identificar padrões de movimento disfuncionais por meio de análise do movimento e, depois, corrigi-los com elementos de treinamento específicos. Isso é importante para a saúde a longo prazo após uma lesão. Um padrão de controle de movimento neuromuscular alterado predispõe a uma segunda lesão do LCA após sua reconstrução; portanto, é vital abordar a disfunção e manter esses princípios (Paterno et al., 2010).

Frequentemente, após uma lesão, o indivíduo aprende uma nova maneira de se mover. O corpo sempre buscará o caminho de menor resistência no que se refere ao movimento, pois ele é metabolicamente o mais eficiente. Um corpo pode se organizar funcionalmente de uma maneira extraordinária, mas o que é metabolicamente mais eficiente pode não ser necessariamente o mais mecanicamente eficiente a longo prazo (Buckthorpe e Roi, 2018).

Compreender essas nuances e como elas podem contribuir para o atraso do "movimento normal" é importante para que possam ser abordadas e corrigidas de forma crítica. A disfunção do movimento pode levar a uma série de problemas. As estratégias de intervenção mais eficazes devem visar a essas deficiências modificáveis para otimizar a competência de controle de movimento.

A Figura 38.5 mostra a técnica ideal para o agachamento unipodal na vista frontal, por exemplo. O alinhamento do joelho não apresenta deslocamento medial (ausência de valgo), não há inclinação pélvica e o tronco permanece vertical. Para que o controle do plano frontal ideal seja exibido, é necessário haver uma base sólida de força (pico de torque) na abdução do quadril, flexão e extensão do joelho, pois isso está correlacionado com menos movimento em valgo (Claiborne et al., 2006).

Aqui estão algumas das disfunções de movimento mais prevalentes para o membro inferior e joelho em particular:

Déficit na estabilidade do membro

A falta de estabilidade do membro refere-se a uma inconsistência da posição do joelho no plano frontal, com deslocamento medial do joelho ou qualquer aparecimento em valgo dinâmico, também conhecido como dominância ligamentar (Di Stasi et al., 2013). Esta cadeia alterada de cinemática da articulação do joelho está geralmente associada a uma queda pélvica contralateral e leve intrarrotação do pé nas manobras de corte (Imwalle et al., 2009). Esse é um fator de risco para uma variedade de patologias de joelho diferentes, como ruptura do LCA, entorse do ligamento colateral medial, carga compartimental medial, rupturas do menisco medial, impacto do coxim adiposo etc.

A Figura 38.6 mostra onde o joelho direito está em posição valgo, com rotação interna do quadril com eversão do pé. O paciente também está adotando uma posição inclinada para frente, sobrecarregando o compartimento anterior da articulação do joelho. Este é um bom exemplo de controle lombopélvico prejudicado.

Como um adendo, a posição do pé é importante na análise do movimento. Embora não seja exibido na Figura 38.6, uma postura de "dedo do pé para dentro" geralmente resulta em aumento da adução do quadril, aumento da abdução do joelho e aumento da rotação interna do joelho (ângulo e momento), todos fatores de risco significativos para uma lesão importante no joelho, como uma ruptura do LCA (Tran et al., 2016).

Déficit na estabilidade pélvica

Isso se refere ao desalinhamento no plano frontal da região pélvica, geralmente visto como uma caminhada pélvica ou queda do quadril (Jamison et al., 2012). Isso é frequentemente observado em combinação com um joelho valgo associado (Sigward e Powers, 2007).

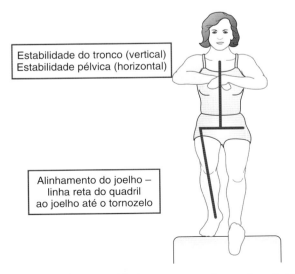

Figura 38.5 Alinhamento ideal para um agachamento unipodal, vista frontal.

389

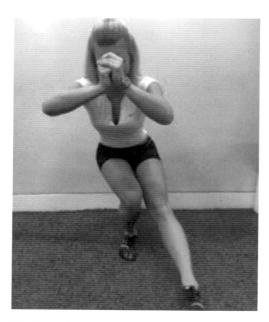

Figura 38.6 Exemplo de valgo dinâmico do joelho do lado direito.

A Figura 38.7 mostra uma perspectiva anterior e posterior, revelando o quadril subindo no lado direito. Há também um pequeno deslocamento medial do joelho. A fraqueza do glúteo médio direito fará com que o quadril esquerdo caia ao se posicionar sobre o membro direito. A Figura 38.8 mostra o sinal de Trendelenburg, que revela fraqueza dos abdutores do quadril esquerdo com queda subsequente na pelve direita.

Déficit na estabilidade do tronco

Isso se refere ao desvio excessivo do tronco em relação à linha mediana com desestabilização proximal (Zazullak et al., 2007). A inclinação ipsilateral do tronco no corte é comumente observada na análise. A inclinação do tronco para o lado direito com um joelho valgo presente na articulação do joelho durante um agachamento unipodal é mostrada na Figura 38.9. A técnica ideal para um agachamento com uma única perna na vista lateral é apresentada na Figura 38.10. O alinhamento do joelho não apresenta deslocamento medial (ausência de valgo), não há inclinação pélvica e o tronco permanece vertical.

Déficit na absorção de choque

Isso se refere à incapacidade do atleta de dissipar cargas, como altas forças de reação do solo, geralmente observadas com alto ângulo do joelho em um *drop jump* e manobras de salto (Leppänen et al., 2017). Isso pode ser medido utilizando uma plataforma de força, que é um auxiliar útil. Posturas eretas tendem a ser comumente vistas aqui e isso pode ser conhecido como a adoção de uma "estratégia de joelho" em que uma aterrissagem mais rígida envolve aumento da extensão do joelho, diminuição da extensão do quadril e, portanto, menos glúteo máximo, como visto na Figura 38.11 (Pollard et al., 2010).

Déficit na estratégia de movimento

O déficit na estratégia de movimento ocorre com relação à cinemática global alterada no plano sagital. A distribuição e a dissipação desiguais de carga costumam ser vistas com esses déficits. Carregar incorretamente para a frente sobre os joelhos é uma falha comum, sendo normal a fraqueza dos grupos musculares posteriores.

A Figura 38.12 revela uma carga excessiva por meio das articulações do joelho, com má posição dele com relação aos dedos dos pés. Isso ocorre apesar de uma postura central e ereta relativamente bem-controladas.

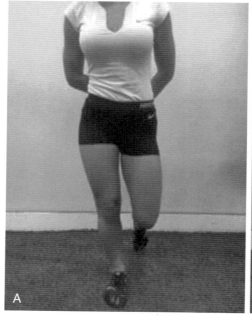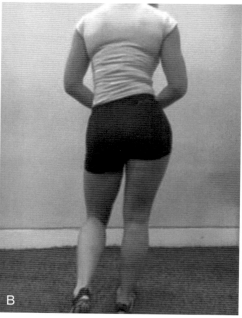

Figura 38.7 Imagens anterior (A) e posterior (B) do quadril subindo no lado direito (observe as ondulações na camiseta).

Análise de Movimento: a Ciência Encontra a Prática | Capítulo | 38 |

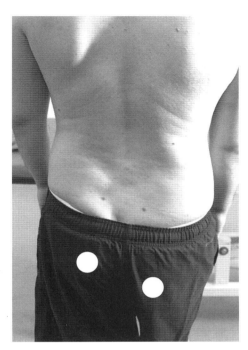

Figura 38.8 Sinal de Trendelenburg. Os círculos brancos destacam os marcos anatômicos das espinhas ilíacas superiores posteriores, que são os principais locais ósseos a serem observados para este sinal.

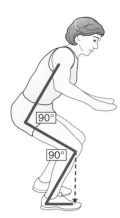

Posição do tronco e joelho – flexão igual do joelho e dobra do quadril é favorável para a abordagem de "estratégia do quadril", conhecida como "dupla flexão"

A posição do joelho em relação aos dedos dos pés é importante

Figura 38.10 Alinhamento ideal para agachamento unipodal, vista lateral.

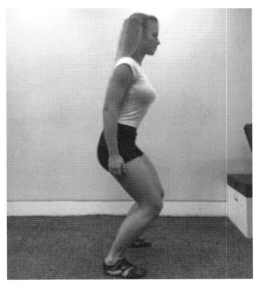

Figura 38.11 Exemplo de padrão de carregamento quádruplo dominante no joelho, em vez de carregar por meio da articulação do quadril e recrutar melhor os glúteos.

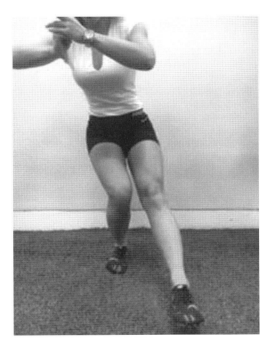

Figura 38.9 Exemplo de tronco inclinado para o mesmo lado da postura valgo do joelho.

Desequilíbrios musculares

A disfunção do movimento pode ser causada por desequilíbrios musculares devido à inibição muscular ou dominância sinérgica resultante (explicada adiante) de um grupo de músculos ou devido a déficits relativos de força (fraqueza, mas função normal).

Um exemplo poderia ser um glúteo máximo fraco e inibido sendo "assistido" pelo músculo bíceps femoral, que pode se tornar hiperativo e dominante, durante a extensão do quadril. Isso pode ser identificado por meio de técnicas de palpação muscular com uma avaliação em decúbito ventral dos músculos isquiotibiais e glúteos. A distinção entre os dois é importante e contribuirá diretamente para o sucesso de um programa de treinamento de movimento.

Se houver inibição, ela precisa ser tratada para treinar um movimento com eficácia. Se um músculo não pode ser ativado devido à inibição, ele não pode ser treinado em sua função e a compensação resultante ocorrerá em movimento. Se o treinamento corretivo não ocorrer, essas compensações serão reforçadas e os padrões de movimento defeituosos permanecerão (Buckthorpe e Roi, 2018).

É essencial garantir que o treinamento de movimento harmonizado seja construído sobre uma base sólida e que o padrão de movimento correto seja utilizado, treinado e desenvolvido em padrões de movimento inconscientes específicos do esporte.

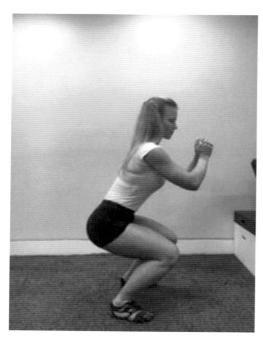

Figura 38.12 Fatores variáveis que podem surgir de padrões de movimento disfuncionais, como carga excessiva e cisalhamento por meio dos joelhos, além dos dedos dos pés.

Um conceito importante aqui é treinar padrões eficazes de movimento seguros e conscientes. Isso pode exigir alguma forma de retreinamento corretivo, se ainda não tiver sido realizado com sucesso no estágio inicial do processo de reabilitação. Portanto, é essencial identificar inicialmente qualquer disfunção subjacente por meio da análise do movimento. Um programa de reeducação do movimento individual precisará ser desenvolvido para considerar os desequilíbrios e um programa corretivo eficaz deverá ser implementado para lidar com isso, como o descrito no exemplo a seguir.

A inibição recíproca descreve o processo dos músculos de um lado de uma articulação relaxando para acomodar a contração do outro lado dessa articulação, como o agonista produz uma ação enquanto o músculo antagonista relaxa (Hamill et al., 2015).

Como exemplo, a rigidez do músculo psoas pode inibir a ativação do glúteo máximo; a inibição recíproca alterada pode contribuir para desequilíbrios musculares e disfunção do movimento, como valgo dinâmico do joelho durante o agachamento unipodal (ver o programa corretivo adiante para mais detalhes). Isso precisa ser abordado para permitir a complexidade do movimento para o fortalecimento funcional e movimentos esportivos.

Aqui está um exemplo de um programa corretivo para lidar com a instabilidade do joelho referida como valgo dinâmico do joelho (um fator de risco significativo para lesão do LCA) (Hewett et al., 2005) durante um padrão de agachamento, que visa o movimento máximo por meio do quadril e articulações do joelho.

Lembre-se de que a estabilidade da articulação do joelho é atribuída a restrições passivas e ativas. As restrições passivas são os ligamentos e a cápsula articular. As restrições ativas são os músculos, que fornecem estabilidade à articulação em movimento. Músculos saudáveis e bem-recrutados são muito importantes para ajudar a reduzir o risco de lesão das restrições passivas de uma articulação, como a do joelho.

Um programa corretivo abordará a vulnerabilidade em um movimento mais lento e controlado inicialmente, antes de introduzir a prática dinâmica. O processo é descrito a seguir:

Identifique os músculos contraídos. Psoas, tensor da fáscia lata (TFL), bíceps femoral, vasto lateral.

Relaxe os músculos contraídos. Liberação de tecido mole, rolo de espuma, alongamento estático ou dinâmico.

Identifique, reative e fortaleça os músculos inibidos ou fracos. Glúteo médio, transverso, multífido, glúteo máximo, vasto medial oblíquo (VMO).

Trate a dominância sinérgica e a inibição recíproca. O músculo dominante sinérgico pode ser o bíceps femoral, que é hiperativo porque o glúteo máximo é inibido pelo músculo psoas, que pode ser curto e tenso. Portanto, precisamos incorporar o amolecimento e o alongamento (flexibilidade) do psoas, liberar o bíceps femoral e isolar o fortalecimento dos músculos glúteos.

Implemente um programa de estabilidade central e lombopélvica. Ativação transversal como exercício *dead bug*, cão-pássaro, ponte, *bear crawl*, *clam* em pé com faixa e outros exercícios fundamentais para direcionar o controle lombopélvico.

Trate o padrão de movimento com exercícios funcionais (localmente e depois globalmente). No caso de joelho valgo dinâmico, o foco será no transverso, multífido, oblíquo interno, glúteo máximo, glúteo médio em termos de fortalecimento, para então progredir para o agachamento com perna dupla, agachamento dividido, *lunges* e agachamentos simples etc.

Vejamos outro exemplo:

Um TFL hiperativo (um flexor do quadril, um rotador interno do fêmur e um abdutor) pode resultar na inibição recíproca do glúteo máximo ou isquiotibiais laterais. Nesses casos, a prática do movimento inconsciente apenas reforçará um padrão de dominância do TFL. O retreinamento deverá incluir a redução da ativação do TFL e/ou aumento da ativação do glúteo máximo e do glúteo médio em movimento.

- Utilize exercícios com uma ativação maior do glúteo médio do que do TFL, como extensão do quadril em pronação ou pontes com uma faixa ao redor dos joelhos para aumentar as forças de abdução
- Uma dica extra é aproveitar as vantagens do potencial do glúteo máximo para inibir reciprocamente o TFL, combinando a abdução do quadril com a extensão do quadril
- Reduzir os graus de liberdade de movimento (p. ex., reduzindo a amplitude de movimento dos exercícios) também pode ajudar. Por exemplo, se a amplitude de abdução do quadril for de 0 a 90°, deitando-se de lado e com a perna esticada, pode-se trabalhar em uma amplitude entre 20 e 60°. Nessa faixa, as fibras do glúteo médio se tornam cada vez mais ativas.

A dominância sinérgica é o processo pelo qual o músculo agonista principal de um movimento é inibido ou fraco e o sinérgico (um músculo auxiliar) se torna o principal contribuinte para o movimento.

Um exemplo de dominância sinérgica é quando a inibição do músculo glúteo máximo precipita a dominância sobrejacente dos isquiotibiais laterais (bíceps femoral em particular) para rotação externa do fêmur e extensão do quadril (Billiet et al., 2018). Isso pode ser identificado por eletromiografia, se disponível, ou por meio de técnicas de palpação muscular. Obviamente, é sempre importante observar que os músculos não são mutuamente exclusivos em relação à contração. Frequentemente, há contração parcial ou cocontração de antagonistas, tensão ou fraqueza do músculo psoas e/ou do reto femoral. Todos eles desempenham um papel no recrutamento, ou inibição, do glúteo máximo.

A dominância sinérgica pode ser um fator contribuinte para uma lesão do LCA (Boxe 38.2). Os isquiotibiais podem ficar sobrecarregados como um rotador externo do quadril, em vez de um extensor do quadril, que é seu movimento principal. Isso pode ser

Análise de Movimento: a Ciência Encontra a Prática — Capítulo 38

avaliado por meio de teste muscular manual padrão. Quando eles trabalham dessa maneira, não agem mais com eficiência como flexores de joelho e, mais importante, como estabilizadores. Essa dominância precisa ser tratada, se presente, antes que o controle do movimento inconsciente seja realizado, caso contrário, a fadiga do tecido e um ciclo de lesão cumulativa podem ocorrer.

Como fazer análise do movimento?

A análise do movimento é uma avaliação do movimento de um indivíduo. Pode combinar a avaliação da biomecânica por um indivíduo treinado ou o uso de tecnologia, como análise de vídeo.

A neurofisiologia também deve ser considerada na análise do movimento. Sua contribuição é difícil de medir, mas as teorias do Isokinetic Medical Group sugerem que, para compreender e eliminar um déficit, é importante estimular o processo de aprendizagem consciente por meio da educação e da revisão da análise de vídeo.

A partir de critérios definidos, uma análise dos movimentos específicos para o esporte é feita, realizando uma avaliação qualitativa (déficit prevalecente) e uma quantitativa baseada em um sistema de pontuação.

Aqui está um exemplo dos movimentos e critérios focados no teste de análise de movimento (TAM) usado pelo Isokinetic Medical Group. É importante ter em mente que essa é uma estratégia para testar o movimento.

Medidas biomecânicas durante a aterrissagem e estabilidade postural predizem a segunda lesão do LCA após a reconstrução do LCA e o RAJ (Paterno et al., 2010). O TAM envolve a avaliação de seis movimentos específicos: agachamento unipodal, desaceleração, *drop jump*, salto frontal, salto lateral e mudança de direção. Cinco critérios são usados para quantificar déficits, incluindo:

- Estabilidade do membro
- Estabilidade da pelve
- Estabilidade do tronco
- Absorção de impacto
- Estratégia de movimento.

Estabilidade do membro

Isso se concentra na capacidade de estabilizar a perna e evitar movimentos que podem causar danos às articulações. Questões biomecânicas como joelho valgo, joelho varo, rotação tibial, pronação e supinação do pé são características de movimento importantes que precisam ser captadas para entender completamente onde a carga excessiva ou insuficiente pode estar ocorrendo para um indivíduo (Khayambashi et al., 2016).

Boxe 38.2 Biomecânica da marcha pós-reconstrução do ligamento cruzado anterior e suas implicações

O que dizem os especialistas sobre as consequências do movimento anormal?

O risco estimado ao longo da vida de osteoartrite (OA) sintomática do joelho após lesão do ligamento cruzado anterior (LCA) (independentemente do tratamento) é de 34% em comparação com 14% em indivíduos não lesionados e o risco de ter uma artroplastia total do joelho é de 22% *versus* 6% (Suter et al., 2017). A prevalência de OA tibiofemoral e patelofemoral em pacientes após lesão do LCA e subsequente reconstrução tem sido relacionada a mudanças específicas na mecânica de aterrissagem, caminhada e marcha em corrida (Culvenor e Crossley, 2016).

Pacientes que sofreram reconstrução do LCA (RLCA) pousam, correm e caminham com ângulos de flexão do joelho e momentos extensores internos do joelho diminuídos (Kline et al., 2016; Roewer et al., 2011). Essa mudança no movimento pode ter implicações para a função a longo prazo e tensões de carregamento da articulação. Erhart-Hledik et al. (2017) encontraram a presença dessas mudanças na marcha (diminuição do ângulo de flexão do joelho e dos movimentos extensores internos) em 2 anos de pós-operatório e predisseram a pontuação do questionário KOOS (resultado funcional) em 8 anos. As mudanças na marcha durante a caminhada parecem ter ocorrido cerca de 4 semanas após a operação (Hadizadeh et al., 2016).

Essas mudanças distintas nos parâmetros cinemáticos e cinéticos (diminuição da flexão do joelho, momento de extensão interna do joelho) também ocorreram durante tarefas de aterrissagem de carga mais elevada (salto para a frente) em pacientes de RLCA que apresentavam sinais radiológicos de OA da articulação patelofemoral nos primeiros 2 anos após a operação (Culvenor et al., 2016). Essas alterações quando vistas na corrida parecem estar associadas a cargas e estresse da articulação patelofemoral aumentados (Herrington et al., 2017), que pode ser o precursor para o desenvolvimento de dor na articulação patelofemoral e OA (Culvenor e Crossley, 2016). Essas mudanças, quando vistas na marcha em corrida após 6 meses, parecem estar relacionadas à força do quadríceps aos 3 meses após a operação (Kline et al., 2016).

A pesquisa atual parece mostrar que os pacientes com RLCA no pós-operatório não conseguem flexionar os joelhos adequadamente e gerar momentos articulares internos apropriados durante a aterrissagem, caminhada e corrida; isso pode estar relacionado à baixa força do quadríceps. A presença desse padrão de movimento parece aumentar as cargas na articulação patelofemoral, o que a pode predispor à degeneração. A presença desse padrão de movimento parece ter implicações significativas para os resultados funcionais a longo prazo.

Com agradecimentos ao Dr. Lee Herrington por esta seção.

Fontes: Culvenor, A., Crossley, K., 2016. Patellofemoral osteoarthritis: are we missing an important source of symptoms after anterior cruciate ligament reconstruction? Journal of Orthopaedic and Sports Physical Therapy 46 (4), 232-234.

Culvenor, A., Perration, L., Guermazi, A., Bryant, A., Whitehead, T., Morris, H., et al., 2016. Knee kinematics and kinetics are associated with early patellofemoral osteoarthritis following anterior cruciate ligament reconstruction. Osteoarthritis & Cartilage 24, 1548-1553.

Erhart-Hledik, J., Chu, C., Asay, J., Andriacchi, T., 2017. Gait mechanics 2 years after anterior cruciate ligament reconstruction are associated with longer-term changes in patient-reported outcomes. Journal of Orthopaedic Research 5 (3), 634-640.

Hadizadeh, M., Amri, S., Mohafez, H., Roohi, S., Mokhtar, A., 2016. Gait analysis of national athletes after anterior cruciate ligament reconstruction following three stages of rehabilitation program: symmetrical perspective. Gait & Posture 48, pp. 152-158.

Herrington, L., Alarifi, S., Jones, R., 2017. Patellofemoral joint loads during running at the time of return to sport in elite athletes with ACL reconstruction. American Journal of Sports Medicine 45, 2812-2816.

Kline, P., Johnson, D., Ireland, M., Noehren, B., 2016. Clinical predictors of knee mechanics at return to sport after ACL reconstruction. Medicine and Science in Sports and Exercise 48 (5), 790-795.

Roewer, B., Di Stasi, S., Synder-Mackler, L., 2011. Quadriceps strength and weight acceptance strategies continue to improve two years after ACL reconstruction. Journal of Biomechanics 44 (10), 1948-1953.

Suter, L., Smith, S., Katz, Englund M., Hunter, D., Frobell, R., et al., 2017. Projecting lifetime risk of symptomatic knee osteoarthritis and total knee replacement in individuals sustaining a complete ACL tear in early adulthood. Arthritis Care & Research 69 (2), 201-208.

Parte | 2 | Aplicação Clínica

Por exemplo, se um joelho está em posição valgo, isso pode levar a forças de compressão excessivas em todo o compartimento lateral do joelho, contrastando com as forças de cisalhamento ou alongamento medialmente; isso pode precipitar uma lesão no ligamento colateral medial do joelho, entre outros problemas.

Estabilidade da pelve

Isso se refere amplamente à capacidade de estabilizar a pelve no plano frontal. Uma função do glúteo médio é estabilizar a pelve e evitar que um lado caia mais que o outro ao caminhar, conhecido como "marcha de Trendelenburg". O glúteo médio funciona como os músculos do manguito rotador externo da articulação do ombro. Quando isso acontece, pode influenciar o movimento pelo resto do corpo e influenciar a dissipação de força pelo quadril, sobrecarregando um lado mais do que o outro.

Estabilidade do tronco

Isso se refere à capacidade de manter o controle do torso em movimento. Lesões do LCA geralmente envolvem uma queda lateral do tronco, que muda o centro de massa.

Absorção de impacto

A absorção de impacto é estimada visualmente por meio do exame da mecânica de pouso e, em particular, verificando até que ponto o atleta pode efetivamente pousar suavemente, dissipando a força pelos músculos. Um fator de risco destacado para lesões do LCA é conhecido como dominância ligamentar (Myer et al., 2004; 2011). É quando a força é absorvida pelo ligamento e/ou articulação em oposição a ser absorvida excentricamente pela unidade do tendão do músculo. "Amolecer" as articulações por flexão nas do quadril e joelho ajudará a dissipar significativamente as cargas no joelho.

Estratégia de movimento

A estratégia de movimento detalha a adoção de padrões de movimento pelo paciente em que favorecem determinados grupos musculares no plano sagital em relação a outros. Por exemplo, a fraqueza do glúteo máximo pode resultar no paciente inclinado para frente, com maior carga sobre os joelhos, adotando assim uma "estratégia do joelho" no lugar de uma "estratégia do quadril" mais correta, em que a carga é feita inicialmente por meio dos músculos posteriores do quadril. Isso está relacionado ao centro de massa, força muscular e produção de torque. Para diminuir a produção da força muscular necessária ou para evitar a dor, pode-se adotar certas posições nos movimentos para utilizar ou evitar preferencialmente determinados grupos musculares. Isso pode ser denominado dominância quádrupla ou evitação do joelho.

Força muscular do quadril

Isso é fundamental para reduzir potenciais lesões no joelho, como mostra o trabalho de Khayambashi et al. (2014). A redução da força do rotador externo do quadril (< 20% do peso corporal) e a redução da força de abdução do quadril (< 35% do peso corporal) estão associadas à predição de lesões do LCA sem contato.

A inclinação anterior ou posterior da pelve também influencia a estabilidade pélvica no plano sagital de movimento. Um fator-chave no treinamento central deve ser treinar a capacidade de resistir a movimentos indesejados (p. ex., melhorar a ativação e o tempo do glúteo médio na aterrissagem com uma perna para ter a força para estabilizar e evitar que a pelve caia para um lado).

A capacidade de resistir ao torque de adução do quadril pela gravidade é crucial.

Isso pode ser direcionado de várias maneiras:

Em *lunge* para trás com placa deslizante resistida, a tração do cabo cria uma força de flexão do quadril contra a qual o glúteo máximo deve se estabilizar. O movimento também imita a ação do quadril de correr e subir escadas. Semelhante à corrida, o corpo deve ser puxado sobre o pé por uma poderosa extensão de quadril. A postura unipodal enfatiza o glúteo médio e as fibras superiores do glúteo máximo (Billiet et al., 2018).

Outros exercícios que induzem uma alta atividade dos glúteos máximo e médio que podem ajudar a traduzir para uma melhor aterrissagem com uma perna são o agachamento com uma perna e o levantamento terra romeno com uma perna (Stastny et al., 2016).

Esses exercícios unipodais requerem extensão concêntrica ou excêntrica do quadril ao longo de uma grande amplitude de movimento e estabilidade pélvica no plano frontal em conjunto com um controle da perna de apoio nos planos frontal e transverso. Isso leva a um alto impulso neural para o glúteo máximo, o glúteo médio e a cadeia posterior em sua totalidade. Praticar a aterrissagem com uma perna enquanto segura um halter leve no lado contralateral provavelmente ajudará no disparo do glúteo médio e na estabilização pélvica, pois essa é uma ótima maneira de contrariar as forças rotacionais e criar fortalecimento do pilar lombopélvico.

Função muscular

A função muscular é amplamente determinada pela arquitetura muscular; compreender essa anatomia é importante para treinar bem o controle do movimento. Por exemplo, o glúteo médio é um músculo muito forte devido a sua área de seção transversal relativamente pequena, devido ao empacotamento de muitas fibras musculares curtas em paralelo. Devido a essa composição, ele não pode produzir forças muito grandes em grandes amplitudes de movimento; essencialmente, estabiliza a pelve e o fêmur, e deve ser treinado e avaliado dessa maneira.

Um exemplo de exercício para isso poderia ser o exercício de *clam* isolado: deite-se de lado, quadris e joelhos dobrados em um ângulo de 45°, calcanhares próximos um do outro; em seguida, execute a abdução do quadril sem rolar a pelve, permanecendo imóvel com os calcanhares juntos. Esse exercício isola o glúteo médio. Pode-se então passar para o *clam* em pé ou em degrau para treiná-lo globalmente.

Análise pós-movimento: treinamento neuromotor direcionado

O movimento é produzido por meio do sistema neuromuscular, que envolve a contração dos músculos por meio de sinais neurais do sistema nervoso central e a produção de força por meio de conexões de tendão ao osso (Hamill et al., 2015). O desenvolvimento da coordenação do movimento não é tão simples quanto fazer os pacientes se movimentarem. Os padrões de movimento antálgico (p. ex., aqueles que se desenvolvem para evitar a dor) podem ser difíceis de corrigir. Além disso, os desequilíbrios musculares subjacentes, antes da lesão ou por causa da lesão, podem alterar a maneira como o corpo se move para "compensar" a fraqueza.

394

Portanto, quando há disfunção do movimento, os padrões corretos de movimento precisam ser redesenvolvidos pelo paciente por meio de um programa corretivo individualizado de *treinamento neuromotor* (TNM) que visa o sistema neuromuscular em sua totalidade. Tendo verificado a disfunção do movimento, o TNM específico deve ser realizado para resolver os problemas identificados no teste de análise do movimento.

O TNM envolve o direcionamento de habilidades motoras, como coordenação, agilidade e propriocepção. O TNM específico, eficaz e sensível pode ajudar a restaurar a função completa e a acelerar um RAJ. Um atleta pode se mover com eficiência após uma lesão, mas também deve aprender a se mover corretamente utilizando o TNM.

A padronização motora ideal é imprescindível após uma lesão no LCA. Uma vez que o LCA foi rompido, há diminuição da entrada somatossensorial (Grooms et al., 2015) e qualidade do movimento alterada bilateralmente (Goerger et al., 2014). A conexão entre o cérebro e os músculos precisa ser retreinada.

O TNM enfatizando a qualidade do controle de movimento deve ajudar a reduzir o potencial de novas lesões ou lesões secundárias no RAJ. Além de ajudar a prevenir novas lesões, o aprimoramento do desempenho pode ocorrer, pois o TNM ajuda a aguçar o mecanismo de *feedfoward*, um componente-chave para manter os atletas em forma e jogando.

Teoria da neuroplasticidade e aplicação prática

Após considerar todos os fatores que podem influenciar a qualidade do padrão motor (Figura 38.13), é importante entender que a neuroplasticidade desempenha um papel importante ao abordar questões de forma prática após a análise do movimento. A neuroplasticidade pode ser definida como a capacidade do cérebro de mudar, remodelar e reorganizar com o objetivo de melhorar a habilidade de se adaptar a novas situações (Demarin et al., 2014).

Doyon e Benali (2005) descreveram um modelo de aprendizagem de uma nova sequência e adaptação motoras em resposta a uma mudança. Ao ser inicialmente ensinado um novo exercício, os processos cognitivos governam a fase chamada de "aprendizado rápido". Outras vias neurais estão envolvidas na segunda etapa, que é conhecida como fase de "aprendizado lento". As fases finais de aprendizagem de uma nova sequência motora são chamadas de "consolidação", "automação" e "retenção", quando o padrão de movimento se torna enraizado no cérebro. Uma vez que cada nova adaptação ocorre, uma nova sequência motora "correta" é criada.

> **Mecanismo de motor *feedforward***
> O papel do mecanismo motor *feedforward* é pré-ativar certos músculos e tendões necessários para tarefas motoras para fornecer o controle de movimento ideal. Isso inclui a ativação dos músculos corretos antes da aterrissagem, mudança de direção ou desaceleração.

Esse modelo teórico foi traduzido na prática clínica para uma aplicação mais prática. Para aprender um novo movimento básico identificado a partir da análise do movimento, é imperativo seguir uma abordagem em fases para aprender um

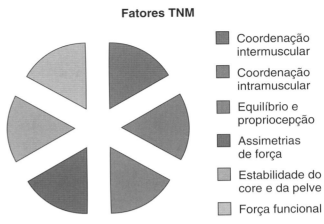

Figura 38.13 Fatores de padrão de movimento que podem contribuir para um padrão motor incorreto. Deve-se desenvolver um programa amplamente individualizado que aborde todos ou alguns desses aspectos. Um foco na taxa de desenvolvimento de força (a rapidez com que a força pode ser produzida), rápida ativação neural e coordenação muscular geral são imperativos. (*Esta figura se encontra reproduzida em cores no Encarte.*)

novo hábito. Isso pode levar de 18 a 254 dias (Lally et al., 2010). A Tabela 38.1 descreve um modelo para ensinar o *drop jump*, como exemplo.

O objetivo desse treinamento é alcançar a retenção a longo prazo de novos padrões motores, os quais devem estar associados a melhores resultados clínicos e funcionais, principalmente com reteste da análise do movimento para todas as lesões.

Conclusão

A vida requer movimento.

Aristóteles (384-322 a.C.), filósofo e cientista grego

Uma abordagem ampla, que analisa o ser em sua totalidade, é necessária para retreinar o movimento antes do RAJ e vários fatores influenciam a competência dele. A disfunção do movimento é um fator significativo nas lesões do LCA, bem como em muitas outras entidades que vemos todos os dias.

A incompetência de movimento pode ter contribuído para a lesão original ou pode ter se desenvolvido por causa dela; portanto, a reeducação do movimento deve ser um aspecto de todos os programas de reabilitação sob medida. O objetivo aqui é treinar os pacientes para serem capazes de se mover com eficiência e segurança antes de retornarem aos movimentos específicos do esporte.

A análise e a correção de um perfil de movimento utilizando TNM seletivamente elaborado, visando a retenção de movimento a longo prazo, é a base para entender como analisar e treinar melhor o movimento. Isso pode ajudar significativamente a melhorar os resultados da reabilitação e a reduzir as taxas de novas lesões.

Agradecimento

Agradecimento especial ao Dr. Matthew Buckthorpe, do Isokinetic Medical Group, que realmente ajudou no desenvolvimento de minha educação nesse campo e neste capítulo.

Parte |2| Aplicação Clínica

Tabela 38.1 **Processo de aprendizagem motora para aplicação prática.**

Racional da fase	Processo
Fase cognitiva	
Desconstruir o movimento disfuncional	Sugestão verbal do que o paciente está fazendo de errado (pode incluir "absorva a carga suavemente, dobre seus quadris e depois os joelhos, não se incline para frente") Vídeo revelando o movimento correto de como executar o *drop jump* corretamente Poucas repetições de alta qualidade *Feedforward* (p. ex., vídeo e dicas durante a execução ajudam a compreender o movimento incorreto do *drop jump* para a educação do paciente)
Fase associativa	
Reconstruir nova tarefa de movimento	Menos instruções (apenas uma ou duas agora, como "manter o peito para cima") Mais repetição, mais prática O *biofeedback* imediato em tempo real continua (vendo cada salto antes do próximo) Estratégias de autocorreção iniciadas (o paciente começa a reconhecer hábitos e abordagens defeituosas por conta própria)
Fase automática	
Automatizar progressivamente o movimento	Sem sugestão Pontos de foco externos (como "empurrar o chão para longe de você") *Biofeedback* atrasado (gravar em vídeo e mostrar depois) Autocorreção mais regular e rigorosa por paciente

Referências bibliográficas

Ardern, C., Taylor, N., Feller, J., Webster, K., 2014. Fifty-five percent to competitive sport following anterior cruciate ligament reconstruction surgery: an updated systematic review and meta-analysis including aspects of physical functioning and contextual factors. British Journal of Sports Medicine 48 (21), 1543-1552.

Bartlett, R., 2007. Introduction to Sports Biomechanics. Routledge, London.

Billiet, L., Swinnen, T., De Vlam, K., Westhovens, R., Van Huffel, S., 2018. Recognition of physical activities from a single arm-worn accelerometer: a multiway approach. Informatics 5, 20.

Buckthorpe, M., Roi, G.S., 2018. The time has come to incorporate a greater focus on rate of force development training in the sports injury rehabilitation process. Muscles, Ligaments and Tendons Journal 7 (3), 435-441.

Claiborne, T.L., Armstrong, C.W., Gandhi, V., Pincivero, D.M., 2006. Relationship between hip and knee strength and knee valgus during a single leg squat. Journal of Applied Biomechanics 22 (1), 41-50.

Clark, M., Lucett, S., Sutton, B., 2013. NASM Essentials Of Corrective Exercise Training. Jones & Bartlett Learning/National Academy of Sports Medicine, Burlington, MA.

Demarin, V., Morovic, S., Bene, R., 2014. Neuroplasticity. Periodicum Biologorum 116 (2), 209-211.

Di Stasi, S., Myer, G.D., Hewett, T.E., 2013. Neuromuscular training to target deficits associated with second anterior cruciate ligament injury. The Journal of Orthopaedic & Sports Physical Therapy 43 (11), 777-A11.

Doyon, J., Benali, H., 2005. Reorganization and plasticity in the adult brain during learning of motor skills. Current Opinions in Neurobiology 15 (2), 161-167.

Goerger, B., Marshall, S., Beutler, A., Blackburn, J., Wilckens, J., Padua, D., 2014. Anterior cruciate ligament injury alters pre-injury lower extremity biomechanics in the injured and uninjured leg: the JUMP-ACL study. British Journal of Sports Medicine 49 (3), 188-195.

Grooms, D., Appelbaum, G., Onate, J., 2015. Neuroplasticity following anterior cruciate ligament injury: a framework for visual–motor training approaches in rehabilitation. Journal of Orthopaedic Sports Physical Therapy 45 (5), 381-393.

Hamill, J., Knutzen, K., Derrick, T.R., 2015. Biomechanical Basis of Human Movement, fourth ed. Lippincott Williams & Wilkins, Philadelphia, PA.

Hewett, T.E., Myer, G.D., Ford, K.R., Heidt Jr., R.S., Colosimo, A.J., McLean, S.G., et al., 2005. Biomechanical measures of neuromuscular control and valgus loading of the knee predict anterior cruciate ligament injury risk in female athletes: a prospective study. American Journal of Sports Medicine 233 (4), 492-501.

Imwalle, L.E., Myer, G.D., Ford, K.R., Hewett, T.E., 2009. Relationship between hip and knee kinematics in athletic women during cutting manoeuvres: a possible link to noncontact anterior cruciate ligament injury and prevention. Journal of Strength Conditioning Research 23 (8), 2223-2230.

Jamison, S.T., Pan, X., Chaudhari, A.M., 2012. Knee moments during run-to-cut maneuvers are associated with lateral trunk positioning. The Journal of Biomechanics 45 (11), 1881-1885.

Khayambashi, K., Fallah, A., Movahedi, A., Bagwell, J., Powers, C., 2014. Posterolateral hip muscle strengthening versus quadriceps strengthening for patellofemoral pain: a comparative control trial. Archives of Physical Medicine and Rehabilitation 95 (5), 900-907.

Khayambashi, K., Ghoddosi, N., Straub, R.K., Powers, C.M., 2016. Hip muscle strength predicts noncontact anterior cruciate ligament injury in male and female athletes: a prospective study. American Journal of Sports Medicine 44 (2), 355-361.

Lally, P., van Jaarsveld, C.H.M., Potts, H.W.W., Wardle, J., 2010. How are habits formed: modelling habit formation in the real world. European Journal of Social Psychology 40, 998-1009.

Leppänen, M., Pasanen, K., Kujala, U.M., 2017. Stiff landings are associated with increased ACL injury risk in young female basketball and floorball players. The American Journal of Sports Medicine 45 (2), 386-393.

Myer, G.D., Ford, K.R., Hewett, T.E., 2011. New method to identify athletes at high risk of ACL injury using clinic-based measurements and freeware computer analysis. The British Journal of Sports Medicine 45 (4), 238-244.

Myer, G.D., Ford, K.R., Hewett, T.E., 2004. Rationale and clinical techniques for anterior cruciate ligament injury prevention among female athletes. Journal of Athletic Training 39 (4), 352-364.

Paterno, M., Schmitt, L., Ford, K., Rauh, M., Myer, G., Huang, B., et al., 2010. Biomechanical measures during landing and postural stability predict second anterior cruciate ligament injury after anterior cruciate ligament reconstruction and return to sport. American Journal of Sports Medicine 38 (10), 1968-1978.

Peh, S.Y., Chow, J.Y., Davids, K., 2011. Focus of attention and its impact on movement behaviour. The Journal of Science and Medicine in Sport 14 (1), 70-78.

Pollard, C.D., Sigward, S.M., Powers, C.M., 2010. Limited hip and knee flexion during landing is associated with increased frontal plane knee motion and moments. Clinical Biomechanics 25 (2), 142-146.

Sigward, S.M., Powers, C.M., 2007. Loading characteristics of females exhibiting excessive valgus moments during cutting. Clinical Biomechanics 22 (7), 827-833.

Stastny, P., Tufano, J.J., Golas, A., Petr, M., 2016. Strengthening the gluteus medius using various bodyweight and resistance exercises. Journal of Strength and Conditioning Research 38 (3), 91-101.

Tran, A.A., Gatewood, C., Harris, A.H.S., Thompson, J.A., Dragoo, J.L., 2016. The effect of foot landing position on biomechanical risk factors associated with anterior cruciate ligament injury. The Journal of Experimental Orthopaedics 3, 13.

Zazulak, B.T., Hewett, T.E., Reeves, N.P., Goldberg, B., Cholewicki, J., 2007. Deficits in neuromuscular control of the trunk predict knee injury risk: a prospective biomechanical–epidemiologic study. American Journal of Sports Medicine 35 (7), 1123-1130.

Capítulo | 39 |

Eficácia do Condicionamento: Roteiro para Otimizar os Resultados na Reabilitação com Base no Desempenho

Claire Minshull

Introdução

Quer estejamos lidando com um atleta profissional de alto desempenho ou com um atleta de esportes recreativos, uma lesão pode significar a indesejável interrupção do treinamento ou desempenho, ou ambos. O objetivo de qualquer programa de reabilitação esportiva subsequente é permitir que o atleta retorne aos esportes com segurança, eficácia e, idealmente, o mais rápido possível.

O desenvolvimento e a implantação de um plano de reabilitação bem-sucedido geralmente requerem que o profissional de reabilitação tenha o conhecimento e o domínio de várias disciplinas diferentes, desde a cinesiologia à força e condicionamento, da psicologia comportamental ao imageamento e ao diagnóstico. Com todos esses requisitos, juntamente com as pressões para fazer o atleta voltar ao esporte rapidamente, alguém pode ser perdoado por deixar algo de fora da lista. Infelizmente, isso às vezes pode significar ignorar alguns dos princípios básicos que impulsionam fundamentalmente a adaptação e, portanto, a recuperação bem-sucedida.

Fora dos domínios do esporte de elite bem-financiado, com recursos abundantes e equipes multi e interprofissionais, muitas vezes há escassez de tempo, experiência, pessoal, equipamento e financiamento. Frequentemente, os profissionais de reabilitação estão limitados a uma única sessão por semana com um atleta, mas o objetivo permanece o mesmo: fazer o atleta voltar ao esporte o mais rápido possível.

Neste capítulo, introduzimos o conceito de eficácia do condicionamento e um processo a seguir para fornecer a melhor oportunidade de atingir os resultados desejados de sua intervenção. Abordamos como estruturar a reabilitação para melhorar a adaptação neuromuscular favorável e explorar como alavancar a ciência para otimizar a eficácia da reabilitação e do condicionamento em estágio final. O objetivo é equipá-lo com mais ferramentas para obter os melhores resultados, mesmo nas condições mais exigentes.

Antes de nos aprofundarmos na eficácia do condicionamento, veremos os fatores fundamentais que determinam a estabilidade articular dinâmica e, portanto, os fatores que queremos influenciar em nossos esforços de reabilitação, usando o joelho como exemplo.

Estabilidade dinâmica da articulação do joelho

A estabilidade da articulação é determinada pela interação complexa de contribuições de estruturas "passivas" e "ativas". As estruturas passivas representam a geometria óssea, meniscos, ligamentos, tendões etc. Embora reconheçamos que não são verdadeiramente passivas, ou seja, possuem tecido sensorial que modula as respostas reflexas (Çabuk e Çabuk, 2016; Solomonow, 2006), a musculatura, que representa o lado "ativo" do modelo, tem um papel maior na estabilização da articulação em condições dinâmicas e, portanto, protege essas estruturas articulares vulneráveis (Figura 39.1). Atividades dinâmicas de intensidade e complexidade crescentes exigem contribuições crescentes das estruturas ativas (p. ex., a musculatura). Por exemplo, estando parados, podemos manter a estabilidade no joelho, "travando-os" por meio do mecanismo de "aparafusar" (Boxe 39.1). No entanto, durante atividades extenuantes envolvendo rápidas acelerações, desacelerações e mudanças direcionais, a carga mecânica da articulação tem o potencial de exceder as capacidades de tração do tecido conectivo; essas forças devem ser neutralizadas de forma eficaz por contribuições da musculatura circundante (Blackburn et al., 2008; Minshull et al., 2012a).

A importância das capacidades neuromusculares para a manutenção da estabilidade articular dinâmica e para evitar lesões sem contato é amplamente reconhecida (Hannah et al., 2014; Hewett et al., 2013). Os parâmetros de desempenho neuromuscular que têm sido usados para estimar o risco de lesão incluem: força muscular, definida como a quantidade máxima de força que pode ser exercida em um único esforço; taxa de desenvolvimento de força (TDF), definida como taxa de aumento da força contrátil; e, precedendo tudo, está o tempo de resposta da musculatura, denominado retardo eletromecânico (REM). REM é definido como o atraso de tempo entre o início da atividade elétrica e o início da produção de força muscular e é determinado por uma série de processos fisiológicos para colocar o músculo em um estado de "prontidão" para produzir força substancial. Quanto mais rápido esses processos ocorrem, mais rápido a força muscular pode ser iniciada e produzida. Obviamente, a padronização resultante das respostas musculares deve ser realizada de maneira controlada e apropriada para a situação. A revisão desse

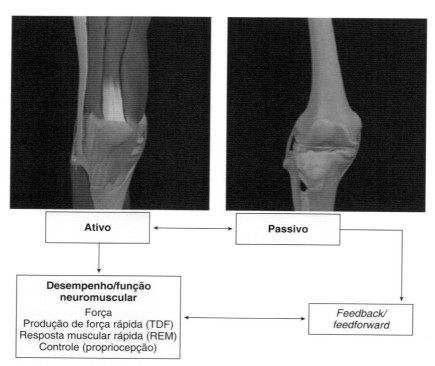

Figura 39.1 Modelo conceitual para estabilidade da articulação do joelho. *REM*, retardo eletromecânico; *TDF*, taxa de desenvolvimento de força. (*Esta figura se encontra reproduzida em cores no Encarte.*)

Boxe 39.1 Mecanismo de "aparafusamento" tibiofemoral

É a rotação entre a tíbia e o fêmur que ocorre no final da extensão do joelho, entre a extensão completa (0°) e 20° de flexão do joelho. A rotação externa da tíbia ocorre durante os graus terminais da extensão do joelho e resulta no aperto de ambos os ligamentos cruzados, o que bloqueia o joelho. A tíbia fica então na posição de estabilidade máxima em relação ao fêmur.

---

desempenho sensorimotor (também chamado de propriocepção) constitui um capítulo em si e está fora do escopo de nosso foco na ativação neuromuscular e na produção de força.

Lesões geralmente acontecem muito rapidamente, em milissegundos (Krosshaug et al., 2007). Assim, a estabilização articular dinâmica bem-sucedida durante o carregamento súbito depende dos parâmetros temporais relacionados com o início, o desenvolvimento e a magnitude da resposta de força muscular (Blackburn et al., 2008; Minshull et al., 2012a), ou seja, a produção de força suficiente para aproveitar essas forças conjuntas prejudiciais muito rapidamente. Isso levanta a questão: qual é a importância relativa da força muscular? Embora a força muscular, ou pico de torque, seja fácil de medir e tenha sido o índice primário usado em vários critérios de retorno ao esporte, como o índice de simetria do membro (Zwolski et al., 2015), podemos estar perdendo informação se focamos apenas na "quantidade máxima de força que pode ser produzida em uma única contração".

Vamos explorar conceitualmente isso usando uma ilustração simples de uma curva força-tempo de uma contração isométrica voluntária máxima (CIVM).

A Figura 39.2 demonstra que o Atleta 2 é mais forte do que o Atleta 1 (ver *asterisco* na curva) durante o teste de extensão máxima do joelho. No entanto, se considerarmos a taxa de produção de força, mesmo que o Atleta 1 seja mais fraco, ele é capaz de "produzir" força muito mais rapidamente, como evidenciado por um gradiente mais acentuado da curva força-tempo. Medido contra uma quantidade arbitrária de força muscular de, por exemplo, 175 N, podemos ver que o Atleta 2 leva quase 200 ms a mais para produzir isso em comparação com o Atleta 1 (ver † na curva). A resposta de emergência, ou seja, a resposta neuromuscular durante ameaças críticas à estabilidade do sistema articular (Minshull et al., 2007), é uma resposta coordenada de vários grupos musculares. Se considerarmos que as lesões do ligamento cruzado anterior (LCA) podem acontecer dentro de 50 ms do contato do pé com o solo (Koga et al., 2010), e que normalmente leva > 300 ms para atingir a força máxima durante uma contração isométrica (Hannah et al., 2014), podemos ver a importância da velocidade da primeira resposta neuromuscular para resistir às ameaças mecânicas à integridade musculoesquelética.

Agora que cobrimos os fundamentos do desempenho neuromuscular, vamos abordar o tópico da eficácia do condicionamento (EC).

Eficácia do condicionamento para reabilitação baseada em desempenho

O que queremos dizer com *eficácia do condicionamento*? Eficácia é "a capacidade de produzir um resultado desejado ou pretendido". Portanto, estamos falando sobre a capacidade de atingir os resultados de desempenho ou reabilitação por meio do condicionamento prescrito – e, claro, seguido (consulte o Capítulo 43 sobre "adesão" do paciente). Um único programa genérico não fornecerá todos os resultados desejados discutidos até agora, como força, TDF, tempos de resposta muscular e desempenho sensorimotor; nem o gerenciamento de atletas "em tempo real" – embora a tentação possa ser grande quando o tempo é curto. Sem um plano sistemático progressivo para atingir resultados específicos, as melhorias incrementais no desempenho começarão a diminuir, assim como seus retornos sobre o investimento.

Alcançar a eficácia do condicionamento (Figura 39.3) requer uma preparação inicial e a determinação de metas (ver seção

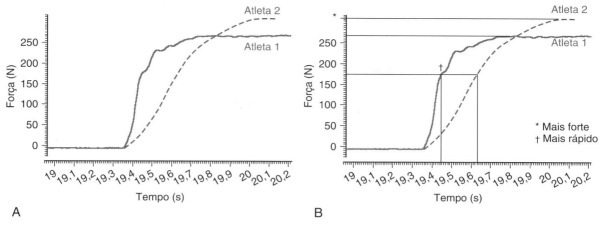

Figura 39.2 Força do músculo quadríceps durante a contração isométrica voluntária máxima (CIVM).

Planejamento e design do programa). Também requer uma compreensão dos princípios básicos que sustentam a adaptação e métodos que garantem que você está entregando o estímulo certo para obter a adaptação fisiológica desejada (ver seção *Abordagem de princípios básicos*). Finalmente, para conseguir um retorno bem-sucedido ao esporte, precisamos desenvolver as capacidades neuromusculares recém-formadas em situações relevantes e imprevisíveis, baseadas no desempenho, para construir resiliência contra lesões futuras (ver seção *Demandas de desempenho e riscos de lesões*).

Planejamento e *design* do programa

Conforme reconhecido anteriormente, um único programa genérico não produzirá vários resultados desejados. Diferentes estímulos neuromusculares e, portanto, adaptações, serão produzidos pela manipulação da quantidade de repetições, séries, carga/intensidade e períodos de descanso dentro de um programa de exercícios.

Para oferecer o programa de reabilitação esportiva mais eficaz, precisamos ter uma visão clara de seu objetivo final. As fases de planejamento estabelecerão múltiplos objetivos a curto prazo, permitindo uma abordagem sistemática e progressiva para atingi-los. O programa pode então ser projetado de maneira ideal para cada uma das partes componentes, de modo que os esforços possam ser investidos com foco nos objetivos. Decisões como a importância da força muscular absoluta em comparação com os tempos de resposta muscular rápida (REM) ou a aptidão cardiovascular precisarão ser feitas em cada fase para aprimorar o foco.

A força muscular é importante para a estabilidade articular dinâmica e as capacidades de absorção de choque; portanto, em indivíduos nos quais a capacidade de força foi drasticamente reduzida, por exemplo, nos frágeis e idosos, ou após lesão prolongada, intervenção cirúrgica e imobilização, a força muscular pode constituir o foco das fases preliminares da reabilitação. No entanto, um atleta de alto desempenho que sofreu uma lesão menos grave e apenas uma ausência limitada do treinamento teve sua capacidade de força reduzida em um grau menor, podendo ser restaurada muito mais rapidamente, com foco principal no estabelecimento de uma rápida velocidade de resposta muscular (REM) e na capacidade de produzir parte de sua força de modo mais veloz (TDF). Na verdade, capacidades neuromusculares temporais comprometidas podem ter constituído um fator de risco para a lesão inicial!

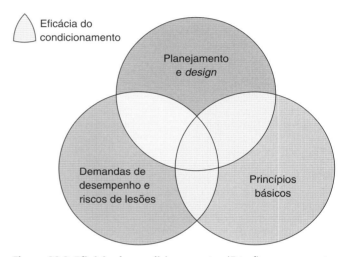

Figura 39.3 Eficácia do condicionamento. (*Esta figura se encontra reproduzida em cores no Encarte.*)

Ameaças à eficácia do condicionamento

Aqui, as ameaças à eficácia do condicionamento são *design* e planejamento inadequados. Isso pode ser simplesmente devido à falta de tempo ou, principalmente, por pensar que não temos tempo suficiente para nos dedicar ao planejamento. Isso significa que a chance de retornos decrescentes aumenta, sendo que os benefícios obtidos diminuem continuamente de acordo com a quantidade de esforço investido. Alguns dos efeitos negativos controláveis resultantes do planejamento impróprio que ameaçam a eficácia do condicionamento são fornecidos a seguir.

Fadiga

Repetições de contrações musculares de alta intensidade ou de sessões de exercício podem causar perdas progressivas de desempenho (Minshull et al., 2012a); por exemplo, uma redução progressiva na força muscular de até 15% foi relatada após uma simulação de uma partida de basquete (Ansdell e Dekerle, 2020). Os mecanismos subjacentes provavelmente significarão que o treinamento em um estado de fadiga terá um impacto negativo no potencial de adaptação.

Considere a sequência de exercícios e, mais importante, os períodos de descanso em cada sessão para maximizar a oportunidade de recuperação e, portanto, a eficácia do condicionamento.

Por exemplo, se o tempo dita que sua sessão deve envolver um componente de fortalecimento muscular, bem como um treinamento de agilidade, como você sequenciará esses exercícios? A ordem dos exercícios intrassessão pode influenciar a magnitude das adaptações fisiológicas. A realização de treinamento de força antes do exercício de resistência pode minimizar a intrusão da fadiga muscular e otimizar a oportunidade de ganhos neuromusculares e cardiovasculares e vice-versa (Coffey e Hawley, 2017). Da mesma maneira, exercícios desafiadores de desempenho sensorimotor em superfícies instáveis, exigindo pivotamento, mudanças direcionais e desafios de equilíbrio, requerem contribuições significativas da capacidade da unidade motora de contração rápida. Preceder o exercício fatigante com repouso insuficiente pode comprometer a capacidade de ativação da unidade motora de contração rápida e proporcionar um risco aumentado de lesão, bem como oportunidade subótima para adaptação.

Efeitos colaterais – dano muscular induzido por exercício

O músculo esquelético é suscetível a danos ultraestruturais após exercícios excêntricos de alta intensidade não habituais. Isso pode ser evidente no atleta que inicia o treinamento, uma partida ou uma reabilitação após um período prolongado de inatividade ou descondicionamento relacionado com lesões (Minshull et al., 2012b). O dano muscular induzido pelo exercício (DMIE) é predominantemente causado pela atividade muscular excêntrica, em que o músculo se alonga enquanto está sob carga, como corrida em declive, a fase de abaixamento durante o exercício de resistência, aterrissagem de um salto etc. As principais consequências funcionais do DMIE incluem reduções prolongadas na força muscular, TDF, e potência e equilíbrio entre 15 e 70% (Power et al., 2012; Sayers e Clarkson, 2001) que atinge o pico 24 a 48 horas pós-exercício (Hyldahl et al., 2014).

O treinamento muscular excêntrico deve formar um componente importante de qualquer programa de reabilitação, uma vez que a maioria das atividades esportivas requer desempenho de alto nível sob essas condições (p. ex., desacelerações, mudanças de direção) e o microtrauma e remodelamento resultantes são importantes para ganhos neuromusculares e mudanças morfológicas. Porém, como no caso da fadiga muscular, é importante considerar o sequenciamento do exercício, principalmente dentro da sequência diária. Devido ao dano preferencial às fibras musculares de contração rápida (Hyldahl et al., 2014), é plausível que uma TDF ou intervenção de treinamento de força muscular provavelmente não produza os mesmos ganhos em um músculo sintomático de dano em comparação com um músculo não danificado, já que a dor pode indicar níveis reduzidos de esforço voluntário. Na ausência de sistemas dinamométricos complexos, avaliações simples de dor muscular de início tardio (DMIT) em uma escala visual analógica e testes funcionais de salto vertical podem ajudar o profissional a monitorar a recuperação.

Técnicas para aumentar a eficácia do condicionamento

Os princípios básicos de treinamento determinarão a eficácia de sua intervenção (i. e., alcançar os resultados que você deseja alcançar). São eles: especificidade, sobrecarga e progressão (Kraemer e Ratamess, 2004) (Figura 39.4). Esses pilares fundamentais estão bem estabelecidos na literatura de desempenho, mas infelizmente não aparecem com tanta frequência nas pesquisas de reabilitação (Minshull e Gleeson, 2017). A aplicação desses princípios garantirá que sua intervenção produzirá o resultado desejado, seja o aumento da força muscular, velocidade de *sprint* ou condicionamento cardiovascular.

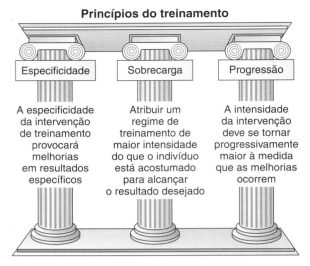

Figura 39.4 Princípios do treinamento.

Especificidade

A especificidade da intervenção de treinamento provocará melhorias em resultados específicos. Após uma lesão, o objetivo pode ser "aumentar a força dos músculos do joelho". No entanto, um objetivo muito mais específico e mensurável seria "aumentar a resistência dos isquiotibiais em 20%".

Sobrecarga

Esse termo se refere a designar um regime de treinamento de maior demanda física do que o indivíduo está acostumado, a fim de atingir o resultado desejado. Isso é determinado pela intensidade do treinamento, volume, repetições, séries, descanso e frequência, que serão abordados na próxima seção.

Progressão

Isso significa que a demanda física da intervenção deve se tornar progressivamente maior à medida que as melhorias ocorrem. Se o objetivo é promover uma adaptação de força, precisamos planejar como manter esse estímulo de fortalecimento à medida que a adaptação ocorre. Aliás, isso não significa aumentar o número de repetições.

Abordagem de princípios básicos

Em uma recente revisão sistemática do treinamento de resistência (em comparação com um controle sem exercício) para o tratamento da osteoartrite do joelho, descobrimos que os princípios básicos de especificidade, sobrecarga e progressão foram aplicados de forma inconsistente e relatados de forma inadequada em todos os estudos elegíveis para revisão (Minshull e Gleeson, 2017).

Digamos que você determinou que uma das principais metas de seu atleta é aumentar a força muscular do quadríceps. Um exercício comumente prescrito, para qualquer articulação, pode ser: 3 séries de 10 a 12 repetições de extensões de joelho com uma faixa de resistência. Esse é *realmente* um exercício de treinamento de força?

A seguir estão mais algumas perguntas:
- Por que a faixa de 10 a 12 repetições?

- O que acontece quando 12 repetições podem ser facilmente realizadas?
- Em relação ao anterior, você aumenta para 20 repetições?
- O que determina a cessação do exercício?

Essa série de perguntas simples realmente desafia a justificativa para a intervenção. Se a eficácia do condicionamento foi devidamente considerada e o programa planejado para atingir os resultados pretendidos, eles resistirão ao escrutínio. No entanto, esse tipo de exercício *não* é um exercício de força muscular *per se*. Isso vai condicionar a resistência muscular, ou seja, a resistência a fadiga por exercícios de longa duração. Embora algumas mudanças na força muscular possam ser alcançadas nas fases iniciais da reabilitação, quando o atleta experimentou atrofia muscular significativa ou é novo no treinamento de resistência, esses efeitos irão estabilizar-se rapidamente. Daí em diante, forças musculares maiores são necessárias para provocar mudanças na força muscular máxima.

Para condicionar o músculo de maneira ideal, nos referimos ao espectro de força-resistência do treinamento de resistência (Peterson et al., 2005) (Figura 39.5). Isso descreve como programas que usam baixas repetições e alta resistência (3 a 5 repetições máximas [RM]) elicitarão a adaptação ideal de força, enquanto o treinamento com altas repetições e baixa resistência (≥ 12RM) promove a resistência muscular (Fleck e Kraemer, 2014). Existem outras maneiras de medir e garantir que o músculo receba sobrecarga suficiente, como usar uma porcentagem calculada de 1RM. No entanto, isso requer um teste máximo de 1RM que o paciente pode não ser capaz de tolerar e é difícil progredir a carga na ausência de supervisão e repetição do teste. Ao atribuir um número de RM (p. ex., 3 a 5), o paciente é capaz de determinar individualmente o que isso representa em termos de carga e progredir independentemente conforme ocorre a adaptação.

Um estudo clássico de Campos et al. (2002) ilustrou isso muito bem. Trinta e dois participantes foram divididos em quatro grupos: um grupo de baixa repetição executando 3 a 5RM para quatro séries de *leg press*, agachamento e extensão de joelho; um grupo de repetição intermediária realizando 9 a 11RM por três séries (mesmos exercícios); um grupo de alta repetição realizando 20 a 28RM por duas séries (mesmos exercícios); e um grupo de controle que não pratica exercícios. Todos os grupos de exercícios realizaram o mesmo volume de treinamento. A força dinâmica máxima (*leg press* 1RM) melhorou significativamente mais para o grupo de baixa repetição (61%) em comparação com os outros grupos de treinamento (36 e 32%). Não surpreendentemente, os maiores ganhos na resistência muscular, medidos como a quantidade de repetições realizadas a 60% 1RM (*leg press*), foram mostrados no grupo de repetições altas (94% *versus* uma perda de 20% no grupo de repetições baixas).

Provavelmente não é aconselhável carregar repentinamente músculos não acostumados ao treinamento de resistência dessa maneira. No entanto, isso mostra que o planejamento e *design* adequados permitem uma abordagem progressiva para o fortalecimento muscular eficaz. A propósito, exatamente os mesmos princípios básicos se aplicam a intervenções para condicionar outros parâmetros neuromusculares.

Reabilitação da taxa de desenvolvimento de força

Como já estabelecemos, TDF é a capacidade de desenvolver rapidamente a força muscular. Os determinantes da TDF incluem o recrutamento de unidades motoras de contração rápida, a rapidez da ciclagem de pontes cruzadas e a rigidez do músculo e do tecido conjuntivo (Maffiuletti et al., 2016). Consequentemente, as melhorias em qualquer um desses fatores são suscetíveis de provocar uma adaptação positiva na TDF. Embora estudos tenham sugerido que várias modalidades podem provocar melhorias na TDF, em indivíduos acostumados a exercícios, resistência de alta carga e treinamento balístico mostraram melhorar a TDF (Bogdanis et al., 2018; Farup et al., 2014).

Reabilitação do retardo eletromecânico

O REM – intervalo de tempo entre o início da atividade elétrica e o início da produção de força – é determinado pelo recrutamento de unidades motoras, a propagação do potencial de ação por meio do músculo e o alongamento do componente elástico em série (as estruturas viscoelásticas incluindo tendão, aponeurose e fibras musculares) (Nordez et al., 2009). Na maioria das circunstâncias, o atraso é determinado principalmente pelo quão "elástico" esse tecido conjuntivo é: quanto mais elástico, mais tempo leva para transmitir a força muscular ao osso. Portanto, o condicionamento eficaz de REM envolverá intervenções para promover a ativação da unidade motora de contração rápida e, talvez mais importante, a rigidez do tecido conjuntivo. As modalidades de exercício incluem treinamento pesado de resistência (Stock et al., 2016).

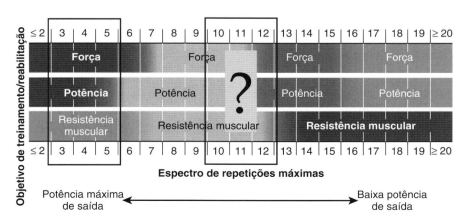

Figura 39.5 Espectro de força-resistência do treinamento de resistência. "Repetições máximas" refere-se ao número de repetições que podem ser realizadas (com a maneira correta) contra uma resistência; 5 RM significa falha em realizar a sexta repetição. (Adaptada de Baechle, T., Earle, R., 2008. Essentials of Strength Training and Conditioning, third ed. Human Kinetics, Champaign, Ill; Fleck, S.J., Kraemer, W.J., 2014. Designing Resistance Training Programmes. fourth ed. Human Kinetics, Champaign, Ill.)

Ameaças à eficácia do condicionamento

As consequências do desuso no manejo de um atleta lesionado incluem perdas de força muscular, área transversal e alterações no impulso neural (Farthing e Zehr, 2014). Estes podem ser exacerbados no membro lesionado por dor e efusão (Fitzgerald, 2005) e são impulsionados pela inibição muscular artrogênica (IMA). A IMA é uma inibição neural contínua que impede o sistema nervoso central de ativar totalmente a musculatura. Isso significa que a ativação muscular máxima não é alcançável e, desse modo, a eficácia de qualquer condicionamento associado que a requeira provavelmente alcançará resultados abaixo do ideal. A seguir, apresentamos três técnicas baseadas em evidências para mitigar a influência da IMA.

Técnicas para aumentar a eficácia do condicionamento

Modo e amplitude da ativação muscular

Pense no modo de ativação muscular. Normalmente segue um padrão concêntrico-excêntrico conforme os músculos se contraem e ficam mais curtos para levantar uma resistência, e então se alongam sob carga para controlar a sua desaceleração. Quais são suas opções se uma resposta inibitória à dor for elicitada? Você consegue identificar em qual momento do movimento a dor é desencadeada? Se estiver relacionado à parte concêntrica, é possível focar somente na parte inferior (excêntrica)? Os protocolos de treinamento de força excêntrica, quando ajustados para a capacidade excêntrica, podem provocar maiores ganhos na força muscular em comparação com o treinamento concêntrico (Roig et al., 2009). Se qualquer contração dinâmica forte não for possível, considere as contrações isométricas. Você pode manipular a amplitude para identificar uma posição articular confortável. Além de induzir alterações neuromusculares na posição articular selecionada, o treinamento isométrico máximo em comprimentos musculares longos demonstrou conferir alterações à força concêntrica, ou seja, sob condições dinâmicas (Noorkõiv et al., 2015).

Velocidade da ativação muscular

A dor é percebida em menos de um segundo após o estímulo ser aplicado e a repetição desse estímulo em 3 segundos aumenta a intensidade da sensação de dor (Barrell e Price, 1975). Portanto, esforços de duração muito curta de ≤ 1 segundo podem ser suficientes para contornar a resposta à dor e seus efeitos inibitórios. Combinado com a técnica de modular o tipo de ativação muscular, você tem a oportunidade de induzir cargas pesadas por um período muito curto. Com descanso suficiente, isso pode fornecer um estímulo eficaz para desenvolver as capacidades de geração de força e velocidade muscular.

Educação cruzada

O que acontece se a dor, derrame ou disfunção for demais para superar? Talvez o membro esteja engessado ou haja restrições clínicas que impeçam exercícios de resistência pesados. O fenômeno da educação cruzada descreve o ganho de força no membro oposto não treinado após o treinamento de resistência unilateral do membro "treinado". Na prática, isso significa que o treinamento de força adequadamente projetado no membro não lesionado pode provocar ganhos ou atenuar o declínio no membro lesionado. Em certas circunstâncias, os ganhos de força podem chegar a 50% do observado para o lado treinado (Farthing e Zehr, 2014).

O efeito da educação cruzada é um fenômeno bem-documentado na literatura de fisiologia e desempenho esportivo. No entanto, é uma técnica pouco utilizada na reabilitação na qual, indiscutivelmente, existem as maiores oportunidades de impacto. Acredita-se que esse fenômeno seja, em parte, devido a uma adaptação neural e "transbordamento" de atividade motora não intencional do córtex motor treinado para o não treinado durante contrações unilaterais fortes. Para uma revisão abrangente do efeito de educação cruzada, consulte Hendy e Lamon (2017). A fim de maximizar os ganhos de força no lado não treinado, a intervenção do treinamento de resistência no lado treinado deve ser de intensidade e volume suficientemente altos e seguir os princípios de especificidade, sobrecarga e progressão. Uma revisão pessoal e qualitativa da literatura relevante mostra que uma dose mínima de 300+ repetições, aderindo a um foco de treinamento de força (carga alta, poucas repetições), é provavelmente necessária. Além disso, uma meta-análise recente relatou o potencial para um efeito ligeiramente maior por meio do treinamento excêntrico (Manca et al., 2017).

Demandas de desempenho e riscos de lesões

O profissional de reabilitação deve compreender as demandas do esporte tanto para as necessidades de desempenho, quanto para construir resiliência contra lesões futuras. Isso torna possível o projeto de exercícios apropriados para promover o desdobramento das capacidades neuromusculares recém-formadas em situações imprevisíveis baseadas no desempenho. Ao planejar o retorno ao jogo, o praticante deve estabelecer quais fatores são mais importantes em qual estágio da reabilitação e, em seguida, garantir que o programa seja projetado para alcançar isso. Aqui, estamos equilibrando a restauração da função, das necessidades de desempenho e da capacidade muscular, juntamente com a compreensão das ameaças impostas pela competição específica do esporte e pelo estresse por exercício baseado em treinamento.

Por exemplo, as demandas de desempenho comuns de *sprint* e esportes de equipe são acelerações rápidas e velocidade em linha reta. No entanto, enquanto o *sprint* envolve pequenas demandas de desempenho em um plano predominantemente sagital em um ambiente previsível, os esportes coletivos envolvem múltiplas acelerações, desacelerações, mudanças de direção e demandas de desempenho multiplanar em um ambiente frequentemente imprevisível. Portanto, os riscos e perfis de lesões são diferentes entre esses esportes, com exceção, talvez, de uma alta incidência de distensões nos isquiotibiais. Assim, os esportes coletivos requerem uma abordagem progressiva adicional para condicionar tempos de resposta muscular rápidos e TDF em vários planos para atenuar com sucesso o carregamento dinâmico durante mudanças direcionais de alta velocidade. Em outro caso, considere as ginastas, que são expostas a muitas aterrissagens de alto impacto durante a saída dos aparelhos, às vezes realizando mais de 200 saídas por semana (Özguven e Berme, 1988). Dado que mais de um terço de todas as lesões sofridas por mulheres jovens competitivas ocorrem durante a saída (Caine et al., 1988), o condicionamento aqui deve se concentrar em aumentar progressivamente a capacidade de resistir e atenuar as forças de reação de uma maneira controlada para manter a estabilidade da articulação.

Um exemplo hipotético da hierarquia de importância dos fatores neuromusculares dentro de um programa de reabilitação do LCA é mostrado na Figura 39.6. Depois de abordar a amplitude de movimento (ADM), a dor e a restauração da marcha na

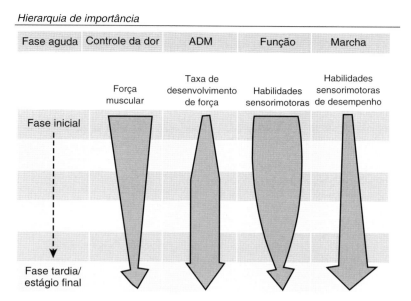

Figura 39.6 Reabilitação do desempenho neuromuscular. Exemplo de hierarquia de importância em um programa de reabilitação baseado em desempenho. *ADM*, amplitude de movimento.

fase aguda do pós-operatório, o foco principal nos estágios iniciais da reabilitação é o desenvolvimento da força e das habilidades sensorimotoras (propriocepção). Conforme a força e o controle são aprimorados, o foco muda para melhorar a produção de força muscular explosiva (TDF), culminando finalmente nas habilidades de desempenho sensorimotoras, nas quais os exercícios dinâmicos são representativos das demandas e ameaças específicas do esporte. Quando chegarmos aos estágios finais de um programa de reabilitação e nos prepararmos para o retorno ao jogo, o atleta terá alcançado os fundamentos necessários em força, produção de força explosiva e desempenho sensorimotor "estático". O foco passa a ser a capacidade de implantá-lo funcionalmente por meio da exposição segura a cenários imprevisíveis e menos estáveis – na verdade, praticando para o cenário de emergência. Um exemplo pode ser a construção de exercícios de mudança direcional de baixa velocidade dentro do ambiente específico de esportes (*i. e.*, no campo, na quadra) para exercícios de mudança direcional de alta velocidade envolvendo tarefas de desempenho e mudanças sutis na estabilidade da superfície.

Uma vez que o retorno ao jogo tenha sido alcançado, a preservação desses ganhos profiláticos ao longo da temporada competitiva requer um plano estruturado que leve em consideração os efeitos físicos agudos de sessões de treinamento e performances únicas, os efeitos colaterais do treinamento sazonal e cronograma de desempenho e a recuperação necessária para a restauração adequada das capacidades neuromusculares. Claramente, cada esporte será diferente no volume e no tipo de demandas físicas (em relação ao rúgbi profissional, ver o Capítulo 37).

Ameaças à eficácia do condicionamento

As ameaças específicas à eficácia do condicionamento são variadas e serão determinadas pela situação específica do esporte. No entanto, a falta de compreensão das demandas de desempenho esportivo e dos riscos de lesões pode influenciar a eficácia de um retorno ao jogo bem-sucedido. Para a preservação contínua dos efeitos profiláticos, existem alguns fatores comuns a serem considerados:

Efeitos cumulativos

Os efeitos cumulativos de treinamento e competição específicos para esportes podem estar relacionados com efeitos intrassessão, como fadiga muscular aguda, ou efeitos entre as sessões, como dano muscular induzido por exercício. Cobrimos alguns dos efeitos deletérios sobre o desempenho e as capacidades neuromusculares na seção anterior.

Carga de treinamento

Este é um grande tópico, que incorpora muitas medidas diferentes de carga. No entanto, uma pesquisa recente focada especificamente na corrida de alta velocidade propõe isso como um fator de risco para lesões. Lembre-se de que esta pesquisa ainda está engatinhando e são necessárias investigações de maior qualidade. No entanto, é interessante notar que grandes volumes de treinamento em altas velocidades e grandes mudanças semanais em corrida de alta velocidade foram correlacionados com o risco de lesões no futebol e no futebol australiano (Malone et al., 2018; Saw et al., 2018).

Técnicas para aumentar a eficácia do condicionamento

Efeito da sessão repetida

O efeito da sessão repetida (SR) refere-se à adaptação pela qual uma única sessão de exercício excêntrico protege contra as consequências das sessões excêntricas subsequentes (Nosaka e Marcelo, 2011), o que significa que, em comparação com a primeira sessão, uma segunda sessão de contrações de alongamento está associada à diminuição da perda de força contrátil, menos dor e redução na quantidade de marcadores indiretos de dano no sangue.

Abordamos os potenciais efeitos prejudiciais do exercício excêntrico e danos musculares associados na seção anterior. No entanto, se planejado corretamente, é possível construir resiliência em seu atleta para episódios futuros. Isso será benéfico para períodos cheios de treinamento e de jogos. Então, quanto e quando?

Aplicação Clínica

Um único episódio de alta intensidade de exercício excêntrico pode resultar em perdas substanciais para o desempenho neuromuscular, incluindo perdas crescentes de força muscular dos isquiotibiais e TDF até 36 e 65%, respectivamente, em 48 horas pós-exercício, e uma resposta DMIT prolongada (Minshull et al., 2012b). Se o atleta realizou exatamente o mesmo exercício novamente dias ou semanas depois, as alterações na força e dor serão comparativamente menores. Naturalmente, o DMIT não é agradável e em uma temporada competitiva pode não ser viável degradar o desempenho dos atletas a tal ponto. Então, quanto é suficiente?

A dose e a intensidade da sessão inicial determinam a duração do efeito protetor: maiores intensidades e doses que provocam maior dano muscular geralmente conferem os efeitos protetores mais longos. No entanto, efeitos de curta duração podem ser alcançados por meio de contrações excêntricas de baixo nível que não provocam nenhuma consequência no desempenho neuromuscular. Por exemplo, contrações excêntricas equivalentes a apenas 10% de CIVM atenuaram significativamente a magnitude do dano muscular induzido por uma sessão subsequente de exercício excêntrico máximo nos flexores e extensores do joelho por até 7 dias (Lin et al., 2015). Portanto, com o planejamento adequado da temporada, episódios de exercícios de resistência excêntrica de baixo nível podem ser usados profilaticamente para atenuar as perdas de desempenho associadas a épocas de demandas de desempenho condensadas. Existem outras maneiras de provocar o efeito SR, como contrações isométricas em músculos longos. No entanto, isso está além do escopo deste capítulo e o leitor pode consultar Nosaka e Marcelo (2011) para uma excelente revisão conduzida por uma autoridade altamente respeitada na área.

Conclusão

Frequentemente, múltiplas demandas concorrentes e restrições de tempo e recursos sabotam a eficácia do condicionamento e, portanto, a capacidade de alcançar um retorno rápido e seguro ao jogo. Aqui está uma estrutura para enfocar seu pensamento e aprimorar suas intervenções – para, em última análise, certificar-se de que seus objetivos desejados e seu plano de reabilitação estão alinhados. Um plano progressivo e sistemático que incorpora os princípios básicos de condicionamento e adaptação é a base para alcançar os resultados da reabilitação. Depois disso, quaisquer novos métodos, técnicas e tecnologias de treinamento podem ser combinados para obter ganhos marginais. Acerte o básico e o resto virá.

Referências bibliográficas

Ansdell, P., Dekerle, J., 2020. Sodium bicarbonate supplementation delays neuromuscular fatigue without changes in performance outcomes during a basketball match simulation protocol. Journal of Strength and Conditioning Research 34 (5), 1369-1375.

Barrell, J.J., Price, D.D., 1975. The perception of first and second pain as a function of psychological set. Perception and Psychophysics 17 (2), 163-166.

Blackburn, J.T., Bell, D.R., Norcross, M.F., Hudson, J.D., Engstrom, L.A., 2008. Comparison of hamstring neuromechanical properties between healthy males and females and the influence of musculotendinous stiffness. Journal of Electromyography and Kinesiology 19, e362-e369.

Bogdanis, G.C., Tsoukos, A., Brown, L.E., Selima, E., Veligekas, P., Spengos, K., et al. 2018. Muscle fiber and performance changes after fast eccentric complex training. Medicine & Science in Sports & Exercise 50 (4), 729-738.

Çabuk, H., Çabuk, F.K., 2016. Mechanoreceptors of the ligaments and tendons around the knee. Clinical Anatomy 29 (6), 789-795.

Caine, D., Cochrane, B., Caine, C., Zemper, E., 1988. An epidemiologic investigation of injuries affecting young competitive female gymnasts. The American Journal of Sports Medicine 17, 811-820.

Campos, G.E., Luecke, T.J., Wendeln, H.K., Toma, K., Hagerman, F.C., Murray, T.F., et al. 2002. Muscular adaptations in response to three different resistance-training regimens: specificity of repetition maximum training zones. European Journal of Applied Physiology 88, 50-60.

Coffey, V.G., Hawley, J.A., 2017. Concurrent exercise training: do opposites distract? The Journal of Physiology 595 (9), 2883-2896.

Farthing, J.P., Zehr, E.P., 2014. Restoring symmetry: clinical applications of cross-education. Exercise and Sport Sciences Reviews 42 (2), 70-75.

Farup, J., Sørensen, H., Kjølhede, T., 2014. Similar changes in muscle fiber phenotype with differentiated consequences for rate of force development: endurance versus resistance training. Human Movement Science 34, 109-119.

Fitzgerald, G.K., 2005. Therapeutic exercise for knee osteoarthritis; considering factors that may influence outcome. Europa Medicophysica 41, 163-171.

Fleck, S.J., Kraemer, W.J., 2014. Designing Resistance Training Programmes, fourth ed. Human Kinetics, Champaign, Ill.

Hannah, R., Minshull, C., Smith, S.L., Folland, J.P., 2014. Longer electromechanical delay impairs hamstrings explosive force versus quadriceps. Medicine & Science in Sports & Exercise 46 (5), 963-972.

Hendy, A.M., Lamon, S., 2017. The cross-education phenomenon: brain and beyond. Frontiers in Physiology 8, 297.

Hewett, T.E., Di Stasi, S.L., Myer, G.D., 2013. Current concepts for injury prevention in athletes after anterior cruciate ligament reconstruction. The American Journal of Sports Medicine 41 (1), 216-224.

Hyldahl, R.D., Hubal, M.J., 2014. Lengthening our perspective: morphological, cellular, and molecular responses to eccentric exercise. Muscle Nerve 49 (2), 155-170.

Koga, H., Nakamae, A., Shima, Y., Iwasa, J., Myklebust, G., Engebretsen, L., et al., 2010. Mechanisms for noncontact anterior cruciate ligament injuries: knee joint kinematics in 10 injury situations from female team handball and basketball. The American Journal of Sports Medicine 38 (11), 2218-2225.

Kraemer, W.J., Ratamess, N.A., 2004. Fundamentals of resistance training: progression and exercise prescription. Medicine & Science in Sports & Exercise 36, 674-688.

Krosshaug, T., Slauterbeck, J.R., Engebretsen, L., Bahr, R., 2007. Analysis of anterior cruciate ligament injury mechanisms: three-dimensional motion reconstruction from video sequences. The Scandinavian Journal of Medicine Science in Sports 17, 508-519.

Lin, M.J., Chen, T.C., Chen, H.L., Wu, B.H., Nosaka, K., 2015. Low-intensity eccentric contractions of the knee extensors and flexors protect against muscle damage. Applied Physiology, Nutrition, and Metabolism 40, 1004-1011.

Maffiuletti, N.A., Aagaard, P., Blazevich, A.J., Folland, J., Tillin, N., Duchateau, J., 2016. Rate of force development: physiological and methodological considerations. European Journal of Applied Physiology 116 (6), 1091-1116.

Malone, S., Owen, A., Mendes, B., Hughes, B., Collins, K., Gabbett, T.J., 2018. High-speed running and sprinting as an injury risk factor in soccer: can well-developed physical qualities reduce the risk? The Journal of Science and Medicine in Sport 21 (3), 257-262.

Manca, A., Dragone, D., Dvir, Z., Deriu, F., 2017. Cross-education of muscular strength following unilateral resistance training: a meta-analysis. European Journal of Applied Physiology 117, 2335-2354.

Minshull, C., Eston, R., Rees, D., Gleeson, N., 2012b. Knee joint neuromuscular activation performance during muscle damage and superimposed fatigue. Journal of Sports Sciences 30 (10), 1015-1024.

Minshull, C., Gleeson, N., Walters-Edwards, M., Eston, R., Rees, D., 2007. Effects of acute fatigue on the volitional and magnetically-evoked electromechanical delay of the knee flexors in males and females. European Journal of Applied Physiology 100, 469-478.

Minshull, C., Eston, R., Bailey, A., Rees, D., Gleeson, N., 2012a. Repeated exercise stress impairs volitional but not magnetically evoked electromechanical delay of the knee flexors. Journal of Sports Sciences 30 (2), 217-225.

Minshull, C., Gleeson, N., 2017. Considerations of the principles of resistance training in exercise studies for the management of knee osteoarthritis: a systematic review. Archives of Physical Medicine and Rehabilitation 98 (9), 1842-1851.

Noorkõiv, M., Nosaka, K., Blazevich, A.J., 2015. Effects of isometric quadriceps strength training at different muscle lengths on dynamic torque production. Journal of Sports Sciences 33 (18), 1952-1961.

Nordez, A., Gallot, T., Catheline, S., Guével, A., Cornu, C., Hug, F., 2009. Electromechanical delay revisited using very high frame rate ultrasound. The Journal of Applied Physiology 106 (6), 1970-1975.

Nosaka, K., Marcelo, A., 2011. Repeated bout effect; research update and future perspective. Brazilian Journal of Biomotricity 5, 5-15.

Özguven, H.N., Berme, N., 1988. An experimental and analytical study of impact forces during human jumping. Journal of Biomechanics 21, 1061-1066.

Peterson, M.D., Rhea, M.R., Alvar, B.R., 2005. Applications of the dose–response for muscular strength development: a review of meta-analytic efficacy and reliability for designing training prescription. Journal of Strength and Conditioning Research 9, 950-958.

Power, G.A., Dalton, B.H., Rice, C.L., Vandervoort, A.A., 2012. Power loss is greater following lengthening contractions in old versus young women. Age (Dordr). 34 (3), 737-750.

Roig, M., O'Brien, K., Kirk, G., Murray, R., McKinnon, P., Shadgan, B., et al. 2009. The effects of eccentric versus concentric resistance training on muscle strength and mass in healthy adults: a systematic review with meta-analysis. The British Journal of Sports Medicine 43 (8), 556-568.

Saw, R., Finch, C.F., Samra, D., Baquie, P., Cardoso, T., Hope, D., et al. 2018. Injuries in Australian rules football: an overview of injury rates, patterns, and mechanisms across all levels of play. The Journal of Science and Medicine in Sport 21 (3), 257-262.

Sayers, S.P., Clarkson, P.M., 2001. Force recovery after eccentric exercise in males and females. European Journal of Applied Physiology 84 (1–2), 122-126.

Solomonow, M., 2006. Sensory-motor control of ligaments and associated neuromuscular disorders. Journal of Electromyography & Kinesiology 16 (6), 549-567.

Stock, M.S., Olinghouse, K.D., Mota, J.A., Drusch, A.S., Thompson, B.J., 2016. Muscle group specific changes in the electromechanical delay following short-term resistance training. The Journal of Science and Medicine in Sport 19 (9), 761-765.

Zwolski, C., Schmitt, L.C., Quatman-Yates, C., Thomas, S., Hewett, T.E., Paterno, M.V., 2015. The influence of quadriceps strength asymmetry on patient-reported function at time of return to sport after anterior cruciate ligament reconstruction. The American Journal of Sports Medicine 43 (9), 2242-2249.

Capítulo | **40** |

Atleta "Versátil": Principais Considerações de Desempenho para o Manejo de Lesões Relacionadas com Tornozelo, Tronco e Tendão em Ginastas do Sexo Feminino

Jason Laird

Introdução

Gerenciar a saúde e o desempenho de atletas de elite é uma tarefa exigente e envolve muitos praticantes que trabalham no esporte, incluindo aqueles que fazem parte de equipes de ciência e medicina do esporte. O fato de os atletas trabalharem no limite do que é fisicamente possível, juntamente com os riscos inerentes à execução repetida de certas tarefas físicas, faz com que manter os atletas livres de lesões e disponíveis para competir seja um trabalho em tempo integral para muitos profissionais em todo o mundo. Devido a uma miríade de fatores, há certos esportes ou ambientes atléticos que representam a extremidade mais desafiadora do espectro quando se trata de gerenciar a saúde e o desempenho do atleta. A ginástica artística feminina (GAF) é um desses ambientes.

Um dos aspectos mais importantes da gestão do desempenho atlético e de lesões é entender o "mundo" dos atletas e como eles interagem com ele. Dado o perfil de idade típico das atletas de GAF, a natureza única dessa modalidade e suas demandas de treinamento, é essencial que os profissionais dessa área estejam cientes dos fatores que podem influenciar uma ginasta. Isso permite que eles resolvam totalmente os problemas que surgem e ajuda a apoiar essas atletas em sua jornada para o sucesso. O objetivo deste capítulo é fornecer ao leitor informações claras e práticas sobre o mundo de uma ginasta, e destacar e reforçar a compreensão dos fatores críticos que influenciam as lesões, a reabilitação, o treinamento e o desempenho esportivo. Isso deve ajudar os profissionais no caminho para auxiliar o sucesso e, com isso, fornecer uma compreensão mais completa da ginasta "versátil".

Perfil de idade típico de ginastas de elite

Um bom ponto de partida para entender a ginasta é conhecer as idades típicas de atletas de nível de elite na GAF. Há uma grande diferença entre a idade dos campeões olímpicos masculinos e femininos da ginástica olímpica, com as mulheres sendo, em média, 7 anos mais novas do que os homens. A idade média das mulheres é de 17 anos e dos homens é de 24 anos.

Fatores-chave que influenciam a saúde na ginástica feminina

Equipe multiprofissional da ginasta

O cuidado holístico da equipe multiprofissional é fundamental no manejo de uma ginasta. Com a variedade de características pessoais, físicas e esportivas associadas à ginástica de elite, é imperativo que uma política de comunicação inclusiva apropriada seja adotada. Na verdade, assim como a equipe de profissionais da saúde e do movimento, pais, treinadores, professores, irmãos e companheiras de equipe podem se combinar para formar a equipe multiprofissional da ginasta em um sentido global. Com a natureza exigente do treinamento de nível de elite e a necessidade de treinamento especializado, o papel do treinador em fornecer apoio autônomo, encorajamento após erros e especialização técnica/tática é fundamental na motivação da atleta, ao mesmo tempo tendo efeito na minimização do risco de lesão (Knight et al., 2010). Ao desenvolver relacionamentos com as principais partes interessadas (talvez os mais importantes sejam os pais e treinadores da ginasta), o profissional pode gerenciar com mais sucesso lesões e ameaças de desempenho, facilitando a equipe multiprofissional para aproximar e garantir que as informações relevantes sejam compreendidas e acionadas por todos.

Crescimento e maturação

Foi sugerido que atletas jovens de elite são particularmente vulneráveis a lesões esportivas devido a processos físicos e fisiológicos de crescimento (Popovic et al., 2012). Os fatores de risco de lesão que são exclusivos da jovem atleta incluem, mas não estão limitados a:

- Vulnerabilidade da placa de crescimento (Frank et al., 2007)
- Pico de velocidade de crescimento, maturidade esquelética e estirão de crescimento na adolescência (Niemeyer et al., 2006)
- Maturidade biológica (Malina et al., 2004)

- Controle postural (Quatman-Yates et al., 2012)
- Volume de treinamento (Loud et al., 2005).

Dado que as ginastas são expostas a programas de treinamento de maior volume e intensidade do que atletas de idade semelhante em outros esportes (Burt et al., 2010), é pertinente que os profissionais estejam totalmente cientes desses fatores de risco relacionados com o crescimento e a maturação. Uma das principais funções de um profissional que trabalha com uma ginasta é fornecer aos principais interessados uma consciência de como esses fatores de risco podem interagir com lesões e desempenho. Além disso, é importante que a equipe de saúde desempenhe um papel proativo ao abordar os fatores de risco modificáveis (em particular, o controle postural e o volume de treinamento) durante esses estágios de crescimento e maturação, ao lado dos pais e do treinador.

Gerenciando a "carga"

Para entender completamente a carga e seu efeito na ginasta, é importante primeiro estar ciente das limitações de tempo percebidas comumente atribuídas ao treinamento dentro da GAF. Com as ginastas femininas sendo elegíveis para a seleção olímpica a partir dos 16 anos, o tempo disponível para introduzir e desenvolver a dificuldade técnica nas rotinas é comparativamente menor do que para os ginastas masculinos, que são elegíveis para competir nas Olimpíadas a partir dos 18 anos. Essa janela de oportunidade relativamente pequena para introduzir e desenvolver conhecimento técnico pode resultar em cargas de volume de treinamento técnico muito alto para ginastas femininas jovens, com o objetivo de maximizar a melhoria de desempenho. Quando a carga é considerada em um sentido mais global, coisas como carga de viagem e carga psicológica também entram em jogo. Dada a idade e o estágio de vida típicos das jovens ginastas de elite, elas geralmente têm uma variedade de tipos de carga para lidar – por exemplo, treinamento em clubes, competições no exterior, trabalhos escolares e provas. Esse conceito de carga global é importante e é necessário buscar informações sobre todos esses fatores ao tentar determinar a melhor forma de afetar a carga e sua relação real com lesões e declínio de desempenho. Conforme indicado por diversos autores (Fry et al., 1991; Kenttä e Hassmén, 1998; Kuipers e Keizer, 1988) e representado na Figura 40.1, um equilíbrio entre a carga e a recuperação é vital; a falta de compreensão desse conceito pode levar a fadiga prolongada, redução da capacidade de aceitar cargas e aumento do risco de lesões e doenças.

Treinamento técnico e preparação física

É fundamental para o desenvolvimento da robustez da ginasta ter a correta estrutura e equilíbrio entre o treinamento técnico e a preparação física. O domínio técnico das rotinas é o resultado desejado e a meta de desempenho das ginastas. No entanto, a maneira como competências físicas robustas podem ajudar a sustentar esses aspectos técnicos é menos tratada e compreendida. É necessário fornecer às ginastas a habilidade de tolerar as altas forças a que são submetidas durante o treinamento e a competição. O treinamento de força e o condicionamento em atletas jovens, especificamente aqueles métodos que visam melhorar a força e as qualidades de potência, têm sido um assunto gerador de discussões e é especialmente controverso em ambientes estéticos como balé e ginástica. No entanto, atualmente há uma abundância de evidências para apoiar o uso de treinamento de resistência em populações jovens (Faigenbaum et al., 2009). Outra consideração importante é a visão controversa de que o aumento da força muscular reduz a aparência estética da rotina de uma ginasta. Pesquisas dentro do balé profissional, entretanto, mostraram que o treinamento de força tem um impacto positivo no desempenho e não altera os componentes estéticos específicos da coxa (Koutedakis e Sharp, 2004). Também é importante observar que o uso de dosagens de treinamento de força apropriadas (p. ex., uma a quatro repetições a 80 a 100% de uma repetição máxima (1RM) por três a quatro séries) pode ter como alvo a força em vez da hipertrofia muscular.

Nutrição

A ginástica é um esporte que requer uma série de atributos físicos, incluindo potência, velocidade e coordenação. Desse modo, é importante que as jovens ginastas consumam energia e nutrientes suficientes para suportar as exigências do seu treino e competição, bem como do crescimento e manutenção dos tecidos

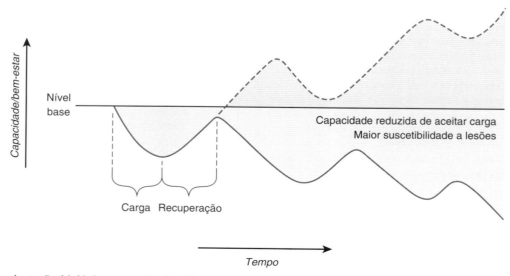

Figura 40.1 Má adaptação biológica por meio de ciclos de carga excessiva e/ou recuperação inadequada. (Adaptada de Soligard, T., Schwellnus, M., Alonso, J.M., Bahr, R., Clarsen, B., Dijkstra, H.P., et al., 2016. How much is too much? (Part 1) International Olympic Committee consensus statement on load in sport and risk of injury. British Journal of Sports Medicine 50 (17), 1030-1041.)

Atleta "Versátil": Principais Considerações de Desempenho para o Manejo de Lesões... **Capítulo | 40 |**

(Sundgot-Borgen et al., 2013). Devido à natureza estética de seu esporte, no entanto, as ginastas parecem estar em maior risco de empregar estratégias de dieta e sobrecarga de treinamento para alcançar um físico mais magro (Siatras e Mameletzi, 2014). Isso pode levar à ingestão inadequada de energia e nutrientes, resultando em efeitos como atraso na menarca, problemas de crescimento ósseo e redução de altura, peso e gordura corporal (Sundgot-Borgen e Garthe, 2011). As recomendações de treinadores e juízes para melhorar o desempenho reduzindo o peso também podem exacerbar esse problema (Sundgot-Borgen e Garthe, 2011). A dieta pode desencadear um efeito cascata de eventos, resultando em: baixa disponibilidade de energia (com ou sem distúrbios alimentares), amenorreia e distúrbios minerais ósseos; isso é denominado "tríade da atleta feminina" e é explicado em detalhes em outra publicação (Brown et al., 2017). Em combinação, essas condições podem predispor as atletas do sexo feminino a um maior risco de doenças e lesões (Triplett e Stone, 2016). Portanto, deve haver um foco contínuo na educação de ginastas, pais e treinadores na otimização da ingestão de energia e nutrientes para apoiar a saúde e o crescimento, melhorar o desempenho e reduzir lesões e doenças. Todos os profissionais que trabalham com jovens ginastas devem ter um papel proativo no compartilhamento de informações e usar o apoio de nutricionistas profissionais devidamente treinados, se necessário.

Estressores psicológicos

Existem numerosos estressores psicológicos que podem desempenhar um papel na vida de uma ginasta. O estresse relacionado à vida é um achado comum na literatura pré-lesão (Kerr e Minden, 1988). Eventos significativos de estresse na vida (experiências que produzem tensão percebida, como começar uma nova escola ou a perda de um membro da família) têm se mostrado altamente preditivos de lesões em atletas (Kerr e Minden, 1988). Estresse e ansiedade podem se manifestar em qualquer ponto ao longo da jornada da ginasta para o sucesso, mas podem ser particularmente significativos quando a ginasta está competindo. O ambiente de competição pode ser desgastante, com grande potencial para estresse e ansiedade, especialmente para indivíduos inexperientes. Algumas ginastas conseguem superar a dificuldade e podem produzir suas melhores performances na frente de juízes, espectadores e sob o escrutínio de câmeras de TV, enquanto outras são incapazes de lidar adequadamente com seus níveis de estresse. Isso pode levar à hostilidade, confusão ou depressão e, em última instância, declínio do desempenho (Massimo e Massimo, 2013).

Existem algumas técnicas importantes para lidar com o estresse que todos os profissionais devem conhecer ao trabalhar com ginastas, pois podem ajudar a prevenir ou apoiar o controle de estressores psicológicos. Essas técnicas incluem imaginação, habilidades de relaxamento, conversa interna positiva, habilidades de concentração e retreinamento de padrões de pensamento

negativo. É importante considerar a opção de encaminhamento a um psicólogo do esporte devidamente treinado (se disponível) para tratar de questões de enfrentamento.

Considerações sobre lesões e reabilitação

Esta seção descreve as lesões comuns na GAF, bem como fornece sugestões quanto ao seu manejo e reabilitação.

Epidemiologia de lesões

Pesquisa epidemiológica de lesões sofridas por ginastas de alto nível nos Jogos Olímpicos (Edouard et al., 2017). A Tabela 40.1 mostra a incidência de lesões em ginastas artísticos masculinos e femininos e destaca um claro aumento na incidência na Rio 2016 em comparação com os dois Jogos anteriores.

Esses resultados, no entanto, podem não nos dar uma imagem verdadeira do cenário de lesões. Existem alguns motivos para ter cuidado com essas descobertas. Houve uma melhora na taxa de conformidade no relato de lesões ao longo desse tempo. Além disso, este estudo foi baseado em uma quantidade relativamente pequena de ginastas. Lesões foram incluídas apenas se tivessem "ocorrido recentemente" durante o treinamento ou competição nos Jogos Olímpicos; dessa forma, esse tipo de vigilância de lesões não fornece informações sobre lesões recorrentes ou por uso excessivo, que representam uma alta proporção de lesões nesse grupo de atletas.

A Figura 40.2 resume os locais de lesão mais comuns de dois artigos recentes (Edouard et al., 2017; Kerr et al., 2015). Lesões no tornozelo, tronco e tendinopatia da perna são as mais frequentemente encontradas na GAF.

Lesões no tornozelo

Além de ser a lesão mais comum, as lesões no tornozelo normalmente causam a maior carga de lesões na GAF. As entorses ligamentares são comuns (Kerr et al., 2015), assim como as lesões que afetam os tendões ao redor do tornozelo e do pé, como o tibial posterior. Problemas na articulação do tornozelo, como lesões osteocondrais e impacto do tornozelo, também foram relatados em ginastas do sexo feminino.

Ao considerar as lesões do tornozelo, é importante observar os mecanismos comuns de lesão e sua relação com o aparelho individual. No que diz respeito ao salto e ao solo, os componentes de decolagem e aterrissagem são frequentemente os precursores de lesões no tornozelo, assim como o fato de que esses componentes se repetem em cargas de alto volume (Marshall et al., 2007). Equipamentos de piso mais macio (como *fast-track* e *tumble-track*) podem ser usados para minimizar as forças de impacto a que uma ginasta é submetida ao longo de uma sessão ou bloco de treinamento. Além disso, os tipos de "acrobacias"

Tabela 40.1 **Incidência de lesões por mil ginastas registradas nos Jogos Olímpicos de 2008, 2012 e 2016.**

Jogos Olímpicos	Incidência total	Incidência entre os homens	Incidência entre as mulheres
Pequim 2008	72,5	62,5	82,5
Londres 2012	76,9	91,8	61,9
Rio 2016	134	93,8	173,5

Adaptada de Edouard, P., Steffen, K., Junge, A., Leglise, M., Soligard, T., Engebretsen, L., 2017. Gymnastics injury incidence during the 2008, 2012 and 2016 Olympic Games: analysis of prospectively collected surveillance data from 963 registered gymnasts during Olympic Games. British Journal of Sports Medicine 52 (7), 475-481.

| Parte | 2 | Aplicação Clínica

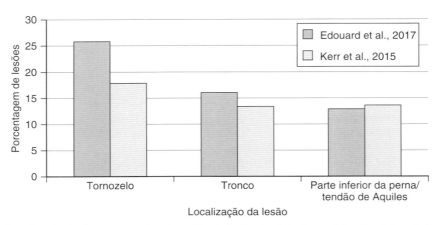

Figura 40.2 Localizações das lesões em estudos de epidemiologia da ginástica artística feminina. (Adaptada de Edouard, P., Steffen, K., Junge, A., Leglise, M., Soligard, T., Engebretsen, L., 2017. Gymnastics injury incidence during the 2008, 2012 and 2016 Olympic Games: analysis of prospectively collected surveillance data from 963 registered gymnasts during Olympic Games. British Journal of Sports Medicine 52 (7), 475-481; Kerr, Z.Y., Hayden, R., Barr, M., Klossner, D.A., Dompier, T.P., 2015. Epidemiology of National Collegiate Athletic Association women's gymnastics injuries, 2009-2010 through 2013-2014. Journal of Athletic Training 50 (08), 870-878.) (*Esta figura se encontra reproduzida em cores no Encarte.*)

que ocorrem na rotina do solo (e, portanto, amplamente praticados) são importantes a serem considerados ao tratar lesões no tornozelo. Aumentar a dificuldade técnica das "acrobacias" geralmente significa uma necessidade de maior potência, altura do salto e cambalhotas/giros no ar. À medida que a dificuldade aumenta, o risco de não concluir totalmente a "acrobacia" ou executá-la incorretamente também aumenta, aumentando a probabilidade de um pouso incorreto.

As aterrissagens curtas são um importante fator de risco para o desenvolvimento de uma lesão no tornozelo e esforços devem ser feitos para (1) reduzir a frequência de aterrissagens curtas, em primeira instância, e (2) promover um sistema robusto de relatórios e gestão visando melhorar o acesso médico a aquelas que sofrem uma lesão relacionada a uma aterrissagem curta.

Barras e traves também requerem uma descida de altura e, portanto, estão sujeitas a uma grande força de pouso. Dada a propensão para as ginastas estarem sujeitas a frequências e forças de salto em altura e pouso durante o treinamento e competição, a mecânica de pouso ideal, bem como a força e capacidade dos membros inferiores devem ser partes essenciais da preparação física de uma ginasta.

Principais considerações em lesões de tornozelo

O relato precoce da lesão no tornozelo é fundamental para permitir à ginasta acesso rápido a cuidados médicos adequados e para ajudar a prevenir quaisquer complicações secundárias à lesão; essa via de comunicação da lesão (desde a ginasta que sofreu uma lesão no tornozelo até o médico responsável sendo informado do incidente) deve ser bem estabelecida antes da lesão. Informações sobre o mecanismo de lesão são fundamentais (aterrissagens curtas e mecanismos de inversão/eversão do tornozelo são comuns nessa população), assim como a localização e a intensidade da dor. Relatos subjetivos de instabilidade devem ser avaliados como uma questão de prioridade na ginasta de elite. Objetivamente, uma avaliação como a medição da dorsiflexão do tornozelo com joelho na parede (Figura 40.3) também pode ajudar a estabelecer qualquer falta de amplitude ou movimento e/ou dor com a posição de dorsiflexão. Além de ser usada como um marcador de avaliação inicial, essa medida também pode ajudar a orientar a progressão por meio de um programa de retorno à ginástica, ajudando a avaliar a amplitude de movimento e sua relação com a carga.

Um papel fundamental do tornozelo da ginasta é produzir força durante as tarefas de corrida e salto. Como consequência, durante os períodos de imobilidade ou descarga (como no pós-operatório), é essencial que os principais grupos musculares mantenham sua capacidade de produzir força por meio de amplitudes seguras de movimento. A fim de prevenir o desgaste muscular e possíveis atrasos nas progressões da reabilitação, as contrações isométricas podem ser utilizadas no estágio inicial. A estimulação muscular (p. ex., Compex) para o complexo da panturrilha, fibular, tibial posterior e tibial anterior também pode ser valiosa. O uso de dinamometria manual ou dinamometria isocinética também pode ajudar a monitorar a força muscular durante o processo de reabilitação, em particular para os inversores e eversores.

Normalmente, os estágios intermediários a tardios do retorno à ginástica após uma lesão no tornozelo devem incluir uma variedade de tarefas de salto e aterrissagem, incluindo o uso de diferentes alturas, velocidades e direções, bem como abordar

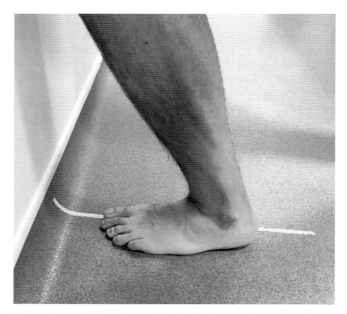

Figura 40.3 Medida da dorsiflexão do tornozelo com joelho na parede.

quaisquer falhas biomecânicas na técnica de aterrissagem. Em particular, pousos para trás devem ser incluídos prontamente, pois essa é a direção de pouso para as habilidades mais comuns relacionadas a mesa, solo e descida de aparelhos. Deve-se ter cuidado para incluir a qualidade dos pousos, e não apenas a quantidade de repetições concluídas. O contato do pé com o trampolim é um componente-chave do aparelho de salto e deve, portanto, progredir de forma constante ao longo de um plano de reabilitação do tornozelo; progressões de impactos de saltos estáticos para impactos após corrida e impactos com o trampolim precisam ser levadas em consideração no processo de projeto de reabilitação. Um programa de corrida/*sprint* progressivo também deve ser projetado para facilitar uma transição suave para um *sprint* de salto completo no final do processo de reabilitação. Estratégias de monitoramento simples, como quantificar impactos (quantidade de pousos por exercício ou por sessão) e distância (quanta corrida em qual intensidade de *sprint*) ajudarão a sobrecarregar progressivamente a ginasta e evitar picos indesejados na carga de treinamento durante o programa de reabilitação.

Lesões no tronco

Lesões no tronco e na coluna lombar são comuns na ginástica e podem afetar a ginasta em particular. As patologias que afetam as ginastas incluem disfunção da articulação facetária, fraturas por estresse/defeitos da pars, lesões de disco e fraturas por compressão vertebral (Kruse e Lemmen, 2009). Dado o nível de flexibilidade, força e posições corporais únicas requeridas para o esporte, há uma variedade de padrões de movimento e posições que precisam ser entendidas ao se considerar lesões de tronco dentro da ginástica, em particular no que diz respeito a aterrissagens, saltos e hiperextensão.

Estudos em biomecânica de técnicas de ginástica mostraram que uma grande quantidade de força é traduzida ao longo da coluna axial durante tarefas como salto a partir do solo, ressalto e aterrissagem (Bruggeman, 1987). As forças verticais foram medidas em 3,4 a 5,6 vezes o peso corporal durante a decolagem para uma habilidade de salto mortal para trás. Essas altas forças devem ser levadas em consideração no manejo de ginastas, em particular com adolescentes que podem ter sistemas musculoesqueléticos imaturos e, consequentemente, são mais suscetíveis a lesões (Engebretsen et al., 2010).

A natureza de certas habilidades dentro da ginástica exige que a atleta tenha uma grande mobilidade da coluna, particularmente em hiperextensão (p. ex., elementos para trás na trave; Figura 40.4). Habilidades como pré-voo de Yurchenko na mesa e elementos de acrobacia para trás incluem hiperextensão de alta velocidade (Bruggemann, 2005) e podem ser fatores contribuintes para patologias da coluna posterior. A repetição envolvida no treinamento desses elementos de hiperextensão pode levar a doenças lombares crônicas. No entanto, a presença de patologia na investigação nem sempre se correlaciona com um histórico de dor lombar (Goldstein et al., 1991; Jackson et al., 1976). Uma compreensão clara da biomecânica da rotina e do cronograma de treinamento de uma ginasta é, portanto, imprescindível para gerenciar com eficácia os distúrbios da coluna lombar nessa população.

Principais considerações em lesões de tronco

A avaliação da dor de tronco e lombar em ginastas deve ser multimodal e incluir elementos subjetivos e objetivos. Os principais recursos para avaliar incluem pontuações subjetivas de dor em

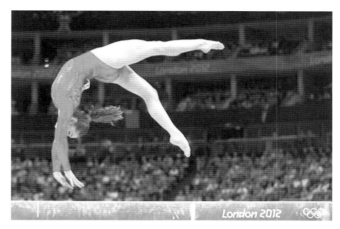

Figura 40.4 A necessidade de mobilidade da coluna é grande em ginastas. Isso é observado em elementos traseiros na trave.

movimentos de extensão e carga axial do tronco (p. ex., pousos), bem como pontuações de dor com atividades da vida diária (escola/trabalho, caminhada etc.). Medidas objetivas, como padrões de movimento combinados da coluna lombar, testes neurodinâmicos e testes de capacidade do tronco, também podem ser úteis. Como mencionado, a presença de patologia na investigação pode ou não combinar com os sintomas atuais de uma ginasta. É importante, portanto, não usar a imagem isoladamente. Discussões robustas com a equipe são necessárias com relação à realização de uma investigação e se algum resultado mudaria o manejo planejado (com base em descobertas subjetivas e objetivas).

Retornar à ginástica após uma lesão no tronco pode oferecer à praticante uma série de desafios. Isso se deve, em parte, ao alto nível funcional exigido no estágio final da reabilitação, quando os elementos finais do treinamento específico para o esporte incluem hiperextensão máxima e aterrissagens de alta força. Patologias relacionadas à extensão (p. ex., uma fratura por estresse da coluna lombar) podem ser gerenciadas com um período de descarga agressivo no estágio inicial e progressão para um programa de carregamento adequado. Este programa de carga deve incluir, na fase final, uma replicação de posições específicas da ginástica com ênfase na força e na capacidade da musculatura do tronco, a fim de lidar com a alta demanda e frequência do treinamento da ginástica. A chave para esta estratégia de reabilitação deve ser a consciência de quando reintroduzir a extensão lombar, a velocidade e a posição de como essa carga ocorre e a manutenção dos principais elos de comunicação com a equipe técnica em torno da reintrodução de elementos técnicos de ginástica ao longo do espectro de reabilitação em relação à dor e à função da ginasta.

Spencer et al. (2016) destacaram e categorizaram habilidades espinais modificáveis; essas informações fornecem uma estrutura para os profissionais usarem ao selecionar os exercícios para as ginastas com base no objetivo e nos resultados físicos pretendidos. A Figura 40.5 mostra o uso de exercícios para a coluna classificados por "resultado físico" (mobilidade, controle motor, capacidade de trabalho, força) e "funcionalidade" (não funcional, funcional). Embora não seja um espectro exato de exercícios, pode auxiliar o raciocínio clínico de um profissional em relação à seleção de exercícios de reabilitação da coluna vertebral. Por exemplo, durante os estágios iniciais de reabilitação após uma fratura por estresse da coluna lombar, pode haver uma ênfase no trabalho de mobilidade sem dor (tanto não funcional

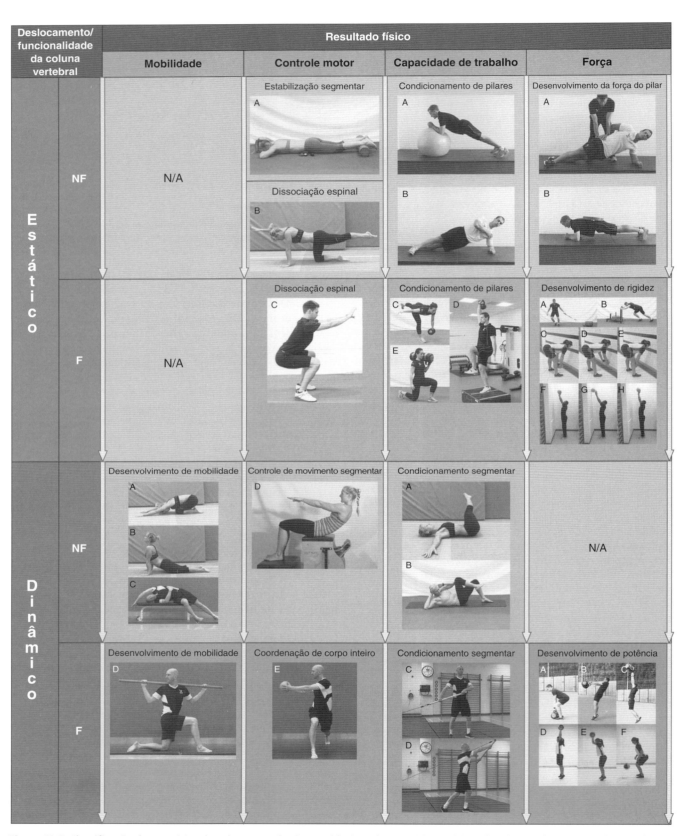

Figura 40.5 Classificação de exercícios da coluna vertebral com objetivos de exercício posicionados dentro do contexto dos resultados físicos pretendidos. *F*, funcional; *N/A*, não aplicável; *NF*, não funcional. (Adaptada de Spencer, S., Wolf, A., Rushton, A., 2016. Spinal-exercise prescription in sport: classifying physical training and rehabilitation by intention and outcome. Journal of Athletic Training, 51 (8), 613-628.)

Atleta "Versátil": Principais Considerações de Desempenho para o Manejo de Lesões...

Capítulo | 40 |

quanto funcional), além de exercícios de controle motor estático e dinâmico.

A força e a potência das pernas são componentes importantes na GAF, em particular para o salto e o aparelho de solo. Os elementos de dificuldade mais alta agora exigem que a ginasta seja mais poderosa no chão e na mesa de salto para ter mais tempo no ar para executar a habilidade. Desse modo, a ginasta moderna tem uma necessidade maior de produzir essa força e potência a fim de manter o nível de dificuldade necessário para vencer no esporte de elite. As estratégias para melhorar a força e a potência das pernas precisam considerar o histórico de lesões da ginasta, bem como sua habilidade técnica em relação aos exercícios selecionados. É importante destacar os altos níveis de carga axial da coluna vertebral inerentes a um esporte de salto e aterrissagem (Bruggeman, 1987). Exercícios utilizando equipamentos como *leg press* e máquinas de extensão/flexão de joelhos podem ajudar a fornecer à ginasta um estímulo adequado e seguro para melhorar a força e a potência. Qualquer que seja o método usado para melhorar a força e a potência das pernas, o ajuste dessas sessões em torno da semana/bloco de treinamento de uma ginasta é imperativo e um diálogo aberto com os treinadores é necessário para maximizar o treinamento e as oportunidades de desenvolvimento.

Tendinopatia de membro inferior

As decolagens e pousos possuem um papel fundamental no desempenho da ginástica, com saltos, rebotes, quedas e descidas constituindo a maior parte da rotina de uma atleta. A força pelo tendão de Aquiles durante um salto para trás foi medida em até 16 vezes o peso corporal (Bruggeman, 1987). Dadas essas forças altas e a frequência com que essas habilidades são treinadas ou executadas, não é surpreendente que a tendinopatia dos membros inferiores (incluindo Aquiles e patela) esteja consistentemente entre as três lesões mais comuns na GAF. Conforme indicado anteriormente, a superfície em que a ginasta pousa pode ser um fator-chave no desenvolvimento de certas lesões. Por exemplo, na preparação para a competição, quando as ginastas realizam uma porcentagem maior de suas rotinas em superfícies mais duras (p. ex., rotinas de solo completas no piso de competição, em vez de com esteiras ou parcialmente em pista rápida/*tumble-track*), há uma tendência para elevar a incidência de distúrbios dos tendões dos membros inferiores, como a tendinopatia de Aquiles.

Principais considerações de reabilitação em lesões de tendão

Por sua própria definição, tendinopatia inclui patologia e dor em um tendão. Essa dor pode inibir a utilização do armazenamento de energia dentro do tendão e levar a um comprometimento da função e do desempenho (Cook e Purdam, 2014). A reabilitação total dessas lesões pode ser lenta; é comum que as ginastas continuem a treinar e competir enquanto apresentam dores contínuas relacionadas à tendinopatia. É importante, entretanto, que o diálogo entre a ginasta, o técnico e a equipe de saúde seja claro e aberto a respeito da dor relacionada à tendinopatia. Durante os períodos em que a ginasta está treinando e competindo com dor, testes simples de monitoramento da dor no tendão podem ser usados para monitorar o padrão de dor e ajudar a ajustar a carga de treinamento da ginasta de forma adequada. O uso de pontuações na escala visual analógica de dor (VAD) com testes como elevação do calcanhar em uma perna (Aquiles) ou agachamento com declínio (patela) pode ser adequado. O uso de imagens para ajudar no tratamento sazonal da tendinopatia não é comum. No entanto, a caracterização do tecido por ultrassom pode oferecer uma maneira de monitorar os tendões no futuro e mais pesquisas são necessárias (Cook e Purdam, 2014).

Tal como acontece com o manejo da tendinopatia em outros esportes, o manejo do tendão de uma ginasta deve começar com a compreensão do estágio da tendinopatia e se o tendão é tolerante ou intolerante à carga. Informações adicionais sobre tendinopatia e seu manejo podem ser encontradas em uma variedade de fontes (Cook e Purdam, 2009; Cook e Purdam, 2012; Scott et al., 2013).

O manejo da tendinopatia de uma ginasta na temporada é uma consideração importante, com muitas apresentações crônicas de tendão nessa população. A reabilitação com exercícios excêntricos de carga pesada pode ser uma estratégia apropriada, dada uma janela de oportunidade de "pré-temporada". No entanto, o uso desse tipo de programa pode não ser apropriado para a ginasta enquanto ela continua treinando e competindo. Isométricos de carga pesada são comuns no manejo da ginasta com tendinopatia sazonal com o objetivo de fornecer um estímulo de carga ao tendão sem associação de dores musculares e tendíneas (Ranson et al., 2016). Modalidades como terapia por ondas de choque extracorpórea e faixas/órteses podem ser adjuvantes benéficos ao modelo de carregamento tradicional. Essas modalidades podem ajudar a preencher a lacuna entre a necessidade de continuar treinando/desempenhando a curto prazo e a realização de um programa de carregamento abrangente, cuja eficácia só pode aparecer a longo prazo.

O uso de medicamentos e injeções para reduzir a dor no tendão em atletas é um tema controverso e que foge ao escopo deste capítulo; mais informações podem ser encontradas em um artigo de Cook e Purdam (2014).

A chave para o manejo da tendinopatia durante a temporada é garantir que o tendão seja submetido à carga adequada em relação ao resto do programa específico de ginástica e que não haja incompatibilidade entre a capacidade de carga do tendão e a carga colocada sobre ele (Cook e Purdam, 2014). Estar ciente do calendário de treinamento e competição da ginasta e ter um diálogo contínuo com o treinador é importante no planejamento de certas fases de reabilitação juntamente com o cronograma de treinamento. Pode ser que durante períodos de treinamento pliométrico intenso (como um aumento no número de saltos mortais completos no piso de competição), outros exercícios focados no tendão podem ser reduzidos em frequência ou intensidade.

Dadas as altas forças exigidas de um tendão durante as tarefas de salto e aterrissagem, é importante que os exercícios destinados a fortalecer o complexo músculo-tendão (mais comumente o tendão da panturrilha-tendão de Aquiles ou tendões do quadríceps-patela) sejam adequadamente carregados. O uso de pesos relativamente pesados (mais de 80% de 1RM da ginasta) é necessário para produzir o resultado de aumentar a produção de força máxima; isso é normalmente feito em três a quatro séries de cinco a oito repetições (Baker, 2014). O uso de equipamento de força externo ou um ginásio de força pode ser necessário para aplicar com segurança essas cargas à ginasta (p. ex., o uso de uma máquina de *leg press* para carregamento isométrico ou excêntrico da panturrilha). Uma vez integrado ao programa semanal de uma ginasta, esse programa de força progressiva pode continuar ao longo da temporada e pode ser reduzido gradualmente nas semanas anteriores à competição.

O princípio da sobrecarga progressiva deve ser usado ao projetar protocolos de retorno ao salto para ginastas. A prescrição de carga, frequência e intensidade dos exercícios pliométricos deve ser sobreposta ao volume geral de treinamento da ginasta para que seja dada consideração à carga somativa das atividades pliométricas. É fácil sobrecarregar o programa de uma ginasta se uma abordagem combinada não for usada. A colaboração com a equipe técnica é fundamental. Os exercícios pliométricos podem ser adicionados assim que o trabalho concêntrico/excêntrico dos membros inferiores estiver livre de dor e a ginasta estiver em boa forma. Testes rápidos, como a capacidade de levantar a panturrilha com uma perna, movimentos de agachamento com uma perna e exercícios de corrida de baixo nível são um bom indicador para a introdução de exercícios pliométricos. Um plano básico de progressão da reabilitação pliométrica está delineado na Figura 40.6.

Resumo

O trabalho com a ginástica proporciona ao profissional um ambiente único para apoiar o desempenho esportivo. O conhecimento do perfil etário das ginastas femininas e as relações entre o crescimento, a maturação e as exigências físicas e psicológicas do esporte são essenciais para que o praticante tenha um impacto positivo no desempenho desse grupo de atletas. O esporte da GAF é muito exigente e em constante mudança. É necessário que os profissionais estejam totalmente informados sobre os principais requisitos técnicos e físicos do esporte, a fim de ajudar a apoiar a ginasta e o treinador a ultrapassar os limites do desempenho físico humano, ao mesmo tempo que minimiza o efeito das lesões.

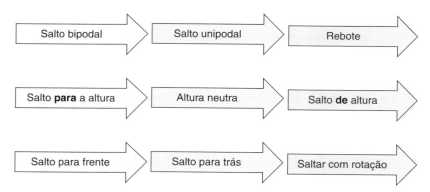

Figura 40.6 Noções básicas de progressão de reabilitação pliométrica para ginastas.

Referências bibliográficas

Baker, D., 2014. Using strength platforms for explosive performance. In: Joyce, D., Lewindon, D. (Eds.), High Performance Training for Sports. Human Kinetics, Champaign, IL, pp. 127-144.

Brown, K.A., Dewoolkar, A.V., Baker, N., Docich, C., 2017. The female athlete triad: special considerations for adolescent female athletes. Translational Pediatrics 6 (3), 144-149.

Bruggeman, G.P., 1987. Biomechanics in gymnastics. Medicine and Sport Science 25, 142-176.

Bruggemann, G.P., 2005. Biomechanical and biological limits in artistic gymnastics. In: Proceedings of the XXIII International Symposium on Biomechanics in Sports. The China Institute of Sport Science, Beijing, China, pp. 22-27.

Burt, L.A., Naughton, G.A., Higham, D.G., Landeo, R., 2010. Training load in pre-pubertal female artistic gymnastics. Science of Gymnastics 2 (3), 5-14.

Cook, J.L., Purdam, C.R., 2009. Is tendon pathology a continuum? A pathology model to explain the clinical presentation of load-induced tendinopathy. British Journal of Sports Medicine 43 (6), 409-416.

Cook, J.L., Purdam, C.R., 2012. Is compressive load a factor in the development of tendinopathy? British Journal of Sports Medicine 46 (3), 163-168.

Cook, J.L., Purdam, C.R., 2014. The challenge of managing tendinopathy in competing athletes. British Journal of Sports Medicine 48 (7), 506-509.

Edouard, P., Steffen, K., Junge, A., Leglise, M., Soligard, T., Engebretsen, L., 2017. Gymnastics injury incidence during the 2008, 2012 and 2016 Olympic Games: analysis of prospectively collected surveillance data from 963 registered gymnasts during Olympic Games. British Journal of Sports Medicine 52 (7), 475-481.

Engebretsen, L., Steffen, K., Bahr, R., Broderick, C., Dvorak, J., Janarv, P., et al., 2010. The International Olympic Committee Consensus statement on age determination in high-level young athletes. British Journal of Sports Medicine 44, 476-484.

Faigenbaum, A.D., Kraemer, W.J., Blimkie, C.J., Jeffreys, I., Micheli, L.J., Nitka, M., et al., 2009. Youth resistance training: updated position statement paper from the national strength and conditioning association. The Journal of Strength & Conditioning Research 23 (5), 60-79.

Frank, J.B., Jarit, G.J., Bravman, J.T., Rosen, J.E., 2007. Lower extremity injuries in the skeletally immature athlete. Journal of the American Academy of Orthopaedic Surgeons 15 (6), 356-366.

Fry, R.W., Morton, A.R., Keast, D., 1991. Overtraining in athletes. An update. Sports Medicine 12, 32-65.

Goldstein, J.D., Berger, P.E., Windler, G.E., Jackson, D.W., 1991. Spine injuries in gymnasts and swimmers. An epidemiologic investigation. The American Journal of Sports Medicine 19, 463-468.

Jackson, D.W., Wiltse, L.L., Cirincoine, R.J., 1976. Spondylolysis in the female gymnast. Clinical Orthopaedics and Related Research 117, 68-73.

Kenttä, G., Hassmén, P., 1998. Overtraining and recovery. A conceptual model. Sports Medicine 26, 1-16.

Kerr, G., Minden, H., 1988. Psychological factors related to the occurrence of athletic injuries. Journal of Sport & Exercise Psychology 10 (2), 167-173.

Kerr, Z.Y., Hayden, R., Barr, M., Klossner, D.A., Dompier, T.P., 2015. Epidemiology of National Collegiate Athletic Association women's gymnastics injuries, 2009-2010 through 2013-2014. Journal of Athletic Training 50 (8), 870-878.

Knight, C.J., Boden, C.M., Holt, N.L., 2010. Junior tennis players' preferences for parental behaviors. Journal of Applied Sport Psychology 22, 377-391.

Koutedakis, Y., Sharp, N.C., 2004. Thigh muscles strength training, dance exercise, dynamometry, and anthropometry in professional ballerinas. The Journal of Strength & Conditioning Research 18 (4), 714-718.

Kruse, D., Lemmen, B., 2009. Spine injuries in the sport of gymnastics. Current Sports Medicine Reports 8 (1), 20-28.

Kuipers, H., Keizer, H.A., 1988. Overtraining in elite athletes. Review and directions for the future. Sports Medicine 6, 79-92.

Loud, K.J., Gordon, C.M., Micheli, L.J., Field, A.E., 2005. Correlates of stress fractures among preadolescent and adolescent girls. Pediatrics 115 (4), 399-406.

Malina, R.M., Bouchard, C., Bar-Or, O., 2004. Growth, Maturation and Physical Activity. Human Kinetics, Champaign, IL.

Marshall, S.W., Covassin, T., Dick, R., Nassar, L.G., Agel, J., 2007. Descriptive epidemiology of collegiate women's gymnastics injuries: national collegiate athletic association injury surveillance system, 1988-1989 through 2003-2004. Journal of Athletic Training 42 (2), 234-240.

Massimo, J., Massimo, S., 2013. Psychological health and well-being. In: Gymnastics Psychology: The Ultimate Guide for Coaches, Gymnasts and Parents. Morgan James Publishing, New York, pp. 134-162.

Niemeyer, P., Weinberg, A., Schmitt, H., Kreuz, P.C., Ewerbeck, V., Kasten, P., 2006. Stress fracture in the juvenile skeletal system. International Journal of Sports Medicine 27 (3), 242-249.

Popovic, N., Bukva, B., Maffulli, N., Caine, D., 2012. The younger athlete. In: Brukne, P., Khan, K., et al. (Eds.), Brukner and Khan's Clinical Sports Medicine, fourth ed. McGraw-Hill Education, Australia, pp. 888-909.

Quatman-Yates, C.C., Quatman, C.E., Meszaros, A.J., Paterno, M.V., Hewett, T.E., 2012. A systematic review of sensorimotor function during adolescence: a developmental stage of increased motor awkwardness? British Journal of Sports Medicine 46 (9), 649-655.

Ranson, C., Joyce, D., McGuiggan, P., 2016. Tendon injuries. In: Joyce, D., Lewindon, D. (Eds.), Sports Injury Prevention and Rehabilitation. Routledge, London, pp. 199-211.

Scott, A., Docking, S., Vicenzino, B., Alfredson, H., Murphy, R., Carr, A.J., et al., 2013. Sports and exercise-related tendinopathies: a review of selected topical issues by participants of the second International Scientific Tendinopathy Symposium (ISTS) Vancouver 2012. British Journal of Sports Medicine 47, 536-544.

Siatras, T., Mameletzi, D., 2014. The female athlete triad in gymnastics. Science of Gymnastics 6 (1), 5-22.

Soligard, T., Schwellnus, M., Alonso, J.M., Bahr, R., Clarsen, B., Dijkstra, H.P., et al., 2016. How much is too much? (Part 1) International Olympic Committee consensus statement on load in sport and risk of injury. British Journal of Sports Medicine 50 (17), 1030-1041.

Spencer, S., Wolf, A., Rushton, A., 2016. Spinal-exercise prescription in sport: classifying physical training and rehabilitation by intention and outcome. Journal of Athletic Training 51 (8), 613-628.

Sundgot-Borgen, J., Garthe, I., 2011. Elite athletes in aesthetic and Olympic weight-class sports and the challenge of body weight and body composition. Journal of Sport Sciences 29 (1), 101-114.

Sundgot-Borgen, J., Garthe, I., Meyer, N., 2013. Energy needs and weight management for gymnasts. In: Caine, D.J., Russell, K., Lim, L. (Eds.), Gymnastics. John Wiley & Sons, Ltd, Chichester, UK, pp. 51-59.

Triplett, N.T., Stone, M., 2016. The female athlete. In: Joyce, D., Lewindon, D. (Eds.), Sports Injury Prevention and Rehabilitation. Routledge, London, pp. 429-435.

Capítulo | 41 |

Introdução à Medicina da Dança

Nick Allen

Introdução

Embora existam muitas semelhanças entre o esporte e a dança, e ainda mais com certos esportes direcionados à estética, também existem numerosas diferenças. Compreender a especificidade da dança pode melhorar o manejo de lesões e os resultados da reabilitação por meio da compreensão das várias demandas impostas aos dançarinos.

Exigências extrínsecas aos dançarinos

Superfícies

Evidências esportivas sugerem que o impacto surge de uma mudança na superfície. A dança é tipicamente apresentada em teatro; entretanto, em sua essência, especialmente na dança contemporânea, uma variedade de superfícies pode ser encontrada. Para grandes companhias de dança, as aulas e os ensaios podem ocorrer em estúdios customizados. As propriedades de redução de força ideais para uma pista de dança foram sugeridas como 60% (Hopper et al., 2013). Dançarinos que assistem a aulas ou ensaiam em salas comunitárias têm menor probabilidade de encontrar superfícies que demonstrem essas propriedades. Do mesmo modo, estruturas com propriedades de redução de força têm menos probabilidade de estar disponíveis em teatros maiores quando se trata de apresentações. Muitos teatros atendem a diversos usos e têm pisos construídos para atender a uma variedade de tipos de apresentações, incluindo ópera, pantomima etc., bem como lidar com uma grande quantidade de cenários.

A superfície do piso também influencia o risco de lesões. O balé é amplamente executado em superfícies de linóleo, que podem variar consideravelmente no coeficiente de atrito, afetando o risco. O coeficiente de atrito pode ser afetado por produtos de limpeza ou transferência da pele dos dançarinos (cremes, óleos de massagem etc.) criando inconsistência em superfícies escorregadias. Alguns dançarinos, especialmente no balé, usam resina para ajudar com sapatilhas de ponta em superfícies escorregadias.

Trabalhando com a indústria, os profissionais da saúde podem examinar a construção do palco e do piso para reduzir esse risco. Trabalhando com dançarinos individualmente, é importante criar elementos de controle imprevisto dentro de seu treinamento. Normalmente, os movimentos dos dançarinos são coreografados para que haja poucos ou nenhum movimento inesperado. O uso de exercícios reacionários como parte de um programa de propriocepção ajudará a apoiar os dançarinos nesta área.

Trajes/sapatos

Os bailarinos normalmente realizam as aulas e a maioria dos ensaios com meia-calça/*collants* ou macacões com sapatilhas, sapatilhas de jazz ou de personagens ou tênis. Dependendo da atuação, seu figurino pode ser pesado, restritivo ou dificultar sua visão (no caso de máscaras e peças para a cabeça). Os dançarinos normalmente têm ensaios gerais antes das apresentações, mas eles podem ser apenas na preparação imediata para um *show*, reduzindo o impacto do treinamento dentro de suas fantasias.

O calçado na dança também pode diferir consideravelmente. No balé, pode-se esperar que os bailarinos dancem nas pontas (Figura 41.1 A) ou com uma perna só nas pontas (Figura 41.1 B). Nessa posição, o suporte de peso normalmente ocorre nas pontas do primeiro e segundo dedos do pé. Esteticamente, alguns dançarinos podem se esforçar para criar um arco longitudinal estendido pela porção medial do pé e aumentar a flexão plantar com a articulação talocrural. O impacto em áreas-chave, como a articulação talocrural navicular e posterior, é notável. A construção de uma sapatilha de ponta é baseada na estética e oferece suporte reduzido. Impulsionados pela estética, alguns dançarinos também "quebram" suas sapatilhas de ponta para ajudar a alcançar essas posições estendidas. Os dançarinos também podem usar sapatos estreitos como parte de seu impulso estético. Na presença de um neuroma de Morton, isso precisa ser considerado. Quando não estão em sapatilhas de ponta, as mulheres podem usar sapatilhas, também usadas por bailarinos. Elas oferecem pouco ou nenhum suporte estrutural. Os dançarinos também podem usar sapatos de jazz que tenham um pouco de sola no calcanhar e no antepé, mas pouco suporte para o arco, permitindo que os dançarinos ainda atinjam sua estética de apontar o pé. Os sapatos dos personagens na dança podem variar consideravelmente, desde sandálias até botas na altura do joelho, com as quais se espera que todos os dançarinos se apresentem.

Os calçados de dançarinos contemporâneos podem variar de pés descalços a tênis e botas pesadas. As dançarinas de salão costumam se apresentar com saltos positivos, enquanto para os dançarinos de salão são usados calçados que lembram sapatos de jazz; eles oferecem algum suporte, mas são projetados para facilitar o movimento no meio do pé.

Adereços/equipamento/iluminação

Devido à variedade de coreografias e papéis apresentados aos bailarinos, existem vários desafios adicionais que podem impactar nas lesões. Devido às demandas e custos associados ao acesso aos principais palcos do teatro, muitos ensaios para as produções acontecerão em estúdios distintos. Às vezes, não há capacidade para incluir cenário nos estúdios, então os dançarinos ensaiarão

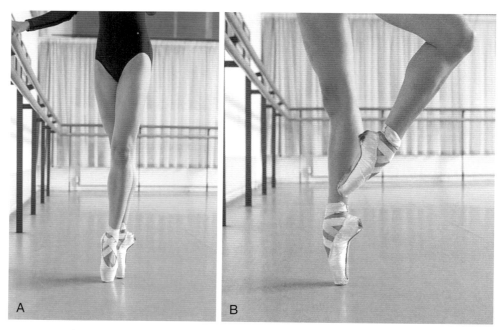

Figura 41.1 A. *En pointe.* B. *Cou-de-pied en pointe.* (Fotógrafo: Ty Singleton.)

na ausência do cenário que precisarão considerar durante as apresentações. Certas apresentações – frequentemente vistas com a dança contemporânea – terão dançarinos se apresentando em altura e isso pode resultar em um aumento de lesões traumáticas. Normalmente, a iluminação nos estúdios é muito boa, enquanto a iluminação durante as apresentações é focada em destacar a apresentação; isso pode mudar as dicas visuais disponíveis para um dançarino (e o que ele está acostumado nos ensaios). O uso de adereços em certas coreografias também requer competência e aquisição de habilidades, como o uso de espadas em produções como *Romeu e Julieta*.

Exigências intrínsecas aos dançarinos

Carga de trabalho

O treinamento em dança é projetado para apoiar o movimento altamente qualificado e eficiente observado nos bailarinos profissionais. O treinamento para bailarinos profissionais começa para valer nas escolas profissionalizantes, quando os alunos ingressam no que poderia ser visto como uma posição de treinamento em tempo integral desde os 11 anos, mas muitos dançaram desde os 3 ou 4 anos em escolas de dança locais. A Figura 41.2 é um exemplo da distribuição relativa dos diferentes aspectos do treinamento realizado em uma escola profissionalizante de dança. Como pode ser visto ao longo do desenvolvimento do dançarino, o treinamento específico da dança é o foco principal, aumentando exponencialmente quando os compromissos escolares terminam. Ao longo do desenvolvimento da dança, a preparação física pode consistir apenas de 1 a 3 horas por semana.

É importante compreender a natureza do treinamento e do desenvolvimento de um dançarino e não fazer suposições sobre as principais variáveis fisiológicas, como força e preparo físico, mesmo para dançarinos de elite.

O processo de desenvolvimento e treinamento responsável por criar o padrão de movimento eficiente que torna o movimento na dança esteticamente agradável também pode criar desafios potenciais para aqueles que procuram apoiar os dançarinos em seu condicionamento e reabilitação. Isso pode incluir a falta de exposição aos programas de treinamento complementar típicos, como treinamento de força, estabilidade do *core* etc., vistos em outros esportes. O tempo investido na educação de dançarinos sobre os objetivos e resultados positivos esperados da reabilitação pode ser uma parte importante do processo e melhora a compreensão e a adesão. Parte dessa educação pode precisar se concentrar nas mudanças estéticas esperadas. Não é incomum que os dançarinos sejam cautelosos com o treinamento de força por medo de hipertrofia ou perda de flexibilidade. É importante que essas áreas sejam discutidas para melhorar a adesão. A falta de formação complementar típica também pode explicar o porquê de pesquisas sobre variáveis fisiológicas como $VO_{2máx}$ e força demonstraram resultados abaixo do esperado (Wyon et al., 2016). Os resultados funcionais notáveis exigidos na dança ilustram que as lições podem ser aprendidas com a dança em torno da obtenção de resultados extraordinários por meio de biomecânica eficiente e padrões de movimento, apesar dos indicadores fisiológicos mais baixos do que o esperado. No entanto, também significa que melhorar certas medidas de desempenho fisiológico é um caminho que pode ser seguido para fornecer aos bailarinos maior resistência contra lesões.

Grandes companhias de balé podem ter o que parece ser um ciclo de temporada típico visto no futebol ou rúgbi de primeira divisão. A temporada começa em agosto e vai até o início do próximo verão. Eles normalmente podem ter um período de folga (até 5 semanas) durante o verão com mais 1 semana no meio da temporada. Companhias menores podem não ter um formato tão consistente e dançarinos podem ter dificuldade para planejar seu condicionamento da mesma maneira. Dançarinos independentes, que trabalham de contrato em contrato, são ainda mais desafiados, pois as pressões financeiras podem levá-los a aceitar contratos em vez de se recuperar de períodos de treinamento.

Uma programação típica em uma grande companhia de balé pode envolver aulas 6 dias por semana, durando cerca de 1 hora a 1 hora e meia. O formato da aula pode variar, mas consistirá basicamente em três áreas principais: barra, centro e saltos. Durante a barra, os dançarinos usarão a barra de parede (ou

Introdução à Medicina da Dança **Capítulo** | **41** |

Idade cronológica	12	13	14	15	16	17	18	19
☐ Treinamento suplementar	2	2	1	1	1	1	1	3
■ Atividades acadêmicas	18	18	18	20	20	10	10	0
■ Dança	19	19	19	17	17	27	27	37

Figura 41.2 Exemplo de carga horária semanal em uma escola profissionalizante de dança. (Adaptada de Injuries and adolescent ballet dancers: Current evidence, epidemiology, and intervention, PhD Thesis, Nico Kolokythas, 2019.) (*Esta figura se encontra reproduzida em cores no Encarte.*)

ocasionalmente barra autônoma) para se apoiar e se estabilizar enquanto passam pelo que pode ser descrito como uma sessão de aquecimento sistemático e ativação neuromuscular por meio da construção de movimento e intensidade usando movimentos de balé (*pliés, relevés* etc.). Durante o centro, eles não usarão mais a barra como apoio e começarão a se mover e girar. Finalmente, progredirão para saltos, novamente de forma incremental de *petit* (pequeno) a *grand* (grande) *jeté* (saltos). A aula serve para apoiar e desenvolver a técnica e a eficiência dos movimentos sinônimos de dança. Por meio de sua construção incremental, pode ser usada como aquecimento e suporte de força e resistência de potência.

Dependendo da época da temporada, a aula pode ser acompanhada por até 6 horas de ensaios. Uma companhia de dança pode ensaiar mais de uma peça por vez devido a restrições de tempo no final da temporada. Os ensaios ainda ocorrerão durante os períodos de atuação, mas serão reduzidos devido aos *shows*. Uma produção em grande escala pode realizar entre sete e nove *shows* por semana, por períodos que se estendem de semanas a meses dependendo dos contratos, com 150 *shows* por ano normalmente realizados por uma companhia de balé de grande escala. Uma produção do West End ou da Broadway pode ser apresentada durante todo o ano e por muitos anos, com os mesmos dançarinos repetindo os mesmos movimentos ano após ano. Dependendo do tamanho da companhia e da duração do *show*, pode haver vários elencos para um *show*.

Se houver apenas um elenco, haverá pressão sobre o dançarino, pois ele estará envolvido em todos os ensaios relevantes, bem como terá a pressão psicológica de saber que não há substituição caso ele não consiga se apresentar devido a uma lesão. Se houver vários elencos, pode significar que a maior parte do trabalho é feita com o primeiro elenco e outros elencos podem não ter o mesmo nível de preparação. Quanto mais bem preparado um dançarino, menor o risco de lesões. Além disso, os dançarinos podem cumprir mais de um papel em um *show*, com alguns dançarinos realizando vários papéis em uma única apresentação. A variação de carga e exposição que isso cria pode aumentar o risco de lesões se o dançarino não estiver suficientemente preparado. Também existe uma variação na intensidade da carga de trabalho entre os diferentes papéis, bem como entre os diferentes programas ou coreografias.

Alguns esportes têm usado dados epidemiológicos para orientar as decisões sobre mudanças de regras para ajudar a reduzir as lesões em seu esporte. Por exemplo, as regras do futebol australiano mudaram a largada/sinalização e, portanto, reduziram a incidência de lesões do ligamento cruzado posterior, enquanto o rúgbi de 15 está constantemente examinando a correlação entre lesões e o *scrum* e áreas de contato para reduzir a prevalência de lesões. Aqueles que trabalham com dança têm a obrigação de construir dados epidemiológicos para melhorar a compreensão dos coreógrafos das possíveis correlações entre o planejamento de desempenho e as taxas de lesões, para que eles possam tomar decisões adequadas que minimizem a ocorrência de lesões. A combinação de intensidade e volume fornece a carga de trabalho relacionada à dança e é uma consideração importante para dançarinos em termos de melhorar o desempenho e desenvolver resistência a lesões.

No esporte, os atletas normalmente se aquecem imediatamente antes da competição, muitas vezes na mesma roupa com a qual competem. No entanto, devido aos requisitos de traje, cabelo e maquiagem das apresentações de dança, a preparação física pode ocorrer mais cedo do que o esperado. Os bailarinos podem ter aulas muitas horas antes do *show* devido à natureza de sua programação de ensaios. Os dançarinos que apoiam *shows* do tipo *West End* podem realizar uma sessão sob a orientação do bailarino principal antes de um *show* como parte de sua preparação para o desempenho, mas, novamente, pode haver restrições de tempo. O momento da preparação da apresentação também pode afetar o horário das refeições, com os dançarinos muitas vezes incapazes de comer no que é considerado um momento ideal antes da apresentação (3 horas antes do *show*). Dada a natureza dinâmica da dança, muitos relutam em comer mais perto de um *show* quando sua programação permite. O uso de *smoothies* caseiros pode ser uma forma de melhorar o desempenho da ingestão nutricional que é mais bem tolerada.

Lesão na dança

Embora existam desafios metodológicos, as revisões sistemáticas indicaram que a incidência de lesões na dança é de 1,3 lesões por 1.000 horas de dança (Tabela 41.1) (Allen et al., 2014). As taxas de lesões no balé são relatadas como mais altas, com até 4,4 lesões por 1.000 horas de dança dadas em uma auditoria de lesão prospectiva (Tabela 41.2) (Allen et al., 2012).

Bronner et al. (2003) conduziram uma extensa pesquisa sobre a incidência de lesões na dança moderna e contemporânea. A pesquisa deles mostrou os benefícios dos cuidados com profissionais de saúde especializados na dança, bem como uma boa análise dos padrões de lesões na dança moderna. Eles relataram uma incidência de lesões em uma companhia de dança moderna de 0,41 lesões por 1.000 horas de dança. Eles relataram que as lesões nas extremidades inferiores respondem por 60% do total de lesões. Destes, 52% estavam no pé e no tornozelo, 24% no joelho, 8% na perna, 8% na coxa e 8% no quadril.

421

Tabela 41.1 Incidência de lesões musculoesqueléticas na dança: uma revisão sistemática.

Tipo de estudos (projeto)	Incidência geral de lesões (observacional)
Quantidade de estudos	29
Limitações	Sérias
Inconsistência	Séria
Resultado indireto	Nenhum desfecho indireto sério detectado
Imprecisão	Sem imprecisão
Viés de publicação	Não detectado
Qualidade	Muito baixa
Incidência de lesões por horas de dança	
Incidência média/1.000 h	1,33
Faixa de incidência/1.000 h	0,18 a 4,7
Intervalo de confiança de 95%	0,20 a 4,35*
Lesões por dançarino/ano	
Número médio de lesões/dançarino/ano	1,93
Faixa de lesões/dançarino/ano	0,05 a 6,83
Intervalo de confiança de 95%	0,29 a 4,5

*Com base em 12 estudos. (Adaptada de Allen, N., Ribbans, W.J., Nevill, A.M., Wyon, M.A., 2014. Musculoskeletal injuries in dance: a systematic review. International Journal of Physical Medicine & Rehabilitation 3 (1), 1-8.)

A dança moderna pode ser categorizada em diferentes gêneros, sendo o hip hop um dos estilos mais populares. O trabalho de Ojofeitimi et al. (2012) sobre o hip hop demonstrou que esta é uma disciplina que os profissionais de saúde da dança precisam estar cientes, com lesões nas extremidades inferiores responsáveis por mais da metade do total de lesões (55%), sendo pé e tornozelo (20%) os mais comumente lesionados de todo o corpo, como no balé. De todas as lesões nessas duas áreas, 48% foram entorses de tornozelo. Em contraste com as lesões de balé, as lesões dos membros superiores representaram 29% do total de lesões. Aqui, as lesões mais comuns na mão foram luxações dos dedos (27%), fraturas nos dedos (22%) e rupturas ligamentares (12%). Os tecidos mais comumente lesionados foram músculo-tendão (29%), seguido por articulação-ligamento (não ósseo) (25%) e estresse/fratura óssea (11%).

Os dançarinos frequentemente registram níveis mais altos de exposição em comparação aos atletas, com dançarinos conhecidos por realizarem 35 horas de atividades relacionadas à dança por semana. Juntamente com a alta quantidade de apresentações, não é surpreendente que haja maior prevalência de lesões por uso excessivo na dança (Figura 41.3).

Dada a confiança dos dançarinos na biomecânica ideal e na proficiência técnica nos padrões de movimento para proteção contra as lesões, as altas taxas de exposição são uma consideração importante ao se desenvolver programas de reabilitação para essa população. Os dançarinos, por meio de suas taxas de exposição tipicamente altas, têm menos tolerância a desvios da norma antes de correr o risco de desenvolver lesões por uso excessivo. Portanto, o que pode parecer uma anomalia biomecânica sutil pode ser prejudicial por meio de carregamentos repetidos durante um período prolongado (Allen et al., 2013).

Terminologia de dança

Parte da avaliação e do manejo bem-sucedido de um dançarino será por meio da compreensão da especificidade de suas necessidades. Parte disso envolve a compreensão da natureza do movimento e da terminologia usada para descrever esses movimentos.

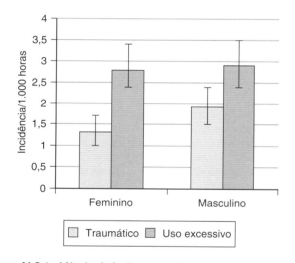

Figura 41.3 Incidência de lesões traumáticas e por excesso de uso em bailarinos profissionais por gênero. (Adaptada de Allen et al., 2012.)

Tabela 41.2 Incidência de lesões em dançarinos de uma companhia de balé profissional ao longo de 1 ano.

	Dançarinas		Dançarinos	
	N° de lesões (% de todas as lesões)	Incidência de lesões/1.000 h de dança (95% IC)	N° de lesões (% de todas as lesões)	Incidência de lesões/1.000 h de dança (95% IC)
Atividade de dança restrita	150 (87)	3,6 (3,1 a 4,2)	147 (80)	3,8 (3,3 a 4,5)
Retirada completa da dança*	22 (13)	0,53 (0,35 a 0,81)	36 (20)	0,94 (0,68 a 1,30)
Todas as lesões	172 (100)	4,1 (3,6 a 4,8)	183 (100)	4,8 (4,1 a 5,5)

*Lesões que exigiram a saída completa das atividades relacionadas à dança como parte da gravidade global. IC, intervalo de confiança. (Adaptada de Allen, N., Nevill, A., Brooks, J., Koutedakis, Y., Wyon, M., 2012. Ballet injuries: injury incidence and severity over 1 year. Journal of Orthopaedic Sports Physical Therapy 42 (9), 781-790.)

A partir da terminologia do balé, é possível encontrar qualquer um desses termos. Muitos se desenvolverão a partir das cinco posições-padrão usadas no balé que se relacionam com a posição das pernas e/ou braços (Figuras 41.4 e 41.5).

Além disso, os dançarinos descreverão a execução de movimentos como *plié* (movimento do tipo agachamento; Figura 41.6), *relevé* (levantamento do calcanhar; Figura 41.7), *développés* (Figura 41.8 A e B), batidas incluindo *tendu* e *glissés* (movimentos dinâmicos das pernas) e *port de bras cambre* (movimentos do tronco em flexão ou extensão com os braços) ou *arabesques* (Figura 41.8 C).

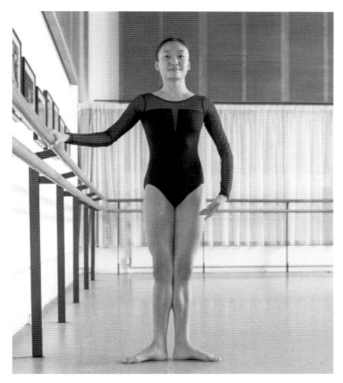

Figura 41.4 Primeira posição dos braços *bras bas*. (Dançarina: Yaoqian Shang; fotógrafo: Ty Singleton.)

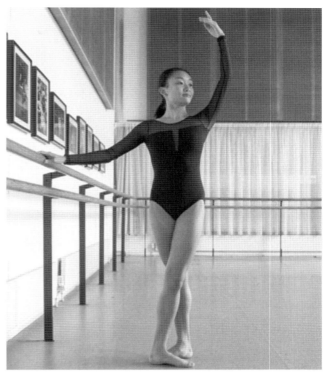

Figura 41.5 Braços na quinta posição. (Dançarina: Yaoqian Shang; fotógrafo: Ty Singleton.)

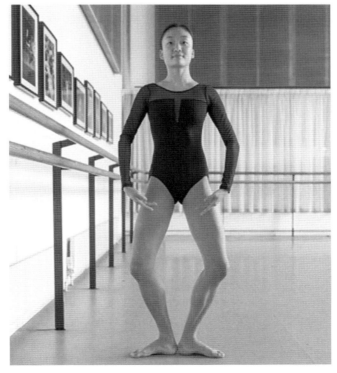

Figura 41.6 *Plié* na primeira posição braços *bras bas*. (Dançarina: Yaoqian Shang; fotógrafo: Ty Singleton.)

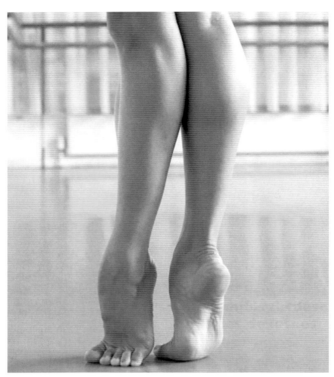

Figura 41.7 Quinta posição en *demi-pointe*. (Dançarina: Yaoqian Shang; fotógrafo: Ty Singleton.)

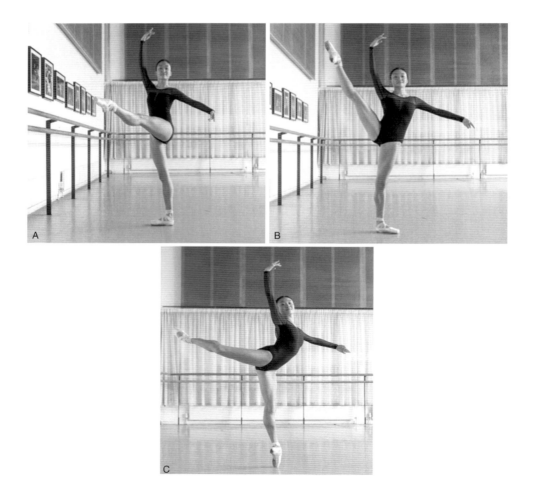

Figura 41.8 A. *Développé devant en croisé.* B. *Développé* na segunda posição. C. *Attitude derrière effacé en pointe*, braços na quarta posição. (Dançarina: Yaoqian Shang; fotógrafo: Ty Singleton.)

Movimentos mais dinâmicos ou balísticos incluem piruetas e *fouettés* (girar), *jeté* e *sissonnes* (saltos, Figura 41.9), e *pas de deux* (parceria/levantar/ser levantado).

Da perspectiva contemporânea, podem ser encontradas mais descrições baseadas em movimento; embora muitos movimentos tenham suas origens no movimento do balé, eles evoluíram e não podem mais ser descritos facilmente usando a mesma terminologia. A dança contemporânea pode envolver mais "trabalho no chão", no qual os dançarinos utilizam o contato com o chão em uma extensão maior do que no balé, sendo que "bater" no chão não é incomum. Esse aspecto do trabalho contemporâneo pode aumentar a incidência de lesões nos membros superiores e até mesmo por concussão. A parceria na dança contemporânea também pode ser diferente. Em vez de executar algumas das linhas mais claras exibidas no balé, os dançarinos contemporâneos são conhecidos por se engajarem em elevações baseadas em impulso, usando rotação e ângulos. Isso permite que eles criem içamentos que podem ser executados por parceiros menores com parceiros maiores. Embora isso apoie a ambição artística, se não for bem executado, introduz uma carga desproporcional e aumenta o risco de lesões.

Reabilitação de um dançarino

A reabilitação de qualquer atleta é um processo multifatorial com inúmeras considerações, incluindo natureza e gravidade da lesão, fatores predisponentes, momento na temporada e carreira, lesão anterior etc. Aplicar a especificidade da dança aos modelos etiológicos tradicionais permite ao profissional formular uma estratégia em torno do processo de reabilitação para considerar algumas áreas não necessariamente vistas em outras populações esportivas.

Ao examinar um paciente, o profissional de saúde formula ideias em torno do diagnóstico da lesão, possíveis fatores causais, bem como os resultados funcionais exigidos pelo atleta ou dançarino para um retorno seguro, incluindo a redução do risco de recorrência.

É importante estabelecer um diagnóstico claro com a compreensão da origem dos sintomas. A diferenciação da origem dos sintomas em químicos (inflamatórios), mecânicos (carga sobre o tecido) ou ambos auxiliarão no processo de manejo e no desenho da reabilitação, pensando inclusive em aspectos relacionados à dor. Nas lesões traumáticas, pode haver uma expectativa de origem química devido ao trauma tecidual de um evento estimulante. Em lesões por excesso de uso, a influência da carga biomecânica no desenvolvimento dos sintomas é mais provável, com uma apresentação combinada de química e mecânica. Em bailarinos, há uma maior prevalência de lesões por excesso de uso. Isso requer que o profissional de saúde examinador realize uma avaliação biomecânica completa para estabelecer a origem e o nexo de causalidade.

Os programas de tratamento de lesões, incluindo reabilitação, são centrados na avaliação do que está impedindo o paciente de realizar tudo o que faria normalmente. É a lesão aguda e a dor/limitação associada a ela? Existe alguma força subjacente ou déficit de potência? Existe uma capacidade funcional limitada devido à falta de treinamento adequado?

O modelo intervencionista híbrido (MIH) é um modelo teórico projetado para permitir que os médicos planejem as estratégias empregadas durante o processo de lesão e reabilitação (Allen et al., 2013) (Figura 41.10). O modelo propõe a implementação de três suportes, a saber: treinamento de base neuromuscular, carga segmentar (incluindo força ou resistência a fadiga em demanda de potência) e integração funcional. A chave para a implementação do MIH é a sequência (neuromuscular seguida de força seguida de integração funcional) e as proporções relativas dos diferentes componentes em cada estágio do episódio de lesão. As proporções relativas são influenciadas pela avaliação do fator limitante atual pelo profissional de saúde.

No estágio inicial de uma lesão aguda, o provável fator limitante é a própria lesão e qualquer dor associada e, portanto, constitui o foco do programa de manejo. Um resultado notável da dor na lesão aguda é o impacto na inibição muscular. Dentro do MIH, a facilitação neuromuscular formaria o maior componente do programa de reabilitação para restaurar e apoiar a ativação muscular durante esse momento-chave. O exercício neuromuscular é normalmente bem tolerado na presença de dor e, portanto, adapta-se bem nos estágios iniciais.

À medida que o paciente progride nos estágios da lesão, o próximo fator limitante e o foco do manejo podem ser a causa da lesão. Aqui, a identificação e o tratamento de qualquer potencial déficit de força ou potência pode ser a maior proporção do desenho do programa. Nesse estágio, o programa ainda começará com exercícios de ativação muscular, mas também incluirá alguns exercícios de ativação funcional no final da sessão.

Nos estágios finais de uma lesão, o foco e o manejo mudam para os requisitos funcionais do atleta para seu retorno seguro ao desempenho ou competição. Uma ativação muscular mais curta e um programa baseado na força serão seguidos por um componente funcionalmente dirigido estendido. Na reabilitação de bailarinos, é importante otimizar a carga como parte dessa preparação e treinamento de resiliência. Esta é uma parte fundamental do componente de integração funcional do MIH. Ele permite a criação de uma carga crônica adequada por meio do programa de reabilitação para construir resistência para os picos inevitáveis na carga de trabalho aguda tipicamente vistos na dança profissional. Ele considera o impacto da carga da carreira, da carga das temporadas anteriores, bem como da carga de treinamento crônica das 4 semanas anteriores. A pesquisa sugeriu que os atletas mais jovens podem ter maior risco de lesões devido à falta de carga de treinamento crônica adequada e os atletas mais velhos podem estar

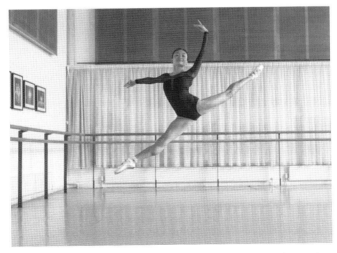

Figura 41.9 *Sissonne* com os braços na quarta posição. (Dançarina: Yaoqian Shang; fotógrafo: Ty Singleton.)

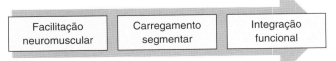

Figura 41.10 Modelo intervencionista híbrido.

mais em risco devido à carga crônica acumulativa excessiva ou lesão anterior que afeta a carga de treinamento. A pesquisa também sugere que picos na carga de trabalho aguda podem resultar em aumento da lesão por estresse ósseo; isso pode ser de particular relevância para dançarinos mais jovens que ainda não possuem a carga de trabalho crônica para se apoiar contra esses picos. Em contraste, a carga de trabalho crônica acumulativa excessiva pode resultar em aumento do risco de alterações patológicas nas superfícies articulares, um problema associado a dançarinos mais velhos e experientes. Todas essas questões devem ser consideradas ao projetar programas de reabilitação para dançarinos.

Critérios de retorno à dança

Ao determinar a adequação de retorno ao jogo na população esportiva, geralmente fica claro quais critérios físicos são necessários para o retorno total, já que a natureza do esporte em questão, embora afetada pela oposição, fornece um grau relativo de consistência. Na dança, devido ao vasto potencial de variação nas demandas fisiológicas de diferentes coreografias e papéis, a decisão de um dançarino de retornar à performance é mais matizada. Requer uma compreensão total do que é exigido no papel ao qual o dançarino retornará. Um retorno gradual pode ser considerado se a função envolvida não exigir capacidade física total; nesse caso, o retorno ao compromisso de desempenho de nível total em um ponto posterior deve ser contingente à conclusão do processo de reabilitação. Como nos esportes, "voltar a jogar" precisa ser uma decisão da equipe que envolva o dançarino, a equipe artística, a clínica e a equipe de condicionamento. A equipe artística pode esclarecer os requisitos físicos do dançarino necessários para os próximos ensaios e papéis desempenhados. É importante entender a perspectiva do dançarino; é importante ter consciência de suas opiniões sobre contratos, desenvolvimento de carreira e pressão de desempenho.

Do ponto de vista clínico, a adaptação de um modelo esportivo comumente usado pode orientar o profissional de saúde no processo de decisão. Na ausência de dados de linha de base pré-temporada, o uso de teste de índice de simetria de membro pode fornecer um ponto de referência útil para lesões de membros superiores e inferiores. Um índice de simetria de membro ≤ 25% dá alguma sugestão de um risco de lesão reduzido com base na literatura de reabilitação do ligamento cruzado anterior e protocolos de retorno ao jogo e ≤ 10% dá uma confiança ainda mais forte de que não haverá déficit de desempenho. Os testes podem ser ajustados para se adequar a patologias específicas, mas para o membro inferior podem incluir:
- Movimento normal:
  - Teste de movimento funcional para avaliar a competência de movimento e controle neuromuscular
- Amplitude de movimento:
  - Amplitude de movimento do quadril (particularmente a rotação interna como um indicador de como os rotadores externos do quadril estão lidando)
  - Joelho na parede – um indicador de simetria para posições funcionais como *plié* e a habilidade de abaixar os calcanhares durante os saltos
- Equilíbrio/propriocepção:
  - Teste de equilíbrio
  - *Biodex* (dinamometria isocinética) – teste atlético unipodal
  - *Hop and hold* – avaliação do controle
- Força muscular:
  - Salto – altura, distância, resistência, simetria (distância em salto único, distância em saltos repetidos, cruzamentos, velocidade sobre distância etc.)
  - Salto – Optojump/plataforma de força (se disponível)

- Força muscular:
  - Joelho, isocinética de extensão/flexão de tornozelo (se disponível).

Outros testes funcionais incluem a participação incremental nas fases da aula (barra, centro e saltos) com trabalho adicional de levantamento/parceria, conforme relevante, mas que deve ser incluído com todos os dançarinos que são obrigados a levantar como parte de sua função para certificar-se de que estão seguros para prosseguir.

Uma parte desafiadora da decisão de voltar à dança gira em torno da avaliação de força e resistência a fadiga em demanda de potência. A natureza da dança pode envolver sessões prolongadas de intervalos de alta intensidade contra trabalhos mais longos e de baixa intensidade. O uso de força repetida (elevações ou elevações repetidas) e exercícios de potência (exercícios pliométricos na *jump box*) com sessões curtas de recuperação pode ajudar na avaliação e preparação. Além disso, a avaliação da carga de treinamento crônica de um papel (um resultado da exposição combinada com a intensidade do treinamento) ajudará a estabelecer a adequação para o retorno a um período de performance, em vez de apenas se o dançarino pode cumprir os requisitos técnicos para um único *show*.

Papel da triagem na dança

O papel da triagem na previsão de lesões é uma área de debate. Há uma falta de consenso quanto ao seu valor na previsão de lesões e, além disso, o que o rastreamento deve implicar. A triagem na dança pode incluir uma análise do estágio básico de condicionamento do dançarino, no qual os programas de melhoria de desempenho e prevenção de lesões podem ser baseados.

Triagem clínica

Os exames médicos padrão usados no esporte, conforme defendidos pelo Comitê Olímpico Internacional como uma Avaliação Periódica da Saúde, ajudarão aqueles que gerenciam os dançarinos (Ljungqvist et al., 2009). O questionamento sobre a frequência do ciclo menstrual e a ingestão alimentar pode fornecer informações sobre o risco potencial associado a déficits relativos de energia. Com exceção do ambiente de salão de baile competitivo, os dançarinos não estão sujeitos aos regulamentos e testes da Agência Mundial Antidopagem. O papel do profissional de saúde deve incluir educar os dançarinos sobre os riscos dos medicamentos para melhorar o desempenho e isso pode ser coberto por meio da triagem médica.

A triagem cardíaca no esporte é uma área em crescimento, com muitos esportes defendendo um eletrocardiograma (ECG) de repouso e histórico familiar antes da participação no alto nível. Faltam pesquisas sobre o risco cardíaco em dançarinos. Seguindo nossa própria pesquisa que incluiu ECG, ecocardiograma e histórico familiar, até que pesquisas adicionais mostrem o contrário, defendemos a necessidade de pelo menos um histórico familiar e ECG de repouso para bailarinos adultos.

Rastreamento musculoesquelético

Avaliações musculoesqueléticas da amplitude de movimento articular e força muscular têm sido empregadas em vários esportes. A pesquisa em esportes sugeriu que a rotação interna reduzida nos ombros e quadris pode estar ligada ao aumento do risco de lesões. Do mesmo modo, a amplitude de movimento aumentada ou excessiva tem sido associada ao risco de lesões por meio da estabilidade diminuída. A hipermobilidade articular generalizada foi encontrada em esportes em que a amplitude de movimento adquirida excede a faixa fisiológica normal. Os dançarinos podem normalmente exceder a gama de movimentos

Introdução à Medicina da Dança **Capítulo** | **41** |

observada na maioria das populações esportivas. Além disso, a pesquisa demonstrou uma prevalência mais alta de transtornos do espectro de hipermobilidade (TEH; formalmente conhecidos como síndromes articulares de hipermobilidade benigna) em escolas profissionalizantes e nos escalões mais baixos de companhias de balé profissional (abaixo do nível principal) em comparação com a população em geral. No entanto, uma análise mais aprofundada mostra uma prevalência mais baixa de TEH nos escalões superiores das companhias de balé profissionais em comparação com a população em geral. Sugeriu-se que a identificação de talentos em dançarinos mais jovens se concentrou em maior flexibilidade ou "facilidade", como visto em pessoas com TEH, mas a capacidade de suportar as demandas físicas de balé de alto nível requer maior estabilidade. No entanto, é importante reconhecer o impacto e aplicar estratégias de manejo adequadas para dançarinos com maior mobilidade. O uso dos critérios de Brighton (Grahame et al., 2000) como uma avaliação de TEH pode auxiliar nas decisões de manejo em torno da natureza dos programas de suporte necessários.

A diferenciação entre TEH e hipermobilidade adquirida é importante do ponto de vista do modelo da saúde, pois o TEH pode impactar na função autonômica, fadiga, dor, taquicardia ortostática postural, funções gastrintestinais, da bexiga ou pélvicas. Além disso, o impacto da amplitude de movimento excessiva é considerável no que diz respeito ao risco de lesões e direcionamento de treino preventivo. A pesquisa demonstrou diferenças posturais notáveis e aumento da dor em 35 indivíduos com TEH em comparação com controles pareados. A articulação do joelho tem se mostrado a com maior risco de hipermobilidade (Booshanam et al., 2011). Foi encontrada uma relação entre hipermobilidade articular generalizada e um histórico de instabilidade glenoumeral (P = 0,23) em recrutas militares (Cameron et al., 2010). Além disso, os pacientes com hipermobilidade têm maior incidência de luxações recorrentes do ombro (60% *versus* 39%) (Muhammad et al., 2013). Finalmente, correlações positivas entre TEH e hérnias de disco lombar também foram relatadas (Aktas et al., 2011).

Teste de movimento

Competência de movimento por meio de teste de movimento normal, como a tela de movimento funcional (TMF), pode ajudar a elucidar onde os dançarinos lutam para controlar certos movimentos "normais" enquanto alcançam níveis notáveis de habilidade em movimentos específicos da dança. No entanto, o nível mais alto de flexibilidade precisa ser considerado na interpretação do teste de movimento normal, em vez de empregar avaliações e análises genéricas tiradas de outras populações esportivas.

A avaliação de alguns movimentos específicos da dança pode agregar valor, mas requer uma boa análise técnica. Por exemplo, pode-se notar que em um *plié* na segunda posição, um dançarino está alcançando sua virada por meio da rotação tibial excessiva em vez da rotação externa do quadril, aumentando assim o risco de lesão no joelho ou na tíbia. Além disso, a simetria pode ser avaliada observando uma mudança no alinhamento por meio dos membros inferiores.

Os testes de condicionamento físico são um desafio no ambiente da dança. Dentro dos esportes, o aprimoramento da tecnologia proporciona um aumento nos testes em campo que mostram boas correlações com variáveis fisiológicas reconhecidas como $\dot{V}O_{2máx}$. O uso de um teste específico para a dança, como o Teste de Aptidão Aeróbica de Dança, desenvolvido pelo Professor Wyon, pode ajudar a fornecer uma análise dos níveis de aptidão física específicos da dança; ele apresenta boas correlações com o $\dot{V}O_{2máx}$ tanto para bailarinos contemporâneos, quanto para bailarinos clássicos (Wyon et al., 2003).

Resumo

O termo "atleta artístico" é adequado para a dança; é o resultado da aptidão artística em um contexto de demandas fisiológicas. A chave para apoiar com sucesso esses atletas notáveis é entender a especificidade de sua disciplina. Isso inclui a aplicação de modificadores de risco por meio da compreensão do risco intrínseco e extrínseco. A utilização de um modelo de reabilitação como o MIH permite que os profissionais de saúde planejem programas que incorporem os aspectos fundamentais do controle neuromuscular, da força e da capacidade funcional necessários para a dança. Voltar para a dança após uma lesão apresenta desafios semelhantes aos do esporte, e testes sistemáticos e estratégias de saída podem reduzir o risco de nova lesão e déficits de desempenho. Tendo na prevenção de lesões um objetivo principal, a utilização de informações obtidas na exibição de dança pode aumentar a base sobre a qual os programas de prevenção de lesões podem ser baseados.

Referências bibliográficas

Aktas, I., Ofluolu, D., Akgün, K., 2011. Relationship between lumbar disc herniation and benign joint hypermobility syndrome. Turkish Journal of Physical Medicine and Rehabilitation 57, 85-88.

Allen, N., Nevill, A., Brooks, J., Koutedakis, Y., Wyon, M., 2012. Ballet injuries: injury incidence and severity over 1 year. Journal of Orthopaedic & Sports Physical Therapy 42 (9), 781-790.

Allen, N., Ribbans, W.J., Nevill, A.M., Wyon, M.A., 2014. Musculoskeletal injuries in dance: a systematic review. International Journal of Physical Medicine & Rehabilitation 3 (1), 1-8.

Allen, N., Nevill, A.M., Brooks, J.H., Koutedakis, Y., Wyon, M.A., 2013. The effect of a comprehensive injury audit program on injury incidence in ballet: a 3-year prospective study. Clinical Journal of Sport Medicine 23 (5), 373-378.

Booshanam, D.S., Cherian, B., Joseph, C.P., Mathew, J., Thomas, R., 2011. Evaluation of posture and pain in persons with benign joint hypermobility syndrome. Rheumatology International 31 (12), 1561-1565.

Bronner, S., Ojofeitimi, S., Rose, D., 2003. Injuries in a modern dance company. Effect of comprehensive management on injury incidence and time loss. The American Journal of Sports Medicine 31 (3), 365-373.

Cameron, K.L., Duffey, M.L., DeBerardino, T.M., Stoneman, P.D., Jones, C.J., Owens, B.D., 2010. Association of generalized joint hypermobility with a history of glenohumeral joint instability. Journal of Athletic Training 45 (3), 253-258.

Grahame, R., Bird, H.A., Child, A., 2000. The revised (Brighton 1998) criteria for the diagnosis of benign joint hypermobility syndrome (BJHS). Journal of Rheumatology 27 (7), 1777-1779.

Hopper, L.S., Allen, N., Wyon, M., Alderson, J.A., Elliott, B.C., Ackland, T.R., 2013. Dance floor mechanical properties and dancer injuries in a touring professional ballet company. Journal of Science and Medicine In Sport / Sports Medicine Australia 17 (1), 29-33.

Ljungqvist, A., Jenoure, P.J., Engebretsen, L., Alonso, J.M., Bahr, R., Clough, A.F., et al., 2009. The International Olympic Committee (IOC) consensus statement on periodic health evaluation of elite athletes March 2009. British Journal of Sports Medicine 43 (9), 631-643.

Muhammad, A.A., Jenkins, P., Ashton, F., Christopher, M.R., 2013. Hypermobility – a risk factor for recurrent shoulder dislocations. British Journal of Sports Medicine 47, e3.

Ojofeitimi, S., Bronner, S., Woo, H., 2012. Injury incidence in hip hop dance. Scandinavian Journal of Medicine & Science in Sports 22 (3), 347-355.

Wyon, M., Redding, E., Abt, G., et.al., 2003. Development, reliability and validity of a multistage dance specific aerobic fitness test (DAFT). Journal of Dance Medicine and Science, 7 (3), 80-84.

Wyon, M., Allen, N., Cloak, R., Needham-Beck, S., 2016. Assessment of maximum aerobic capacity and anaerobic threshold of elite ballet dancers. Medical Problems of Performing Artists 31 (3), 145-150.

Seção | 2 | Considerações Práticas

Capítulo | 42 |

Preparação para Responder a uma Emergência

Natalie Shur, Paulina Czubacka, Jim Moxon, Rohi Shah, Tom Hallas e Johnny Wilson

Preparação para ação de emergência

Os membros da equipe do departamento médico que trabalham no esporte profissional têm segundos para tomar uma decisão que pode ter um impacto significativo na saúde do jogador. A exposição a eventos traumáticos e com risco de morte pode não ser uma ocorrência comum no esporte, mas quando eles surgem, a equipe médica no local precisa estar pronta para reagir imediatamente e de maneira coordenada para gerenciar a situação emergencial. Os médicos devem possuir as ferramentas certas para o trabalho – seja uma entorse de tornozelo ou uma parada cardíaca. O Protocolo de Ação de Emergência (PAE) deve ser constantemente revisado; a exposição a certos eventos deve levar à reflexão e, quando apropriado, à implementação de mudanças para desenvolver a prática. A medicina esportiva está evoluindo diariamente, movida pela discussão, pelo compartilhamento de práticas e pela cooperação de equipes médicas adversárias em caso de traumas graves no campo de jogo (CDJ). O objetivo deste capítulo é fornecer uma visão sobre o trabalho diário do departamento médico no esporte profissional, discutindo os seguintes aspectos:
- PAE
- Equipamentos e consumíveis usados diariamente por prestadores de cuidados médicos no esporte profissional
- Considerações para a prescrição e a administração de medicamentos em ambientes esportivos
- Processo de extricação (salvamento da vítima) para cenários de emergência
- Processo de transferência
- *Debriefing*, que irá melhorar a prática
- Qualificações de primeiros socorros de emergência necessárias.

Protocolo de Ação de Emergência

Fundamentos

O PAE incorpora a noção de que qualquer provedor de auxílio emergencial, dada a prática e a preparação adequadas, deve ser capaz de avaliar e lidar com segurança com a maioria dos cenários clínicos de emergência. Eles são uma parte crítica para garantir a segurança do atleta durante o treinamento e a competição. No entanto, quando surgem circunstâncias que estão fora da norma convencional, a utilização de uma abordagem sistemática de *vias respiratórias (airway), respiração (breathing), circulação, deficiência, exposição* (A-E) ajudará a avaliar, identificar e tratar atletas com lesões potencialmente fatais. Esses são os princípios fundamentais ensinados em qualquer curso de resposta à emergência pré-hospitalar, e o treinamento é frequentemente um pré-requisito para trabalhar no ambiente esportivo.

Sabe-se bem que os praticantes de esportes não lidam com lesões que ameacem os membros ou a vida diariamente, visto que os atletas são normalmente considerados a coorte mais saudável da população em geral. Quando surgem situações de emergência, geralmente há um evento traumático causador em oposição a um problema patológico subjacente. Portanto, quando patologias clínicas perigosas ocorrem inesperadamente, pânico, pessoal e treinamento incompetentes, equipamentos inadequados ou simplesmente planejamento e preparação inadequados podem levar a resultados fatais. Frequentemente, a causa subjacente é multifatorial, ou seja, o modelo do queijo suíço (Reason, 2000). Isso destaca a importância de ter uma rotina sistemática e bem praticada para lidar com qualquer emergência.

Os cursos de emergência podem fornecer uma base e delinear um sistema de gestão. No entanto, a menos que seja praticado, utilizado e atualizado rotineiramente, esse fundamento se perde facilmente. A natureza caótica dos dias de jogo, agravada pelas pressões do jogador e da gestão, muitas vezes faz com que o PAE seja um acordo verbal rápido entre os provedores e, às vezes, o time visitante pode ser completamente excluído desse plano. A maioria dos ambientes esportivos são atividades altamente visíveis e divulgadas, com o manejo de cada incidente sob escrutínio. As falhas são frequentemente enfatizadas na mídia, destacando a necessidade de lidar com as emergências de forma sistemática e eficiente.

Guia para o Protocolo de Ação de Emergência

Uma tentativa de abordar o PAE no ambiente dinâmico de eventos esportivos é a implementação do "quadro PAE" (Figura 42.1)

Parte | 2 | Aplicação Clínica

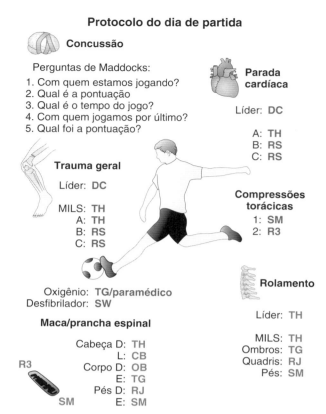

Figura 42.1 Exemplo de placa de Protocolo de Ação de Emergência para referência ao conduzir instruções para a equipe médica antes de eventos esportivos (as siglas correspondem às iniciais dos nomes de uma equipe hipotética).

por Shah et al. (2018). Esse quadro projetado para fins específicos define as funções dos membros da equipe no caso de uma emergência. Um intervalo dedicado para isso deve ocorrer antes de cada partida em casa, designando e revisando claramente as funções individuais. Isso varia de cenários gerais de trauma, em que um único membro gerencia as vias respiratórias com estabilização da coluna cervical, até cenários com maior risco de morte, em que os membros da equipe recebem funções específicas para as vias respiratórias, respiração e circulação. Isso segue até o manejo isolado do membro em trauma ou torção de um paciente antes da extricação. Um líder de equipe designado deve estar fora da movimentação para supervisionar o cenário.

O treinamento de simulação de rotina, que replica prováveis cenários de emergência da vida real antes de uma partida, permite que a equipe pratique o trabalho em sincronia e se torne eficiente em termos de tempo. Isso também permite que os membros da equipe reflitam sobre seu desempenho e identifiquem as áreas a serem melhoradas (Figura 42.2).

Com o aumento da conscientização sobre patologias cardíacas, incluindo parada cardíaca súbita (PCS), ter um protocolo estrito com funções A-E designadas permite intervenções em que o tempo é um fator crítico. No caso de um colapso não traumático, a PCS deve ser presumida e, portanto, a aplicação precoce de um desfibrilador e a realização de compressões torácicas eficazes são essenciais, mudando efetivamente a abordagem clássica A-B-C (vias respiratórias [*airway*], respiração [*breathing*], circulação) para uma abordagem C-A-B (circulação, vias respiratórias [*airway*], respiração [*breathing*]). O quadro PAE é responsável por designar qual membro da equipe iniciará as compressões torácicas, aplicará um desfibrilador e obterá acesso venoso para administração de medicamentos. A sessão específica antes de um evento esportivo é um momento importante para se comunicar e envolver as equipes paramédicas, líderes de equipes externas ou qualquer pessoal prestando atendimento de emergência no dia, para designar sua função específica durante uma emergência. A disponibilidade da ambulância deve ser conhecida antes do evento, incluindo o tempo de chegada ao local ou, se estiver no local, onde deve ficar.

O material impresso destacando a disponibilidade e a localização do equipamento no local, saídas de emergência, detalhes de contato de emergência e o departamento de acidente e emergência hospitalar mais próximo deve estar prontamente disponível e distribuído aos líderes da equipe visitante. Enquanto o quadro PAE fornece um lembrete visual simples de funções pré-designadas, simplesmente ter um momento antes de qualquer evento esportivo para discutir e alocar funções garante que uma equipe possa trabalhar com eficiência e como uma unidade.

A preparação do dia do jogo reforça e adapta de muitas maneiras os princípios básicos ensinados em cursos de resposta à emergência. No entanto, a menos que praticado de forma rotineira, os principais aspectos da prestação de cuidados de emergência podem ser facilmente negligenciados e mal executados. A criação de uma etapa organizacional simples com uma sessão dedicada antes de um evento esportivo pode ajudar a criar uma abordagem sistemática para lidar de forma eficaz com emergências médicas.

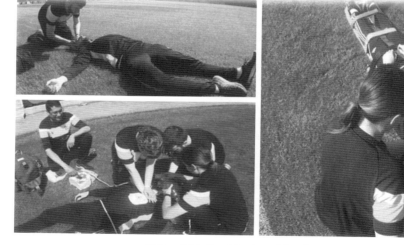

Figura 42.2 Cenário de prática de emergência: parada cardíaca.

Preparação para Responder a uma Emergência **Capítulo** | 42 |

Conteúdo do *kit* médico e da sacola de viagem

Kit médico

O equipamento que um médico carrega ao lado do campo deve ser suficiente para lidar com qualquer emergência, caso ela aconteça. A comunicação com os paramédicos e a equipe médica geral antes de qualquer evento é fundamental para identificar quais

equipamentos cada um carrega e é responsável. A Tabela 42.1 apresenta os equipamentos essenciais, com a justificativa, que o médico deve carregar nos dias de jogos para eventos esportivos.

Kit do fisioterapeuta

Cada profissional da saúde deve estar ciente do que é necessário em sua bolsa "de campo". Alguns países podem ter legislações ou recomendações específicas, assim como os times podem determinar em protocolo, em sua equipe, quais são os itens que cada *kit*

Tabela 42.1 **Equipamento recomendado exigido em um *kit* médico do lado do campo.**

Sistema	Equipamento	Justificativa
Via respiratória e respiração	Vias respiratórias orofaríngeas e nasofaríngeas, seleção de tamanhos	Adjuntos das vias respiratórias
	Máscara de bolso	Equipamento de proteção pessoal
	Bolsa-máscara-válvula (ambu)	Ventilação
	Máscara sem *rebreather*	Para entrega de oxigênio de alto fluxo
	Kit de sucção portátil	Remover secreções
	Oxímetro de pulso	Medição de saturação de oxigênio
	Tanque de oxigênio	Hipoxia
	Fórceps de Magill	Obstrução por corpo estranho
	Gel lubrificante	Lubrificar os acessórios das vias respiratórias antes da inserção
Circulação	Desfibrilador externo automatizado	Parada cardíaca
	Estetoscópio	Auscultação
	Esfigmomanômetro	Medição da pressão arterial
	Cânula intravenosa e conjuntos de administração	Estabelecer acesso intravenoso para fluidos/medicamentos
	Ligante pélvico	Fratura pélvica
	Lixeira de objetos cortantes	Eliminação de perfurocortantes
	Gaze estéril	Hemostasia para cortes/abrasões
Disfunção	Monitor de glicose sanguínea	Avaliação rápida de glicose sanguínea
	Lanterna de caneta	Avaliação do tamanho da pupila/avaliação orofaríngea
Tratamento de feridas	*Steristrips*	Fechamento de ferida
	Cola para feridas	Fechamento de ferida
	Suturas	Fechamento de ferida
	Tampões nasais	Epistaxe
Outros	Acesso intraósseo	Se não for possível estabelecer o acesso IV
	Kit de cricotireoidotomia	Se incapaz de proteger as vias respiratórias usando adjuvantes
	Luvas	Equipamento de proteção pessoal
	Termômetro	Medição de temperatura
	Câmara do nebulizador para máscara sem respirador	Distribuir salbutamol nebulizado em caso de broncospasmo

IV, intravenoso.

431

deve conter, criando uma *checklist* própria. Atualmente, é uma prática comum ter grandes bolsas de corrida contendo equipamentos não essenciais ao cuidar de um jogador ao lado do campo.

A principal preocupação ao atender o jogador ao lado do campo é o manejo das vias respiratórias, respiração e circulação do atleta e isso deve ser refletido pelo conteúdo das bolsas do médico e do fisioterapeuta. A Figura 42.3 apresenta um exemplo de conteúdo para a bolsa "de campo" de um fisioterapeuta e a Tabela 42.2 lista o equipamento que prepara o médico adequadamente para esses cenários de emergência. Todas as peças de equipamento dentro de uma bolsa devem ser fundamentadas e conter peças exigidas pelo corpo clínico que rege o esporte em questão.

Durante o ano do calendário esportivo, a maioria dos profissionais de saúde esportiva viajam para longe de suas instalações regulares. Isso requer um planejamento meticuloso para permitir ao médico realizar tratamentos regulares, bem como lidar com situações de emergência enquanto estiver ausente. Se viajar longas distâncias no exterior, pode ser necessário fornecer certos equipamentos (p. ex., gases comprimidos e desfibrilador externo automático [DEA]) antes da viagem, pois podem não ser autorizados a serem transferidos em um avião. O clima também desempenha um papel importante na preparação para uma viagem fora, pois os atletas podem ser expostos a temperaturas extremas. Se os jogadores precisarem de certos tipos de medicamentos, o médico deve se assegurar de levar o suficiente para a duração da viagem. Um exemplo de lista de equipamentos para uma mala de viagem é apresentado na Figura 42.4 e na Tabela 42.3.

Os dias de jogo podem ser dias atarefados no departamento médico. Portanto, certos consumíveis podem ser colocados no vestiário para permitir que os próprios jogadores gerenciem as fitas, os cuidados com as bolhas, o enrolamento de espuma e o alongamento para a preparação antes da partida (Figura 42.5).

Prescrição

Ao fornecer suporte médico durante eventos esportivos, os médicos precisarão ter acesso a uma extensa lista de medicamentos para gerenciar a maioria das situações médicas, caso elas surjam. Um profissional deve ser capaz de justificar todos os itens em sua mochila. Se você não sabe por que um item está na sua bolsa, ou não se sente confortável em prescrevê-lo, livre-se dele. A Tabela 42.4 representa um guia para os medicamentos recomendados para se ter acesso; entretanto, esta lista será influenciada pelo histórico médico de seus atletas.

O uso de medicamentos em atletas tem ganhado atenção nos últimos anos. As evidências sugerem que atletas de alto nível usam medicamentos antiasmáticos, anti-histamínicos, anti-inflamatórios não esteroides (AINEs) e antibióticos orais com significativamente mais frequência do que controles da mesma idade (Alaranta et al., 2008). É vital prescrever esses medicamentos criteriosamente para reduzir o risco de efeitos colaterais, que podem afetar negativamente o desempenho. Os médicos devem se familiarizar com a lista de substâncias proibidas da Agência Mundial Antidoping (WADA, do inglês *World Anti-Doping Agency*), que é atualizada a cada mês de janeiro. Incentive os jogadores a consultar um médico experiente da equipe antes de administrar suplementos ou quando prescritos por outro profissional, visto que nem todos os médicos estão cientes da lista da WADA. Deve-se ter cuidado para observar não apenas os medicamentos proibidos, mas aqueles que têm um limite de dose, por exemplo, salbutamol. Se medicamentos proibidos são necessários em uma situação de emergência, um pedido de isenção de uso terapêutico (IUT) deve ser feito na primeira oportunidade disponível.

A prescrição em um ambiente de alto desempenho apresenta vários desafios. Os jogadores costumam solicitar analgesia. Frequentemente, analgesia é administrada profilaticamente pelos jogadores, apesar de não apresentarem dor ou lesão; alguns podem depender disso como apoio psicológico antes dos jogos. Os jogadores podem pedir dosagem inadequada ou formulações de analgesia para problemas menores de dor. Em geral, recomendamos evitar AINE nas primeiras 48 horas após uma lesão, pois pode estimular mais sangramento (Lippi et al., 2006).

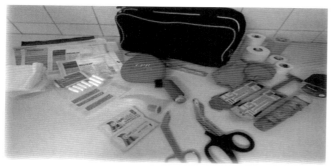

Figura 42.3 Exemplo de equipamento para bolsa "de campo" do fisioterapeuta no Reino Unido.

Tabela 42.2 Equipamento recomendado exigido em um *kit* de fisioterapeuta ao lado do campo.

Vias respiratórias e respiração	Circulação	Outros
Adjunto da via respiratória orofaríngea: usado para abrir e manter as vias respiratórias do atleta *Lubrificante das vias respiratórias*: ajuda na aplicação do adjunto das vias respiratórias *Máscara de RCP*: cria uma vedação para respirações mais eficazes e evita o contato direto atleta-médico *Cânula IV*: usada para descompressão de um pneumotórax suspeito *Inalador para asma (se necessário)*: transportado na bolsa se houver jogadores asmáticos na equipe; usado para aliviar os sintomas	*Curativo para trauma*: usado para grandes sangramentos *Botões nasais*: usados para sangramentos nasais *Vaselina*: usada para ajudar a parar/prevenir o sangramento de pequenos cortes *Gaze*: usada para compressão para ajudar a parar o sangramento *Toalhetes com álcool e solução salina*: usados para limpar feridas *Curativos*: aplicados em feridas para manter a compressão e reduzir o risco de infecção *Fita*: AAE para aplicar compressão extra e segurar o curativo aplicado na ferida no lugar	*Luvas*: usadas para reduzir o risco de infecção *Navalha*: para retirar os pelos para aplicação de DEA *Tesoura de corte de tufo*: para remover roupas/botas/fita para expor a área *Fita*: AAE, óxido de zinco: tala de dedo, fita de articulação *Epipen*: usado para administrar epinefrina em caso de choque anafilático *Soro fisiológico*: usado para limpar um olho/remover a sujeira do olho *Lentes de contato (se necessário)*: quando os atletas usam lentes durante eventos esportivos

RCP, reanimação cardiopulmonar; *DEA*, desfibrilador externo automático; *AAE*, atadura adesiva elástica; *IV*, intravenosa.

Preparação para Responder a uma Emergência **Capítulo** | 42 |

Tabela 42.3 **Exemplo de equipamento para uma bolsa de viagem para um médico esportivo.**

Consumíveis do dia do jogo	*Deep Heat®*, *Vick Vaporub®*, pinças, tesouras para unhas, tesouras para tufos, tesouras para ataduras em bolha, protetores para os dedos dos pés
Tratamento de feridas	Botões nasais, emplastros adesivos, curativo militar, curativos de iodo, curativos *Jelonet®*, fitas esterilizadas, tapa-olho, curativo para os dedos, curativo triangular, curativos adesivos de tamanhos variados, toalhetes de limpeza de feridas, cápsulas de solução salina
Consumíveis	*TubiGrip®* (vários tamanhos), toalhetes de limpeza de superfície, divisórias de dedo do pé, tratamento para bolhas na segunda pele, *Hypafix®*, cera de massagem, creme de massagem, caixa para perfurocortantes, gaze não estéril, agulhas de acupuntura de tamanhos variados, vaselina, luvas nitrílicas P/M/G, protetor solar, creme pós-sol, *spray* de iodo, *spray* de pré-fita, *spray* para remoção de fita, *spray* para congelamento de feridas, repelente de insetos, pó de talco
Ajuda de emergência/consumíveis	AOF, ANF, lubrificante para vias respiratórias, baterias DEA, máscara de RCP, MVB, máscara sem respirador, nebulizador, cânula IV, manta metálica, navalha
Fita	*Underwrap®*, óxido de zinco 2,5/3,5/5 cm, fita adesiva elástica 5/7,5 cm, fita cinesiológica
Outros	Sacos de gelo, sacos de lixo clínico, cintos de segurança, enchimento de espuma, fita métrica, *TheraBands®*, formulários em caso de emergência (I.C.E), formulários, formulários PCST5, formulários de incidentes de emergência, PAE para um local, caneta, marcador permanente, medidor de pressão arterial

DEA, desfibrilador externo automático; *MVB*, máscara de válvula de bolsa; *RCP*, reanimação cardiopulmonar; *IV*, intravenoso; *ANF*, adjuvantes das vias respiratórias nasofaríngeas; *AOF*, adjuvantes das vias respiratórias orofaríngeas; *PAE*, Protocolo de Ação de Emergência.

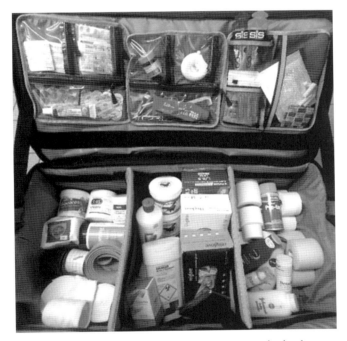

Figura 42.4 Exemplo de equipamento em uma mala de viagem.

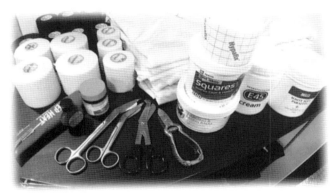

Figura 42.5 Consumíveis colocados no vestiário.

a população em geral. Um meio termo nessa situação pode ser a prescrição de altas doses de vitamina C e zinco, visto que a maioria das ITRS são de origem viral (NICE, 2008). Assim, pode-se reduzir a prescrição desnecessária de antibióticos, enquanto os jogadores e treinadores sentem que os sintomas estão sendo levados a sério e tratados de forma adequada.

Os médicos são frequentemente abordados por funcionários que não jogam para obter medicamentos ou tratamento. Embora possa ser tentador ajudar os colegas, se o tratamento médico de funcionários não jogadores não for uma obrigação contratual, é ético prestar cuidados a indivíduos de maneira informal? Alguns considerariam que os médicos não deveriam, em hipótese alguma, prescrever medicamentos fora de suas obrigações contratuais. Outros podem restringi-lo ao fornecimento de medicamentos sem receita. Seria prudente envolver o Departamento de Recursos Humanos do clube esportivo para esclarecer os acordos contratuais antes de prescrever para qualquer equipe não esportiva. A equipe de fisioterapia também pode ser abordada para fornecer medicamentos. A menos que sejam fisioterapeutas prescritores registrados, os fisioterapeutas não estão autorizados a prescrever medicamentos. No entanto, em um ambiente de equipe de apoio, é permitido ao médico orientar as prescrições com protocolos claros para a administração de medicamentos por outra equipe, com anotações precisas. Por fim, todos os

Os jogadores podem solicitar comprimidos para dormir devido à insônia ou ao nervosismo antes de uma grande partida. Os sedativos são muito viciantes e podem permanecer no sistema por 48 horas após a ingestão, o que pode afetar o desempenho e o tempo de reação. Boa educação sobre higiene do sono adequada e medidas conservadoras devem ser incentivadas sempre que possível. Os profissionais de saúde devem explorar as razões pelas quais os jogadores solicitam certos sedativos ou analgésicos fortes, aconselhando o paciente sobre alternativas. É preciso cuidar para não criar dependência.

Quando os jogadores apresentam sintomas de infecção do trato respiratório superior (ITRS), pode haver pressão para tratar com antibióticos; essa também é uma expectativa comum entre

433

Parte | 2 | Aplicação Clínica

Tabela 42.4 **Medicamentos sugeridos para os médicos terem ao lado do campo.**

Grupo	Medicamento	Indicação
Emergência	Epinefrina 1:1000 500 microgramas Epipen 1:1000 300 microgramas IM	Anafilaxia
	Epinefrina 1:10.000 1 mg IV	Parada cardíaca
	Amiodarona	Parada cardíaca
	Benzodiazepínicos – midazolam bucal	Apreensão
	Hidrocortisona	Anafilaxia
	Glucagon	Hipoglicemia
	Gel de glicose concentrado – *Hypostop®*	Hipoglicemia
	Oxigênio	Parada cardíaca, hipoxia, lesão grave
	Ácido acetilsalicílico 300 mg	Infarto do miocárdio
	Spray sublingual de nitroglicerina (NTG)	Angina
	Anti-histamínico – clorfeniramina	Anafilaxia
	Agonistas β_2 inalados de curta ação – salbutamol + câmara de aeração	Asma/broncoconstrição
Geral	Antibióticos – incluindo penicilina, amplo espectro não penicilina, tópico	Infecção
	Analgesia – paracetamol, AINE, ácido acetilsalicílico, parenteral	Dor
	Anestesia – lidocaína (incluindo tópica), bupivacaína	Procedimentos, por exemplo, sutura
	Água estéril	Irrigação de feridas
	Proclorperazina (parenteral)	Vômito
Respiratório/ONG	Esteroides inalatórios	Asma
	Pomada antibiótica – cloranfenicol	Conjuntivite
	Naseptin®	Epistaxe recorrente
Gastrintestinal	Antiácidos	Dispepsia
	Loperamida	Diarreia
	Laxantes, por exemplo, *senna®*	Prisão de ventre
	Antiespasmódico, por exemplo, mebeverina	Espasmo intestinal

ONG, ouvido, nariz e garganta; *IM*, intramuscular; *IV*, intravenoso; *AINE*, anti-inflamatórios não esteroides.

medicamentos devem ser armazenados com segurança em um armário adequado e trancado, com acesso limitado aos membros apropriados da equipe.

Extricação

Equipamentos essenciais para diferentes tipos de extricação devem estar disponíveis ao lado do campo e incluir uma prancha longa/espinal com blocos de cabeça e tiras, um colar cervical, uma maca com sistema de bloqueio de cabeça e tiras, uma maca tipo cesto, uma seleção de talas de fratura e uma tala Kendrick (Figura 42.6).

Extricação para lesões não espinais ou parada cardíaca

No caso de uma lesão do tecido mole, o jogador deve ser questionado se consegue sair do CDJ. Se o jogador acreditar que não consegue sair do campo, a equipe médica apoiará o jogador com a utilização da técnica de extricação adequada. Por exemplo, com suspeita de fratura ou lesão ligamentar, pode-se apoiar manualmente o membro afetado com/sem imobilização (dependendo da lesão) e o jogador pode receber ajuda de outros membros da equipe médica para garantir uma transferência segura para o dispositivo de extricação.

No caso de uma suspeita de concussão, a equipe médica deverá considerar a possibilidade de remoção do atleta do jogo, pensando em sua saúde e segurança. No entanto, apenas em circunstâncias em que o jogador não tem capacidade para tomar uma decisão sobre os seus cuidados que essa decisão é tomada pelo médico assistente.

No caso de uma parada cardíaca, para eficiência de tempo, o jogador pode ser transferido diretamente para o dispositivo do tipo *scoop* que se abre ao transferir o jogador para um carrinho de ambulância. O atleta pode ser levantado no dispositivo *scoop* que se abre pela equipe médica que posicionará cabeça, ombros,

Extricação para lesões na coluna vertebral

Temos dois dispositivos de imobilização da coluna – prancha longa e concha. A experiência pessoal levou à avaliação de suas vantagens/desvantagens relativas mostradas na Tabela 42.5.

Um jogador será rolado com quatro pessoas, liderado pelo primeiro respondente do lado do campo que fornecerá estabilização manual em linha (MILS, do inglês *manual in-line stabilization*). Três membros rolarão os ombros, quadris e pés (três braços por cima, três por baixo). Um membro designado irá, então, inserir a prancha ou concha nas costas do jogador e o jogador é rebaixado ao comando do líder. Se uma prancha longa estiver sendo usada, o jogador será reposicionado novamente com o comando do líder. Os blocos de cabeça e tiras serão inseridos enquanto o líder estiver em MILS até que os blocos de cabeça sejam colocados. Se possível, nomeie outra pessoa não envolvida com o rolamento do jogador para preparar as correias do cinto de segurança ou aranha para uma aplicação rápida e fácil. Amarre dos ombros até os pés, garantindo que as alças estejam niveladas em ambos os lados e que a tensão seja igual durante a aplicação das alças. As amarras do tipo aranha podem não alcançar os pés do jogador, dependendo da altura (Hanson e Carlin, 2012).

Transferência

Uma transferência efetiva é vital no ambiente da medicina esportiva e de exercício, onde a transferência de cuidados frequentemente ocorre. No entanto, essa é uma habilidade difícil de dominar. Neste cenário, a transferência pode ocorrer quando o primeiro a responder no CDJ é acompanhado por membros da equipe médica, se um jogador é transferido do CDJ para a ambulância ou na admissão ao hospital. A duração da transferência dependerá da situação, mas geralmente deve incluir informações suficientes para que o novo cuidador assuma os cuidados com segurança.

Existem várias ferramentas que foram projetadas para garantir uma transferência eficaz. Elas fornecem uma estrutura padronizada para comunicação factual concisa entre prestadores de cuidados de saúde, garantindo que todas as informações importantes sejam transmitidas (Leonard et al., 2004). Isso inclui o SBAR (Figura 42.7), frequentemente usado no ambiente de atenção secundária, e o ATMIST, proposto no ambiente de medicina do futebol.

Embora um não seja necessariamente superior ao outro, o importante é ter um sistema que seja usado de forma consistente.

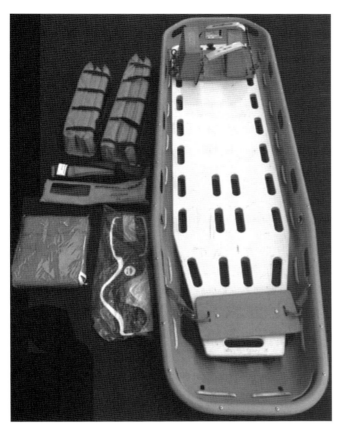

Figura 42.6 Equipamento de extricação lateral incluindo *(sentido horário, a partir do canto superior esquerdo)* talas de fratura, prancha longa e concha com blocos de cabeça e tiras, colar cervical, cobertor e cinto tipo aranha.

quadris e pés. O jogador será levantado o suficiente para fornecer espaço para o dispositivo deslizar por baixo e o atleta é então abaixado para dentro do dispositivo. As tiras do tipo aranha são usadas para prender o jogador na prancha; a parte superior da cinta (cinta em Y) não é usada no cenário de parada cardíaca, pois obstruirá as pás do desfibrilador e as compressões torácicas. A pessoa que apoia a cabeça deve liderar o cenário, de modo que a extricação coordenada ocorra com o mínimo de perturbação nos ferimentos.

Tabela 42.5 **Vantagens e desvantagens dos dispositivos prancha longa e concha.**

Equipamento	Prancha longa	Concha
Vantagens	Rígido para maior suporte Pode ser usado para transportar por distâncias adicionais Pode acomodar melhor uma variedade de tamanhos de jogadores Pode prender cinto de segurança/alças tipo aranha O jogador só é rolado uma vez Compatível com raios X	Comprimento ajustável Pode ser dividido em dois para que o jogador possa ser "inclinado" em vez de rolado Compatível com raios X e ressonância magnética, portanto, o jogador não precisa ser transferido para outro dispositivo e pode ir direto para o exame de imagem
Desvantagens	Normalmente, o reajuste da posição de um jogador na prancha é necessário antes da imobilização Não é compatível com ressonância magnética, então o jogador precisará ser transferido	Pode ser muito curto para jogadores mais altos, mesmo no comprimento máximo Estreito Deve ser usado apenas para transferência para o cesto, pois não é tão rígido quanto uma prancha longa Forma uma grande lacuna da base do suporte do torso até o suporte dos pés quando em comprimento máximo

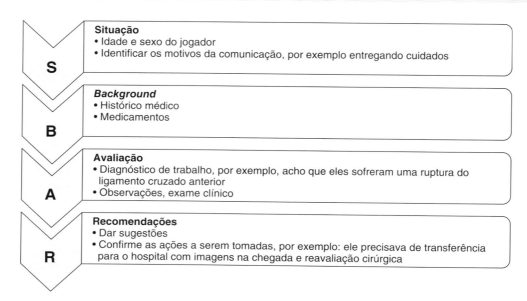

Figura 42.7 Algoritmo SBAR para estruturação de transferência.

Os problemas de comunicação e colaboração têm se mostrado os mais fortes preditores de danos à saúde (Leonard et al., 2004). Portanto, uma transferência efetiva é essencial para garantir que informações críticas não sejam omitidas. Os benefícios de uma transferência correta incluem melhor tomada de decisão pelo profissional que recebe o caso, priorização de tarefas, melhor experiência do paciente e melhor gerenciamento do tempo (Eggins e Slade, 2015).

As principais informações que devem ser comunicadas em um ambiente de medicina esportiva incluem:

1. Detalhes básicos do paciente.
2. Informações sobre a lesão ou doença.
3. Sinais e sintomas.
4. Antecedentes, como qualquer histórico médico anterior que possa ser relevante.
5. Informações de avaliação clínica, por exemplo, sinais vitais, impressão clínica.
6. Qualquer intervenção que você tenha realizado.

Se houver qualquer lesão em um membro, o estado neurovascular deve ser sempre comunicado e o tempo em que os pulsos etc., foram perdidos, se inicialmente presentes. Os jogadores podem precisar de cirurgia na admissão ao hospital; portanto, outras informações importantes a ser entregues incluem quando eles comeram e beberam pela última vez, pois será importante para o planejamento da anestesia.

Debriefing

Um *debriefing* da equipe é um diálogo facilitado ou orientado que ocorre entre os membros da equipe para revisar e refletir sobre seu desempenho (Lyons et al., 2015). O *debriefing* é uma ferramenta útil para avaliar eventos a fim de identificar áreas de boas práticas e áreas para melhorias. No entanto, essa ferramenta também tem sido empregada como um método para refletir sobre os eventos após um incidente crítico, como uma parada cardíaca. De fato, grande parte da literatura relacionada ao *debriefing* gira em torno de incidentes críticos. Nessas circunstâncias, esse processo permite que os indivíduos discutam o desempenho de cada um e em nível de equipe, identifiquem os erros cometidos e desenvolvam um plano para melhorar sua próxima atuação (Salas et al., 2008). Várias ferramentas foram desenvolvidas para fornecer uma estrutura para o *debriefing*, dentre elas o SHARP, uma ferramenta de *feedback* de cinco etapas (Ahmed et al., 2013), mostradas na Figura 42.8.

No cenário de esportes de elite, muitas vezes há o fardo adicional de se tomar decisões sob o escrutínio de fãs e câmeras de TV. Além disso, pode haver conflitos entre os interesses de saúde de um indivíduo e os do clube, por exemplo, com decisões de retorno ao jogo. Pode haver complexidade adicional ao cobrir jogos fora ou trabalhar no exterior, tendo que lidar com um novo ambiente com equipes ou instalações diferentes. Todos esses aspectos tornam ainda mais importante o engajamento no *debriefing*, para processar as habilidades complexas de tomada de decisão e melhorar o planejamento para cenários semelhantes no futuro. Além disso, o *debriefing* pode identificar áreas que podem se beneficiar da auditoria – para reavaliar e melhorar o plano de ação de emergência para um determinado cenário.

Qualificações para ajuda de emergência

A maioria dos profissionais de saúde entra no ambiente esportivo com a experiência de trabalhar em um hospital, clínica geral ou clínicas comunitárias. Quando nos deparamos com situações de emergência nesses ambientes, geralmente há um bom acesso ao

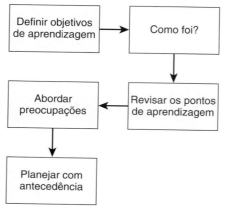

Figura 42.8 Ferramenta de *debriefing* SHARP.

Preparação para Responder a uma Emergência Capítulo | 42 |

apoio dos colegas profissionais de saúde, equipamentos médicos e um ambiente controlado, longe do olhar do público em geral, da mídia e de outros pacientes.

Isso contrasta fortemente ao trabalhar com profissionais do esporte, em que se pode deparar com o gerenciamento de situações de risco de vida e membros, muitas vezes em más condições climáticas, com suporte médico e equipamentos limitados, sob o escrutínio da mídia e do público em geral. Ao trabalhar ao lado de pessoas que têm interesse no resultado de suas ações e decisões, esses colegas geralmente não têm conhecimento médico e podem buscar influenciar as decisões médicas no interesse de ganhar um jogo.

O treinamento em atendimento de emergência no esporte visa proteger os jogadores e os profissionais de saúde. Nessas situações, médicos e fisioterapeutas não agem de acordo com o princípio do "bom samaritano", mas de acordo com a lei comum. Portanto, o padrão de atendimento médico deve ser mais alto quando prestado por um indivíduo com treinamento médico (Advanced Trauma Medical Management in Football, 2017).

A Football Association insiste que qualquer profissional de saúde que trabalhe com faixas etárias acima de 16 anos na Premier League, English Football League e Women's Super League deve concluir o curso intitulado *Advanced Trauma Medical Management in Football* (ATMMiF). Os candidatos devem preencher a leitura do pré-curso e um questionário de múltipla escolha. Isso é seguido por um curso intensivo de 2 dias composto por uma mistura de ensino didático, sessões interativas e práticas baseadas em cenários sobre uma série de competências, como gerenciamento de vias respiratórias no futebol (Advanced Trauma Medical Management in Football, 2017). O curso também fornece ensino sobre planejamento de ações de emergência, ciclos de auditoria e procedimentos operacionais padrão, como gerenciamento de jogadores inconscientes.

Há uma variedade de outros cursos de ajuda de emergência baseados em esportes que foram endossados pela Faculdade de Atendimento Pré-Hospitalar do Royal College of Surgeons de Edimburgo e pela Faculdade de Medicina do Esporte e Exercício, que são considerados equivalentes ao ATMMiF. Estes são:

- Gestão Médica de Emergência em Esportes Individuais e de Equipe (EMMITS, do inglês *Emergency Medical Management in Individual and Team Sports*)
- Princípios Padrão de Reanimação e Trauma nos Esportes (SPORTS, do inglês *Standard Principals of Resuscitation and Trauma in Sports*)
- Gestão Médica Imediata no Campo do Jogo (IMMFP, *Immediate Medical Management on the Field of Play*)

- Cuidados Imediatos no Esporte (ICS, do inglês *Immediate Care in Sport*)
- Habilidades Médicas Cardíacas e de Campo (SCRUMCAPS, *Medical Cardiac and Pitch Side Skills*).

Os cursos de socorro de emergência são um componente vital do treinamento para profissionais de saúde. Eles não apenas fornecem as competências médicas baseadas na prática, mas também fornecem orientações valiosas sobre a governança clínica e uma oportunidade de interagir com outras pessoas que trabalham em ambientes esportivos.

Conclusão

O planejamento de ações de emergência é fundamental para fornecer cuidados médicos seguros e eficazes e primeiros socorros em um ambiente esportivo. Para garantir um ambiente de trabalho eficiente, onde cada membro da equipe médica está ciente de suas funções e responsabilidades, o "quadro PAE" apresentado neste capítulo pode ser implementado e servir como um lembrete visual. Para manter o conjunto de habilidades desenvolvido em cursos e eventos de DPC, os médicos devem praticar os cenários regularmente. Ter um PAE e praticar os cenários de trauma e extricação ajudará a reduzir o risco de erros e minimizará o atraso no atendimento. Uma boa comunicação é vital para o PAE. É essencial ter um sistema de transferência em vigor para que o socorrista comunique suas descobertas e diagnóstico ao resto da equipe. Além disso, a reflexão sobre cada cenário no campo deve ser realizada para permitir a aprendizagem entre pares de uma maneira construtiva. Para fornecer o padrão de cuidado apropriado, o conteúdo da bolsa "de campo", da bolsa para traumas e da bolsa de viagem deve estar de acordo com as diretrizes disponíveis para determinados esportes e satisfazer as necessidades médicas do jogador ou equipe de jogo. O equipamento usado deve ser regularmente verificado, reparado e documentado.

Agradecimentos

Gostaríamos de agradecer a Dean Chatterjee, Stephanie Makin e Rebecca Johnston por suas contribuições, visão e experiência úteis na elaboração deste capítulo.

Referências bibliográficas

Ahmed, M., Arora, S., Russ, S., Darzi, A., Vincent, C., Sevdalis, N., 2013. Operation debrief: a SHARP improvement in performance feedback in the operating room. Annals of Surgery 258 (6), 958-963.

Alaranta, A., Alaranta, H., Helenius, I., 2008. Use of prescription drugs in athletes. Sports Medicine 38 (6), 449-463.

Eggins, S., Slade, D., 2015. Communication in clinical handover: improving the safety and quality of the patient experience. Journal of Public Health Research 4 (3), 666.

Hanson, J.R., Carlin, B., 2012. Sports prehospital-immediate care and spinal injury: not a car crash in sight. British journal of sports medicine, 46 (16), 1097-1101.

Leonard, M., Graham, S., Bonacum, D., 2004. The human factor: the critical importance of effective teamwork and communication in providing safe care. Quality and Safety in Health Care 13 (Suppl. 1), i85-i90.

Lippi, G., Franchini, M., Guidi, G.C., Kean, W.F., 2006. Non-steroidal anti-inflammatory drugs in athletes. British Journal of Sports Medicine 40 (8), 661-662;discussion 2-3.

Lyons, R., Lazzara, E.H., Benishek, L.E., Zajac, S., Gregory, M., Sonesh, S.C., Salas, E., 2015. Enhancing the effectiveness of team debriefings in

medical simulation: More best practices. The Joint Commission Journal on Quality and Patient Safety, 41 (3), 115-125.

NICE Short Clinical Guidelines Technical Team, 2008. Respiratory Tract Infections – Antibiotic Prescribing. Prescribing of Antibiotics for Self-Limiting Respiratory Tract Infections in Adults and Children in Primary Care. National Institute for Health and Clinical Excellence, London.

Reason, J., 2000. Human error: models and management. British Medical Journal 320 (7237), 768-770.

Salas, E., Klein, C., King, H., Salisbury, M., Augenstein, J.S., Birnbach, D.J., et al., 2008. Debriefing medical teams: 12 evidence-based best practices and tips. Joint Commission Journal on Quality and Patient Safety / Joint Commission Resources 34 (9), 518-527.

Shah, R., Chatterjee, A.D., Wilson, J., 2018. Creating a model of best practice: the match day emergency action protocol. British Journal of Sports Medicine 52 (23), 1535-1536.

The Football Association, FA Level 5. Advanced Trauma Medical Management in Football (ATMMiF) course. http://www.thefa.com/learning/courses/the-fa-level-5-advanced-trauma-medical-management-in-football.

Capítulo | **43** |

O Que é Reabilitação sem Aceitação do Paciente? Importância da Psicologia na Reabilitação de Lesões Esportivas

Anna Waters

Introdução

Quando atletas lesionados se encontram pela primeira vez com seus profissionais de medicina esportiva (PME), geralmente a primeira pergunta feita é: "Quando posso voltar ao meu esporte e competir novamente?". A resposta depende não apenas da lesão do atleta, mas também da sua resposta à sua lesão, da sua capacidade de lidar com o impacto emocional potencial da lesão, da sua confiança e da comunicação com sua equipe de reabilitação e o quanto eles acreditam no programa de reabilitação e aderem a ele. Finalmente, no ponto de retorno ao jogo, a confiança do atleta na sua habilidade, confiança na parte do corpo lesionada e na capacidade de lidar com possíveis problemas de nova lesão são todos fatores cruciais para determinar a prontidão de um atleta para retornar ao esporte.

Há alguns anos, conheci um jóquei que fraturou a tíbia e a fíbula durante a queda de um cavalo. Ao longo de sua reabilitação, ele estava bem adiantado com relação ao seu programa e já estava de volta a um cavalo muito tempo antes do seu PME ou consultor avisá-lo que estava apto para fazê-lo. Ele acelerou todo o seu tempo de recuperação para estar em forma o suficiente para retornar à corrida. Curiosamente, quando seu consultor o classificou como apto para competir novamente alguns dias depois, ele me ligou e reservou para me ver. Descobriu-se que de repente ele havia perdido completamente a confiança para correr. Ao se deparar com a realidade da corrida de cavalos novamente, ele deixou de se esforçar para quebrar todos os recordes em termos de tempo de recuperação e ficou dominado por temores de novas lesões e dúvidas sobre sua capacidade de montar. Ele continuou ligando para o seu agente a fim de cancelar sua corrida de retorno. Em vez disso, resolvemos os seus medos e as suas preocupações.

Esse é um cenário relativamente comum, resultado de não processar e abordar as questões psicológicas no início e durante o processo de reabilitação, de modo que quando o atleta é considerado clinicamente apto para retornar ao esporte, ele não está psicologicamente pronto. Para esse jóquei, todos (incluindo sua equipe de reabilitação) pensaram que ele estava lidando muito bem com sua reabilitação. No entanto, ao se concentrar tão intensamente em acelerar sua reabilitação, ele evitou lidar com sua resposta emocional e psicológica, e teve que lidar com ela quando confrontado com a realidade de retornar às corridas de cavalos.

Em seguida, qual a importância que você acredita que a psicologia do esporte tem no campo da medicina esportiva? Como um PME lendo isso, quanto você entende sobre o papel da psicologia em seu trabalho com pacientes diariamente? Você acredita que está bem equipado para lidar com os aspectos psicológicos da reabilitação de lesões esportivas e retorno ao esporte?

Os resultados da pesquisa sugerem que, embora a psicologia do esporte tenha sido identificada como importante pelos PMEs, a maioria acredita estar despreparada e sem treinamento para lidar com os fatores psicológicos na reabilitação de lesões esportivas. Vamos explorar um resumo das principais descobertas nessa área.

Mann et al. (2007) examinaram a compreensão dos médicos do esporte sobre as questões psicológicas em pacientes atletas. Eles descobriram que os médicos encontram com frequência problemas psicológicos nesse grupo de pacientes. Portanto, é necessário que os PMEs tenham ferramentas para facilitar a avaliação desses problemas e uma maior comunicação entre os psicólogos do esporte e os praticantes da medicina esportiva.

Arvinen-Barrow e seus colegas conduziram vários estudos de pesquisa examinando a compreensão e o uso da psicologia do esporte por fisioterapeutas do Reino Unido em seu trabalho. Em particular, eles observaram que, apesar de uma crença geral dos PMEs de que as estratégias psicossociais são importantes para aumentar a eficácia da reabilitação de lesões (Arvinen-Barrow et al., 2007; 2014; Hemmings e Povey, 2002; Larson et al., 1996) e evidências que essas abordagens são eficazes (Beneka et al., 2007; Flint, 1998a; Ievleva e Orlick, 1991), muitos não acreditam que tenham a compreensão e o treinamento necessários para serem capazes de implementar essas estratégias (Hamson-Utley et al., 2008; Stiller-Ostrowski e Hamson-Utley, 2010). Em consonância com outros pesquisadores, Arvinen-Barrow et al. (2007) recomendam que uma maior colaboração entre psicólogos do esporte e fisioterapeutas nesse cenário clínico seria benéfica.

Nos últimos 30 anos, pesquisas examinaram e identificaram a importância dos fatores psicológicos nas lesões esportivas e na reabilitação. Esse conjunto de pesquisas destaca o impacto psicológico que uma lesão pode ter sobre os atletas (Heil, 1993; Ray e Wiese-Bjornstal, 1999; Taylor e Taylor, 1997). Modelos foram desenvolvidos para levar em conta as respostas psicológicas dos atletas a lesões (Walker et al., 2007; Wiese-Bjornstal et al., 1998). Em paralelo, habilidades e intervenções psicológicas foram desenvolvidas para facilitar a velocidade de recuperação

Parte | 2 | Aplicação Clínica

e o retorno bem-sucedido dos atletas ao jogo (Ievleva e Orlick, 1991; Kamphoff et al., 2010; Williams e Scherzer, 2010).

Pesquisas recentes em psicologia do esporte identificaram alguns resultados interessantes de particular relevância para os PMEs. Por exemplo, Ardern et al. (2013) descobriram que certas respostas psicológicas chave medeiam a pré-cirurgia e 4 meses após a cirurgia significativamente previram o retorno ao jogo 12 meses após a reconstrução do ligamento cruzado anterior. Esse achado com resultados de pesquisas anteriores (Brand e Nyland, 2009; McCullough et al., 2012), fornece evidências que sugerem que fatores psicológicos são importantes para o retorno ao esporte e que podem ter sido sub-reconhecidos até o momento.

Embora as descobertas dessas pesquisas sejam interessantes, como elas impactam a prática clínica? Existem lacunas entre as descobertas significativas da pesquisa em psicologia do esporte e sua aplicação em contextos do mundo real. Pela literatura conduzida até o momento, isso parece ser em particular verdadeiro no que diz respeito à ligação entre a pesquisa em psicologia do esporte e as equipes de medicina do esporte.

Apesar da importância dos fatores psicológicos na medicina esportiva, ainda existe uma falta de compreensão teórica em muitos ambientes clínicos, formas estruturadas insuficientes para os PMEs trabalharem com psicólogos do esporte e uma ausência de formas práticas claras de integrar a psicologia do esporte em uma equipe de medicina esportiva. Este capítulo abordará essas áreas e as seguintes questões:

- Fornecer informações sobre as respostas psicológicas dos atletas a lesões
- Examinar a adesão à reabilitação de lesões
- Introduzir métodos para melhorar a adesão à reabilitação em atletas
- Apresentar algumas das habilidades e ferramentas da psicologia do esporte que podem ser integradas ao trabalho dos PMEs com atletas lesionados.

O conteúdo apresentado se relaciona bem com o Capítulo 39 sobre a eficácia do condicionamento. O leitor é referido a esse capítulo como um excelente roteiro para os fundamentos da adaptação neuromuscular e princípios básicos de treinamento ao estruturar sessões de reabilitação. Combinado com as sugestões feitas neste capítulo, fornece uma base holística sobre a qual desenvolver planos de intervenção para seus clientes.

Respostas psicológicas a lesões

Os atletas apresentam uma variedade de respostas psicológicas a lesões e diversos fatores afetam essa resposta. Por exemplo, seu nível de participação no esporte, gravidade da lesão, momento na temporada e experiência anterior com lesão. É importante para os PMEs obter *insight* e compreensão das respostas psicológicas úteis e inúteis que os atletas podem exibir e ter isso em mente ao desenvolver e entregar programas de intervenção para atletas lesionados.

Resposta positiva

A discussão em torno da resposta psicológica a lesões esportivas geralmente se concentra na resposta negativa. No entanto, a lesão pode ser um evento positivo para alguns atletas; por exemplo, se um atleta está tendo uma temporada difícil e com baixo desempenho, a lesão pode oferecer uma fuga bem-vinda ou interromper o treinamento intensivo.

Muitos atletas experimentam benefícios emocionais positivos decorrentes de lesões esportivas. Udry (1997) examinou

as consequências positivas das lesões conduzindo entrevistas retrospectivas com 21 atletas lesionados da equipe de esqui dos EUA. Ela descobriu que 95% dos atletas relataram uma ou mais consequências positivas de suas lesões. Elas foram agrupadas em três categorias gerais: crescimento pessoal (p. ex., "Aprendi como ajudar outros esquiadores lesionados", "Aprendi diferentes lados de mim mesmo"); melhorias de desempenho com base psicológica (p. ex., "Tornei-me mentalmente mais resistente", "Ela (lesão) me deu uma maior ética de trabalho"); e desenvolvimento físico-técnico (p. ex., "Aprendi a esquiar tecnicamente melhor", "Aprendi o que meu corpo pode aguentar").

Udry (1999) acrescenta que nem todos os atletas lesionados terão benefícios positivos com as lesões e que os PMEs que trabalham com esses atletas podem ajudar a facilitar o processo pelo qual eles obtêm consequências positivas de suas lesões e sugeriu cinco recomendações de como isso pode ser feito (Boxe 43.1).

Modelos de resposta psicológica de atletas a lesões

Modelos teóricos foram desenvolvidos para demonstrar e oferecer informações sobre as reações psicológicas que os atletas experimentam quando lesionados. É útil para os PMEs considerar a resposta individual do atleta à lesão e, em seguida, refletir sobre como essas respostas se encaixam em um modelo validado. Kolt (2004a) sugere que esse processo permite ao PME interpretar porque muitas reações acontecem e como elas podem impactar no processo de reabilitação. Em particular, os modelos de resposta ao luto e de avaliação cognitiva têm sido amplamente adotados.

Modelos de resposta ao luto

Modelos de resposta ao luto ou de estágio foram retirados de outras áreas de pesquisa, como o processo de morte, e aplicados ao contexto de lesões esportivas (Mueller e Ryan, 1991). O modelo de Kübler Ross (1969) foi desenvolvido para explicar perdas significativas (como a morte de um membro da família ou ente

---

Boxe 43.1 Para facilitar consequências positivas de lesões atléticas

1. Reconhecer que obter consequências positivas exige esforço. O atleta não deve assumir passivamente que consequências positivas ocorrerão, ele deve trabalhar duro para que isso aconteça.
2. Reconhecer que diferentes estratégias de resolução de problemas podem ser usadas, por exemplo, converter uma situação negativa em positiva ou encorajar o atleta a renunciar a papéis problemáticos.
3. Reconhecer que a ressignificação pode não ocorrer imediatamente. Os atletas podem exigir uma quantidade considerável de tempo para serem capazes de contrabalançar os aspectos negativos de suas lesões.
4. Evitar vitimização secundária. Certifique-se de que as pessoas não banalizem ou minimizem as experiências de atletas lesionados.
5. Reconhecer que as consequências positivas das lesões podem se estender além do atleta individual. As lesões afetarão as pessoas próximas ao atleta lesionado, por isso é importante ajudá-los a também contrabalançar o impacto negativo das lesões.

Adaptado de Udry, E., 1999. The paradox of injuries: unexpected positive consequences. In: Pargman, D., (Ed.), Psychological Bases of Sport Injuries, second ed. Fitness Information Technology, Morgantown, WV, pp. 79-88.

O Que é Reabilitação sem Aceitação do Paciente? Importância da Psicologia na Reabilitação...

querido) e sugere que as pessoas progridem por cinco estágios de luto: negação, raiva, barganha, depressão e aceitação. Esse modelo foi sugerido para se relacionar com lesões esportivas, uma vez que os atletas podem experimentar uma sensação de perda de si por causa da lesão (Gordon, 1991; Macci e Crossman, 1996).

A literatura sobre lesões esportivas demonstra algum suporte para os modelos de luto (McDonald e Hardy, 1990; Mueller e Ryan, 1991). A crítica inclui que os modelos assumem que a lesão representa uma forma de perda para o atleta e, portanto, requer luto (Walker e Heaney, 2013). Em segundo lugar, esses modelos não conseguem captar um elemento-chave da lesão esportiva que são as diferenças individuais na resposta à lesão (Evans e Hardy, 1995; Harris, 2003; Walker et al., 2007). No mundo da psicologia do esporte, é geralmente aceito que as respostas a lesões são vistas de maneira flexível, reconhecendo a singularidade de cada atleta. Weinberg e Gould (2011) sugerem que todos os atletas têm uma resposta típica a lesões, mas a velocidade e a facilidade com que progridem variam amplamente.

Modelo integrado de resposta a lesões esportivas e reabilitação

A segunda categoria principal de resposta psicológica aos modelos de lesão são os de avaliação cognitiva, que se baseiam nas teorias de estresse, enfrentamento e responsividade emocional. O modelo integrado de resposta a lesões esportivas e reabilitação é indiscutivelmente o mais aceito e bem desenvolvido na literatura de psicologia do esporte (Anderson et al., 2004; Kolt e McEvoy, 2003; Walker et al., 2007).

O modelo integrado (Figura 43.1) sugere que a resposta de um atleta a uma lesão esportiva é influenciada por variáveis pré-lesão, como personalidade, histórico de estressores, recursos de enfrentamento e intervenções preventivas, bem como variáveis pós-lesão (Wiese-Bjornstal et al., 1998). Como pode ser visto na Figura 43.1, durante as fases pós-lesão, a maneira como o atleta avalia a lesão influencia sua resposta comportamental (p. ex., seu uso de apoio social, suas habilidades psicológicas e sua adesão à reabilitação), suas respostas emocionais (p. ex., medo do desconhecido, frustração ou atitude positiva) e os resultados psicossociais e físicos. O modelo reconhece a interação entre a avaliação cognitiva e as respostas emocionais e comportamentais como um processo cíclico bidirecional e dinâmico, que por sua vez tem um efeito nos resultados de recuperação física e psicológica. Nesse modelo, características pessoais (p. ex., histórico de lesões, tolerância à dor, habilidades de enfrentamento) e fatores situacionais (p. ex., tipo de esporte, influências do treinador, dinâmica familiar, ambiente de reabilitação) são sugeridos como tendo impacto direto nas avaliações cognitivas.

Esse modelo oferece aos PMEs uma estrutura útil para a compreensão dos aspectos psicológicos de lesões esportivas e reabilitação e pode ser utilizado para ajudar a desenvolver planos de intervenção individualizados para cada atleta.

Modelo do chimpanzé

Nos últimos 3 anos, tenho trabalhado com o professor Steve Peters utilizando seu modelo de chimpanzé (Peters, 2012). Esse modelo simplifica muito a neurociência e explica como a mente pode ser vista como tendo três equipes, cada uma com sua própria agenda e maneira de trabalhar.

O *humano* (você) se baseia, sobretudo, no lobo frontal, que está associado ao pensamento lógico e trabalha com fatos e verdades. O *chimpanzé* é uma máquina pensante emocional independente que trabalha com sentimentos e impressões baseados sobretudo no sistema límbico. Esse sistema é encontrado na parte inferior

do cérebro; ele combina funções mentais superiores e emoções primitivas em um único sistema, frequentemente conhecido como sistema nervoso emocional. Não é apenas responsável por nossas vidas emocionais, mas também pelo aprendizado e pela memória. O sistema límbico inclui a amígdala, o hipocampo, o tálamo, o hipotálamo e os gânglios da base (Figuras. 43.2 e 43.3).

Há também o *computador*, espalhado por todo o cérebro, que é uma área de armazenamento de pensamentos e comportamentos programados. É importante notar que um modelo não é um fato científico puro ou uma hipótese. É apenas uma representação simples para auxiliar na compreensão e nos ajudar a usar a ciência. O professor Peters desenvolveu o modelo com base em sua experiência de 30 anos trabalhando como psiquiatra e ensinando neurociência para estudantes de medicina na Sheffield University. Apesar da enorme popularidade do modelo em um amplo espectro de campos e disciplinas, o seu valor ainda não foi comprovado por meio de pesquisas científicas.

Em meu trabalho utilizando o modelo do chimpanzé com esportistas lesionados, descobri que ele permite que as pessoas entendam como sua mente funciona e como seu cérebro único está respondendo ao processo de lesão e reabilitação. Aprender a distinguir entre o pensamento emocional e o lógico/racional sobre a lesão pode ser uma maneira útil de começar a gerenciar as respostas individuais. A parte do cérebro do chimpanzé acha difícil lidar com a realidade e expressa pensamentos emocionais sobre a lesão ("Por que isso aconteceu comigo?", "Nunca vou voltar para onde estava", "Não é justo"), enquanto a parte humana do cérebro aceita e entende a lesão de forma relativamente rápida e pode então começar a trabalhar nos planos de enfrentamento, planos de reabilitação e processos.

No exemplo do jóquei de corrida de cavalos no início desse capítulo, a parte humana de seu cérebro aceitou a lesão, mas seu chimpanzé ficou obcecado em voltar a cavalgar o mais rápido possível e isso o distraiu do processamento de suas respostas emocionais à lesão. Quebrar recordes para se recuperar o mais rápido possível tornou-se um desafio emocionante para seu chimpanzé. Porém, ao se deparar com a realidade de ter que cavalgar novamente, seu chimpanzé entrou em pânico e toda a emoção que não havia sido expressa no início e durante a reabilitação veio à tona e teve que ser processada e tratada naquele momento.

Adesão à reabilitação de lesões

Conforme definido por Meichenbaum e Turk (1987), a adesão é um "envolvimento colaborativo voluntário ativo do paciente em um curso de comportamento mutuamente aceitável para produzir um resultado preventivo ou terapêutico desejado". Para o PME, a adesão pode envolver comportamentos como cumprir as instruções dos profissionais da saúde, comparecer e estar ativamente envolvido em sessões de reabilitação, evitar comportamentos potencialmente prejudiciais, realizar exercícios de reabilitação em casa, completar crioterapia e prescrições de saúde em casa.

Apesar de parecer óbvio que a adesão é crucial para o sucesso da reabilitação de atletas lesionados, há uma falta de evidências empíricas para apoiar essa noção. Um estudo de Brewer (1998) indicou que dependendo de como a adesão aos programas de reabilitação de lesões esportivas foi medida, taxas variando de 40 a 91% foram registradas. Os resultados de Taylor e May (1996) indicam que a não adesão para atividades domiciliares é de 54 a 60%. Relativamente poucos estudos forneceram evidências de que níveis mais altos de adesão estavam relacionados com melhores resultados de lesões esportivas (Brewer et al., 2000; Kolt e McEvoy, 2003; Schoo, 2002).

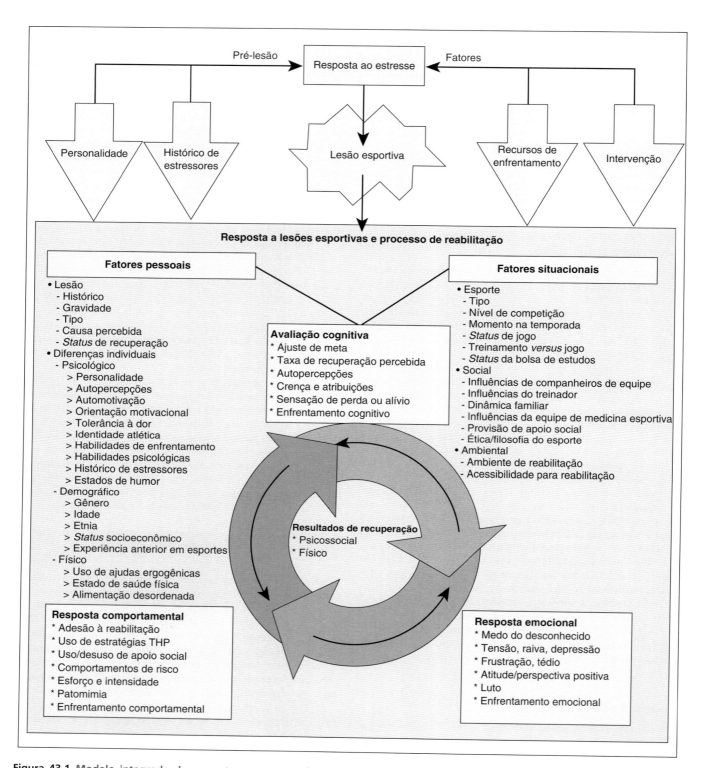

Figura 43.1 Modelo integrado de resposta ao estresse da lesão. *THP*, treinamento de habilidades psicológicas. (Adaptada de Wiese-Bjornstal, D.M., Smith, A.M., Shaffer, S.M., Morrey, M.A., 1998. An integrated model of response to sports injury: psychological and sociological dynamics. Journal of Applied Sport Psychology 10, 46-69.)

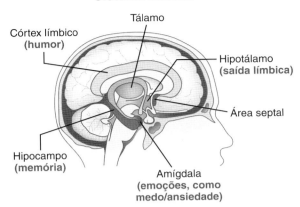

Figura 43.2 Sistema límbico. (*Esta figura se encontra reproduzida em cores no Encarte.*)

Métodos para melhorar a adesão à reabilitação em atletas

O modelo integrado demonstra como vários fatores situacionais, pessoais e emocionais podem impactar na adesão à reabilitação. Ele fornece uma maneira útil de compreender a importância de tratar cada atleta como um indivíduo e como é vital obter uma visão de uma variedade de fatores em todos os aspectos da vida do atleta, todos os quais podem impactar em sua capacidade de aderir aos seu programa de reabilitação.

Para o PME, pode ser interessante notar que vários fatores contextuais foram encontrados para estar relacionados com uma maior adesão. Esses incluem maior crença na eficácia do tratamento (Duda et al., 1989; Taylor e May, 1996), conforto do ambiente de reabilitação (Brewer et al., 1999), conveniência do agendamento da reabilitação (Fields et al., 1995), percepção de esforço durante exercícios de reabilitação (Brewer et al., 1999) e expectativa do profissional de reabilitação em relação à adesão do paciente (Taylor e May, 1996). Um estudo realizado por Fisher e Hoisington (1993) descobriu que os pacientes relataram que ter profissionais da saúde que eram atenciosos, honestos e encorajadores os ajudava no processo de reabilitação.

Em uma revisão da literatura sobre adesão a programas de reabilitação de lesões esportivas, Levy et al. (2006) concluíram que os PMEs devem empregar várias estratégias para melhorar o comportamento de reabilitação. Isso incluiu o estabelecimento de metas, o uso de diários, o desenvolvimento de planos de ação, o aprimoramento de crenças e capacidades em relação às modalidades de reabilitação e o uso de planilhas decisórias.

Kolt (2004b) descreve uma variedade de métodos para aumentar a adesão à reabilitação em atletas, seis dos quais estão resumidos no Boxe 43.2.

Habilidades de psicologia do esporte para integrar em sua prática

Kolt e Andersen (2004) constataram que para que as intervenções psicológicas sejam bem recebidas por um atleta, elas precisam ser realizadas pelo PME de modo que apareçam como parte integrante e esperada da reabilitação. É importante para o PME estar confiante na eficácia das habilidades e em sua própria capacidade de ensiná-las. A palavra-chave é "habilidade". A seguir estão as *habilidades* da psicologia do esporte e, como qualquer habilidade de reabilitação física, levam tempo e prática para serem benéficas. Alguns atletas podem utilizar as habilidades da psicologia do esporte antes da lesão; nesse caso, eles simplesmente precisam ser orientados na adaptação para uso na reabilitação. Para atletas que não estão familiarizados com essas habilidades, o PME precisará educá-lo sobre os benefícios das habilidades e ensiná-las por meio de um plano de intervenção estruturado.

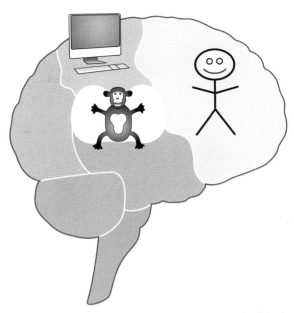

Figura 43.3 Cérebro do chimpanzé. (© Steve Peters and Jeff Battista)

Definição de metas

O estabelecimento de metas é uma técnica iniciada por Locke (1968) e é uma das intervenções psicológicas mais populares no

---

Boxe 43.2 Métodos para melhorar a adesão à reabilitação em atletas

1. *Educação* – dedicar tempo para educar os clientes sobre suas lesões, a lógica por trás das abordagens de tratamento e gerenciamento de ferimentos e estabelecer expectativas realistas.
2. *Criação de comunicação e relacionamento* – muito importante para estabelecer um relacionamento e se comunicar de maneira adequada para todos. Isso precisa ser aprendido com a experiência, não com os livros didáticos.
3. *Apoio social* – por meio de grupos de apoio a lesões e modelos de pares recomendados para a reabilitação de lesões esportivas. A modelagem de pares envolve conectar um atleta lesionado com um atleta que passou por uma reabilitação bem-sucedida e voltou ao funcionamento pré-lesão.
4. *Estabelecimento e cumprimento de metas* – constatou-se que o estabelecimento de metas específicas de reabilitação resulta em maior tempo gasto com exercícios de reabilitação e maior compreensão do programa de reabilitação. Veja mais sugestões sobre o estabelecimento de metas posteriormente nesse capítulo.
5. *Eficácia do tratamento e adaptação dos programas de reabilitação* – importante adaptar o programa às necessidades do indivíduo. Para construir a eficácia do tratamento nos clientes, os PMEs precisam garantir que o cliente possa realizar as tarefas de reabilitação atribuídas e que as tarefas sejam significativas e valiosas para o indivíduo.
6. *Responsabilidade do atleta* – os atletas gostam de se sentir responsáveis por sua reabilitação e esse senso de controle pode aumentar o comprometimento e a adesão. Os PMEs podem usar abordagens que estimulem algum nível de independência para os clientes.

esporte. É frequentemente utilizada por atletas para promover o desempenho (Weinberg e Gould, 2011) e, para muitos, o estabelecimento de metas é parte integrante do treinamento diário. O processo de definição de metas pode ajudar os atletas a entender onde estão atualmente e também aonde querem chegar. Locke (1968) sugeriu que o estabelecimento de metas impacta o desempenho de quatro maneiras: concentra a atenção, mobiliza esforço em proporção às demandas da tarefa, aumenta a persistência e encoraja o indivíduo a desenvolver estratégias para atingir seus objetivos. A literatura sobre reabilitação de lesões esportivas identificou o estabelecimento de metas para ter vários benefícios para o atleta. Três tipos de metas foram identificados e se tornaram populares na literatura da psicologia do esporte. São eles: metas de resultado, metas de desempenho e metas de processo (Hardy et al., 1996).

Metas de resultado. Elas se concentram no resultado de um evento, como ganhar uma medalha de ouro ou um resultado específico de uma competição e, desse modo, envolvem comparação interpessoal. Uma meta de resultado não está no controle do atleta. Um exemplo de meta de resultado na reabilitação poderia ser:

- Retorno bem-sucedido ao nível anterior de desempenho esportivo
- Ganhar uma medalha de ouro nas próximas Olimpíadas.

Metas de desempenho. Estão relacionadas com metas estatísticas pessoais sobre o desempenho anterior pessoal do próprio atleta. Assim, elas estão mais sob o controle do atleta do que as metas de resultados, mas ainda não estão sob controle completo. Por exemplo, uma meta de desempenho em reabilitação pode ser conseguir recuperar 50% da amplitude de movimento de um membro lesionado. Outros exemplos podem ser:

- Recuperar a estabilidade em uma parte do corpo com incrementos percentuais específicos
- Recuperar a confiança em uma parte do corpo lesionada com incrementos percentuais específicos
- Ser capaz de agachar uma quantidade específica de peso na academia
- Ser capaz de correr uma certa distância e/ou velocidade.

Metas de processo. Elas estão relacionadas às metas de desempenho e concentram-se nas ações ou tarefas que o atleta precisa realizar para atingir o resultado de desempenho desejado. As metas do processo devem ser tarefas ou ações que estão sob o controle do atleta. Na reabilitação, exemplos de metas de processo podem ser:

- Completar exercícios específicos para melhorar a amplitude de movimento
- Participar de todas as cinco sessões de reabilitação na academia a cada semana
- Focar em um movimento específico durante um exercício de reabilitação
- Fazer os alongamentos recomendados pelo PME.

De acordo com Cox (2007), quando metas de resultado, de desempenho e de processo são empregadas em conjunto, os atletas têm muito mais chance de experimentar melhorias de desempenho e desenvolvimento psicológico do que quando alguma é empregada isoladamente (p. ex., metas de resultado). Por exemplo, você inicialmente define uma meta de resultado, define metas de desempenho para ajudá-lo a atingir sua meta de resultado e, em seguida, processa as metas para se concentrar nos processos em que precisa se envolver para atingir suas metas de desempenho.

Metas a curto prazo foram a técnica de psicologia do esporte mais utilizada e relatada pelos fisioterapeutas no estudo de Arvinen-Barrow et al. (2007). No entanto, o estudo identificou que, embora os fisioterapeutas definam metas físicas diárias, bem como metas gerais de recuperação, essas metas eram em grande parte ordenadas pelo fisioterapeuta; como resultado, os atletas tinham pouca ou nenhuma propriedade das metas. Para que o estabelecimento de metas seja eficaz, é vital que o atleta esteja envolvido no processo de definição de metas. Arvinen-Barrow et al. (2010) sugerem que, como os fisioterapeutas são especialistas nos aspectos físicos do processo de cura, sua opinião deve ser a principal a ser considerada; entretanto, é imperativo que o atleta faça parte ativamente do processo (Boxe 43.3).

Relaxamento

Simplesmente inspirar, expirar e relaxar por alguns minutos pode ter um impacto significativo no desempenho. Observando alguns atletas famosos, é fácil ver Johnny Wilkinson, por exemplo, respirando fundo algumas vezes, relaxando e concentrando-se antes de bater um pênalti. Cristiano Ronaldo é mais um bom exemplo de jogador que, na hora de cobrar um pênalti, alinha seu remate, respira fundo e espera até estar concentrado e pronto para chutar o pênalti. Ser capaz de relaxar e se concentrar não acontece da noite para o dia, mas pode ser praticado e desenvolvido de maneira eficaz com o tempo.

A literatura da psicologia do esporte identificou dois tipos de relaxamento, ambos aplicáveis a atletas saudáveis e com lesões (Boxe 43.4). São eles os relaxamentos físico (somático) e mental (cognitivo) (Flint, 1998b). O principal objetivo do relaxamento físico é liberar a tensão do corpo e a técnica mais comumente usada no esporte é o relaxamento muscular progressivo (RMP) (Jacobson, 1938). O objetivo do relaxamento mental é focar na mente, em vez do corpo, com a ideia de que uma mente relaxada pode levar a um corpo relaxado e as técnicas mais comuns incluem o treinamento autogênico (Schultz e Luthe, 1969), o controle da respiração e a resposta de relaxamento (Benson, 2000). O treinamento de relaxamento pode ser usado para aliviar a dor e o estresse, que muitas vezes podem ser proeminentes durante a reabilitação de lesões.

Boxe 43.3 Pontos-chave para o estabelecimento de metas

- Comece o processo de definição de metas em conversa com o atleta
- Defina metas específicas (a tendência comum é definir metas vagas)
- Inclua metas de resultado, desempenho e processo
- Defina metas de desempenho e de processo com o atleta em torno de parâmetros psicológicos, como: confiança na parte do corpo lesionada, motivação, comprometimento, adesão, ansiedade etc
- Garanta o acordo entre o PME e os atletas sobre as estratégias de realização de metas
- Escreva as metas
- Forneça suporte de meta para os atletas
- Incorpore objetivos nas sessões de reabilitação
- Lembre-se de revisar e modificar as metas regularmente.

Boxe 43.4 Pontos-chave para o relaxamento

- O relaxamento é útil em todo o processo de lesão
- O relaxamento pode ajudar os atletas a lidar com a dor, o estresse e a ansiedade associados ao processo de lesão
- O relaxamento pode ajudar os atletas a obterem uma sensação de controle sobre sua dor e sua reabilitação
- É útil educar o atleta sobre os benefícios do relaxamento
- Certifique-se de que existe uma estrutura para o treinamento de relaxamento
- Meça a eficácia do relaxamento.

Relaxamento muscular progressivo

O RMP visa ensinar ao indivíduo como é relaxar os músculos, contraindo os grupos musculares, por sua vez, e depois relaxando-os. Dessa maneira, os atletas aprendem a ter consciência de como é a sensação dos músculos quando estão tensos e, então, o que podem fazer para relaxá-los. Por meio da prática, os atletas podem aprender a reconhecer a diferença entre músculos tensos e relaxados.

O RMP é um bom exercício para fazer inicialmente quando um atleta está lesionado, porque a tensão muscular contribui para o aumento da experiência de dor. Tensionar e relaxar ativamente os músculos dá aos atletas uma sensação de controle sobre o controle da dor e das lesões. As primeiras sessões de RMP podem durar até 30 minutos e é recomendado que os atletas sigam um roteiro para 16 grupos musculares. Estudos demonstraram uma variedade de benefícios do RMP, incluindo redução da ansiedade somática (Kolt et al., 2002; Maynard et al., 1995), dor reumática (Stenstrom et al., 1996) e tensão muscular (Lehrer, 1982).

Resposta de relaxamento

Benson (2000) popularizou uma maneira científica de relaxamento com base no relaxamento meditativo, mas sem o elemento espiritual e chamou-lhe "a resposta de relaxamento". Existem quatro elementos principais para a resposta de relaxamento:
1. Um lugar tranquilo para minimizar as distrações.
2. Uma posição confortável que pode ser mantida.
3. Escolher um único pensamento ou palavra para focar a atenção, por exemplo, "acalmar" ou "relaxar", que não estimula os pensamentos; a palavra é repetida na expiração.
4. Uma atitude passiva; isso significa permitir que pensamentos e imagens passem por sua mente sem se envolver com eles.

A resposta de relaxamento ensina os atletas a aquietar a mente, concentrar-se e reduzir a tensão muscular. A resposta de relaxamento pode ajudar os atletas a obter um maior senso de controle sobre a dor e o processo de reabilitação (Taylor e Taylor, 1998).

Imagens mentais

As imagens mentais, ou visualização, é uma das habilidades mais úteis para usar durante a reabilitação. Imagem refere-se a criar ou recriar uma experiência na mente (Weinburg e Gould, 2011) (Figura 43.4). Há uma grande quantidade de evidências para apoiar o uso de imagens por atletas saudáveis (Arvinen-Barrow et al., 2008), e sua aplicação na recuperação de lesões esportivas está bem documentada na literatura. Apesar disso, as imagens mentais parecem ser as menos favorecidas pelos PMEs. Isso pode ser devido à falta de compreensão quanto aos seus benefícios e, possivelmente, uma percepção errônea do que uma intervenção de imagens mentais acarreta (Arvinen-Barrow et al., 2010).

Estudos de pesquisa descobriram que quatro tipos de imagens podem ser úteis durante o processo de reabilitação (Boxe 43.5).

Imagens curativas. O atleta imagina a cicatrização da parte do corpo lesionada (p. ex., imaginando o tecido rompido cicatrizando em conjunto, uma ruptura em um osso cicatrizando em um osso forte e saudável).

Tratamento da dor. O atleta se distrai da dor se imaginando deitado na praia, por exemplo. Ievleva e Orlick (1991) sugerem imaginar a dor sendo lavada, ou ver cores frias correndo pela dor para reduzi-la (p. ex., vendo azuis frios correndo pela área, imaginando a dor deixando o corpo).

Processo de reabilitação. O atleta se imagina realizando os processos que precisa completar para se recuperar totalmente (p. ex., exercícios específicos na academia, superando desafios e contratempos, aderindo ao programa de reabilitação).

Desempenho. Imagens do atleta realizando habilidades específicas do esporte (p. ex., imagem de exercícios de treinamento ou um desempenho de competição).

Suporte social

O suporte social facilita o enfrentamento. De acordo com Weinberg e Gould (2011), pode ajudar a reduzir o estresse, melhorar o humor, aumentar a motivação para a reabilitação e melhorar a adesão ao tratamento. Na literatura da psicologia do esporte, o suporte social é considerado parte integrante do processo de enfrentamento para atletas lesionados (Bianco, 2001; Podlog e Eklund, 2007). O Boxe 43.6 descreve alguns aspectos-chave desse processo.

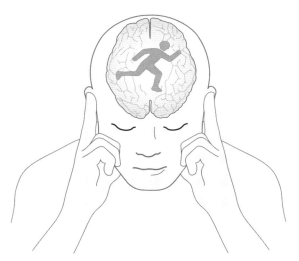

Figura 43.4 Imagens mentais.

Boxe 43.5 Pontos-chave para imagens/visualizações mentais

- Incentivar o uso de imagens de cura e controle da dor na parte inicial do processo de reabilitação
- Incentivar o uso de imagens do processo de reabilitação durante a fase de reabilitação/recuperação
- Incentivar o uso de imagens de desempenho durante todo o processo de reabilitação, mas em particular durante o retorno à fase de atividade completa
- Medir a capacidade e eficácia das imagens dos atletas.

Boxe 43.6 Pontos-chave para o suporte social

- Inicialmente, o suporte informativo é muito importante para que o atleta entenda a natureza de sua lesão. Também é importante fornecer escuta e apoio emocional
- Durante a fase de reabilitação, a necessidade de suporte social é maior quando a recuperação é lenta. O atleta também pode se beneficiar de desafio emocional, suporte técnico e suporte motivacional
- Durante a fase de retorno à atividade plena, o suporte social pode precisar se concentrar na construção da confiança e motivação do atleta para o retorno ao jogo
- Os resultados da pesquisa sugerem que os atletas recorrem aos PMEs para obter suporte informativo e à família e amigos para obter suporte emocional.

Parte | 2 | Aplicação Clínica

Família, amigos e companheiros de equipe podem ter dificuldade em compreender o impacto que uma lesão pode ter no atleta. Se a lesão for uma ameaça à carreira, os membros de apoio podem se sentir desconfortáveis ao falar sobre o esporte para o atleta lesionado (Petitpas e Danish, 1995). Do mesmo modo, pode ser mais fácil para os membros da equipe de apoio falar sobre os aspectos físicos e práticos da reabilitação de lesões, em vez dos sentimentos do atleta. Quando isso acontece, o atleta pode não ter a oportunidade de discutir como está se sentindo em relação à lesão e pode perder uma parte importante de seu ajuste psicológico à lesão (Petitpas e Danish, 1995).

Ao trabalhar com atletas lesionados, é importante considerar o tipo de suporte social que o atleta pode estar recebendo. Existem várias formas de suporte social, incluindo apoio de escuta, apoio emocional, desafio emocional, apreciação da tarefa, desafio da tarefa, confirmação da realidade, assistência material e assistência pessoal (Richman et al., 1993).

Os atletas de um estudo de Arvinen-Barrow e colegas de 2014 relataram que presumiram que os PMEs sabem como eles se sentem, então não sentiram necessidade de explicar. Na verdade, apenas o atleta conhece sua dor individual ou como está se sentindo. Portanto, é vital que os PMEs iniciem uma linha aberta de comunicação sobre sentimentos e dores psicológicas com os atletas com quem trabalham, perguntando sobre isso.

Compreensão de quando encaminhar

Uma habilidade chave para um PME é saber quando é hora de encaminhar um atleta para o psicólogo do esporte ou outro consultor de saúde mental. Harris (2005) destaca a importância de os fisioterapeutas estarem atentos à competência pessoal no que diz respeito ao uso de intervenções psicológicas e saber quando é a hora de encaminhá-las. Os PMEs que estabelecem um relacionamento com um atleta estão em uma boa posição para detectar os sinais de advertência se esse indivíduo estiver lutando para lidar com a lesão. Geralmente, quando os atletas se sentem compreendidos, é muito mais provável que falem sobre seus medos, preocupações e ansiedades. O Boxe 43.7 mostra as áreas identificadas por Petitpas e Danish (1995) como sinais de ajuste insuficiente e, se você vir uma ou várias delas, seria aconselhável encaminhar o atleta.

> **Boxe 43.7 Sinais de mau ajuste**
>
> - Sentimentos de raiva, confusão ou apatia
> - Falta de engajamento com a reabilitação
> - Perguntar obsessivamente: "Quando poderei jogar de novo?"
> - Falta de crença no processo de reabilitação
> - Negação, por exemplo, "Essa lesão não é séria"
> - Um histórico de voltar muito cedo de uma lesão
> - Gabar-se de realizações
> - Afastamento de outras pessoas significativas
> - Concentrar-se em pequenas queixas físicas
> - Dependência do fisioterapeuta
> - Culpa por decepcionar a equipe
> - Mudanças rápidas de humor ou mudanças repentinas de comportamento
> - Sentimento de impotência impactando a lesão.

Adaptado de Petitpas, A., Danish, A., 1995. Caring for injured athletes. In: Murphy, S., (Ed.), Sport Psychology Interventions. Human Kinetics, Champaign, IL, pp. 255-281.

Conclusão

Esse capítulo o conduziu em uma jornada pela psicologia da reabilitação de lesões esportivas, começando com a observação de seu papel na medicina esportiva, depois explorando as respostas psicológicas às lesões esportivas e, em seguida, examinando a adesão e as estratégias práticas para aumentá-la; finalmente, examinamos quatro habilidades psicológicas que podem ser ensinadas para ajudar atletas lesionados. A mensagem principal que gostaria de deixar é a importância de tratar cada atleta como um indivíduo único, que você pode conhecer e ajudar em sua jornada de reabilitação. Dois atletas não responderão e lidarão com a mesma lesão da mesma maneira. Cada vez que um novo cliente entra pela minha porta, meu trabalho é obter *insights* sobre o cérebro único dessa pessoa. Lembre-se do jóquei no início do capítulo; parecia que ele estava lidando excepcionalmente bem com sua reabilitação, mas o impacto emocional o atingiu no ponto de retorno ao esporte. Nunca tome as coisas pelo valor nominal. Reserve um tempo para ouvir seus clientes, fazer as perguntas certas e desenvolver planos de intervenção individuais para cada pessoa.

Referências bibliográficas

Anderson, A.G., White, A., McKay, J., 2004. Athletes' emotional response to injury. In: Lavallee, D., Thatcher, J., Jones, M. (Eds.), Coping and Emotion in Sport. Nova Science, New York, pp. 207-221.

Ardern, C.L., Taylor, N.F., Feller, J.A., Whitehead, T.S., Webster, K.E., 2013. Psychological responses matter in returning to preinjury level of sport after anterior cruciate ligament reconstruction surgery. The American Journal of Sports Medicine 41 (7), 1549-1558.

Arvinen-Barrow, M., Hemmings, B., Weigand, D., Becker, C.A., Booth, L., 2007. Views of chartered physiotherapists on the psychological content of their practice: a national follow-up survey in the UK. Journal of Sports Rehabilitation 16 (2), 111-121.

Arvinen-Barrow, M., Massey, W.V., Hemmings, B., 2014. Role of sport medicine professionals in addressing psychosocial aspects of sport-injury rehabilitation: professional athletes views. Journal of Athletic Training 49 (6), 764-772.

Arvinen-Barrow, M., Penny, G., Hemmings, B., Corr, S., 2010. UK chartered physiotherapists' personal experiences in using psychological interventions with injured athletes: an interpretative phenomenological analysis. Psychology of Sport and Exercise 11 (1), 58-66.

Arvinen-Barrow, M., Weigand, D.A., Thomas, S., Hemmings, B., Walley, M., 2008. The use of imagery across competitive levels and time of season: a cross-sectional study amongst synchronized skaters in Finland. European Journal of Sport Sciences 8 (3), 135-142.

Beneka, A., Malliou, P., Bebetsos, E., Gioftsidou, A., Pafis, G., Godolias, G., 2007. Appropriate Counselling Techniques for Specific Components of the Rehabilitation Plan: A Review of the literature. Physical Training, August 2012. Available at: https://ejmas.com/pt/2007pt/ptart_beneka_0707.html.

Benson, H., 2000. The Relaxation Response. HarperCollins, New York.

Bianco, T., 2001. Social support and recovery from sport injury: elite skiers share their experiences. Research Quarterly for Exercise & Sport 72, 376-388.

Brand, E., Nyland, J., 2009. Patient outcomes following anterior cruciate ligament reconstruction: the influence of psychological factors. Orthopedics 32, 335-341.

Brewer, B.W., 1998. Adherence to sport injury rehabilitation programs. Journal of Applied Sport Psychology 10, 70-82.

Brewer, B.W., Daly, J.M., Van Raalte, J.L., Petitpas, A.J., Sklar, J.H., 1999. A psychometric evaluation of the rehabilitation adherence questionnaire. Journal of Sport & Exercise Psychology 21, 167-173.

Brewer, B.W., Van Raalte, J.L., Cornelius, A.E., Petitpas, A.J., Sklar, J.H., Pohlman, M.H., et al., 2000. Psychological factors, rehabilitation outcome following anterior cruciate ligament reconstruction. Rehabilitation Psychology 45, 20-37.

Cox, R.H., 2007. Sport Psychology: Concepts and Application, sixth ed. McGraw-Hill, Boston, MA.

Duda, J.L., Smart, A.E., Tappe, M.L., 1989. Predictors of adherence in the rehabilitation of athletic injuries: an application of personal investment theory. Journal of Sport & Exercise Psychology 11, 367-381.

Evans, L., Hardy, L., 1995. Sport injury and grief response: a review. Journal of Sport & Exercise Psychology 17, 227-245.

Fields, J., Murphey, M., Horodyski, M., Stopka, C., 1995. Factors associated with adherence to sport injury rehabilitation in college-age athletes. Journal of Sport Rehabilitation 4, 172-180.

Fisher, A.C., Hoisington, L.L., 1993. Injured athletes' attitudes and judgments towards rehabilitation adherence. Journal of Athletic Training 28 (1), 48-53.

Flint, F.A., 1998a. Integrating sports psychology and sports medicine in research: the dilemmas. Journal of Applied Sport Psychology 10, 83-102.

Flint, F.A., 1998b. Specialized psychological interventions. In: Flint, F.A. (Ed.), Psychology of Sports Injury. Human Kinetics, Leeds, UK, pp. 29-50.

Gordon, S., Milios, D., Grove, R., 1991. Psychological aspects of the recovery process from sport injury: the perspective of sport physiotherapist. Australian Journal of Science and Medicine in Sport 23 (2), 53-60.

Hamson-Utley, J.J., Martin, S., Walters, J., 2008. Athletic trainers' and physical therapists' perceptions of the effectiveness of psychological skills within sport injury rehabilitation programs. Journal of Athletic Training 43 (3), 258-264.

Hardy, L., Jones, G., Gould, D., 1996. Understanding Psychological Preparation for Sport: Theory and Practice for Elite Performers. Wiley, Chichester, UK.

Harris, L., 2005. Perceptions and attitudes of athletic training and students toward a course addressing psychological issues in rehabilitation. Journal Of Allied Health 34, 101-109.

Harris, L.L., 2003. Integrating and analysing psychosocial and stage theories to challenge the development of the injured collegiate athlete. Journal of Athletic Training 38 (1), 75-82.

Heil, J., 1993. Psychology of Sport Injury. Human Kinetics, Champaign, IL.

Hemmings, B., Povey, L., 2002. Views of chartered physiotherapists on the psychological content of their practise: a preliminary study in the United Kingdom. British Journal of Sports Medicine 36 (1), 61-64.

Ievleva, L., Orlick, T., 1991. Mental links to enhanced healing: an exploratory study. The Sport Psychologist 5, 25-40.

Jacobson, E., 1938. Progressive Relaxation. University of Chicago Press, Chicago, IL.

Kamphoff, C., Hamson-Utley, J.J., Antoine, B., Knutson, B., Thomae, J., Hoenig, C., 2010. Athletic training students perceptions of the importance and effectiveness of psychological skills within sport injury rehabilitation. Athletic Training Education Journal 5 (3), 109-116.

Kolt, G.S., 2004a. Psychology of injury and rehabilitation. In: Kolt, G.S., Snyder-Mackler, L. (Eds.), Physical Therapies in Sport and Exercise. Churchill Livingstone, London, pp. 165-183.

Kolt, G.S., 2004b. Injury from sport, exercise and physical activity. In: Kolt, G.S., Andersen, M.B. (Eds.), Psychology in the Physical and Manual Therapies. Churchill Livingstone Inc., Philadelphia, PA, pp. 247-267.

Kolt, G.S., Andersen, M.B., 2004. Psychology in the Physical and Manual Therapies. Churchill Livingstone Inc, Philadelphia, PA.

Kolt, G.S., McEvoy, J.F., 2003. Adherence to rehabilitation in patients with lower back pain. Manual Therapy 8, 110-116.

Kolt, G.S., Gill, S., Keating, J., 2002. An examination of the multi-process theory: the effects of two relaxation techniques on state anxiety. [Abstract]. Australian Journal of Psychology 54 (Suppl.), 39.

Kübler-Ross, E., 1969. On Death and Dying. MacMillan, London.

Larson, G.A., Starkey, C., Zaichkowsky, L.D., 1996. Psychological aspects of athletic injuries as perceived by athletic trainers. The Sport Psychologist 10, 37-47.

Lehrer, P.M., 1982. How to relax and how not to relax: a re-evaluation of the work of Edmund Jacobson. Behaviour Research and Therapy 20, 417-428.

Levy, A.R., Pullman, R.C.J., Clough, P.J., McNaughton, L.R., 2006. Adherence to sports injury rehabilitation programmes: a conceptual review. Research in Sports Medicine 14, 149-162.

Locke, E.A., 1968. Towards a theory of task motivation incentives. Organizational Behavior & Human Performance 3, 157-189.

Macci, R., Crossman, J., 1996. After the fall: reflections of injured classical ballet dancers. Journal of Sport Behaviour 19, 221-234.

Mann, B.J., Grana, W.A., Indelicato, P.A., O'Neill, D.F., George, S.Z., 2007. A survey of sports medicine physicians regarding psychological issues in patient-athletes. The American Journal of Sports Medicine 35 (12), 2140-2147.

Maynard, I.W., Hemmings, B., Warwick-Evans, L., 1995. The effects of a somatic intervention strategy on competitive state anxiety and performance in semi-professional soccer players. The Sport Psychologist 9, 51-64.

McCullough, K.A., Phelps, K.D., Spindler, K.P., Matava, M.J., Dunn, W.R., Parker, R.D., et al., 2012. Return to high school and college-level football after anterior cruciate ligament reconstruction. The American Journal of Sports Medicine 40, 2523-2529.

McDonald, S.A., Hardy, C.J., 1990. Affective response patterns of the injured athlete: an exploratory analysis. The Sport Psychologist 4, 261-274.

Meichenbaum, D., Turk, D.C., 1987. Facilitating Treatment Adherence. Plenum, New York.

Mueller, F.O., Ryan, A. (Eds.), 1991. The Sports Medicine Team and Athletic Injury Prevention. Davis, Philadelphia, PA.

Peters, S., 2012. The Chimp Paradox. Random House, London.

Petitpas, A., Danish, A., 1995. Caring for injured athletes. In: Murphy, S. (Ed.), Sport Psychology Interventions. Human Kinetics, Champaign, IL, pp. 255-281.

Podlog, L., Eklund, R.C., 2007. Psychosocial consideration of the return to sport following injury. Journal of Applied Sport Psychology 19, 207-225.

Ray, R., Wiese-Bjornstall, D.M., 1999. Counseling in Sports Medicine. Human Kinetics, Champaign, IL.

Richman, J.M., Rosenfeld, L.B., Hardy, C.J., 1993. The Social Support Survey: a validation study of a clinical measure of the social support process. Research on Social Work Practice 3, 288-311.

Schoo, A.M., 2002. Exercise Performance in Older People with Osteoarthritis: Relationships between Exercise Adherence Correctness of Exercise Performance and Associated pain. Unpublished Doctoral Dissertation. La Trobe University, Bundoora, Australia.

Schultz, L., Luthe, W., 1969. Autogenic Methods, 1. Grune and Stratton, New York.

Stenstrom, C.H., Arge, B., Sundbom, A., 1996. Dynamic training versus relaxation training as home exercise for patients with inflammatory rheumatic diseases: a ransomised controlled study. Scandinavian Journal of Rheumatology 25, 28-33.

Stiller-Ostrowski, J.L., Hamson-Utley, J.J., 2010. Athletic trainers' educational satisfaction and technique use within the psychosocial intervention and referral content area. Athletic Training Education Journal 5 (1), 4-11.

Taylor, A.H., May, S., 1996. Threat and cooing appraisals as determinants of compliance with sports injury rehabilitation: an application of protection motivation theory. Journal of Sports Science 14, 471-482.

Taylor, J., Taylor, S., 1997. Psychological Approaches to Sports Injury Rehabilitation. Aspen, Gaithersburg, MD.

Taylor, J., Taylor, S., 1998. Pain education and management in the rehabilitation from sports injury. The Sport Psychologist 12, 68-88.

Udry, E., 1997. Coping and social support among injured athletes following surgery. Journal of Sport & Exercise Psychology 19, 71-90.

Udry, E., 1999. The paradox of injuries: Unexpected positive consequences. In: Pargman, D. (Ed.), Psychological Bases of Sport Injuries, second ed. Fitness Information Technology, Morgantown, WV, pp. 79-88.

Walker, N., Heaney, C., 2013. Psychological response to injury. In: Arvinen-Barrow, M., Walker, N. (Eds.), The Psychology of Sport Injury and Rehabilitation. Routledge, London, pp. 23-40.

Walker, N., Thatcher, J., Lavallee, D., 2007. Psychological responses to injury in competitive sport: a critical review. Journal of the Royal Society for the Promotion of Health, the 127 (4), 174-180.

Weinberg, R.S., Gould, D., 2011. Foundations of Sport and Exercise Psychology, fifth ed. Human Kinetics, Champaign, IL.

Wiese-Bjornstal, D.M., Smith, A.M., Shaffer, S.M., Morrey, M.A., 1998. An integrated model of response to sports injury: psychological and sociological dynamics. Journal of Applied Sport Psychology 10, 46-69.

Williams, J.M., Scherzer, C.B., 2010. Injury risk and rehabilitation: psychological considerations. In: Williams, J.M. (Ed.), Applied Sport Psychology: Personal Growth to Peak Performance. McGraw-Hill, New York, pp. 512-541.

Índice Alfabético

A

Abordagem(ns)
- baseadas em campo as vantagens de testar o $\dot{V}O_{2máx}$, 114
- de sistemas multimodais, 177

Absorção
- de impacto, 394
- de luz pelos tecidos, 58

Ação
- muscular, 22
- - concêntrica, 22
- - excêntrica, 22
- - isométrica, 22
- sinérgica, 388

Aceleração, 188, 350

Acetilcolina, 4

Acompanhamento, 388
- durante os anos de especialização, 346

Acoplamento excitação-contração, 4

Actina e miosina, 2

Acupuntura, 264, 269, 273
- chinesa tradicional, 105
- médica ocidental, 105

Adaptações
- morfológicas, 9
- musculares, 7
- - ao treinamento de resistência, 7, 8
- neurais, 8
- para esportes *overhead*, 360

Adereços/equipamento/iluminação para dança, 419

Adesão à reabilitação de lesões, 441

Adição de mionúcleos, 10

Agentes
- anti-inflamatórios, 256
- eletrofísicos, 53

Agilidade, 188, 342

Agonista, 2, 388

Alimentos funcionais, 79

Alinhamento
- da crista ilíaca, 171
- do ombro, 171
- espinal, 171
- filosófico e de treinamento, 378

Alongamento excêntrico dos isquiotibiais, 182

Alterações no senso de posição articular, 70

Ambiente(s), 308
- de baixa carga, 13

Ameaças à eficácia do condicionamento, 401, 404, 405

Amplitude de movimento, 218, 220, 246
- ativa (ADMA), 227
- - assistida (ADMAA), 227
- de rotação na articulação glenoumeral, 360
- do antebraço, 267
- do cotovelo, 362
- do punho, 263

Analgesia por acupuntura, 105, 106
- aplicação e mecanismos, 105
- efeito de camadas, 106
- fisiologia da, 105
- inflamação e cura, 108

Análise
- biomecânica/de movimento, 28
- das necessidades, 28, 29
- de lesões, 28
- de movimento, 385, 393
- fisiológica, 28
- pós-movimento, 394

Anatomia
- da região inguinal, 135
- do cotovelo, 251
- dos ossos longos pediátricos, 315

Angiogênese, 8

Antagonista, 2, 388

Anti-inflamatórios, 274
- e terapia de injeção, 266, 269

Aplicação de ultrassom em relação ao reparo tecidual, 54

Apófise, 315

Apofisite
- da base do quinto metatarso, 325
- de tração, 323
- - do tubérculo tibial, 324
- do calcâneo, 324
- do polo inferior da patela, 324

Apoios isométricos de perna dupla, 203

Aptidão aeróbica geral, 352

Aquecimento tecidual, 56

Área transversal, 25

Arquitetura muscular, 25

Arranjo(s)
- de fascículos penados, 2
- fusiforme, 2
- musculares, 2

Arremesso biomecânica do, 252

Articulação(ões)
- carpometacarpal lesões da, 266, 267
- do joelho, estabilidade dinâmica da, 399
- do quadril, 159, 160
- esternoclavicular, 246
- glenoumeral, 246
- - frouxidão e instabilidade da, 248
- MCF, 270
- púbica e adutores, 141
- radiocapitelar, 252
- radioulnar proximal, 252
- ulno-umeral, 252

Artrite séptica, 329

Artrocinemática, 218, 220

Artrograma por ressonância magnética, 249

Artropatias inflamatórias e terapia a *laser*, 59

Ativação isométrica do manguito rotador, 227, 230

Atleta *overhead*, 357
- lesionado, 364

Aumento da força e potência musculares, 26

Avaliação
- clínica
- - de insuficiências sensorimotoras, 217
- - e planejamento de tratamento no jovem jogador de futebol, 308
- da extensão do tronco, 173
- da flexão do tronco, 172
- da maturidade biológica, 310
- de risco da coluna cervical em um contexto esportivo, 277
- do atleta *overhead* lesionado, 364
- do controle oculomotor, 282
- do desenvolvimento dos pelos genitais/ púbicos, 310
- do ombro esportivo, 243
- fisiológica de $\dot{V}O_{2máx}$, 112
- fora do campo do ombro esportivo, 245
- funcional, 249
- no campo do ombro esportivo, 244
- objetiva, observacional e comportamental, 308
- optocinética, 283
- subjetiva, 308

Avulsão, 137, 138
- da espinha tibial, 320
- do tubérculo tibial, 320

B

Balance Error Scoring System, 219

Bandagem, 309

Banho de contraste, 81

Biobanding, 311

Biogênese mitocondrial, 8

Biomecânica
- articular, 5
- da atividade overhead, 357
- da marcha pós-reconstrução do ligamento cruzado anterior, 393
- das lesões esportivas, 41
- do arremesso, 252

Boxe, 261

Braço do momento, 5

C

Cabeça do fêmur, 159

Cadeia cinética, 89
- tronco e membro inferior, 362

Calcificação, 137

Calor, 371
- específico, 67
- latente de fusão, 67

Capacidade de força, 141

Cápsula
- articular, 15
- da articulação do quadril, 160

Índice Alfabético

Carga, 13
- de trabalho, 420
- de treinamento, 405
- - e repetições, 31
Cartilagem articular, 14
Células
- da substância cinza periaquadutal, 106
- do trato anterolateral, 106
Células-satélite, 2, 10
Cereja ácida Montmorency, 79, 80
Chute, 143
Cicatrização de feridas fisiologia da, 156
Ciclo
- de alongamento-encurtamento, 4, 22
- de *feedback*, 381
Cinética e cinemática da tarefa esportiva, 143
Cirurgia de reconstrução da virilha
esquerda, 155
Classificação
- de lesões em tecidos moles, 369
- de Salter-Harris de fraturas fisárias, 315, 316
Coativação/cocontração, 388
Colisões, 350
Coluna cervical, 277, 286
Complexo
- hipotalâmico hipofisário, 106
- lombopélvico-quadril, 183
- piramidal-ligamento púbico anterior-adutor
longo, 142
Compressão, 371
Comprimento do músculo, 25
Concussão, 291
Condicionamento, 21, 399
- em pés, 227
- específico do futebol, 301
- *off-feet*, 227
- para a batalha do momentum, 349
- técnicas para aumentar a eficácia do, 402,
404, 405
Condições pediátricas graves, 323
Condução, 66
Consumo máximo de oxigênio, 111
Contração
- concêntrica, 388
- excêntrica, 388
- isométrica, 388
- muscular, 2, 5
Contranutação sacral, 173
Controle
- deslizante de isquiotibiais em uma prancha
deslizante, 180
- neuromuscular
- - do movimento, 1
- - e neurodinâmica, 184
- oculomotor, 282
Convecção, 66
Convergência do sistema nervoso central, 90
Conversão, 67
Coordenação olho-cabeça, 283
Corrida(s), 143, 350
- assistidas, 187
- de alta velocidade, 188, 345
- de trenó, 187
- em piscina, 184
- resistidas, 187
Cotovelo esportivo, 251
Crescimento, 409
- e maturação, 310
- ósseo, 315
Criação
- de um ambiente seguro, 312
- dessas passagens, 354
Crioterapia, 65
- aplicações ao lado do campo a
aplicação de, 71

- base científica, 67
- contraindicações para, 74
- de corpo inteiro, 72, 82
- - e fisiologia, 72
- - e lesão, 73
- - e patologias sistêmicas, 74
- - e psicologia, 73
- - e recuperação, 73
- dose-resposta, 68
- e compressão, 71
- modalidades e métodos de, 70
- perigos, contraindicações e relatos de
eventos adversos para, 74
Critérios de retorno à dança, 426
Curva comprimento-tensão, 145

D

Dano muscular induzido pelo
exercício, 80, 402
Debriefing, 436
Déficit
- na absorção de choque, 390
- na estabilidade
- - do membro, 389
- - do tronco, 390
- - pélvica, 389
- na estratégia de movimento, 390
Definição de metas, 443
Deformação biomecânica, 90
Deformidade
- do ombro, 245
- plástica, 317
Demandas
- de desempenho e riscos de lesões, 404
- específicas, 350
- gerais, 350
Densidade energética, 59
Departamento de ciência e medicina do
esporte, 308
Derrame, 137
Desaceleração, 188
Descoloração (vermelhidão), 371
Desempenho, 445
- de resistência, 111
Desenvolvimento
- atlético a longo prazo, 309
- de força/potência, 299, 304
- de qualidades
- - de velocidade
- - - em crianças, 341
- - - em meninos e meninas, 344
- - específicas, 27
Desequilíbrio, 280
- muscular, 388, 391
Desuso, 13
Determinantes fisiológicos para o
desempenho de resistência, 111
Diáfise, 315
Diagramas de corpo livre, 388
Dinamometria portátil, 198
Disfunção
- arterial cervical, 278
- do movimento, 389
- lombopélvica, 169
- - avaliação, 170
- - - visual e observação, 170
- - histórico do paciente, 170
- - papel do exame de imagem, 175
- - prevenção, 174
- - resultados da avaliação, 174
- sensorimotora, 281
Dissecção da artéria
- carótida interna, 278
- vertebral, 278

Dissociação cabeça-corpo, 283
Distensão, 137
Doença
- de Freiberg, 326
- de Iselin, 325
- de Köhler, 326
- de Legg-Calvé-Perthes, 325
- de Osgood-Schlatter, 324
- de Scheuermann, 326
- de Sever, 324
Domínio sinérgico, 388
Dor, 371
- de cabeça e tontura, 277
- e instabilidade nas articulações
acromioclaviculares, 247
- específica, 364
- inespecífica, 364
- lombar no adolescente, 328
- muscular de início retardado, 25
- na articulação
- - do tornozelo, 217
- - sacroilíaca, 171
- na fisioterapia esportiva, 87
- na virilha, 141
- - incidência, 151
- neuropática, 107
- no braço de arremesso, 357
- no quadril relacionada à articulação
do quadril, 163
- nociplástica, 91
- plantar no calcanhar, 222
- tratamento da, 445
Doses terapêuticas, 59

E

Edema da articulação do tornozelo, 217
Educação cruzada, 404
Efeitos
- colaterais, 402
- cumulativos, 405
- da idade relativa, 311
- da musculatura tensa no alinhamento
da pelve, 171
- da sessão repetida, 405
- do resfriamento
- - no músculo, 69
- - no sentido da posição articular, 70
Eficácia do condicionamento, 399
- para reabilitação baseada em
desempenho, 400
Eixo
- frontal ou anteroposterior, 386
- transversal ou horizontal sagital, 386
- vertical ou longitudinal, 386
Eletroacupuntura, 108
Eletrocardiograma de repouso de 12
derivações, 338
Eletroterapia, 53, 269, 273
- modalidades de, 264
Elevação, 372
- ativa da perna reta, 174
- passiva da perna reta, 174
Embasamento, 72
Endomísio, 1
Energia para o movimento, 2
Entorse lateral do tornozelo, 41, 215
- avaliação clínica, 216
- - fratura, 216
- - ligamentos, 216
- descrição do caso, 215
- epidemiologia, 215
- mecanismo da lesão, 215

450

Índice Alfabético

Epicondilite lateral, 255
- fisioterapia, 256
- tratamento(s)
- - biológicos, 256
- - cirúrgico, 257
Epicondilite medial, 257
Epífise, 315
- femoral superior desviada, 327
Epimísio, 1
Equação(ões)
- de Fick, 111
- de predição sem exercício, 119
- - quantificação do $\dot{V}O_{2máx}$, 119
Equilíbrio
- postural estático e dinâmico, 218, 221
- térmico, 66
Equipe multiprofissional
- da ginasta, 409
- e abordagem centrada no atleta, 307
Escala(s)
- de dor, 308
- numérica de classificação de dor "semáforo", 217
Escápula, 360
Esforços repetidos de alta intensidade, 354
Especificidade, 26, 179, 402
Espectro de desuso após lesão esportiva, 13
Espondilólise, 328
Espondilolistese, 328
Esporte-específico com retorno à fase de corrida, 147
Estabilidade
- da pelve, 394
- dinâmica da articulação do joelho, 399
- do membro, 393
- do olhar, 283
- do tronco, 394
Estado cognitivo-emocional-social, 93, 94
Estágio(s)
- de coleta de dados, 349
- de comparação, 349
- de implementação, 349
- de previsão, 349
- de reabilitação, 373
- - de pré-alta, 374
Esteira Alterg, 198
Estimulação
- local, 88, 90
- química, 90
Estímulo do treinamento de resistência, 7
Estratégia de movimento, 394
Estresse
- ósseo e tecido não contrátil, 147
- térmico, 65
- /tensão, 193
Estressores psicológicos, 411
Estrutura do músculo esquelético, 1
Evaporação, 67
Evento cardíaco no atleta jovem, 335
Exame
- clínico do ombro esportivo, 244
- objetivo de dor na virilha, 141
Execução, 388
Exercício(s)
- de assistência, 31
- de cadeia cinética
- - aberta (CCA), 227, 235, 236
- - fechada (CCF), 227, 232
- - de controle neuromuscular
- - mergulhador, 185
- - moinho de vento, 185
- de *core*, 31

- de *endurance* do manguito rotador, 227
- de força
- - excêntrica do manguito rotador, 227, 236
- - máxima da parte superior do corpo (PSC), 227
- de potência, 31
- de resistência, 7
- - da musculatura do manguito rotador, 230
- horizontais do tipo horizontal *push*, 237
- nórdico de isquiotibiais, 181, 182
- pliométricos, 183
- usados no programa de intervenção de fortalecimento do pescoço, 284
- utilizando o peso corporal, 23
- verticais do tipo vertical *push*, 237
Exigências
- extrínsecas aos dançarinos, 419
- intrínsecas aos dançarinos, 420
Extensão do tronco, 173
Extricação, 434
- para lesões
- - na coluna vertebral, 435
- - não espinais ou parada cardíaca, 434

F

Fadiga, 7, 401
- central, 10, 11
- durante exercício(s)
- - muito intensos, 10
- - prolongado de resistência, 11
- muscular, 10
- periférica, 10
Faixa de resistência/banda elástica, 187
Fáscia, 1
Fascículos, 1
Fase(s)
- aguda, 369
- crônica, 370
- de diversão e de aprender a treinar, 342
- de elevação/aceleração, 360
- de redução, 303
- de remodelamento do reparo, 55
- de sobrecarga
- - de treinamento, 303
- - do jogo, 303
- de treinabilidade acelerada, 341
- do movimento, 387
- proliferativa, 54
- subaguda, 369
Fator(es)
- agravantes, 244
- de predisposição, 94
- que afetam a força muscular, 22
- que confundem e limitam as alterações crônicas no $\dot{V}O_{2máx}$, 120
Feridas abertas e terapia a *laser*, 59
Fibras
- amielínicas do tipo C, 106
- musculares, 1
- no músculo esquelético, 3
Filamentos finos e grossos, 2
Filosofia
- de treinamento de força, 377
- do Chelsea FC, 208
Filtro de diagnóstico, 243
Fise/placa epifisária, 315
Flexão
- do tronco, 172
- lateral do tronco, 173
Flexibilidade, 195
Fluxo de força
- de rúgbi, 378

- fundamental, 377
- geral, 378
Força(s), 21
- da articulação glenoumeral, 361
- da parte superior do corpo, 236
- excêntrica do manguito rotador, 232
- explosiva, 183, 378
- função de mão, 263, 267, 271
- isométrica, 28
- lombopélvica-quadril, 183
- máxima, 31, 378
- muscular, 5
- - da articulação do tornozelo, 218, 221
- - do quadril, 394
- - importância da, 21
- - reativa, 378
- - do manguito rotador, 227, 238
Fotobioativação, 58
Fotobiomodulação, 57, 58
Fratura(s)
- da eminência tibial, 320
- em fivela (torus), 317
- em galho verde, 317
- incompletas, 317
- por avulsão, 319
- - apofisária, 317
- - - pélvica, 318
- - do calcâneo, 321
- por estresse, 204
Frequência
- cardíaca e prescrições de sessões de treinamento, 346
- de disparo, 22
- de treinamento, 28
Frouxidão
- e instabilidade da articulação glenoumeral, 248
- generalizada, 248
Função
- da virilha no esporte, 143
- motora do pescoço, 283
- muscular, 394
- - e miocinemática, 142

G

Gelo
- e compressão, 264, 269, 273
- triturado/em cubos/umedecido, 71
Gerenciamento do atleta *overhead*, 357
- lesionado, 365
- total, 362
Gestão
- durante a temporada, 363
- entre temporadas, 362
Giro, 188
Glicólise, 2
Golpe de força, 2
Guardiões da cultura e valores do clube, 308
Guia para o protocolo de ação de emergência, 429

H

Habilidades
- de contato, 227, 239
- de psicologia do esporte, 443
- específicas de esporte e posição, 238
- /reabilitação específicas do esporte/posição, 227
Hematomas, 245
Hidratação e seus efeitos na elasticidade muscular, 196
Hidroterapia, 184

Índice Alfabético

Hipertrofia muscular, 9, 31
Homeostase térmica, 65
Hook test, 248
Hormônio adrenocorticotrófico, 106

I

Idade
- biológica ou esquelética, 310
- como preditor de patologia, 243
- cronológica, 310
- psicológica, 311
Identificação precoce de patologia grave, 243
Iliopsoas, 167
Imageamento por ressonância magnética, 311
Imagens
- curativas, 445
- mentais, 445
Imersão em água fria, 71, 81
Imobilização, 13
Impacto, 350
- anterior do tornozelo, 222
- femoroacetabular, 154, 328
- interno, 47
- posterior do tornozelo, 222
Impulso de quadril bipodal e unipodal, 181
Inadequações de força, 195
Incapacidade do paciente resultante de doença do tornozelo, 43
Inchaço, 371
- da articulação do tornozelo, 217
- no ombro, 245
Incidência de rupturas e o calendário do futebol, 194
Inclinação sacral, 173
Individualidade, 27
Infecções ósseas e articulares, 329
Inflamação, 54
- aguda, 369, 371
- crônica, 370, 371
- subaguda, 371
Influências regionais, 89
Inibição recíproca, 388
Instabilidade
- aguda do cotovelo, 253
- do cotovelo, 252
- - crônica, 254
- do ombro, 48, 49
- do tornozelo crônica, 222
- em valgo, 255
- rotatória posterolateral, 254
Insuficiência(s)
- ativa, 388
- passiva, 388
- sensorimotoras, 216, 217
Integração de volta ao treinamento completo, 147
Interação *laser*-tecido, 58

K

Kit
- do fisioterapeuta, 431
- médico, 431

L

Lábio acetabular, 159
Lançamento resistido, 248
Laser, aplicações clínicas, 59
Lei
- de Hooke, 146
- de Wolff/Davis, 146

Lesão(ões)
- agudas, 371
- - e crônicas na virilha, 139
- cerebral traumática, 279
- - leve, 291
- - - ao lado do campo reconhecimento imediato da, 292
- - - tratamento de, 295
- comuns no joelho, 210
- da articulação carpometacarpal, 266, 267
- de adutor, 153
- de banda sagital, 262, 263
- - apresentação/testagem para, 262
- de canto posterolateral, 211
- de menisco, 211
- de tecido mole e terapia a *laser*, 59
- de tornozelo, 412
- do ligamento
- - colateral
- - - medial, 210
- - - ulnar, 270
- - - - na base do polegar, 270
- - cruzado anterior, 43, 210
- - - anatomia, 44
- - - consequências, 46
- - - mecanismos de lesão e fatores de risco, 44
- - - medidas de resultado, 46
- - - tratamento, 45
- - - triagem e prevenção, 44
- dos isquiotibiais, 177
- - classificação de, 178
- - exigências anatômicas esportivas, 177
- - filosofia de reabilitação para a melhora de desempenho, 178
- - melhora da habilidade atlética, 178
- - métricas de resultado, 189
- - otimização do envolvimento do atleta, 178
- - reabilitação
- - - adequada, 178
- - - de desempenho, 178
- - - redução do risco de lesões futuras, 178
- - - retorno ao jogo, 189
- em tecidos moles
- - classificação de, 369
- - tratamento e manejo de, 369
- epidemiologia de, 411
- esportivas, 13
- - biomecânica das, 41
- - na virilha tratamento cirúrgico de, 151
- musculoesquelética de membro inferior, 215
- na cabeça
- - avaliação clínica, 292
- - diagnóstico e manejo, 291
- - investigações, 294
- - manejo, 291
- - - agudo, 295
- - sinais de alerta, 292
- - sintomas, 291
- - - crônicos/persistentes, 295
- - tratamento de lesão cerebral traumática leve, 295
- na dança, 421
- na virilha, 131
- - apresentação e diagnóstico, 152
- - cintilografia óssea com radionuclídeo, 153
- - cirurgia, 154
- - controvérsias, 156
- - diagnóstico, 140
- - - diferencial, 154
- - diferenças crônicas/agudas na apresentação crônica, 145
- - equipe multiprofissional, 156
- - estágios do manejo no contexto agudo, 145

- - etiologia, 139, 152
- - fase
- - - de condicionamento/remodelamento do tecido, 145
- - - de sangramento, 145
- - - inflamatória, 145
- - ferramenta de exclusão, 131
- - fisiologia da cicatrização de feridas, 156
- - imagem de ultrassonografia em, 131
- - incidência e epidemiologia, 139
- - indicações para a cirurgia, 154
- - intervenção médica/farmacoterapia, 143
- - radiografia simples, 153
- - reabilitação, 143, 156
- - reconstrução da virilha, 155
- - ressonância magnética, 153
- - resultado e recorrência, 156
- - rupturas de espessura total *versus* parcial, 132
- - sinais, 153
- - sintomas, 152
- - técnica cirúrgica, 154
- - tempo ideal para fazer o exame, 131
- - tenotomia do adutor, 155
- - tomografia computadorizada, 132
- - ultrassonografia, 133, 153
- nas mãos e nos punhos, 261
- no joelho, 207
- - epidemiologia, 207
- - estrutura de tratamento, 208
- - filosofia do departamento médico do Chelsea FC, 207
- - intervenções direcionadas "específicas para o joelho", 209
- - métodos de progressão funcional, 208
- - reabilitação em campo, 212
- - unidade de prevenção de lesões do Chelsea FC, 213
- no ombro, 47
- - de categorias 1 e 2, 227
- - de categorias 3 e 4, 227
- no tornozelo, 41, 411
- - efeitos da reabilitação na incidência e recorrência, 43
- - epidemiologia, 41
- - incapacidade do paciente resultante de doença do tornozelo, 43
- - mecanismo e apresentação clínica, 41
- - protocolos
- - - de reabilitação do tornozelo, 42
- - - de treinamento de força, 42
- - no tronco, 413
- - por estresse do osso púbico, 154
- - que ocorrem na mão e no punho no boxe, 261
- SLAP, 248
Levantamento
- da panturrilha
- - com peso corporal em uma perna, 202
- - de perna dupla com peso corporal, 201
- - do joelho
- - - com as duas pernas dobradas, 201
- - - dobrado em uma única perna com peso corporal, 202
- de peso, 23
- terra
- - isométrico, 179
- - romeno de uma perna
- - - com barra, 179
- - - com propulsão do joelho e supino frontal, 180
Ligamento, 15
- de Bigelow, 160

Índice Alfabético

- do cotovelo, 252
- iliofemoral, 160
- isquiofemoral, 160
- pubofemoral, 160
- redondo, 160
Localização da dor, 244

M

Macrociclo, 33
Manejo deficiente da carga de treinamento, 197
Manguito rotador, 223, 246
Máquina
- Keizer, 203
- Smith, 203
Marcadores de avaliação visual da postura, 171
Massa muscular, 171
Massagem de tecidos moles, 99
Maturação, 409
Maturidade biológica, 310
Mecânica
- do pé, 196
- muscular, 4
Mecanismo
- de "aparafusamento" tibiofemoral, 400
- de analgesia por acupuntura, 107
- de início, 243
- de motor *feedforward*, 395
Mecanorreceptores, 282
Mecanotransdução, 9
Medicina da dança, 419
Metáfise, 315
Metas
- de desempenho, 444
- de processo, 444
- de resultado, 444
Métodos
- Bateman, 247
- de corrida resistidos, 187
- de progressão funcional, 208
- para determinar a carga de treinamento, 32
- para melhorar a adesão à reabilitação em atletas, 443
- que utilizam medidas antropométricas, 310
Microestrutura, 2, 3
Miofibrilas, 2
Miosite ossificante, 138
Mitocôndrias, 2
Mobilizações
- articulares, 264
- de tecidos moles, 264, 269, 273
Modalidades de exercício e $\dot{V}O_{2máx}$, 113
Modelo(s)
- de análise, 387
- de análise de movimento, 388
- de periodização adaptativa, 376
- de raciocínio de dor e movimento, 88
- de regressão/progressão, 237
- de resposta
- - ao luto, 440
- - psicológica de atletas a lesões, 440
- de treinamento de força, 377
- determinísticos, 388
- do chimpanzé, 441
- integrado de resposta a lesões esportivas e reabilitação, 441
- mecânico do músculo, 25, 26
Modificação
- de Marsh da técnica de Gilmore, 155
- pelos receptores musculares e tendíneos, 22
Modo e amplitude da ativação muscular, 404

Modulação central, 91, 94
Módulo de Young, 146
Monitoramento da resposta da frequência cardíaca, 346
Morte súbita cardíaca, 335
- condições cardíacas relacionadas, 336
- desenho do programa de triagem, 337
- em atletas, 336
- histórico médico e exame físico, 337
Movimento
- ocular de perseguição suave (posição neutra), 282
- sacádico dos olhos, 282
Mudança de direção, 143, 350
- e agilidade, 187
Múltiplas funções de membros da equipe multiprofissional, 313
Músculo(s)
- abdominal, 142
- adutor, 142
- bipenados, 2
- esquelético, 1, 16
- forma e função do, 1
- inteiros, 1
- que cruzam a articulação do cotovelo, 252
- que produzem o movimento, 386

N

Neurociência, 88
Neurodinâmica, 185
Neurofisiologia, 250
Neuropatodinâmica, 89
Nocicepção, 88
Nós dos dedos, 262
Nutação sacral, 173
Nutrição, 410

O

Observação, 245
Ocupação (esporte), 244
Ombro(s), 47
- avaliação, 224
- do adolescente, 226
- esportivo, 243
- - exame clínico do, 244
- - fora do campo do, 245
- - no campo do, 244
- - papel da imagem no, 224
- saudáveis, 223
Ondas de choque, 60
Ordem do exercício, 31
Órtese para epicondilite lateral, 256
Ossos, 14
- do cotovelo, 251
- em crescimento, 315, 323
- - diagnóstico e tratamento, 316
- - ferramentas de decisão clínica de fratura, 317
- - fraturas
- - - crônicas que afetam a placa de crescimento, 317
- - - por avulsão apofisária, 317
- - sinais e sintomas, 315
- - tratamento de fratura, 317
Osteocinemática, 218, 220
Osteocondrite dissecante, 325
Osteocondrose, 323
- articular, 325
- fisária, 326
- não articulares, 323
Osteologia, 251
Osteomielite aguda, 329

Osteosarcoma, 330
Otimização do processo
- de monitoramento, 381
- de planejamento, 379
- de revisão, 382
- de treinamento, 381

P

Palpação, 173, 246
- nas articulações acromioclaviculares, 247
Paradigma de fadiga-aptidão, 34
Paraquedas, 187
Passagens de significância, 353
Patologias
- musculoesqueléticas que causam dor na virilha, 140
- não musculoesqueléticas que causam dor na virilha, 141
Patomecânica da atividade *overhead*, 357
Pelve, 169, 170
Perda
- de função, 371
- de massa muscular, 245
Perfil de idade típico de ginastas de elite, 409
Perimísio, 1
Periodização
- do treinamento, 33
- para um velocista de pista, 30
- tática, 378, 379
Período fora da temporada, 299
Periósteo, 315
Pescoço, 277
Pico de esforço fisiológico, 114
Piores cenários, 353
Planejamento
- da reabilitação, 309
- e design do programa, 401
Plano(s)
- e eixos do movimento, 386
- frontal, 386
- horizontal ou transversal, 386
- sagital, 386
Plasma rico em plaquetas, 210
Plasticidade dependente de atividade, 92, 94
Pliometria, 183, 345
- de alto limiar, 183
- de baixo limiar, 183
Ponte cruzada, 2
Pontuação de Beighton, 248
Posição
- da cabeça e do pescoço, 171
- de teste do joelho à parede, 195
- do joelho, 171
Postura
- do pé, 171
- marcadores de avaliação visual, 171
Potência, 32
- muscular, 5, 27
Potenciação pós-ativação, 25
Potenciais de ação, 4
Pré-síncope, 280
Pré-temporada, 301, 302
Preparação, 387
- para ação de emergência, 429
- pré-torneio, 312
Prescrição
- de exercícios, 31, 345, 432
- - para promover aumentos em $\dot{V}O_{2máx}$, 120
- de treinamento físico $\dot{V}O_{2máx}$, 119
Primeiros socorros, 313
Princípios de reabilitação, 21

453

Índice Alfabético

Processamento central para a produção da dor, 88
Processo de reabilitação, 445
Produção de força, 27
Programa
- de força durante a temporada, 375
- de treinamento fora de temporada, 300
- excêntrico de isquiotibiais fora da temporada, 300
Progressão, 402
Projetando um treino de "força", 28
Proliferação, 54
Prono, 173
Propriedades contráteis do músculo, 3
Propriocepção, 232
Proteínas contráteis, 2
Protocolo(s)
- Alterg, 198
- de ação de emergência, 429
- de adutor, 133
- de reabilitação do tornozelo, 42
- de teste para garantir uma determinação precisa do $\dot{V}O_{2máx}$, 114
- de treinamento de força, 42
Psicologia na reabilitação de lesões esportivas, 439
Pull-up
- horizontal, 237
- vertical, 238

Q

Quadril, 159
- esportivo, 159
- estrutura, 159
- forma da articulação, 159
- função, 160
- mecânica periarticular e microinstabilidade, 160
- movimento no esporte, 162
- patologia, 163
- radiologia, 164
- reabilitação, 164
- retorno à atividade/esporte, 163
Qualidades de velocidade em atletas jovens, 341
Qualificações para ajuda de emergência, 436
Queda de joelho dobrado, 141

R

Rabdomiossarcoma, 330
Radiação térmica, 67
Radiofrequência
- aplicações de, 55
- de ondas não curtas, 57
Radiografia(s)
- de punho e mão, 310
- simples, 249
- - lesões na virilha, 132
Rastreamento musculoesquelético, 426
Reabilitação, 264, 269, 273
- com base no desempenho, 399
- da taxa de desenvolvimento de força, 403
- de desempenho, 183
- - exposição à corrida, 184
- - para lesões dos isquiotibiais, 177
- de estágio intermediário, 373
- de força de isquiotibiais, 179
- de um dançarino, 425
- do ombro
- - lesionado, 226
- - manejo durante a temporada, 240
- - medidas de resultado, 239

- - no rúgbi, 223
- - reintegração e retorno ao desempenho, 239
- do retardo eletromecânico, 403
- do tornozelo do jogador de futebol, 216
- em estágio
- - inicial, 373
- - tardio, 373
- em ginásio para o retorno ao jogo, 199
- em lesões de tendão, 415
- esportiva integrada, 94
- para os nós dos dedos, 266
- sem aceitação do paciente, 439
Reação de fosfocreatina, 2
Reconstrução da virilha, 155
Recrutamento da unidade motora, 22
Recuperação, 32
- esportiva e atlética, 79
- esportiva e atlética fisiologia da, 79
Redução da atividade, 373
Reflexos, 282
Reformulação da relação entre dor
- e dano ao tecido, 87
- e movimento, 88
Região
- do quadril, 136
- femoral, 134
- inguinal, 134
- lombopélvica, 169
Regras
- de pé e tornozelo de Ottawa, 317
- do joelho de Ottawa, 317
Regulação
- do *turnover* (renovação) da proteína muscular, 9
- transcricional, 9
Relação(ões)
- comprimento-tensão, 388
- - do músculo esquelético, 4
- - e força-velocidade, 4
- dose-resposta e $\dot{V}O_{2máx}$, 120
- entre as temperaturas da superfície da pele e do tecido profundo, 69
- força-velocidade, 4, 26
Relaxamento, 444
- muscular progressivo, 445
Remodelamento, 55
Rendimentos decrescentes, 27
Repetição máxima, 32
Resfriamento, 372
Resistência muscular, 27, 32
Resposta(s)
- adaptativas, 8
- de relaxamento, 445
- de sinalização intracelular, 10
- positiva, 440
- psicológicas a lesões, 440
Ressonância magnética, 249
- de ligamento cruzado anterior intacto e ruptura do ligamento cruzado anterior do joelho, 45
- lesões na virilha, 132
Retorno
- ao jogo, 238
- às habilidades de contato, 239
Reversibilidade, 27
Risco potencial específico do esporte, 244
Rotinas divididas, 28
Roupas de compressão, 80
Rúgbi, 223, 227
Ruptura, 137
- /avulsões de tendão, 258
- da virilha, 151
- do adutor, 137

- do bíceps, 248
- do ligamento cruzado anterior, 43
- do manguito rotador, 47
- do peitoral maior, 247
- do tendão
- - de Aquiles, 222
- - do bíceps distal, 258
- - do tríceps, 258
- muscular
- - avaliação e uso de imagens radiológicas, 194
- - causas
- - - comumente consideradas, 195
- - - menos consideradas, 196
- - dos músculos gastrocnêmio e sóleo em jogadores de futebol profissional, 193
- - reabilitação, 197
- - sinais de alerta, 204

S

Salto, 203
Salvaguarda, 312
Sangue e aspiração, 249
Sarcolema, 2
Sarcoma(s), 330
- de Ewing, 330
Sarcômeros, 2
Sarcoplasma, 2
Saúde
- mental, 286
- na ginástica feminina, 409
- óssea, 330
Seleção de exercícios, 31, 179
Sensibilidade óssea, 246
Sensibilização central, 91
Sentido de posição articular, 232
Sinal
- de atraso da rotação externa, 247
- de Trendelenburg, 391
- do sulco, 248
- eletromiográfico, 9
Síndrome
- de LCTL, 291
- de Sinding-Larsen-Johansson, 324
- do encarceramento da artéria poplítea, 204
- do quadril com ressalto, 164
- do seio do tarso, 222
Sínfise púbica, 154
Sintomas
- de instabilidade, 243
- neurológicos, 244
Sistema(s)
- capsular-ligamentar, 160
- cardiorrespiratório, 16
- de controle postural, 283
- miofascial, 160
- nervoso
- - central, 1
- - periférico, 1
- - simpático, 282
Sobrecarga, 26, 402
- progressiva, 33, 179
Somação, 5
Sono, 83
Sprint, 188
Star Excursion Balance Test, 220
Subcarga, 303
Superfícies na dança, 419
Supino nesta posição, 173
Suporte social, 445
Suspeita de dor
- inguinal na virilha, 134

Índice Alfabético

- na virilha relacionada com o
- - adutor, 133
- - quadril, 135

T

Técnicas de proteção do ligamento colateral ulnar, 273
Tecnologia GPS, 349
- papel no condicionamento, 353
- papel no planejamento, 352
- para estratégias de condicionamento, 349
Tendinopatia, 136
- adutora, 136
- de Aquiles
- - da porção média, 222
- - de inserção, 222
- de membro inferior, 415
- do bíceps proximal, 248
Tenotomia do adutor, 155
Teoria
- da neuroplasticidade, 395
- do filamento deslizante para a contração muscular, 2
Terapia
- a *laser*, 57
- - de baixo nível, 58
- - para o alívio da dor, 59
- com banho de contraste, 81
- de injeção, 274
- de microcorrente, 60
- manual, 99, 264, 269, 273
- - efeitos
- - - mecânicos, 100
- - - na dor, 99
- - - no controle motor, 101
- - fisiologia da, 99
- por exercícios, 264, 273
- por ondas
- - curtas pulsadas, 55
- - - efeitos clínico, 56
- - de choque, 60
- - - focada e radial, 60
Terminologia de dança, 422
Termômetro digital portátil, 69
Teste(s)
- *belly press*, 247
- cinéticos, 172
- de "batidas de tesoura", 141
- de 1RM, 32
- de apreensão e realocação, 248
- de *astrand-ryhming*, 118, 119
- de caminhada, 118
- de capacidade de trabalho muscular/ resistência da panturrilha, 197
- de cegonha, 173
- de ciclismo submáximo, 118
- de compressão, 141
- - ativa de O'Brien, 248

- de corrida, 118
- de Cozens, 255
- de escada, 118
- de estabilidade da extremidade superior de cadeia cinética fechada, 249
- de estresse da sínfise púbica, 141
- de extensão do quadril, 173
- de gancho, 248
- de Gerber, 247
- de Gillet, 173
- de instabilidade, 247
- de Jerk, 248
- de lata
- - cheia, 247
- - vazia (Jobe), 247
- de movimento, 427
- de provocação resistida, 141
- de retirada, 247
- de rotação externa isométrica, 247
- de Thomas para a flexão do quadril, 141
- de torção do pescoço com perseguição suave, 282
- diferenciais para o pescoço e triagem neurológica, 249
- do abraço de urso, 247
- do cachecol (*scarf test*), 247
- do joelho à parede/teste de afundo com suporte de peso, 197
- do *pivot-shift* lateral, 254
- *ekblom-bak*, 119
- em decúbito dorsal deitado, 174
- em pé, 172
- laboratoriais, 249
- para quantificação de $\dot{V}O_{2máx}$, 116
Tetania, 5
Tomografia computadorizada, 249
Tontura, 280
- cervicogênica, 280
- contínua, 279
Tornozelo esportivo, 215
Trabalho na academia aspectos práticos do, 312
Trajes/sapatos os bailarinos, 419
Transferência, 435
- de calor, 66
Transição da fase fora da temporada para a pré-temporada, 302
Transporte, 312
Trato
- dorsolateral, 106
- espinotalâmico, 106
Treinamento
- com carga, 145
- - do adutor, 146
- - em musculatura abdominal, 146
- com kettlebell, 25
- com peso(s)
- - em aparelho, 23
- - livres, 23

- complexo/contraste, 24
- de agilidade, 188, 343
- de equilíbrio, 42
- de força global, 283
- de resistência, 345
- - na dor no pescoço, 285
- - variável, 24
- do sistema sensorimotor do pescoço, 286
- excêntrico, 24
- intervalado de alta intensidade (HIIT), 120
- isométrico, 283
- neuromotor direcionado, 394
- pliométrico, 23
- - para o pescoço, 285
- técnico e preparação física, 410
Triagem
- cardíaca pré-participação em atletas, 338
- clínica, 426
- na dança, 426
Triângulo
- na virilha, 164
- Stanmore, 48
Trombose venosa profunda, 204
Tumor(es), 204
- diagnosticados erroneamente como lesões musculoesqueléticas, 330

U

Ultrassom
- efeitos e usos não térmicos do, 54
- pulsado de baixa intensidade e cicatrização de fraturas, 55
- terapêutico, 53
- usos clínicos da terapia de, 54
Ultrassonografia, 249
Uso de órteses, 196

V

Velocidade, 341, 350
- da ativação muscular, 404
- de contração, 26
Vermelhidão, 246
Vertigem, 280
- objetiva, 280
- subjetiva, 280
Vestimenta com peso, 187
Viagem com crianças em idade escolar, 312
Virilha
- de Gilmore, 151
- função no esporte, 143
$\dot{V}O_{2máx}$ e sua associação
- com a saúde ideal, 112
- com desempenho esportivo ideal, 111
Volumes e intensidades de corrida, 300

Y

Y-teste, 220